W9-AXT-996

Current Issues in Nursing

Edited by

Joanne Comi McCloskey
Distinguished Professor, College of Nursing
The University of Iowa
Adjunct Associate Director of Nursing
The University of Iowa Hospitals and Clinics
Iowa City, Iowa

Helen Kennedy Grace
Vice President-Program
W.K. Kellogg Foundation
Battle Creek, Michigan

Fourth Edition

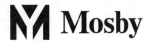 Mosby

St. Louis Baltimore Boston Chicago London Madrid Philadelphia Sydney Toronto

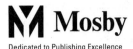

Dedicated to Publishing Excellence

Editor: N. Darlene Como
Assistant Editor: Barbara M. Carroll
Project Manager: Mark Spann
Designer: David Zielinski

Fourth Edition

Copyright © 1994 by Mosby–Year Book, Inc.

Previous editions copyrighted 1981, 1985, 1990

All rights reserved. No part of this publication may be reproduced, stored in a retrieval system, or transmitted, in any form or by any means, electronic, mechanical, photocopying, recording, or otherwise, without prior written permission from the publisher.

Permission to photocopy or reproduce solely for internal or personal use is permitted for libraries or other users registered with the Copyright Clearance Center, provided that the base fee of $4.00 per chapter plus $.10 per page is paid directly to the Copyright Clearance Center, 27 Congress Street, Salem, MA 01970. This consent does not extend to other kinds of copying, such as copying for general distribution, for advertising or promotional purposes, for creating new collected works, or for resale.

Printed in the United States of America
Composition by Carlisle Communications, Ltd.
Printing/Binding by Maple-Vail–Binghamton

Mosby–Year Book, Inc.
11830 Westline Industrial Drive
St. Louis, Missouri 63146

Library of Congress Cataloging in Publication Data

Current issues in nursing / edited by Joanne Comi McCloskey, Helen
   Kennedy Grace. — 4th ed.
      p.   cm.
   Includes bibliographical references and index.
   ISBN 0-8016-6954-5
   1. Nursing.   2. Nursing—United States.   3. Nursing—Social
aspects.   4. Nursing—Social aspects—United States.   I. McCloskey,
Joanne Comi.   II. Grace, Helen K.
   [DNLM: 1. Nursing. 2. Nursing Theory. 3. Education, Nursing.
4. Ethics, Nursing. WY 16 C976 1994]
RT63.C87   1994
610.73—dc20
DNLM/DLC
for Library of Congress   93–46173
                                    CIP

95 96 97 98 / 9 8 7 6 5 4 3 2

Contributors

Genrose J. Alfano, RN, MA, FAAN
Consultant
Freeport, New York

Linda K. Amos, RN, EdD, FAAN
Dean and Professor
University of Utah
College of Nursing
Salt Lake City, Utah

Carole A. Anderson, RN, PhD, FAAN
Dean and Professor
College of Nursing
The Ohio State University
Columbus, Ohio

JoAnn Appleyard, RN, PhD
Regional Director of Nursing
Fhp Health Care
Cerritos, California

Susan M. Awbrey, PhD
Associate Professor
Oakland University
School of Education and Human Services
Rochester, Michigan

Ferial A. M. Aly, RN, PhD
Dean and Professor
Faculty of Nursing
University of Alexandria
Alexandria, Egypt

Judith G. Baggs, RN, PhD
Clinical Nurse Researcher
Strong Memorial Hospital
Assistant Professor of Clinical Nursing
School of Nursing
University of Rochester
Rochester, New York

Geraldine Polly Bednash, RN, PhD, FAAN
Executive Director
American Association of Colleges of Nursing
Washington, D.C.

Leah F. Binder, BA
Director of Public Relations
National League for Nursing
Washington, D.C.

Gillian Biscoe, RN, RM, BHA, MSc, FCNA FCN(NSW)
Chief Executive
ACT Department of Health
Canberra, Australian Capital Territory, Australia

Mary A. Blegen, RN, PhD
Associate Professor
College of Nursing
The University of Iowa
Iowa City, Iowa

Janice M. Brencick, RN, MS
Doctoral Student
University of Colorado Health Sciences Center
Denver, Colorado

Pamela J. Brink, RN, PhD, FAAN
Professor and Associate Dean, Research
Faculty of Nursing
University of Alberta
Edmonton, Alberta, Canada

Roslyn McCallister Brock, MHSA
Program Associate—Health Programming
W.K. Kellogg Foundation
Battle Creek, Michigan

Barbara Brodie, RN, PhD, FAAN
Professor
School of Nursing
University of Virginia
Charlottesville, Virginia

Kathleen Coen Buckwalter, RN, PhD, FAAN
Professor
College of Nursing
The University of Iowa
Iowa City, Iowa

Maureen McCormac Bueno, RN, PhD
Director, Nursing Systems
Robert Wood Johnson University Hospital
New Brunswick, New Jersey

Gloria M. Bulechek, RN, PhD
Associate Professor
College of Nursing
The University of Iowa
Iowa City, Iowa

Paulette Burns, PhD, RN
Assistant Professor and
Division Director, Tulsa Campus
College of Nursing
University of Oklahoma
Tulsa, Oklahoma

Cecelia Capuzzi, RN, PhD
Associate Professor
School of Nursing
Oregon Health Sciences University
Portland, Oregon

Lynda Juall Carpenito, RN, MSN
President
LJC Consultants Inc.
Mickleton, New Jersey

Martha A. Carpenter, RN, PhD
Assistant Professor
College of Nursing
The University of Iowa
Iowa City, Iowa

Patricia T. Castiglia, RN, PhD, PNP, C
Dean
College of Nursing and Allied Health
The University of Texas at El Paso
El Paso, Texas

Roseni Rosângela Chompré
Director Nursing Development Program
Assistant Professor of the School of Nursing
The Federal University of Minas Gerais
Luxemburgo, Belo Horizonte, Brasil

Maria Auxiliadora C. Christofaro
Assistant Professor of the School of Nursing
The Federal University of Minas Gerais
Luxemburgo, Belo Horizonte, Brasil

June Clark, RN, PhD, RH, FRCN
Professor of Nursing and Head of School
of Health Care Studies
Middlesex University
Queensway, Enfield, England

Ann Faas Collard, RN, PhD, FAAN, C
Senior Research Associate
Institute for Health Policy
Brandeis University
Waltham, Massachusetts

Joyce Colling, RN, PhD, FAAN
Professor and Chair
Community Health Care Systems Department
School of Nursing
Oregon Health Sciences University
Portland, Oregon

Colleen Conway-Welch, RN, PhD, FAAN, CNM
Professor and Dean
School of Nursing
Vanderbilt University
Nashville, Tennessee

Perle Slavik Cowen, RN, PhD
Assistant Professor
College of Nursing
The University of Iowa
Iowa City, Iowa

Connie R. Curran, RN, EdD, FAAN
Consultant and Professor
University of Illinois
Chicago, Illinois

Carolyne Kahle Davis, RN, PhD
National Health Care Advisor
Ernst and Young
Washington, D.C.

Susan L. Dean-Baar, RN, PhD, CRRN
Assistant Professor
School of Nursing
University of Wisconsin–Milwaukee
Milwaukee, Wisconsin

Vivien De Back, RN, PhD, FAAN
Clinical Professor
School of Nursing
and
Nursing Education Fellow
University of Wisconsin–Milwaukee
Eastern Europe
Project HOPE
Milwaukee, Wisconsin

Elizabeth C. Devine, RN, PhD, FAAN
Associate Professor
School of Nursing
University of Wisconsin–Milwaukee
Milwaukee, Wisconsin

Donna Diers, RN, MSN, FAAN
The Annie W. Goodrich Professor
Chair, Adult Health Division
Director, Policy Studies
Yale University School of Nursing
Lecturer, School of Public Health
Yale University School of Medicine
New Haven, Connecticut

Elizabeth O. Dietz, RN, EdD, C
Professor/Nurse Practitioner
San Jose State University
San Jose, California

Sr. Rosemary Donley, RN, PhD, FAAN
Executive Vice President
The Catholic University of America
Washington, D.C.

Eunice K. M. Ernst, MPH, CNM
Executive Director
National Association of Childbearing Centers
Perkiomenville, Pennsylvania

Claire M. Fagin, RN, PhD, FAAN
Professor, School of Nursing
University of Pennsylvania
Philadelphia, Pennsylvania

Sharon S. Farley, RN, PhD
Associate Professor and Director,
Rural Elderly Enhancement Program
School of Nursing
Auburn University at Montgomery
Montgomery, Alabama

Mary V. Fenton, RN, DrPH
Dean and Professor
The University of Texas Medical Branch
School of Nursing at Galveston
Galveston, Texas

Sharon L. Firlit, RN, PhD
Associate Chief Nursing Service/Education
Department of Veterans Affairs
Edward Hines, Jr., Hospital
Hines, Illinois
and
Instructor, Clinical Faculty
Niehoff School of Nursing
Loyola University
Chicago, Illinois

Sr. Mary Jean Flaherty, RN, PhD, FAAN
Dean, School of Nursing
The Catholic University of America
Washington, D.C.

Lyndia Flanagan, MA
Consultant
American Nurses Association
Washington, D.C.

Patricia R. Forni, RN, PhD, FAAN
Dean
College of Nursing
The University of Oklahoma
Health Sciences Center
Oklahoma City, Oklahoma

David Anthony Forrester, RN, PhD
Professor and Associate Dean,
Academic Affairs and Research
and
Director, Center for Nursing Research
University of Medicine and Dentistry of New Jersey
School of Nursing
Newark, New Jersey

Virginia Kliner Fowkes, FNP, MHS
Director, Primary Care Associate Program
Stanford Area Health Education Center
Division of Family and Community Medicine
Stanford University School of Medicine
Palo Alto, California

Maryann F. Fralic, RN, DrPh, FAAN
Vice President for Nursing
The Johns Hopkins Hospital
Baltimore, Maryland
Formerly:
Senior Vice President, Nursing
Robert Wood Johnson University Hospital
New Brunswick, New Jersey

Sara T. Fry, RN, PhD, FAAN
Associate Professor
University of Maryland at Baltimore
School of Nursing
Baltimore, Maryland

Betty S. Furuta, RN, MS
Assistant Dean, Student and International Academic
Services
Assistant Clinical Professor
Department of Mental Health, Community, and
Administrative Nursing
School of Nursing
University of California, San Francisco
San Francisco, California

Sr. Lucia Gamroth, RN, PhD
Research Associate
Benedictine Nursing Center
Mt. Angel, Oregon
and
Instructor, Community Health Care Systems
Oregon Health Sciences University
School of Nursing
Portland, Oregon

Helen Kennedy Grace, RN, PhD, FAAN
Vice President-Program
W. K. Kellogg Foundation
Battle Creek, Michigan

Judith R. Graves, RN, PhD, FAAN
Professor
University of Utah
College of Nursing
Salt Lake City, Utah

Edward J. Halloran, RN, PhD, FAAN
Associate Professor
School of Nursing
The University of North Carolina at Chapel Hill
Chapel Hill, North Carolina

Donna Sullivan Havens, RN, PhD
Assistant Professor
School of Nursing
Duke University
Durham, North Carolina

Sue Thomas Hegyvary, RN, PhD, FAAN
Professor and Dean
School of Nursing
University of Washington
Seattle, Washington

Linda C. Hodges, RN, EdD
Dean and Professor
University of Arkansas for Medical Sciences
College of Nursing
Little Rock, Arkansas

Constance A. Holleran, RN, MSN, FAAN
Executive Director
International Council of Nurses
Geneva, Switzerland

Diane Gardner Huber, RN, PhD
Associate Professor
College of Nursing
The University of Iowa
Iowa City, Iowa
and
Adjunct Director of Nursing
Mercy Hospital
Iowa City, Iowa

Mary Louise Icenhour, RN, PhD
Assistant Professor
School of Nursing
Duke University
Durham, North Carolina

Marguerite M. Jackson, RN, MS, FAAN, CIC
Administrative Director
Medical Center Epidemiology Unit
University of California, San Diego
San Diego, California

Sonia Jaimovich, RN, MPH
Associate Professor
School of Nursing
Catholic University of Chile
Santiago, Chile

Lucille A. Joel, RN, EdD, FAAN
Professor and Director
Teaching Nursing Home
College of Nursing
Rutgers, The State University of New Jersey
Newark, New Jersey

Marion Johnson, RN, PhD
Associate Professor
College of Nursing
The University of Iowa
Iowa City, Iowa
and
Adjunct Associate Administrator
Mercy Medical Center
Cedar Rapids, Iowa

Karen Sue Kauffman, RN, PhD
Assistant Professor
Frances Payne Bolton School of Nursing
Case Western Reserve University
Cleveland, Ohio

Catherine Kelleher, RN, ScD
Assistant Professor, School of Nursing
Joint Appointment, Oncology, School of Medicine
The Johns Hopkins University
Baltimore, Maryland

Janet C. Ross Kerr, RN, PhD
Professor
Faculty of Nursing
The University of Alberta
Edmonton, Alberta, Canada

Shaké Ketefian, RN, EdD, FAAN
Professor, and Director of the Doctoral Program
University of Michigan
School of Nursing
Ann Arbor, Michigan

Diane K. Kjervik, RN, JD, FAAN
Professor
The University of Texas at Austin
School of Nursing
Austin, Texas

Robert J. Kus, RN, PhD
St. Mary's Seminary
Wickliffe, Ohio

Ilta Lange, RN, MS
Director, Outpatient Clinic
Catholic University Hospital
and
Assistant Professor
School of Nursing
Catholic University of Chile
Santiago, Chile

Cynthia L. Lenz, RN, PhD
Senior Vice President and
Chief Operating Officer
Health First, Clinics Division
Knoxville, Tennessee

Juliene G. Lipson, RN, PhD, FAAN
Associate Professor
Department of Mental Health, Community, and
Administrative Nursing
School of Nursing
University of California, San Francisco
San Francisco, California

Maxine E. Loomis, RN, PhD, FAAN, CS
Distinguished Professor Emeritus
University of South Carolina
College of Nursing
Columbia, South Carolina

Sally Peck Lundeen, RN, PhD, FAAN
Director, Nursing Center
University of Wisconsin–Milwaukee
Milwaukee, Wisconsin

Meridean L. Maas, RN, PhD, FAAN
Associate Professor
Area Chair, Organizations and Systems
College of Nursing
The University of Iowa
Iowa City, Iowa
and
Adjunct Associate Executive in Nursing
Iowa Veterans Home
Marshalltown, Iowa

Catherine Malloy, RN, DrPH, C
Professor and Associate Dean for Academic Programs
George Mason University
School of Nursing
Fairfax, Virginia

Pamela Maraldo, RN, PhD, FAAN
President
Planned Parenthood Federation of America
New York, New York

Karen Martin, RN, MSN, FAAN
Health Care Consultant
Omaha, Nebraska

Hans O. Mauksch, PhD
Professor Emeritus
University of Missouri at Columbia
Columbia, Missouri
and
Lecturer
University of Georgia
Athens, Georgia

Joanne Comi McCloskey, RN, PhD, FAAN
Distinguished Professor
College of Nursing
The University of Iowa
and
Adjunct Associate Director of Nursing
The University of Iowa Hospitals and Clinics
Iowa City, Iowa

Diana C. McPherson, RN, BSN, CIC
Senior Nurse Epidemiologist
Medical Center Epidemiology Unit
University of California, San Diego
San Diego, California

Phyllis D. Meadows, RN, MSN
Program Associate
W.K. Kellogg Foundation
Detroit, Michigan

Anamaria Vaz de Assis Medina, MS
Autonomous Consultant
School of Nursing
Federal University of Minas Gerais
Luxemburgo, Belo Horizonte, Brasil

Afaf I. Meleis, RN, PhD, DrPS (hon), FAAN
Professor
Department of Mental Health, Community, and
Administrative Nursing
School of Nursing
University of California, San Francisco
San Francisco, California

Janet Mentink, FNP, PhD, C
Director
Family Nurse Practitioner and Physician Assistant Program
Department of Family Medicine
School of Medicine
University of California at Davis
Davis, California

Mary Etta Mills, RN, ScD
Associate Professor
Chair, Department of Education, Administration, and
Health Policy
School of Nursing
University of Maryland
Baltimore, Maryland

Maria Mitchell, RN, MS, PNP
President and Chief Operating Officer
Community Health Accreditation Program, Inc.
New York, New York

Mary D. Naylor, RN, PhD, FAAN
Associate Dean
Killebrew/Censits Term
Professor of Undergraduate Education
School of Nursing
University of Pennsylvania
Philadelphia, Pennsylvania

Margo C. Neal, RN, MN
Vice President and Publisher
Nursecom, Inc.
Malibu, California

Karen S. O'Connor, RN, MA
Director
Department of Practice, Economics and Policy
American Nurses Association, Inc.
Washington, D.C.

Virginia M. Ohlson, RN, PhD, FAAN
Professor Emeritus
University of Illinois at Chicago
College of Nursing
Chicago, Illinois

Ellen F. Olshansky, RN, DNSc, ARNP, C
Associate Professor and Coordinator
Women's Health Care Nurse Practitioner Program
Department of Parent and Child Nursing
School of Nursing
University of Washington
Seattle, Washington

Patricia M. Ostmoe, RN, PhD
Professor and Dean
School of Nursing
University of Wisconsin–Eau Claire
Eau Claire, Wisconsin

Rebecca Partridge, RN, PhD
Coordinator of Hospital Quality Assurance
Department of Nursing
Stanford University Hospital
Stanford, California

Adele W. Pike, RN, MSN
Clinical Nurse Specialist
Beth Israel Hospital
Boston, Massachusetts

Gaye W. Poteet, RN, PhD
Consultant and Lecturer
Management Development Enterprises
Galveston, Texas

Richard W. Redman, RN, PhD
Associate Professor, and
Director, Division of Nursing and Health Systems
Administration
The University of Michigan
School of Nursing
Ann Arbor, Michigan

Barbara Robertson, RNRM, D.Litt et Phil
Professor and Head
Department of Nursing Education
University of the Witwatersrand
Johannesburg, South Africa

Marilyn L. Rothert, RN, PhD, FAAN
Acting Dean and Professor
Michigan State University
College of Nursing
East Lansing, Michigan

Polly Ryan, RN, PhD
Research Nursing, Department of Nursing
Milwaukee County Medical Complex Hospital
Milwaukee, Wisconsin

Marla E. Salmon, RN, ScD, FAAN
Director
Division of Nursing
Department of Health and Human Services
Rockville, Maryland

Janet C. Scherubel, RN, PhD, CCRN
Assistant to the Director
Nursing Services Research and Support
Nursing Affairs
Rush-Presbyterian-St. Luke's Medical Center
Chicago, Illinois

Carole A. Shea, RN, PhD
Associate Dean and Graduate Director
College of Nursing
Northeastern University
Boston, Massachusetts

Susan Sherman, RN, MA
Professor and Head
Department of Nursing
Community College of Philadelphia
Project Administrator
The Community College–Nursing Home Partnership
Philadelphia, Pennsylvania

Roy L. Simpson, RN
Corporate Director, Nursing Affairs
HealthQuest
Atlanta, Georgia

Joy Smith, RN, BSN
Director of Nursing
Benedictine Nursing Center
Mt. Angel, Oregon

Linda S. Smith, RN, MS
Nursing Instructor
Gateway Technical College
Kenosha, Wisconsin

Janet Specht, RN, C, MA
Doctoral Student
The University of Iowa
Iowa City, Iowa

Richard B. Splane, PhD, LLD
Professor Emeritus
University of British Columbia
and
Consultant, Social Policy
Splane Associates
Vancouver, British Columbia, Canada

Verna Huffman Splane, RN, MPH, LLD
Associate Professor
Faculty of Nursing
University of Alberta
Edmonton, Alberta, Canada
and
Consultant, International Nursing
Splane Associates
Vancouver, British Columbia, Canada

Margaret J. Stafford, RN, MSN, FAAN
Adjunct Faculty
University of Illinois and Loyola University
Chicago, Illinois

Nancy A. Stotts, RN, EdD
Associate Professor
Department of Physiological Nursing
University of California, San Francisco
San Francisco, California

Maureen Beirne Streff, RN, MS, CS
Certified Psychiatric Clinical Specialist
Streff Associates
Acton, Massachusetts
and
Lobbyist and Public Relations Specialist
Nurses United for Responsible Services
Cambridge, Massachusetts

Neville E. Strumpf, RN, PhD, FAAN, C
Doris Schwartz Term Professor and Director
Gerontological Nurse Clinician Program
School of Nursing
University of Pennsylvania
Philadelphia, Pennsylvania

Margretta Madden Styles, RN, EdD, FAAN
Professor Emerita
University of California, San Francisco
San Francisco, California

Elizabeth A. Swanson, RN, PhD
Associate Professor
College of Nursing
The University of Iowa
Iowa City, Iowa

Sandra S. Sweeney, RN, PhD
Professor, Nursing Systems
University of Wisconsin–Eau Claire
Eau Claire, Wisconsin

Geraldine J. Talarczyk, RN, EdD
Associate Professor and Associate Dean for Academic
Affairs
Michigan State University
College of Nursing
East Lansing, Michigan

Starla Tate, RN, MNSc
Instructor of Nursing
University of Arkansas for Medical Sciences
College of Nursing
Little Rock, Arkansas

Barbara Volk Tebbitt, RN, MS
Consultant in Health Care and Nursing Administration
Shoreview, Minnesota

Cheryl Bagley Thompson, RN, PhD, CS
Assistant Professor, Nursing Informatics
University of Utah
College of Nursing
Salt Lake City, Utah

Marita G. Titler, RN, PhD
Associate Director of Nursing Research
University of Iowa Hospitals and Clinics
Iowa City, Iowa

Pamela A. Triolo, RN, PhD
Chief Nursing Officer
University Hospital
and
Associate Dean
College of Nursing
University of Nebraska Medical Center
Omaha, Nebraska

Toni Tripp-Reimer, RN, PhD, FAAN
Professor and Director
Office for Nursing Research Development and Utilization
College of Nursing
The University of Iowa
Iowa City, Iowa

Susan M. Tucker, RN, MSN, PHN
Director of Nursing, MCH/SNF
Kaiser Permanente Medical Center
Panorama City, California

Judith J. Warren, RN, PhD
Associate Professor
College of Nursing
University of Nebraska Medical Center
and
Assistant Director of Nursing Research
University of Nebraska Hospital
Omaha, Nebraska

Verle Waters, RN, MA
Dean Emeritus
Ohlone College
Project Consultant
The Community College–Nursing Home Partnership
Fremont, California

Glenn Webster, PhD
Associate Professor of Philosophy
and
Adjunct Associate Professor of Nursing
University of Colorado at Denver
Denver, Colorado

Kay Weiler, RN, JD
Assistant Professor
College of Nursing
The University of Iowa
Iowa City, Iowa

John M. Welton, RN, MSN
Doctoral Student
School of Nursing
The University of North Carolina at Chapel Hill
Chapel Hill, North Carolina

Harriet H. Werley, RN, PhD, FAAN
Distinguished Professor, Emerita
School of Nursing
University of Wisconsin–Milwaukee
Milwaukee, Wisconsin

Karen E. Witt, RN, MSN
Associate Professor, Nursing Systems
University of Wisconsin–Eau Claire
Eau Claire, Wisconsin

Karen S. Wulff, RN, EdD
Executive Staff Specialist and Clinical Director
Swedish Medical Center
Seattle, Washington

Carolyn J. Yocom, RN, PhD
Director of Research Services
National Council of State Boards of Nursing
Chicago, Illinois

Karen Zander, RN, MS, CS
Principal
The Center for Case Management, Inc.
South Natick, Massachusetts

CeCelia R. Zorn, RN, PhD
Assistant Professor
School of Nursing
University of Wisconsin–Eau Claire
Eau Claire, Wisconsin

Preface

Nursing, worldwide, is a profession undergoing rapid change. The changes in nursing are related to the changes in society: in the wake of the women's movement, nurses have become more personally and politically assertive; more flexible education patterns and government's increasing financial support for education have led to an acceptance of university education for nurses, advanced degrees, and the generation of new nursing knowledge; automation and increasing technology have caused specialization. Nursing is also influenced greatly by the changes in health care: an aging society with more chronic health care problems has promoted the nursing specialty of gerontology with more attention to the problems of long-term care and nursing homes; prospective payment and cost containment efforts in health care have created concerns in nursing about cost of services and about new ways to structure the delivery of health care to be more efficient; AIDS and the care of these patients raised issues related to ethics, nursing knowledge, and practice. And more than ever, amidst all the change, nurses are practicing independently, expanding their roles, and requesting equal participation in the important decisions affecting patient care and health care policy.

In periods of rapid change, decisions must often be made quickly. With many issues confronting such a large and diverse profession, there is danger that decisions will be made without full knowledge or without sufficient opportunity to discuss and debate. Or worse yet, issues may be ignored and decisions not made. The purpose of this book is to provide a forum for knowledgeable debate on the important issues that concern all of today's nurses so that intelligent decision making can occur.

As in the previous editions, the issues are identified and addressed in 12 sections (parts): definitions of nursing, nursing knowledge, changing education, changing practice, quality assurance, governance, health care reform, health care costs, personal and professional assertiveness, role conflict, cultural diversity, and ethics. As in previous editions, each section includes an *overview* of the section, a *debate* chapter, and several *viewpoint* chapters. Try as we might to keep the content

at a reasonable length, the growing complexity of nursing is demonstrated in the growth of the volumes. In the first edition, we had 75 chapters, in the second, 84, in the third, 89 and, in this edition, 103. Of the 103 chapters in this edition, only 2 are reprints from the third edition, 45 are updates from the third edition, and 56 are totally new. Most of the updated chapters are so much revised that they are not comparable to the previous versions. All the chapters are original pieces written for this book. To our knowledge, only two the chapters have been published elsewhere, and that was with our permission. We have continued a feature that was introduced with the third edition, concluding each section with a chapter written from an international perspective.

Among the new content topics for this edition are: patient outcomes, use of nursing assistants, computer-based patient record, total quality management, standards and guidelines, shared governance, nursing's agenda for health care reform, hospital work redesign, risk of exposure to bloodborne pathogens, child abuse, and advance directives. In addition to a good deal of new content, changes in this edition include a different first section, the expansion of the previous section on government intervention to a section now called health care reform, and the expansion of the previous section called cost-effectiveness to a section now called health care costs. While its title remains the same as in this edition, Part One, Definitions of Nursing, is totally new. The previous edition's first section's content on nursing theory is now included in the second section on nursing knowledge. Now, Part One provides an overview of the facts and issues about specific groups of nurses and serves as an introduction to the rest of the book. Chapters are included about staff nurses, advanced nurse practitioners, nurse administrators, nursing faculty, nurse researchers, nurse entrepreneurs, and international nursing leaders.

Each section begins with an **overview** where we introduce the theme for the section and briefly describe each of the chapters in it. The section overviews, which highlight some of the important points in each chapter and raise some related issues, assist readers to select chapters for in-depth reading.

Following the overview, each section includes a **debate** chapter, featuring the pros and cons of one of the problematic issues in nursing. A listing of the titles of debate chapters in the edition gives some idea of the scope of the issues:

- What is nursing?
- Is nursing research used in practice?
- Diversity in nursing education: Does it help or hinder the profession?
- Should nurses use assistants?
- How can we assure health care quality?
- Does nursing have the power to change the health care system?
- Solving the health care dilemma: What will work?
- Can health care costs be contained?
- Career development: Its status in nursing
- Can there be one nursing organization?
- Cultural diversity in nursing: How much can we tolerate?
- Do we have health care rationing?

In the first edition, the debate chapters were a result of master's students' participation in an issues course at the University of Illinois College of Nursing. (The editors were both on faculty at Illinois at the time.) The chapters were based on actual oral debates that took place in class. For each debate a small group of from two to five students were asked to choose a topic, make up a reading list for advance distribution, and present all sides of the issue in a debate format to the rest of the class. Each group was instructed to stress the facts and research findings and to be as creative in presentation as possible. The approach was intellectual but the mood was fun. Several groups conducted their own surveys of class knowledge and opinions prior to class. Others dressed for and acted out parts. For example, in one class a physician assistant and nurse practitioner dressed exactly alike in their lab coats and stethoscopes, and in another the students played the parts of nursing deans to argue out the merits of a PhD or a DN program.

Each group was required to state its debate topic in a debate form; the same topic could lead to several debates. For example, the topic, expanded role, resulted in one group in a debate titled "Should Nurses Practice Dependently, Independently, or Interdependently?" and in another group resulted in a debate titled "Nurse Practitioners or Physician Assistants?" In a two-hour course, one hour was allocated for the debate presentation and one hour for questions and debate with the rest of the class.

Some of the class debates were written up and were published in the first edition. In the second, third, and fourth editions we have kept the same format, as we think debates are an excellent teaching mode for this content. Students who debate the material, as well as their audience, are involved in sorting out the complicated issues surrounding the debate. Many times, just knowing all the facts leads to effective decision making; at other times, it leads to the knowledge of what further research is needed before effective decision making can occur.

The bulk of the book is composed of **viewpoint** chapters. In these, each author gives her or his own view and critical analysis of one particular aspect of the section's general topic. Viewpoints are those of the individual authors and may involve their taking a controversial stand, presenting a case study or results of some research, reviewing the past and current status of a topic, or outlining problems and future directions. The viewpoint chapters differ from the debate chapters as the words viewpoint and debate differ: the viewpoint chapters, for the most part, offer only one side or one aspect of an issue. It is hoped that the viewpoint chapters provide material and ideas for other debates, that readers will agree or take issue, that after reading a viewpoint they will be stimulated to think and seek out more information.

It is impossible to list all the many viewpoints here but a sample list of titles will, we hope, make you eager to read these and more.

- Clinical nurse specialists and nurse practitioners: Who are they, what do they do, and what challenges do they face?
- Patient classification schemas: Do we still need them?
- Community college–nursing home partnerships
- Flextime and self-scheduling: Benefits and difficulties
- Death of the care plan
- How can the quality of nursing practice be measured?
- Nursing and consumerism: How can we get decision making closer to the consumer?
- The costs of cocaine (crack) exposure: A broader perspective
- Feminism: The new look in nursing
- Entering collegial relationships: The demise of nurse as victim
- Increasing the pool of minority students
- The evolving HIV-AIDS pandemic: A study in stigmatization and its ethical challenges for nursing

Each of the sections ends with an international chapter. Reading of these chapters will expand the horizons of all nurses. Their titles are:

- International nursing leaders: Who are they, what do they do, and what challenges do they face?
- The international classification of nursing
- Development of models in international exchange to upgrade nursing education
- Primary health care in developing countries
- Selfcare as a concept to guide quality nursing practice in Latin American countries
- International nursing: The role of the International Council of Nurses and the World Health Organization
- The Canadian health care system: Overview and issues

- Who pays for the costs of care in other countries?
- Nursing in Russia: Impact of recent political changes
- Traditional roles for women and the impact on nursing services in Brazil
- Woman's health: A global perspective
- What are the ethical issues from a worldwide viewpoint?

As its size suggests, the book offers a fairly complete analysis of all of today's important nursing issues. Careful reading, thought, and debate today promote good decisions, actions, and achievements tomorrow.

Joanne Comi McCloskey
Helen Kennedy Grace

WHO IS THIS BOOK FOR?

This book is appropriate for several audiences. First, it is an ideal text for a senior level undergraduate or graduate level issues course. Faculty who are teaching courses designed to help associate degree and diploma RNs make the transition to the university will also find this particularly useful. An instructor using this text could easily have a class orally present the debates written here or could structure a whole new set of debates using the readings as source material.

Second, this book is useful as a core book for a graduate curriculum. There is something here that fits with most graduate nursing courses. For example, the section on nursing knowledge is appropriate for nursing theory course, the section on education for education courses, the sections on practice, quality assurance, and health care reform for nursing administration and clinical specialization

courses, the section on personal and professional assertiveness for leadership classes, and so on. By picking and choosing from the numerous viewpoints, every class in the graduate curriculum can benefit from the use of this book. In addition, by using one text throughout the curriculum, there is financial savings for the individual student and consistency in expectations from the faculty.

Third, the book is of interest to all nurses or nonnurses interested in developments in the profession of nursing. The book is an excellent source of information about nursing and about the issues confronting the profession. The chapters are written by subject experts and include many well known nursing leaders. The book is stimulating and envigorating and the challenges within will revitalize and energize the reader. It would make a good gift for a new RN or for a nurse returning to graduate school.

Acknowledgments

Every book, especially one of this size that involves so many authors, takes many people to finish the job. For help with the fourth edition, we wish to thank, in particular, four:

Linda Duncan, Executive Editor, Mosby–Year Book, who initiated the book and provided good feedback on the proposed table of contents. Shortly after we began, she undertook new responsibilities that removed her from the day-to-day operations of this book, but she has continued to lend her support.

Darlene Como, Executive Editor, Mosby–Year Book, who took over the book from Linda, and who has been very supportive and helpful in its production. She guided the book through all of the various production steps and her good taste is evident in its look.

Jennifer Clougherty, Program Associate at the University of Iowa, who did all the administrative work related to the book. Her excellent organization and communication skills made it possible for two busy people to add a book to their workloads.

Terry Stanton, Manager, Carlisle Publishers Services, who directed the copy editing and composition of the book. He had endless patience to be sure things were done right and looked good.

We also want to thank all of our authors. As the results demonstrate, each of them took seriously the task. Yes, there were a few who needed several reminders to respond, but as their chapters demonstrate they are a very responsible and knowledgeable group of people.

Finally, we are grateful for the continued support and enthusiasm for this book from the nursing community, both in the United States and other countries. We hope that this edition continues to meet your needs.

Contents

ONE   **DEFINITIONS OF NURSING**

OVERVIEW: The Richness of Nursing 2
Joanne Comi McCloskey, Helen Kennedy Grace

DEBATE

1   What Is Nursing? 5
Donna Diers

VIEWPOINTS

2   Staff Nurses: Who Are They, What Do They Do, and What Challenges Do They Face? 15
Lyndia Flanagan

3   Clinical Nurse Specialists and Nurse Practitioners: Who Are They, What Do They Do, and What Challenges Do They Face? 19
Margaret J. Stafford, JoAnn Appleyard

4   Nurse Administrators: Who Are They, What Do They Do, and What Challenges Do They Face? 26
Barbara Volk Tebbitt

5   Nursing Faculty: Who Are They, What Do They Do, and What Challenges Do They Face? 32
Carole Anderson

6   Nurse Researchers: Who Are They, What Do They Do, and What Challenges Do They Face? 38
Nancy A. Stotts

7   Nurse Entrepreneurs: Who Are They, What Do They Do, and What Challenges Do They Face? 43
Lynda Juall Carpenito, Margo C. Neal

8   International Nursing Leaders: Who Are They, What Do They Do, and What Challenges Do They Face? 49
Verna Huffman Splane, Richard B. Splane

TWO   **NURSING KNOWLEDGE**

OVERVIEW: The Connecting Link 58
Joanne Comi McCloskey, Helen Kennedy Grace

DEBATE

9   Is Nursing Research Used in Practice? 61
Kay Weiler, Kathleen Coen Buckwalter, Marita G. Titler

VIEWPOINTS

10   The Nursing Theory–Nursing Practice Connection 76
     Sharon L. Firlit
11   The Primacy of Practice in Nursing 82
     Janice Brencick, Glenn Webster
12   The Nursing Theory–Nursing Research Connection 87
     Mary A. Blegen, Toni Tripp-Reimer
13   The Reorganization of Nursing Knowledge 92
     Maxine Loomis
14   Patient Classification Schemas: Do We Still Need Them? 104
     Catherine Kelleher
15   Why the Nursing Minimum Data Set (NMDS)? 113
     Harriet H. Werley, Polly Ryan, CeCelia R. Zorn, Elizabeth Devine
16   Nursing Diagnosis Taxonomy Development: Overview and Issues 123
     Judith J. Warren
17   Nursing Intervention Classification (NIC): Defining Nursing Care 129
     Gloria M. Bulechek, Joanne Comi McCloskey
18   Nursing-Focused Patient Outcomes: Challenge for the Nineties 136
     Marion Johnson, Meridean Maas
19   The International Classification of Nursing 143
     June Clark

THREE   CHANGING EDUCATION

OVERVIEW: The Need for Educational Reform 150
Joanne Comi McCloskey, Helen Kennedy Grace

DEBATE

20   Diversity in Nursing Education: Does It Help or Hinder the Profession? 153
     Vivien De Back

VIEWPOINTS

21   Recruitment of Students into Nursing 158
     Mary D. Naylor
22   The Changing Pool of Students 163
     Geraldine Polly Bednash
23   Partnerships in Nursing Education: Expanding the Boundaries 170
     Marilyn L. Rothert, Geraldine J. Talarczyk, Susan M. Awbrey
24   Community College–Nursing Home Partnerships 177
     Susan Sherman, Verle Waters
25   Graduate Education: Making the Right Choice 182
     Gaye W. Poteet, Linda C. Hodges, Starla Tate
26   The Changing Face of Graduate Education: A Viewpoint 188
     Shaké Ketefian, Richard W. Redman
27   National Initiatives for Change 196
     Colleen Conway-Welch

28   Development of Models of International Exchange to Upgrade Nursing Education 202
      Mary V. Fenton

FOUR   CHANGING PRACTICE

OVERVIEW: Change Creates Opportunities 208
Joanne Comi McCloskey, Helen Kennedy Grace

DEBATE

29   Should Nurses Use Assistants? 212
      Elizabeth O. Dietz

VIEWPOINTS

30   Changes in the Hospital As a Place of Practice 220
      Lucille A. Joel
31   Developing Community Partnerships: Shifting Power from Health Professionals to Citizens 226
      Sharon Farley
32   Leadership for Change in Public and Community Health Nursing 233
      Marla E. Salmon
33   Midwifery: A Nursing Challenge 241
      Eunice K. M. Ernst
34   Long-Term Care: Meeting Obligations to the Elderly 248
      Neville E. Strumpf, Karen Sue Kauffman
35   Nurses and Case Management: To Control or to Collaborate? 254
      Karen Zander
36   Flextime and Self-Scheduling: Benefits and Difficulties 261
      Karen S. Wulff
37   Death of the Care Plan 267
      Susan M. Tucker
38   The Computer-Based Patient Record and How It Will Affect the Nurse's Practice 270
      Roy Simpson
39   Primary Health Care in Developing Countries 276
      Barbara Robertson

FIVE   QUALITY IMPROVEMENT

OVERVIEW: Multifaceted Approaches to Quality Improvement 284
Joanne Comi McCloskey, Helen Kennedy Grace

DEBATE

40   How Can We Assure Health Care Quality? 287
      Maria Mitchell

VIEWPOINTS

41   Measuring Quality: A Systematic Integrative Approach 295
Linda C. Hodges, Mary Louise Icenhour, Starla Tate

42   Quality Assurance in Long-Term Care 303
Lucia Gamroth, Joy Smith

43   The Status of Quality Assurance in Home Health Care 310
Joyce Colling

44   Standards and Guidelines: How Do They Assure Quality? 316
Susan L. Dean-Baar

45   TQM/CQI: What Is It? Does It Work? 321
Pamela Klauer Triolo

46   Nursing Certification: A Matter for the Professional Organization 327
Gloria M. Bulechek, Meridean L. Maas

47   Validating Clinical Competence: Old and New Approaches 336
Carolyn J. Yocom

48   How Can the Quality of Nursing Practice Be Measured? 342
Karen Martin

49   Self-Care As a Concept to Guide Quality Nursing Practice in Latin American Countries 350
Ilta Lange, Sonia Jaimovich

SIX   GOVERNANCE

OVERVIEW: Shedding Dependency 358
Joanne Comi McCloskey, Helen Kennedy Grace

DEBATE

50   Does Nursing Have the Power to Change the Health Care System? 361
Sandra S. Sweeney, Karen E. Witt

VIEWPOINTS

51   Why Are We Seeing More Unionization? 373
Karen S. O'Connor

52   Community Nursing Centers: Implications for Health Care Reform 382
Sally Peck Lundeen

53   A Guide to Nursing Organizations: What They Are and How to Choose Them 388
Sue Thomas Hegyvary

54   Faculty Governance and Strong Deans: Are They Compatible? 393
Patricia M. Ostmoe

55   Shared Governance in Nursing: What Is Shared, Who Governs, and Who Benefits? 398
Meridean L. Maas, Janet P. Specht

56   International Nursing: The Role of the International Council of Nurses and the World Health Organization 407
Virginia M. Ohlson, Margretta Madden Styles

SEVEN   **HEALTH CARE REFORM**

OVERVIEW: The Role of Nursing in Achieving Health Care Reform 418
Joanne Comi McCloskey, Helen Kennedy Grace

DEBATE

57   Solving the Health Care Dilemma: What Will Work? 420
       Helen Kennedy Grace, Roslyn McCallister Brock

VIEWPOINTS

58   Nursing's Agenda for Health Care Reform 426
       Pamela J. Maraldo
59   Financing of Health Care and Its Impact on Nursing 432
       Carolyne Kahle Davis
60   Third-Party Reimbursement Issues for Advanced Practice Nurses in the '90s 437
       Maureen Beirne Streff
61   Nursing and Consumerism: How Can We Get Decision Making Closer to the
       Consumer? 450
       Claire M. Fagin, Leah F. Binder
62   Work Redesign: The Key to True Health Care Reform 460
       Connie R. Curran
63   The Canadian Health Care System: Overview and Issues 467
       Janet C. Ross Kerr

EIGHT   **HEALTH CARE COSTS**

OVERVIEW: Nursing's Part In Health Care Costs 474
Joanne Comi McCloskey, Helen Kennedy Grace

DEBATE

64   Can Health Care Costs Be Contained? 477
       Helen Kennedy Grace

VIEWPOINTS

65   Costing Out Nursing Services: Is It Happening? 483
       Janet C. Scherubel
66   Balancing Cost and Quality: A Model for Action 490
       Maureen McCormac Bueno, Maryann F. Fralic
67   Long-Term Care Overpriced and Underrated 501
       Genrose J. Alfano
68   Paying for Health Care: Trends, Issues and Future Directions 506
       Ann F. Collard
69   The Costs of Safety Precautions to Reduce Risk of Exposure to Bloodborne
       Pathogens 515
       Diana C. McPherson, Marguerite M. Jackson
70   The Costs of Cocaine (Crack) Exposure: A Broader Perspective 522
       Phyllis D. Meadows

71 Are Nurses Getting Paid What They Are Worth? 528
Donna Sullivan Havens, Mary Etta Mills

72 How Can Nursing Decrease the Costs of Nursing Education? 534
Patricia R. Forni, Paulette Burns

73 Who Pays for the Costs of Care in Other Countries? 541
Gillian Biscoe

NINE PERSONAL AND PROFESSIONAL ASSERTIVENESS

OVERVIEW: The Winds of Change 546
Joanne Comi McCloskey, Helen Kennedy Grace

DEBATE

74 Career Development: Its Status in Nursing 549
Elizabeth Swanson

VIEWPOINTS

75 Nursing's Quest for Professionalism 559
Barbara Brodie

76 Strategies for Changing Nursing's Image 566
Rosemary Donley, Mary Jean Flaherty

77 Feminism: The New Look in Nursing 572
Carole A. Shea

78 Collaboration Between Nurses and Physicians: What Is It? Does It Exist? 580
Judith G. Baggs

79 Multidisciplinary Community-Based Education and Practice 586
Cynthia L. Lenz

80 Nursing in Russia: Impact of Recent Political Changes 595
Linda S. Smith

TEN ROLE CONFLICT

OVERVIEW: Choosing Our Conflicts 604
Joanne Comi McCloskey, Helen Kennedy Grace

DEBATE

81 Can There Be One Nursing Organization? 607
Rebecca Partridge

VIEWPOINTS

82 Has the Frontline Nurse Been Abandoned? 616
Hans O. Mauksch

83 What Are the Sources of Stress for Nurses? 623
Diane Gardner Huber

84 Nurses and Physician Assistants: Issues and Challenges 632
Virginia Kliner Fowkes, Janet Mentink

85 Entering Collegial Relationships: The Demise of Nurse as Victim 638
Adele W. Pike

86 Conflict and Nursing Professionalization 643
Marion Johnson

87 Traditional Roles for Women and the Impact on Nursing Services in Brazil 650
Roseni Rosângela Chompré, Anamaria Vaz de Assis Medina, Maria Auxiliadora C. Christofaro

ELEVEN   **CULTURAL DIVERSITY**

OVERVIEW: Addressing the Imbalances 656
Joanne Comi McCloskey, Helen Kennedy Grace

DEBATE

88 Cultural Diversity in Nursing: How Much Can We Tolerate? 658
Pamela J. Brink

VIEWPOINTS

89 Cultural Diversity in the Student Body Revisited 665
Betty S. Furuta, Juliene G. Lipson

90 Nurses and Unpopular Clients 671
Robert J. Kus

91 Increasing the Pool of Minority Students 676
Patricia T. Castiglia

92 Why Aren't There More Men in Nursing? 683
Edward J. Halloran, John M. Welton

93 Woman's Health: A Global Perspective 692
Afaf I. Meleis, Ferial A. M. Aly

TWELVE   **ETHICS**

OVERVIEW: Ethics of Caring Decisions 702
Joanne Comi McCloskey, Helen Kennedy Grace

DEBATE

94 Do We Have Health Care Rationing? 705
Sara T. Fry

VIEWPOINTS

95 The Oregon Model of Decision Making and Its Implications for Nursing Practice 711
Cecelia Capuzzi

96 Indigent Care 718
Catherine Malloy

97   The Evolving HIV-AIDS Pandemic: A Study in Stigmatization and Its Ethical Challenges for Nursing 725
David Anthony Forrester

98   Child Abuse: What Is Nursing's Role? 731
Perle Slavik Cowen

99   Maintaining Personhood in the Context of Assisted Reproductive Technology 742
Ellen F. Olshansky

100   Knowledge Technology: Costs, Benefits, and Ethical Considerations 746
Cheryl Bagley Thompson, Linda K. Amos, Judith R. Graves

101   Advance Directives: Implications for Nursing 752
Diane K. Kjervik

102   Tutor or Tyrant? 758
Martha A. Carpenter

103   What Are the Ethical Issues from a Worldwide Viewpoint? 763
Constance A. Holleran

Concluding Notes and Future Directions 769
Joanne Comi McCloskey, Helen Kennedy Grace

Index 771

PART ONE

DEFINITIONS OF NURSING

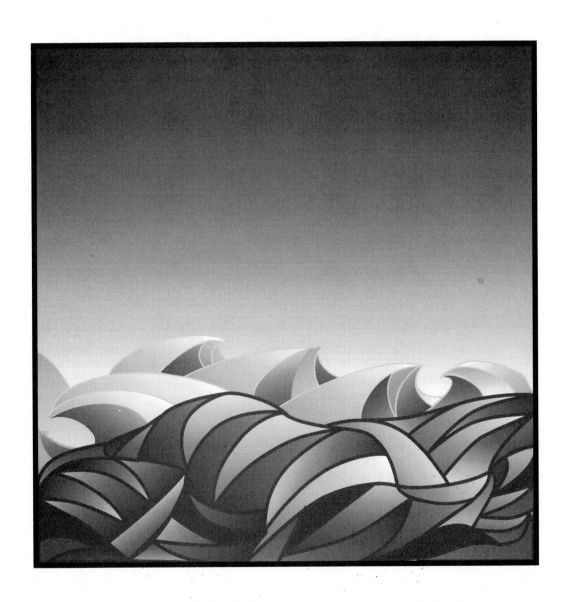

The richness of nursing

JOANNE COMI McCLOSKEY, HELEN KENNEDY GRACE

Nursing is a career rich in opportunity and variety. Entering the profession gives one an enormous choice of type of work and kind of setting. Nurses work in hospitals, homes, hospices, nursing homes, industries, doctors' offices, neighborhood health centers, private practices, schools, universities, government agencies, professional associations, and insurance companies. Education for nurses is as varied as work settings, ranging from a two-year associate degree and a three-year diploma to master's and doctoral degrees. Most nurses stay in nursing and change jobs several times over the course of their professional careers. The incredible variety of work and workers is the source of many of the issues that confront the profession. This section serves as an introduction to the issues discussed in the rest of the book. Many of the key positions in nursing are discussed here in separate chapters.

What is nursing? In the opening chapter Diers examines nursing's long-time search for a definition of nursing. She begins by looking at dictionary definitions, then definitions in law. This exercise illustrates the need to evaluate definitions according to the purposes and times for which they are written. Diers then moves to examine the nursing definitions of Nightingale and Henderson because these are important background works. Theories of nursing then are reviewed as another source of nursing definitions. Diers concludes that the definitional question is a political and legal one, not a conceptual one. She stresses that we need to strive continually to broaden our definitional boundaries. What we need, she says, is description more than definition. In a field so enormous and so complex we should not be surprised or distressed that we cannot condense this into a simple short definition. Diers says that a description of our ever-changing and complex role goes further to answer the question, What is nursing? than any of the definitions put forth

over the years. Meaningful descriptions would help convey the picture that "we do it all."

We do much of it as staff nurses working in hospitals. In the first viewpoint chapter Flanagan overviews the role and challenges for the staff nurse. Approximately two thirds of the 2 million nurses work in hospitals in the United States, and most work as staff nurses. Today's typical staff nurse is older, however, and has more education than in the past. This more stable and mature work force is more vocal in expressing the frustrations of the job. Using data obtained from a 1991 Opinion Research nationwide study of staff nurses, Flanagan says that staff nurses want to provide the best nursing care possible but that circumstances make it difficult. Nurses today function in a more stressful environment than earlier generations of nurses did. Job stressors are many and include inadequate staffing, little voice in workplace decision making, constant interruptions, lack of support, paperwork, high noise levels, and inadequate compensation. The greatest challenge facing staff nurses, she says, is the need to achieve control of the environment in which nursing is practiced. While nurses have begun to take action to strengthen nursing's influence, the pressures are increasing. In the future nurses will need more skills in the areas of strategic planning, marketing, cost containment, and ethics. Continuous change in health care will continue to make nursing a challenging and high-pressure job. Various challenges confronting nurses in practice are discussed in Part Four, titled "Changing Practice," and elsewhere in this book.

Challenged by their jobs, many staff nurses return to school to get advanced degrees and more knowledge that will help them make the needed reforms in their work settings. Many nurses who go on for advanced degrees become specialized in a clinical area of practice. Two types of specialized clinical practitioners are the clinical specialist and the nurse practitioner. Stafford and Appleyard review the origins of both and outline the functions and roles of each. Profiles of six clinical specialists who function in different specialties demonstrate the wide variety of depth and expertise. The authors then discuss a recent trend that may lead to the merger of the two roles and the single title of advanced practitioner.

Reimbursement for services is a major issue for these nurses. The independence of advanced nurse practitioners is thwarted when regulatory agencies and state and federal legislative bodies use the term *supervision* rather than *collaboration* to describe the interdependent relationship between physician and nurse. Clinical specialists and nurse practitioners face many challenges, but their potential impact as a united group should be strong enough to both meet the challenges and make a valuable contribution to health care.

Next, Tebbitt discusses the challenging job of the nurse administrator. A brief look at the past begins with Nightingale, who defined the major role of the nurse administrator as education of others who care for the acutely ill. As time went on, the roles of education and administration were separated. Today's nurse executive has 10 major roles: figurehead, leader, liaison, monitor, disseminator, spokesperson, entrepreneur, disturbance handler, resource allocator, and negotiator. Tebbitt also discusses six functions of the nurse executive: planner, implementer, coordinator, arbitrator, guide, and image setter. Tebbitt says that the role of tomorrow's nurse executive will be less remedial or corrective and more entrepreneurial or innovative. She outlines six challenges facing tomorrow's nurse executives. Success in the future, she says, will be measured by staff growth and satisfaction.

Faculty and the challenges they face are addressed next. Anderson profiles the estimated 19,000 nursing faculty members working in more than 1600 programs. Nursing, she says, has two types of faculty members: one who is master's prepared, teaching mostly clinical courses in a diploma or associate degree program, and the other more likely to possess the doctorate, employed by a college or university, and expected to integrate teaching, research, and service. While progress has been made in doctoral preparation of faculty, still fewer than half of those teaching in baccalaureate- and higher-degree programs have doctorates. Anderson says that this noncomparability of credentials coupled with the lower status of a female occupation marginalizes academic nurses. Without power and influence

academic nurses become angry and distrustful, which in turn causes academic men in other disciplines to further isolate them. Anderson overviews the various faculty roles and identifies the challenges facing nursing faculty. One challenge is the need for new models for undergraduate clinical teaching. Another is to ensure that our programs meet the needs of students but are rigorous and of high quality. She challenges faculty to work to eliminate practices that do not enhance the goal to become full participants in the academy. Among the poor practices she lists are team teaching and harsh treatment of students. This chapter raises many issues that need to be discussed and debated widely. It is an excellent introduction to issues in changing education.

Research in nursing has increased tremendously in the past decade. Stotts uses a research approach to describe nurse researchers, what they study, and the challenges they face. She reviewed studies published in three nursing research journals as a representative sample. Her analysis demonstrates that most of the recently published nursing research is clinical research. Small sample sizes are an issue in many of these studies. Nurse researchers use a variety of methodologies, and much research is done with a group of investigators. She found little evidence, however, of established programs of research. Another important issue is that of clinical significance versus statistical significance. The fairly large number of studies focusing on instrument development and refinement reflects, says Stotts, the maturing of the field. This chapter provides an introduction to the nature of nursing research. Students and beginning researchers will want to seek out experienced researchers for further discussion about the research process and challenges. Part Two, on nursing knowledge, provides more information and detail about some of the processes involved in building a science of nursing.

Perhaps the most nontraditional role in nursing is the entrepreneur. Carpenito and Neal say that nurse entrepreneurs include a variety of people who are self-employed or pursing careers that include consulting, writing, editing, owning staffing agencies, giving workshops, or providing patient care. Entrepreneurs seek to "make a difference for a profit." They say that the growth of entrepreneurship in nursing parallels the women's movement. Using their own experience as successful entrepreneurs and those of 17 colleagues whom they queried, Carpenito and Neal discuss a number of issues. Both the pros and cons of being self-employed are discussed. The pros include the freedom to do one's own thing and the flexible work hours. The cons include financial worries and isolation from colleagues. Excellent tips are given on how to start your own business. The chapter provides a very helpful orientation to the work and concerns of nurse entrepreneurs.

The last chapter in the section focuses on nurses in leadership positions at the international level. In the beginning of their chapter, Splane and Splane overview the international leadership of Florence Nightingale and the early leaders of the International Council of Nurses (ICN). They then use what they call a tricolumn base to analyze current international leadership. The three columns are the International Council of Nurses (ICN), the nurses in leadership positions within governments of the various nations (chief nursing officers), and nursing involvement in the World Health Organization. In 1985 the ICN began to award a prize to honor an international leader. The chapter authors do an excellent job of identifying past and present international nursing leaders. They give examples of nursing leadership in the World Health Organization, which they say has had "a limited perspective on nursing." It is at this level that nurses from many countries find common ground to influence international health policy.

Around the world it is the nursing leaders who are shaping the future of nursing and health care. Nurse leaders can be found working in a variety of positions and places. Nurse practitioners, administrators, faculty members, researchers, and entrepreneurs are joining hands to better define nursing's impact on health care. They continue to face many challenges, discussed in the rest of this book, but their united efforts are making nursing strong.

CHAPTER 1

Debate

What is nursing?

DONNA DIERS

Nursing does not suffer from lack of attempted definition. A good deal of expensive theoretical and political energy has been consumed by trying to isolate the core and the boundaries of the practice and the discipline, but agreement has yet to be achieved.

In this chapter the search for definition is examined. The intent is not to resolve the debate by providing a new definition. Rather, the purposes, parameters and policy consequences of this search are examined with a beady eye. Why define nursing—to what purpose and end? If we do not know what nursing *is,* how can we justify teaching it, or studying it or making decisions about it in a policy framework?

DICTIONARY DEFINITIONS

Dictionaries are published reports of common usage including linguistic derivation and part of speech—noun, verb, etc. That is all they are; they are not by themselves the definitive source. In the first edition of the *Random House Dictionary, to nurse* means to foster or cherish ("to nurse one's meager talents"); to treat or handle with adroit care ("to nurse one's nest egg"); to bring up, train or nurture; to clasp or handle carefully or fondly ("to nurse a memento"); to preserve ("to nurse a drink").[31] *Nurse* suggests attendance and service; its antonym is neglect.

Note that these definitions are of the transitive verb form. The gerund—nursing—derives from it and thus there is no definition of *nursing*. In the noun form, at least in this dictionary, a *nurse* is "a person, especially a woman [sic], who takes care of the sick or infirm; a woman [sic] who has the general care of a child or children; a woman [sic] employed to suckle an infant; or any fostering agency or influence." A delightfully

obscure meaning in billiards says a nurse is the act of maintaining the position of billiard balls in preparation for a carom.

Because dictionaries record common meaning, that meaning can and does change. It is encouraging to note that in the 1992 collegiate version of *Random House,* the first meaning of *nurse* is "a person formally educated in the care of the sick or infirm, especially a registered nurse"[32]—surely some progress even if they have not learned to capitalize the title.

There is no common lexical dictionary definition of nur*sing;* for that, one must turn to *Taber's Cyclopedic Medical Dictionary,*[39] which, despite its name, is compiled for nurses and allied health professionals. There one finds several columns about the noun, beginning with, "An individual who provides health care"[39] (not very clarifying). Whoever wrote this section then tries to get a grip on it:

The extent of participation [in health care] varies from simple patient care tasks to the most expert professional techniques necessary in acute life-threatening situations. The ability of a nurse to function in making self-directed judgments and to act independently will depend on his or her professional background, motivation and opportunity for professional development. . . . The roles of nurses constantly change in response to the growth of biomedical knowledge, changes in patterns of demand for health services, and the evolution of professional relationships among nurses, physicians and other health professionals.[39]

Subsequent paragraphs distinguish among types of nurses: charge nurse, community health, flight, general duty, graduate, head, licensed practical, private duty, registered, school, anesthetist, midwife, and practitioner. But when we come to nur*sing,* it is "scientific care of the sick by a graduate, registered nurse" but "loosely applied to any care of the sick."[39]

Congress weighed in when the staff of the Subcommittee on Health and the Environment of the House Committee on Interstate and Foreign Commerce produced their *Discursive Dictionary of Health Care*[38] to help members of Congress find their way through the minefield of healthspeak. Here a nurse is "an individual whose primary responsibility is the provision of nursing care,"[38] and nursing care is

... care intended to assist an individual, sick or well, in the performance of those activities contributing to health or its recovery (or to peaceful death) that he would perform unaided if he had the necessary strength, will or knowledge.[38]

This definition borrows from Virginia Henderson, to whom we will return shortly.

The purpose of dictionary definitions is simply to record derivation and common usage, not to distinguish nursing from anything else. There is no political agenda for dictionary definitions, except to the extent that common meaning reflects political realities. Since dictionaries are produced for the public, they portray the lay meaning of words.

DEFINITION IN THE LAW

Legal definitions contained in nurse practice acts exist to protect the public and protect the *title*. The U.S. Constitution delegates to the states police powers to protect the public, in the case of practice acts, from the unauthorized or unqualified practice of the profession. These acts are not enabling acts. They are restrictive, defining (more or less vaguely) the outer limits of authorized practice and quite clearly defining qualifications for using the legal title Registered Nurse (or Licensed Practical [Vocational] Nurse, Nurse Practitioner, Nurse-midwife, depending on state law). Licensing laws and their definitions are regulatory. They do not protect the nurse's practice from the charge of practicing medicine without a license or malpractice, although with clever legal assistance, practice acts may be used to *win* a court case.[36]

Practice acts are interpreted by state agencies, by boards of nursing under various titles, by interpretive statements in regulations or declaratory rulings, and by ad hoc interpretations by a board or sometimes even the staff. Further refinement of definitions of nursing come from rulings of attorneys general when requested by the board of nursing. Thus first-assisting in surgery may be interpreted by the board of nursing as within the defined practice of nursing in one state but not in another.

North Carolina became the first state to pass a licensing law, in 1903, and like many subsequent acts in other states, it was intended to protect the title, not to define the practice. The early statutes were certification statutes, permissive rather than mandatory. In general they permitted anyone to perform legally the functions of a nurse, even for compensation, but only licensed individuals could use the RN title.[16] The early acts were criticized by organized medicine and hospital associations for creating a nursing shortage by requiring registration and restricting the use of the title. Connecticut's legislature dealt with this problem interestingly. In 1907 an amendment to the Nurse Practice Act created a board of appeals to which nurses denied certification by the Nursing Board could turn. The appeals board consisted entirely of physicians, and their decisions were binding on the Nursing Board. As Hadley notes, ". . . the appeal board allowed the medical establishment to ensure that there would be an ample supply of nurses able to work at lower wages. . . ."[16]

New York deserves the distinction of first *defining* nursing in law, in 1938. The New York State Nurses Association (NYSNA) argued that "No practice can be controlled unless it is defined."[12] Control was sought over unlicensed or otherwise unqualified individuals trading on the title *nurse* and, it could be assumed, taking work away from those who were licensed.

In this regard, nursing is not different from other licensed professions, including medicine. Licensure is usually sought by the profession to protect its own interests, as a study by Andrews[4] of medical licensure laws often amusingly points out. By very broadly defining medicine, for example, almost anyone's practice, including a mother's, may be captured within it. See, for example, the Michigan definition of medical practice:

"Practice of medicine" means the diagnosis, treatment, prevention, cure, or relieving of a human disease, ailment, defect, complaint, or other physical or mental condition, by attendance, advice, device, diagnostic test, or other means, or offering, undertaking, attempting to do, or holding oneself out as able to do, any of these acts.[4]

The act of defining the work of a profession within the law, then, is a political act, and the resulting definitions must be read in that context. A compelling instance is the way the notion of diagnosis has been inserted in nursing practice acts. Idaho slipped the diagnosing function into its practice act first by legislating an exception to the part of the statute that prohibited unauthorized diagnosis and treatment.[5] New York, however, redefined nursing:

The practice of the profession of nursing . . . is defined as diagnosing and treating human responses to actual or potential health problems through such services as case finding, health teaching, health counseling and provision of care supportive to the restorative of life and well-being.[12]

The New York State Nurses Association was advised by its counsel that the diagnostic privilege was the sine qua non of independent practice.[12] The "human responses" modifier slips around "disease," which is central to medical practice acts. As a legislative memorandum (drafted by NYSNA) that accompanied the original bill notes,

Inclusion . . . of the diagnostic function would authorize the nursing practitioner to make *nursing diagnoses,* **not** medical diagnoses. Whereas the diagnostic function as an intellectual process is central to the practice of any number of professions, including medicine and nursing, the *focus* of this function varies among these professions. For example, the focus in medicine is the nature and degree of pathology or deviation from normalcy; within nursing the focus is the *individual's response* to an actual or potential health problem and the nursing needs arising from such responses.[12] (emphasis in original)

Thus, the attempt to broaden the definition of nursing to include diagnosis had, on the advice of one person, to consider the reality of physician opposition and what emerged was a semantic sleight-of-hand that, it can be argued, does not match modern nursing practice, even in less-than-expanded roles. The political reality was the need to build a fence between medicine and nursing; the problem was that this very real concern translated into defining the outer boundaries of nursing in a way ("human responses") that limited expansion and economic progress.

The publication and wide distribution of the American Nurses Association (ANA) monograph *Nursing: A Social Policy Statement*[1] has had the effect of codifying a definition of nursing based on New York State's definition: "Nursing is the diagnosis and treatment of human responses to actual or potential health problems," as if there were some national consensus. The slippage from a politically motivated set of phrases to this definition whose purpose is different—"to reflect . . . the influence of nursing theory that is part of nursing's evolution"[1]—further underscores the need to examine definitions according to their purpose. The purpose of the ANA document was to define the nature and scope of nursing practice to serve as a basis for ANA policy regarding credentialing and the establishment of qualifications for entry into nursing practice.[1] Control is still the issue: control of the entrée into nursing and control of those within it to assure that nurses do nursing, not something else.

Perhaps the ANA's right hand did not know what its left hand was doing, for in 1981 the ANA suggested language of nurse practice acts read:

The practice of nursing means the performance for compensation of professional services requiring substantial specialized knowledge of the biological, physical, behavioral, psychological and sociological sciences and of nursing theory as the basis for assessment, diagnosis, planning, intervention and evaluation in the promotion and maintenance of health; the casefinding and management of illness, injury or infirmity; the restoration of optimum function; or the achievement of a dignified death. Nursing practice includes but is not limited to administration, teaching, counseling, supervision, delegation, and evaluation of practice and execution of the medical regimen including the administration of medications and treatments prescribed by any person authorized by state law to prescribe. Each registered nurse is directly accountable and responsible to the consumer for quality of nursing care rendered.[2]

Note the exclusion of human responses and "actual or potential health problems." This suggested definition follows from the ANA's policy position, which advocates a single license to practice professional nursing without separate or additional licensure for specialized practice. Thus, the definition is designed to be inclusive enough to contain advanced practice and to keep the Association poised to speak both to basic and advanced nursing practice issues (and members).

The landmark case, *Sermchief v. Gonzales,*[36] turned on the language of the nurse practice act in Missouri, which is very close to the ANA suggested language. In *Sermchief,* the Supreme Court of Missouri determined that the acts of two nurse practitioners did indeed constitute the practice of nursing, not the practice of medicine, under Missouri law (including prescribing under standing orders and protocols). One might conclude, that the obfuscatory language of the New York act and the ANA's *Social Policy Statement* was not, in a legal sense, necessary after all.

By 1990, the ANA's suggested language for nurse practice acts had changed in an interestingly subtle way to "the practice of nursing means the performance of services for compensation in the provision of diagnosis and treatment of human responses to health or illness."[3] This change from "health problems" in the *Social Policy Statement* to "health and illness" broadened the target of nursing practice and still slithered away from boldly stating that nurses diagnose and treat disease (a "human response" to health could . . . er . . . be disease). The 1990 version also widens nursing's scope to include case management, establishing standards of practice, directing practice, and collaboration.

But nursing is no more real in legal definition than it is in dictionaries. The legal definition in practice acts is a political issue, not a theoretical or conceptual one. What emerges from the political process is often compromise. The "suggested language" quoted above has the advantage of being only suggested and not yet subject to the wear and tear of political negotiations, which is why it can be read as more expansive than many legal definitions of nursing. And, like dictionary definitions, legal ones can change and do.

NIGHTINGALE AND HENDERSON

A careful examination of Florence Nightingale's and Virginia Henderson's definitions of nursing is in order since they are the underpinnings of much of today's search for roots.

In *Notes on Nursing—What It Is and What It Is Not,* Florence Nightingale writes, "I use the word *nursing* for want of a better," and ". . . a nurse means any person in charge of the personal health of another."[28]

A marginal note in the printed original volume and later facsimile editions says, "Nursing ought to assist the reparative process," for Nightingale believed that ". . . all disease at some period or other of its course, is more or less a reparative process . . ." and that

. . . the symptoms or the sufferings generally considered to be inevitable and incidental to the disease are very often not symptoms of the disease at all but of something quite different—of the want of fresh air, or of light, or of warmth, or of quiet, or of cleanliness or of punctuality and care in the administration of diet, of each of or all of these.[28]

The furthest she goes toward definition is to say,

It [the word *nursing*] has been limited to signify little more than the administration of medicines and the application of poultices. It ought to signify the proper use of fresh air, light, warmth, cleanliness, quiet, and the proper selection and administration of diet—all at the least expense of vital power to the patient.[28]

The often-quoted definition of nursing attributed to Nightingale comes much later in the book in a discussion of what medicine or surgery can do and what nature can:

It is often thought that medicine is the curative process. It is no such thing; medicine is the surgery of functions, as surgery proper is that of limbs and organs. Neither can do anything but remove obstructions; neither can cure; nature alone cures.[28]

And thus, ". . . what nursing has to do . . . is to put the patient in the best condition for nature to act upon

him."[28] But this is not a definition of nursing; read in context, it is a somewhat offhand statement of nursing's function or goal.

Virginia Henderson's definition is of the unique *function* of the nurse, which she deliberately calls not a definition, but a "personal concept":

The unique function of the nurse is to assist the individual, sick or well, in the performance of those activities contributing to health or its recovery (or to peaceful death) that he would perform unaided if he had the necessary strength, will or knowledge. And to do this in such a way as to help him gain independence as rapidly as possible.[17]

Henderson is careful to say in the immediately following sentences that this is not all there is to nursing and that this statement was never intended to define the entire discipline. This statement is about the *unique* function of the nursing: ". . . this aspect of her work . . . she initiates and controls; of this she is master."[17] For Henderson, this unique function is the core of nursing from which all other things spring and which must be protected. "No one . . . should make such heavy demands on another member [of the medical team] that any one of them is unable to perform his or her unique function."[17] In a passage so lovely that it is almost poetry, Henderson translates this unique function:

[The nurse] is temporarily the consciousness of the unconscious, the love of life for the suicidal, the leg of the amputee, the eyes of the newly blind, a means of locomotion for the infant, knowledge and confidence for the young mother, the [voice] for those too weak or withdrawn to speak.[17]

In these activities the nurse is and, as Henderson argues, should be an independent practitioner ". . . able to make independent judgments as long as he or she is not diagnosing, prescribing treatment for disease, or making a prognosis, for these are the physician's functions."[17] Reflecting on these statements 30 years after they were first published, Henderson revises her emphasis:

Today I see the role of nurses as givers of "primary health care," as those who diagnose and treat when a doctor is unavailable, even as the midwife functions in the absence of an obstetrician. Nurses may be the general (medical) practitioners of tomorrow.

The modification in my concept of nursing since I wrote . . . in 1966 suggests a different emphasis. . . . I recognize now, as I think the majority of health care providers recognize, that registered nurses . . . are the major providers of primary care. Obstetrical nurses, or midwives, have been universally recognized worldwide as the providers of primary care for mothers and newborns. They diagnose and treat as well as "care."[18]

Nightingale wrote *Notes on Nursing* as a kind of Red Cross handbook for home nursing to explain the laws of the human body as she understood them and thus how the nursing functions could affect health. She wrote to make conscious the implicit knowledge that women in particular had, especially of diet and cleanliness, so that all women who "nursed" could be better prepared. But she also was writing a political treatise to enlist others in her mission.

Henderson devised her "personal concept" to help her understand her own experience, and she advocated that all nurses develop their own:

... I would urge every nurse to develop her own concept, otherwise she is merely imitating others or acting under authority. In my own case I felt as though I were steering an uncharted course until I resolved certain doubts about my true function.[18]

Both of these definitions go not to what nursing *is* but rather what nursing *does*. That is a distinction to keep in mind as we dig deeper into the definitional trench.

THEORIES AND DEFINITIONS

This is neither the time nor the place to analyze fully the various theoretical perspectives that might constitute another source of definition of nursing. That work has been done (and done and done again) and is usefully summarized by Afaf Meleis.[24]

In the heady 1960s there were what can only be seen in retrospect as two parallel but essentially unrelated areas of development of the field. First, there was the explosion of words, sentences, paragraphs, and papers posing various positions on what nursing is and what, therefore, nursing theory (later "nursing science") ought to be. And, second, there was the expanding role of nurses in specialty practice addressed in the next section.

Many of the outpourings about nursing theory were done by the first wave of nurses seeking doctoral degrees—in other disciplines primarily, since there were few doctoral programs in nursing. Leslie Nicoll's[27] remarkable compilation of many of these early theory pieces with contemporary comments by the original authors shows the commitment nurses had to figuring out what nursing was, often in the face of questions by the sociologists or psychologists on their dissertation committees.

This was also the time during which nursing began to move with deliberate speed into the universities,

and when postbasic programs grew and flowered. It was necessary for nursing faculties to justify what was particularly and peculiarly nursing in these graduate programs, that which would mark nursing and its knowledge as intellectual and as different from applied to anything else. What resulted was what Virginia Henderson actually had advocated—personal conceptions—but those conceptions were not about the practice of nursing, they were about the "discipline." The National League for Nursing helped reify these personal conceptions by imposing an accreditation criterion that specified that schools of nursing must have a "conceptual framework" to guide the curricula. Many apparently read that criterion as requiring the imposition or adoption of Somebody's personal conception as the overarching model for the curriculum, and we can now laugh at some of the crimes committed in the name of professionalizing nursing. (My favorite was a graduate curriculum in one unnamed school of nursing in which whole courses were based on one *clause* in one sentence of Dorothea Orem's work.)

There were theories about the content of nursing—Rogers' "science of unitary man," Roy's adaptation theory, Orem's theory of self-care deficits, and so on. It was never clear, however, whether these theories were *about* nursing, *for* nursing, *of* nursing. And, as later reflection pointed out,[13] these theories were really conceptual models that all had the same domains in more or less specificity: person, environment, health, and nursing. "Nursing" in these contexts was more or less the glue that held the whole thing together—often without much specificity because the theories dealt more with the nature of human beings in sickness and health than about what we are supposed to do about that. Thus, for Martha Rogers, for example, the goal of nursing was to bring and promote symphonic interaction between human beings and their environment through participation in a process of change[24] to "strengthen the coherence and integrity of the human field and to direct and redirect patterning of the human and environmental fields."[33] And nursing was simply the "learned profession" that did not, whatever that was. For Imogene King, nursing was called for when individuals could not function in their roles and was ". . . a process of human interaction between nurse and client whereby each perceives the other in the situation and, through communication, they set goals, explore means and agree on means to achieve goals."[19] For Joyce Travelbee, nursing was about finding meaning in experience to produce hope.[40] And so on.

The purpose of these grand theories and conceptual models was to develop the discipline, particularly the academic part of the discipline, to provide some structure to the research and perhaps to stake out turf that would be uniquely nursing, not in opposition to medicine but as different from applied social science. To be academically viable, however, these conceptual models had to look like other theoretical models in other disciplines. Because the other disciplines did not practice, they did not offer a precedent for including concepts about delivering a personal service, and thus the nursing conceptual models did not either. There was, however, a less-than-entirely-explicit agenda that if we would all just do the research guided by whatever conceptual model under whatever theoretical emphasis, then we would finally know what nursing *is*.

At the same time, another set of theories about nursing theory was evolving. These metatheoretical notions were not content-specific. They were about what nursing knowledge ought to look like as theory and how nursing knowledge could and should be built. There were implicit definitions of nursing in these theoretical meanderings. The clearest was in the work of philosophers Dickoff and James,[6,7] who said that since nursing is a practice discipline, nursing's theory had to encompass things such as values and goals. Theory, they said, was a "mental invention to some purpose,"[6] and when that purpose was to guide or prescribe practice, the theory had to take a different form.

There is an assumption here and in the related work of Wald and Leonard[42] that we know what practice *is;* we just need to understand what within it works. The "practice theorists" had no need for definition since the work grew from practice and was shaped by practice.

But much of this work was remote from the other driving definitional force: the expanding role of nursing.

ADVANCED PRACTICE AS DEFINITIONAL PROBLEM

The work of the nursing theorists can be read as attempts to define the core of nursing or at least the core concepts. When nursing began to expand in the 1960s, the question of nursing's boundaries became the hot topic.

Barbara Resnick[23] is generally acknowledged as the first nurse practitioner, at least in the United States. Her work occurred as part of a clinical trial of the efficacy of nursing in the management (no hint of "diagnosis" or "treatment") of chronically ill adults.

Charles Lewis, MD, who was her partner in this work, wrote later of how controversial it was for a nurse to take on this *independent* role,[22] a role that reads today as very conservative.

Expanding the nursing role was legitimized by the *Report of the Secretary's Commission*,[41] chaired by Rozella Schlotfeldt. The report defined "primary care" as first contact, continuing and coordinated care that nurses surely could provide. The report does not deal in any depth with what was, by 1971, already common in hospital intensive care units. The expansion of nursing's boundaries was a twofold expansion: into independent functioning without physician direction and into providing certain services, especially physical examination, diagnosis, and treatment, that had been "formerly medicine."[11]

While the movement of nurses into primary care practice as nurse practitioners generated considerable controversy, nurses as nurse-midwives and nurse anesthetists had expanded their roles long before the 1960s[9] with much the same internal and external controversy about whether what they did was "really" nursing. The fire came both in and outside nursing for nurse practitioners as it had for the earlier specialties. Part of the problem was that at exactly the same time nurses moved into primary care, physicians created their own assistants. Thus, Martha Rogers was moved to write that nurse practitioners were wolves in sheep's clothing and ought to just admit that they were filling in for doctors.[34] Loretta Ford[15] has written poignantly of the discrimination both from nursing and medicine against her pediatric nurse practitioner training program.

Ford was clear from the beginning that her concept of the nurse practitioner role grew from a base in community health nursing, where nurses had long functioned independently and had managed illness alone. The growth of intensive care in hospitals quickly legitimized what nurses had been doing all along in caring for acutely ill people when everyone else had gone home. Very soon, research showed that nurses could clearly do the work,[35,37] and over time enough evidence accumulated to conclude that the performance of nurse practitioners, in productivity and quality, was at least equal to if not better than that of physicians.[29]

Yet questions remain about whether the work of advanced practice, as it is coming to be called, is delegated medical functions or within nursing's boundaries. The definitional question, however, is a political and legal one, not a conceptual one, and it is increasingly becoming an economic question as well.

Political and legal ground has a tendency to shift. What was incomprehensible as nursing yesterday becomes routine tomorrow. As the U.S. health care policy framework turns ever more rapidly toward issues of cost and quality, the practice of professionals looks different. Nurse practitioners grew up in an era of physician shortage, so it was all right for nurses to substitute. Hospitals now are creating new positions for nurses to fill in some instances where house staff are not available. The same questions about whether this is more of the "physician dumping syndrome" are raised.[38]

When nurses' roles expanded, the suspicion was that nurse practitioners would no longer think of themselves as nurses, but rather as minidoctors. The language of the policy makers reinforced that notion: "midlevel" practitioners, halfway between real nurses and doctors, with nothing to call their own. This did not happen, and someone could do an interesting dissertation on why it did not.

Nursing roles have expanded because the talent is there and because there is a need, whether the need is for people to manage the care of the chronically mentally ill,[20] manage the care of rape victims, including testifying in court,[21] or devise and manage care for patients awaiting heart transplants. When nurses do it, it is nursing.

FROM DEFINITION TO DESCRIPTION

At the heart of the search for definition in nursing is the woeful recognition that nursing is so badly understood by the public, policy makers, professional colleagues, and health care administrators. In spite of over 100 years of rhetoric, some of it quite elegant, nursing remains a mystery to those outside it.[8]

What we ache for is not definition, it is description—what the work is and what it is like to do it.

Nursing is two things: the care of the sick, or the potentially sick, and the tending of the entire environment within which care happens.

Nurses deal with the most basic of human needs: feeding, heartbreak, warmth, elimination, suffering, loneliness, birth and death. Our hands get dirty, our uniforms stained, and our psyches eroded by daily contact with human beings in need—people crying, immobilized, angry, frightened, depressed and only occasionally joyful. We live with the outcome of a diagnosis made or missed; the crisis of faith in a higher being or a physician; the knowledge of decline, dis-

ability, permanent change, death, and the consciousness of our own mortality. We must be graceful over vomitus and effluvia, and dignified as we change the dressing, pack the wound, debride the decubitus and give out the bad news. With our hands and eyes we touch the lives of others and are admitted to the privacy of their inner space without even asking.[10]

We must know anatomy and physiology, pharmacology and biochemistry, social psychology, ethics, data analysis, management, and administrative science. We must know how to find, use, clean, and repair the equipment. We have to know how the heating system works, who really knows how to make the elevator come to the floor, and what the phone number for diagnostic radiology really is (it is not under *x* or *d* or *r*; it is under *i*—imaging). We have to be able to read a chart and a nursing or medical journal with equal facility. We have to know shortcuts and priority setting, the personalities of the surgical team, how to get the house staff to cooperate, and how to provide expert testimony in a malpractice suit.

. . . when a person says, "I am going to *nurse* my cold," he hastens to arrange this environment so that he can be as free as possible from stress and takes all means at his disposal to increase his comfort. On the other hand, when he says, "I am *doctoring* my cold," we know that he is not only relying on his own inner natural resources, but also on the products of medical science—pills, inhalers and the like.[30] (emphasis in original)

In one typical university teaching hospital, data from two general medical units over a three-month period showed 109 different diagnostic-related groups (DRGs) for about 500 patients.[14] Patient conditions ranged from stroke, with all its variations for the reversible to the catastrophic, to gastrointestinal bleeding, to infections of all kinds, to cancer, to out-of-control diabetes and everything in between.

What makes this kind of nursing difficult is not just the sheer physical work of helping people in and out of beds and wheelchairs, turning, lifting, pulling, tucking, feeding, carrying, reaching. It is not even the teaching, comforting, rubbing, bathing, careful listening, or endless documenting. It is not even the 500 different personalities and the 500 families. What is wearing even in a well-staffed and well-equipped hospital is the enormous amount of information it takes to care for people. To know that in this patient, one has to remember all one ever knew about ketoacidosis. To know that, in this other one, the rate of flow of the IV must be monitored closely because in this elderly person with kidney disease and emphysema the possibility of sending him into pulmonary edema is real. And in this one, the blood loss has produced dizziness and confusion and she cannot be left alone to fall out of bed. And in this one, the toxic effects of the poisons administered to chase his cancer have made him susceptible to any adventuresome bacterium, which would kill him.

A 25-year old man came for a scheduled visit [to a nurse practitioner] "just for a physical exam" because public service announcements on TV suggested that a routine exam was overdue for him. Three times during the interview he mentioned a childhood "heart murmur" which he had been told he had "outgrown." When asked, "How did you hope I could help you today?" he replied, "Just check for that heart murmur I used to have." Then he explained that his younger sister had died five months earlier of sudden, unexplained, but probably cardiac death. His sister had also had a heart murmur during childhood, and she too had been told some years earlier that she had outgrown it. As the patient was describing his sister's death, it became clear that he feared the same fate, and his fear more than anything explained the visit.[25]

It is not difficult to find descriptions of nursing nor to make up one's own out of last week's work. If the question "What is nursing?" is genuinely asked by the genuinely curious, then description might go further than definition.

CONCLUSION

Why is the question "What is nursing?" even raised, especially in the 1990s?

Dictionary, legal, and conceptual definitions abound. Are not they enough?

Surely they are not; otherwise the question would not still be the first-order heading for this first part of this book.

Nursing does not defy definition; it is simply so huge that it cannot be distilled satisfactorily into one or two pithy sentences. That is made out to be the fault of the discipline, that we cannot rest on the way other disciplines define themselves. But do they?

The social sciences are coming to wonder about their own definitions in these times of cutbacks in university funding and federal grants. What *is*, for example, sociology these days? It used to be the study of social groups, but now what is the boundary between sociology and organizational behavior, or political science? Psychology used to be the study of intrapersonal processes, but now it is also psychoimmunology and psychobiology and who knows what else.

Medicine (but never doctoring) seems not to worry about what its definition is. Anything physicians wish to define as medicine is medicine, except when it is in medicine's interest to decide that what was formerly medicine might now be done by others, and the extreme example closest to hand is abortion. In 1991 the American College of Obstetricians and Gynecologists (ACOG) and the National Abortion Federation (NAF) published the results of a symposium on abortion providers. One finding was that "trained midlevel clinicians" (PAs, nurse practitioners, and certified nurse-midwives) are "qualified to perform first trimester abortions under the supervision of a physician."[26] So long as it is "under the supervision" of a physician, one could conclude that it is still medical practice, whether it is abortion, primary care, or giving medications. But this semantic dance went away in nurse practice acts 20 years ago. Whether nurses wish to take on any new function is a different question. This is not an issue of definition; it is an issue of control, including economic control, for if something must be done "under supervision," then it cannot be billed separately. And guess who collects the dough.

These are semantic and legal fine hairs. Nursing has grown its own fine hairs when, for example, the use of International Classification of Diseases (ICD) codes to label patient problems are thought to be somehow the practice of medicine. ICD codes were originally invented for public health statistical interests to record and track causes of death. They are not owned by the American Medical Association. They are merely a very long set of labels of physiology, anatomical, and sometimes sociological names for things.

The boundary question is when does nursing leave off and something else start? More interesting is what the analysis in this chapter has, it is to be hoped, made clear: that there is a giant hole in nursing's conceptual work. There is hardly anything in the intellectual literature in nursing, other than standards of practice that are, in their own way, conceptual work that deals with specialty practice.

Inside nursing, the debate is about generalization versus specialization, and that, like every other thread to this theme, is both a political and conceptual issue—and increasingly an economic one too as hospitals begin to push for cross-training of nurses so that they may do more than one specialty.

What nursing *is* will not be resolved by arguing, by research, by conceptual handstands; it is not possible to know whether when a tree falls in the empty forest it makes any noise. It will be resolved, if at all, by recognizing that nursing changes very fast for all kinds of reasons and that those changes redefine the field as fast as we can write about it.

The changes occur now mostly in the clinical arena; they used to happen in the academic world. Generations of nursing faculty have now taught generations of nursing students in all kinds of educational programs to make the trills of innovation in the practice environment. If that is now confusing, and makes us question what nursing is, we should take that as a tribute.

Nurses run hospitals, home care agencies, nursing homes, and school health services. We serve on hospital boards and health planning agencies; we work in political campaigns and run for public office; we analyze and make public policy; we teach our own and other people's students; we do research, write books, articles, and best-selling fiction; we organize to support causes from legalizing birth control to AIDS funding to putting a statue of a woman at the Vietnam Memorial.

There are over 2 million nurses in the United States. In a field so enormous, it is not surprising that there might be confusion about what nursing is.

We do it all.

REFERENCES

1. American Nurses Association. (1980). *Nursing: A social policy statement.* Kansas City, Mo: Author.
2. American Nurses Association. (1981). *Suggested state legislation.* Kansas City, Mo: Author.
3. American Nurses Association. (1990). *Suggested state legislation.* Kansas City, Mo: Author.
4. Andrews, L. B. (1983). *Deregulating doctoring.* Emmaus, Pa: People's Medical Society.
5. Bullough, B. (Ed.). (1980). *The law and the expanding nursing role.* Philadelphia: F. A. Davis.
6. Dickoff, J., & James, P. (1968). A theory of theories: A position paper. *Nursing Research, 17,* 197-203.
7. Dickoff, J., James, P., & Weidenbach, E. (1968). Theory in a practice discipline: Part I: Practice oriented theory. *Nursing Research, 17,* 415-435.
8. Diers, D. (1988). The mystery of nursing. In *Final report of the Secretary's Commission on Nursing: Vol. II.* Washington, D.C.: U.S. Government Printing Office.
9. Diers, D. (1992). Nurse-midwives and nurse anesthetists: The cutting edge in specialist practice. In L. H. Aiken & C. M. Fagin (Eds.), *Charting nursing's future—Agenda for the 1990's* (pp. 159-180). Philadelphia: J. B. Lippincott.
10. Diers, D., & Evans, D. (1980). Excellence in nursing. *Image: The Journal of Nursing Scholarship, 12,* 27-38.
11. Diers, D., & Molde, S. (1983). Nurses in primary care: The new gatekeepers. *American Journal of Nursing, 83,* 742-745.
12. Driscoll, V. M. (1976). *Legitimizing the profession of nursing: The distinct mission of the New York State Nurses Association.* Albany, N.Y.: Foundation of the New York State Nurses Association.
13. Fawcett, J. (1980). A framework for analysis and evaluation of conceptual models of nursing. *Nurse Educator, 5,* 10-14.
14. Flood, S., & Diers, D. (1988). Nurse staffing, patient outcome and cost. *Nursing Management, 19,* 34-53.
15. Ford, L. C. (1982). Nurse practitioners: History of a new idea and predictions for the future. In L. H. Aiken (Ed.), *Nursing in the 1980's* (pp. 231-248). Philadelphia: J. B. Lippincott.
16. Hadley, E. H. (1989). Nurses and prescriptive authority: A legal and economic analysis. *American Journal of Law & Medicine, 15,* 245-300.
17. Henderson, V. A. (1961). *Basic principles of nursing care.* London: International Council of Nurses.
18. Henderson, V. A. (1991). *The nature of nursing—Reflections after 25 years.* New York: National League for Nursing.
19. King, I. M. (1981). *A theory for nursing: Systems, concepts, process.* New York: John Wiley & Sons.
20. Krauss, J. B., & Slavinsky, A. T. (1982). *The chronically mentally ill and the community.* Boston: Blackwell Scientific.
21. Ledray, L. (1992). The sexual assault nurse clinician: A fifteen-year experience in Minneapolis; the sexual assault examination: Overview and lessons learned on one program. *Journal of Emergency Nursing, 18,* 217-232.
22. Lewis, C. E. (1982). Nurse practitioners and the physician surplus. In L. H. Aiken (Ed.), *Nursing in the 1980's* (pp. 249-266). Philadelphia: J. B. Lippincott.
23. Lewis, C. E., & Resnick, B. A. (1967). Nurse clinics and progressive ambulatory patient care. *New England Journal of Medicine, 277,* 1236-1241.
24. Meleis, A. I. (1991). *Theoretical nursing: Development and progress* (2nd ed.). Philadelphia: J. B. Lippincott.
25. Molde, S., & Baker, D. (1985). Explaining primary care visits. *Image: The Journal of Nursing Scholarship, 17,* 72-76.
26. National Abortion Federation & American College of Obstetricians and Gynecologists. (1991). *Who will provide abortions? Ensuring the availability of qualified practitioners.* Washington, D.C.: National Abortion Federation.
27. Nicoll, L. H. (Ed.). (1986). *Perspectives on nursing theory.* Boston: Little, Brown.
28. Nightingale, F. (1859/1946). *Notes on nursing—what it is and what it is not.* Philadelphia: J. B. Lippincott.
29. Office of Technology Assessment. (1986). *Nurse practitioners, physician assistants, and certified nurse-midwives: A policy analysis.* Washington, D.C.: U.S. Government Printing Office.
30. Orlando, I. J. (1961). *The dynamic nurse-patient relationship.* New York: G. P. Putnam's Sons.
31. *Random House Dictionary.* (1966). New York: Random House.
32. *Random House Collegiate Dictionary.* (1992). New York: Random House.
33. Rogers, M. (1970). *An introduction to the theoretical basis of nursing.* Philadelphia: F. A. Davis.
34. Rogers, M. (1975). Euphemisms in nursing's future. *Image: The Journal of Nursing Scholarship, 7,* 3-9.
35. Schulman, J., & Wood, C. (1972). Experience of a nurse practitioner in a general medical clinic. *Journal of the American Medical Association, 219,* 1453-1461.
36. *Sermchief v. Gonzales,* 660 S.W. 2d 683.
37. Spitzer, W. O., Sackett, D. L., Sibley, J. C., Roberts, R. S., Gent, M., Kergin, D. J., Hackett, B. C., & Olnyich, A. (1974). The Burlington randomized trial of the nurse practitioner. *New England Journal of Medicine, 290,* 251-256.

38. Subcommittee on Health and the Environment, U.S. House of Representatives. (1976). *A discursive dictionary of health care.* Washington, D.C.: U.S. Government Printing Office.

39. Thomas, C. L. (Ed.). (1981). *Taber's cyclopedic medical dictionary.* Philadelphia: F. A. Davis.

40. Travelbee, J. (1966). *Interpersonal aspects of nursing.* Philadelphia: F. A. Davis.

41. U.S. Department of Health, Education and Welfare. (1971). *Report of the Secretary's Committee to Study Extended Role of Nurses—Extending the scope of nursing practice.* (Pub. No. HSM 73-2037). Washington, D.C.: U.S. Government Printing Office.

42. Wald, F. S., & Leonard, R. C. (1964). Towards development of nursing practice theory. *Nursing Research, 13,* 309-313.

CHAPTER 2

Viewpoints

Staff nurses

Who are they, what do they do, and what challenges do they face?

LYNDIA FLANAGAN

Over the past 25 years, there have been profound changes both in the demands for health care services and in the ways in which services are delivered. Most notably, hospitalization has come to be viewed as part of a continuum of care rather than as the primary site of treatment. While the emergence of alternative delivery systems has created new and different career and employment opportunities for nurses, hospitals remain the primary worksite for registered nurses (RNs). According to the most current data, more than two thirds (67.9%) of registered nurses work in hospitals. Moreover, about two thirds of all employed RNs hold staff nurse positions or "general duty" nursing jobs.

DEMOGRAPHIC DATA

Many observers contend that today's staff nurse population represents a work force with greater experience, expertise, efficiency, and stability than earlier generations. A number of factors influence this assessment, including the average age and level of education of the nursing population.

The registered nurse population is growing older. Like the general population, the RN work force seems to mirror the pattern of the "baby boom" generation.[11] Twenty-five years ago, the largest portion of staff nurses (RNs performing direct patient care) was under the age of 30. By 1977, data revealed that the median age of employed registered nurses had climbed to 38 years of age. Preliminary analysis of the most recent National Sample Survey of RNs indicates that the av-

erage age of RNs in March 1988 was 42.[15] This "graying" of the work force is further confirmed by the fact that, in 1991, the median age of staff nurses responding to a nationwide survey sponsored by the American Nurses Association (ANA) was 35 to 44.[17] It is suggested that the older-age profile of RNs allows for nursing services to build a more highly expert and stable work force.[18]

At the same time that the staff nurse population has been aging, the level of education has also changed. In 1977, the nursing diploma was the highest nursing-related educational credential of the majority of nurses (67%). Only 18% held baccalaureates in nursing and 11%, associate degrees. By 1988, however, less than 40% reported a nursing diploma as the highest level of educational preparation. The majority of RNs held either an associate degree or baccalaureate in nursing (25% and 27%, respectively).[11]

While demographics, such as age and educational preparation, are fundamental to any work force profile, such data reflect only one dimension of the population's characteristics. To fully understand today's staff nurse population, it is equally important to take a closer look at what motivates these individuals to enter nursing, what is most important to them in their work, and how they are responding to challenges and changes in the workplace.

MOTIVATION FOR CAREER CHOICE

In 1991, the American Nurses Association enlisted the assistance of the Opinion Research Division of

Fleishman-Hillard, Inc. to conduct a survey of registered nurses. The survey targeted hospital nurses located in the 50 states and the District of Columbia. Staff nurses and special assignment nurses (ER, ICU, OR) comprised 91% of the sample.

This nationwide mail survey of 1,193 RNs, conducted between March 22 and April 15, 1991, resulted in the first major examination of staff nurse attitudes about nursing and workplace issues in the 1990s.[1] Among the insight gleaned from this survey is basic information about why staff nurses enter nursing and what is most and least important to them in working as nurses.

The motivation for choosing nursing as a career clearly has not changed dramatically over the years. A desire to help people (71%) and an interest in health care (63%) were the leading reasons that survey respondents became nurses. Moreover, the prospect of job opportunities was reported as a primary reason almost twice as often as a good income (44% versus 23%). The desire to be a professional was selected by 43% of the respondents as the primary reason for becoming a registered nurse.[17]

Given this perspective, it is not surprising that the survey also revealed that patient care and professional issues dominate the list of workplace concerns. From a list of 19 work-related factors, respondents assigned the greatest importance to the following: providing quality patient care (89%); caring about patients' best interests (77%); being treated as a professional (65%); adequate staffing (60%); safe working environment (57%); and letting RNs do what RNs are taught to do (56%). Far less importance was assigned to such considerations as working with new technology, health care benefits, time off on holidays, child care and elder care assistance, and opportunities for overtime.[3]

A number of studies indicate that the number-one priority of staff nurses is quality patient care. Most of these studies also document the challenges and frustrations that staff nurses experience in an industry that is undergoing dramatic changes.[6,7,8,9,14,16] This type of information provides insight into yet another facet or dimension of the profile of today's staff nurse—the roles they perform and the level of job satisfaction they experience.

CHANGING AND EXPANDING ROLES

In a 1976 edition of *Professional Nursing: Foundations, Perspectives, and Relationships*, Notter and Spalding noted that the general staff nurse, "perhaps more than any other nurse," had to be "alert to changing medical and health care practices and the newer demands made on nurses."[13] They emphasized that a staff nurse needed to be willing to accept change and to be able to see the broadening scope of his or her job. The wisdom of this advice cannot be ignored.

Alterations in population characteristics, scientific and technological advancements, changing disease patterns, and increasingly diverse lifestyles have resulted in demands for a type of health care that was virtually nonexistent one or two decades ago. Increased patient acuity and earlier discharges characterize the "sicker and quicker" reality of the prospective payment system. Individuals who are being hospitalized tend to be more seriously ill, yet their length of stay is shorter. Patients who would have been cared for in intensive care units only a few years ago are now assigned to regular medical-surgical units. And older patients, more critically ill than ever before, are requiring increased nursing skill and nursing time.[2]

Further compounding the demands placed on staff nurses today is the shift in focus from caring for a patient to providing a service to a customer. There is general consensus within the industry that patients are acting more like customers and that this change represents a significant shift in the patient's power.[2] Nurses describe patients as more questioning, less trusting, more knowledgeable, more demanding of high-quality service and care, more cost-conscious, and more willing to shop around.

When asked about how these and other factors affect the delivery of nursing care, staff nurses tend to offer four basic observations:

- Hospital nursing has become more complex.
- There is an ever-present need to stay current with medical and technological advancements.
- Nurses are expected to assume greater responsibilities, especially with regard to coordination of care and patient education.
- Nurses must manage a wider range of duties, including more nonnursing functions.

LEVEL OF JOB SATISFACTION

When asked about how they feel about the work they are doing, staff nurses respond with one common theme: they want to provide the best nursing care possible, *but* circumstances make it extremely difficult.

The following comments, gathered through a series of interviews, are characteristic of the concerns expressed by staff nurses all across the country:

"There's a tremendous education that we've had to pick up and deal with for patients. So the whole aspect of nursing has become very difficult and, while enjoyable, it's been very hard for nurses to carry that out."

"As we are required to spend more time to treat the patients that are sicker, our time is being consumed more and more by paperwork responsibilities and administrative functions that are better left to other people. So it puts us in a professional conflict between our bond to the patient and the need for patient care and our job to perform duties in other areas of nursing."

"You find yourself sometimes in a situation as the only RN over five or ten other people for a patient load that's tremendously high. If you truly want to deliver quality patient care, you find yourself not being able to do that and it's very frustrating."

In light of the ongoing shortages of nurses and other health personnel, several studies have examined the quality of the work environment in hospitals and explored those factors that seem to foster job satisfaction. In general, these studies have confirmed the need to improve the working conditions of staff nurses and have drawn attention to the importance of such factors as nurse-patient ratios, support services, involvement in decision making, level of compensation, amount of paperwork, opportunity for professional development, and respect received from hospital management and physicians.[7,8,9,10,16]

While new and innovative strategies are being implemented to attract and retain nurses in the work force, there is still room for improvement in the quality of the work environment. Clearly, there continues to be a tension between what is most important to nurses and what they perceive they are getting from their employers in terms of support and recognition. In the 1991 survey of staff nurse attitudes, for example, respondents were asked to assign importance to workplace concerns and to rank the strengths and weaknesses of their hospitals. Analysis of this information revealed gaps between what was important to the nurses and hospital performance in the areas of adequate staffing, respect, professionalism, and quality patient care.[3]

STRESSFUL WORK ENVIRONMENT

What does all of this mean with regard to a description or profile of the staff nurse population? It means that no explanation would be complete without the acknowledgment that these nurses function in a more highly stressful environment than earlier generations. The list of job stressors cited by staff nurses is long and varied. It includes inadequate staffing/personnel shortages; constant interruptions; lack of support or help from peers; pressure to document and complete paperwork; unattractive or disorganized work areas; high or constant noise levels; inability to find supplies and/or secure information; no voice in workplace decision making; significant changes in the organization and delivery of services; lack of respect from other health care professionals; conflict between the service orientation of nursing and the business focus of the industry; inadequate compensation; and the grief associated with the death of patients.[4,7,10,12] Given these and other concerns, it is not surprising that staff nurses frequently report feelings of being "used up" at the end of the work day, emotionally drained from work, frustrated by work, fatigued when having to get up and go to work, and burned out.[1] How staff nurses cope with these feelings and other symptoms of job stress will greatly affect how this segment of the work force is perceived in the future.

FUTURE CHALLENGES

Staff nurses are involved in more high-stress situations than ever before. They daily experience a wide range of situations that raise serious professional issues, pose ethical dilemmas, challenge value systems, trigger communication breakdowns, and/or cause confrontation.

By far the greatest challenge facing staff nurses today is the need to achieve effective control of the environment in which nursing is practiced and services are offered. One dimension of control in the workplace comes from the expertise required to practice nursing. Another equally important dimension of control comes from the individual skills necessary to manage stressful situations and to engage in problem solving and decision making in the workplace.[2]

All nurses are aware of the physiological and emotional reactions to stress as well as the measures necessary to reduce and/or alleviate various stress responses. While nurses are trained to observe stress symptoms in others, they do not always apply the same insight to themselves. The changing dynamics of the industry, the increasing demands for health care, adverse employment conditions, and the nature of nursing as a service-oriented, predominantly female profession all contribute to the tensions and conflicts nurses experience on a daily basis. As individuals, nurses need to be sensitive to their personal levels of tolerance for different types of stress and to develop an effective stress management plan that considers the whole person (physical, emotional, intellectual, social, and spiritual needs). By developing a self-care philosophy, nurses can enhance both their professional and personal well-being.

Maximizing involvement in workplace decision making also is essential for nurses to ensure the delivery of quality nursing care and to foster job satisfaction. More and more nurses have begun to take action to strengthen nursing's influence, particularly in hospital settings. Some of these strategies include decentralization of nursing services, negotiation of bargaining agreements that provide for special committees to address professional and practice concerns, and creation of self-governance systems. Through the growing volume of literature on the empowerment of nursing, staff nurses need to stay apprised of these and other trends and their potential impact on nurse involvement in workplace decision making.

As the 21st century approaches, there is every indication that staff nurses will face increasing pressures. As bottom-line solvency continues to be a driving force in the health care industry, the nursing profession will be expected to find new and creative ways to deliver quality nursing care that is more cost effective. Industry analysts agree that the future funding of services and programs will be based primarily on the ability of the services/programs to show a cost/benefit relationship. Greater attention will focus on the relationship between process and outcome. As a result, nurses will need to develop greater insight and ability in such areas as strategic planning, marketing, cost containment, and cost accounting management. They also will be expected to utilize centralized information systems that integrate financial information with clinical and statistical data.[2]

Ethical considerations will also demand more attention. The major ethical issues confronting health care professionals have been identified as the quality of life versus the sanctity of life, the right to live versus the right to die, informed consent, confidentiality, rights of children, unethical behavior of other practitioners, role conflict, and the allocation of scarce resources.[5] Although many of these issues have become the subjects of legislation or court rulings, this action has not lessened the potential for conflicts.

In short, the health care industry will continue to undergo dramatic changes for some time. As a result, staff nurses will continue to be confronted with a broad range of opportunities and challenges that test their skills and abilities.

REFERENCES

1. American Nurses Association. (1991, July 1). Inadequate staffing threatens patient care, nurses say. *American Nurses Association News,* p. 1.
2. Flanagan, L. (1990). *Survival skills in the workplace, what every nurse should know.* Kansas City, Mo: American Nurses Association.
3. Fleishman-Hillard Inc. (1991, May). *Opportunities for growth, a report to the American Nurses Association.*
4. Gallagher, D. (1989). Is stress ripping nurses apart? *Imprint, 36*(2), 59-63.
5. Kelly, L. Y. (1987). *The nursing experience—trends, challenges, and transitions.* New York: Macmillan.
6. Kramer, M. (1974). *Reality shock: Why nurses leave nursing.* St Louis: Mosby.
7. Kramer, M., & Schmalenberg, C. (1991). Job satisfaction and retention, insights for the 90s, Part 1. *Nursing 91, 21*(3), 50-55.
8. Kramer, M., & Schmalenberg, C. (1991). Job satisfaction and retention, insights for the 90s, Part 2. *Nursing 91, 21*(4), 51-55.
9. McClure, M. L., et al. (1983). *Magnet hospitals: attraction and retention of professional nurses.* Kansas City, Mo: American Nurses Association.
10. McCranie, E., Lambert, V., & Lambert, C. (1987). Work stress, hardiness and burnout among hospital staff nurses. *Nursing Research, 36*(6), 374-377.
11. McKibbin, R. C. (1990). *The nursing shortage and the 1990s.* Kansas City, Mo: American Nurses Association.
12. McLean, A. (1979). *Work stress.* Reading, Mass: Addison-Wesley.
13. Notter, L. E., & Spalding, E. K. (1976). *Professional nursing—foundations, perspectives and relationships.* Philadelphia: J. B. Lippincott.
14. Schmalenberg, C., & Kramer, M. (1979). *Coping with reality shock: The voices of experience.* Rockville, Md: Aspen Systems Corporation.
15. U.S. Department of Health and Human Services. (1990). *The registered nurse population—1988.* Washington, D.C.: Author.
16. Wandelt, M. A., Pierce, P. M., & Widdowson, R. R. (1981). Why nurses leave nursing and what can be done about it. *American Journal of Nursing, 81*(1), 72-77.
17. Yeast, C. (1991). Nurses—who are we and what motivates us. *The American Nurse, 23*(9), 10.
18. Young, W. B. (1989). Taking advantage of the older age profile of today's registered nurses. *Nursing and Health Care, 10*(4), 189-191.

CHAPTER 3

Clinical nurse specialists and nurse practitioners

Who are they, what do they do, and what challenges do they face?

MARGARET STAFFORD, JOANN APPLEYARD

Specialization has been articulated as "a mark of the advancement of the nursing profession."[4] The clinical nurse specialist (CNS) and nurse practitioner (NP) roles were developed in response to this advancement. The profession needed clinical practitioners who could focus on a specific segment of the whole of nursing by acquiring in-depth knowledge and advanced skills in a defined area of practice.[4]

Historically, there are two significant differences between the prototype CNS and NP: the primary reasons for their becoming and the educational requirements for their respective roles.[14,25] On the other hand, they share a common element: a continuing commitment to clinical practice—a practice that demands expert knowledge and skill and includes the direct and continuous care of sick patients, as well as health promotion for clients who are well.

At this point in time, major issues that affect the CNS and NP are being debated, such as: (1) their merger (of sorts) into one entity; (2) the regulatory process that legitimizes their advanced practice; (3) prescriptive authority; and (4) compensation for their services. This chapter will profile the CNS and NP,* identifying their impact on the health care system and discussing related concepts and issues.

HISTORICAL ORIGIN OF THE CNS

There have always been "specialists" in nursing who acquired specialized knowledge and skill through prac-

tice and on-the-job instruction. During the 1930s and 1940s many nurses also attended short-term postgraduate educational programs sponsored by hospitals and became the specialists in their particular fields.[12,22] But the modern CNS emerged in response to the recognized need to improve the quality of patient care and the clinical *practice* of professional nursing, primarily in the acute care setting.[8,21,28,38,41,47]

Nursing care had deteriorated seriously during and immediately after World War II. A significant factor related to this decline was the dramatic decrease in the number of registered nurses practicing in hospitals.[43] Many nurses returning from the war used the GI bill to go back to school and become teachers or administrators, and a number of nurses were no longer content to work in the paternalistic environment of the hospital, where low salaries and substandard working conditions were the norm.[12]

The "quick fix" (replacing RNs with less qualified health care providers) to the acute nursing shortage and substandard patient care failed to address nurses' concerns. In spite of emerging technology and increased complexity of care, hospitals continued to use war-time measures to fill the gap: volunteers became paid nurses' aides, and vocational (practical) nurses were introduced to provide the major part of direct care for patients.[8,12,33,42,46] Team nursing was introduced, but it further fragmented patient care and frustrated the registered nurses, who continued to leave hospitals.[12] In our experience, the registered nurse felt devalued because others with less education and professionalism took over the nursing care of patients,

---

*The American Nurses Association lists 25,000 to 30,000 NPs and "about" 40,000 CNSs with advanced degrees.

while the professional nurse "nursed" the desk. And the development of shortened programs in hospital diploma schools as well as associate degree programs in community colleges contributed little to the recognized need for *increased* knowledge and skill at the bedside.

In 1947, a National Nursing Council (representing the American Nurses Association and other health care organizations) obtained a grant from the Carnegie Foundation and commissioned Esther Lucille Brown to study and determine how professional nursing schools could meet the demand for nursing services. One result of the study was Brown's publication on *Nursing for the Future*[9] in which she strongly proposed that basic schools of nursing be in universities and colleges but that:

> . . . provisions for the development of some specialists within clinical nursing has been viewed in this report as necessary, if the base on which nursing service rests is to be strengthened, and if the profession is to look forward to a sound healthy development.[9]

The now famous Williamsburg Conference of nurse educators, which put into motion the first master's-prepared psychiatric CNS,[36] followed this report. In 1961 Frances Reiter presented a paper enunciating her concept of the nurse clinician, which is virtually synonymous with the CNS of today—"one . . . who consistently demonstrates a high degree of clinical judgement and an advanced level of competence in the performance of nursing care in a clinical area of specialization."[41]

During the decade of the 1960s, publications expressing the need for clinical nursing to keep abreast of the knowledge explosion in both technological and behavioral sciences[8] flourished. Federal funding was obtained to support this "need," and by the early 1960s, programs to prepare clinical nurse specialists were in place in many areas of clinical practice.[25] In 1966, a change in the structure of the American Nurses Association to include divisions of clinical practice gave further impetus to the development of master's-prepared clinicians.[12,25]

PROFILES OF THE CLINICAL NURSE SPECIALIST
Who they are

The criteria for specialists in nursing practice were identified in ANA's *Social Policy Statement* as "a nurse who, through study and supervised practice at the graduate level (master's or doctorate), has become expert in a defined area of knowledge and practice in a selected clinical area of nursing."[2] Hamric and Taylor suggest that the development of this "expert" results from a "complex and emotional process." Their study describes seven identifiable phases of development but indicates that movement from phase to phase occurs in a highly fluid, individual fashion.[23] For purposes of this discussion, the focus will be on the experienced CNS who has reached an advanced "phase" of practice and has successfully integrated the various components of the role.

Organizational placement of the CNS

Clinical nurse specialists are found primarily in institutional settings, typically in staff positions. However, many and varied organizational arrangements are described in the literature.[43] The advantages and disadvantages of line versus staff accountability have been discussed elsewhere[5,22] and will not be dealt with here other than to present a bias predicated on years of successful experience as a CNS in a "staff" position and dialogue with CNSs in "line" positions. The success of this staff role, however, is contingent upon reciprocal trust and respect and, as identified by Brown,[10] a sharing of responsibility and authority between the CNS and the person to whom the CNS is administratively accountable.

Regardless of organizational placement and reporting mechanisms, the CNS usually works from a "home base" and is available for consultation from other units.[28] Many clinical nurse specialists have clinical faculty appointments, and some full-time faculty members carry part-time CNS appointments. The common element, however, is the direct and continuous involvement with patients and families with emphasis on a nursing versus a medical care model.

Functions of the CNS, what they do

Expert clinical practice is the sine quo non of the CNS. Practice (actual ongoing experience with patients and families) provides the content and directs participation in various subroles such as clinical research, consultation, teaching and leadership/administration.[22] This concept is exemplified by the following CNS leaders with excerpts from their activities. These examples, gleaned for the most part from personal contact and interaction, are not intended to be all-inclusive but rather to provide the reader with some insight into what Fralic refers to as "nursing's precious resource."[17]

• Nancy Burke is a CNS in psychiatric mental health nursing. She maintains a private practice, is a consultant to the department of psychiatry in a university hospital, has an adjunct appointment in the college of nursing, and maintains a collaborative practice with her psychiatrist husband. Her activities include liaison work with family members of hospitalized patients, seeing them in the hospital and office and calling them at least weekly to keep them apprised of the patient's progress and involving them as indicated in the plans for therapy. As a certified psychodramatist, Nancy conducts four psychodrama groups per week. In her group at the university she has medical residents, nursing students, and myriad others as participant observers " . . . who never fail to get involved."

• Meg Gulanick's practice as a CNS has evolved from expert care of critically ill patients to CNS director of the cardiac rehabilitation program at a large medical center's acute care facility. Meg has been the preceptor for some 48 graduate nursing students and one PhD candidate. She maintains that her contributions to nursing diagnosis literature (six books, two in their second editions and one in its third edition) and to nursing research derive their credibility from her patient care experiences.

• Kristin Kleinschmidt is the CNS for the cardiac care unit (CCU) and cardiac clinic of a large Veterans Administration hospital. She does informal teaching in CCU several times a week, is a consultant and resource person to the cardiology units, and conducts critical care and ECG classes on a routine basis. In the clinic, she works with a cardiologist and cardiac technician to provide a cost-effective team approach to comprehensive care. She is responsible for the follow-up care of patients with intractable dysrhythmias, cardiac pacemakers, and internal cardiac defibrillators (ICD), with clinical privileges to modify/program patients' pacemakers and ICDs as indicated. Kris has written extensively on pacemaker therapy and has presented numerous lectures related to ICD and pacemaker interventions. She has also developed a significant administrative leadership subrole as a member or chair of several nursing/hospitalwide committees.

• Ann Henrick provides primary nursing care to patients and their families in a heart failure research clinic. She also is the coordinator, co-investigator (with a physician colleague) and, in some instances, the principle investigator of research protocols related to this high-risk patient population. Clinical privileges to admit patients to the hospital, to modify their drug regimen, and to order and perform diagnostic tests are granted to Ann from the Medical/Nursing Executive

Committee of the hospital. However, her ability to teach patients the basics that affect their energy level, to encourage and assist them in modifying their diet and exercise patterns and in accepting the challenge of monitoring their own progress—all of these optimal patient outcomes—provide the real authority for her practice.

• Kathleen Perry functions in a hospital-based home care program, giving nursing care to four to five "older" patients and families on an ongoing basis. She has explored and studied the diagnostic statement, Knowledge Deficit, a recurring problem for this patient population. She likewise has identified the potential for serious negative patient outcomes in the presence of care giver stress, a phenomenon she currently is addressing as a PhD candidate in nursing. She believes her involvement as a clinical preceptor offers students a "knowledge embedded in practice" that enhances their ability to function in the CNS role. Kathy advises staff nurses in her agency on ethical and professional issues as they move forward in their state nurses' association's professional bargaining unit activities.

• Virginia (Ginny) T. Williams, one of the first CNSs to "hang out her shingle," has been in "family nursing" for 17 years in a small rural town. Her approach to independent practice is based on a philosophy of nursing that encompasses such concepts as caring, coping, and contracting, as well as autonomy, accountability, and availability. She contracts with patients and/or their family members to give or provide for short- and long-term nursing care in the home and often arranges respite care for the care giver. Ginny usually has a graduate student with her as she makes her calls and is a ready resource person for nurse researchers and faculty.[49]

• And then there is Joyce Waterman Taylor, CNS emerita in neurosciences. Joyce has not only implemented all of the subroles in a highly qualitative fashion, but also has expanded and incorporated additional competencies. She believes strongly that primary nursing (my patient, my nurse) is the way to improve care for all patients and to provide job satisfaction for nurses. In all of her work settings, she has introduced and taught the concepts of primary nursing within a holistic framework. And, for Joyce, collaborative practice also is an article of faith; she consistently develops and nurtures collaborative relationships with physicians and other disciplines. Her widely published work on the outcomes of care and outcome standards led to her appointment to several national and local committees and task forces. Joyce has been singled out by her peers and colleagues as the quintessential clinical nurse specialist.

ORIGINS OF THE NURSE PRACTITIONER ROLE

The 1960s were characterized by social change, including a political emphasis on health care as a right for all citizens. Access to all levels of health care services was seen as a particular problem, and the NP role was developed to help meet the demand for primary care services. The first formal education program for NPs was established in 1965 at the University of Colorado School of Nursing to prepare registered nurses to deliver primary care to children in underserved communities.[20] By 1975, practitioner programs had proliferated, and NPs were being trained in a variety of medical fields, including obstetrics and gynecology, internal medicine, pediatrics, geriatrics, and family practice. During that first decade, educational programs tended to be nondegree, certificate programs that were one year or less in length. Many of these programs were funded by the federal government in an effort to prepare more primary care providers for underserved populations. Since 1975, the nondegree programs have decreased substantially, and most NPs are now educated in graduate programs leading to a master's degree in nursing.[37]

National certification for NPs was first established in the mid-1970s by the National Certification Board of Pediatric Nurse Practitioners and Nurses. The American Nurses Association (American Nurses Credentialing Center) soon followed suit, establishing national certification for NPs in gerontology, pediatrics, adult health, family health, and school health. NPs in neonatology, obstetrics, and gynecology are certified by the National Certification Corporation for Obstetric, Gynecologic, and Neonatal Nursing Specialties. Most NPs today are certified by one of these national organizations. Increasingly, certification is a requirement for employment, and in some states it is a requirement by the state licensing board.

WHO ARE NPs AND WHAT DO THEY DO?

NPs are educated to perform a broad spectrum of primary care interventions, including health assessment, risk appraisal, health education and counseling,

diagnosis and management of acute minor illnesses and injuries, and management of chronic conditions. Although most NPs work in primary care settings, such as physicians' offices, health maintenance organizations (HMOs), and community or public health clinics, increasing numbers are employed in hospitals, nursing homes, schools, industrial settings, and home health agencies.[37] In all of these settings NPs provide the essential health care services described above with emphasis on health promotion and disease prevention activities.[30]

Taking into account the basic primary care practice divisions of internal medicine, pediatrics, family practice, obstetrics and gynecology, and geriatrics, NPs tend to perform as generalists rather than as specialists in terms of clinical practice. This means that they focus on broad health concerns within a given division of practice rather than concentrating on a particular body system or a set of related diseases. Exceptions to this are those NPs who work as employees or as partners to physicians in specialty practice. In these speciality settings, the roles of NPs and CNSs are quite similar and may be considered interchangable.

SPECIFIC ROLE ISSUES FOR NURSE PRACTITIONERS

The literature on NPs is voluminous, and a review by Koch, Pazaki, and Campbell[27] categorizes five major topics: NP roles, educational issues, evaluation, legal issues, and the evolving health care crisis. One major concern that has been debated repeatedly during the past 20 years is whether NPs function as physician substitutes or as nurses in advanced practice roles.[6,7,15,16,32,48] The differences between physician and nursing roles involve issues of nursing autonomy and paradigm disparities about the nature of health care.[1]

Historically, nurses have tended to view their focus as "caring," while physicians have directed their efforts toward "curing."[31] Traditionally, nurses have assisted physicians in the "cure" of patients by following orders and using their nursing skills and knowledge to "care" for patients and their families. Caring involved activities such as bathing, feeding, and providing skin care and passive exercise for a bedridden patient. It also involved listening, counseling, teaching, and coordinating interventions from multiple health care providers. Curing involved specific activities directed toward the diagnosis and treatment of disease. When nurses followed physician orders in carrying out diagnostic tests or in administering treatments to patients, they were participating in the curative aspect of health care. When they assessed and provided for patient and/or family needs for emotional support and health teaching or guidance, they were participating in the caring component.

The historical view was that nursing practice was both dependent upon medical practice and independent from it, and the independent functions tended to be those on the caring end of the continuum. Thus, nursing autonomy was more related to caring interventions than to curative ones. The development of advanced nursing practice roles has changed this circumstance. NPs daily perform interventions aimed at curing acute minor illnesses and injuries. While carrying out these interventions, they assess their patients' responses to health problems and initiate appropriate teaching and counseling to help them manage treatment plans and prevent recurrences or secondary problems.

As indicated above, caring and curing are not mutually exclusive concepts. Rather, they are part of a continuum, and both physicians and nurses carry out activities in these arenas. Both caring and curative interventions are necessary in primary care, and there is convincing evidence that NPs effectively combine these practice components in their roles.[29,44,51] Although NPs carry out health care activities that used to be primarily in the physician's domain, they are performing these activities as nurses with a significant emphasis on the responses and needs of the whole patient and family.

THE CNS AND NP IN TRANSITION
Merging the two ANA councils

Several studies, papers, and intense dialogue with members of ANA's CNS and NP councils indicated more similarities than differences between the CNS and NP.[18,19,24,26,45] Thus, the two councils merged into a single Council of Nurses in Advanced Practice (CNAP).[40] The educational requirements (master's or doctorate) and role development now are well established.[3] And although the issue of a singular title at this time is still being debated,[26] the concept of both groups being identified as advanced practitioners is widely accepted.[19]

Regulation and reimbursement issues

The inconsistencies of the regulation and professional certification of nurses in advanced practice from state

to state prompted the National Council of State Boards of Nursing (NCSBN) in March of 1992 to propose a second license for nurses seeking reimbursement and prescriptive authority.[34] The profession's historical view (which is *still* valid) is that the responsibility and accountability for defining specialty nursing practice and its qualifications rest with the profession.[2] Formal meetings between the NCSBN and the ANA are taking place to examine alternative mechanisms (other than licensure) to regulate *advanced* practice. And ANA has begun a deliberate process with organized nursing through the Nursing Organization Liaison Forum (NOLF) and other specialty organizations to revisit *Nursing: A Social Policy Statement* as it pertains specifically to specialization.[3,11,40] It is incumbent upon all advanced practitioners to be actively and cohesively involved in ANA's and the state nurses' associations' collaborative efforts to:

- Protect the public and nursing's autonomous control of advanced nursing practice.
- Increase the adherence of nurses in advanced practice to national standards of certification and peer review.
- Introduce requirements for uniform mandatory reimbursement to reflect adequately advanced practitioners' worth.
- Eliminate barriers that restrict consumer access to services of qualified advanced practitioners.
- Build a national and state database on advanced practitioners including their scope of practice, location, cost, and outcomes of their care.[3]

CURRENT MANDATES/CHALLENGES

There are substantial barriers to the practice of NP and some CNS roles because of the overlap between traditional medical and nursing functions. This is especially true in settings where nurses attempt to provide comprehensive primary care services. Although most state nursing practice acts enacted during the past 20 years have been updated to include some kind of legal authority for advanced nursing practice, the statutory language varies widely, from very broad mention of specialty practice to specific definitions of scope of practice.[39] By 1992, NPs in 40 states had some legal authority to prescribe medicines, but again the language varies widely.[39] In many states NP prescribing privileges are dependent upon physician or pharmacist approval, where in other states NPs may independently prescribe all kinds of drugs, including controlled substances.

The issue of independence is a major problem for both nurse practitioners and physicians. From the inception of the NP role, it was intended that some of the interventions involving diagnosis and treatment of disease be carried out in collaboration with physicians or, as organized medicine asserts, *under physician supervision*.

The independent practice of nurses is a politically charged arena, with organized medicine firmly against all efforts of nurses to be recognized as independent health care providers who receive direct reimbursement for their services. When regulatory agencies and state and federal legislative bodies use the term *supervision* rather than *collaboration* to describe the interdependent relationship between physicians and nurses, organized medicine can claim that nursing practice is completely dependent upon medical practice and that physicians should receive all direct reimbursement for health care services delivered by nurses outside of institutional settings. Nurses must continue to work diligently to educate legislators, regulators, and the general public about the independent aspects of nursing practice that are broadly defined in all nursing practice acts. It is also necessary to remind these groups that nurses do practice under their own licenses and that nurses' licenses are not contingent upon physicians' licenses.

An operational definition of the concept of collaboration was adopted in 1992 by the ANA Congress on Nursing Practice:

Collaboration means a collegial working relationship with another health care provider in the provision of (to supply) patient care. Collaborative practice requires (may include) the discussion of patient diagnosis and cooperation in the management and delivery of care. Each collaborator is available to the other for consultation either in person or by communication device, but need not be physically present on the premises at the time the actions are performed. The patient-designated health care provider is responsible for the overall direction and management of patient care.[4]

This definition should be used as a basis for all discussions or negotiations where the issue is "physician supervision" of nursing practice.

The individual accomplishments of CNSs and NPs are prelude to their potential collective positive impact on the health care of individuals and families and on health care policy in general. To this end, they must sustain and enhance their significant roles in the following initiatives:

- Nursing's agenda for health care reform
- Federal government's agenda to improve the effectiveness and appropriateness of health care services through their Agency for Health Care Policy and Research (AHCPR)
- Nursing's taxonomy development and related scientific studies

It is likewise crucial that nurses in advanced practice: (1) continue to demonstrate their cost effectiveness in cost-driven hospital and clinic environments; (2) increase their presence in extended care/nursing home facilities; (3) advance theory and research-based clinical practice models that demonstrate a high quality of patient care and reflect measurable, nurse-sensitive patient outcomes; and (4) help other health professionals, health care consumers, and public servants recognize the contribution being made by nurses in advanced practices.[13,50]

REFERENCES

1. Allen, M. (1977). Comparative theories of the expanded role in nursing and implications for nursing practice: A working paper. *Nursing Papers, 9*(2), 38-45.
2. American Nurses Association. (1980). *Nursing: A social policy statement.* Kansas City, Mo: Author.
3. American Nurses Association. (1992). *House of delegates report: 1992 convention, Las Vegas, Nev.* (pp. 235-240). Kansas City, Mo: Author.
4. American Nurses Association. (1992). *House of delegates report: 1992 convention, Las Vegas, Nev.* (pp. 104-120). Kansas City, Mo: Author.
5. Baird, S. B., & Prouty, M. P. (1989). Administratively enhancing CNS contribution. In A. B. Hamrick & J. A. Spross (Eds.), *The clinical nurse specialist in theory and practice* (2nd ed., pp. 262-264). Philadelphia: W. B. Saunders.
6. Bates, B. (1970). Doctor and nurse: changing roles and relations. *New England Journal of Medicine, 283*(3), 129-134.
7. Bates, B. (1974). Twelve paradoxes: A message for nurse practitioners. *Nursing Outlook, 22*(11), 686-688.
8. Berlinger, M. R. (1973). The preparation and roles of the clinical nurse specialist. In J. P. Riehl & J. W. McVay (Eds.), *The clinical nurse specialist: interpretations* (pp. 100-107). New York: Appleton-Century-Crofts.
9. Brown, E. L. (1948). *Nursing for the future.* New York: Russel Sage Foundation.
10. Brown, S. J. (1989). Supportive supervision of the CNS. In A. B. Hamrick & J. A. Spross (Eds.), *The clinical nurse specialist in theory and practice* (2nd ed.). Philadelphia: W. B. Saunders.
11. Cronenwett, L. R. (July 14, 1992). *A report to CNAP members from the chairperson, Congress of Nursing Practice,* Kansas City, Mo: American Nurses Association.
12. Donahue, M. P. (1985). *Nursing the finest art.* St Louis: Mosby.
13. Donovan, C. T. (1985). Clinical nurse specialist practice in an acute care setting. In K. E. Barnard & G. R. Smith (Eds.), *Faculty practice in action.* Kansas City, Mo: American Academy of Nursing.

14. Elder, R. G., & Bullough, B. (1990). Nurse practitioners and clinical nurse specialists: Are the roles merging? *Clinical Nurse Specialist, 4*(2), 78-84.

15. Edmunds, M. (1979, September/October). Junior doctoring. *Nurse Practitioner,* 8-46.

16. Edmunds, M. W., & Ruth, M. V. (1991). NPs who replace physicians: Role expansion or exploitation? *Nurse Practitioner, 16*(9), 46, 49.

17. Fralic, M. F. (1988). Executive development, Nursing precious resource: The clinical nurse specialist. *Journal of Nursing Administration, 18*(2) 5-6.

18. Forbes, K. E. (1990). Merge!!! *Momentum 8*(31).

19. Forbes, K. E., Rafson, J., Spross, J. A., & Kozlowski, I. (1990). The clinical nurse specialist and nurse practitioner: Core curriculum survey results. *Clinical Nurse Specialist, 4*(2), 63-66.

20. Ford, L. C., & Silver, H. K. (1967). The expanded role of the nurse in child care. *Nursing Outlook, 15*(8).

21. Georgopoulous, B., & Christman, L. (1970). The clinical nurse specialist: A role model. *American Journal of Nursing, 70*(5), 1030-1039.

22. Hamrick, A. B. (1989). History and overview of the CNS role. In A. B. Hamrick & J. A. Spross (Eds.), *The clinical nurse specialist in theory and practice* (2d ed., pp. 3-18). Philadelphia: W. B. Saunders.

23. Hamrick, A. B., & Taylor, J. W. (1989). Role development of the CNS. In A. B. Hamrick & J. A. Spross (Eds.), *The clinical nurse specialist in theory and practice* (2nd ed., pp. 6-39). Philadelphia: W. B. Saunders.

24. Hockenberry, E. M., & Hodgson, W. (1991). Merging advanced practice roles: The NP and CNS. *Journal of Pediatric Health, 5*(3), 158-159.

25. Hoeffer, B., & Murphy, S. (1984). Specialization in nursing practice. In *Issues in professional nursing practice, Part 2* (pp. 1-5). Kansas City, Mo: American Nurses Association.

26. Kitzman, H. J. (1989). The CNS and NP. In A. B. Hamrick & J. A. Spross (Eds.), *The clinical nurse specialist in theory and practice* (2nd ed.). Philadelphia: W. B. Saunders.

27. Koch, L. W., Pazaki, S. H., & Campbell, J. D. (1992). The first 20 years of nurse practitioner literature: An evolution of joint practice issues. *Nurse Practitioner, 17*(2), 62-71.

28. Koetters, L. (1989). Clinical practice and direct patient care. In A. B. Hamrick, & J. A. Spross (Eds.), *The clinical nurse specialist in theory and practice* (2nd ed.). Philadelphia: W. B. Saunders.

29. Leininger, M. M., Little, D. E., & Carnevali, D. (1972). Primex the professional nurse, responsible, accountable, reaching out and taking an active, frontline position in primary health care. *American Journal of Nursing, 72*(7), 1274-1277.

30. Lewis, C. E., & Resnik, B. A. (1985). Nurse clinics and progressive ambulatory patient care. *New England Journal of Medicine, 277*(23), 1236-1241.

31. Linn, L. S. (1974). Care vs cure: How the nurse practitioner views the patient. *Nursing Outlook, 22*(10), 641-644.

32. Mauksch, I. G., & Rogers, M. E. (1975). Nursing is coming of age . . . through the practitioner movement. *American Journal of Nursing, 75*(10), 1834-1843.

33. McClure, M. L. (1990). Introduction. In I. E. Goertzen (Ed.), *Differentiating nursing practice into the twenty-first century.* Selected papers from the 18th annual meeting and 1990 conference of the American Academy of Nursing, Charleston, South Carolina, October 14-15. Kansas City, Mo: American Academy of Nursing.

34. National Council of State Boards of Nursing, Inc. (1991). Advanced nursing practice survey results. *Issues, 12*(2).

35. National Council of State Boards of Nursing, Inc. (1992). Position paper on the licensure of Advanced Nursing Practice, May 18, 1992, National Council of the State Board of Nursing, Inc.

36. National League for Nursing. (1958). *The education of the clinical specialist in psychiatric nursing.* New York: Author.

37. Office of Technology Assessment. (1986). Nurse practitioners, physician assistants, and certified nurse-midwives: A policy analysis. *Health Technology Case Study 37.* Washington, D.C.: Congress of the United States.

38. Padilla, G. (1973). Clinical specialist research: Evaluation and recommendations, conclusions and implications. In J. P. Riehl & J. W. McVay (Eds.), *The clinical nurse specialist: Interpretations* (pp. 283-334). New York: Appleton-Century-Crofts.

39. Pearson, L. J. (1992). 1991-92 update: How each state stands on legislative issues affecting advanced nursing practice. *Nurse Practitioner, 17*(1), 14-23.

40. Pokorny, B. E., & Barnard, K. E. (1992). ANA to revise nursing statement. *The American Nurse, 24*(5), 6.

41. Reiter, F. (1961). Improvement of nursing practice. In J.P. Riehl & J.W. McVay, (Eds.), *The clinical nurse specialist: Interpretations.* New York: Appleton-Century-Crofts.

42. Reiter, F. (1966). The clinical nursing approach. *Nursing Forum, 5*(1), 42.

43. Sample, S. A. (1987). Justifying and structuring the CNS role within a nursing organization. In A. B. Hamrick & J. A. Spross (Eds.), *The clinical nurse specialist in theory and practice* (2nd ed., pp. 251-260). Philadelphia: W. B. Saunders.

44. Simborg, D. W., Starfield, B. H., & Horn, S. D. (1978). Physicians and non-physician health practitioners: The characteristics of their practices and their relationships, *American Journal of Public Health, 68*(1), 44-48.

45. Sparacino, P., & Denand, A. (1986). Specialization in advanced nursing practice [Editorial]. *Council of Primary Health Care Nurse Practitioners/Council of Clinical Nurse Specialists Newsletter, 4*(2).

46. Stafford, M. J. (1988). Margaret Stafford. In T. M. Schorr & A. Zimmerman (Eds.), *Making choices, taking chances: Nurse leaders tell their stories.* St Louis: Mosby.

47. Vaughan, M. (1968). Difficult task: Defining role of the clinical specialist. *Hospital Topics, 5*(18), 93-94.

48. Weston, J. (1975). Whither the "nurse" in nurse practitioner? *Nursing Outlook, 23*(3), 148-152.

49. Williams, V., & Oudt, B. (1988). Virginia T. Williams. In T. M. Schorr & A. Zimmerman (Eds.), *Making choices, taking chances: Nurse leaders tell their stories* (pp. 394-400). St Louis: Mosby.

50. Wright, J. E. (1990). Joining forces for the good of our clients. *Clinical Nurse Specialist, 4*(2), 76-77.

51. Yedida, M. J. (1981). *Delivering primary health care nurse practitioners at work.* Boston: Auburn House.

CHAPTER 4

Nurse administrators

Who are they, what do they do, and what challenges do they face?

BARBARA VOLK TEBBITT

Top nurse administrators come in assortments ranging from rare Stradivarius to country fiddles; from vintage wines to home-brew; and from vibrating VWs to reticent Rolls Royces. Top level nurse executives demonstrate behavioral patterns ranging from the classical X pattern of being understanding, warm, and friendly to the Y pattern of being businesslike, efficient, and responsible and on down the alphabet to the Z pattern of being imaginative, stimulating, enthusiastic, and resurgent.

— Anonymous

Much ado has been made in the last decade about the dynamic changes and demands in health care, technology, and regulations and the consequent complexity of the nurse administrator's role. To better understand the role and functions of nurse administrators today, as well as the future challenges individuals in these positions will face, it is helpful to take a brief look at our past.

"Nightingale's Perspective of Nursing Administration"[9] reflects the applicability of Florence Nightingale's mid-1880s concepts and theories to nurse administrators today. In her time, Nightingale defined the major role of a nurse administrator (then called superintendent) to be education of others in the care of the ill. She espoused the individual characteristics of conciseness and decisiveness along with imagination and wit. Nightingale was committed to intelligent discipline and strength of character for nurse administrators, also acknowledging a need for collaboration, tact, and sensibility. Her emphasis was on the need for personal lifelong learning.

Nightingale described hospitals as an "intermediate stage of civilization" and the science of administration as "the driest, most technical, and the most difficult." In her writing she spoke of the need for the nurse admin-istrator to have authority for all clinical or nursing practice, administration, and education. Nightingale understood effective administration to begin with knowledge of disease, health, and the nursing needs of those requiring care. She used data and statistics to continuously monitor and improve patient outcomes with the understanding and belief such diligence would eventually assure health and wellness in society. She introduced the first principles of personnel administration and had an acute awareness of the economics of health care prevalent in her time. The core of Nightingale's 50-plus books, pamphlets, and reports and her 15,000-plus letters synchronize the practical and theoretical, qualitative with quantitative data, and clinical practice and administration.[9] This sense of harmonizing and balancing care delivery, program development, and resource management was Nightingale's philosophy on administration and continues true today.

Perhaps the major change in nursing administration between the mid-1800s and the early to mid-1900s was distinguishing the roles of administration and education, resulting in separate individuals to direct schools of nursing, their educational standards, and accrediting practices.[5] Since the mid-1950s numerous national projects and studies have addressed the changing societal, economic, and environmental demands on the role and functions of the nurse administrator. These changes stimulated the evolution of numerous profiles of nurse administrator roles and administrative titles and refocused required and desirable nursing leadership knowledge and behaviors.[5] As responsibilities and priorities for the role and position of the nurse administrator have evolved, criteria for preparation have been addressed and revised by multiple accrediting agencies and professional organizations, most notably the Joint Commission on Accreditation of Healthcare Organizations (JCAHO) and, most recently, the American Organization of Nurse Executives (AONE).

THE NURSE ADMINISTRATOR TODAY

The above-noted groups are in agreement that the nurse administrator for the 1990s (whom they now call "nurse executive"):

- Will be a registered nurse
- Will be responsible for the administration and management of the nursing organization, whether that be a department or division
- Will be accountable for defining the discipline of nursing and for developing nursing practice standards that will be adhered to wherever nursing is practiced throughout the organization
- Will be a member of the senior administrative team of the organization and as such will be responsible for participating in setting the strategic direction and planning for the organization
- Will be qualified by advanced education and management experience to demonstrate competence to meet these responsibilities[2,13]

To demonstrate what this advanced education and management expertise should incorporate and entail, it is necessary to address the roles and functions of the nurse executive today in greater detail.

Roles of the nurse executive

The 10 major roles nurse executives play in health care today remain as identified for those of any executive by Mintzberg and specifically applied to nurse administrators by Stevens more than a decade ago. They are:

1. *Figurehead* serving both as symbolic and formal head of nursing in the organization
2. *Leader* by directing associates to goal achievement through provision of a self-motivating environment
3. *Liaison* through building communications networks both within and outside of the organization
4. *Monitor* by continually scanning the external and internal environment to keep abreast of changes in health care that may require redirection of planning or work efforts
5. *Disseminator* in sharing and distributing information relating to nursing throughout the organization and/or community

6. *Spokesperson* by addressing the key publics in speaking for nursing
7. *Entrepreneur* in looking for improvement opportunities in the workplace and taking initiative in new projects and developments
8. *Disturbance handler* by mediating and resolving disagreements among teams and/or work groups
9. *Resource allocator* determining how nursing resources will be distributed and
10. *Negotiator* by managing formal and informal work-related issues with both internal and external groups[17,24]

Functions of the nurse executive

The 10 major role components for the nurse executive identified above hold true irrespective of the job or position title, the size, or the location of the health care institution. They remain—as in the time of Nightingale—technical and difficult and, to some nurse administrators, demanding and frustrating. However, they are rarely referred to as "the driest," but rather as exciting and stimulating by most nurse executives today.

These role components may and do differ in specific activities and time requirements from large to small institutions; however, there is great similarity in the overall role functions of nurse executives.[21,23,26]

This similarity minimally includes specific functions as planner, implementer, coordinator, arbitrator, guide, and image setter.[25] Activities and expectations within these individual functions are delineated under each area; however, they are not meant to be all inclusive.

As planner, the nurse executive participates in developing, implementing and evaluating the organization's vision, values, strategic direction, goals, and objectives and interprets the role of nursing in the organization's strategic plan. In so doing the nurse executive speaks the language of both administration and nursing and is aware of public policy's influence on the organization's and nursing's financial well-being. This awareness supports the need to continually assess the external and internal environment for factors that potentially affect the organization's and nursing's policies and programs. The nurse executive participates in the organization's financial forecasting and planning and articulates nursing's contributions to the organization's financial viability, as well as the resources necessary for effective patient care delivery. He or she also formulates nursing's vision and values, mission, philosophy, goals, and objectives, integrates them with those of the organization, and establishes and executes a financial plan for nursing. The nurse executive defines nursing standards of care and practice wherever nursing is practiced or provided within the organization and develops, implements, and evaluates nursing policies and programs to determine and allocate financial, human, material, and informational resources required. In addition, the executive participates in an organizationwide assessment of management information and database needs to provide an information system for clinical, management, and administrative decision making and supports the most beneficial and affordable integration of nursing's information system into the organization's overall system. He or she also participates in development of organizationwide continuous quality improvement methodologies and provides mechanisms for nursing staff to participate in planning, financial, quality improvement, and education activities and processes both within the organization and within nursing per se.

As an implementer, the nurse executive works with nursing, medical, and administrative staff to develop clinical programs of care that reflect available resources and an assessed community or customer need and interprets the standards of care into the nursing process or practice both by establishing and maintaining a suitable and caring environment and by designing, evaluating, and maintaining an effective nursing practice model and care delivery system. In addition, the executive maintains policies, procedures, standards, and programs based on regular evaluation incorporating the criteria for quality, productivity, and customer and staff satisfaction.

As a coordinator, the nurse executive assumes responsibility for universal quality of nursing care and practice rendered within the organization and links nursing services vertically and horizontally by seeking opportunities for cooperative efforts with other departments, disciplines, and agencies. In addition he or she ensures prudent utilization of all resources while assuring patient safety and adequate resources are available for providing nursing care and provides direction in analyzing and maintaining nursing's compliance with regulations and legislation.

As an arbitrator, the nurse executive relates with nursing and medical staff, department heads, and administration, contributes directly to administrative problem solving and decision making, and responds to nursing staff concerns regarding biomedical, ethical, and/or legal issues. He or she also develops mechanisms to facilitate productive goal-related outcomes

with other disciplines and departments and defines and negotiates dependent, interdependent, and independent roles and functions for nursing practice within the organization.

As a guide, the nurse executive adapts leadership style to changing situations and competencies of staff; solves problems with staff, makes decisions, and delegates authority; and sets expectations for, coaches/counsels, develops, disciplines, or terminates staff (may do so for select positions only, depending on size and complexity of the organization). In addition, the executive encourages and rewards staff to participate in development, implementation, and evaluation of nursing policies and programs; develops effective evaluation mechanisms and systems; and responds to personal and professional development and education needs of nursing staff.

As an image setter, the nurse executive creates and manages the values and culture of the nursing organization, develops the nursing services image for/to nursing staff, and identifies staffing requirements in type and amount. He or she also defines characteristics or qualifications for desired applicants, develops policies and programs consistent with recruitment and retention of qualified nursing staff considering factors external to the organization, and employs and deploys staff (may do so for select positions only).[4,16]

Role behaviors of the nurse executive

Role behaviors of the nurse executive, which are distinct from functions, are unique to the individual nurse executive and are frequently most contingent upon the following conditions. First is the health care organization's environment. What is its economic base—profit or nonprofit? What are the sources of capital and operating funds? Is the facility new or old? What are the available technology and staff, bed size and percent occupancy, and types of patients—acuity and mix? Other issues such as organizational structure and relationships, and medical staff, governing body, and community involvement are important also.[8] Other influencing factors include the clinical practice setting (e.g., existing nursing standards, roles, responsibilities, and functions) and the personal constitution of the nurse executive (e.g., aptitude, attitude, maturation, values, motivation, needs, personality, and past experiences).[1]

Most nurse executives today would agree that the more positive and supportive the organizational environment and practice setting, the greater the opportunity for the nurse executive to achieve personal effectiveness in the most flexible, conscientious, efficient, responsible, and responsive manner possible.

CHALLENGE FOR TOMORROW'S NURSE EXECUTIVE

Never before in the history of health care or nursing has there been such an emphasis on quality, performance, productivity, results, and consumer and employee satisfaction. A newly found competence and commitment, a sense of collegiality and social presence, personal integrity, confidence and courage in risk taking, and a sense of well-being and self-actualization will be keys to survival and success for future executives.

The role of tomorrow's nurse executive will be less remedial or corrective as well as less maintenance oriented in pursuit of organizational or divisional balance. Rather, the role will be more entrepreneurial or proactive and innovative as the nurse executive searches for new potential and opportunities for products, programs, and services in the face of constant environmental uncertainty and ambiguity.[3,7,10,12]

Daily functions of the nurse executive will include interacting with the health care marketplace; negotiating with the internal and external environments; expanding political influence; refining, stabilizing and harmonizing interests and demands of nursing's constituencies; and brokering, bridging, and linking organizational and nursing gaps by anticipating both short- and long-term actions and decisions.

The above-identified personal characteristics, roles, and functions will be essential to meet the following environmental and organizational challenges facing tomorrow's nurse executives.

Challenge 1: Being knowledgeable of and accessing information to more accurately predict and manage future organizational change

Being knowledgeable means the nurse executive is at the "cutting edge" of the current literature regarding health care, nursing, and business trends. In addition, it will be an expectation that the nurse executive know and be involved in the politics of business, health care, and professional organizations. This will enhance the nurse executive's effective utilization of local, state, regional, and national networks when anticipating or planning change. Within the organization, the nurse executive will need to be well appraised of decision making occurring at the governing body, administrative, and medical staff levels, whether that be in defining vision and mission, quality of care, strategic planning, financial viability, reducing risk and liability, policy and service development, community relations, or organizational growth.[6,19] It is the nurse executive's responsibility to constantly reappraise the nexus or linkage nursing has to the rest of the organization. The role of spokesperson for nursing in any areas requiring change in care or practice will be critical to the governing body/administration/medical staff triad and to maintaining the credibility of nursing and the nurse executive in the organization.

Challenge 2: Setting the organization's agenda for the future

This challenge is threefold. First, leaders of health care organizations will need to begin to focus more closely on their communities and the needs of their specific constituencies when setting their strategic direction and their organizational goals to better reflect their association with their communities. Second, leaders of health care organizations and health care providers also will need to refocus from a disease orientation to a more holistic perspective on healing through the connection and interplay of the mind, body, spirit, and emotions. Third, health care organizations will become much more culturally diversified. As a result, it will become imperative to know other's beliefs and values to understand what people will need to "buy into" to change their former mindsets.

For the nurse executive this means thinking larger, broader, and leaner in the constant search to find the most appropriate and best fit for nursing within the organization and the community. This will require the ability to move large organizations of individuals rapidly by changing perspectives rather than purpose and by optimizing opportunities.[11,18]

Challenge 3: Understanding the interrelationships and patterns in solving complex problems

As specialization and diversification continue to be integrated in health care, little will remain straightforward and simple. Every health care organization and nurse executive within it will need to generate a process to integrate information and translate its applicability to the organization's internal and external environment quickly and reliably to add cohesion, validity, and viability to management and administrative functions.

Nurse executives will need to carefully apply defined and clear methods, models, plans, and strategies to implement and accomplish goals. Greater consideration will need to be given to interrelationships among programs, products, services, organizational structure, culture, administrative style, work climate, and management practices. The effectiveness of forecasting and planning will depend heavily on what kind of fiscal and human resources are available; how clearly the roles of individuals and teams are defined; whether standards for responsibility, accountability, and authority are set; and the degree to which systems are supportive of work methods necessary for goal achievement.

Information will no longer be solely sufficient for alternative generation in problem solving as in the past. The nurse executive's personal capabilities and claimant groups' expectations, experience and interest in, knowledge of, and skill in problem solving, as well as organizational constraints, needs, resources, and priorities will be critical factors for understanding interrelationships and patterns in solving complex problems.

Challenge 4: Facilitating and supporting research to maximize human potential and fiscal resources

Healthcare delivery will become even more dynamic, complex, challenging, and difficult in the next decade and century. Confronted with this rapidly changing economic environment and practice setting, the nurse executive will have a newly found responsibility to improve the quality, cost effectiveness, and efficiency of patient care through research of systems, services, programs, and policies.[22]

Critical dimensions of care provided by nurses and those influenced by and related to nursing will surface. Opportunities will exist for introducing interactive models of research investigating technological innovations in patient care delivery, health promotion, health maintenance, illness prevention, and holistic care. Continuous quality improvement efforts, policy issues, and ethics will reveal additional opportunities for collaboration and cooperative research efforts with other departments or agencies. Discussion, study, analysis, and controlled comparisons of nursing care and management, as well as their importance in health care delivery, will necessitate the introduction of multisite studies to a much greater degree than has been true in the past.[15]

Research in nursing and nursing administration will need to set a futuristic course of action to maximize the creative potential of scarce human and fiscal resources. In setting such a course, researchers in nursing will need to move away from the past emphasis on identifying traits and studying the interrelationships of those traits for personal effectiveness toward participation of nursing staff in cooperative inquiry and action research for the purpose of bringing about improvements and change not only in care delivery, but also in the workplace and the organization as a whole.[20]

Challenge 5: Creating an empowered work environment — or making and implementing decisions through others

Although decisions are no longer arrived at arbitrarily or autonomously by effective nurse executives today, the need for collaboration through staff involvement in the planning and problem-solving processes will be even more imperative in the future. Leadership will not be measured in terms of the leadership exercised but rather in the leadership evoked, since it is through the staff that many of the nurse executive's responsibilities will be met. Leadership will not be measured in the power exercised over others, but in terms of the power released in others through the nurse executive's ability to influence the structure in which staff work and so facilitate change of their attitudes and behaviors. Leadership will not be measured in goals defined and direction given by the nurse executive, but in terms of the plan of action and goals staff members work out for themselves with the nurse executive's help. Lastly, leadership will not be measured by service and projects completed by the nurse executive, but in terms of growth in competence, sense of responsibility, and personal satisfaction felt among the staff; that is, in how well the nurse executive gets the staff to care and to share a sense of common purpose through planning with and rewarding them.

These expectations will impact the nurse executive personally by forcing a change from policy maker and directive issuer to leader, coach, and guide — to create a climate of creativity that translates theoretical verbiage into "how to's" by bridging the gap between what the staff knows and what the staff does. Through this process the nurse executive will become role model not only of nursing, but also of the organization at large.

In conclusion, success of the nurse executive in the future will depend upon:

- Defining a vision that stretches the thoughts, actions, and capacities of the nursing staff beyond today's realities

- Focusing on results that are essential and strategic both personally and organizationally
- Thinking and linking micro (individual), macro (organizational) and mega (societal) needs and results
- Defining the results to be accomplished and demonstrating what accomplishment will mean and the conditions under which accomplishment will be observed by others
- Identifying specifically what is needed to achieve the desired results
- Concentrating on strengths rather than limitations by focusing efforts on performance that will yield the greatest payoffs
- Moving beyond what is known, found acceptable or comfortable and conventional,[14] and, most importantly,
- Presenting oneself as authentic, confidence-inspiring, approachable, predictable, accountable, and professional

REFERENCES

1. Adams, C. (1990). Leadership behavior of chief nurse executives. *Nursing Management, 21*(8), 36-39.
2. American Hospital Association. (1990). Role and function of the hospital nurse executive. In *Management advisory* (pp. 1–3). Chicago: American Organization of Nurse Executives.
3. Bolster, C. J., & Petit, B. (1990). Quest for health care value will drive nontraditional opportunities for patient care executives. *Aspen's Advisor for Nurse Executives, 5*(7), 4-7.
4. Brown, C. L., & Schultz, P. R. (1991). Outcomes of power development in work relationships. *The Journal of Nursing Administration, 21*(2), 35-39.
5. Erickson, E. (1980). The nursing service director 1880-1980. *The Journal of Nursing Administration, 10*(4), 6-12.
6. Flarey, D. (1991). The nurse executive and the governing body synergy for a new era. *The Journal of Nursing Administration, 21*(12), 11-17.
7. Fralic, M. F. (1992). Nurse executive practice—into the next millennium: From limbo dancer to pole vaulter. *The Journal of Nursing Administration, 22*(2), 15-16.
8. Fralix, P. (1989). Administrative positioning of the nurse executive. *Aspen's Advisor For Nurse Executives, 4*(11), 5-6.
9. Henry, B., Woods, S., & Nagelkerk, J. (1990). Nightingale's perspective of nursing administration. *Nursing and Health Care, 11*(4), 201-205.
10. Johnson, J., & Bergmann, C. L. (1988). Nursing managers at the broker's table: The nurse executive's role. *The Journal of Nursing Administration, 18*(6), 18-21.
11. Johnson, L. (1990). Strategic managment: A new dimension of the nurse executive's role. *The Journal of Nursing Administration, 20*(9), 7-10.
12. Johnson, P. T. (1989). Normative power of chief executive nurses. *Image: The Journal of Nursing Scholarship, 21*(3), 162-167.
13. Joint Commission on Accreditation of Healthcare Organizations. (1992). *Accreditation manual for hospitals* (pp. 79-84). Chicago: Author.
14. Kaufman, R. (1992). 6 steps to strategic success. *Training & Development Journal, 46*(5), 107-112.
15. McDaniel, C. (1990). Nursing administration research as a paradigm reflection. *Nursing and Health Care, 11*(4), 191-193.
16. Miller, K. L. (1987). The human care perspective in nursing administration. *The Journal of Nursing Administration, 17*(2), 10-12.
17. Mintzberg, H. (1975). The manager's job: Folklore and fact. *Harvard Business Review, 53*(4), 49-61.
18. Murphy, M. (1988). Nurse executives: Becoming first-string players. *Aspen's Advisor for Nurse Executives, 3*(9), 7-8.
19. Nitta, D. E., & Spicer, J. G. (1989). The nurse executive's responsibility to the governing board. *Aspen's Advisor for Nurse Executives, 4*(11), 6-8.
20. Parker, M. E., Gordon, S. C., & Brannon, P. T. (1992). Involving nursing staff in research: A non-traditional approach. *The Journal of Nursing Administration, 22*(4), 58-63.
21. Pilette, P. C., & Kirby, K. K. (1991). Expectations and responsibilities of the nursing director role. *Nursing Management, 22*(3), 77-80.
22. Rosswurm, M. A. (1992). A research-based practice model in a hospital setting. *The Journal of Nursing Administration, 22*(3), 57-60.
23. Sorrentino, E. A. (1992). Profiling a chief nursing officer. *Nursing Management, 23*(3), 32-34.
24. Stevens, B. J. (1981). The role of the nurse executive. *The Journal of Nursing Administration, 11*(2), 19-23.
25. Tebbitt, B. V. (1990). *Nursing services: Internal functions and responsibilities.* Course 1, Unit 8, Hospital Administration (pp. 56-62). Minneapolis: University of Minnesota.
26. Ulrich, B. (1985). Time management for the nurse executive. *Nursing Economic$, 3*(4), 318-323.

CHAPTER 5

Nursing faculty

Who are they, what do they do, and what challenges do they face?

CAROLE A. ANDERSON

WHO ARE THE FACULTY?

More than 1,600 nursing programs in this country employ an estimated 22,000 full- ($n = 18,853$) and part-time ($n = 3488$) faculty members. Of these, 9.8% work in diploma programs, 50.5% in associate degree programs, and 39.7% in baccalaureate and higher degree programs.[5] Most faculty work full time, but there is an increasing trend toward the use of part-time faculty in response to fluctuating enrollments and diminishing financial resources.

The doctoral degree is the commonly expected and accepted entry-level credential for teaching in colleges and universities, but in nursing all faculty still fall far short of being doctorally prepared. Nevertheless, there is a growing trend toward a better educated faculty. In 1992, 21.4% of nursing faculty were doctorally prepared, a favorable improvement when compared with only 3% in 1972, and 10.6% in 1984.[5] Yet these numbers are still far lower than the level of doctoral preparation of faculty in other professional programs. Not surprisingly, the largest percentage of doctorally prepared faculty (43%) is found in baccalaureate and higher degree programs.[1]

The vast majority (91%) of faculty teaching in nursing programs are nurses. Diploma programs have the highest percentage (3.3%) of nonnurse faculty.[5] Most nursing faculty are women, only 8.5% are members of a minority group,[5] and 49.2% of faculty teaching in colleges and universities are untenured.[1]

The reasons for a less educated nursing faculty are found in our heritage and history. Nursing education's heritage began in hospitals, not in colleges and universities. Hospital-based (diploma) educational programs were the norm for the first half of the century, and although the first baccalaureate program was started in the early 1900s, for the first half of this century the vast majority of nurses continued to be prepared in diploma schools. Vocational education (diploma) was perhaps appropriate for those earlier times when society deemed the education of women unnecessary and even undesirable.

However, times and women have changed. Women now constitute over half of college freshmen and in 1986 were awarded 51% of the bachelor's, 50% of the master's, and 35% of the doctoral degrees.[7] Nursing education, however, developed relatively slowly in institutions of higher education and even today continues to lag far behind other major professions. It was not until World War II that the number of baccalaureate programs began to significantly increase.

A new type of nursing education program was developed during the 1950s: the associate degree (AD). This program was designed to prepare a technical nurse to complement the professional nurse who was prepared in a college or university. Today, AD programs represent a majority (50.5%) of all nursing programs. In 1989-91, AD programs graduated almost two and one-half times the number of graduates from baccalaureate programs.

For the past 30 years considerable discussion has centered on what "entry" credential is needed for beginning nursing practice. The debate persists today despite official resolutions from all the major nursing organizations declaring that the baccalaureate *should* be the entry-level preparation for professional practice. Nurses continue to have the lowest level of required educational preparation of *all* health professionals. As an illustration, medicine, optometry, dentistry, and veterinary medicine all require a minimum of four years of postbaccalaureate education plus additional years in specialty training. Pharmacy is quickly moving from the baccalaureate to the doctoral (PharmD) as the entry-level preparation. Occupational and physical therapy, dietetics, and medical technology all require the baccalaureate degree.

Given our history and the present-day reality that only 39.7% of nursing's educational programs are in colleges and universities, it is easy to understand that nursing's faculty profile, even today, would most likely parallel that found in vocational and technical institutions. This may be appropriate for diploma and AD programs, given the goals of the parent institution, but the situation in colleges and universities is quite different. In these institutions, nursing programs are seriously compromised because their faculties are so dissimilar from other faculties on their campuses. Furthermore, within the nursing unit itself, the faculty is split into two factions: those with and those without doctorates—a divisive and provocative arrangement.

In colleges and universities, faculty who are not doctorally prepared typically teach at the undergraduate level and are especially involved in undergraduate clinical teaching. Historically, the relatively few number of faculty with doctorates were assigned to the graduate program since most universities require the doctorate for the granting of graduate-level faculty status.

Doctoral education for nurse faculty has an interesting history. Until very recently, most nurses obtained their doctoral work in nonnursing fields (primarily education). But in 1988, approximately 36% of nurse faculty with doctorates had received them in nursing. This fact is most likely a function of the increase in the number of doctoral programs in nursing from 14 in 1973 to 54 in 1991.[2]

How do all of these facts and figures combine to make a profile of nursing faculty that answers the question: Who are the faculty in nursing education? And perhaps there is a more important question: What are the implications of that profile for the future of nursing education?

To begin, nursing does not have a single "typical" faculty member because of the diversity of parent institutions in which nursing programs reside. Rather, two faculty profiles emerge. The typical nurse faculty member teaching in a diploma or associate degree program is a nonminority woman prepared at the master's level who devotes the majority of her time to teaching undergraduates in both the classroom and clinical setting. The faculty role is confined to only one dimension of the academic role: teaching.[5]

On the other hand, a typical faculty member teaching in a college or university is also a nonminority woman but is much more likely to possess the doctorate (43%). Her teaching is most likely concentrated in the graduate program, and she is also expected to fulfill all three requirements of the academic role: teaching, research/scholarship, and service. Only very recently have doctorally prepared faculty carried responsibilities in both the undergraduate and graduate programs. (In 1990-91, 25.2% taught at both levels.[1])

So, unlike other disciplines, nursing as an academic discipline is characterized by wide variation in the types and kinds of faculty teaching in our various programs. Today, it is likely that only in the major research universities that offer the full range of academic programs, including the doctorate ($n = 50+$), is there greater uniformity of academic preparation found among the nursing faculty; and these faculty also enjoy greater comparability to their faculty colleagues in other academic disciplines. Several implications emerge from the current faculty profile in nursing centered on two major factors: noncomparability of credentials and female dominance.

Noncomparability of credentials

Because nursing faculty on the whole are not as fully and comparably prepared as faculty found in other academic disciplines they, de facto, occupy a marginal social status within the college/university. Faculty with marginal status are not full participants in the life of the academy and are denied a reference group that represents the diversity of the institution. Furthermore, knowing that they are "less" qualified than their colleagues, nursing faculty tend to isolate themselves in their own department/college and become further removed from valuable sources of information and opportunities to influence campus events.

Higher education is uniquely characterized by its system of faculty governance. Colleges and universities are, in their essence, a collection of people: the faculty. The life blood of the institution is the faculty. It is the faculty who generate the reputation and attract the best students and whose opinions guide the course of action. Faculty who do not fully participate in this governance are, by definition, set apart from institutional life. To the extent that this is true for nursing faculty, the nursing program is made vulnerable because it lacks a strong, fully empowered faculty.

Female dominance

Nursing has always been and continues to be a female-dominated profession. In a very real sense, nursing as a profession can be viewed as a microcosm of women's issues in this country. Women's history is nursing's history! Nursing's development both as a profession and as an academic discipline has been shaped by this powerful fact. Yet, ironically, we, the profession, do not address this issue, and nurses do not consistently identify with the goals, objectives, and strategies of the women's movement. Rather, nurses tend to relate their position as nursing faculty to the particular institutional setting rather than to their personal and psychological development and deemed social status as women. The most recent data on women in higher education[5] indicate that although the number of women faculty is growing, the proportion of women has remained steady at about one fourth of the total college and university faculty and that the greatest increase has been at the entry, assistant professor level. Compared to their male colleagues, women are clustered in the lower academic ranks, a smaller percentage achieve tenure, and women earn lower average salaries at every rank. The most disheartening fact is that precious little has changed in this profile over the past 20 years. The overall conclusion is that it is still difficult for women to succeed in the academy. Why?

Aisenberg and Harrington studied two groups of academic women: those who had left their positions and those who had tenure. They found similar themes in both groups:

Essentially, they are themes that depict an experience of professional marginality and of exclusion from the centers of professional authority. Taken together, the stories reveal a continuum of outsiderness—literal in the case of the deflected women but nonetheless real for the tenured women as well.[3]

Central to Aisenberg and Harrington's explanation of what happens to academic women is what they call the "marriage plot" that defines marriage as being the goal for all women and, in turn, the ways in which a woman should behave in order to meet her goal. Because this has been the paradigm for women for so long, these authors argue that women cannot ignore it or rid themselves of it as a guide for their behavior and as a measure of their success.[3] As a result, women, just like men, face the same overall task of becoming expert professionals, but in addition a woman must also deal with a whole set of other demands and expectations that relegate her pursuit of a career as secondary to other roles of wife/mother and also to her male partner's career.

For many female faculty, this conflict is carried into their daily lives, and they find themselves faced with a continuous struggle rooted in the desire to be "womanly" as society defines "woman" and "successful" as her profession defines success. Couple this personal conflict with the reality that the typical academic institution's policies and practices, the very fabric of the culture of higher education, have been crafted by and for men. The result is a climate in which women find it difficult to thrive and achieve. Recent studies on various campuses across this country attest to a climate that makes it difficult for women to advance within professorial ranks and to high-level administrative posts that offer the opportunity to influence policy and improve the climate.

In a profound way, then, this marginal status for academic women is compounded for nursing faculty who do not possess the same credentials as other women faculty. Quite realistically, their disenfranchisement/marginality is made even greater.

Interesting behavior patterns emerge when individuals are placed in positions without power and influence and are dominated by groups that deny them membership. Anger, resentment, and distrust are common, as are futility and frustration and diminished pleasure derived from one's work. At times these forces create paradoxical behaviors, such as a sense of entitlement, to compensate for the oppression. These discomforting behaviors are interpreted by men in negative ways that cause them to isolate women further.

Because nursing faculty are predominately women, slightly different internal patterns of behavior emerge, but in many ways these patterns parallel those described above: doctorally prepared faculty are the "privileged class," and nondoctorally prepared faculty are marginalized and made ineligible for membership in the elite group. Master's-prepared faculty are often motivated to pursue doctoral education in order to gain membership in the more prestigious group, which more often than not means that they do not have to teach undergraduate clinical courses.

WHAT DO FACULTY DO?

In differing proportions faculty teach, do research, publish, and provide service to the institution and the profession. To accomplish these varied tasks, faculty need to acquire the very best graduate education. Ideally, they should also possess the desire to further develop and strengthen a set of personal characteristics that Schoenfeld and Magnan (in a delightful and enormously useful book called *Mentor in a Manual*[6]) identify as being necessary to succeed in academe. These characteristics include: knowledge (information, data, theories, concepts, facts); skills (technical, scientific, communication, information retrieval, analysis and synthesis); and insight (wisdom, vision) and values.[6]

Teaching

A successful teacher possesses a thorough command of the subject matter being taught, which requires that faculty must continuously strive to expand their knowledge base in a world of rapidly changing information. This requires a commitment to continuous learning that goes beyond rhetoric to the investment of substantial time, energy, and money in one's own development as a teacher.

Successful teachers are those who convey a liking and deep respect for students that in turn creates an environment conducive to learning. Good teachers are able to present material in an objective and well-organized manner, convey a sense of excitement for the material, and stimulate students to want to learn more. Successful teachers vary their teaching methodologies according to the characteristics of the class (e.g., large lecture, small seminar), understand and use state-of-the-art teaching methods, and evaluate student learning in an objective manner. The very best teachers truly enjoy teaching and their students and have learned to balance those duties with their other responsibilities.

Through the advising process, teachers help students identify their interests and make decisions about their futures.

Research and scholarship

Some institutions claim teaching to be their primary and almost exclusive mission, which means that very little research or scholarship are required of faculty. However, even these institutions are increasingly requiring at least a modest level of research and scholarship. Junior faculty are wise to devote considerable effort in determining the precise expectations for teaching, research, and scholarship to be used as a guide for setting priorities.

Research training is the primary objective of doctoral education. Although nursing has typically re-

quired knowledge of the research process as part of the required courses in the master's program, the depth of knowledge and skills necessary to actually conduct research are acquired in a doctoral program. Research in nursing focused on the development of knowledge that provides the foundation for clinical practice. Consequently, research should focus on clinical phenomena. In 1988, the National Center for Nursing Research (NCNR) was established within the National Institutes for Health (NIH) to provide nursing with increased access to federal support for research.

In 1991, the U.S. Surgeon General published *Health Care 2000*, the objectives for the nation's health for the year 2000. These objectives serve as guiding principles for the delineation of research priorities within the NIH (including the NCNR) for the rest of the decade. Essentially, this document outlines the nation's most pressing health care problems and sets out objectives to improve the nation's health. Nursing research has the potential to make significant contributions to this agenda, and nursing faculty need to focus their programs of research in these areas as a way of establishing nursing as a research discipline capable of making a difference in the lives of those for whom we care: our patients. Over the past five years, the NCNR has used expert panels to develop a research agenda for nursing that sets priorities for the science of nursing. This agenda includes the study of low birth weight infants, information systems, symptom management, nursing care delivery systems, long-term care, health promotion, and AIDS.

Service

Faculty provide service to the nursing department/college, the parent institution, and the profession. This service takes many forms, but a major mechanism for the provision of service is the system of faculty governance, usually through some type of committee structure.

In its simplest form, faculty governance is the authority and control possessed by the faculty to make decisions in curriculum, degree requirements, subject matter and methods of instruction, student policies as they relate to the educational process, and faculty status, including appointments, promotion, and tenure. Faculty governance is a critical part of the faculty role that should not be taken lightly since it is, in its truest sense, the heart of the university.

Faculty contribute to the profession in a variety of ways. Faculty are members of professional organizations and provide service to them in the form of membership on committees and boards. Faculty also provide continuing education through different organizations that serve the profession.

Nursing faculty may also provide service to the institution through clinical practice. Such service may be part of the faculty role, but it may also be undertaken on a volunteer basis. The extent to which faculty do or do not practice affects their credibility as teachers. Unfortunately, many nursing faculty have become far removed from the realities of contemporary practice, which diminishes not only their teaching but also their research since they are not well positioned to identify relevant and significant clinical problems to investigate. This reality is one of the most important challenges facing nursing faculty today.

Although service is an expected part of the faculty role, faculty must guard against spending too much time doing it. Committee work can be very seductive and can also consume inordinate amounts of time. Faculty must remember that their *primary* mission is teaching and research and strive to limit their service activities not only to that which is expected but also to that which informs their teaching and scholarship.

CHALLENGES FACING NURSING FACULTY

The greatest challenge facing nursing faculty in colleges and universities is to become full participants in the academy by contributing fully to the goals of the institution through their teaching, research, and service. Nursing faculty need to design and teach in excellent academic programs based on a knowledge of higher education and its standards, the discipline of nursing, and the needs of a health care system of both today *and* tomorrow.

Nursing, as a relative newcomer to higher education, can ill afford the risk of mediocre- or poor-quality educational programs. The decade of the 1990s is developing as a time in which higher education will face particularly difficult fiscal challenges. In this type of environment, only the *very best* will survive. Decisions will have to be made to preserve quality programs that will in the long run preserve the institution itself. Nursing programs in major research universities may be particularly vulnerable; on the whole, their research profile does not parallel that of their colleagues, and, in looking at the data, it is apparent that the AD is *really* the entry-level degree for nursing.

In the mid-1980s nursing programs were faced with dramatic enrollment declines. In response to these declines, many nursing programs very quickly designed a variety of program offerings as a means of attracting students, thereby preserving themselves. Many of these programs are quite innovative and long overdue, but many also challenge commonly accepted educational standards. As much as these can, in the short run, preserve nursing programs, they will in the long run contribute to their demise if they lack quality that is comparable to the parent institution. As an example, Leininger[4] writes of her concern that doctoral programs in nursing may reflect a culture of mediocrity. Her concern derives from the fact that there has been a rapid proliferation in the number of doctoral programs and that many of them lack sufficient numbers of qualified faculty, are without a foundation of faculty research, and suffer from unstable leadership. Leininger's concerns, to the extent that they are true, should raise considerable alarm because the products of these programs are our future faculty. A culture of mediocrity will handicap them enormously in their ability to fulfill a faculty role.

Nursing faculty need to learn the norms that guide faculty work, particularly those related to self-governance. Faculty must become knowledgeable by reading widely and regularly about higher education (e.g., *The Chronicle of Higher Education*), fully understand the goals of their own institutions, and know its system for advancement (know what is expected). Faculty especially must understand that colleges and universities are a meritocracy and that the *products* of their effort are what is valued and rewarded. Especially relevant are the products of research and scholarship.

Nursing faculty must make substantial efforts to bridge the historical schism between nursing service and nursing education. Collaborative efforts contribute to the enhancement of quality in both sectors. Nursing faculty must also increase and keep their knowledge of current clinical practice in order to design and implement high-quality programs, especially at the baccalaureate and master's levels.

Finding ways to stay abreast of current clinical care without having to spend 14 to 16 hours per week teaching undergraduate clinical courses is especially challenging for faculty who teach in major research universities. Because these universities define themselves by their heavy involvement in research, their standards for promotion and advancement expect faculty to be active scholars and researchers. For many years, nursing faculty were treated as an exception to this requirement. But this is no longer true. Doctorally prepared faculty must develop and maintain programs of research and scholarship. However, this becomes very difficult to do if a faculty member is assigned, on a regular basis, to undergraduate clinical teaching. The time commitment is just too great. New models must be developed that utilize other types of instructional personnel. Such models include utilization of teaching assistants, clinical faculty, clinical specialists, and staff nurse preceptors. The challenge is to find a way to effectively utilize doctoral faculty in the teaching of undergraduates without burdening them with the direct clinical supervision aspect of that teaching. Nursing's success as a research discipline is unequivocally linked to meeting this challenge.

Nursing faculty are challenged to develop insight into their own history as nurses, faculty, and women and to confront the conflicts derived from each to be successful in their careers and personal life. As identified by Schoenfeld and Magnan,[6] traits related to achievement in a faculty role include integrity, maturity, will, self-discipline, flexibility, confidence, endurance, decisiveness, coolness under stress, initiative, justice, compassion, sense of humor, creativity, humility, and tact. Developing these characteristics and traits may present substantial challenges for nursing faculty because some are counter to traits considered desirable for women and because models are lacking for others that have not been part of nursing's culture.

And finally, nursing faculty must actively pursue the elimination of those policies, practices, values, and norms that interfere with their own goals as well as goals for excellence. Examples of practices that need elimination include large, cumbersome committee structures; commitment to the *process* of education at the expense of the product; teaching facts rather than principles and concepts; harsh and punitive treatment of students contributing to a reputation for "eating our young"; the absence of a norm for postdoctoral training; devaluing undergraduate instruction; and, finally, team teaching that makes it difficult for individuals to develop strong pedagogical skills and a sense of accountability and responsibility.

Being a faculty member is not an easy job. It requires the very best that one has to offer. It also affords a wealth of opportunity especially to shape the future of the profession and to contribute in meaningful ways to the solution of major health care problems. Becoming a faculty member is not for everyone. It should be reserved for the very best, the brightest, and the most promising. Our students, our future, deserve no less.

REFERENCES

1. American Association of Colleges of Nursing. (1990). *A data base for graduate education in nursing.* Washington, D.C.: Author.
2. American Association of Colleges of Nursing. (1992). *1991-92 enrollment and graduation.* Washington, D.C.: Author.
3. Aisenberg, N., & Harrington, M. (1988). *Women of academe: Outsiders in the sacred grove.* Amherst: University of Massachusetts Press.
4. Leininger, M. (1985). Current doctoral nursing education: A culture of mediocrity or excellence? In J. C. McCloskey and H. K. Grace (Eds.), *Current issues in nursing* (2nd ed., pp. 219-235). St Louis: Mosby.
5. National League for Nursing. (1992). *Nursing data review: 1992.* New York: Author.
6. Schoenfeld, A. C., & Magnan, R. (1992). *Mentor in a manual.* Madison, Wis: Magna.
7. Touchton, J. G., & Davis, L. (1991). *Fact book on women in higher education.* New York: American Council on Education.

CHAPTER 6

Nurse researchers

Who are they, what do they do, and what challenges do they face?

NANCY A. STOTTS

Nurse researchers are individuals who identify important questions about issues in nursing theory and/or practice and seek to answer these questions using a variety of research methods. The ultimate goal of the nurse researcher is to develop the scientific basis for nursing practice.[5] Although vast advances have been made in the development of nursing science over the past few decades, the fact remains that the evolution of science as a discipline and practice is an ongoing process.

The typical research process begins with identification of a significant researchable problem and development of a research proposal. The researcher submits the grant proposal for funding, and a panel of researchers reviews the proposal for its scientific merit. Once funded, the researcher oversees and conducts the study. When completed, the researcher analyzes the findings and draws conclusions, which are disseminated at scientific meetings and through publication in scholarly journals. The process is not over, however, as the researcher goes on to identify new questions that arise out of the completed study and the steps of the research process are repeated. Throughout the career of the researcher, this conceptualization-conduct-dissemination cycle is repeated and produces a focused program of research.

Research is rarely the sole activity of the nurse researcher. Nurse scientists today usually have a faculty or clinical appointment that has a variety of additional role expectations. As a faculty member, one has teaching and university/community service to complete and professional competence to maintain. Those with clinical appointments have practice and administrative re-

sponsibilities. As experts in their field, many are peer reviewers for journals and federal and private grant funding sources. In addition, most are active in scientific and professional organizations. The common denominator of the researcher, however, is research, and examining what they publish is one approach to understanding who nurse researchers are.

To determine who the nurse researchers are, what they do, and what challenges they face, I reviewed two years of research in three major journals. Two years were selected as a brief but representative sample, and the period from July 1990 to July 1992 was chosen because it was the most recent. The three journals selected were *Nursing Research, Western Journal of Nursing Research,* and *Research in Nursing and Health.* They were picked because they are peer reviewed, research focused, and are not identified as specialty focused. Columns dedicated to a specific topic were not included in this analysis. The remainder of this chapter will address who nurse researchers are and what issues they face based on this review.

THE NATURE OF THE RESEARCH

The studies published were examined to determine whether they were bench research, clinical research, studies of nurses/students, instrumentation/methodological studies, or theoretical papers. Of a total of 265 journal articles reviewed, 2 (0.8%) were bench research, 171 (64.5%) were clinical research, 33 (12.5%) were studies of nurses/students, 46 (17.3%) were instrumentation/methodological studies, and 13 (4.9%) were theory/review papers (Fig. 6-1). Examples of articles in each category are

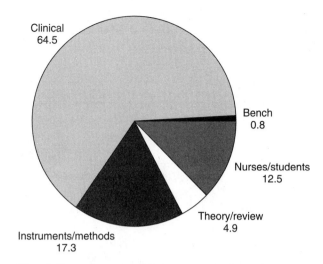

Clinical
64.5

Bench
0.8

Nurses/students
12.5

Theory/review
4.9

Instruments/methods
17.3

Fig. 6-1 Percent of types of research published.

EXAMPLES OF ARTICLES CLASSIFIED AS BENCH RESEARCH, CLINICAL RESEARCH, RESEARCH ON NURSES/STUDENTS, INSTRUMENTATION/METHODOLOGICAL ARTICLES, AND THEORY PAPERS

Bench research

Endotracheal Suctioning-induced Heart Rate Alterations[7]

Clinical research

Holistic Health Patterning in Multiple Sclerosis[6]

The Urine Stream Interruption Test and Pelvic Muscle Function[16]

Research on nurses/students

"Half a Loaf Is Better than No Bread": Public Health Nursing and Physicians in Ontario, 1920-1925[17]

Nurses' Risk Taking Regarding HIV Transmission in the Workplace[9]

Instrumentation/methodology

The IPR Inventory: Development and Psychometric Characteristics[18]

Uncertainty in Illness Theory: A Replication of the Mediating Effects of Mastery and Coping[10]

Theory articles

An Analysis of the Pragmatic Consequences of Holism for Nursing[1]

---

listed in the box above. The three journals reviewed vary in the number of articles published in each of these areas (Fig. 6-2).

These data show that the majority of studies published are clinical studies. There is a paucity of bench research reported in the journals reviewed, indicating either that there is little bench work completed in nursing or that it is reported in other journals.

The heavy emphasis on instrument development and methodological concerns reflects the ongoing struggle within the helping sciences to find a means to capture the phenomena under study. Work on new instruments and refinement of existing instruments is important to nursing science and reflects the maturing of the field. Of importance is the fact that negative and positive results are reported.

STUDY SAMPLE

When the clinical studies were examined, the majority (84.2%) addressed the adult population, some (12.9%) focused on the child/neonate alone, while a small percentage (2.9%) explored the adult-child population. Those papers that used a sample of adult-child either examined each independently or how they interacted. The oldest old, the preterm infant, and all ages in the middle were addressed in the clinical research reported.

The samples examined crossed the health-illness spectrum. They were organized by age, condition, disease, and location on the health-illness trajectory. The box on page 40 provides examples of various study samples included in research published during this two-year period.

Clear from the researchers' discussion of the findings, limitations, and recommendations for further research were important methodological issues. The issue of small sample size was one of the themes. More sharing is needed about strategies nurse researchers use to recruit and retain samples. Of special concern because of the burden of participating in a study are those subjects who are ill, emotionally distressed, or for some reason considered a vulnerable population (e.g., comatose patients, prisoners). Oberst[14] addresses this issue and raises the important question of how a community of scholars might deal with a manuscript that has a small sample size but addresses a potentially important question.

SUBSTANTIVE CONTENT OF THE RESEARCH

The topics of the clinical research varied widely. The substantive focus of the studies could be classified as

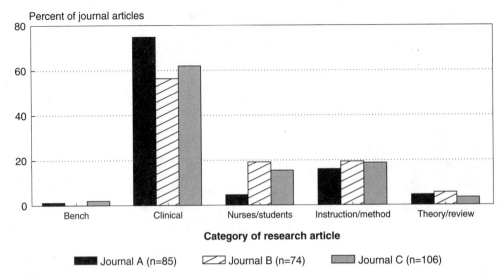

Fig. 6-2 Percent of research articles by category in three journals.

using the person, environment, health, nursing paradigm. Examples of topics studied using this schemata are provided in the box on this page (*right*). What is clear from this review is that nurse researchers address a broad variety of topics. The ability to cluster them is limited and determines whether they address identified priorities or not.

STUDY DESIGN

Designs used for the studies included both qualitative and quantitative techniques. Quantitative methods employed predominated and included descriptive studies, quasiexperimental studies, repeated measures designs, and true experiments. An important issue is whether the appropriate method was used to answer the questions raised. This question reflects a growing awareness of this issue in the field.

COLLABORATION

The question then was raised whether the research conducted was collaborative or by a single researcher. Of the clinical and bench studies reviewed ($n = 173$), 50 (28.9%) were authored by one investigator.

These data show that the majority of research was conducted by groups of researchers (>70%), suggesting collaborative work and the building of the science by a team of researchers. This approach is important in

---

EXAMPLES OF STUDY SAMPLES INCLUDED IN CLINICAL RESEARCH REVIEWED

Heart transplant patients[2]
Multiple sclerosis[6]
Newborns[3]
Nursing home residents[11]
Nursing students[4]
Women[16]

EXAMPLES OF CLINICAL RESEARCH TOPICS CLASSIFIED CATEGORIZED USING THE PERSON, ENVIRONMENT, HEALTH, NURSING PARADIGM

Person
Preterm Infants' Physiologic Response to Early Parent Touch[8]

Environment
Desire for Control and Choice of Antiemetic Treatment for Cancer Chemotherapy[19]

Health
Responses to Chronic Illness: Analysis of Psychological and Physiological Adaptation[15]

Nursing
Lesbian Phobia in Nursing Students[4]

the field because it allows individuals to bring deep and diverse perspectives to a topic so that richness in theory and design can be brought to the project. However, the continued publication of articles by a single individual suggests continued dialogue needs to take place to address the significant divergence from the model of how science is built in most other fields.

BUILDING A PROGRAM OF RESEARCH

To determine whether researchers were conducting a series of studies to build a program of research or not, I reviewed the references at the end of studies. Only in a limited number of cases[10] did the studies cited show the report was submitted as part of a larger or ongoing program of research. These data indicate that much work is early in the researcher's career or is a single study unrelated to the major direction of the individual's research. In addition, from the studies reviewed it appears that there is a limited number of established programs of research. Development of nursing science will require continued attention to this area.

UTILIZATION OF FINDINGS

The issue of clinical utilization or applicability of findings is a theme in these research reports. The ability to transfer content to the clinical area would be stronger if clinical significance and statistical significance were discussed explicitly in each research report. As a discipline, nursing has not established criteria for clinical significance with various treatments and populations, so there is not a standard against which to judge this important criterion.[12] Only with increased dialogue can a comparative standard be agreed upon and established.

In addition, not all findings could or should be used to direct practice.[13] It is a dilemma for both the researcher and the practitioner to understand which nursing interventions work and which do not. The parallel might be drawn between nursing and pharmaceutical intervention. No one would expect every drug to work, yet nurses are surprised when nursing research shows a "no effect" response. It is important that both the research and practitioner accept this reality.

OTHER ISSUES

One of the strategies used by editors of these journals to address important issues in nursing research is to add a column, department, or section on the topic. Among the issues addressed in this way are ethics, strategies of teaching nursing research, research utilization, and cultural sensitivity. Such an approach allows the salient features to be explicated as the basis for discussion and resolution.

SUMMARY

This review was designed to capture who nurse researchers are and what issues challenge them. To accomplish this goal, I examined articles published over a recent two-year period in three major research journals. Data showed that researchers most often study adult patients using quantitative research designs. Topics addressed are quite broad, reflecting the diversity in nursing. Among the issues that often challenge nurse researchers are the quantitative/qualitative dilemma, collaboration, how to build a program of research, and how and when findings should be transferred to practice.

REFERENCES

1. Allen, C. E. (1991). An analysis of the pragmatic consequences of holism for nursing. *Western Journal of Nursing Research, 13*(2), 256-272.
2. Bohachick, P., Anton, B. B., Wooldridge, P. J., Kormos, R. L., Armitage, J. M., Hardesty, R. L., & Griffith, B. P. (1992). Psychosocial outcomes six months after cardiac transplant surgery: A preliminary report. *Research in Nursing and Health, 15*(3), 165-173.
3. Brown, L., Arnold, L., Charsha, D., Allison, D., & Klein, H. (1990). Transcutaneous bilirubinometer: An instrument for clinical research. *Nursing Research, 39*(4), 241-243.
4. Eliason, M. J., & Randall, C. E. (1991). Lesbian phobia in nursing students. *Western Journal of Nursing Research, 13*(3), 363-374.
5. Gennaro, S., & Vessey, J. (1991). Making practice perfect. *Nursing Research, 40*(5), 259.
6. Glick, E. E., & Bugg, A. (1992). Holistic health patterning in multiple sclerosis. *Research in Nursing and Health, 15*(3), 175-185.
7. Gunderson, P. L., Stone, K. S., & Hamlin, R. L. (1991). Endotracheal suctioning-induced heart rate alterations. *Nursing Research, 40*(3), 139-143.
8. Harrison, L. L., Leeper, J., & Yoon, M. (1991). Preterm infants' physiologic response to early parent touch. *Western Journal of Nursing Research, 13*(6), 698-707.
9. McNabb, K., & Keller, M. L. (1991). Nurses' risk taking regarding HIV transmission in the workplace. *Western Journal of Nursing Research, 13*(6), 732-745.
10. Mishel, M. H., Padilla, G., Grant, M., & Sorenson, D. S. (1991). Uncertainty in illness theory: A replication of the mediating effects of mastery and coping. *Nursing Research, 40*(4), 236-240.
11. Munroe, D. J. (1990). The influence of registered nurse staffing on quality of nursing home care. *Research in Nursing and Health, 13*(4), 263-270.

12. Oberst, M. T. (1991). The research-practice linkage in nursing research journals. *Research in Nursing and Health, 14*(6), iii-iv.

13. Oberst, M. T. (1991). The generalizability and clinical application dilemma. *Research in Nursing and Health, 14*(6), iii-iv.

14. Oberst, M. T. (1992). On small samples and good ideas. *Research in Nursing and Health, 15,* 163-64.

15. Pollock, S. E., Christian, B. J., & Sands, D. (1990). Responses to chronic illness: Analysis of psychological and physiological adaptation. *Nursing Research, 39*(5), 300-304.

16. Sampselle, C. M., & DeLancey J. O. (1992). The urine stream interruption test and pelvic muscle function. *Nursing Research, 41*(2), 73-77.

17. Stuart, M. (1992). "Half a loaf is better than no bread": Public health nursing and physicians in Ontario, 1920-1925. *Nursing Research, 41*(1), 21-27.

18. Tilden, V. P., Nelson, C. A., & May, B. A. (1990). Use of qualitative methods to enhance content validity. *Nursing Research, 39*(3), 172-5.

19. Wallston, K. A., Smith, R. A., King, J. E., Smith, M. S., Rye, P., & Burish, T. G. (1991). Desire for control and choice of antiemetic treatment for cancer chemotherapy. *Western Journal of Nursing Research, 13*(1), 12-23.

CHAPTER 7

Nurse entrepreneurs

Who are they, what do they do, and what challenges do they face?

LYNDA JUALL CARPENITO, MARGO C. NEAL

What is an entrepreneur? Webster's[8] defines an entrepreneur as "one who organizes, manages, and assumes the risks of a business or enterprise." Herron and Herron see the essence of entrepreneurship as "innovation through reallocation or reconfiguration of resources ... [and] an awareness of or alertness to the opportunity to do so for the purpose of creating benefit."[4]

A "common sense" of nurse entrepreneurs has not included the traditional role of "private duty nurse" or even nurse therapists. Certainly, nurses in these roles were and are entrepreneurial. Today, the common accepted definition of nurse entrepreneurs refers to someone who is self-employed in either a nonclinical mode—for example, consultant, educator, editor, writer—or in a clinical role—for example, nurse practitioners or nurse therapists.

Nurse entrepreneurs have grown and developed over the past decade, although there were a few nurses who pursued nontraditional careers in the 1970s. For example, Jean Steele set up a joint practice in Boston, and Margo Neal was one of the first nurses to provide continuing education workshops nationally. In the late 1970s and early 1980s, nurse entrepreneurs were a relatively new phenomenon; in the 1990s, they have become a permanent part of the nursing landscape. This nontraditional role for nurses is supported by many graduate schools that invite nurse entrepreneurs to speak to their students. Another indication of the permanency of this role is its listing as a role option in nursing in a survey conducted by Aydelotte, Hardy, and Hope,[1] which was published by the ANA. The growth of nurse entrepreneurs appears to parallel the women's movement toward greater equality of the genders. It also parallels the increasing number of men in the profession and nurses with advanced degrees.

Where are the outlets for nurses who are highly educated to do specialized assessments, identify and evaluate patient outcomes, and make treatment decisions? Universities take the majority; hospitals and other health agencies take fewer. The constricting economic climate in hospitals mandates employing few of these advanced practitioners. If the economic climate in hospitals were different, would this highly educated group of nurses work in them? Or would they opt for roles where they perceive they would have the potential for internal control of what they do and greater economic benefit?

Shoultz, Hatcher, and Hurrell state that the growing edges of a new paradigm in nursing "are to be found not within the well-developed or established boundaries of the profession, the old paradigm, but on the edges, at the point of interprofessional and community contact."[7] This is a time of chaos and needed change in the healthcare system. It is a time to focus on preventive care, and nurses, by emphasizing the wellness model, can have a piece of the pie; it is a time to be proactive, not reactive.[7]

WHO ARE THEY, WHAT DO THEY DO?

In a guest editorial in the *Journal of Continuing Education,* Keough wrote, "In a field as diversified as nursing, each of us should be able to find career satisfaction."[5] A career is an occupation that one follows as one's life's work. It represents a progressive course of action a person takes to achieve one's

---

EXAMPLES OF SERVICES PROVIDED BY CONSULTANTS

Accreditation and regulatory compliance

Organizational development
Case management
Communications
Computer information management
Cost containment
Evaluation
Quality management
Planning & forecasting
Home health services
Discharge planning
Resource management
Educational programs

Employee relations

Classification systems
Risk management
Recruitment & retention
Staff development
Delivery systems
Documentation systems
Research program development
Staffing & scheduling
    Standards
    Management development
    Fiscal management

From: Directory of Consultants. (1992). *Journal of Nursing Administration, 22* (7/8), p. 75.

---

professional goals. Entrepreneurs organize, manage, and assume the risk to achieve their goals. They seek to make a difference for a profit.

The exact number of entrepreneurs in nursing is unknown. What is known is that the group is very diverse and provides a multitude of services. For example, entrepreneurs serve as consultants for risk management or provide direct client services, such as nurse practitioners, or produce and market a product, such as uniforms or software. For the past several years the *Journal of Nursing Administration* has published an annual list of consultants and, more recently, *Perspectives in Psychiatric Care* has started to publish a comparable list for nurse therapists in private practice. The *Journal of Nursing Administration's* 1992 *Directory of Consultants* lists more than 400 consultants and the services they provide.[2] The box above lists examples of the variety of services provided.

In addition to the services noted in the box, nurses have created companies that provide air ambulance service, home health care, temporary staffing, uniforms and client hospital gowns, pediatric surgical preparation kits, educational toys, corporate employee health programs, child care, elder care, editorial services, and emergency management training. Other nurse-run businesses provide direct client services, such as chronic pain management, breastfeeding counseling, health teaching, enterostomal therapy, family therapy, parenting classes, and home adaption with a neurological disability.

To determine characteristics, work style, benefits, and problems of entrepreneurs, we surveyed a convenience sample of 20 nurse entrepreneurs; the return rate was 85%, ($n = 17$). A listing of the respondents appears in Table 7-1.

WHAT ARE THE CHARACTERISTICS OF SUCCESSFUL ENTREPRENEURS?

Not everyone wants to be an entrepreneur, and not everyone who attempts self-employment will be successful. In 1985, the Center for Entrepreneurial Management surveyed its 2,500 members in an attempt to develop a profile of an entrepreneur. The box on page 46 presents characteristics found to be present in the entrepreneurs surveyed. Examine the list in the box, and check those characteristics that best describe you. How many characteristics of a successful entrepreneur do you have?

Drucker writes, "Entrepreneurs always search for change, respond to it, and exploit it as an opportunity."[3] In our survey, several entrepreneurs emphasized the need to have good interpersonal skills (Dolan, Fishman, Gostel, Puetz). Hall Johnson emphasized good listening skills as a method to generate marketable ideas. Burgess wrote that one had to be "open to changing as the market requires and to look down the road as to what is changing and developing a response, while focusing on what needs to be done now."

The majority of the respondents said that entrepreneurs should be creative, humorous, flexible, and enthusiastic. Alfaro-LeFevre expands on the above by adding curiosity, humility, and persistence. When faced with problems or failure, one needs the ability to face rejection and stand back (Milazzo) and to have "thick skin" (Porter-O'Grady). Manthey emphasizes that one needs a "strong desire to keep moving forward in personal growth and willingness to change." All respon-

Table 7-1 Survey Respondents

Roberta Abruzzese Consultant RELSA Garden City, N.Y.	Suzanne Hall Johnson Director Hall Johnson Communication, Inc. Lakewood, Colo.
Rosalinda Alfaro-LeFevre President N.D.N.P. Consultants Malvern, Pa.	Marie Manthey President Creative Nursing Management, Inc. Minneapolis, Minn.
Christine Bolwell Owner Diskovery Saratoga, Calif.	Vicki L. Milazzo President Medical-Legal Consulting Institute, Inc. Houston, Texas
Connie Burgess President Connie Burgess & Associates Long Beach, Calif.	Tim Porter-O'Grady Senior Partner, CEO Tim Porter-O'Grady Inc. Atlanta, Ga.
Rose Mary Carroll-Johnson Editor Nursing Diagnosis, Oncology Nursing Forum Valencia, Calif.	Belinda E. Puetz President, CEO Belinda E. Puetz & Associates, Inc. Pensacola, Fla.
Mariam B. Dolan President Heritage Home Health Bristol, N.H.	Roxane Spitzer-Lehmann President S/L Associates San Diego, Calif.
Dorothy J. Fishman President Fishman Associates Farmington, Conn.	Ann VanSlyck President VanSlyck & Associates, Inc. Phoenix, Ariz.
Roberta Gostel President Healthcare Multimedia Design Richmond, Va.	Sylvia Weber Psychiatric Nurse Clinical Specialist Counseling & Mental Health Services Cranston, R.I.
Sandra Jansen President Birth Plus Los Angeles, Calif.	

dents agreed that an entrepreneur must be a self-starter, self-disciplined, "driven," and have a lot of energy. Carroll-Johnson describes the need to have the willingness to invest money in anticipation of long-term gains. Jansen wrote that one needed bravery to give up the familiar financial security. In response to the question What are the forces that led you to start your own business? two respondents reported termination from their positions, and two reported unsatisfactory work situations. Since the profile mentioned earlier listed termination from position or resignation from an unsatisfactory position as characteristics of en-

trepreneurs, it would be interesting to ask those surveyed, Were you happy in your position before starting your business?

When asked, What is the best aspect of being self-employed? several respondents cited being their own boss, enjoying the freedom, and reaping the benefits of their hard work. Manthey replied, "Being able to stretch yourself as far as you can go without hitting a wall put up by someone else." Weber wrote, "I can be as creative as I want without needing to get everything I do approved by a board, boss, etc." Carroll-Johnson liked the flexibility to be able to take a few hours

---

CHARACTERISTICS OF SUCCESSFUL ENTREPRENEURS

- Have been fired from a job
- One or both parents were self-employed
- Had a business, e.g., babysitting, yard work, baking before the age of twenty
- Is the oldest child in the family
- Has a bachelor's or master's degree
- Wanted to start a business to work primarily for themselves
- Tends to fall in love too quickly with new ideas
- Very organized
- Extroverted
- Enjoys people

From: Mancuso, J. (1985). *The entrepreneur's quiz.* New York: Center for Entrepreneurial Management.

---

during the day to work at her child's school. Bolwell said that the best aspect of being self-employed was also the most difficult, that is, "having the ability to self-determine goals and approaches to achieving those goals." One of this chapter's authors (Carpenito) likes the freedom to choose her direction and focus but suffers from taking on too many projects. Spitzer-Lehmann enjoys assisting many organizations and the freedom from politics.

WHAT ARE THE CHALLENGES?

Most entrepreneurs will agree that those not self-employed usually view entrepreneurs as having all this freedom to decide if they want to work today and, if so, when and at what. Others have an impression that self-employed persons work fewer hours than their company-employed counterparts. Respondents to our survey reported working a range of 4 to 18 hours a day, with only one reporting 4 hours. Nine of the 15 reported usually working six days. Weekends were viewed as very productive because of fewer interruptions, e.g., telephone, staff.

When asked, How many vacation days did you have last year? one respondent said none and one reported one day. Of the 13 remaining, 7 took two weeks, 3 took four weeks, 1 took six weeks, and 1 vacationed two months. Milazzo wrote, "The real challenge is not to let your business pervade your personal life." Most entrepreneurs report difficulty turning off their creative thinking when they walk out of their office. Carpenito

found that an office in her home made her home no longer a place of respite.

In addition to days worked, entrepreneurs often do not count the time involved in traveling. For example, if a person travels for work for one week, travel time takes Sunday and Friday evenings; thus two of the three weekend evenings are gone.

Inherent in every business are the activities, personnel, equipment, and supplies necessary to accomplish the business goals. When employed by someone else, most nurses are primarily concerned with their work activities. They utilize personnel, supplies, and equipment but may not be aware of their cost. Several respondents said that they had anticipated big expenses for copiers, computers, and fax machines but were surprised at the "little things" required to set up an office, such as paper products, postage, phone calls, and office supplies. In addition, they were surprised about the cost of taxes, legal fees, professional services (printing, editing), unemployment compensation, health insurance, airfares, and marketing. What previously were called benefits, that is, sick time, vacation, health insurance, are now a business expense. No income is earned when you are on vacation.

The question What is the downside about being self-employed? evoked some interesting responses. One respondent described the impositions made on her time by phone calls or requests by friends and relatives for rides to appointments because "she is always available and not really working."

Fear of financial failure, an uneven income, and the uncertainty of one's income next year was cited by most respondents. One respondent said, "You can't pass the buck," while another reported the difficulty of letting go at the end of the day. Four respondents reported the "loneliness" of being self-employed, the isolation from colleagues, and the lack of office atmosphere.

The statement Describe one business experience which was a nightmare yielded descriptions of several situations that future entrepreneurs will probably experience. One respondent replied, "When faced with the first cancellation of a seminar, I immediately concluded my venture was a total failure, when in fact I had been canceled because the RNs went on strike." Another described consulting at a hospital that had just recently been unionized so that "When I showed up I was everybody's bait; nothing was going to change them. Everything I did was sabotaged." Another respondent wrote, "In the past when I have met with

WHY DO YOU WANT TO START YOUR OWN BUSINESS?

1. It seems like a good idea.
2. You want to try something new.
3. It's something you've had in mind for a long time.
4. You think you'll have more free time than now.
5. It's the thing to do.
6. You need a challenge.
7. It sounds like fun.
8. You're fed up with your present system.
9. You want to be independent.
10. You want to do things your way.

CFOs or CEOs and another person is present who is not a nurse, they automatically turn to the other person as if I couldn't possibly understand the 'business issues' because I am a nurse." One respondent reported that when she decided to start her business, her director of nursing wrote her a letter warning her that she would fail "as most nurses do."

STARTING YOUR OWN BUSINESS

In a review of the literature on risk taking as a crucial component of entrepreneurship, Herron and Herron concluded that although early management studies seemed to support that belief, more recent studies "hold that risk-taking propensity is not a distinguishing characteristic of entrepreneurs." Herron and Herron state that "the empirical management literature strongly suggests that need for achievement is crucial to the decision to become an entrepreneur."[4]

Nevertheless, there are many risks with which to be dealt. There are financial risks. (Can I derive sufficient income from the enterprise? Will I be able to sustain the services I provide? Will my practice be successful? grow?) And there are the psychological risks. (Do I see myself as an independent practitioner? Will I be able to work on an individual basis versus part of a team? Will I succeed? Can I do it?)

One of the best ways to find the answers to these questions is to do your homework. For example, ask yourself why you want to start your own business. The box above lists some questions that you need to answer honestly to yourself. Like any working position, being an entrepreneur has many rewards, but it also involves hard work and long hours; it can bring moments of great elation offset by despair. In short, it is not a panacea to all problems in other work areas. It does, however, provide an opportunity for creativity and an internal locus of control over one's work.

Once you are clear as to why you want to be an entrepreneur, you need to go through some other checklists (the box on page 48). The next step is to write a business plan. The actual writing of the plan is very important because it forces you to focus on your goals, objectives, and means of achieving them. Like any good plan or budget your business plan will be a guide. It is important that it be flexible to allow you to take advantage of unforseen opportunities, which always appear.

Many books and articles are readily available to help you write a business plan. At a minimum, the plan should include the purpose of your business, your specific goals and objectives, a definition of your products/services, a financial forecast of proposed expenditures and income for the first 6 months (in detail) and for the first 3 years (in less detail), and initial funding resources. It also needs to include your plans for initial funding resources.

A crucial part of any business plan is the marketing component. In our experience, this is the most difficult aspect for nurses. Going from the position of an employee—where the direct marketing is done by others—to an entrepreneurial status—where the individual must do the marketing—is difficult. This transition is a little like going to a non-English-speaking country without an interpreter and armed with only a few words of the new language.

A marketing plan is essential unless, of course, you are one of those fortunate few who have people sitting on their doorstep begging to buy their services. If so, lucky you. Otherwise, consider these questions:

- How will you tell your target market about your business?
- Why do you think people will buy what you are selling?
- Who and what are your competitors, and how will you differentiate yourself from them?
- What are the features of your services/products and what benefits will they provide?
- What will you charge?

Students often ask how a person comes up with new ideas. The question recalls to us a friend who was an art director in an ad agency. She always said, "The more creative you are, the more creative you become." That

---

PLANNING AND EVALUATING ECONOMIC OPPORTUNITY

What services/products will you provide?

Will they be the same as others now available?
- How will yours differ?
- What is your rationale for choosing them?
- Will you start with one service/product or several?
- What are your qualifications to provide these services or produce the product?
- Are your services something that people need? or want? or both?

Who is your target market?

Hospitals? Schools? Individuals? Organizations? Why should they buy from you?
- You're a nice person and you deserve a chance.
- You're just starting out and need a break.
- You have a sound product.
- You have a service not available elsewhere.

Who are your competitors and what are they selling? How will these services/products generate income for you?

---

is how you come up with new ideas. They emerge. You are automatically on alert to new ways of doing things, of looking for an unmet need. Then you check it out, ask questions, weigh the risks and opportunity, and make plans.

SUMMARY

For would-be entrepreneurs, Alfaro-LeFevre advises to "have a clear vision of what you want to do" and "to look at false starts as stepping stones to getting there rather than signs to give up." Several respondents (Abruzzese, Puetz, Manthey, Burgess, VanSlyck) advise neophyte entrepreneurs to have the financial resources to make it through the hard times of the first year or two. VanSlyck also advises to hire talented staff. Bur-

gess suggests that you know your product well, know how you are going to sell it, and expand slowly. Weber advises to set a plan with target dates and then to triple the time line on the dates.

Because entrepreneurs are responsible for their successes and failures, Gostel recommends that you learn as much as you can about yourself before starting your own business: What is your work style? What are your peak- and low-energy periods during the day? Plan activities according to energy levels; for example, answer mail during low-energy periods. Porter-O'Grady responded with, "Stick it out through the tough first two years," and "the client always comes first." And Milazzo poignantly advises to "go for your dream and be sure you can pursue something you are genuinely passionate about. Money should not be your motivation!" And finally, as expressed by Burgess, "It is mine. The autonomy, the accountability, the decisions, the relationships with clients are all up to me. So the good decisions as well as the poor ones are my responsibility. I am responsible for my successes. It constantly stretches my creativity."

REFERENCES

1. Aydelotte, M., Hardy, M., & Hope, K. (1988). *Nurses in private practice: Characteristics, organizational arrangements, and reimbursement policy.* Kansas City, Mo: American Nurses Foundation.
2. Directory of Consultants. (1992). *Journal of Nursing Administration, 22*(7/8), 74-136.
3. Drucker, P. F. (1985). *Innovation and entrepreneurship.* New York: Harper & Row.
4. Herron, D., & Herron, L. (1991). Entrepreneurial nursing as a conceptual basis for in-hospital nursing practice models. *Nursing Economic$, 9,* 310-316.
5. Keough, J. (1977). Guest editorial. *Journal of Continuing Education, 11*(3), 4.
6. Mancuso, J. (1985). *The entrepreneur's quiz.* New York: Center for Entrepreneurial Management.
7. Shoultz, J. Hatcher, P., & Hurrell, M. (1992). Growing edges of a new paradigm: The future of nursing in the health of the nation. *Nursing Outlook,* 40, 57-61.
8. *Webster's new collegiate dictionary.* (1977). Springfield, Mass: G&C Merriam.

CHAPTER 8

International nursing leaders

Who are they, what do they do, and what challenges do they face?

VERNA HUFFMAN SPLANE, RICHARD B. SPLANE

Nursing is undergoing rapid change throughout all countries in the world, yet the accelerating mobility of nurses and the expanding range of nursing endeavors worldwide will depend on a greater understanding of international aspects of health care. Albeit frequently unrecognized and unacknowledged by their peers nurses who exhibit leadership qualities and assume international leadership roles are a vital part of our past and present, and they must be a part of our future.

Our intent in this chapter is to focus on the international nursing leaders, past and present, who come within the scope of an international study we are undertaking, together with our direct observation of and linkages with some notable examples of international nursing leaders of today and of the recent past.[18] Our study started out to be an inquiry about present-day nursing leaders holding senior positions in national governments. It was dramatically and very productively enlarged when we discovered that to do justice to the subject, which we had begun to call the chief nursing officer (CNO) movement, we needed to probe its roots. The roots proved to be remarkably deep, implanted indeed in what Bullough, Bullough, and Stanton have called "the Nightingale Era, 1850 to 1910."[4] It was in that era that we discovered the first international nursing leaders worthy of close study and emulation. As we came to know who they were, we also discovered what they did and the challenges they faced. Because their lives are firmly framed in the past and because much research has been and is being done about them, we can hold them in an ideally stable and focused perspective with a view to eliciting such insights as they may offer on the present and the future.

FLORENCE NIGHTINGALE AND HER CHALLENGES

We begin at the point in 1854 when the telegraphed reports to the *London Times* on the scandalous treatment of the wounded and dying in the Crimea and in the Scutari barracks brought Florence Nightingale from genteel obscurity onto the world stage, where her Crimean and post-Crimean achievements would keep her throughout her lifetime.

Florence Nightingale's standing as an international nursing leader is unchallengeable, even if her self-imposed immobility kept her in one part of the world for half of her unceasingly creative career. Her influence during that part of her life was largely based on what she wrote, to whom she wrote, and to whom she granted audience. Nonetheless, the breadth of her contacts and networks was global. Many were within the British Empire, then at its zenith, and a goodly number centered on India, the jewel in the imperial crown, to which no viceroy departed London without consulting Miss Nightingale.[20] But her network spread beyond the Empire, reaching parts of the Orient, all of Europe, the Middle East, Australia, and the Americas, where she was greatly revered, sometimes to the point of idolatry. And, of some importance in the present context, was Florence Nightingale's practice of identifying leadership potential in young nurses and dispatching them, somewhat imperiously at times, to numerous locations where leadership was acutely needed.

To ask what challenges Florence Nightingale faced and what she did about them is to call for yet another two-volume biography. In the simplest terms, she was challenged by every contemporary obstacle to human health and well-being, and what she did was to attack them systematically and unrelentingly, believing that "never to know that you are beaten is the way to victory."[6] Poor nursing and nonexistent nursing were the obstacles to human well-being, and she was convinced she had a mission to confront these obstacles and overcome them. And from that conviction emerged the genesis of modern nursing. Nursing, however, was not her central interest, nor was a voluntary hospital, like St. Thomas', representative of the means she employed to promote her main objectives. Described as "nursing's most astute political operator,"[7] she focused rather on legislatures and the public service. More specifically, she channeled her energies and skills toward the British Parliament at Westminster and on those who would carry out the laws it enacted: the civil and military bureaucracy. It was thus mainly to public policy that she looked for the attainment of her broad range of social goals.

Early leaders in ICN

In addition to Florence Nightingale, the early international nursing leaders who are the initial focus of this review are those who created the International Council of Nurses (ICN). For the purposes of this chapter, six are selected as representatives of international nursing leadership in the era.

• **Ethel Bedford Fenwick** of Great Britain was the prime mover in the formation of the ICN and served as its first president. Her contributions to nursing both nationally and internationally stand in the annals of British nursing second only to those of Florence Nightingale. Her nursing commitments were to improved education and training, to its testing by examination under public auspices, and to state registration of those achieving the approved standards. Only by such means, she believed, could the welfare of the patient and of the general public be safeguarded and the level of nursing raised to a professional level.[3] Her devotion to the registration cause and to other means of advancing nursing, coupled with her lobbying and organizational skills, extended far beyond the Nightingale Era, but it was in the earlier period that she and her work for nursing were linked to her "active support of the whole feminist movement and the battle for women's suffrage."[3] In the words of Daisy Bridges, "she sought indefatigably to raise the status of women in general, and of nurses in particular." For her, "the nurse question is the woman question."[3]

• **Lavinia Lloyd Dock**, a renowned American nursing leader, became the first honorary secretary of ICN, holding the position from 1900 to 1923. It would be difficult to overstate the dimensions of her contributions to the Council and to the whole field of nursing. She drew from her own resources the means to cross the Atlantic repeatedly to conduct the business of ICN. It was mainly on ICN's behalf that she also maintained a voluminous correspondence with nursing organizations and individual nurses around the world. A byproduct of the direct and documentary data she thereby secured, however, became a major source for the monumental history that she set out to write with a no less distinguished and versatile colleague, Adelaide Nutting, who was concurrently principal of the Johns Hopkins School of Nurses and president of the American Federation of Nurses.

On the fly leaf of the 1907 edition of their history, Lavinia Dock gives an indication of the range of her networks through mentioning three or four of her working and honorary positions: secretary of the American Federation of Nurses; honorary member of both the Matrons' Council of Great Britain and Ireland, and of the German Nurses Association; a member of the Nurses' Settlement, New York.

The Nurses' Settlement was a component of the renowned Henry Street Settlement. There as "a feminist and a suffragist"[3] she was linked with the settlement's founder, Lillian Wald, and thereby with movements for peace, social and economic justice, and health as a basic human right. The communal endeavors headed by those two remarkable women and their associates can be viewed as a harbinger, in the Nightingale Era, of the primary health care movement of our time.[1]

• **Agnes Karll**, third president of ICN (1909 to 1912), was also the founding president of the German Nurses Association. She came on the international stage as hostess at two of the early Congresses (Berlin in 1904 and Cologne in 1912) and as a leader in advancing courageous positions taken against longstanding obstacles to the progress of nursing: the dominance of religious institutions and of physicians; the reluctant inclusion of male nurses; and the debasing working conditions to which the great body of nurses was subjected. Associated with her in welcoming the Congress participants were representatives of the German Woman Suffrage Association and the Association of Men Nurses of Berlin.[3] As a nurse who worked for causes that were destined to be under repeated attack in many countries as well as her own, Agnes Karll merits a revered place in the history of nursing.

• **Charlotte Gordon Norrie**, a Danish suffragist, played an important role in the founding meetings of the ICN and was also a founder of the Union of Danish Nurses. She is perhaps best remembered as the first in a succession of outstanding Danish nurses: Henny Tscherning, ICN's longest reigning president (1915 to 1922); Christianne Reimann, successor to Lavinia Dock as the second honorary secretary of ICN and later its first executive secretary; and Eli Magnussen, whose long life, beginning in the Nightingale Era and extending into the 1990s, has been distinguished by notable service with the ICN, the World Health Organization, and a range of nursing endeavors in her own country. In World War II, her courageous work in occupied Denmark led to imprisonment by Nazi invaders and very nearly made her a second Edith Cavell.

• **Mary Agnes Snively**, a Canadian member of ICN's Provisional Committee in 1900, became the Council's first treasurer and, with Lavinia Dock, the organizer of ICN's first Congress, held in Buffalo in 1901. She is also seen as a Canadian representative of the remarkable exchange across the international border with the United States, of women who became highly influential nursing leaders in one or other of the two countries. Among many examples of Canadians who as young women crossed the border to distinguished careers in the United States were Isobel Hampton (Robb), Adelaide Nutting, and Isobel Stewart. Eunice Dyke, a Canadian nurse who returned to Canada from Johns Hopkins to become an internationally recognized leader in public health nursing, was an early example of scores of international nurses who would receive part of their nursing education in the United States. Mary Agnes Snively was also an example of this phenomenon, having been appointed on her graduation from the Bellevue Hospital in New York to a lifetime of nursing leadership as Lady Superintendent of the Toronto General Hospital and first president of what became the Canadian Nurses Association.

• **Grace Neill** had the distinction of presenting the first paper at the historic Nursing Section of the meeting of the International Council of Women (ICW) in London in 1899. It was from that meeting that the International Council of Nurses emerged, modeling itself on the ICW and continuing to carry into its narrower focus a comparable commitment to women's issues, notably those relating to women's right to the franchise and to stand for election to office.

Grace Neill happened to be in London on this celebrated occasion on business from her position in New Zealand. Grace Neill, alone among the founders of ICN, "held the enviable position of an enfranchised woman!"[3] This Scottish-born nurse had received her nursing training in London and had been Lady Superintendent at a hospital in Manchester before emigrating first to Australia and then to the country with the world's most advanced social policy, New Zealand. That young British dominion had extended the franchise to women in 1893, and in 1895 had appointed a woman, Grace Neill, to a senior position in government. Her achievements in the position included improvements in all aspects of nursing education and practice, the establishment of maternity homes, and the winning of legislation for the registration of nurses in 1901 and for midwives in 1904. In our study,[18] we identify Grace Neill as the first chief nursing officer in a national ministry of health and an exemplary model for those who would, in many countries, receive comparable appointments during the next hundred years.

THE CHALLENGES FACING THE EARLY LEADERS

The foregoing review of a sampling of the international nursing leaders of the Nightingale Era has sought to identify two categories of challenges: those having to do with nursing as a calling or profession and those relating to nursing as a human service that functions within and assumes some responsibility for the sociopolitical communities (from parochial to global) of which it is a part.

A formidable array of challenges confronted nursing as a respectable calling and as an emerging profession. Not long before the arrival of Florence Nightingale, nursing had only begun to emerge from what Nutting and Dock vividly describe as the dark period of nursing when "the condition of the nursing art, the well being of the patient, and the status of the nurse all sank to an indescribable level of degradation."[15] Clearly the work of bringing nursing to recognized professional standards would prove to be an unending challenge.

The second group of challenges facing the international nurses of the Nightingale Era extended beyond nursing to women's issues to parliamentary democracy and, as exemplified by the nurses of the Henry Street Settlement, to issues of social justice and war and peace. Many of the challenges were feminist challenges that became blurred in the following decades before they were brought forward again in more recent times.

AN ANALYTICAL TRIAD

In moving our focus forward from the Nightingale Era through the intervening periods to the 1990s, we find it useful to have a tricolumn base for our analysis: the first of the three columns is a movement—the chief nursing officer movement; the second is the ICN. The third, unlike the first two, which had their beginnings in the Nightingale Era, is the new international institution or group of institutions that emerged at the end of World War II, namely the United Nations and its specialized agencies, notably the World Health Organization (WHO).

This triad is seen to consist of two institutions (the ICN and WHO) that are clearly international in nature, linked with a movement that appears to be confined to national frontiers. The case for the inclusion of the CNO movement in the triad is based on the assertion that nursing leadership is needed within national governments for the optimal development of broad and effective nursing initiatives internationally.

Chief Nursing Officers (CNOs) in National Ministries of Health: One column of the triad

Our study of the CNO movement revealed, as noted earlier, that its roots were to be found in the Nightingale Era. The movement made slow growth until World War II (1939 to 1945), but during the first quarter century following the war there was a remarkable confluence of favorable forces that brought about a golden age of CNO development. Foremost among the favorable influences was the WHO itself, expressed through the resolutions of its governing body, the World Health Assembly (WHA); the support of the first two Directors-General, Dr. Brock Chisholm of Canada and Dr. M.G. Candau of Brazil; the outstanding work of the nursing leaders in Geneva and the regions; and the body of nursing advisors and consultants serving in all parts of the world.

The CNO movement also received substantial support from Britain. The example of the strong CNO position in London from World War II and the influence of the Colonial Office and later the Commonwealth Office reinforced support for the CNO position by nursing and also by medical groups in virtually all of the Commonwealth countries.

Examples abound of international nursing leadership related to the CNO movement stretching from the Nightingale era to the present. A large measure of credit must be ascribed to the charitable foundations: the Rockefeller, Carnegie, and W. K. Kellogg Foundations; The League of Red Cross Societies; and the Florence Nightingale International Fund. Similarly, credit needs to be accorded to national governments and nongovernmental agencies for giving their senior nurses leave to carry international assignments and to be on national delegations to international meetings.

Examples of the latter date from the first meeting of the World Health Assembly, when the first woman and the first nurse to address the Assembly was Lucile Petry (Leone), the chief nursing officer and assistant surgeon general of the United States.[14] Numerous other CNOs since that time have been on their country's WHO delegations and have carried leadership roles on WHO's expert committees and technical discussions. The earliest examples are Tehmina Adranvala, India; Mary Lambie, New Zealand; Venny Snellman, Finland; Rosa Pinheiro, Brazil; and Docciah Kisseih, Ghana.[21] More recently the number of CNOs on national delegations has increased and the United Kingdom has the distinction of having its CNOs from 1949 to 1993 (Elizabeth Cockayne, Kathleen Raven, Phyllis Friend, Anne Poole and Yvonne Moores) as key figures on nearly all of its delegations.[16]

As many as half of the sovereign states of the world have, at various times, had CNOs serving as focal points for nursing in their national ministries of health. The growth has been uneven, and the positions have often been, and continue to be, vulnerable. The findings of our study[18] suggest, however, that a number of contemporary factors strengthen the case for the establishment and retention of the CNO position when it is filled by a well-qualified nurse capable of effective performance in respect both to domestic and international nursing issues.

The continuing role of the ICN: The second column of the triad

The importance of the ICN as the generator, rallying point, and vehicle for international nursing leadership was amply illustrated in the earlier era. The promise demonstrated then has been maintained for what is almost a century of remarkable performance in promoting the development of nursing as a profession and contributing to the health and well-being of the human family.

The growth of ICN from 8 national associations in membership with only a few hundred individual members in 1910, to 110 national member associations embracing some 1 million nurses in 1993 has been ac-

Table 8-1 Presidents of the International Council of Nurses

Name	Country	Year
Ethel Gordon Bedford Fenwick	United Kingdom	1900-1904
Susan McGahey	Australia	1904-1909
Agnes Karll	Germany	1909-1912
Annie Goodrich	United States	1912-1915
Henny Tscherning	Denmark	1915-1922
Sophie Mannerheim	Finland	1922-1925
Nina Gage	China	1925-1929
Leonie Chaptal	France	1929-1933
Alicia Lloyd Still	United Kingdom	1933-1937
Effie Taylor	United States	1937-1947
Gerda Hojer	Sweden	1947-1953
Marie Bihet	Belgium	1953-1957
Agnes Ohlson	United States	1957-1961
Alice Clamageran	France	1961-1965
Alice Girard	Canada	1965-1969
Margarethe Kruse	Denmark	1969-1973
Dorothy Cornelius	United States	1973-1977
Olive Anstey	Australia	1977-1981
E. Muringo Kiereini	Kenya	1981-1985
Nelly Garzon	Colombia	1985-1989
Mo-Im-Kim	Korea	1989-1993
Margretta Madsen Styles	United States	1993-1997

Source: Annual Reports, ICN.

Table 8-2 Executive Directors of the International Council of Nurses*

Name	Country	Year
Lavinia Dock	United States	1900-1922
Christianne Reimann	Denmark	1922-1934
Anna Schwarzenberg	Austria	1934-1947
Daisy Bridges	United Kingdom	1948-1961
Helen Nussbaum	Switzerland	1961-1967
Sheila Quinn	United Kingdom	1967-1970
Adele Herwitz	United States	1970-1976
Barbara Fawkes	United Kingdom	1977-1978
Winnifred Logan	United Kingdom	1979-1981
Constance Holleran	United States	1981-

Source: Annual Reports, ICN.
*The title has changed a number of times and has included executive secretary, general secretary, and executive director.

companied by a proportionate increase in nurses who have displayed leadership qualities expressed in significant aspects of international work.

The problem in any discussion of international nursing leadership is to decide the degree and quality of leadership that merits identification in a hypothetical Who's Who in Nursing Leadership. This is especially difficult in respect to the ICN, which has had 22 presidents (Table 8-1) and 10 executive directors (Table 8-2). However, their election or appointment offers sufficient evidence of the role they have played or are playing to ensure their standing as international leaders.

The position of executive director of ICN evolved from its volunteer and unpaid status at the beginning to its preeminence today. The council has been remarkably successful in recruiting executive directors capable of sustaining the international nursing leadership that has been the hallmark of ICN.

A complete compendium of international nursing leaders associated with the ICN would be far more extensive than those presented in Tables 8-1 and 8-2 and would include outstanding vice presidents, per-

sons who have contributed strongly in the Council of National Representatives (the body that sets overall policy for the organization and elects the board of directors), and chairpersons, as well as many members of major committees, notably the highly important Professional Services Committee.

ICN's leadership award. ICN has been keenly aware of the importance of honoring the profession's leaders in various ways, the most significant being through the rigorously selective granting of the Christianne Reimann Award. This highly prized award, which includes a substantial sum of money, serves to keep alive the memory of the lifetime contributions of Christianne Reimann, as well as the generous bequest left in her will. The award, looked upon as a type of Nobel Prize for nursing, was first received in 1985 by Virginia Henderson of the United States. It was a recognition of an American nurse internationally recognized as a lecturer, researcher, educator, and author of *Basic Principles of Nursing Care,* a book that has enjoyed unparalleled influence in nursing education, having been translated into some 26 languages.[8] In 1989 the award was presented to Dame Nita Barrow, whose various roles have included service as the CNO in Jamaica; leadership in the formation of various Caribbean nursing associations; senior roles in the secretariat of the World Council of Churches and as one of its presidents; president of the International Federation of Adult Education; world president of the Young Women's Christian Association; head of the forum at the Women's Year events in Nairobi in 1987; member of the Eminent Person's Group on a reconciliation mission to

South Africa in 1989; and, most recently, governor-general of her native Barbados. Dame Sheila Quinn of the United Kingdom received the award at the 20th Quadrennial Congress of the ICN in Madrid in June 1993. Dame Sheila has an outstanding record of service to international nursing, having served as a consultant to and the executive director and the first vice president of ICN; the president of the Standing Committee of Nurses of the European Community; and president of the Royal College of Nursing.

The World Health Organization and nursing leadership: The third column of the triad

Nursing in the World Health Organization (WHO) from 1948 to 1972 was comprised of a nursing unit headed by a chief nursing officer in the Geneva headquarters; regional nursing officers in the six regions with offices located in Alexandria, Brazzaville, Copenhagen, New Delhi, Manila, and Washington; and nursing advisors and consultants, seldom exceeding 200, throughout the system. During WHO's first quarter century, the contribution of this small complement of select nurses working in collaboration with other positive forces transformed the state of nursing worldwide.

This chapter can do little more in respect to the leadership of the CNOs in Geneva than identify them and give their countries of origin. In the period 1948 to 1972, they were: Olive Baggallay, the United Kingdom, 1948 to 1954; Lyle Creelman, Canada, who had first been appointed as a nursing consultant in 1949 and whose period as CNO, reaching from 1954 to 1968, extended her tenure in WHO to nearly 20 highly influential years; Lily Turnbull, Canada, 1968 to 1972, who, following the elimination of the CNO position, served from 1972 to 1975 in WHO's Health Manpower Division.[17]

Regional nursing officers and scores of advisors and consultants who worked with national counterparts on long- and short-term appointments were of crucial importance to the advancement of nursing, midwifery, nursing specializations, and auxiliary nursing. Although it must be both arbitrary and incomplete, some sampling is called for of international nurses, past and present, serving in WHO's six regions between 1950 and 1992.

- Region of the Americas: Agnes Chagas, United States and Brazil; Esther Lipton, United States; Margaret Cammaert, Canada; Maricel Manfredi, Colombia; Sandra Land, United States

- African Region: Louise Bell, United Kingdom; Dorothy Potts, Canada; Aena Konde, Zaire; Sybil Misse, Cameroon
- South East Asia Region: Doris Pederson, New Zealand; Dorothy Hall, Canada; Amelia Mangay Maglacas, Philippines; Saiyud Niyomviphat, Thailand; Sally Birch, United States
- Eastern Mediterranean Region: Eli Magnussen, Denmark; Inger Götshe, Denmark; Dorothy Potts, Canada; Enaam Abou Youssef, Egypt
- Western Pacific Region: Elizabeth Hill, United States; Lily Turnbull, Canada; Lourdeo Verderesi, Brazil; Theresa Miller, United States
- European Region: Fernanda Alves Diniz, Portugal; Maria Tito de Moreas, Portugal; Dorothy Hall, Canada; Marie Farrell, United States; Elisabeth Stussi, France; Jane Salvage, United Kingdom[19]

Some comment is required on the earlier reference to the elimination of the CNO position in the Geneva headquarters in 1972 and the transference of the nurses from the nursing unit to functional programs within the organization. This move, and comparable moves that weakened the nursing programs in the regions, was officially rationalized as a measure to merge separate professional programs within a framework of more comprehensive programs for the strengthening of health services.

Whatever the motive, the effect of the move was to weaken nursing not only within but beyond WHO. In a number of countries, persons in authority, who were averse to the advances nursing had made and the status it had attained, used the WHO example as grounds for eliminating the CNO position and downgrading nursing. It is not to be implied that WHO did not continue after 1972 to be an important, if weakened, force for the advancement of nursing. What may be stated is that although the World Health Assembly continued at various times to express its recognition of the importance of nursing and midwifery, this has not been adequately reflected in the actions of the secretariat.

The situation at the Geneva headquarters, which had been so adversely affected by the elimination of the CNO position in 1972, was ultimately improved during the tenure of Amelia Mangay Maglacas, a highly qualified nurse from the Philippines who was appointed scientist. In her 14 years in Geneva, from 1975 to 1989, she had the difficult task of restoring the nursing presence in the Geneva headquarters. By the mid-1980s her position had been renamed chief scientist for nursing and she, along with the nursing world, generally had the satisfaction of hearing nursing described by Dr. Halfdan Mahler, the director general of WHO, as "the most positive force in all of the health field for the implementation of the primary health care strategy."[22] Before she left her post in Geneva, she had initiated the establishment of a global network of WHO collaborating centers in nursing, a highly promising source of future international nursing leaders.

On her retirement as chief scientist for nursing, Amelia Maglacas left her successor, Miriam Hirschfeld of Israel, a significantly stronger status for nursing in WHO than she had found on her arrival. There continued, however, to be the challenging task of dealing with the full mandate of the position within a secretariat evincing only a limited perspective on the profession.

THE TRIAD AT WORK: TWO EXAMPLES

The three entities of the triad, WHO, ICN, and the CNO movement, evidence common international goals and the capacity for constructive collaborative endeavors. A notable example of such collaboration reached its dramatic climax at the 1992 meeting of the World Health Assembly. It was the latest episode in the 20-year campaign by the nursing profession to have nursing within WHO recover the status, resources, and mandate for worldwide service that it possessed from 1948 to 1972.

A WHA nursing resolution adopted in 1989 had called for measures that would strengthen nursing and midwifery through concrete action by nursing organizations, national governments, and, of crucial importance to the whole undertaking, by the director general of WHO (since 1987, Dr. Hiroshi Nakajima) and other senior members of the secretariat.[9]

A report of the director general that showed lack of progress on the 1989 resolution prompted Constance Holleran, executive director of ICN (which is in official relationship with WHO), to meet with the executive board of WHO and present a strong statement outlining the concern of ICN on the lack of action on the resolution.[10] This initiative caused the triad network to prepare a resolution for the WHA meeting in May 1992. Entitled "Strengthening Nursing and Midwifery in Support of Strategies for Health for All,"[13] it called for the establishment of a Global Nursing Advisory Committee. The resolution had the support of 50 countries, and its impending adoption seemed to represent the successful culmination of an important stage in the continuing campaign.

However, as debate on the resolution was concluding, a senior official of the secretariat stated that the proposals in the resolution would not be given WHO's financial and organizational support. It was at that point that Dame Anne Poole, the eminent chief nursing officer of the United Kingdom and a member of her country's delegation, made a dramatic intervention on the floor of the General Assembly that brought about a complete reversal of the secretariat's negative decision: an Advisory Committee was authorized by the director general and every cooperation promised for the implementation of its recommendations.[12]

A further instance of collaboration by members of the triad was the Commonwealth Meeting of Chief Nursing Officers and National Nurses Associations convened in Malta in September 1992 at the request of the Commonwealth Ministers of Health.[5] Organized by the Commonwealth Foundation, the meeting had representatives from 41 Commonwealth countries. Completing the representation of the triad, in what was seen as a meeting of historic importance, were Constance Holleran, ICN, and Miriam Herschfeld, WHO. A major goal of the meeting was to prepare for the consideration of the Commonwealth Ministers of Health meeting in October 1992 a document on the state of nursing in the Commonwealth and the steps to be taken for nursing to achieve its full potential in support of Health For All by the year 2000 and beyond. The document will undoubtedly elicit wider interest and attain broader influence.

These two instances illustrate how nursing leaders, governmental and nongovernmental, are able to collaborate to influence public policy. They indicate that nurses are progressively learning how governments operate and how they can be influenced if the appropriate strategies are employed, including the strategy of persistence, akin to Florence Nightingale's refusal to admit defeat. And, of key importance, these examples indicate the need for nurses and nursing organizations at every level to define their goals and to work together for their achievement.

The importance of public policy reflected in the work of the triad and evident in the work of the international nursing leaders in the Nightingale Era is resuming a high degree of priority in the work of many nursing organizations. It was prominent in the 19th Quadrennial Congress of the ICN in South Korea in

1989, especially in the addresses of Baroness Caroline Cox of the United Kingdom[9] and of Dame Nita Barrow of Barbados.[2] And, significantly, a major topic for discussion at the 20th ICN Congress in Madrid in 1993 is "Nurses in Ministries of Health: Influence, Power and Politics."[11]

BEYOND THE TRIAD: OTHER LEADERS, OTHER TASKS

The approach to international nursing leadership taken in this chapter has not ventured beyond the sociopolitical channels outlined at the outset. That the field of international nursing and the corps of international nursing leaders extends far more broadly is acknowledged. International nursing leaders come from national and subnational nursing associations, from universities, institutes, WHO collaborating centers, nursing associations organized along the lines of religious faith, and other types of professional groupings, including the Sigma Theta Tau International Honor Society of Nursing. Their work extends to international conferences, workshops, bilateral and multilateral undertakings, and specialist nursing groups. They are to the fore, as well, in other undertakings that clearly involve public policy: the unending and vital question of the regulation of nurses and the complex issues of defining and monitoring nursing standards to deal with the increasing cross border mobility of nurses.

A closing comment: It is encouraging to know that international nursing leadership has flourished to the point that a single chapter can only touch on one of its numerous aspects.

REFERENCES

1. Anderson, E. T. (1991). Editorial: A call for transformation. *Public Health Nursing, 8,* 1-2.
2. Barrow, N. R. (1989). Nursing, a new tomorrow [Keynote address]. In *Nineteenth Quadrennial Congress of the ICN, Seoul, South Korea, 1989.* Geneva: International Council of Nurses.
3. Bridges, D. (1967). *A history of the International Council of Nurses 1899-1964: The first sixty-five years.* Philadelphia and Toronto: J. B. Lippincott.
4. Bullough, V., Bullough, B., & Stanton, M. (Eds.). (1990). *Florence Nightingale and her era: A collection of new scholarship.* New York: Garland.
5. Commonwealth Foundation. (1992, September 7-10). *Meeting of commonwealth chief nursing officers and professional associations: Challenges and opportunities.* Malta: Author.
6. Cook, E. (1913). *The life of Florence Nightingale.* (Vols. I & II). London: Macmillan.
7. Cox, C. (1989). *Forging nursing's future: A sociopolitical perspective.* An address presented at the Nineteenth Quadrennial Congress of the ICN, Seoul, South Korea. Geneva: International Council of Nurses.
8. Henderson, V. (1961). *Basic principles of nursing care.* London: International Council of Nurses.
9. International Council of Nurses. (1989). 1989 WHA resolution 42:27, Strengthening of the role of nursing and midwifery personnel in support of the strategy for health for all. *International Nursing Review, 36,* 4.
10. International Council of Nurses. (1992). ICN statement to the WHO executive board, 22 January, 1992. *International Nursing Review, 39,* 2.
11. International Council of Nurses. (1992). ICN's 20th Quadrennial Congress "U for Q," Madrid, Spain, 20-25 June, 1993. *Preliminary program.* Geneva: Author.
12. International Council of Nurses. (1992). Nursing demonstrates cohesion at World Health Assembly. *International Nursing Review,* 4.
13. International Council of Nurses. (1992). Resolution WHA 45.5, Forty-fifth World Health Assembly, 4-15 May, 1992. Strengthening nursing and midwifery in support of strategies for health for all. *International Nursing Review, 39,* 4.
14. Leone, L. P. (1987). An interview with Dr. Lucile Petry Leone by R. B. and V. Splane. San Francisco.
15. Nutting, A., & Dock, L. (1907). *A history of nursing: The evolution of nursing from the earliest times to the foundation of the first English and American training schools for nurses.* New York & London: G. B. Putnam's Sons.
16. Splane, R. B., & Splane V. H. (1985). Taped interviews with Dame Elizabeth Cockayne, Cobham, 1985; Dame Kathleen Raven, London, 1985; Dame Phyllis Friend, London, 1985; Dame Anne Poole, London; Yvonne Moores, London, 1986.
17. Splane, R. B., & Splane V. H. (1986). Interview with Lily Turnbull, CNO, WHO, 1968-72. Saskatoon, Canada.
18. Splane, R. B., Splane V. (1993). *Chief nursing officers in national ministries of health: Focal points for nursing leadership.* San Francisco: University of California, San Francisco.
19. Splane, R. B., & Splane V. H. (1992). Telephone interviews with Dr. Lyle Creelman, Vancouver; Dr. Miriam Hirschfeldt, Geneva; Ms. Maricel Manfredi, Washington, D.C. (Present and former Chief Nursing Officers in WHO).
20. Strachey, L. (1935). *Eminent Victorians.* New York & London: Harcourt Brace Jovanovich.
21. World Health Organization. (1950). Expert committee on nursing: Report on the first session. 20-26 February, 1950. *Technical Report Series,* No. 24. Geneva: Author.
22. World Health Organization. (1985, January 14). Geneva: Author.

PART TWO

NURSING KNOWLEDGE

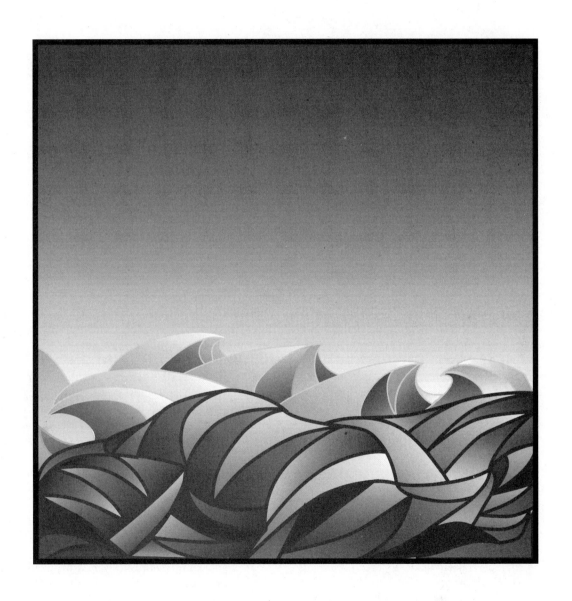

The connecting link

JOANNE COMI McCLOSKEY, HELEN KENNEDY GRACE

The connectedness of nursing has been a concern over the years. At some points, the practice of nursing appeared to be almost totally divorced from nursing research. Nursing education, which draws upon research for its body of knowledge, sometimes bridged the gap between research and practice, but, all too frequently, nursing education drew its content primarily from the theoreticians and researchers while students had to practice in a world far removed from what they were learning in the classroom. Once out of nursing educational programs, nurses tend to leave research/theoretical models behind them as they coped with the "real world" of practice. This section shows dramatic evidence of the progress being made in bridging the worlds of nursing research and practice from a number of perspectives.

In the debate (Chapter 9), Weiler, Buckwalter, and Titler pose the question "Is nursing research used in practice?" Noting that it was only in the 1980s that the majority of nursing research had applicability to nursing practice rather than to other themes such as educational research, the authors argue that considerable progress is being made and that the profession is committed to research-based practice. Support for this thesis is drawn from the following observations:

1. Professional organizations' recognition of the importance of research in their mission statements and in sponsorship of conferences to report research
2. Increased emphasis on approaches to getting nursing research integrated and used in practice
3. Advances that have been made in preparation of nurses to use research
4. Efforts to reduce barriers to research dissemination, such as continuing education programs and nursing journals that inform practicing nurses about recent advances in nursing knowledge

Despite the evidence of these advances, the authors note that there is considerable progress yet to be made. Large numbers of practicing nurses have had minimal preparation in nursing research as part of their basic education. Nurses rarely have had experience in participating in research studies as part of their preparation and thus have little understanding of the process and the potential value to their practice. Researchers contribute to the problem by the way in which they sometimes report their findings. Use of jargon, unclear research reports, lag time in publication, and lack of replication studies are factors that contribute to the problem. Another factor is the lack of support for integration of nursing research into practice within the organizational frameworks in which nurses work. Considerable work is being done to change the organizational environments to legitimize nursing research as an integral part of nursing practice.

Addressing the continuity between theory and practice, in Chapter 10 Firlit reviews the progression in development of theoretical constructs in the field and supports the view that the essence of nursing is "caring in the human experience." With this as the anchoring point, it is then argued that practice is the base for the development and its validation of nursing theory. Nursing administrators are challenged to create an environment of theory-based nursing practice.

In Chapter 11 Brencick and Webster continue the discussion of the primacy of practice in nursing. In this chapter they first clarify the differences between a theoretical science and its preoccupation with knowing what is and a practice profession with its concern for changing what is. They assert that these are two separate goals that should not be confused: The practicing professional uses knowledge from the sciences to effect change, but the goal of practice is not the advancement of science. They contend that the controversy over whether there is a "science of nursing" can be resolved by understanding the relationships between science and nursing. Science emphasizes the attempt to gain knowledge of the general or repeatable, while nursing practice is concerned with the individual. Practice draws upon knowledge of the general, but its major focus is upon changing the condition or status of the patient, not with simply knowing what is. The authors suggest that nurses might argue that nursing is a science on political grounds, noting that to be a science carries with it a certain amount of prestige in our society. However, they conclude the core of the profession of nursing is clinical practice.

The connection between theory and research is addressed next, in Chapter 12, by Blegen and Tripp-Reimer. They show that nursing theory and nursing research have developed separately. Theoretical developments in nursing have served to differentiate the discipline from medicine and to provide curriculum models to distinguish nursing education from medical education. The authors show that, for a long time, research in nursing was not concerned with developing a body of nursing knowledge. The authors say, however, that the focus of nursing on the metatheory level has not been useful for advancing nursing science. Midlevel theory is needed to articulate with nursing research. The establishment of nursing doctoral programs should facilitate the connectedness of nursing theory and research. The advancement of nursing science, argue the authors, depends on an interplay between theory and research. Our studies need both.

Chapter 13 turns to the organization of nursing knowledge, where Loomis likens nursing research to the exploration of "the other side of silence"—the patient side. Retracing the historical development of nursing knowledge, Loomis notes the steady progression toward clinical research. Recent conferences and large-scale research projects have focused upon classification systems for nursing practice. Concluding this extensive review, the author proposes a new classificatory system based on a definition of nursing that acknowledges two distinct realms, illness and health, and that defines nursing as the science of health and healing. With this as a framework a new model for the development of nursing science is proposed. Nursing science is divided into two categories, the study of clinical nursing therapeutics and the study of the social issues in relation to nursing. Relationships between human responses and nursing interventions are viewed as especially important.

The next four chapters (Chapters 14 through 17) focus on the burgeoning field of nursing classificatory systems. Kelleher provides a comprehensive overview of the approaches used in developing classificatory systems. Early techniques were focused upon patient classification as a means of projecting nursing staffing, with staffing levels adjusted to the level of the illness. With the advent of diagnostic-related groups this focus was changed to length-of-stay variables. Improvements in patient classificatory systems could be made by use of predictive models based on stay, by capturing characteristics unique to stages of illness that correlate with nursing demand, and by use of a standardized set of patient characteristics that correlate with nursing work.

The Nursing Minimum Data Set (NMDS) is one of these systems. The NMDS is a standardized approach that facilitates the abstraction of essential core, minimum data to describe nursing practice intended for use in any and all settings where nursing care is provided. In Chapter 15, Werley et al. detail the background in the development of the NMDS; summarize its purposes; outline the benefits to nursing education, practice and administration; advocate the NMDS as a source of information for shaping health policy; and summarize the issues related to full implementation and use of the NMDS. While the NMDS system has been developed, the difficulty in obtaining funding for putting the system into full-scale implementation impedes realizing its full potential. The authors encourage broadscale use of the NMDS and involvement and commitment of nursing toward use of the minimum data set to describe nursing as a means of developing a database for practice-related nursing research.

A complimentary approach to developing a standardized language for describing nursing is that of those involved in development of the nursing diagnosis taxonomy. Tracing the development of the North American Nursing Diagnosis Association's (NANDA) classification system from the 1970s, Warren describes the inherent difficulties in Chapter 16. Lack of a single framework for classifying the phenomena in nursing, validation of the taxonomy, and integration of use of the taxonomies into the nursing field are some of the challenges. The purposes for constructing a taxonomy are to:

1. Describe the structure and relationships of objects between each other
2. Generate hypotheses that describe the relationships between objects

3. Achieve an economy of memory and to facilitate communication
4. Ease the manipulation of observations

In Chapter 17, noting that the work of nurses is little understood and that the impact of nursing care is virtually invisible, Bulechek and McCloskey describe the work being done in compiling the Nursing Interventions Classification (NIC). Following extensive review of the literature and an expert ranking process, 336 nursing interventions were identified and, through use of a hierarchical clustering technique, 26 groups of interventions and 6 supergroups, called domains, have been identified. NIC complements the work that has been done in nursing diagnosis in contributing to the creation of an universal language for nursing.

Nursing-focused patient outcomes for evaluation of health care effectiveness is advanced by Johnson as the challenge for the 1990s. Concerns over cost, quality, and distribution of resources are contributing to this focus. Research is essential to making the relationships between costs and benefits of approaches to care. Outcomes of patient care are increasingly being correlated with structure and process of the care provided. This focus on outcome measures poses a number of conceptual issues that need to be clarified. These include:

1. Definitional issues regarding the desired outcomes
2. The object of an intervention—a single patient, a family, or a community
3. The desired patient state and whose definition should apply
4. Timing of the outcome measurement

The challenge for nursing is to take the prior work that has been done and focus upon the development of nursing-sensitive outcome measures. This will require considerable work in addressing the interface between the various classificatory systems described in the four articles addressing this issue.

Concluding this section is the importance of an international classificatory system for nursing addressed by Clark. Hampton-Robb recognized the importance of a universal nursing language as early as 1909. Eighty years later, in the 1989 Council of National Representatives to the International Council of Nurses, the necessity for an International Classification for Nursing Practice was recognized by a resolution proposing this development. In Chapter 18 Clark addresses some of the complexities of developing a universal language for nursing and notes that arguments for the development of a classificatory system as a means of creating a nursing science have not resulted in much progress. However, she predicts that concerns for the cost of health care and computerization will move the field forward. Building on beginning efforts around the world, the International Classification for Nursing Practice is embarking upon this enormous task.

Ironically, the linkage of nursing research to practice is increasingly being driven by political and economic forces, in contrast to the earlier concerns for development of a "nursing science." From this perspective it is important to revisit the Brencick and Webster chapter, which makes the distinction between a science and a profession. The classificatory systems that are developing, while driven by economic and political forces and propelled by the informatics revolution, are creating a new momentum for nursing research. The practice of nursing is rapidly becoming the driving force for nursing research. This change represents a dramatic shift over the past decade and holds forth a bright promise for the future.

CHAPTER 9

Debate

Is nursing research used in practice?

KAY WEILER, KATHLEEN COEN BUCKWALTER, MARITA G. TITLER

The conduct, utilization, and dissemination of research is an ongoing concern to the nursing profession, and the development of a scientific base for practice is regarded as essential for quality patient care.[86] As noted in a previous edition of this chapter,[120] numerous position papers and editorials have been written extolling the virtues of research to practice, and many nursing organizations and accrediting bodies have outlined the importance of research in practice. However, major areas of concern remain. For example, is nursing research sufficiently encouraged and professionally supported? Is nursing research accessible, usable, and relevant? Are research-based interventions, policies, and procedures improving patient care?

Early in the history of the profession, Nightingale combined dedicated patient care with vigorous research. Regrettably, Nightingale's groundwork of documentation, classification, and verification was not sustained. Rather, nurses focused on other ways of learning, such as tradition, reference to authority, experience, trial and error, and on nursing education and the delivery of services, while other professions addressed clinical questions now considered appropriate for nursing inquiry.[19] Although the journal *Nursing Research* was established in 1952 to provide nurses with new knowledge based on research and to inform them about ongoing research,[31] it took nearly 25 years before the journal could claim that the majority of its articles were applicable to clinical practice.[8,20]

More recently, the profession has once again embraced Nightingale's ideals as evidenced by the establishment and increasing stature of the National Institute of Nursing Research; the commitment of the American Nurses Association (ANA) to standards for organized nursing services and standards of clinical nursing practice that support the use of research findings in practice; and the development (by an interdisciplinary panel of health care professionals and a consumer representative, with strong nursing input and leadership) and dissemination of the Agency for Health Care Policy and Research's (AHCPR) Clinical Practice Guidelines. Moreover, the development of several research utilization models have advanced the use of nursing research in practice. Among them are the Conduct and Utilization of Research in Nursing [CURN] project; the Western Interstate Commission for Higher Education [WICHE]; the Nursing Child Assessment Satellite Training [NCAST] project; the Stetler-Marram model; the Dracup-Breu model; the Quality Assurance Model Using Research [QAMUR] model; the Goode model; the Horn model; and the international vision of Sigma Theta Tau and publication of their *Actions for the 1990s.*

An increasing number of clinical specialty organizations (e.g., Association of Critical Care Nurses, the National Association of Pediatric Nurse Associates and Practitioners, and the National Association of Transplant Coordinators) now offer grants to support the conduct and utilization of research. Also, private foundations such as Robert Wood Johnson and the Pew Memorial Trust provide grant monies to practice agencies and academic centers for research related to redesigning the delivery of nursing care. In addition, the Joint Commission for Accreditation of Healthcare Organizations (JCAHO) requires that policies, procedures, standards of patient care, and standards of nursing practice be developed from current scientific knowledge.[64]

These developments testify to the profession's renewed commitment to research-based practice and

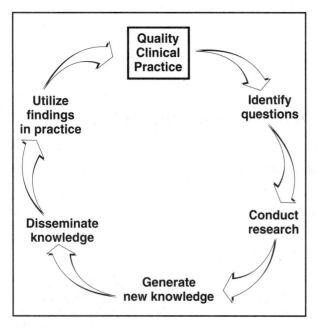

Fig. 9-1 Research process.

provide tangible evidence that integrating nursing research into the practice setting is valued by specialty groups, professional organizations, and funding agencies. However, this effort, although a step in the right direction, does not enable us to state unequivocally that we have significantly advanced the profession's utilization and dissemination of validated research findings.

CHAPTER OVERVIEW AND DEFINITIONS

The purpose of this chapter is to update the debate about whether nursing research is used in practice or not. It examines issues related to the utilization and dissemination of knowledge generated by nursing research and addresses the question, Are research findings influencing the nature and quality of patient care? As dictated by the debate format, we reflect on this issue and present arguments both for and against the question.

Utilization and dissemination are closely related and integrated aspects of the research process (see Fig. 9-1). For purposes of this chapter, *utilization* is defined as "the actual, systematic implementation of a scientifically sound, research-based innovation in a health care setting with an accompanying process to assess the outcome(s) of the clinical change."[97] As a process, it

consists of first critically analyzing the literature, then selecting and implementing appropriate interventions, and finally evaluating the outcome.[57] We use the term *dissemination* to refer to "any systematic effort that is directed towards making the essentials of reported research available to nurses in clinical practice in a style that facilitates consideration of practice. Dissemination efforts may take various forms such as publications, conferences, consultation, or inservice education programs,"[97] as well as topic-focused journal clubs.

We contend that although the profession has made significant strides in recent years, the issues surrounding utilization and dissemination of research in nursing practice are still unresolved and lend themselves to further discussion. Therefore, we will highlight barriers to and strategies for integrating nursing research in the practice setting.

As we revised this chapter, we have considered related issues set forth by Horsley[58] and invite the reader to do the same: "Who is responsible for the complex set of activities involved in using research practice? The individual nurse, the organization, or both? What factors influence the use of research in practice? What constitutes successful utilization of research in practice? Does nursing research make a difference in practice, and if so, what difference does it make?"

ARGUMENTS THAT SUPPORT THAT RESEARCH IS BEING USED IN PRACTICE

The four factors that have most contributed to the use of nursing research in practice are: (1) changes in the conceptualization of nursing and the value of research; (2) development and testing of models for utilization of nursing research; (3) advances in the preparation of nurses to use research; and (4) minimizing barriers to research dissemination and use.

Changes in the conceptualization of nursing and the value of research

Changes in the conceptualization of nursing and the importance of research to nursing practice have occurred primarily in the areas of professional direction, support, and nurturance, as highlighted below in examples from selected professional and federal organizations.

American Nurses Association (ANA). The ANA's professional commitment to nursing research has remained constant over the past three decades. However, the suggested application of research directives to patient care, nursing interventions, and general public health care policy has changed with an expanded vision of the application of nursing research. In 1962, the ANA "Blueprint for Research in Nursing"[6] suggested six major areas of nursing research. Notably, the document stressed the importance of comparing cost assessment for nursing interventions but did not emphasize clinical research.[121]

By 1985, the ANA *Directions for Nursing Research: Toward the Twenty-first Century* identified research goals, stated strategies for goal attainment, and minimum criteria to be achieved in the 1990s. In 1988, the ANA *Standards for Organized Nursing Services* emphasized the importance of research utilization based on the rationale that "the continuing advancement of nursing practice and administration depends on the ongoing availability and utilization of a valid and current knowledge base."[4] Standard VIII states, "Within organized nursing services, research in nursing, health, and nursing systems are facilitated; research findings are disseminated; and support is provided for integration of these findings into the delivery of nursing care and administration." Most recently, in the 1991 *Standards of Clinical Nursing Practice,* the standards of professional performance (Standard VII Research) state, "The nurse uses research findings in practice."[5] Measurement criteria relate to nurses' use of research-based interventions and participation in research activities appropriate to their educational level, position, and practice setting. Thus, the ANA has set forth both goals and strategies related to developing a scientific base for practice, which includes facilitating the establishment of the profession's research agenda, supporting research to describe and/or measure the quality and cost effectiveness of nursing interventions, and demonstrating quality outcomes of various organizational models and financial arrangements for nursing services.[12]

Sigma Theta Tau. As the professional honorary society, Sigma Theta Tau has taken a leadership role in supporting the development, dissemination, and utilization of nursing knowledge as set forth in the opening paragraph of the society's mission statement. Two of the four major goals of the organization are relevant to this discussion and include: knowledge dissemination and knowledge utilization along with knowledge development and resource development. Goals for the 1991 to 1993 biennium include, "Clinical databases will be developed so that the dissemination of scientific information will assist in bridging the gap between nursing research and nursing prac-

tice."[117] Similar objectives and activities are noted as essential components of the Research Committee's Action Plan for 1989 to 1991.[107]

To facilitate this goal, the society sponsors regional research utilization conferences that explore methods of promoting both research development and utilization in diverse settings and enhance discussion among nursing administrators, educators, and clinicians. Sigma Theta Tau also gives regional awards for utilization of research that honor an individual or group who has influenced research-based nursing practice through an innovation or through the provision of leadership towards a research-based innovation.[44] Further, they invite the submission of abstracts specific to nursing research for the International State of the Science Congress, which also serves as a forum for discussion of research conduct, utilization, and strategies to facilitate use of research findings in practice settings.

Agency for Health Care Policy and Research (AHCPR). Nurses are working collaboratively with physicians and consumers to establish clinical practice guidelines. The recently established AHCPR, formerly the National Center for Health Services Research and Health Care Technology Assessment (NCHSR), has a mission "to enhance the quality of patient care services through improved knowledge that can be used in meeting society's health care needs."[1] The AHCPR awards grants, available for nurses, for conferences and workshops that foster the exchange of information on innovations in health care delivery and technology and developing and improving methods of disseminating findings and information resulting from health services research activities of AHCPR. The agency also supports efforts to disseminate and adopt practice guidelines and clinical research findings, and health services research data-related products.

American Association of Critical-Care Nurses (AACN). The AACN exemplifies the commitment of specialty organizations to research in practice as reflected in their outcome standards and the priorities the organization has set for research, which include both contextual and patient-centered areas of research.[2,76] The recent completion of the national multicentered study known as the Thunder Project resulted in staff being involved in research conduction and seeing the effects of their efforts in answering an important clinical research question. The purpose of the research was to evaluate the effect of heparinized and nonheparinized flush solutions on the patency of arterial lines.

AACN is also committed to research utilization. It has appointed a research utilization task force to assist staff nurses' incorporation of research findings in practice and to investigate mechanisms for dissemination of research utilization information.

Demonstration of economic value of research

Nursing interventions, protocols, and outcomes are increasingly based on systematic data collection and analysis. Justification of nursing actions has been fostered by demands from both consumer and quality assurance sectors. Despite insufficient financial support (5 cents for every $1,000 of gross hospital revenues), nursing research is making significant contributions to the health care system and the economic value of using nursing research can be demonstrated.[27,34,35,51,52,87,90,94,106] By formulating cost and quality indicators to measure nursing research utilization, nurse executives and clinical researchers can and have demonstrated that research-based practice saves health care dollars.[46,47,115]

Models for utilization of nursing research

At present there are numerous approaches to the utilization process based on different theories of knowledge. Examples of these models of research utilization include the CURN project, WICHE, the NCAST project, the Stetler-Marram model, the Dracup-Breu model, the QAMUR model, the Goode model, and the Horn model. These models have been developed to facilitate the use of scientific nursing knowledge in clinical practice settings.[29,46,57,59,67,74,109,119] All of these projects have emphasized utilizing and disseminating research findings for the practicing nurse.

Early utilization models. The Regional Program for Nursing Research Development was an early demonstration project designed to develop models to overcome barriers to research utilization.[74] Another utilization program (NCAST) was actually a series of three training projects carried out over 10 years.[67] One of the best-known early models was the CURN project. The primary objective of this project was to develop and test a model to facilitate the use of scientific nursing knowledge in clinical practice settings.[59]

Stetler and Marram[109] developed a three-phase model for evaluation of research findings for application in clinical settings that provides another useful framework. Theory stages in this model included: (1) validation—critical examination of research to de-

termine strengths and weaknesses; (2) comparative evaluation—assessing the desirability and feasibility of research for a particular setting; and (3) decision making—defining the most appropriate type of application of the research finding. Hefferin, Horsley, and Ventura[53] propose the addition of a fourth phase to this model. This step entails evaluation of the proposed practice change using pretest and posttest strategies. A significant feature of their recommendation is relating "both the degree and direction of this effect to the appropriate theoretical basis for the change."[53]

The Dracup-Breu model uses a six-step methodology to devise solutions to specific clinical practice problems. These steps include: identification of the problem, review and critique of appropriate research literature, establishing objectives, analyzing the setting and devising a plan, implementation of the plan, and evaluation of outcomes.[29]

More recent utilization models. The QAMUR model is based on the CURN model but combines quality assurance and research utilization as well as the conduct of research. Another aspect of this model is the inclusion of publication of research findings that enhances the scientific knowledge base for practice.[119]

An excellent example of personal interest and commitment to research-based practice is reported by Goode, Lovett, Hayes, and Butcher.[46] The Goode model is derived from systems theory, incorporating interaction between the system and the environment. Elements of the model include input, throughput, output, and feedback/evaluation (Fig. 9-2). Goode and her colleagues reported three nursing protocols developed from identified patient care needs based upon professional research implemented to meet the needs of their specific patient population and evaluated to determine whether they were achieving the desired results or not. This report demonstrates the potential patient benefits and personal rewards that nurses involved in research utilization may experience, such as mutual beliefs in the need for research utilization, a recognition that the research process is framing quality patient care, and increased personal and professional self-concept in the ability to critique and utilize the research process.

The final model to be discussed is somewhat different in that it is an organizational model for research utilization. The Horn model[57] uses a building block process that emphasizes interaction between the components of organizational commitment, change agents, planned change process, and outcomes of research-based practice (See Fig. 9-3).

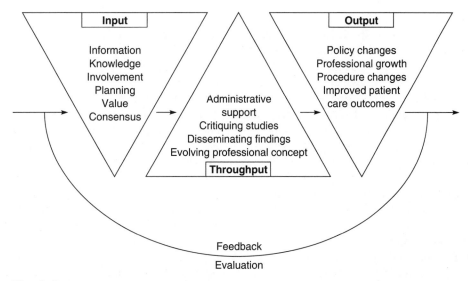

Fig. 9-2 The Goode Model. A systems theory model for using new research-based knowledge. *(From: Goode, C.J., Lovett, M.K., Hayes, J.E., & Butcher, L.A. [1987]. Use of research-based knowledge in clinical practice.* Journal of Nursing Administration, 17, *p. 11. Used with permission.)*

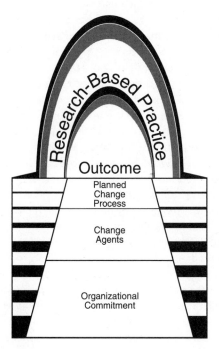

Fig. 9-3 The Horn Model. *(From: Horn Video Productions. [1989]. Research utilization: A process of organizational change. Ida Grove, Iowa. Used with permission.)*

Advances in the preparation of nurses to use research

The National League for Nursing[91] endorsed the position that the preparation of nurses to conduct research generally belongs at the doctoral level. There are currently 54 nursing education programs that offer a doctoral program in nursing, up from 45 programs in 1987.[92] An important emphasis of these programs is the development of a strong cadre of nurse scientists.[62] Further, some doctoral programs (e.g., The University of Iowa College of Nursing[113]) now require research residencies, during which a doctoral student may serve, for example, as an "apprentice" to an established nurse researcher based in a clinical setting whose responsibility for research encompasses both clinical and administrative areas. This residency provides first-hand experience on how the role of the clinical nurse researcher is operationalized and what strategies can be used to implement research-based changes in practice. Time management in the role and the importance of creating a positive research climate can be realized.

The majority of baccalaureate nursing programs now include content related to nursing research in their curricula.[30,114] There is increasing educational emphasis on the skills of reading research reports critically and critiquing the results. Teaching methods and tools have been developed to better assist students in evaluating research and applying research findings, including innovative computer-assisted instructional programs.[56] Nursing students are also being taught to use research findings as a basis for interventions. Similarly, more master's-level research courses are incorporating content related to the utilization of nursing research. This is an important development in that master's-prepared clinical nursing specialists are in a key position to initiate and support changes in practice based on research.[22] In keeping with curricular shifts toward the understanding and use of research, an increasing number of research citations are found in nursing texts.

Jacox[62] has identified additional factors indicating that nurses are becoming increasingly competent to design, conduct, and use nursing research. These factors include an increase in the expected role of nursing faculty members to conduct and publish research findings; the number of nurse researchers in clinical agencies; the number of nurses belonging to the ANA Council of Nurse Researchers; the level of federal funding for nursing research and training; the number of research proposals submitted to the Division of Nursing and the National Center for Nursing Research; and the proportion of current nursing research which is related to clinical practice.

Minimizing barriers to research dissemination and use

Major strides have been made in recent years to minimize barriers to the use of research in nursing practice. Haller, Reynolds, and Horsley's[50] criteria to determine whether research is ready for use in practice include: (1) the need for replication to provide greater confidence in the reliability and validity of findings, which usually means more than one study in a research base; (2) examination of each study's scientific merit, especially validity, reliability, generalizability, and statistical significance; (3) determination of any potential risks to patients.

Once these criteria have been met, the next hurdle to overcome is the transmission of the information to nurses who need it and can use it in their daily practice. This is not an easy hurdle, but it has been aided by more continuing education programs related to research utilization and increased avenues for the publication and dissemination of nursing research to practitioners.

Continuing education programs are an effective means to inform nurses about models of research utilization and provide an opportunity for the identification of potential areas of application of research findings. One popular format for these projects has been a long-term (i.e., 2 to 3 year) continuing education model, featuring several 2- to 3-day conferences held within a discrete geographic region. These projects offer a combination of formal presentations related to theories, models and methods of research utilization, and expert consultation/guidance for participants, who are expected to apply the knowledge and skills acquired through the conduct of a research utilization project in their home settings. Eligible participants include those nurses with master's or doctoral degrees in a position to implement research-based change in practice and management, to integrate research-based knowledge in curricula, and to teach research utilization content.[24,43]

Another mechanism for disseminating research findings for practice is the professional literature. The "central function of journals is to provide current information related to practice, trends, and issues affecting a discipline."[118] The breadth and diversity of nursing make dissemination of research difficult. However, the increased number of specialty journals presenting research reports,[111,112] the publication of research-based articles in the nonrefereed journals traditionally subscribed to by clinicians,[85] the development of a computerized nursing index for research,[121] and, most recently the Virginia Henderson International Library at Sigma Theta Tau International headquarters should make targeting and retrieval of research much easier.

Innovative publications that assist in the dissemination of research information to practitioners are appearing. The *Annual Review of Nursing Research* is approaching its 10th year and dramatically demonstrates the scope and amount of nursing research. Until 1990, *The Research Review: Studies for Nursing Practice* provided abstracts of research reports, scientific updates, and new and noteworthy research projects. A similar publication, *Nursing Scan in Research: Applications for Clinical Practice,* currently serves this function.

In 1988, *Applied Nursing Research (ANR)*,[39] a journal devoted to the advancement of nursing as a research-based profession, appeared. *ANR* focuses on the clinical implications of nursing research and integrates scientifically documented information in a readable manner for nurses in a variety of settings—practice, education, research, and management. Rather than emphasizing methodological or analytical strategies, this journal highlights the clinical applications of research. In keeping with this purpose, every manuscript submitted is jointly reviewed by a clinician and a researcher. In addition to original manuscripts, *ANR* features research briefs, columns devoted to clinical problems and methods, and an "ask an expert" section, where practicing nurses can voice ideas of clinical problems or potential innovations they would like to see studied by nurse researchers.

The most recent journal of this nature is *Clinical Nursing Research*. Begun in 1992, the journal is intended for clinical practitioners and researchers, and the writing style is understandable. The journal includes research reports and encourages the publication of replication studies.[122]

The advent of journals such as *Clinical Nursing Research* and *ANR*, designed as forums for all professional nurses, should help to bridge the gap between research and practice and enhance research utilization in practice settings. Subscribing to professional journals, attending research meetings, and active involvement in professional and specialty organizations are all behaviors that reflect nurses' commitment to professional practice.

Other evidence that barriers to the conduct and utilization of research are gradually eroding include: more positive attitudes about research by clinicians, increasing institutional and administrative support for nursing research, and the establishment of more nursing research positions in clinical settings.[23,103,105] A subgroup of nurse researchers in clinical settings formed within the Council of Nurse Researchers convenes at CNR meetings to network and discuss issues of such positions in clinical practice. The presence of an established clinical nurse researcher in the practice setting provides nurses with a person who can: (1) facilitate the identification of scientific knowledge useful in practice; (2) develop research-focused meetings and discussion groups to promote the implementation of findings; and (3) identify current and potentially researchable problems relevant to nursing practice, administration, and education.[25,73,116] Further, nondoctorally prepared nurses can contribute to the use of research in practice in a variety of ways, such as by systematically documenting their patient care problems, decreasing organizational barriers, disseminating research findings to their colleagues, and serving as role models in the transfer of research-based knowledge into practice.[22,23,98]

Increased collaboration between nurses in service and academic settings is yet another effort to decrease barriers to the utilization and dissemination of research. For example, the Nursing Consortium for Research in Practice at Stanford University Hospital offers nurses from a variety of service agencies the chance to become involved in research through consultation, workshops, and participation in multisite studies.[99,100,101]

Discussion – state of the science

In 1975 the Western Interstate Commission for Higher Education (WICHE) conducted a nationwide Delphi survey to determine in part whether research was being used in practice or not. In response to the question "What items are the most important areas of research value for the profession?" 3 of the top 4 answers were related to the use of research:

1. Determine means for greater utilization of research in practice
2. Determine effective means of communicating, evaluating, and implementing change in practice
3. Establish the relationship between clinical nursing research and quality care[81]

Krone and Loomis[71] maintain that the use of research findings can be enhanced by actually getting nurses involved in various aspects of the research process. For this involvement to be most effective, they recommend that it be related to problems of personal interest and concern to the clinician.

Davis[25] effectively argues that organizational and cultural factors play a significant role in the introduction of nursing research into clinical settings. She suggests that we must build into the system some rewards for using and conducting research, such as pay increases, promotions, paid leaves, and funded travel to attend research conferences. Again, administrative support for research-related activities cannot be underrated.

In analyzing the utilization of nursing research, Horsley[58] has identified that research may be used in the development of new studies, the generation of new theories, the testing of presented theories, or the verification or documentation for changes in practice (Fig. 9-4). Horsley has defined the research utilization model to identify research components and research products for practicing nurses and nursing students. The model identifies potential areas of investigation and calls for innovative instructional strategies for nursing students and an extension of the projects directed toward practicing nurses. The list of issues regarding research utilization in practice is long; however, in 1985 Horsley concluded "the list of validated solutions is essentially blank."[58]

Barnard[9] suggests that nurse researchers have recognized a responsibility to go beyond just reporting

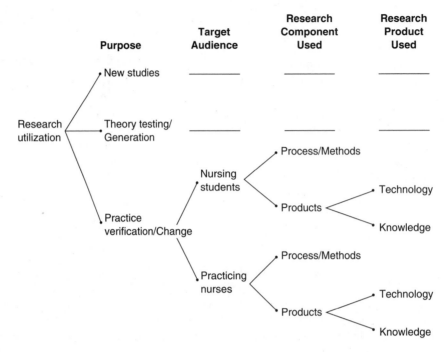

Fig. 9-4 Relationship between research utilization and the use of research in practice. *(From: Horsley J.A. [1985] Using research in practice: The current context.* Western Journal of Nursing Research, 7, p. 135. *Reprinted by permission of Sage Publications, Inc.)*

their findings. The research process can be viewed as extending through to the actual implementation phase.[72] The burden for implementation is no longer borne by the staff nurse alone. Nurse researchers are sharing the responsibility for transmitting their results into practice, and a number of projects have been developed and funded that deal explicitly with the translation of research findings into practice.[10,54,79]

Brett reported a study of fourteen nursing research findings and the extent to which nurses used these selected research findings. She found that "The majority of nurses were aware of the average innovation, were persuaded about it, and used the average innovation at least sometimes."[15] None of the innovations ranked in the "unaware" stage; however, only one innovation was in the "always use" stage. In this study, there were statistically significant relationships between a nurse's knowledge of research-based interventions and the hours a week spent reading professional literature, reading *Nursing Research,* and reading *RN* journal.[15] This suggests that nursing journals convey information being integrated into clinical practice.

A replication of the Brett study by Coyle and Sokop found a significant relationship between the nurse's knowledge of research-based interventions and atten-

dance at conferences where research results were presented, reading of *Heart and Lung,* and job satisfaction. As with Brett's findings, there was no statistically significant relationship between "level of education, years of nursing experience, professional membership, time spent in continuing education, current pursuit of a degree, completion of a nursing research class, or hours spent in reading professional literature."[21]

The accumulation of research evidence in selected (certainly not all) areas of nursing science has gone beyond the ability of most clinicians to read and synthesize this evidence in a meaningful way. As the amount of research evidence in nursing continues to grow, comprehensive, integrated reviews are needed to synthesize large amounts of evidence and to present it in easily understandable summaries of the research literature for users. Quantitative methods have been developed and refined which summarize the results of research studies[45] and help clinicians answer the important question, Do we know anything?, especially with regard to the effectiveness of various kinds of nursing treatments. For example, one development that has aided practitioners in their decisions regarding adoptability of a particular intervention or treatment is in the realm of statistical methods for metaanalysis, which can extract estimates of effect size and magnitude from the data given in research reports.

A number of metaanalyses have been conducted related to nursing problems, and the interested reader is referred to selected examples in the nursing literature by Olson, Heater, and Becker[93] for a review of nursing interventions on children and parents; Engle and Graney[33] for a refinement of gerontological nursing research and theory; Heater, Becker, and Olson[52] on nursing interventions and patient outcomes; Hathaway[51] on the effects of preoperative instruction on postoperative outcomes; Devine[26] for effects of psychoeducational care for adult surgical patients; Burkhardt[18] on the effects of therapy on the mental health of the elderly; and Goode et al.[47] on the effects of heparin flush and saline flush.

All the factors discussed above share common elements and have value in terms of helping nurses to use research in their practice. As nurses become more aware of these approaches and adopt a strategy that is comfortable for them and relevant to their practice setting, the profession will move toward its goal of research-based practice with theoretical underpinnings from nursing and other professions. There is hope that Bloch's model[13] for conceptualizing nursing research and science, in which dissemination and use of findings into education and practice is the outcome, may indeed become an undebatable reality.

In summary, there is evidence that research is increasingly being used in practice. Nursing has made a good beginning and has laid the foundation that will eventually lead to a scientific basis for practice. However, at present not enough research is getting translated to practice settings. That which is being used is taking too long in the translation process, as discussed next, in arguments against the statement that research is being used in practice.

ARGUMENTS THAT DO NOT SUPPORT THE USE OF RESEARCH IN PRACTICE

Nursing has suffered from the view that nurses are technical caregivers and not scientists and, further, that there is a paucity of researchable problems within nursing. Many nurses are regarded as having a "doer" worker orientation rather than a view of themselves as scholars and creative thinkers.[36,68,116] This view leads to a devaluation of nursing knowledge and diminished accountability for data-based practice. Three factors that have inhibited or delayed the transmission of nurs-

ing research into practice are: (1) values and qualifications of practicing nurses; (2) process of research implementation; and (3) organizational factors.

Values and qualifications of practicing nurses

Most nurses lack the preparation necessary to evaluate and implement research in their own environments.[3,36,63,89] Although many baccalaureate programs now include some orientation to research, more course content is needed. Most practicing nurses have not had courses in nursing research, and in fact the majority of current practitioners are either diploma- or associate degree-prepared and may not be qualified to understand, critically evaluate, and implement research findings.[66,68] Furthermore, these nurses tend to read clinical journals that do not provide access to research findings.[68,85,111,118] Circulation statistics show that most nurses depend on one of four journals (*Nursing '90, RN, Nursing Management,* and *Image*).[112] On the positive side, the arrival of *Image* as the nursing journal with the fourth-largest circulation indicates that more nurses are reading relevant and timely nursing research reports.

The small percentage of nurses with graduate-level preparation suggests that it is unrealistic to depend solely on them to translate research into practice. Even if master's-prepared nurses want to implement the research protocols that they have learned, barriers still exist because the practice setting does not support the pursuit or implementation of research-based interventions. In most environments, there is no established clinical nurse research director or committee that provides an effective means of reviewing research protocols for scientific merit. Often, the essential collaboration with other clinical researchers—persons skilled in the process of drafting research proposals and committed to scientific rigor in clinical practice—is lacking, as are the processes available to assist nursing clinical researchers in successfully applying for and receiving institutional review board approval.[11,32]

Beyond consideration of the educational preparation of nurses are other factors related to their socialization, attitudes toward research, and orientation to nursing. Hunt[60] concluded that relevant research findings are not put into practice because practitioners: (1) do not know about them; (2) do not understand them; (3) do not believe them; (4) do not know how to apply them; or (5) are not allowed to use them. Dracup and Weinberg[28] identified yet another reason for the gap between nursing practice and research: Many nurse researchers are *not* practicing clinicians and, therefore, frequently identify research problems with little relevance for practice. This view is supported by McBride, Diers, and Schmidt[84] who concluded that "no matter how good the nursing research, it will affect practice only when it deals with phenomena that are seen as problems by practitioners." They further caution researchers from going "back into the ivory tower" to congratulate themselves on their nursing practice research.

Greenwood was more emphatic in describing the crux of the problem: "*Clinical nurses do not perceive research findings as relevant to their practice.* And further, they do not perceive them as relevant to their practice because frequently they *are not* relevant to their practice."[48]

Process of research implementation

Rogers[102] has identified four elements in the process of research dissemination or diffusion: (*a*) the innovation—the idea, practice or object new to the potential adopter; (*b*) the communication channel—the means by which one individual shares an innovation with another; (*c*) time—the time it takes an individual to move from first knowledge of an innovation to its adoption or rejection; and (*d*) the social system—the set of interrelated units that are engaged in joint problem solving to accomplish a common goal.[41]

Integrating research into practice is not an easy task. The process requires not only education and intellectual capacity but also judgment, discipline, and perseverance.[36] However, insufficient numbers of practitioners have been exposed to and use the available guidelines on how to use research or how to critique the literature for application of research in their own clinical settings.[109] Regrettably, the isolation of research from practice documented by Ketefian[65] continues to some degree today, and nurses still have difficulty locating, reviewing, and analyzing research findings useful in their practice.[15,21,53] More studies need to include concrete suggestions for the use of the findings in the practice setting.

Nursing research reports also contribute to the barriers encountered in the implementation of their results. For example, methodological investigations are scarce; data sources are limited and need to consider a wide variety of data forms (e.g., records, archives, observational techniques, unobtrusive measures, longitudinal studies). Nursing needs to change the pervasive

attitude that all research must be experimental or quasi-experimental to be meaningful. Case study methods and qualitative investigations are equally valuable to the profession. Most importantly, the research activities need to indicate a systematic building of a science for nursing practice.[17]

Other barriers to the implementation of research include: research jargon perceived as foreign or unusable by many clinicians;[82,104] research reports that are not clear or are disorganized; a substantial time lag in publication of research findings that may be as long as several years;[88] and a tremendous lack of replication studies necessary to validate clinical findings.[37,53] Similarly, Haller and Reynolds[49] suggest replication and construct validity are important criteria for the use of research findings in practice. Rather than building discrete knowledge bases through systematic study of various content areas, current research efforts tend to be diffuse and unfocused.

Even when these barriers are absent or have been overcome, there may be barriers to the clinical implementation of the research. The practice setting may not offer clear guidelines for the establishment and evaluation of the research instruments; there may not be realistic timetables for the development, implementation, or evaluation of research protocols; or the essential collaboration between the nursing department and the institutional review board may not facilitate nursing research.[69]

Organizational factors

To assess clinician's perceptions of the barriers to utilization of research findings in practice, Funk, Champagne, Wiese, and Tornquist[42] developed the BARRIERS scale, which has 4 subscales: (1) "characteristics of the nurse, that is, the nurse's research values, skills, and awareness; (2) characteristics of the setting, that is, barriers and limitations perceived in the work setting; (3) characteristics of the research, such as its methodological soundness and the appropriateness of conclusions drawn from the research; and (4) characteristics of the presentation of the research and its accessibility."[42]

The two greatest barriers were identified in the setting and included that the nurse did not believe that he or she had enough authority to change the patient care procedures and that there was not enough time on the job to implement new ideas. All of the 8 characteristics of the work setting were ranked by the participants as among the top 10 barriers to utilization of nursing research.[42]

Additional organizational barriers may occur in the development of the research-based practice, including: a poorly articulated plan for the establishment of the clinical research position; an absence of or inadequate communication between the clinical nurse researcher (CNR), and the administrative and staff members of the department; and the costs associated with the research, such as secretarial support, statistical consultation, or staff release time.[95]

Staff nurses within the organization may become barriers to research utilization if they do not perceive that they have the authority to participate in the definition and modification of their practice based on research or if they feel powerless to effect changes in their clinical setting. Institutional support is a critical factor in the conduct and use of research, and the nurse executive is in a particularly influential role.[32,46,53] For successful implementation of research findings, nursing service administrators must demonstrate a genuine commitment to research, which entails development of self, staff, and resources.[53,69] However, not all nurse executives have exhibited that essential commitment to nursing research.

STRATEGIES FOR INCREASING USE OF RESEARCH IN PRACTICE

The nursing profession is acutely aware of the problems discussed above, and a number of ways to facilitate the translation of nursing research into practice have been advanced.

Several authors have discussed the value of disseminating the results of nursing research and offer suggestions to achieve this goal. Recommended strategies to bring research findings to the attention of practicing nurses include satellite communication modes,[67] marketing strategies,[16,38] and organizational mechanisms.[25] The consortium approach is also effective in facilities where both library and financial resources are scarce and where sharing information is desired.[123]

Davis[25] addressed issues surrounding the incorporation of research findings into practice and cited the need to recognize the organizational and cultural aspects of nursing practice that influence the research environment. Specific suggestions for incorporating research into the organizational setting include: establishment of research committees; using consultant services for the development and implementation of clinical research; using a currently employed clinical nurse specialist to develop and carry out research; developing collaboration with nurse scientists and academic programs; appointment of a full-time or part-time nurse researcher; and creating a nursing research department or division.[69]

The role of the nurse executive may be a critical factor to the effective utilization of research within the institution.[69] If nurse executives want to foster research-based practice then their attitudes, policy statements, and actions must demonstrate and communicate their professional commitment to research-based interventions.[14,40,70,95,96,98,108] Nurse executives may demonstrate their commitment by fostering an environment that recognizes and rewards clinical research. They may also play a key role in the development of nursing research by establishing nursing research departments or divisions with clearly delineated areas of responsibility and authority, defined channels of communication, and specific responsibilities for reporting.[7,78,83,105]

Other modifications in organizational expectations need to be developed. The addition of research as an element of the position description for nurses at all levels and specifically for clinical nurse specialists is indicated.[75] Informational mechanisms need to be established to provide clinicians with opportunities to discuss research findings, new ideas, and views regarding possible testing protocols.[9,43] In particular, employment of nurse researchers by clinical facilities could promote the conduct and use of research. More institutions are establishing this role.[69] Although many positive changes are underway, institutional support for nursing research to date is not widespread, and scientific knowledge has not yet become the basis for nursing practice.

Organizational mechanisms that legitimize research activity, such as released clinical time for research and recognition through the formal reward system, need to be established. Fugleberg[40] asserted that there should be a specific performance criteria for all nursing managers to encourage research in the practice setting. She also maintained that if all nursing staff were encouraged to assist graduate student research, general staff interest in nursing would increase. Networking has been cited as a method of sharing resources and providing educational offerings that would stimulate staff interest in nursing research.[61] Analysis of quality assurance programs has been another method of providing research in a practical, applicable way.[77] Most of these strategies have been predicated on the notion of planned change.

Planned change

Hersey and Blanchard[55] presented two models for change: directive and participative. They found the latter approach more appropriate for implementing change with regard to nursing research in clinical settings, with one modification. Rather than concentrating initially on making new knowledge available to clinicians, we have found it more effective to first begin working on attitudinal changes. That is, developing a positive attitude and a commitment among clinicians in the direction of the desired change promotes the use of research findings in their particular setting. Involvement of an individual nurse or group of nurses in helping to determine the methods by which research will be reviewed and translated into practice is particularly effective and is analogous to group participation in problem solving. Translating commitment into behavior is not an easy task. It is helpful to identify respected clinicians who may already be familiar with and value research and to attempt to gain their active support for using more research in practice. If this is accomplished, organizational change may be facilitated by getting other nurses to pattern their behavior after the clinicians they admire and perceive to be leaders.

In examining the change process, Kurt Lewin[80] identified three phases: unfreezing, changing, and refreezing. Stevenson[110] has put forth Lewin's framework as one that is effective in developing staff research potential and overcoming resistance to research. Briefly, Lewin's three phases are as follows:

1. Unfreezing involves breaking down the old traditions and customs to make way for new alternatives. This might entail motivating nurses to abandon their usual approach to practice based on intuition and to substitute a desire to provide patient care based on tested theories and knowledge about human responses to health and illness.
2. Changing requires new patterns of behavior acquired through the mechanisms of identification and internalization. For example, nurse researchers who serve as models of the desired behaviors may be introduced to the clinical setting (identification), or the staff nurses could be placed in situations that require them to use research findings in their practice to function successfully (internalization).
3. Refreezing is the process by which the newly acquired behaviors become integrated into the nurse's personality and work role. Even when new behaviors such as use of research findings are adopted, the behaviors must be reinforced and sustained or they will be extinguished.

CONCLUSION

In summary, there is general agreement that the conduct of clinical research and the translation and dissemination of relevant research findings into practice are important professional objectives. Research values and activities appear well accepted in many professional arenas, and there is increasing evidence of the presence of such activities and values in the practice setting. The degree to which these objectives are being addressed is evident in part by the amount of current literature devoted to topics related to nursing research; the strong endorsement of research by professional organizations; the number of nursing research conferences, journals, and texts; the increasing number of clinical nurse researchers; and the amount of federal funding available for the conduct, utilization, and dissemination of research. While reports of individual efforts to promote a positive research environment are plentiful, it also is evident that research values and activities have not been fully translated into practice.

The implementation of research findings in clinical practice with the subsequent goal of maintaining a research-based practice is promoted as one of the major movements toward the achievement of full professional status. Since the last edition of this chapter was published, the balance has shifted in favor of the utilization and dissemination of nursing research in practice. It is interesting to note that most of the citations indicating that nursing research is not being used were from the 1970s and 1980s. Thus, progress has been made toward an affirmative answer to the question Is nursing research used in practice? However, there is still more work to be done.

REFERENCES

1. Agency for Health Care Policy and Research. (1991). *Center of general health services intramural research, annotated bibliography, long-term care studies.* Rockville, Md: Author.
2. American Association of Critical-Care Nurses. (1991). *AACN announces research priorities.* AACN Press Release. Aliso Viejo, California, November 21.
3. American Nurses Association. (1985). *Directions for nursing research: Toward the twenty-first century.* Kansas City, Mo: Author.
4. American Nurses Association. (1988). *Standards for organized nursing services.* Kansas City, Mo: Author.

5. American Nurses Association. (1991). *Standards of clinical nursing practice*. Kansas City, Mo: Author.

6. American Nurses Association Committee on Research and Studies. (1962). ANA blueprint for research in nursing. *American Journal of Nursing, 62,* 69-71.

7. American Organization of Nurse Executives. (1985). Strategies: Integration of nursing research into the practice setting. In *Nurse executive management strategies* (pp. 1-11). Chicago: American Hospital Association.

8. Baer, E. D. (1987). 'A cooperative venture' in pursuit of professional status: A research journal for nursing. *Nursing Research, 36,* 18-25.

9. Barnard, K. E. (1982). The research cycle: Nursing, the profession, the discipline. *Western Journal of Nursing Research, 4,* 1-12.

10. Barnard, K. E., & Eyres, S. J. (Eds.). (1979). *Child health assessment: Part 2. The first year of life* (DHEW Pub No. HRA 79-25). Washington, D.C.: U.S. Government Printing Office.

11. Bartos, B., Sexton, P. R., & Taggart, J. A. (1991). The institutional research review board. In M. A. Mateo & K. T. Kirchhoff (Eds.), *Conducting and using nursing research in the clinical setting* (pp. 31-41). Baltimore: Williams and Wilkins.

12. Bergstrom, N. (1991). Scientific base for nursing practice is the goal of the ANA, Council of Nurse Researchers.

13. Bloch, D. (1981). A conceptualization of nursing research and nursing science. In J. C. McCloskey & H. K. Grace (Eds.), *Current issues in nursing* (pp. 81-93). Cambridge, Mass: Blackwell Scientific.

14. Bolton, L. B. (1991). Resources for research. In M. A. Mateo & K. T. Kirchhoff (Eds.), *Conducting and using nursing research in the clinical setting* (pp. 22-30). Baltimore: Williams and Wilkins.

15. Brett, J. L. L. (1987). Use of nursing practice research findings. *Nursing Research, 36,* 344-349.

16. Brooten, D. A. (1982). Is soft sell enough? *Nursing Research, 31,* 195.

17. Brown, J. S., Tanner, C. A., & Padrick, K. P. (1984). Nursing's search for scientific knowledge. *Nursing Research, 33,* 26-32.

18. Burkhardt, C. S. (1987). The effect of therapy on the mental health of the elderly. *Research in Nursing and Health, 10,* 277-285.

19. Carnegie, M. E. (1974). The shifting of research emphasis and investigators. *Nursing Research, 23,* 195.

20. Carnegie, M. E. (1976). The editor's report—1976 [Editorial]. *Nursing Research, 25,* 3.

21. Coyle, L. A., & Sokop, A. G. (1990). Innovation adoption behavior among nurses. *Nursing Research, 39,* 176-180.

22. Cronenwett, L. R. (1986). Research contributions of clinical nurse specialists. *Journal of Nursing Administration, 16,* 6-7.

23. Cronenwett, L. R. (1986). Selecting a nurse researcher. *Journal of Nursing Administration, 16,* 7-8.

24. Cronenwett, L. R., & Stetler, C. (1986). Proposal submitted to Division of Nursing, USPHS, Special Projects Grants, Nov. 1.

25. Davis, M. Z. (1981). Promoting nursing research in the clinical setting. *Journal of Nursing Administration, 11,* 22-27.

26. Devine, E. C. (1992). The what, why and how of meta-analysis. Presented at Advanced Quatitative Methods Institute, St. Mary's College, Md, July 27.

27. Devine, E. C., & Cook, T. D. (1986). Clinical and cost-saving effects of psychoeducational interventions with surgical patients: A metaanalysis. *Research in Nursing and Health, 9,* 89-105.

28. Dracup, K., & Weinberg, S. L. (1983). Another case for nursing research. *Heart and Lung, 12,* 3.

29. Dracup, K. A., & Breu, C. S. (1977). Strengthening practice through research utilization. In M. V. Batey (Ed.), *Communicating nursing research* (pp. 339-353). Boulder, Co: Western Interstate Commission for Higher Education.

30. Duffy, M. E. (1987). The research process in baccalaureate nursing education: A ten-year review. *Image: The Journal of Nursing Scholarship, 19,* 87-91.

31. Editorial. (1952). A new magazine for nurses, *American Journal of Nursing, 52,* 664.

32. Egan, E. C., McElmurry, B. J., & Jameson, H. M. (1981). Practice-based research: Assessing your department's readiness. *Journal of Nursing Administration, 11,* 26-32.

33. Engle, V. F., & Graney, M. J. (1990). Meta-analysis for the refinement of gerontological nursing research and theory. *Journal of Gerontological Nursing, 16*(9), 12-15.

34. Fagin, C. M. (1982). The economic value of nursing research. *American Journal of Nursing, 82,* 1844-1849.

35. Fagin, C. M. (1990). Nursing's value proves itself. *American Journal of Nursing, 90*(10), 17-30.

36. Fawcett, J. (1979). Integrating research into the faculty workload. *Nursing Outlook, 27,* 259-262.

37. Fawcett, J. (1983). Contemporary nursing research: Its relevance for nursing practice. In N. L. Chaska (Ed.), *The nursing profession: A time to speak* (pp. 169-182). New York: McGraw-Hill.

38. Fine, R. B. (1980). Marketing nursing research. *Journal of Nursing Administration, 10*(11), 21-23.

39. Fitzpatrick, J. J. (Ed.). (1988). *Applied nursing research*. Philadelphia: W. B. Saunders.

40. Fugleberg, B. B. (1986). Nursing research in the practice setting. *Nursing Administration Quarterly, 11,* 38-42.

41. Funk, S. G., Champagne, M. T., Wiese, R. A., & Tornquist, E. M. (1991). BARRIERS: The barriers to research utilization scale. *Applied Nursing Research, 4,* 39-45.

42. Funk, S. G., Champagne, M. T., Wiese, R. A., & Tornquist, E. M. (1991). Barriers to using research findings in practice: The clinician's perspective. *Applied Nursing Research, 4,* 90-95.

43. Funk, S. G., Tornquist, E. M., Champagne, M. T., & Wiese, R. A. (1992). *Key aspects of elder care*. New York: Springer.

44. Germain, C. P. (1991). Regional awards for utilization of research in nursing practice. *Reflections,* (Summer/Fall), 12.

45. Glass, G. V., McGaw, B., & Smith, M. L. (1976). Primary, secondary, and meta-analysis of research. *Educational Researcher, 5,* 3-8.

46. Goode, C. J., Lovett, M. K., Hayes, J. E., & Butcher, L. A. (1987). Use of research-based knowledge in clinical practice. *Journal of Nursing Administration, 17,* 11-18.

47. Goode, C. J., Titler, M., Rakel, B., Ones, D. S., Kleiber C., Small, S., & Triolo, P. K. (1991). A meta-analysis of effects of heparin flush and saline flush: Quality and cost implications. *Nursing Research, 40,* 324-329.

48. Greenwood, J. (1984). Nursing research: A position paper. *Journal of Advanced Nursing, 9,* 77-82.

49. Haller, K. B., & Reynolds, M. A. (1986). Using research in practice: A case for replication in nursing—part 2. *Western Journal of Nursing Research, 8*(2), 249-252.

50. Haller, K. B., Reynolds, M. A., & Horsley, J. A. (1979). Developing research-based innovation protocols: Process, criteria and issues. *Research in Nursing and Health, 2,* 45-51.

51. Hathway, D. (1986). Effect of preoperative instruction on postoperative outcomes: A meta-analysis. *Nursing Research, 35,* 269-275.

52. Heater, B. S., Becker, A. M., & Olson, R. K. (1988). Nursing interventions and patient outcomes: A meta-analysis of studies. *Nursing Research, 37,* 303-307.

53. Hefferin, E. A., Horsley, J. A., & Ventura, M. R. (1982). Promoting research-based nursing: The nurse administrator's role. *Journal of Nursing Administration, 12,* 34-41.

54. Henry, B., Moody, L. E., Pendergast, J. F., O'Donnell, J., Hutchinson, S. A., & Scully, G. (1987). Delineation of nursing administration research priorities. *Nursing Research, 36,* 309-314.

55. Hersey, P., & Blanchard, K. H. (1988). *Management of organizational behavior* (5th ed.). Englewood Cliffs, N.J.: Prentice-Hall.

56. Holzemer, W. L., Slaughter, R. E., Chambers, D. B., Dulock, H. L., & Paul, S. M. (1990). *Introduction to research: A computer-based tutorial (CBT) for nurses and other health-care professionals.* San Francisco: University of California School of Nursing.

57. Horn Video Productions. (1989). *Research utilization: A process of organizational change.* Ida Grove, Iowa.

58. Horsley, J. A. (1985). Using research in practice: The current context. *Western Journal of Nursing Research, 7,* 135-9.

59. Horsley, J. A., Crane, J., Crabtree, M. K., & Wood, D. J. (1983). *Using research to improve nursing practice: A guide.* CURN Project. New York: Grune & Stratton.

60. Hunt, J. (1981). Indicators for nursing practice: The use of research findings. *Journal of Advanced Nursing, 6,* 189-194.

61. Hunt, V., Stark, J. L., Fisher, F., Hegedus, K., Joy, L., & Woldum, K. (1983). Networking: A managerial strategy for research development in a service setting. *Journal of Nursing Administration, 13,* 27-32.

62. Jacox, A. (1986). The coming of age of nursing research. *Nursing Outlook, 34,* 276-281.

63. Jacox, A. (1974). Nursing research and the clinician. *Nursing Outlook, 22,* 382-385.

64. Joint Commission on Accreditation of Healthcare Organizations. (1991). *1992 Joint Commission accreditation manual for hospitals. Volume II, Scoring guidelines.* Oakbrook Terrace, Ill: Author.

65. Ketefian, S. (1975). Application of selected nursing research findings into nursing practice: A pilot study. *Nursing Research, 24,* 89-92.

66. Ketefian, S. (1980). Using research in practice: Selected issues in the translation of research to nursing practice. *Western Journal of Nursing Research, 2,* 429-431.

67. King, D., Barnard, K. E., & Hoehn, R. (1981). Disseminating the results of nursing research. *Nursing Outlook, 29,* 164-9.

68. Kirchhoff, K. T. (1983). Should staff nurses be expected to use research? *Western Journal of Nursing Research, 5,* 245-247.

69. Kirchhoff, K. T., & Titler, M. G. (in press). Responsibilities of nurse executives in conducting and using research in the practice setting. In *Nursing management desk reference: Concept, strategies and skills.*

70. Knafl, K. A., Hagle, M. E., Bevis, M. E., Faux, S. A., & Kirchhoff, K. T. (1989). How researchers and administrators view the role of the clinical nurse researcher. *Western Journal of Nursing Research, 11,* 583-592.

71. Krone, K. P., & Loomis, M. E. (1982). Developing practice-relevant research: A model that worked. *Journal of Nursing Administration, 12,* 38-41.

72. Krueger, J. C. (1979). A vital link in the nursing research cycle. *Western Journal of Nursing Research, 1,* 148-152.

73. Krueger, J. C. (1982). A survey of research utilization in community health nursing. *Western Journal of Nursing Research, 4,* 244-248.

74. Krueger, J. C., Nelson, A. H., & Wolanin, M. O. (1978). *Nursing research: Development, collaboration, and utilization.* Germantown, Md: Aspen.

75. Kruse, L. C., Scheffel, A. L., Buckwalter, K. C., & Stolley, J. M. (1992). Research promotion in hospital nursing service setting. *The Iowa Nurse Reporter, 6*(2), 5, 12.

76. Kuhn, R. C. (1990). *AACN outcome standards for nursing care of the critically ill.* Laguna Niguel, Calif: American Association of Critical-Care Nurses.

77. Larson, E. (1983). Combining nursing quality assurance and research programs. *Journal of Nursing Administration, 13,* 32-5.

78. Lawson, L. (1987). Developing a research structure within the nursing department. *Journal of Nursing Administration, 17*(11), 6-7.

79. Lewandowski, L. A., & Kositsky, A. N. (1983). Research priorities for critical care nursing: A study by the American Association of Critical-Care Nurses. *Heart and Lung, 12,* 35-44.

80. Lewin, K. (1951). *Field theory in social sciences* (pp. 188-232). New York: Harper and Row.

81. Lindeman, C. A. (1975). Priorities in clinical nursing research. *Nursing Outlook, 23,* 693-8.

82. Ludeman, R. (1980). The language and importance of nursing research. *Western Journal of Nursing Research, 2,* 432-434.

83. MacKay, R. C., Grantham, M. A., & Ross, S. E. M. (1984). Building a hospital nursing research department. *Journal of Nursing Administration, 14*(7 & 8), 23-27.

84. McBride, M. A., Diers, D., & Schmidt, R. L. (1970). Nurse-researcher: The crucial hyphen. *American Journal of Nursing, 70,* 1256-1260.

85. McCloskey, J. C., & Buckwalter, K. C. (1982). Publishing in non-refereed journals is not only o.k. it's necessary. *Western Journal of Nursing Research, 4,* 255-6.

86. McClure M. L. (1981). Promoting practice-based research: A critical need. *Journal of Nursing Administration, 11*(11), 66-70.

87. McGrath, S. (1990). The cost-effectiveness of nurse practitioners. *Nurse Practitioner, 15*(7), 40-42.

88. Mercer, R. T. (1984). Nursing research: The bridge to excellence in practice. *Image: The Journal of Nursing Scholarship, 16,* 47-51.

89. Murdough, C., Kramer, M., & Schmalenberg, C. E. (1981). The teaching of nursing research: A survey report. *Nursing Education, 6,* 28-35.

90. Neidlinger, S. H., Scroggins, K., & Kennedy, L. M. (1987). Cost evaluation of discharge planning for hospitalized elderly. *Nursing Economic$, 5,* 225-230.

91. NLN Council of Baccalaureate and Higher Degree Programs. (1987). *Doctoral programs in nursing 1986-87* (NLN Pub No. 15-1448). New York: Author.

92. Nursing Doctoral Program in the United States. (1991). *Reflections,* Summer/Fall, 23-24.

93. Olson, R. K., Heater, B. S., & Becker, A. M. (1990). A meta-analysis of the effects of nursing interventions on children and parents. *MCN: American Journal of Maternal-Child Nursing, 15,* 104-108.

94. Peterson, F. Y., & Kirchhoff, K. T. (1991). Analysis of the research about heparinized versus nonheparinized vascular lines. *Heart and Lung, 20,* 631-640.

95. Pettengill, M. M., Knafl, K. A., Bevis, M. E., & Kirchhoff, K. T. (1988). Nursing research in midwestern hospitals. *Western Journal of Nursing Research, 10,* 705-717.

96. Pranulis, M. F., & Driever, M. J. (1990). A conceptual framework for analyzing influences on research productivity in clinical settings. *Western Journal of Nursing Research, 12,* 563-565.

97. Regional utilization of research in nursing practice award. (1992). In *Sigma Theta Tau International awards information book.* Indianapolis: Sigma Theta Tau International.

98. Rempusheski, V. F. (1991). Incorporating research role and practice role. *Applied Nursing Research, 4(1),* 46-48.

99. Rizzuto, C., & Mitchell, M. (1988). Research in service settings: Part I: Consortium project outcomes. *Journal of Nursing Administration, 18(2),* 32-37.

100. Rizzuto, C., & Mitchell, M. (1988). Research in service settings: Part II: Consortium project. *Journal of Nursing Administration, 18(3),* 19-24.

101. Rizzuto, C., & Mitchell, M. (1990). Outcomes of research consortium project. *Journal of Nursing Administration, 20(4),* 13-17.

102. Rogers, E. M. (1983). *Diffusion of innovations.* New York: The Free Press.

103. Rosswurm, M. A. (1992). A research-based practice model in a hospital setting. *Journal of Nursing Administration, 22(3),* 57-60.

104. Schrader, E. S. (1979). Gobbledygook as a barrier to research. *Association of Operating Room Nurses Journal, 30,* 13-14.

105. Schutzenhofer, K. K. (1991). Scholarly pursuit in the clinical setting: An obligation of professional nursing. *Journal of Professional Nursing, 7(1),* 10-15.

106. Schwartz R., Moody, L., Yarandi, H., & Anderson, G. C. (1987). A meta-analysis of critical outcome variables in nonnutritive sucking in preterm infants. *Nursing Research, 36,* 292-295.

107. Sigma Theta Tau. (1991). *Actions for the 1990's.* Indianapolis: Sigma Theta Tau International.

108. Snyder-Halpern, R. (1991). Attributes of service-based nursing research programs useful for decision-making. *Nursing Administration Quarterly, 15(4),* 82-84.

109. Stetler, C. B., & Marram, G. (1976). Evaluating research findings for applicability in practice. *Nursing Outlook, 24,* 559-563.

110. Stevenson, J. S. (1980). Developing staff research potential: Overcoming nurse resistance to research. In L. Machan (Ed.), *The practitioner-teacher role: Practice what you teach* (pp. 73-78). Wakefield, Mass: Nursing Resources.

111. Swanson, E., & McCloskey, J. C. (1986). Publishing opportunities for nurses. *Nursing Outlook, 34,* 227-235.

112. Swanson, E. A., McCloskey, J. C., & Bodensteiner, A. (1991). Publishing opportunities for nurses: A comparison of 92 U.S. journals. *Image: The Journal of Nursing Scholarship, 23(1),* 33-38.

113. The University of Iowa College of Nursing. (1991). *The PhD in nursing course descriptions.* Iowa City, Iowa: Author.

114. Thomas, B., & Price, M. M. (1980). Research preparation in baccalaureate nursing education. *Nursing Research, 29,* 259-261.

115. Titler, M. G., Goode, C. J., & Mathis, S. (1992). Nursing research in times of economic cutbacks: Implications for nurse administrators. In M. Johnson (Ed.), *Series on nursing administration* (Vol. 4, pp. 167-182). St Louis: Mosby.

116. Todd, A. H., & Gortner, S. R. (1982). Researchmanship: Removing obstacles to research in the clinical setting. *Western Journal of Nursing Research, 4,* 329-333.

117. Vaughan-Wrobel, B. C. (1991). *Presidential charge.* Indianapolis, Ind: Sigma Theta Tau International.

118. Vaz, D. (1986). An investigation of the usage of the periodical literature of nursing by staff nurses and nursing administrators. *Journal of Continuing Education in Nursing, 17,* 22-6.

119. Watson, C. A., Bulechek, G. M., & McCloskey, J. A. (1987). QAMUR: A quality assurance model using research. *Journal of Nursing Quality Assurance, 2(1),* 21-27.

120. Weiler, K., & Buckwalter, K. C. (1990). Is nursing research used in practice? In J. C. McCloskey & H. K. Grace (Eds.), *Current issues in nursing* (pp. 45-57). St Louis: Mosby.

121. Werley, H. H., & Westlake, S. K. (1985). Impact of nursing research on public policy: An examination of ANA research priority statements. *Journal of Professional Nursing, 1,* 148-156.

122. Wood, M. J., & Hayes, P. (Eds.). (1992). Clinical nursing research: An international journal. *Sage Periodicals Press, 1* (2).

123. Zalar, M. K., Welches, L. J., & Walker, D. D. (1985). Nursing consortium approach to increase research in service settings. *Journal of Nursing Administration, 15,* 36-41.

CHAPTER 10

Viewpoints

The nursing theory–nursing practice connection

SHARON L. FIRLIT

There is growing support for fostering a closer link between nursing theory and nursing practice. Before documenting the premise that nursing theory and nursing practice are mutually interdependent, the relationship of nursing theory and nursing practice to the philosophical foundation of the discipline of nursing is reviewed. Following a supportive argument relating to the interaction between nursing theory and nursing practice, means to strengthen this connection are discussed.

PHILOSOPHICAL BASIS
Nursing's metaparadigm

The metaparadigm of any discipline is its identification of overall areas of interest. A metaparadigm reflects the *philosophical orientation* or worldview espoused by members of a discipline. This gestalt forms the foundation and boundaries for inquiry and knowledge (theory) development within the profession.

The metaparadigm of nursing continues to evolve. In 1980, Flaskerud and Halloran documented consensus within the nursing profession for the central concepts of person, environment, health, and nursing.[17] In 1984, Fawcett[15] formalized these concepts along with three recurring themes originally identified by Donaldson and Crowley in 1978[14] as the metaparadigm of nursing. However, alternative metaparadigms have been proposed. In 1985, Meleis[26] identified seven central nursing phenomena: client, health, environment, interaction, nursing process, transition, and nursing therapeutics. In an analysis of the philosophical roots of four contemporary nursing theories, Sarter[36] identified seven shared themes that contribute to the development of a metaparadigm for nursing. They are process, evolution of consciousness, self-transcendence, open systems, harmony, relativity of space-time, pattern, and holism.

Within the past decade, there has been emphasis in nursing on the concepts of health and caring. In a 1991 article Newman, Sime, and Corcoran-Perry submit that the focus of the discipline of nursing is "*caring in the human health experience.*"[28] This metaparadigm holds promise for the future since it clearly reflects nursing's belief and value regarding the profession's social commitment, nature of service, and area of responsibility for knowledge development.

Knowledge is developed within a discipline based on one or more paradigms. Each paradigm represents a distinctive view or reality within which the metaparadigm phenomena are explicated. Furthermore, each paradigm reflects a research tradition in which methods of investigation or ways of knowing are specified. Therefore, each paradigm contains metaphysical and epistemological beliefs that guide inquiry related to the metaparadigm phenomena.

Newman et al.[28] identify three current perspectives extant in nursing literature as: particulate-deterministic, interactive-integrative, and unitary-transformative. Each differs in its assumptions regarding phenomena, change, relationships, and research methodology. Fawcett[15] considers conceptual models in nursing as paradigms because they each represent a distinctive frame of reference. Examples include King's[21] open system model, Rogers's[34] life process model, and Roy's[35] adaptation model.

Nursing theory

A theory is a statement about the relationship(s) of specifically defined concepts that describe, explain, or predict some phenomenon, and, in professional disciplines, prescribe action.[4,12,26] Nursing theories specify relations among variables derived from the central concepts of nursing's metaparadigm. The way variables are defined is dependent on the paradigm or conceptual framework used by the theorist.

Conceptual models of nursing have generated nursing theories.[21,24,35] Each of these theories has addressed one or more concepts within the model. An example is King's theory of goal attainment which was derived from the concept of interpersonal systems in her conceptual framework.[21] The theory describes the nature of nurse-client interactions that lead to the achievement of goals. Characteristics of the interaction that are specifically defined are perception, communication, transaction, self, role, stress, growth and development, and time and space. A list of propositions, some dealing with process, others dealing with outcome, indicates the predictive value of the concepts in the theory.

Models and theories from other disciplines have also contributed to the development of nursing theory. Walker and Avant[44] identify this approach to theory building as derivation. When derivation is used in nursing theory development, concepts or other components of the original theory or model are redefined or adapted to the nursing metaparadigm. Using this approach, Roy[35] derived the concept of adaptation from Helson's adaptation level theory, and Benner[5] described the stages of nursing practice based on a model of skill acquisition developed by Dreyfus and Dreyfus.

Nursing theories have also been based on broad paradigms or worldviews shared by a variety of disciplines. For example, theories of psychotherapy, education, and other social sciences have been founded on the phenomenological tradition.[11] Paterson and Zderad[31] used this approach, which seeks to understand meanings of human experiences in developing their humanistic nursing practice theory. It was also used by Benner[6] for describing seven domains of nursing practice. Along with naturalistic inquiry, it comprises the human science paradigm discussed by Watson.[45]

Nursing practice

Nursing practice is something more than the application of theoretical knowledge. Donaldson and Crowley[14] state that "clinical practice is always to some extent empirical, pragmatic, intuitive, and artistic." Carper[8] identifies four fundamental patterns of knowledge in nursing care and concludes that nursing practice "depends on the scientific knowledge of human behavior in health and in illness, the aesthetic perception of significant human experiences, a personal understanding of the unique individuality of the self and the capacity to make choices within concrete situations involving particular moral judgments." Elaborating on Carper's work, Chinn and Kramer[9] propose that aesthetics, the art of nursing, is the foundation for the integration of all patterns of knowing. Johnson defines nursing art as "the ability to nurse well . . . the practical know-how that an individual nurse has in a particular situation, which is used to achieve a particular result."[20]

Frameworks have been identified to guide practitioners in integrating various ways of knowing within clinical situations. The model for situation-producing nursing theories proposed by Dickoff, James, and Wiedenbach constitutes "conceptualization of the *relations* that must exist between, on one hand, whatever predictive theories are required and, on the other hand, other things and theories necessary to produce situations of the kind deemed professionally good by the practice discipline in question."[13] So, aesthetic, existential, and moral knowledge are used in addition to the consideration of empirical or scientific theories to identify frameworks. Other frameworks include Shotter's theory of personal action discussed by Clarke[10] and Kuypers' metatheory for practice.[22] In essence, these authors propose that nurses use some model, often unconsciously, to choose theories, adopt them, and integrate them with other knowledge derived from the clinical situation in providing nursing care (goal-directed action). Therefore, explication of this underlying framework may be in itself a theory that can be used to further guide nursing practice.

Although these theories may explain how nurses use knowledge in their practice, controversy over the unique nature of nursing practice continues. The definition of nursing stated in the American Nurses Association's *Social Policy Statement,* "the diagnosis and treatment of human responses to actual and potential health problems,"[3] has been criticized by Schlotfeldt[37] and Orlando.[29] From a panel discussion of six nursing leaders, Smith[40] reports no consensus for what makes nursing unique. While Smith concludes that this "disagreement is heartening,"[40] others would differ with her view, holding that a fundamental, philosophical agreement about the nature of nursing is paramount for the viability of the profession.

Recently, the concepts of health and caring have received increased attention as distinguishing characteristics of nursing practice. Caring has been identified as the essence of nursing.[6,23,45] Since the days of Florence Nightingale, health has been central to nursing. Current theorists specify that health in nursing means the human health experience.[30,32,33] Newman et al. unite these concepts and propose that the focus of nursing is *"caring in the human health experience."*[28]

I believe this statement reflects the unique nature of nursing practice, one that nurses can relate to as relevant to any practice specialty. Caring can be demonstrated as a human trait, as a moral imperative or ideal, as an affect, as an interpersonal relationship, and as a therapeutic intervention.[27] Birth, growth and development, wellness, illness, and death can be synthesized within the ongoing human health experience. Support for and internalization of this statement as the focus of the discipline and the nature of nursing has potential for differentiating nursing from other health care disciplines and empowering its role in society.

THE NURSING THEORY-PRACTICE INTERACTION

Arguments supportive of the interdependence between nursing theory and nursing practice may be categorized into those that view nursing practice as necessary for theory development and theory validation and those that reflect application of theory in practice.

Practice as a basis for nursing theory development

"Theory is born in practice, is refined in research, and must and can return to practice."[12] When this contention was made, only "embryos of nursing theory" existed.[12] Over the past 25 years, however, numerous theories have been developed. Furthermore, resources contributing to theory development are expanding. These include the recognition and integration of different patterns of knowing, the acceptance of multiple philosophical and methodological perspectives, and the increase in doctorally prepared nurses who can facilitate theory advancement.[19]

Carper[8] demonstrated that the body of knowledge that serves as the rationale for nursing practice includes empirical, aesthetic, ethical, and personal knowledge patterns. In the past, only the empirical (scientific) mode has been valued in nursing theory development. However, growing acceptance of each of these patterns as necessary for full knowledge development holds promise for a stronger nursing theory–nursing practice bond. Nurse scientists have already begun to look more openly at the type of knowledge that can be derived from the study of clinical practice. In Benner's[5] study of nursing practice, all four patterns of knowing were documented as components of expert nursing care. Agan[1] studied holistic nursing practice and described the use of intuitive knowing, an aspect of personal knowledge. Clarke[10] proposed that if nursing theory is anchored within the reality of nursing practice, nursing actions and ethical issues assume importance. Thus, using nursing practice as a basis for theory development promotes not only a broader view of reality but also an increased relevance of theory to practice. As Benner contends:

Adequate description of practical knowledge is essential to the development and extension of nursing theory. . . . There is much to learn and appreciate as practicing nurses uncover common meanings acquired as a result of helping, coaching, and intervening in the significantly human events that comprise the art and science of nursing.[5]

Validation of nursing theory in practice

Although arduous and complex, the theory validation process is the essence of the theory-practice relationship.[9] This activity involves the empirical testing of theoretical propositions in the practice setting. Theory testing also provides better feedback to refine theory so that it better represents reality. If repeated results provide evidence of a theory's accuracy, the theory is valid.

Although there has been an increase in research studies based on conceptual models of nursing, Silva[39] contends that little progress has been made in the actual testing of these models. She recommends that nurse theorists follow through with a systematic program of theory testing making explicit key assumptions, propositions, and hypotheses that need to be tested. Examples of theorists who have done so are King[21] and Roy.[35]

Dickoff et al.[13] discuss testing theory in terms of its coherency, palatability, and feasibility claims. In arguing for the importance of theory testing, they maintain that:

Unless within his limits man makes such an attempt, he is forever compelled to act without the light of theory and so to remain at the level of inarticulate art—a position having grave consequences for educating an adequate number of able practitioners, as well as for the quality of practice. Or else he must dumbly follow a theory of dubious validity.[13]

Numerous nursing models and theories are in the process of being tested. The practical validation of a theory is a process that requires concerted effort over a period of time. Because validation of nursing theories takes place within clinical settings, practicing nurses are involved with testing and collection of the data used to verify the theory in question. Thus, practitioners have input into the process of confirming or refining a theory. They provide a vital link in the nursing theory-practice connection.

Application of nursing theory in practice

Although nursing theories may not be fully validated, they serve as a guide to practice for many nurses. In justifying the application of a theory in practice, Chinn and Kramer[9] advise that the following prerequisites be considered:

1. The goals of the theory should be examined and compared with the outcomes or goals judged to be of value in nursing practice
2. The circumstances under which the theory is expected to apply should be congruent with the situation in which the theory actually will be applied
3. Comparison should be made between the variables important in the construction of the theory and variables recognized to be directly influencing the practice situation
4. The relationships within the theory should provide sufficient explanation to provide a basis for planning and implementing nursing actions
5. There should be evidence from actual research that supports the validity of the theory
6. The potential for observing and recording factors that are relevant to the theory's application should be assessed

Ideally, each of these prerequisites should be met before proceeding with application. However, Chinn and Kramer[9] propose that the practitioner is justified in applying the theory if most of the prerequisites are met. If prerequisites are not met, they recommend using a research approach to document the results of the application.

Nursing literature is replete with examples of practicing nurses applying nursing theory. Nurses from the University of Michigan hospitals developed and use an assessment tool derived from the modeling and role-modeling nursing theory.[7] Graduates of the McGill University School of Nursing have applied the McGill model of nursing (a practice-derived model) in ambulatory care, intensive care, and community health.[18] In Winstead-Fry's[46] compendium, various nurses describe how they have applied one of eight different nursing theories. Uys[43] contends that conceptual models of nursing are more like philosophies than theories. They each provide a particular perspective or view of nursing that often becomes an unconscious approach to practice. This is reflected in one nurse's comment: "I don't consciously decide to use Orlando's theory. Rather, it is a way of thinking, a way of responding that is integrated into my total practice."[38]

STRENGTHENING THE NURSING THEORY-PRACTICE BOND

In the past, the connection between nursing theory and nursing practice has been questioned. An earlier article summarizes arguments that refute the nature and relevance of nursing theory to nursing practice.[16] Recent literature fosters a closer link between nursing theory and nursing practice, but further action is needed to strengthen this bond.

Administrative support

Nurse administrators are challenged to create an environment supportive of theory-based nursing practice to empower nurses and promote nursing as a profession.[2,25,41] When a theory has been accepted as the basis for nursing practice in an agency, it is incorporated within the philosophy of nursing, organizational structure, standards of practice, documentation methods, and outcome-oriented performance improvement activities. Nursing practice based on a comprehensive and valid nursing theory clarifies the role of the nurse and the contribution of nursing service to the mission and goals of the organization. Furthermore, nursing practice based on nursing theory promotes autonomy and control over practice.

When deciding to use single or multiple theories for guiding nursing practice in an organization, several issues need to be considered.[42] First, the theory or theories must be congruent with the agency's mission and goals. Second, the diversity of patient populations and/or outcomes may require different approaches. However, the use of multiple theories in an organization can be costly from the standpoint of duplication of standard operating procedures and decentralized staff education. Furthermore, communication within nursing and nonnursing personnel may be compromised by the use of more than one theory. A single theory approach provides consistent, explicit direction for staff and is easier to interpret to physicians and administrators. Finally, overall knowledge of nursing theory by nursing staff is considered. If the staff as a whole is unfamiliar with nursing theories, education, application, and impact on care may be facilitated by the selection of a single theory.

Education and research support

While graduate education in nursing provides a knowledge base in nursing theory and research methods, the majority of the nursing population lacks exposure to information about conceptual models and nursing theories. Many excellent articles on nursing theory-based practice applications and theory testing have been published in *Advances in Nursing Science, Journal of Advanced Nursing,* and *Nursing Science Quarterly,* which are seldom read by staff nurses. There is a need for theorists and researchers to prepare articles for clinical specialty journals and more commonly read journals such as the *American Journal of Nursing* and *Nursing 94.* Nurse educators and advanced practitioners in health care settings need to disseminate and help interpret to their staff current literature on nursing theories and conceptual frameworks. When a nursing service has adopted a nursing theory on which to base its practice, the theorist should be consulted to assist with implementation. We are truly fortunate to have so many of our theorists still alive and willing to collaborate with practicing nurses to apply and refine their theories.

Science and technology have created health experiences that did not exist 50 years ago. As we look into the 21st century, nursing as a profession can and will survive only if it responds to the health experiences of humankind. In doing so, scientific, aesthetic, personal, and ethical knowledge must be integrated in providing care to individuals, families, and communities. The explication of this integration is nursing theory that originates in practice and guides practice. Thus, nursing theory is connected to nursing practice, waiting to be fully developed.

REFERENCES

1. Agan, R. D. (1987). Intuitive knowing as a dimension of nursing. *Advances in Nursing Science, 10*(1), 63-70.
2. Allison, S. E., Mclaughlin, K., & Walker, D. (1991). Nursing theory: A tool to put nursing back into nursing administration. *Nursing Administration Quarterly, 15*(3), 72-78.
3. American Nurses Association. (1980). *Nursing: A social policy statement.* Kansas City, Mo: Author.
4. Argyris, C., & Schon, D. A. (1974). *Theory and practice: Increasing professional effectiveness.* San Francisco: Jossey-Bass.
5. Benner, P. (1984). *From novice to expert: Excellence and power in clinical nursing practice.* Menlo Park, Calif: Addison-Wesley.
6. Benner, P., & Wrubel, J. (1989). *The primacy of caring.* Menlo Park, Calif: Addison-Wesley.
7. Campbell, J., Finch, D., Allport, D., Erickson, H. C., & Swain, M. A. (1985). A theoretical approach to nursing assessment. *Journal of Advanced Nursing, 10,* 111-115.
8. Carper, B. A. (1978). Fundamentals of knowing in nursing. *Advances in Nursing Science, 1*(1), 13-23.
9. Chinn, P. L., & Kramer, M. K. (1991). *Theory and nursing: A systematic approach* (3rd ed.). St Louis: Mosby.
10. Clarke, M. (1986). Action and reflection: Practice and theory in nursing. *The Journal of Advanced Nursing, 11,* 3-11.
11. Cohen, M. Z. (1987). A historical overview of the phenomenological movement. *Image: The Journal of Nursing Scholarship, 19*(1), 31-34.
12. Dickoff, J., James, P., & Wiedenbach, E. (1968). Theory in a practice discipline: Part I. Practice oriented theory. *Nursing Research, 17*(5), 415-435.
13. Dickoff, J., James, P., & Wiedenbach, E. (1968). Theory in a practice discipline: Part II. Practice oriented research. *Nursing Research, 17*(6), 545-554.
14. Donaldson, S. K., & Crowley, D. M. (1978). The discipline of nursing. *Nursing Outlook, 26*(2), 113-120.
15. Fawcett, J. (1984). The metaparadigm of nursing: Present status and future refinements. *Image: The Journal of Nursing Scholarship, 16*(3), 84-87.
16. Firlit, S. L. (1990). Nursing theory and nursing practice: Do they connect? In J. C. McCloskey and H. K. Grace (Eds.), *Current issues in nursing* (3rd ed.). St Louis: Mosby.
17. Flaskerud, J. H., & Halloran, E. J. (1980). Areas of agreement in nursing theory development. *Advances in Nursing Science, 3*(1), 1-7.
18. Gottlieb, L., & Rowat, K. (1987). The McGill model of nursing: A practice-derived model. *Advances in Nursing Science, 9*(4), 51-61.
19. Jennings, B. M. (1987). Nursing theory development: Successes and challenges. *Journal of Advanced Nursing, 12,* 63-67.
20. Johnson, J. L. (1991). Nursing science: Basic, applied or practical? Implications for the art of nursing. *Advances in Nursing Science, 14*(1), 7-16.
21. King, I. M. (1981). *A theory for nursing: Systems, concepts, process.* New York: John Wiley & Sons.
22. Kristjanson, L. J., Tamblyn, R., & Kuypers, J. A. (1987). A model to guide development and application of multiple nursing theories. *Journal of Advanced Nursing, 12,* 523-529.
23. Leininger, M. (Ed.). (1984). *Care: The essence of nursing and health.* Thorofare, N.J.: Slack.
24. Malinski, V. M. (Ed.). (1986). *Explorations on Martha Rogers' science of unitary human beings.* Norwalk, Conn: Appleton-Century-Crofts.
25. Mayberry, A. (1991). Merging nursing theories, models and nursing practice: More than an administrative challenge. *Nursing Administration Quarterly, 15*(3), 44-53.
26. Meleis, A. I. (1985). *Theoretical nursing: Development and progress.* Philadelphia: J. B. Lippincott.
27. Morse, J. M., Solberg, S. M., Neander, W. L., Bottorff, J. L., & Johnson, J. L. (1990). Concepts of caring and caring as a concept. *Advances in Nursing Science, 13*(1), 1-14.

28. Newman, M. A., Sime, A. M., & Corcoran-Perry, S. A. (1991). The focus of the discipline of nursing. *Advances in Nursing Science, 14*(1), 1-6.

29. Orlando, I. J. (1987). Nursing in the 21st century: Alternative paths. *Journal of Advanced Nursing, 12,* 405-412.

30. Parse, R. R. (1981). *Man-living-health: A theory of nursing.* New York: John Wiley & Sons.

31. Paterson, J. G., & Zderad, L. T. (1976). *Humanistic nursing.* New York: John Wiley & Sons.

32. Pender, N. J. (1990). Expressing health through lifestyle patterns. *Nursing Science Quarterly, 3*(3), 115-122.

33. Phillips, J. R. (1990). The different views of health. *Nursing Science Quarterly, 3*(3), 103-104.

34. Rogers, M. (1980). Nursing: A science of unitary man. In J. P. Riehl & C. Roy (Eds.), *Conceptual models for nursing practice* (2nd ed.). New York: Appleton-Century-Crofts.

35. Roy, C., & Roberts, S. L. (1981). *Theory construction in nursing: An adaptation model.* Englewood Cliffs, N.J.: Prentice-Hall.

36. Sarter, B. (1988). Philosophical sources of nursing theory. *Nursing Science Quarterly, 1*(2), 52-59.

37. Schlotfeldt, R. (1987). Defining nursing: A historic controversy. *Nursing Research, 36*(1), 64-67.

38. Schmiedling, N. J. (1986). Orlando's theory. In P. Winstead-Fry (Ed.), *Case studies in nursing theory.* New York: National League for Nursing.

39. Silva, M. C. (1987). Conceptual models of nursing. In J. J. Fitzpatrick & R. L. Taunton (Eds.), *Annual review of nursing research* (Vol. 5). New York: Springer.

40. Smith, M. J. (1988). Perspectives on nursing science. *Nursing Science Quarterly, 1*(2), 80-85.

41. Sorrentino, E. A. (1991). Making theories work for you. *Nursing Administration Quarterly, 15*(3), 54-59.

42. Stevens, B. J. (1984). *Nursing theory: Analysis, application, evaluation* (2nd ed.). Boston: Little, Brown.

43. Uys, L. R. (1987). Foundational studies in nursing. *Journal of Advanced Nursing, 12,* 275-280.

44. Walker, L. O., & Avant, K. C. (1983). *Strategies for theory construction in nursing.* Norwalk, Conn: Appleton-Century-Crofts.

45. Watson, J. (1985). *Nursing: Human science and human care.* Norwalk, Conn: Appleton-Century-Crofts.

46. Winstead-Fry, P., (Ed.). (1986). *Case studies in nursing.* New York: National League for Nursing.

CHAPTER 11

The primacy of practice in nursing

JANICE BRENCICK, GLENN WEBSTER

The argument in this chapter is consistent with the argument of "Nursing and the Philosophy of Science," published in the third edition of *Current Issues in Nursing*.[9] In that chapter an attempt was made to shed light on the controversy over whether and in what sense nursing is science. It was argued that nursing in the primary sense is a profession that makes use of the sciences. The distinction between science, discipline, and profession was examined along with the medieval historical ground for the notion of an academic discipline.[9]

TOOLS USED IN THIS CHAPTER

In this chapter, we pursue clarification of the concept of nursing by bringing several philosophical distinctions and other tools to bear on the current controversies surrounding the nature of nursing. Among the distinctions and tools is the distinction between primary and secondary meanings of a term or concept as employed by Aristotle and some medieval philosophers. The key notion here is that a term or concept may have a number of different but relatable meanings, with some being primary and others secondary. For example, in the phrases *a healthy person, a healthy complexion,* and *a healthy diet,* the meaning of *healthy* changes from phrase to phrase. But there is a primary sense: *healthy* as used in the phrase *healthy person,* for the other senses can be explained in terms of this sense.

A second tool is the distinction between the individual or nonrepeatable and the general or repeatable and the bearing this distinction has on controversies over the primary sense of the word *science.* Both the classical Greeks and many seventeenth-century thinkers believed that science to be science must be concerned with the general and not the particular.[1] Both history and nursing are concerned with the particular.

A third tool in supporting the primacy of nursing practice over nursing theory, nursing sciences, nursing education, and nursing administration is the Bergsonian distinction between intuitions and concepts.[2] Henri Bergson maintained that concepts were dead or fossilized intuitions; without intuitions there would be no concepts. A claim can be made that the source of intuitions needed for concepts in nursing is nursing practice.

Finally, Collingwood's distinction between ordinary science as concerned with the general and the science of history with its concern for knowledge of the individual or particular is of special relevance both to controversies about the primary meaning of "science" and to the situation of nursing in particular.[3] Both history and nursing are concerned ultimately with the particular, though both make use of knowledge of the general.

PROFESSION VERSUS SCIENCE

The distinction between a profession or practice, with its concern with creating new conditions and changing what is, and the preoccupation of theoretical science, with knowing what already is regardless of its value or desirability, remains in the background as fundamental to both this chapter and its predecessor. No profession wants to be limited by having to obey the conditions needed to be a science. Effecting changes in conditions and advancing knowledge are two separate goals that must not be confused because they are often incompatible. The scientist as a scientist only wants to know, he does not want to effect changes. To the contrary, the practicing professional is using knowledge acquired from the sciences to effect changes, and though success in effecting changes often provides indirect confirmation of the knowledge claims of the sciences employed, the goal of the professional is not the advancement of science but success in effecting changes.

The distinctions between profession and science and between the different types of science need to be drawn clearly enough for intelligibility, but in order not to be misapplied, it is necessary to blur those boundaries to make the conceptual map more representative of the actual territory.[10] The uses of two terms—*science* and *nursing* are central to the present discussion. Both terms have a family of uses or meanings rather than a single meaning. Furthermore, both terms can be construed to be "analogous" or "equivocally equivocal" after the pattern of *healthy* as examined by Aristotle in Book Delta of his *Metaphysics*.[1] This is not a result of faulty use of language but is a characteristic usually found in natural languages, such as English. The word or concept *nursing* shifts in meaning in the phrases *nursing profession, nursing care, nursing practice, nursing education, nursing administration, nursing science, nursing theory,* etc. It is the position of the present paper that the primary meaning of *nursing* is to be found in such phrases as *nursing care* and *nursing practice* and that relative to these meanings the other meanings are secondary, just as *healthy* in the phrase *a healthy person* is primary relative to its sense in the phrases *healthy diet* and *healthy complexion.*

THE PRIMARY MEANINGS OF SCIENCE AND NURSING

Much of the controversy concerning whether nursing is a science can be avoided by being clear about the relations between the two families of meanings—science and nursing. There are secondary meanings of both terms in which it is correct to say that "nursing is a science." But in the primary meanings of both terms "nursing is a science" is an incorrect or false statement, for nursing is a profession and the professions are not sciences in the primary meaning of *science.*

The primary meanings of science are meanings associated with such endeavors as physics, chemistry, biology, and other empirical sciences *where the major emphasis is on the attempt to gain knowledge of the general or repeatable aspects of major classes of actual entities within the real or actual world* in the respective domains of these disciplines. That the knowledge is tentative and fallible, rather than absolute and certain, taints even these uses of the term science with paradox, for science to be science the knowledge that is obtained should be certain.[4]

But to choose the "exact sciences," which are limited to certain branches of mathematics, such as geometry and arithmetic, and to symbolic logic, as primary is judged by most to be more paradoxical and less true; for though certainty is achieved in these disciplines, the knowledge is not about anything sufficiently real or substantial. These disciplines can be judged science in a sense that is primary relative to the sense in which physics is science. For science to be science, it must be about something fully real; for nursing theory to be nursing theory, it must be about nursing practice or some direct derivative of nursing practice. There are sciences whose domain is the deficiently real, but these are sciences in some secondary sense.

For a discipline to be accepted as science in the primary sense, its knowledge claims must be supportable by evidence and reason, and it must be knowledge of the more fully real, even though the knowledge is tentative and the reality only partially understood. The problem of the nature of the human sciences will not be addressed at any length here. Though some have claimed that nursing is a human science,[5,7,8] this poses a compound problem: It is not clear that there are (as yet) human sciences other than history, most are uncomfortable in granting that history is science in the primary sense, and nursing in its primary sense is not a science, and a fortiori not a human science.

However, the profession and practice of nursing might benefit greatly from the development of human sciences that do not as yet exist, and these might well deserve to be called "nursing sciences" because nursing would both create and use them. Nursing would create them because of its discovery that knowledge not supplied by any of the existing sciences is needed for nursing practice. However, these sciences would more properly be "sciences in service to nursing" than "nursing sciences," for they are apt to be of use to other professions than nursing and will stand as sciences on their own merits, as is the case with the so-called "medical sciences." For example, anatomy is independent of medicine and is used by both nursing and medicine, as well as by teenagers interested in knowing more about their own bodies.

HISTORY AND NURSING

History is sufficiently representative of the human sciences so that brief attention to the sense in which history is a science is helpful to the discussion of science and nursing. Furthermore, insofar as nursing is concerned with the care of a particular individual or a particular community at a particular time and place, nursing needs science of the particular and science of the general. The nursing sciences alluded to in the preceding paragraph might differ from history only in their tighter focus on some particular individual or community, a tighter focus motivated by the needs for the care of this particular individual or community.

History in the human science sense is used by the nurse to deduce the nature and origin of the patient's problem in order to intervene not just in the present, but in such a manner as to prevent future recurrences of the problem. The taking of a client history in nursing can be facilitated by the nurse learning to do more "scientific" history. The historian is never content to rely on a single source, on verbal or written reports only, but uses the oral reports as evidence for the construction of a narrative that will raise further questions to be answered by physical evidence, such as lab reports and reports of other people than the primary source.[3] The better the narrative, the better the questions, the more extensive becomes the corroborating evidence; for the better understood an historical event or particular patient becomes, the more connections develop between that event or patient and the rest of the contemporary world. In comparing nursing and history, it must be remembered that the historian simply wants to know or understand; the practicing nurse wants to know in order to facilitate changes in the condition of the patient.

One actual example from nursing practice illustrates the usefulness of history for nursing: an elderly patient fell in her home and broke her hip. Without a careful patient history, the attending physician attributed the fall to the patient simply getting old and consequently he wanted to place the patient in a nursing home. But a more careful case history by her nurse revealed that the patient had a worn-out pair of slippers that had long since lost their tread and, in addition, a throw carpet similarly bereft of antiskid protection. These were the causes of the fall, rather than her simply getting old. Otherwise, the patient was in full charge of her faculties, more responsible in many respects than many younger people. A few simple changes—new slippers and a better rug—postponed going to the nursing home indefinitely.

The problem with history, so far as it might claim to be a science in the primary sense, is that the historian is not trying to know the general or repeatable. The historian is trying to justify knowledge claims about particular human actions in a particular place at a particular time. In his history of Roman Britain, R. G. Collingwood[3] was concerned with the construction of what is referred to on contemporary maps as Hadrian's Wall, stretching from the Solway Firth on the west to the coast on the east, forming the boundary between England and Scotland during Roman times.

The construction of a patient history by a nurse is similar to the attempt to perfect a narrative of happenings in Hadrian's time by Collingwood. The difference between the nurse and the historian is that even historical knowledge in nursing is ancillary to care in a manner analogous to that in which knowledge of the general was ancillary to the development of historical knowledge for the historian. The practicing nurse used her knowledge that the patient's fall was caused by poor slippers and carpet to make simple changes that helped prevent future falls, thus avoiding the need to curtail the patient's freedom by placing her in a nursing home. The historian in contrast was content to understand Hadrian's purpose in the construction of his wall. Perhaps such knowledge might be useful to contemporary military strategists, but that was of no concern to the historian.

THE MEANINGS OF *SCIENCE*

Because of nursing practice's focus on the particular, nursing shares with history a controversy over whether there can be science of the particular. A comparison of what Collingwood was doing in Roman Britain with what Erwin Hubble was doing in his *Realm of the Nebulae* sheds some light on the controversy over whether history is science in the primary sense. Both writers were scientists in the sense of examining and weighing the evidence in favor of particular narratives or stories concerning some part of the actual world. Collingwood was concerned with the effects of past human actions in the second century of the Christian Era on the boundary between Scotland and England. Erwin Hubble, in contrast, was concerned with the behavior of all galaxies within the observable universe—that they all moved apart from one another with velocities that increased in proportion to distances. This difference does not seem as significant as their attempt to know and to use the best reasons and evidence for answering their questions about the domain under examination. We side with Collingwood because of nursing's need for science of the particular in addition to science of the general. We support the claims of history to be science in a primary sense.

However this dispute is finally settled; nursing practice needs both science of the particular, as in the case of histories, and science of the general, as in the case of theories about infection, respiration, etc., to effect changes that ameliorate present problems and forestall the occurrence of future problems. Whether or not the seventeenth-century fascination with knowledge of nature under the aspect of eternity was a mistake is not relevant to nursing's needs in the care of patients in the late twentieth century. But the success of nursing practice will add some credence to the claims of history and other human sciences to be science in the primary sense, for nursing is finding the human sciences, history, anthropology, sociology, and etymology to be at least as useful to nursing practice as such natural sciences as biology, physiology, and anatomy.

Science has secondary meanings relative to the above meanings. The professions, including engineering, can be construed to be sciences in secondary senses—secondary because viewing "know how" as knowledge is possible because of the clearer understanding we have of knowledge in the case of *knowledge that.* *Techne* (art in the sense of craft) and *praxis* (action) are sciences in senses secondary to the sense of science in *episteme* (knowledge). In the Greek world view, *episteme* was possible only of the eternal or the general, which was a major historical cause of the prejudice in favor of limiting science in the primary sense to the study of nature under the aspect of eternity. *Techne* and *praxis* by contrast are concerned with the changeable, temporal, and particular. But *techne* is *techne* not because it is a science of the particular, like history, but because it is concerned with changing things, creating things, rather than with just knowing what already is. Hence, *techne* and *praxis* are two steps removed from science in the primary sense.

The caring that is primary to nursing is an instance of *techne* rather than *episteme.* Nursing practice is concerned with changing the condition or status of the client, not with simply knowing what it is. Furthermore, like history and unlike physics, nursing is concerned in the first instance with the individual, with the particular client or community. In nursing, as in history, the general is ancillary to the individual; knowledge of the general is used to facilitate knowledge of the individual. But nursing, unlike any of the sciences, is concerned with changing things rather than with just knowing what is (or was).

Nursing in its primary sense, nursing practice, escapes the criticism of Feuerbach and Marx that "the philosophers have only *interpreted* the world, in various ways; the point, however, is to *change* it."[6] But nursing in its primary sense is science only in one of science's secondary senses. But that this is so is the truth in the claim of some that nursing is a science and perhaps a human science. But it is better to say that nursing uses human science rather than it is a human science, for nursing practice makes use of all of the sciences, both of the general and the particular, of the physical and the human.

Why have many nurses been concerned to classify nursing as a science? Among many factors several pressures have been exerted in this direction. First, the National Science Foundation is better funded than the National Endowment for the Humanities. It is monetarily better to be a science, especially a physical science. Second, science, especially science of the general after the fashion of Newtonian physics, has enjoyed high prestige for the past several centuries. In the struggle to elevate the status of nursing, association with the physical sciences is tempting, as it has been for medicine.

But neither medicine nor nursing is a science in the primary sense. The professions of medicine, nursing, and engineering are consumers of science. There may be nursing sciences or medical sciences, in the sense of sciences of special interest or importance to these respective professions, but these sciences will not be "nursing" or "medical" in a primary sense; they will always be something else such as history or etiology.

THE PRIMACY OF PRACTICE

Combining insights from Aristotle, R. G. Collingwood, and Henri Bergson, it is possible to generate several straightforward arguments for the primacy of practice within nursing. Nursing education is called *nursing* education because it is needed to produce new nurses for the practice of nursing. Nursing administration is *nursing* administration because of its concern with facilitating the practice of nursing. Nursing theory is *nursing* theory because it is reflection on the practice of nursing. And so it is for each of the other secondary meanings of nursing; they are meanings of nursing because of their relationship to the practice of nursing. In nursing practice, we find the primary meaning of nursing that grounds the entire family of secondary meanings.

Another argument for the primacy of nursing follows the lines of a similar argument concerning history and the philosophy of history used by R. G. Collingwood in the introduction to his *Idea of History*. There he observed that two conditions are necessary for doing adequate philosophy of history. To be a good philosopher of history, one must be both a philosopher on the one hand, and a practicing historian on the other hand; for philosophy of history is reflection on the science of history. Unless one is a historian, there is nothing concrete to reflect upon. The reflective thinking needed for *philosophy* of history is second level thinking about the thinking of the scientific historian.[3]

In nursing theory and the philosophy of nursing the same conditions exist as necessary for good theory and philosophy of nursing. The *intuitions* that are the sources of the concepts needed for theory and philosophy occur in nursing practice. These intuitions are in their first instances experiences of the unique and nonrepeatable; for instance, a caring moment, a successful intervention, with a particular patient in a unique situation.

In Henri Bergson's philosophy, concepts are dead or dying intuitions, for at best they preserve some repeatable aspect of the nonrepeatable.[2] And this repeatable aspect remains meaningful only so long as the nonrepeatable source, though past is still present. Without new intuitions as sources for the regeneration of the concepts, the concepts soon lose their meaningfulness through a fading of the past. Good theory is not possible without practice, and the point of theory is the enhancement of practice. One initially comes to nursing practice already possessing theories or a philoso-phy, but these are originally not *nursing* theories or philosophy. A living relationship to practice is necessary to make theories *nursing* theories. Practice is the core of the profession of nursing and the source of all of the concepts of nursing. Hence, clinical practice is essential to all other aspects of nursing.

REFERENCES

1. Aristotle. (1933). *Aristotle XVII: Metaphysics I-IX* (Hugh Tredennick, Trans.). Cambridge, Mass: Harvard University Press (Loeb Classical Library).
2. Bergson, H. (1935). *The two sources of morality and religion.* New York: Holt, Rinehart & Winston.
3. Collingwood, R. G. (1946). *The idea of history.* Oxford: Clarendon Press.
4. Descartes. (1641). Meditations on first philosophy. In E. Anscombe & P. Geach, *Descartes: Philosophical writings.* London: Thomas Nelson & Sons, 1954.
5. Leininger, M. (1984). *Care: The essence of nursing and health.* Thorofare, N.J.: Charles B. Slack.
6. Marx, K. (1959). In L. S. Fever (Ed.), *Marx & Engels: Basic writings on politics & philosophy.* Garden City, N.Y.: Doubleday (Anchor Books).
7. Parse, R. R. (1981). *Man-living-health: A theory of nursing.* New York: John Wiley & Sons.
8. Watson, J. (1988). *Nursing: Human science and human care.* New York: National League for Nursing.
9. Webster, G. A. (1990). Nursing and the philosophy of science. In J. C. McCloskey & H. K. Grace (Eds.), *Current issues in nursing* (3rd ed., pp. 12-16). St Louis: Mosby.
10. Webster, G. A., & Brencick, J. M. (in press). *Nomenclature and classification systems: Ten years later.* Proceedings of the Tenth Conference on Nursing Diagnoses. NANDA.

CHAPTER 12

The nursing theory–nursing research connection

MARY A. BLEGEN, TONI TRIPP-REIMER

In any discipline, science is the result of the interplay between the process of inquiry (research) and the product of knowledge (theory). The purpose of research is to build knowledge in a discipline through the generation or testing of theory. In nursing the relationship between research and theory has not been well understood. In this chapter, an overview of the historical context in which nursing theory and research emerged as separate entities is presented, myths regarding nursing theory are identified, and the nature of the relationship between theory and research is examined. The purpose of this endeavor is to examine popular myths regarding nursing theory while also providing a perspective for the advancement of nursing science.

HISTORY OF THE INTERFACE OF NURSING THEORY AND RESEARCH

Theory and research were first integrated in the works of Nightingale. Her treatise *Notes on Nursing* (first published in 1859) is now widely considered to be the first writing in nursing theory. In this monograph and elsewhere, Nightingale widely identified the need to organize nursing knowledge through observation, recording, and statistical inferences. Furthermore, she supported her theoretical positions through research. For example, when officials of the India office were not forthcoming with a request for mortality and morbidity rates of the British army in India, Nightingale devised an extensive questionnaire and sent it to 200 British stations in India. The problem the questionnaire addressed was the need for sanitary reform in India. In 14 sections, the questionnaire included such topics as the topography, climate, diet, and burial patterns. Nightingale collated the results, summarized the descriptive statistics, prepared graphs, and interpreted the results.[34] These efforts are illustrative of what is considered to be the first efforts in nursing research. They were informed by and reinforced her conceptualizations of the importance of sanitation for the health of the troops.

However, after this initial integration, theory and research developed separately. This is illustrated in Harris's[17] review of 152 doctoral studies (1928-1959) by nurse authors, in which she found only two that suggested having a theoretical basis for nursing research. Factors promoting the separate evolution of research and theory in nursing are presented below.

THE EMERGENCE OF NURSING THEORY

Immediately after Nightingale, most writings on nursing were in the form of procedural recommendations or admonitions. For example, in 1898, in *Nursing: Its Principles and Practice,* Hampton [15] included coverage of such topics as ward supplies, beds, sick room hygiene, baths, and diet.

Conceptual or theoretical developments in nursing for three quarters of the past century were written predominantly to define and differentiate the discipline. In the first part of the 20th century a few definitional statements could be found in the works of pioneers such as Goodrich[14] and Hampton.[15] Many of these early statements focused on nursing's functions and its expanding role. They emphasized nursing's social mandate as not only caring for the sick, but also preventing illness through health education. Harmer, for example, defined the object of nursing as "not only to cure the sick and heal the wounded, but to . . . prevent disease and to preserve health."[16]

Some[14] also were part of a call for nursing education to increasingly be placed in university settings. The movement toward university education was given impetus through the report of the Committee for the Study of Nursing Education[13] and later by the Brown[3] report. While the Goldmark report stressed the need of a broad liberal education for nurses, the Brown report responded affirmatively to two pressing questions of nursing of that day: Can nursing develop a specific content of its own? Will nurse educators ever engage in any considerable amount of research and writing, which for some universities is the hallmark of the right to be included within the fraternity of higher education?[3]

Midcentury writings on conceptualizations of nursing had multiple purposes. They were statements, devised in large part, for the purpose of delineating a separate professional identity from medicine. The development of early conceptual models of nursing[29,30] were both reflective of and contributed to a movement toward an autonomous discipline. Many of these early models reflected the need, as Ujhely noted, "to answer the questions 'What is nursing?' and 'What is unique in nursing?' "[37] The answer increasingly was framed[1] as a movement away from a focus on disease and procedures (which had been met through a functional nursing approach) toward an interpersonally based problem-solving approach focusing on comprehensive nursing (care of the whole patient). In addition, these models served to guide curricula as schools of nursing increasingly moved away from the medical model toward something uniquely nursing.

These conceptual pioneers drew on their experiences in university settings where social and psychological sciences were increasingly important. Many[30,35,37] focused on the interpersonal aspects of care, giving increased attention to social dynamics. In the 1960s, theoretical formulations became increasingly self-conscious. At this time, several national conferences were held, primarily sponsored by the Public Health Service Division of Nursing. These conferences, held between 1967 and 1970, included the Symposium on Theory Development in Nursing held at Case Western Reserve University, three Nursing Theory Conferences held at the University of Kansas, and two conferences on the Nature of Nursing Science at the University of Colorado. At each of these sessions, leaders in the disciplines of nursing, behavioral sciences, and philosophy discussed metatheoretical issues about the discipline of nursing. Papers and discussions focused on the nature of practice theory, the necessity for theory, criteria for theory evaluation, and the relative merits of theory outside of nursing. These conferences laid the foundation for the direction of theory development in nursing for the subsequent two decades.

The National League of Nursing also contributed to the proliferation of nursing conceptual models. In 1972, the League established an explicit mandate that nursing curricula should be based on a conceptual framework in order to be accredited.[26] This fostered the development and concretization of nursing conceptual models. The models that emerged were very important to the development of an autonomous discipline. The evolution of nursing theory from brief definitions and philosophical statements to the emergence of broad relatively nonspecific conceptual models served to differentiate nursing practice from medical practice. They were useful to that end.

Later models, while still concerned with defining and delineating the scope of nursing, also were used as frameworks for curricula in collegiate schools of nursing.[18,20,27] These models provided a broad orientation to the field, which was and is primarily useful in the education of undergraduate students. These students, as well as beginning practitioners, may use the models as templates to cognitively organize their nursing care. However, the structure provided by these models is generally abandoned as practitioners gain clinical expertise.

However, with regard to the relationship between theory and research, this approach currently provides blocks to progress. Although the formulations are useful for defining the discipline and for teaching undergraduate students, they are too nonspecific to be suitable for testing. The broad orientation provided by these models is not appropriate for framing or interpreting research.

The theory level appropriate for advancing nursing science is mid-range theory. Theory at this level is a system of statements about the relationship between two or more concepts defined at a moderate level of abstraction. Mid-range theory attempts to describe, explain, or predict circumscribed phenomena. For example, Mishel's[23,24] Illness Uncertainty Theory predicts clients' response to illness on the basis of their understanding the facts of their illness and treatment plan.

Mid-range theory, the level appropriate for a relationship with research, is rarely discussed in texts on theory development. These texts[5,11,12,31] perpetuate the importance of the broader conceptual models. It is also noteworthy that these texts, in focusing on analysis and evaluation of nursing models, rarely identify the utility of the models for research. When mid-range theories are identified, they are often criticized for lack of clarity or completeness (e.g., discussion of Barnard in Marriner-Tomey[22]).

THE FABRICATION OF THE NURSING PARADIGM

In its efforts to be taken seriously as a science, nursing looked to philosophy and sociology of science to determine appropriate disciplinary characteristics. Unfortunately, this assistance led to an overly analytical approach to the development of the discipline, which can be illustrated in the evolution of the "myth of the nursing paradigm."

In the 1960s and 1970s, a very popular topic was Kuhn's[21,33] discussion of paradigms and scientific revolutions. Kuhn proposed that a discipline's paradigm is a way of delineating and viewing phenomena that fall within the scope of a discipline. Furthermore, the paradigm guides the methodology of the discipline. Kuhn also termed this the metaparadigm or disciplinary matrix.

The emergence of the myth

In 1975, the results of a survey of baccalaureate curricula indicated that four "subconcepts" were the most commonly identified components taught in nursing: man, society, health, and nursing.[38] Referring to the survey three years later, Fawcett[9] noted that person, environment, health, and nursing were the concepts specifying the phenomena of interest to nursing science. In 1984, she declared that they constituted the paradigm (or metaparadigm) of nursing.[10]

However, this was an overly simplistic and uncritical perspective on paradigms. Three of the four concepts (person, environment, and health) are also of interest to other disciplines (such as epidemiology, medical social work, medicine, dentistry, pharmacy, and psychology). Further, while other disciplines' perspectives of these concepts may differ from that of nursing, nursing itself also shows considerable variation in its approaches to these constructs. Consequently, neither the constructs themselves, nor their particular formulation is unique to nursing.

THE EMERGENCE OF NURSING RESEARCH

After Nightingale's time, research conducted by nurses was quite rare. The *American Journal of Nursing* was initiated in 1900 and contained case studies as well as a few practice focused research reports.[6] However, the most significant research of the period concerned educational and professional issues and were sponsored by private organizations, such as the Rockefeller Foundation[13] and the Russell Sage Foundation.[3]

The first journal of nursing science, *Nursing Research,* was initiated in 1952. In early years, nursing research focused on education and characteristics of nurses rather than on aspects of nursing diagnoses and interventions. Clinical topics were generally neglected. Newman, for example, categorized articles published in *Nursing Research* from 1952 to 1968.[28] Predominant research of the time focused on roles and characteristics of nurses; only 12% of the articles addressed nursing process or human behavior. However, in subsequent years the proportion of structural to clinical research has shifted. From 1968 to 1972, the proportion of articles emphasizing the functions and characteristics of nurses decreased to 24%, and articles investigating aspects of nursing practice and human behavior rose to 36%. By 1976, nearly half of the articles published were categorized as clinical studies;[4] this increased to over 75% by 1990.[36] A clear trend of articles reported in *Nursing Research* indicates a movement from research emphasizing nursing education and nursing roles to that focused on clinical practice.

Significant foundation and public support of research training and funding also emerged during the 1950s. In the middle of that decade, the Commonwealth Fund provided financial support to the National League for Nursing for research training, the American Nurses Foundation (a grant award unit) was established as an arm of the American Nurses Association, and the U.S. Public Health Service established the Nursing Grants and Fellowships Program, which provided funds for research projects and predoctoral training. Shortly after these events in 1957, the Walter Reed Army Institute of Research established its division of nursing research, which fostered the development and productivity of a core of nurse investigators. Other initiatives to promote nursing research and training include the Faculty Research Development Grant program (1959-1966), the Research Development Program, and the Nurse Scientist Program.

Until the mid-1950s most doctorally prepared nurses received their terminal degrees in the field of education. Subsequently, nurses were encouraged to obtain doctoral degrees in natural and social sciences through the Nurse Scientist Program initiated in 1962.

As nurses received doctoral degrees in other sciences, considerable debate was generated regarding the appropriateness of "borrowed" versus "unique" theories.

However, nursing was not preparing its own doctorates. The first nursing PhD program was initiated at the University of Pittsburgh in 1954 (in maternal-child nursing), and a DNS in psychiatric nursing at Boston University was begun in 1960. Since that time, more than 50 schools have established doctoral programs in nursing. With preparation in both the content and methods of the discipline, new students can more readily integrate the discipline's theory and research.

The late 1970s saw a proliferation of journals dedicated to nursing research and science, including *Research in Nursing and Health, The Western Journal of Nursing Research,* and *Advances in Nursing Science.* In the next decade initiation of the *Annual Review of Nursing Research* in 1983 indicated that there was a sufficiently large body of research to be synthesized in an integrated research review. "State of the Science" articles in *Image* attested the same.

The National Center for Nursing Research was authorized as a component of the National Institutes of Health in 1985 and was formally established in 1986. Components of the NCNR are Health Promotion/Disease Prevention; Acute and Chronic Illness; and Nursing Systems. The center's mission is the "conduct and support of, and dissemination of information respecting, basic and clinical nursing research, training, and other programs in patient care research." The mandate clearly has shifted from that on nurses and nursing education to nursing practice and patient care. Further, support of the center clearly indicates nursing has come of age as a health science.

TOWARD BUILDING THE SCIENCE OF NURSING

The science of nursing has matured as a result of the interplay of theory and research. The interdependence of these two dimensions has been previously noted.[2,8] However, the nature and necessity of this relationship have not received sufficient acceptance. Evidence of slow acceptance includes the publication of atheoretical research, as well as a continued emphasis on the conceptual models of nursing rather than on mid-range theory construction.

Over a quarter of a century ago, Schwab[32] depicted an important relationship between theory and research. In delineating the components of the structure of a discipline, Schwab noted that there are two major elements: the substantive structure and the syntactical structure. The substantive structure comprises the content and concepts underlying the discipline. Syntactical structure includes modes of inquiry, canons of evidence, and the natural history of data from interpretation through conclusion. The relationship between the substantive and syntactical structure (theory and research) is symbiotic and mutually reinforcing. In fact, the existence of one is contingent, in the long term, on the development of the other.

The importance of the relationship between theory and research has been recognized in nursing. The attempts to specify the linkage between nursing theory and research have used hierarchical levels of theory development and increasing levels of control in research designs; that is, descriptive theory and exploratory research, explanatory theory and descriptive (correlational) research, predictive theory and experimental research, and prescriptive theory and randomized clinical trials.[7,19,25] These formulations work, to a certain extent, because there is a rough correspondence between the level of a theory and the level of a research design generating or testing that theory. However, prescribing research designs to correspond discretely with each of these levels of theory is inappropriate.

Previous attempts to provide guidance for linking theory and research[25] have been helpful but are too broad to direct most research. Theory as a whole is still the most important driving force behind the research plan, but specific linkages between theory and a particular project are provided by two additional considerations: the nature of the phenomena being investigated and the particular piece of the theory being developed.

The linkage between the theory and the research is formed through the decisions made about the research problem and the purpose of the project. These decisions about research problem and purpose are made on the basis of present knowledge (theory) and the nature of the phenomenon. The statement of the research problem is a specification of the knowledge needed in that area, the piece of the theory that will be developed. The purpose of the research project identifies how that project will provide the knowledge, the design that will be used.

Research without theory results in discrete, disparate, particularistic data. While these data may be useful within a unique setting to solve a unique problem, they do not add to the accumulated knowledge of a science.

Similarly, theory without research is mental massage; while not unpleasant, this exercise is a waste of scientific resources.

REFERENCES

1. Abdellah, F. G., Beland, I. L., Martin, S., & Matheney, R. V. (1960). *Patient-centered approaches to nursing.* New York: Macmillan.
2. Benoliel, J. Q. (1977). The interaction between theory and research. *Nursing Outlook, 25,* 108-113.
3. Brown, E. L. (1948). *Nursing for the future.* New York: Russell Sage.
4. Carnegie, M. (1977). Editor's report. *Nursing Research, 26, 3.*
5. Chinn, P. L., & Kramer, M. K. (1991). *Theory and nursing: A systematic approach* (3rd ed.). St Louis: Mosby.
6. Clayton, S. L. (1927). Standardizing nursing techniques, its advantages and disadvantages. *American Journal of Nursing, 27,* 939-943.
7. Diers, D. (1979). *Research in nursing practice.* Philadelphia: J. B. Lippicott.
8. Fawcett, J. (1978). The relationship between theory and research: A double helix. *Advances in Nursing Science, 1*(1), 49-62.
9. Fawcett, J. (1978). The "What" of theory development. In The National League for Nursing (Ed.), *Theory development: What, why, how?* New York: National League for Nursing.
10. Fawcett, J. (1984). The metaparadigm of nursing: Present status and future refinements. *Image: The Journal of Nursing Scholarship, 16,* 84-89.
11. Fawcett, J. (1989). *Analysis and reevaluation of conceptual models of nursing.* Philadelphia: F. A. Davis.
12. Fitzpatrick, J. J., & Whall, A. L. (Eds.). (1989). *Conceptual models of nursing.* Norwalk, Conn: Appleton and Lange.
13. Goldmark, J. (1923). *Nursing and nursing education in the United States: Landmark report.* New York: Macmillan.
14. Goodrich, A. W. (1932; 1912 orig). The need for orientation. *The social and ethical significance of nursing.* New York: Macmillan.
15. Hampton, I. H. (1898). *Nursing: Its principles and practice for hospitals and private use.* Cleveland: Koechert.
16. Harmer, B. (1922). *Textbook of the principles and practice of nursing.* New York: Macmillan.
17. Harris, M. I. (1971). Theorybuilding in nursing. *Image: The Journal of Nursing Scholarship, 4*(1), 6-10.
18. Hawkins, J. W. (1983). Historical development of models of nursing practice. In J. A. Thibodeua (Ed.), *Nursing models: Analysis and evaluation* (pp. 27-42). Monterey, Calif: Wadsworth.
19. Hinshaw, A. S. (1979). Problems in doing research. *Western Journal of Nursing Research, 3,* 251-253.
20. King, I. M. (1981). *Toward a theory for nursing.* New York: John Wiley & Sons.
21. Kuhn, T. S. (1962). *The structure of scientific revolutions.* Chicago: University of Chicago Press.
22. Marriner-Tomey, A. (1986). *Nursing theorists and their work.* St Louis: Mosby.
23. Mishel, M. H. (1981). The measurement of uncertainty in illness. *Nursing Research, 30,* 258-263.
24. Mishel, M. H. (1984). Perceived uncertainty and stress in illness. *Research in Nursing and Health, 7,* 163-171.
25. Moody, L. E. (1990). *Advancing nursing science through research.* Newbury Park, Calif: Sage.
26. National League for Nursing. (1972). *Criteria for the appraisal of baccalaureate and higher degree programs in nursing.* New York: Author.
27. Neuman, B. (1982). *The Neuman systems model: Application to nursing education and practice.* Norwalk, Conn: Appleton-Century-Crofts.
28. Newman, M. (1972). Nursing's theoretical evolution. *Nursing Outlook, 20,* 449-453.
29. Orlando, I. (1961). *The dynamic nurse-patient relationship.* New York: Putnam.
30. Peplau, H. (1952). *Interpersonal relations in nursing.* New York: Putnam.
31. Riehl-Sisca, J. (1989). *Conceptual models for nursing practice.* Norwalk, Conn: Appleton-Century-Crofts.
32. Schwab, J. (1964). Structure of the disciplines: Meanings and significances. In G. W. Ford & L. Pugna (Eds.), *The structure of knowledge and the curriculum.* Chicago: Rand McNally.
33. Shapere, D. (1977). Scientific theories and their domains. In F. Suppe (Ed.), *The structure of scientific theories.* Chicago: University of Illinois Press.
34. Smith, F. B. (1982). *Florence Nightingale: Reputation and power.* London: Croom Helm.
35. Travelbee, J. (1966). *Interpersonal aspects of nursing.* Philadelphia: F. A. Davis.
36. Tripp-Reimer, T. (1991). Class notes (November). Theory construction in nursing, The University of Iowa College of Nursing. Iowa City, Iowa.
37. Ujhely, G. B. (1968). *Determinants of the nurse-patient relationship.* New York: Springer.
38. Yura, H., & Torres, G. (1975). Today's conceptual framework within baccalaureate nursing programs. In National League for Nursing (Ed.), *Conceptual framework: Its meaning and function.* New York: National League for Nursing.

CHAPTER 13

The reorganization of nursing knowledge

MAXINE E. LOOMIS

If we had a keen vision and feeling of all ordinary human life, it would be like hearing the grass grow and the squirrel's heart beat, and we should die of that roar which lies on the other side of silence.
GEORGE ELIOT[10]

Science must be understood as a social phenomenon, a gutsy human enterprise, not the work of robots programmed to collect pure information. Science, since people must do it, is a socially imbedded activity. It progresses by hunch, vision, and intuition. Much of its change through time does not record a closer approach to absolute truth, but the alteration of cultural contexts that influence it so strongly.
STEPHEN JAY GOULD[14]

Many nursing scientists and theoreticians are currently working to assist the profession to examine and value "the other side of silence." They are giving voice to questions, such as: What do patients do to help themselves get well or feel better? How do patients manage chronic health problems? How do nurses care about and for patients? This qualitative approach is being conducted against a backdrop of personal and political reform in the health care system, a canvas upon which nursing is being viewed in its social context.

Nursing leaders provide the initial structure within which students learn and nurses practice. This structure must resemble current reality enough to be credible, yet it must challenge that reality to further and improve the practice of nursing. An initial review of the various systems used to categorize nursing research and nursing practice will be followed by a discussion of the structure of the discipline of nursing. Finally, a recent model is presented in an attempt to explore the similarities and differences between the science and practice of nursing.

CLASSIFICATION OF NURSING RESEARCH

Research means to search or investigate thoroughly. It is a process of investigation or experimentation aimed at the discovery and interpretation of facts, the revision of accepted theories or laws in the light of new facts, or the practical application of such new or revised theories or laws. Research provides the bridge between the academic discipline of nursing science and the professional practice of nursing therapeutics. Research should be either theory testing or theory generating in nature, and this union of research and theory should provide the foundation for nursing practice.

Major trends in nursing research have been documented by Roberts;[38] Brown;[5] Simmons and Henderson;[44] Abdellah;[1] Notter;[35] Gortner, Bloch, and Phillips;[12] and Gortner and Nahm.[13] These reviews produced a clear lineage of the progress of nursing research over the past decades.

Despite the relative paucity of nursing research at that time, Simmons and Henderson[44] developed a comprehensive list of categories that included historical, philosophical, and cultural studies; issues related to the conduct of research (facilities, personnel, support, and method); and categories that can be grouped into the broad areas of nursing practice, education, and administration.

As nursing research progressed, Abdellah[1] developed a comprehensive classification of research projects in nursing supported by the United States Public Health Service (USPHS) from 1955 to 1968 (see box at right). The 167 grants distributed across the following categories reflect the goals of the USPHS at the time: health care personnel in nursing (22.1%); measurement of patient care systems (15.6%); the nurse role and its impact on patient care systems (15.5%); organizations of patient care systems and their impact on the delivery of health services (15.5%); faculty research development grants (11.3%); clinical research of problems related to nursing practice (7%); health communication systems affecting patient care (6%); model and theory development (6%); and health economic systems affecting patient care (1%).

Gortner, Block, and Phillips[12] elaborated the subcategories of building a science of practice and an artistry of practice, establishing structures for optimal delivery of care, developing methodology, and application of research findings in their review of the contributions of nursing research to patient care (see the box on page 94). Gortner and Nahm[13] presented a historical overview of nursing research in the United States that included developments in nursing education and nursing practice research, as well as the development of research resources.

In its 25th anniversary year, *Nursing Research* published 5 articles reviewing the history of clinical nursing research from 1952 through 1975 by specialty area. Barnard and Neal[4] reviewed 78 manuscripts from *Nursing Research* from 1952 to 1976, the ANA *Clinical Conference Series* from 1965 to 1973, and the WICHE *Communicating Nursing Research* series from 1968 to 1973 that related to maternal-child health (see the box on page 94). They reported studies in the following categories: care of the sick or hospitalized child (23%), childrearing (18%), special populations (12.8%), childbearing (11.5%), nurse's role (10.3%), and breast care and breast-feeding (6.4%). Their approach was based on human growth and development, recognizing deviations from the norm and the role of the nurse.

Highriter[17] reviewed 115 community health nursing articles obtained through a MEDLARS worldwide

CLASSIFICATION OF USPHS-SUPPORTED RESEARCH PROJECTS IN NURSING, 1955-1968

	No.	%
1. Clinical research of problems related to nursing practice	12	7
(cardiac nursing, nursing in chronic illness, intensive care nursing, mental health and psychiatric nursing, parent-child health nursing, rehabilitation nursing, cancer nursing, medical-surgical nursing)		
2. Model and theory development	10	6
(application of models and theories)		
3. Measurement of patient care systems	26	15.6
(methodologies used to measure quality patient care, quality of nursing care—criteria of nursing practice)		
4. Organizations of patient care systems and their impact on the delivery of health services	25	15.5
(hospital-based studies, outpatient and extra-hospital-based studies)		
5. The nurse role and its impact on patient care systems	26	15.5
(role behaviors, clinical nurse specialist role)		
6. Health economic systems affecting patient care	2	1
7. Health care personnel in nursing	37	22.1
(recruitment, selection, and evaluation; research in nursing education programs—teaching methods and curricula; the professionalization process in nursing; historical research)		
8. Health communications systems	10	6
(research conferences, tools for research)		
9. Faculty research development grants	19	11.3
TOTAL	167	100 %

From: Abdellah, F. G. (1970). Overview of nursing research 1955-1968, Parts 1, 2, and 3. *Nursing Research, 19,* 6-17, 151-162, 239-252. Copyright 1970 The American Journal of Nursing Company. Used with permission. All rights reserved.

CONTRIBUTIONS OF NURSING RESEARCH TO PATIENT CARE

1. Building a science of practice
2. Refining the artistry of practice (clinical therapeutics)
3. Establishing structures for optimal patient care
4. Developing methodology
5. Application of research findings

From: Gortner, S. R., Bloch, D., & Phillips, T. R. (1976, March/April). Contributions of nursing research to patient care. *Journal of Nursing Administration*, p. 23.

THE HISTORY OF CLINICAL NURSING RESEARCH, 1952-1975

Maternal-child nursing research	No.	%
1. Care of the sick or hospitalized child	18	23
2. Childrearing	14	18
3. Newborn, term, and premature infants	13	18
4. Special populations	10	12.8
5. Childbearing	9	11.5
6. Nurse's role	8	10.3
7. Breast care and breast-feeding	5	6.4
TOTAL	77	100

From: Barnard, K. E., & Neal, M. V. (1977). Maternal-child nursing research: Review of the past and strategies for the future. *Nursing Research, 26,* p. 193. Copyright 1977 The American Journal of Nursing Company. Used with permission. All rights reserved.

---

search and published from 1972 through 1976 (see the box top right). Her report included review and methodology studies (31.3%), service evaluation studies (24.4%), client need assessment (13%), service description studies (13%), community health nursing education (11.3%), and attitude studies (7%). These categories reflect an emphasis on delivery systems and client aggregates. Ellis[9] summarized the most prevalent medical-surgical nursing studies (see the box above, right). These included over 200 such studies published in *Nursing Research* from 1952 through 1975 and involved preoperative and postoperative teaching, patients with cardiac disease, and patients with diabetes mellitus. A secondary set of studies of patients with tuberculosis, neurologic or orthopedic problems, or pulmonary or gastrointestinal disorders was also cited. Emphasis in this body of research was on patient condition.

THE HISTORY OF CLINICAL NURSING RESEARCH, 1952-1975

Community health nursing research	No.	%
1. Service evaluation	28	24.4
2. Client need assessment	15	13
3. Service description studies	15	13
4. Community health nursing education	13	11.3
5. Attitude studies	8	7
6. Study reviews and methodology	36	31.3
TOTAL	115	100

From: Highriter, M. E. (1977). The status of community health nursing research. *Nursing Research, 26,* p. 183. Copyright 1977 The American Journal of Nursing Company. Used with permission. All rights reserved.

THE HISTORY OF CLINICAL NURSING RESEARCH, 1952-1975

Medical-surgical nursing research
1. *Most prevalent*
   A. Preoperative or postoperative nursing care
   B. Patients with cardiac disease
   C. Patients with diabetes mellitus
2. *Next most frequently studied*
   A. Patients with tuberculosis
   B. Patients with neurologic or orthopedic problems
   C. Patients with pulmonary disorders
   D. Patients with gastrointestinal disorders

From: Ellis, R. (1977). Failabilities, fragments and frames: Contemplation on 25 years of research in medical-surgical nursing. *Nursing Research, 26,* p. 177. Copyright 1977 The American Journal of Nursing Company. Used with permission. All rights reserved.

THE HISTORY OF CLINICAL NURSING RESEARCH, 1952-1975

Gerontological nursing research
1. Psychosocial characteristics and nursing needs of the elderly
2. Attitudes of nursing personnel toward the elderly
3. Psychosocial nursing interventions to meet needs of the elderly

From: Gunter, L. M., & Miller, J. C. (1977). Toward a nursing gerontology. *Nursing Research, 26,* p. 208. Copyright 1977 The American Journal of Nursing Company. Used with permission. All rights reserved.

> **THE HISTORY OF CLINICAL NURSING RESEARCH, 1952-1975**
>
> **Psychiatric nursing research**
> 1. Studies of the person
> 2. Studies of interpersonal relationships
> 3. Studies of the social system

From: Sills, G. M. (1977). Research in the field of psychiatric nursing. *Nursing Research, 26*, p. 201. Copyright 1977 The American Journal of Nursing Company. Used with permission. All rights reserved.

Gunter and Miller[15] organized their review of nursing gerontology research by critical concept issues in what was then an emerging field of study (see the box on page 94). Sills's review of research in psychiatric nursing[42] included 310 research endeavors (see the box above). The research was analyzed according to historical and theoretical trends in psychotherapy: the person (a trend occurring before World War II), the relationship (a trend dominant from 1945 to 1955), and the social system (from 1955 through 1977). Finally, O'Connell, and Duffey[36] conducted an analysis of the research in nursing practiced published in *Nursing Research* from 1970 through 1975 (see the box on page 96). Their sample of 88 studies was classified along a number of dimensions, including investigator characteristics, study content, and research methods. Study content was specifically classified according to the general diagnostic category of the subjects (primarily reflecting traditional medical specialty areas), the procedure or technique investigated, the specific needs of patients addressed in the research (including physical and nonphysical needs), and the state of condition of the subject.

Sigma Theta Tau recently revised the research topic category system used in compiling its *Directory of Nurse Researchers.*[41] The box on page 97 contains descriptive information about the Sigma Theta Tau member research and the current research topics. The timeliness of this topic was also emphasized by the inclusion of a well-attended symposium, "The development of a taxonomy for nursing research," sponsored by the American Nurses Association's Cabinet on Nursing Research, at the 1987 International Nursing Research conference in Arlington, Virginia.

More recent research reviews include those reported by Brown, Tanner, and Padrick[6] and Lindsey,[20,21] Loomis,[23] Silva,[43] and Moody et al.[31] Brown, Tanner, and

Padrick[6] analyzed a random sample of 137 studies reported in *Nursing Research, Research in Nursing and Health, Western Journal of Nursing Research,* and the *International Journal of Nursing Studies, 1952-1980.* Loomis[23] described the content in nursing doctoral dissertations from 1976 to 1982 using two models based on the ANA Social Policy Statement:[2] a model of clinical nursing and a model of social issues in nursing. Silva[43] examined the degree to which nursing theories were tested in 62 empirical research studies. Moody et al.[31] analyzed 720 articles in six major refereed journals (1977 to 1986) to determine the type of research and its relevance for clinical practice. All of these reviews report major changes in the type of research conducted and in the theoretical and clinical practice implications for nursing.

Moody et al.[31] provide perhaps the best summary of the content of current clinical research. The investigators conclude that:

1. All studies reviewed had relevance for practice:
   a. two thirds of the studies were focused on assessment.
   b. one third of the studies addressed nursing interventions.
2. The percentage of nurses as first authors has increased.
3. Funding of published research over the decade has increased.
4. The use of research hypotheses did not increase over the decade.
5. Slightly more than half (51%) of the studies had some identifiable theoretical perspective. However, in only 13% was there a relationship between the theory and research design.
6. The use of nursing conceptual models increased significantly in the past five years similar to Silva's[43] findings.
7. Theories from the behavioral and social sciences continue to provide the conceptual basis for the majority of nursing research.
8. Adult health continues to be the most frequent clinical nursing research focus.
9. Nonprobability sampling was the most frequent sampling method utilized.
10. The most frequently studied NANDA diagnoses were: knowledge deficit, anxiety, coping, health maintenance, parenting, and noncompliance.
11. Eighty percent of the studies built on past findings and 75% related study findings to previous research.

RESEARCH IN NURSING PRACTICE,
1970-1975

Procedure or technique
1. Monitoring techniques
2. Physical care techniques
3. Psychiatric treatments
4. Teaching techniques
5. Assessment techniques
6. Organization of staff

Specific needs of patients

Physical needs
1. Food and nutrition
2. Rest and sleep
3. Cleanliness
4. Exercise
5. Elimination
6. Respiration
7. Relief of pain
8. Protection
9. Medication

Nonphysical needs
1. Emotional support
2. Communication
3. Recreation
4. Religious
5. Family

Status
1. Inpatients
2. Outpatients
3. Healthy client

Age
1. Neonates
2. Children
3. 18 through 64 years
4. 65 and over

Specific patient states
1. Anorexia
2. Anxiety and fear
3. Bedridden
4. Dying
5. Fever
6. Healthy
7. Hyperactivity or hypoactivity
8. Incontinence or constipation
9. Infection, inflammation
10. Insomnia
11. Malnutrition
12. Nausea
13. Pain or distress
14. Prematurity
15. Preoperative or postoperative states
16. Reactions to nursing
17. Psychological maladaptation
18. Shock
19. Unconsciousness

From: O'Connell, K. A., & Duffey, M. (1978). Research in nursing practice: Its present scope. In N. C. Chaska (Ed.), *The nursing profession: Views through the mist.* New York: McGraw-Hill.

12. In 1986, 45% of the studies were descriptive, whereas Brown et al. (1984) found that 25% of the 1980 sample to be descriptive.
13. Partial or complete reliability data were reported by 46% of the studies, and 43% addressed validity.

CLASSIFICATION OF NURSING PRACTICE

To date there has been little similarity in the systems used to classify general or specialty areas of nursing practice. Marek[28] attempted to classify existing outcomes reported in the nursing literature. Donaldson and Crowley[8] provided the discipline of nursing with a general direction that is still relevant 15 years later. They proposed that

From its perspective, nursing studies the wholeness or health of humans, recognizing that humans are in continuous interaction with their environments. Nursing's perspective evolves from the practical aim of optimizing human environments for health. Examples of major conceptualizations in nursing deal with:

1. Distinctions between human and nonhuman beings
2. Distinctions between living and nonliving beings
3. Nature of environments and human-environmental interactions from cellular to societal levels
4. Illness versus health and well-being

**SIGMA THETA TAU INTERNATIONAL
DIRECTORY OF NURSE RESEARCHERS,
Third Edition, 1990**

1. **Clinical topics**
   Environment
   Health
   Unhealthy Behaviors

2. **Nursing care activities**
   Nursing Process
   Focus of Assessment/Diagnosis
   Psychosocial

3. **Person**
   Cultural/Transcultural Focus
   Developmental Focus
   Pathophysiological Focus
   Psychological Focus
   Psychopathological Focus
   Social Focus

4. **Educational studies**

5. **Health care delivery**
   Health Systems Research
   Organizational Research

6. **Historical studies**

7. **Methodological studies**

8. **Philosophical perspective**

9. **Professional issues**
   Descriptive Information
   Researchers by Geographic Location
   Researchers by Language
   Researchers by Nursing Model/Theory
   Researchers by Animal Subjects Species

From: Sigma Theta Tau International. (1990). *Directory of nurse
researchers* (3rd ed.). Indianapolis: Author. Used with permission.

---

5. Functioning of the whole human organism versus functioning of the parts
6. Levels of functioning of whole organisms
7. Human characteristics and natural processes, such as consciousness, abstraction; adaptation and healing; growth; change; self-determination; development; aging; dying; reproducing; drive satisfaction; and relating

The concepts of person, environment, health, and nursing were used by University Microfilms International in developing their classification of nursing-related dissertations. The major categories were age-related client groupings (including family and community as clients), nurses and the nursing profession, and methodological issues.

A 1989 conference sponsored by the University of South Carolina College of Nursing engaged experts from across the country in a discussion of human responses: classification, diagnoses, interventions, and outcomes. The purpose of this conference was to provide a forum for conceptual advancement of the process components of nursing practice.[25] Papers presented were by Dr. Kathryn Barnard on the "Classification of Human Responses," Dr. Ada Lindsey[22] on "Approaches to Identification and Labeling of Human Responses," Dr. Joanne McCloskey[30] on the "Classification of Nursing Interventions," and Dr. Norma Lang and Karen Marek[19] on the "Classification of Patient Outcomes."

Conference participants agreed about the importance of developing classificatory systems for nursing practice. The professional advancement of the discipline of nursing depends on a consistent language by which we can communicate our activities, be they practice, research, or theory development. Our conceptual understanding will be reflected in the categories we identify and use to define our phenomena of concern for purposes of nursing science, reimbursement, and inclusion in health care legislation.[25]

Authors of the ANA publication *Classification Systems for Describing Nursing Practice*[3] assert that "nursing must be able to name itself and to describe what it does in order to function effectively in a world where digitalized information is used to establish everything from DRGs to cardiac output." The publication goes on to chronicle the efforts of the North American Nursing Diagnosis Association (NANDA) to develop nursing diagnoses, a taxonomy for the classification of nursing diagnoses, and the work by Loomis et al.[26] and O'Toole and Loomis[37] on the classification of human responses in psychiatric mental health nursing. Activity at the University of Wisconsin–Milwaukee to develop outcome measures of nursing care and the home and community health care classification project conducted at the Visiting Nurse Association of Omaha under Karen Martin's leadership are also reviewed. In this same publication, Saba and Werley and Zorn make compelling cases for a uniform nursing information system and the Nursing Minimum Data Set, respectively.

The North American Nursing Diagnosis Association is the forerunner in the development of nursing diagnoses to guide nursing practice. Since 1973, NANDA

NANDA TAXONOMY II, DRAFT I (WORKING DRAFT) 1-15-90

Human response pattern	Level
Choosing	2. Coping, Impaired
	3. Coping, Compromised
Communicating	2. Verbal Communication, Impaired
	3. Dysreflexia
Exchanging	2. Body Temperature, Altered: Risk
	3. Airway Clearance, Impaired
Feeling	2. Anxiety
	3. Fatigue
Knowing	2.
	3.
Moving	2. Home Maintentance Management, Impaired
	3. Activity Intolerance
Perceiving	2. Sensory Perception, Altered
	3. Body Image Disturbance
Relating	2. Role Performance, Altered
	3. Parental Role Conflict
Valuing	2. Sexual Function, Altered
	3.

From: *NANDA nursing diagnoses and classifications.* Used with permission.

members have committed their energies to the development of nursing diagnoses and more recently toward the development of a taxonomy for the classification of these diagnoses. NANDA's progress can be traced from an original alphabetized listing of approved nursing diagnoses to the current goal of inclusion in the ICD Code of medical diagnoses. All of the NANDA-approved nursing diagnoses[34] include a definition of the diagnosis, defining characteristics, and related factors. For example, chronic low self-esteem is defined as "longstanding negative self-evaluation/feelings about self or self capabilities." Defining characteristics include longstanding or chronic "self negating verbalization; expression of shame/guilt; evaluates self unable to deal with events; rationalizes away/rejects positive feedback and exaggerates negative feedback about self; hesitant to try new things/situations." But what if these defining characteristics are related to a recent divorce? While the NANDA Taxonomy labels these behaviors as defining characteristics of the diagnosis, they might also be regarded as human responses, in which case the health problem is defined by the human response(s). Logic suggests that intervention and amelioration of the human response(s), by definition, removes or cures the health problem (see the box above.)

The classification of Nursing Interventions project at the University of Iowa College of Nursing is a large 6-year project funded by the National Center for Nursing Research, the College of Nursing at the University of Iowa, and the Rockefeller Foundation. The primary goal of the project staff is to build and validate a taxonomy of nursing interventions that will include all of the direct-care treatment activities that nurses perform on behalf of patients.

The project staff has adopted Bulechek and McCloskey's[7] definition of a nursing intervention:

A nursing intervention is any direct-care treatment that a nurse performs on behalf of a client. These treatments include nurse-initiated treatments resulting from nursing diagnoses, physician-initiated treatments resulting from medical diagnoses, and performance of the daily essential functions for the client who cannot do these.

Therefore, their work includes:

1. Nurse-initiated treatment behaviors in response to nursing diagnoses
2. Physician-initiated treatment behaviors in response to medical diagnoses

---

EXAMPLE OF ONE INTERVENTION FROM NIC

Anticipatory guidance

Definition:

Preparation of patient for an anticipated developmental and/or situational crisis

Activities:

Assist the patient to identify possible upcoming, developmental, and/or situational crisis, and the effects the crisis may have on personal and family life

Instruct about normal development and behavior as appropriate

Provide information on realistic expectations related to the patient's behavior

Determine the patient's usual methods of problem-solving

Assist the patient to decide how the problem will be solved

Assist the patient to decide who will solve the problem

Utilize case examples to enhance the patient's problem-solving skills as appropriate

Assist the patient to identify available resources and options for course of action as appropriate

Rehearse techniques needed to cope with upcoming developmental milestone or situational crisis with the patient as appropriate

Assist the patient to adapt to anticipated role changes

Provide a ready reference for the patient (i.e., educational materials/pamphlets) as appropriate

Suggest books/literature for the patient to read as appropriate

Refer the patient to community agencies as appropriate

Schedule visits at strategic developmental/situational points

Schedule extra visits for patient with concerns or difficulties

Schedule follow-up phone calls to evaluate success or reinforcement needs

Provide the patient with a phone number to call for assistance if necessary

Include the family/significant others as appropriate

Background readings:

Denehy, J. A. (1990). Anticipatory guidance. In M. J. Craft & J. A. Denehy (Eds.), *Nursing interventions for infants and children* (pp. 53-68). Philadelphia: W. B. Saunders.

Rakel, B. A. (1992, June). Interventions related to patient teaching. In G. M. Bulechek & J. C. McCloskey (Eds.), *Symposium on nursing interventions* (pp. 289-602). Nursing Clinics of North America.

Schulman, J. L., & Hanley, K. K. (1987). *Anticipatory guidance: An idea whose time has come.* Baltimore: Williams and Wilkins.

Smith, C. E. (1987). Using the teaching process to determine what to teach and how to evaluate learning. In C. E. Smith (Ed.), *Patient education: Nurses in partnership with other health professionals* (pp. 61-95). Philadelphia: W. B. Saunders.

From: Iowa Intervention Project. (1992). In J. C. McCloskey & G. M. Bulechek (Eds.), *Nursing interventions classification (NIC)*. St Louis: Mosby.

---

3. Daily essential function behaviors that may not relate to either medical or nursing diagnoses but are done by the nurse for patients who cannot do these for themselves

The Nursing Interventions Classification (NIC)[18] consists of 336 interventions, each with a label name, definition, activities that a nurse performs to carry out the interventions, and background readings (see the example of Anticipatory Guidance, page 99). The current NIC is proposed as a first draft for clinical use and evaluation. The next draft (NIC II) will include revisions based on feedback from users as well as a taxonomic structure that groups interventions according to their similarities and differences.

Current concerns of the project staff include (1) a need to expand the NANDA diagnosis taxonomy to make it more comprehensive of the human responses treated by nurses and (2) concerns about the need to include aggregates such as communities in the NIC classification. While work on developing classification systems for nursing diagnoses and nursing interventions are proceeding along parallel courses, their conceptual and political activities are by no means mutually exclusive. Indeed, their activities and the efforts of those developing the Omaha System should soon converge to provide a comprehensive picture.

The Omaha System[29] was developed during a series of three research contracts between the VNA of Omaha and the Division of Nursing, Public Health Service, U.S. Department of Health and Human Services between 1975 to 1986. Project activities included development and testing of a Problem Classification Scheme, field testing of the Problem Classification Scheme, development of an expected outcome-outcome criteria scheme, testing, and revision of the Problem Classifi-

---

PROBLEM CLASSIFICATION SCHEME: OMAHA SYSTEM

Environmental domain

Problem
01. Income
02. Sanitation
03. Residence
04. Neighborhood/Workplace safety
05. Other

Psychosocial domain

Problem
06. Communication with community resources
07. Social contact
08. Role change
09. Interpersonal relationship
10. Spiritual distress
11. Grief
12. Emotional stability
13. Human sexuality
14. Caretaking/parenting
15. Neglected child/adult
16. Abused child/adult
17. Growth and development
18. Other

Physiological domain

Problem
19. Hearing
20. Vision
21. Speech and language
22. Dentition
23. Cognition
24. Pain
25. Consciousness
26. Integument
27. Neuro-musculo-skeletal function
28. Respiration
29. Circulation
30. Digestion-hydration
31. Bowel function
32. Genito-urinary function
33. Antepartum/postpartum
34. Other

Health related behaviors domain

Problem
35. Nutrition
36. Sleep and rest patterns
37. Physical activity
38. Personal hygiene
39. Substance use
40. Family planning
41. Health care supervision
42. Prescribed medication regimen
43. Technical procedure
44. Other

From: Martin, K. S., & Scheet, N. J. (1992). *The Omaha System: Applications for community health nursing.* Philadelphia, Pa: W. B. Saunders. Used with permission.

cation Scheme, and testing of a problem rating scale for outcomes and interventions. This work is unique because of the clinical research focus determined as important and productive by the staff in a service setting.

The purpose of the Problem Classification Scheme is to offer community health nurses an orderly method for identifying, labeling, and organizing concerns addressed during professional practice. The 40 nursing diagnoses represent matters of difficulty and concern that historically, presently, or potentially adversely affect any aspect of the client's well-being. Client problems represent health-related matters that nurses are licensed to diagnose and treat; problems are amendable to nursing interventions.[29] However, problems are focused on the individual and immediate family or social system and do not attend to larger aggregates such as communities.

Although the Problem Classification Scheme is intended to be used within the nurse-client relationship and as just one element of the nursing process, its basic structure is outlined in the box above to illustrate the focus of the Omaha System for addressing nursing practice in the community. Each problem includes a definition, a list of modifiers, and a list of signs and symptoms. For example, Problem 08, role change, is defined as movement from, or addition of, one set of expected behavior characteristics for another. Modifiers include health promotion, potential impairment, impairment, family, and individual. Signs/symptoms include (1) involuntary reversal of traditional male/female roles, (2) involuntary reversal of dependent/independent roles, (3) assumes new role, (4) loses previous roles, and (5) other. As with the defining characteristics of the NANDA diagnostic system, the signs and symptoms of the Omaha System are also human responses whose re-

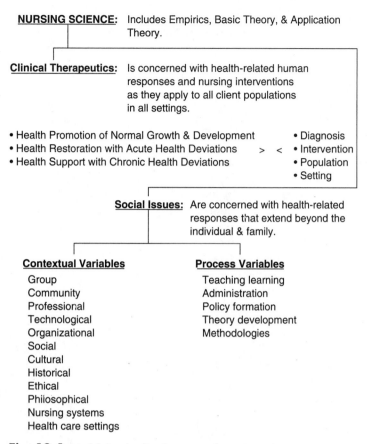

Fig. 13-1 Model for the development of nursing science.

versal or amelioration should constitute evidence of a cure.

The above examples serve to illustrate the difficulties associated with the lack of a holistic approach to life and health problems. There is no way, given a linear model, to clearly separate health problems from nursing diagnoses from defining characteristics from human responses. They are all wrapped together in one clinical, human package. In fact, health problems are also human responses from a holistic perspective.

THE DEVELOPMENT OF A METASYSTEM FOR CLASSIFICATION

So where does all this lead? It is clear that the clinical, theoretical, research, and political/economic dimensions of nursing must converge. The Model for the Development of Nursing Science (Fig. 13-1) contains a structure by which such a consensus can occur. Hall and Allen[16] have proposed a definition of nursing that acknowledges the two distinct realms of illness and

health: "Nursing is concerned with the phenomena of human responses to illness and health." More recently Schlotfeldt[40] asserted that "Nursing is the appraisal and the enhancement of the health status, health assets, and health potentials of human beings." This definition focuses the discipline of nursing entirely on health.

The model with which I am currently working to classify nursing science is based on a series of new assumptions and definitions. The primary definitional change is that nursing is the science of health and healing. Nursing science includes empiric, basic theory, and application theory. Therefore, all professional nurses should be engaged in the activity of nursing science. Nursing science is subdivided into (1) the study of clinical nursing therapeutics and (2) the study of social issues in relation to nursing.

Clinical therapeutics is concerned with health-related human responses and nursing interventions as they apply to all client populations in all private and public settings. Clinical therapeutics is conceptualized along several interrelated dimensions: human responses and related nursing interventions, client populations, and private and community settings. These dimensions correspond with nursing's metaparadigm concepts of health, nursing, person, and environment in a set of relationships that emphasizes the relationship between health and nursing interventions.

The relationship between human responses and nursing interventions is especially important. Health promotion interventions must be studied and implemented in light of what is considered to be normal growth and development for selected client populations within a specific health environment. Health-restoring interventions are directed toward the human responses of individuals and families to acute health deviations. Health-supporting interventions are directed toward the human responses of individuals and families to chronic health deviations. Of course, in the real world of clinical practice, a combination of preventative, restorative, and supportive interventions might be required for clients in acute episodes of chronic illnesses.

Social issues in nursing are concerned with health-related responses that extend beyond the individual and family. It is important to acknowledge and develop our understanding of the various contexts in which we nurses practice health and healing and the various processes by which we attempt to influence the health of individuals, families, groups, and societies. We must continue to research the interface between the science of health and healing and derived theories from the humanities and social sciences in order to understand and influence health in the larger political, social, and international context.

SUMMARY

Nursing: A Social Policy Statement[2] provided a definition of nursing that has launched the profession into the last 20 years of the century.

All nurses practicing with patients and with persons seeking health address the phenomena that form the core of nursing practice. Variations within nursing practice resulting from differences in level of education, extent of experience, and competence occur in regard to the following:
- Assessment of data collection
- Analysis of data
- Breadth and depth of knowledge base, especially clinical, psychosocial, and patho/physiological theories relating to nursing diagnosis and treatment
- The range of nursing techniques

- Need for, kind, and extent of supervision by other nurses in practice
- Evaluation of effects of practice
- Identification of relationships among phenomena, nursing actions, and effects (outcomes for the patients)[2]

That is our purpose and challenge.

It is time for the voice of the mother to be heard in education.[32]

REFERENCES

1. Abdellah, F. G. (1970). Overview of nursing research 1955-1968. Parts 1, 2, and 3. *Nursing Research, 19,* 6-17, 151-162, 239-252.
2. American Nurses Association. (1980). *Nursing: A social policy statement.* Kansas City, Mo: Author.
3. American Nurses Association. (1988). *Classification systems for describing nursing practice.* Kansas City, Mo: Author.
4. Barnard, K. E., & Neal, M. V. (1977). Maternal-child nursing research: Review of the past and strategies for the future. *Nursing Research, 26,* 193-200.
5. Brown, A. F. (1958). *Research in nursing.* Philadelphia: W. B. Saunders.
6. Brown, J. S., Tanner, C. A., & Padrick, K. P. (1984). Nursing's search for scientific knowledge. *Nursing Research, 33,* 26-32.
7. Bulechek, G. M., & McCloskey, J. C. (1989). Nursing interventions: Treatments for potential diagnoses. In R. M. Carroll-Johnson (Ed.), *Proceedings of the eighth conference,* NANDA (pp. 23-30). Philadelphia: J. B. Lippincott.
8. Donaldson, S. K., & Crowley, D. M. (1978). The discipline of nursing. *Nursing Outlook, 26,* 113-120.
9. Ellis, R. (1977). Fallibilities, fragments and frames: Contemplation on 25 years of research in medical-surgical nursing. *Nursing Research, 26,* 177-182.
10. Eliot, G. (1985). *Middlemarch.* New York: Penguin Books. Originally published 1871-72.
11. Fitzpatrick, J. J. (1991). Taxonomy II: Definitions and development. In *Classification of nursing diagnoses: Proceedings of the ninth conference.* Philadelphia: J. B. Lippincott.
12. Gortner, S. R., Bloch, D., & Phillips, T. R. (1976, March/April). Contributions of nursing research to patient care. *Journal of Nursing Administration,* 23-28.
13. Gortner, S. R., & Nahm, H. (1977). An overview of nursing research in the United States. *Nursing Research, 26,* 10-33.
14. Gould, S. J. (1981). *The mismeasure of man.* New York: W. W. Norton.
15. Gunter, L. M., & Miller, J. C. (1977). Toward a nursing gerontology. *Nursing Research, 26,* 208-220.
16. Hall, B. A., & Allen, J. D. (1986). Sharpening nursing's focus by focusing on health. *Nursing and Health Care, 7*(6), 315-320.
17. Highriter, M. E. (1977). The status of community health nursing research. *Nursing Research, 26,* 183-192.
18. Iowa Intervention Project. (1992). In J. C. McCloskey & G. M. Bulechek (Eds.), *Nursing interventions classification (NIC).* St Louis: Mosby.
19. Lang, N. M., & Marek, K. D. (1990). The classification of patient outcomes. *Journal of Professional Nursing, 6,* 3.
20. Lindsey, A. M. (1982). Phenomena and physiological variables of relevance to nursing: Review of a decade of work: Part I. *Western Journal of Nursing Research, 4*(4), 343-364.

21. Lindsey, A. M. (1983). Phenomena and physiological variables of relevance to nursing: Review of a decade of work: Part II. *Western Journal of Nursing Research, 5*(1), 41-63.

22. Lindsey, A. M. (1990). Identification and labeling of human responses. *Journal of Professional Nursing, 6*(3).

23. Loomis, M. E. (1985). Emerging content in nursing: An analysis of dissertation abstracts and titles: 1976-1982. *Nursing Research, 34*, 113-119.

24. Loomis, M. E. (1985). Emerging nursing knowledge. In J. C. McCloskey and H. K. Grace (Eds.), *Current issues in nursing* (2nd ed.). Boston: Blackwell Scientific Publications.

25. Loomis, M. E., & Herman, J. (1990). Nursing classification systems—Discussion and future directions. Summary. *Journal of Professional Nursing, 6*(3), 141-142, 164-166.

26. Loomis, M. E., O'Toole, A. W., Brown, M. S., Pothier, P., West, P., & Wilson, H. S. (1987). Development of a classification system for psychiatric/mental health nursing: Individual response class. *Archives of Psychiatric Nursing, 1*(1).

27. Loomis, M. E., & Wood, D. J. (1983) Cure: The potential outcome of nursing care. *Image: The Journal of Nursing Scholarship, 15*(1), 4-7.

28. Marek, K. D. (1989). The measurement of patient outcomes. *Journal of Quality Assurance, 4*, 1-9.

29. Martin, K. S., & Scheet, N. J. (1992). *The Omaha System: Applications for community health nursing.* Philadelphia: W. B. Saunders.

30. McCloskey, J. C., Bulechek, G. M., Cohen, M. L., Craft, M. J., Crossley, J. D., Denehy, J. A., Glick, O. J., Kruckeberg, T., Maas, M., Prophet, C. M., & Tripp-Reimer, T. (1990). Classification of nursing interventions. *Journal of Professional Nursing, 6, 3.*

31. Moody, L. E., Wilson, M. E., Smyth, K., Schwartz, R., Tittle, M., & Van Cott, M. L. (1988). Analysis of a decade of nursing practice research: 1977-1986. *Nursing Research, 37*(6), 374-379.

32. Noddings, N. (1984). *Caring.* Berkeley, Calif: University of California Press.

33. North American Nursing Diagnosis Association. (1989). *Taxonomy I revised.* St Louis: Mosby.

34. North American Nursing Diagnosis Association. (1991). *Classification of nursing diagnoses: Proceedings of the ninth conference.* Philadelphia: J. B. Lippincott.

35. Notter, L. E. (1974). *Essentials of nursing research.* New York: Springer.

36. O'Connell, K. A., & Duffey, M. (1978). Research in nursing practice: Its present scope. In N. C. Chaska (Ed.), *The nursing profession: Views through the mist.* New York: McGraw-Hill.

37. O'Toole, A. W., & Loomis, M. E. (1989). Revision of the phenomena of concern for psychiatric mental health nursing. *Archives of Psychiatric Nursing, 3,* 5.

38. Roberts, M. M. (1954). *American nursing: History and interpretation.* New York: Macmillan.

39. Rose, R. (1970). *The dynamics of public policy.* Beverly Hills, Calif: Sage.

40. Schlotfeldt, R. M. (1987). Defining nursing: A historic controversy. *Nursing Research, 36,* 64-67.

41. Sigma Theta Tau International. (1990). *Directory of nurse researchers* (3rd ed.). Indianapolis: Author.

42. Sills, G. M. (1977). Research in the field of psychiatric nursing. *Nursing Research, 26,* 201-207.

43. Silva, M. C. (1986). Research testing nursing theory: State of the art. *Advances in Nursing Science, 9*(1), 1-11.

44. Simmons, L. W., & Henderson, V. (1964). *Nursing research: Survey and assessment.* New York: Appleton-Century-Crofts.

CHAPTER 14

Patient classification schemas

Do we still need them?

CATHERINE KELLEHER

The nursing profession has temporarily lost its strategic advantage in the measurement of variation in hospital resource use and has not made much headway in the non-acute settings where care is increasingly shifted in efforts at health care reform. In the acute care realm, nursing can regain vanguard status if it jettisons methodological holdovers from the pre cost-containment era when patient classifications for nurse staffing were first introduced and if it explicitly reconsiders all facets of these tools including purpose, content, format, and their timing. In other service settings, the profession's lack of progress reflects the state of the art, leaving plenty of opportunity to do pioneer work in classification of patients for planning and staffing, as well as quality assessment and reimbursement of care.

In the late 1950s and early 1960s, when techniques were developed to monitor daily needs of acute care patients, the profession had center stage. The first methods developed were patient classifications for nurse staffing.[14,15,94,95,96] Care was paid for based on daily per-diem costs, and nursing dependency was the principal correlate. This remained so until 1983, when the federal government introduced per-case prospective payment for acute care Medicare patients based on diagnostic-related groups (DRGs), and other government and private payers followed suit. Length of stay replaced the specific day as the resource variable of interest, and diagnosis replaced nursing dependency as chief correlate.[19,23,85]

Predictably, in the mid 1980s, methodologists switched focus to classifications based on stay rather than day and to production of illness severity,[40,57] and health status measures[56] to account for variations in length of stay unexplained by DRGs.

In response to changed times, nurses in service and research are actively making headway in several pertinent ways. Some invest efforts in new purposes for acute care patient classifications originally designed for nurse staffing. They range from research and policy,[79] to more concrete applications, such as costing and billing for nursing services,[20,50,81,82] and tracking patterns of demand to better plan for care.[19] Others concentrate on fundamentals needed for interfacility comparisons, such as standardized nursing language,[29] nursing minimum data sets,[93] taxonomies of nursing diagnoses,[68] and interventions[11] to be used as counterparts to medically based DRGs. Only a few institutions are looking at the specific content and format of current acute care classifications and considering major revamping;[10,73-75] no one toys with timing or the dailiness aspect.

Drawbacks to acute care methodologies have almost the status of litany. Aydelotte[4] and Giovannetti[26] have produced the classic critiques in the field; despite their pre-DRG publication, they are relevant today because most acute care classifications were developed pre-DRG. A more recent critique by Lampe[50] takes into account the impact of the new cost containment environment and the variations in the methodologies designed to capture acute care nursing costs.

In brief, the two main areas in which acute care classifications are thought to seriously fall short are in scantiness of description of nursing work and patient state and noncomparability across settings because of the customization of even ready-made tools to fit hospital-specific needs, which prevents inter-hospital comparison of nursing intensity and the use of nursing intensity as a severity adjustment for care. Need for major makeover in acute care tools is implied in these critiques, but there are few explicit suggestions for where and how to start.[46] The point of this chapter is to champion only three:

- To rethink the tradition of rating patients for each day of stay and consider predictive models based on stay rather than day
- To discontinue the custom of collecting the same content from day to day, and substitute a three-part format, i.e., admission, daily, and discharge checklists, each designed to capture characteristics unique to that phase of stay, and that are correlates of nursing demand common across the continuum of care
- To replace current contents, a pastiche of patient condition and nurse work, with a standardized set of patient characteristics, such as the demographic, severity, and health status measures used in studies to improve DRG reimbursement and evaluate quality and effectiveness of care

A brief history of acute and long-term care methodologies (the most developed so far), an overview of what little has been done in classification on the home and ambulatory care front, and relevant advances in measurement of illness severity and health status will be discussed in this chapter.

SOME HISTORY OF PATIENT CLASSIFICATIONS FOR NURSE STAFFING
Acute care

The late 1950s and early 1960s[12,22] were the heyday of progressive patient care. The idea was to provide a thrifty mix of services by reorganizing patients by illness severity and associated demands for medical and nursing care—not by clinical specialty and room type.[89] This ethos gave impetus to nurse staffing studies to advance beyond head count, or census, to care intensity level as the basis for bed and nurse demand.[31,32]

Pioneers at the time tackled two sets of overlapping prediction problems: nursing workload at the nursing unit level and patient readiness for transfer, a concept fundamental to progressive patient care.

The workload problem centered on prediction of changes in demand for nurses by patients cared for via the customary way by keeping them in the same place for all phases of stay. It was tackled by Flagle and colleagues at the Johns Hopkins Hospital in Baltimore, Maryland; their product—controlled variable staffing—included the basic methodologies for patient classification and subsequent nurse manpower allocation in use to this day.[14,15,22,95,96]

In contrast to workload prediction, in which the patient stayed put, readiness for transfer required detection of patient readiness to move on, that is, actual bodily removal to another specialized nursing unit providing a different level of care. In the full-service hospital, service ran from intensive-, intermediate-, and self-, to long-term and home care; the latter rendered on discharge from the facility-based stay.

Strategies for prediction of patient transfer were first developed at Manchester Memorial Hospital in Manchester, Connecticut, the pilot site used to produce guidelines for operationalizing progressive patient care, including nurse staffing methodologies by Flagle's team, who were called in to further develop their techniques.[87,89]

Daily classification of patients took early root. Flagle, from the start, focused on predicting next-day demand for nurses based on current-day status, a time frame eminently sensible since the activity was funded by hospital administrators who focused on daily operation, and at the time, patient bills were paid per diem not per case.

The tenetlike status of daily classification was reinforced by the backdrop of progressive patient care, the essence of which was constant movement of patients through a tiered system. To do this right—i.e., to transfer, or discharge, patients as soon as they were ready—it was vital to monitor patients daily so as not to miss reporting changes in status.

To make transitions from level to level possible, a uniform minimum set of characteristics had to be settled upon that was common to all patients but present in degrees distinctive enough that patients could be grouped into categories that differed in demand for nursing time and skill. To accomplish this, checklists with the same content for every stay were used for staffing methodologies.

While this fixed format had its place, it blinded users to the richer potential of a system at its heart designed to detect signals of change or their absence. Opportunities were lost for systematic capture of characteristics of patients who deviated from the expected smooth transition from higher to lower levels and the implications for fine-tuning care delivery. In actuality, patients could enter the tiered system at any particular level and stay put at that level for the entire hospital stay. Other types of truncations and fluctuations could occur, but the chance to study the patterns and associated patient correlates was missed for the focus on the levels.

Several other traditions settled in—most a product of the times. First, interhospital comparisons were not of compelling interest, in part because of the primitive state of available information systems that precluded large-scale analysis. Consequently, particulars of the checklists used to sort patients into care levels were, for the most part, hospital specific, and the daily data were routinely thrown out. Second, activities of daily living, rather than diagnostic information, were the critical indicators used to differentiate care levels. Third, levels of care best discriminated were intensive versus intermediate. Despite the vision of true integration of all levels of care in the progressive patient care model, long-term care and home care were given short shrift, a fact reflected in the slow growth of classification systems in each of these areas.

Long-term care

In the mid 1960s, the first work on patient classifications for nurse staffing in long-term care began and was modeled on acute care methodologies with special emphasis on activities of daily living.[12]

In 1963, Katz published his now classic *Index of Activities of Daily Living,* an eight-category index claimed to validly and reliably measure degree of dependency across all diagnoses.[44] This generic attribute was a methodologic advance, but much work remained because Katz and colleagues did not take the next step and correlate levels of dependency with demand for nursing care.

By the late 1960s, knowledge of the methodological handicaps to be overcome had accrued,[62,63,64] and teams based at Harvard, Case Western Reserve, Johns Hopkins, and Syracuse University Research Corporation joined to create standardized approaches to long-term-care patient classification, including language, procedures, and a data collection tool known as the Collaborative Patient Assessment Instrument, a breakthrough instrument that fostered across facility comparisons and collection of sociodemographic and medical risk factor data believed to complement activities of daily living as measures of need for care.[42] On the heels of this effort, researchers at Johns Hopkins and the National Center for Health Statistics jointly sponsored a conference which took place in 1975 and led to the development of the Long-Term Health Care Minimum Data Set—a core set of data about providers, services, clients, and costs recommended for national use.[25,86] The advances notwithstanding, most long-term-care data collection and analysis continued to be site specific, and the data were rarely saved.

Not much new occurred until the early 1980s, when DRGs were introduced for acute care reimbursement.

Mavericks in long-term care embraced the per-case mindset and grouper methodology used to create DRGs and developed the prototype for the Resource Utilization Groups (RUGs) classification, which is now up to RUGs III,[13,80] and RUGs-T18 in terms of refinement.[24]

Synergistic with the effort of refining RUGs was the Omnibus Reconciliation Act of 1987 mandate for a national resident assessment instrument for use by 1990, with full implementation by April 1992, in all nursing homes qualified for federal reimbursement. A consortium including RUGs developers and investigators at the Research Triangle Institute, Brown University, and the Hebrew Rehabilitation Center for the Aged produced the required instrument—the Minimum Data Set for Resident Assessment and Care Screening—that consists of 300 items that measure the 13 domains mandated for comprehensive assessment at admission, then annually, and whenever significant changes in resident status may merit reassessment.[66] A modified version of the instrument, the Minimum Data Set Plus, is being used in conjunction with RUGs III in a three-year Health Care Financing Administration sponsored multistate prospective Medicare/Medicaid Nursing Home Case Mix and Quality (NHCMQ) demonstration project scheduled to begin in summer 1993.

While RUGs III was developed specifically for use in the NHCMQ demonstration, RUGs-like systems are being used, or considered, as the basis for reimbursement reform for nursing home care in more than 20 states.[72,91]

Best efforts to date indicate that RUGs-like systems do well in explaining cost per diem but not total costs or length of stay, because the great variability in duration of stay and factors are not yet well understood. Consensus is that while it is currently necessary to make do with per-diem models, researchers should continue to experiment with mixed models that incorporate both daily intensity and length of stay caps to foster incentives for shortened episodes and more cost-effective policies for admission and discharge.[24,80]

The basic RUGs consists simply of three types of measures, an activities-of-daily-living index, a set of services and problems typical of nursing home residents, and a clinical group hierarchy based on care demand that in RUGs III includes the following subgroups: special rehabilitation, extensive care, special care, clinically complex, impaired cognition behavioral problems, and reduced physical function. Patients are first assigned to a clinical subgroup and, once there, to an individual RUG based on degree of dependency in activities of daily living and related problems and service need. In all, there are 44 individual mutually exclusive RUG groups in RUGs III.[13]

As RUGs and its adaptations are increasingly scrutinized, suggestions for supplementation are beginning to be offered, for example, the inclusion of an explicit measure of cognitive function because its impairment has been found to be a significant resource indicator even after controlling for RUGs.[72] Others have taken cues from state-of-the-art severity of illness measures used as adjustments for DRGs in acute care and recommended use of baseline data collected on admission to predict resource use for the entire stay.[53]

To date, demand for nursing and nurse staffing have not been the central focus of RUGs-like schemes with the exception of RUGs III, which has taken explicit account of types of nursing providers and nursing care delivered, though details have not been published.[13] Instead, the thrust has been to identify determinants of overall costs and high cost subsets, including nursing and auxiliary services, such as rehabilitation therapy. Determinants of nursing costs have differed from those for auxiliary and total costs, and the best predictors for nursing have been activities of daily living.[24]

Home and ambulatory care

RUGs-HHC, an adaptation of RUGs II for home health care, has been adapted by some payers to reimburse for care, and several researchers are experimenting with variations on RUGs-HHC.[9,58,83]

In the ambulatory care setting, a number of classifications have recently been developed, but none are in routine use.[65,84,90] Ambulatory Visit Groups, produced by the developers of DRGs, are of the most recent of the classifications and a serious contender of available outpatient methods for use in prospective payment for outpatient visits.[5] However, none of these classifications have an express focus on nursing demand.

Nurse staffing models in home[36,59,60,71] and outpatient care[37,41,48,69,78,88] are in a nascent state. The traditional approach of predicting shift or next-day demand is not readily adaptable to visit-based systems in which the work itself is ill-defined, making it difficult to isolate a set of predictive characteristics for nursing demand.[33]

In any case, there is little information to readily model as data in home and outpatient settings are generally collected on a nonstandardized, sporadic basis and rarely stored for long.[1,61] The likelihood of prospective payment in home and outpatient settings has

provoked interest in remedying this deficiency. Progress has been made in the form of the 1989 recommendations for a uniform ambulatory care data set, but the recommendations have been so recent that there is still little data by which to go.[67]

ILLNESS SEVERITY AND HEALTH STATUS MEASURES

Illness severity measures really took off with the introduction of DRGs. There is extensive descriptive and critical literature regarding these measures, their frequent revisions, and their limitations as adjustments for DRGs.[3,38,39,76]

In contrast, health status measures have a longer developmental history. There has been a surge in the past 20 years,[6,7,43] intensified in the past 10 years,[55,56] as they are looked at to fill gaps in length of stay variations unexplained by DRGs and illness severity adjustments. They are also increasingly applied in related investigations in cost-quality tradeoffs[56,70,92] and outcomes of care.[35,51,54,77] But they are not yet the everyday tools that nursing classifications are, although much work is being done to facilitate their routine use in clinical settings.[2,17,21,27,34]

Illness severity and health status methodologists are remarkably prolific. The nursing profession would do well to keep abreast of advances and use the best in revamping patient classifications for nurse staffing. In a previous publication,[46] I recommended the substitution of illness severity and health status measures for current contents of staffing classifications, so details will not be repeated here.

As to two other suggestions for reform of timing and format of current nursing tools, some comparisons are needed regarding the state of the art in collection of nursing intensity versus illness severity data.

While the convention in nursing is to do daily ratings and to use the same tool throughout the stay, for illness severity the custom is to use discharge abstract or medical record data, as displayed in Table 14-1, and to focus on admission, discharge, or daily collection, not all three (Table 14-2).

Recently, there has been a trend to move from retrospective data collection based on discharge abstract or medical record data to prospective collection of admission data, with options for mid-stay review that give the opportunity to investigate patterns of clinical course, i.e., whether the patient improves, stays the same, or gets worse.[38,92]

Table 14-1   Comparison of Data Sources for Selected Illness Severity Measures

	Medical record	Discharge abstract
Acute Physiology and Chronic Health Evaluation III (APACHE III)	X	
MedisGroups	X	
Computerized Severity of Illness (CSI)	X	
SysteMetrics Computerized Disease Staging		X
Patient Management Categories (PMCs)		X
RAND Sickness-at-Admission Scale*	X	
RAND Discharge Impairment Measures*	X	

*Disease specific measures constructed for selected conditions: Congestive heart failure, acute myocardial infarction, cerebrovascular accident, pneumonia, hip fracture.

Concomitant with the trend to periodic daily rating is a push to restrict data collection to the beginning and end points of stay, that is, admission[45,47] or discharge,[16,49] and to build indexes to predict mortality, or readmission, as well as length of stay and costs.

In contrast, in nursing to date, only one attempt has been made to predict average daily or total nursing demand from admission data only.[8] No one has tested discharge information only or tried to determine if such closely spaced assessments as daily are really needed.

More empirical work is needed to determine who needs to be rated daily or not and to determine the best mix of complementary admission and discharge information that will parsimoniously predict nursing demand. Table 14-3 presents ideas for new data elements.

SUMMARY

"The right patient, in the right bed, with the right services, at the right time"[30] was the central slogan of progressive patient care. Nurse staffing methodologies were integral to realization of these goals that entailed quick detection of readiness for transfer to different levels of care within and across settings, a technique as valuable today as it was radical back then because integrated care systems are considered the keystone to health care reform. Nurses also were trailblazers in use of health status measures in that activities of daily living were and are the chief discriminators of nursing demand in acute inpatient classifications designed for nurse staffing.

We have a heritage to live up to but should not rest on tradition. Our acute care methodologies need makeovers in a number of areas, and some options to consider include having curtailed daily ratings and ratings tailored to the specific phases of hospital stay, and using standardized illness severity and health status measures as proxies for nursing acuity.

Table 14-2   Comparison of Data Collection Strategies By Phase of Hospital Stay: Nurse Staffing Classifications Versus Selected Illness Severity Measures

	Phase of hospital stay			
	Admission	In-hospital		Discharge
		Periodic	Daily	
Nurse Staffing Classifications			X	
Illness Severity Measures				
Acute Physiology and Chronic Health Evaluation III (APACHE III)	X			
MedisGroups	X	X		
Computerized Severity of Illness (CSI)	X	X		X
SysteMetrics Computerized Disease Staging				X
Patient Management Categories (PMCs)				X
RAND Sickness-At-Admission Scale*				X
RAND Discharge Impairment Measures*				X

*Disease specific measures constructed for selected conditions: Congestive heart failure, acute myocardial infarction, cerebrovascular accident, pneumonia, hip fracture.

Table 14-3 Revamping Nurse Staffing Classifications for Acute Care: Some Patient Clinical and Personal Characteristics to Consider By Phase of Hospitalization

Characteristic	Hospital phase		
	Admission	**In-hospital**	**Discharge**
Routinely available			
Clinical	Age*		Discharge disposition*
	Admission urgency		DRG
	Admission source		
Personal	Sex*		
	Race*		
	Marital status†		
	ZIP code*‡		
	Source of payment*		
Special effort to collect			
Clinical	Baseline health status	Daily or periodic health status	Discharge health status
	Physical	measures	measures
	Cognitive		
	Emotional		
	Baseline illness severity	Daily or periodic illness	Discharge illness severity
	measure	severity measure	measure
Personal	Social support measure		
	Perceived need for services		
	measure		
	Selected elements from a		
	cultural assessment tool		

*Comparable element in the Nursing Minimum Data Set (NMDS).
†Proxy for social support.
‡Used to calculate home-hospital distance, an indicator of potential discharge delay if patient resides far away.

Even more of a breakthrough would be patient classifications predictive of nursing demand that are serviceable across site. Such generic systems are reasonable to entertain since many conditions once meriting hospitalization are now treated elsewhere, while those who are actually hospitalized are more acutely ill and are discharged quicker to post acute care. This scenario makes it likely that, with minor modifications, acute care classifications would be predictive off-site, a hunch underscored by the thumbnail sketches presented earlier of efforts at out-of-hospital classification of resource demand which consistently report the importance of activities of daily living which also are core determinants in current acute care nursing tools. Successful development of patient classifications predictive of demand for nursing which are generic in regard to site would be a landmark accomplishment. Despite the insistent call for unified patient data systems to facilitate efficient management of resources in integrated care, few such systems currently exist.

Patient classification schemas: Do we still need them? Yes, we do. We need them to do what they do

well right now, which is to provide inpatient-based rationale for inpatient staffing useful in everyday decisions regarding nurse-patient ratios and tradeoffs in cost and quality of care. We need them to improve in terms of standardization across settings to facilitate inter-hospital comparisons, particularly for use in quality assessment and for isolating nursing from hotel costs to build a case for reimbursement of the nursing component of care. And we need them for professional status to obtain a foothold if not to regain the leadership role the profession once had in systematic measurement of resource variation to efficiently plan and provide good care across all service sites.

REFERENCES

1. Agency for Health Care Policy and Research. (1991). *Report to Congress: The feasibility of linking research-related data bases to federal and non-federal medical administrative data bases* (AHCPR Pub. No. 91-0003). Rockville, Md: U.S. Department of Health and Human Services.
2. Applegate, W. B., Blass, J. P., & Williams, T. F. (1990). Instruments for the functional assessment of older patients. *Current Concepts in Geriatrics, 322*(17), 1207-1214.

3. Aronow, D. B. (1988). Severity of illness measurement: Applications in quality assurance and utilization review. *Medical Care Review, 45*(2), 339-366.

4. Aydelotte, M. K. (1973). *Nurse staffing methodology: A review and critique of selected literature* (DHEW Pub. No. 73-433). Washington, D.C.: U.S. Government Printing Office.

5. Averill, R. F., Goldfield, N. I., McGuire, T. E., Bender, J. A., Mullins, R. L., & Gregg, L. W. (1991). *Design and evaluation of a prospective payment system for ambulatory care.* (Health Care Financing Administration Agreement No. 17-C-99369/1-02). Wallingford, Conn: 3M Health Information Systems.

6. Bergner, M. (1985). Measurement of health status. *Medical Care, 23*(5), 696-704.

7. Bergner, M., & Rothman, M. L. (1987). Health status measures: An overview and guide for selection. *Annual Review of Public Health, 8,* 191-210.

8. Bostrom, J. (1992). Early determinants of required nursing care hours in the acute care setting. *Inquiry, 29,* 99-104.

9. Branch, L. G., & Goldberg, H. B. (1993). A preliminary case mix classification system for Medicare home health clients. *Medical Care, 31*(4), 309-321.

10. Buckle, J. M., Horn, S. D., & Simpson, R. L. (1991). Nursing care classification: A conceptual model. *Applied Nursing Research, 4*(3), 100-106.

11. Bulechek, G. M., & McCloskey, J. C. (1990). Nursing intervention taxonomy development. In J. C. McCloskey & H. K. Grace (Eds.), *Current issues in nursing* (pp. 23-28). St. Louis: Mosby.

12. Cavaiola, L. J., & Young, J. P. (1980). An integrated system for patient assessment and classification and nurse staff allocation for long-term care facilities. *Health Services Research, 15*(3), 281-306.

13. Clauser, S. B., & Fries, B. E. (1992). Nursing home resident assessment and case mix classification: Cross national perspectives. *Health Care Financing Review, 13*(4), 135-155.

14. Connor, R. J. (1961a). Effective use of nursing resources: A research report. *Hospitals, J.A.H.A., 35*(9), 30-39.

15. Connor, R. J. (1961b). A work sampling study of variations in nursing workload. *Hospitals, J.A.H.A., 35*(9), 40-41, 111.

16. Corrigan, J. M., & Martin, J. B. (1992). Identification of factors associated with hospital readmission and development of a predictive model. *Health Services Research, 27*(1), 81-101.

17. Deyo, R. A., & Carter, W. B. (1992). Strategies for improving and expanding the application of health status measures in clinical settings. *Medical Care, 30*(Suppl. 5), MS176-186.

18. Dick, R. S., & Steen, E. B. (Eds.). (1991). *The computer-based patient record. An essential technology for health care.* Washington, D.C.: National Academy Press.

19. Diers, D. (1992). Diagnostic-related groups and the measurement of nursing. In L. Aiken & C. Fagin (Eds.), *Charting nursing's future. Agenda for the 1990s* (pp. 139-156). Philadelphia: J. B. Lippincott.

20. Eckhart, J. G. (1993). Costing out nursing services: Examining the research. *Nursing Economic$, 11*(2), 91-98.

21. Feinstein, A. R. (1992). Benefits and obstacles for development of health status assessment measures in clinical settings. *Medical Care, 30* (Suppl. 5), MS50-MS56.

22. Flagle, C. D. (1960). The problem of organization for hospital inpatient care. *Proceedings of the sixth international meeting, the Institute of Management Sciences* (pp. 275-287). London: Pergamon.

23. Flagle, C. D. (1992). The integrated health care system: Reflection and projection. *Journal of the Society for Health Systems, 3*(4), 16-24.

24. Fries, B. E., Schneider, D. P., Foley, W. J., & Dowling, M. (1989). Case mix classification of Medicare residents in skilled nursing facilities: Resource utilization groups (RUGs-T18). *Medical Care, 37,* 843-858.

25. Gilford, D. M. (Ed.). (1988). *The aging population in the twenty-first century.* Washington, D.C.: National Academy Press.

26. Giovannetti, P. (1978). *Patient classification systems and their uses: A description and analysis* (DHEW Pub. No. [HRA] 78-82). Springfield, Va: National Technical Information Service.

27. Golden, W. E. (1992). Health status measurement. Implementation strategies. *Medical Care, 30* (Suppl. 5), MS187-MS195.

28. Greenfield, S., & Nelson, E. C. (1992). Recent developments and future issues in the use of health status assessment measures in clinical settings. *Medical Care, 30* (Suppl. 5), MS23-MS41.

29. Grobe, S. J. (1990). Nursing intervention lexicon and taxonomy study: Language and classification methods. *Advances in Nursing Science, 13*(2), 22-33.

30. Haldeman, J. C. (1964). Elements of progressive patient care. In L. E. Weeks & J. R. Griffith (Eds.), *Progressive patient care: An anthology* (pp. 1-13). Ann Arbor, Mich: The University of Michigan.

31. Haldeman, J. C., & Abdellah, F. G. (1959a). Concepts of progressive patient care (part 1 of 2). *Hospitals, J.A.H.A., 33,* 38-42, 142-143.

32. Haldeman, J. C., & Abdellah, F. G. (1959b). Concepts of progressive patient care (part 2 of 2). *Hospitals, J.A.H.A., 33,* 41-46.

33. Hastings, C. E. (1987). Classification issues in ambulatory care nursing. *Journal of Ambulatory Care Management, 10*(3), 50-64.

34. Hedrick, S. C., Barrand, N., Deyo, R., Haber, P., James, K., Metter, J., Mor, V., Scanlon, W., Weissert, W., & Williams, M. (1991). Working group recommendations: Measuring outcomes of care in geriatric evaluation and management units. *Journal of the American Geriatrics Society, 39* (Suppl.), 48S-52S.

35. Heithoff, K. A., & Lohr, K. N. (Eds.). (1990). *Effectiveness and outcomes in health care.* Washington, D.C.: National Academy Press.

36. Helberg, J. L. (1989). Reliability of the nursing classification index for home healthcare. *Nursing Management, 20*(3), 48-56.

37. Hoffman, F., & Wakefield, D. S. (1986). Ambulatory care patient classification. *Journal of Nursing Administration, 16*(4), 23-30.

38. Iezzoni, L. I. (1989). Measuring the severity of illness and case mix. In N. Goldfield & D. B. Nash (Eds.), *Providing quality care* (pp. 70-105). Philadelphia: American College of Physicians.

39. Iezzoni, L. I. (1990). Severity of illness measures. Comments and caveats. *Medical Care, 28*(9), 757-761.

40. Iezzoni, L. I., Schwartz, M., & Restuccia, J. (1991). The role of severity information in health policy debates: A survey of state and regional concerns. *Inquiry, 28,* 117-128.

41. Johnson, J. M. (1989). Quantifying an ambulatory care patient classification instrument. *Journal of Nursing Administration, 19*(11), 36-42.

42. Jones, E. W., McNitt, B. J., & McKnight, E. M. (1973). *Patient classification for long term care: User's manual.* (DHEW Publication No. [HRA] 74-3107). Washington, D.C.: Department of Health, Education and Welfare.

43. Katz, S. (Ed.). (1987). The Portugal conference: Measuring quality of life and functional status in clinical and epidemiological research. *Journal of Chronic Diseases, 40*(6), 459-650.

44. Katz, S., Ford, A. B., Moskowitz, R. W., Jackson, B. A., & Jaffe, M. W. (1963). Studies of illness in the aged. The index of ADL: A standardized measure of biological and psychosocial function. *Journal of the American Medical Association, 185*(12), 94-99.

45. Keeler, E. B., Kahn, K. L., Draper, D., Sherwood, M. J., Rubenstein, L. V., Reinisch, E. J., Kosecoff, J., & Brook, R. H. (1990). Changes in sickness at admission following the introduction of the prospective payment system. *Journal of the American Medical Association, 264*(15), 1962-1968.

46. Kelleher, C. (1992). Validated indexes: Key to nursing acuity standardization. *Nursing Economic$, 10*(1), 31-37.

47. Knaus, W. A., Wagner, D. P., Draper, E. A., Zimmerman, J. E., Bergner, M., Bastos, P. G., Sirio, C. A., Murphy, D. J., Lotring, T., Damiano, A., & Harrell, F. E. (1991). The APACHE III prognostic system. Risk prediction of hospital mortality for critically ill hospitalized adults. *Chest, 100,* 619-636.

48. Koerner, B. L. (1987). Clarifying the role of nursing in ambulatory care. *Journal Ambulatory Care Management, 10*(3), 1-7.

49. Kosecoff, J., Kahn, K. L., Rogers, W. H., Reinisch, E. J., Sherwood, M. J., Rubenstein, L. V., Draper, D., Roth, C. P., Chew, C., & Brook, R. H. (1990). Prospective payment system and impairment at discharge: The 'quicker-and-sicker' story revisited. *Journal of the American Medical Association, 264*(15), 1980-1983.

50. Lampe, S. (1987). *Costing hospital nursing services: A review of the literature* (DHHS Pub. No. [HRSA] HRP-0907983). Springfield, Va: National Technical Information Service.

51. Lansky, D., Butler, J. B. V., & Waller, F. T. (1992). Using health status measures in the hospital setting: From acute care to "outcomes management." *Medical Care, 30* (Suppl. 5), MS57-MS73.

52. Lee, S., & Dichter, B. (Eds.). (1992). *MDS & multistate nursing home case mix and quality demonstration training manual.* Natick, Mass: Eliot Press.

53. Liu, K., Coughlin, T., & McBride, T. (1991). Predicting nursing-home admission and length of stay. A duration analysis. *Medical Care, 29*(2), 125-141.

54. Lohr, K. N. (1988). Outcome measurement: Concepts and questions. *Inquiry, 25,* 37-50.

55. Lohr, K. N. (Ed.). (1989). Advances in health status assessment: Conference proceedings. *Medical Care, 27*(Suppl. 3), S1-S294.

56. Lohr, K. N. (Ed.). (1992). Advances in health status assessment. Fostering the application of health status measures in clinical settings: Proceedings of a conference. *Medical Care, 30*(Suppl. 5).

57. Mackenzie, T., Willan, A. R., & the Case Mix Research Group. (1991). *Patient classification systems: An evaluation of the state of the art. Vol. 1* (HCFA Agreement No. 17-C-99133/F-02). Kingston, Ontario: Queens University.

58. Manton, K. G., & Hausner, T. (1987). A multidimensional approach to case mix for home health services. *Health Care Financing Review, 8*(4), 37-54.

59. Martin, K. (1988). Research in home care. *Nursing Clinics of North America, 23*(2), 373-385.

60. Martin, K. S., & Scheet, N. J. (1989). Nursing diagnosis in home health. The Omaha system. In I. M. Martinson & A. Widmer (Eds.), *Home health care nursing* (pp. 67-72). Philadelphia: W. B. Saunders.

61. Matson, T. A., & McDougall, M. D. (Eds.). (1990). *Information systems for ambulatory care.* Chicago: American Hospital Association Publishing.

62. McKnight, E. M. (1967a). *Nursing home research study—Phase I: Quantitative measurement of nursing services.* Denver: Colorado State Department of Public Health.

63. McKnight, E. M. (1967b). *Nursing home research study—Phases II and III: Staff utilization—nursing activities in nursing homes* (Prepared under contract with Division of Nursing, U.S. Department of Health, Education and Welfare). Denver: U.S. Department of Health, Education and Welfare.

64. McKnight, E. M., & Steorts, R. C. (1967). *Nursing home simulation model user's manual.* Santa Monica, Calif: Consolidated Analysis Centers, Inc.

65. Mohr, P., Menzin, J., & Griffiths, S. (1989). *A review of private sector payment methodologies for hospital outpatient services. Final report* (Cooperative Agreement No. 99-C-99168/3-01). Chevy Chase, Md: Project HOPE Center for Health Affairs, HCFA.

66. Morris, N., Howes, C., Fries, B. E., Phillips, C. D., Mor, V., Katz, S., Murphy, K., Drugovich, M. L., & Friedlob, A. S. (1990). Designing the national resident assessment instrument for nursing homes. *The Gerontologist, 30*(3), 293-307.

67. National Committee on Vital and Health Statistics, Subcommittee on Ambulatory and Hospital Care Statistics. (1992). *Proposed revision to the uniform hospital discharge data set. (Final Report).* Hyattsville, Md: Author.

68. North American Nursing Diagnosis Association. (1989). *Taxonomy 1 revised-1989.* St Louis: Author.

69. Parrinello, K. M., & Witzel, P. A. (1990). Analysis of ambulatory nursing practice. *Nursing Economic$, 8*(5), 322-328.

70. Patrick, D. L., & Erickson, P. (1988). Assessing health-related quality of life for clinical decision making. In S. R. Walker & R. M. Rosser (Eds.), *Quality of life: Assessment and application* (pp. 9-49). Lancaster, England: MTP Press.

71. Peters, D. A. (1988). Development of a community health intensity rating scale. *Nursing Research, 37*(4), 202-207.

72. Phillips, C. D., & Hawes, C. (1992). Nursing home case-mix classification and residents suffering from cognitive impairment: RUGs-II and cognition in the Texas case-mix data base. *Medical Care, 30*(2), 105-116.

73. Prescott, P. A. (1991). Nursing intensity: Needed today for more than staffing. *Nursing Economic$, 9*(6), 409-414.

74. Reitz, J. (1985a). Toward a comprehensive nursing intensity index: Part I development. *Nursing Management, 16*(8), 21-30.

75. Reitz, J. (1985b). Toward a comprehensive nursing intensity index: Part II testing. *Nursing Management, 16*(9), 31-42.

76. Rosko, M. D. (1988). DRGs and severity of illness measures: An analysis of patient classification systems. *Journal of Medical Systems, 12*(4), 257-274.

77. Salive, M. E., Mayfield, J., & Weissman, N. (1990). Patient outcomes research teams and the agency for health care policy and research. *Health Services Research, 25*(5), 697-708.

78. Schade, J. G., & Austin, J. K. (1992). Quantifying ambulatory care activities by time and complexity. *Nursing Economic$, 10*(3), 183-192.

79. Scherubel, J. C. (Ed.), & Shaffer, F. A. (Series Ed.). (1988). *Patients and purse strings II* (NLN Pub. No. 20-2191). New York: National League for Nursing.

80. Schneider, D. P., Fries, B. E., Foley, W. J., Desmond, M., & Gormley, W. J. (1988). Case mix for nursing home payment: Resource utilization groups, version II. *Health Care Financing Review,* (Annual suppl.), 39-48.

81. Shaffer, F. A. (Ed.). (1985). *Costing out nursing: Pricing our product* (NLN Pub. No. 20-1982). New York: National League for Nursing.

82. Shaffer, F. A. (Ed.). (1986). *Patients and purse strings: Patient classification and cost management* (NLN Pub. No. 20-2155). New York: National League for Nursing.

83. Smith, M. E., Baker, R., Branch, L. G., Walls, R. C., Grimes, R. M., Karklins, J. M., Kashner, M., Burrage, R., Parks, A., Rogers, P., Saczuk, A., & Wagster-Weare, M. (1992). Case-mix groups for VA hospital-based home care. *Medical Care, 30*(1), 1-16.

84. Starfield, B. H., Weiner, J. P., Mumford, L. M., & Steinwachs, D. M. (1991). Ambulatory care groups: A categorization of diagnoses for research and management. *Health Services Research, 26*(1), 53-74.

85. Thompson, J. D. (1984). The measurement of nursing intensity. *Health Care Financing Review,* (Annual Suppl.), 47-55.

86. U.S. Department of Health and Human Services. (1980). *Report of the National Committee on Vital and Health Statistics. Long-term Health Care, minimum data set* (DHHS Pub. No. (PHS) 80-1158). Hyattsville, Md: Office of Health Research, Statistics, and Technology, National Center for Health Statistics.

87. U.S. Public Health Service. (1962). *Elements of progressive patient care* (PHS Publication No. 930-C-1). Washington, D.C.: U.S. Government Printing Office.

88. Verran, J. A. (1986). Testing a classification instrument for the ambulatory care setting. *Research in Nursing and Health, 9,* 279-287.

89. Weeks, L. E., & Griffith, J. R. (Eds.). (1964). *Progressive patient care, an anthology.* Ann Arbor, Mich: University of Michigan.

90. Weiner, J. P., Starfield, B. H., Steinwachs, D. M., & Mumford, L. M. (1991). Development and application of a population-oriented measure of ambulatory care case-mix. *Medical Care, 29*(5), 452-472.

91. Weissert, W. G., & Musliner, M. C. (1992). Case mix adjusted nursing home reimbursement: A critical review of evidence. *The Milbank Quarterly, 70*(3), 455-490.

92. Welch, C. E., III, & Grover, P. L. (1991). An overview of quality assurance. *Medical Care, 29* (Suppl. 8), AS8-AS28.

93. Werley, H., & Lang, N. (Eds.). (1988). *Identification of the nursing minimum data set.* New York: Springer.

94. Young, J. P. (1962, October). *A method to meet inpatient care needs.* (Report to the U.S. Public Health Service, Department of Health, Education, and Welfare). Baltimore, Md: Johns Hopkins University.

95. Young, J. P., & Wolfe, H. (1965a). Staffing the nursing unit—Part I: Controlled variable staffing. *Nursing Research, 14*(3), 236-243.

96. Young, J. P., & Wolfe, H. (1965b). Staffing the nursing unit—Part II: The multiple assignment technique. *Nursing Research, 14*(4), 299-303.

CHAPTER 15

Why the Nursing Minimum Data Set (NMDS)?

HARRIET H. WERLEY, POLLY RYAN, CECELIA R. ZORN, ELIZABETH C. DEVINE

The Nursing Minimum Data Set (NMDS) is a standardized approach that facilitates the abstraction of essential, core minimum data to describe nursing practice. It is intended for use in any and all settings where nursing care is provided. The NMDS is unique in that it is the only data set whereby the practice of *nursing* can be described, resulting in a nursing database. Widespread use of the NMDS will facilitate the description, comparison, and evaluation of nursing practice across settings—locally, regionally, nationally, and internationally. In addition, use of the NMDS will enable linkage of nursing data with health care data already being collected in various health care settings, such as hospitals, ambulatory care settings, home health care agencies, nursing homes, and other long-term care facilities. Such linkages will enable nurses to access additional data for correlational and predictive purposes, while other health professionals can have access to nursing data. To achieve this, however, elements of the NMDS must be included as an inherent part of all computerized nursing information systems (NISs).

Built on earlier work in the 1970s,[49] the development of the NMDS in 1985 was nursing's initial effort to establish uniform standards for the collection of comparable, minimum, essential core nursing data. In 1991, the American Nurses Association (ANA)[3] recognized the NMDS as the minimum data elements to be included in any data set or patient record. In addition, the ANA Resolution No. 24[2] was passed unanimously by the 1986 House of Delegates. This resolution supported research and development of computerized nursing information systems (NISs).

The recent ANA recognition of the NMDS certainly is timely when considered in light of the recent Pew Commission Report[36] on future trends in health care and expectations for the health professions' practitioners in 2005. The authors of the Pew Commission Report predicted a future trend in the health care industry to be increasingly coordinated care in an attempt to improve the efficiency and effectiveness of the health care system. The coordinated care system "will develop mechanisms to continually and systematically measure outcomes, improve quality, encourage practitioner accountability, and standardize patterns of practice."[36] One result of the movement toward coordinated care will be diversification in the mix of providers in addition to the roles these providers will play in the delivery of health care. More curative and preventive services will be delivered in lower cost settings. The proliferation of alternative care delivery systems will lead to increasingly complex and diversified organizations.

Because of the changing diversity and complexity of health care systems and the changing mix in providers, nurses will assume greater responsibilities for case management and provision of services for direct reimbursement. The Pew Commission recommended the following competencies for future health care providers: (*a*) the ability to manage information, (*b*) the ability to accommodate expanded accountability, (*c*) the ability to participate in coordinated care both on a client level and on a systems level, and (*d*) the ability to ensure cost-effective and appropriate care.

The implementation of the NMDS will help to achieve these competencies for health care practitioners in the future as a system that builds partially upon databases currently in use. It could be used to help to estimate the relative value of health care services across settings and among increasingly diverse and complex systems. In addition, if data were available that demonstrated the cost-effectiveness of nurse-managed clinics in alleviating problems with access to health care, this would help to convince policy makers of the need to fund such services.

Clearly, future trends are forecasting the need for all health care providers to accept accountability for the cost effectiveness of the services they provide. In nursing, this can be facilitated by a coordinated database resulting from the use of the NMDS.

Although the NMDS concept, development, purposes, and elements have been presented in numerous publications nationally and internationally,[41-48,50-52] they bear repeating here. Calls and letters are received daily from national and international health professionals requesting information about the NMDS; many of these individuals are just discovering this work.

BACKGROUND
Concept

The NMDS is based on the concept of the Uniform Minimum Health Data Sets (UMHDSs). A UMHDS has been defined as "a minimum set of items of information with uniform definitions and categories, concerning a specific aspect or dimension of the health care system which meets the essential needs of multiple data users."[18] The concept was developed in 1969 from efforts to identify national health data standards and guidelines.[28,29,31] Several different UMHDSs have been developed in the areas of long-term care, hospital discharge, and ambulatory care.[32-34] The Uniform Hospital Discharge Data Set (UHDDS) is in widespread use today because it is mandated for all Medicare patients.[18-20] But the UHDDS has been studied for several years by the National Committee on Vital and Health Statistics (NCVHS) Subcommittee on Ambulatory and Hospital Care Statistics.[35] Some important changes are being recommended in the Subcommittee's report and the NCVHS chair's letter to the Assistant Secretary for Health for consideration and action. The suggested number of items has been increased slightly, to a total of 20. The long-term and the ambulatory care data sets[14,16,27] have undergone revision and are being tested. However, none of these data sets contain data that describe nursing practice.

At the 1969 Conference on Hospital Discharge Abstract Systems, several criteria were set forth for the development of minimum health data sets.[30,31] These were as follows: (*a*) data items included in the set must be useful to most if not all potential users, such as health care professionals and administrators; planning, regulatory, and legislative bodies at local, state, and federal levels; insurance agencies; and the research community; (*b*) items selected must be those that can be collected readily with reasonable accuracy; (*c*) items should not duplicate data available from other sources;

and (*d*) confidentiality of health care information should be protected.

Built on the concept of the UMHDSs, the NMDS was nursing's first attempt to standardize the collection of essential nursing data. By adapting the definition given for a UMHDS, the NMDS is defined as a minimum set of items of information with uniform definitions and categories concerning the specific dimension of nursing, which meets the information needs of multiple data users in the health care system. The NMDS includes those specific items of information used on a regular basis by the majority of nurses across all types of settings in the delivery of care.

Development

In 1985, following earlier work that had been done at the University of Illinois in 1977,[49] the NMDS was developed consensually through the efforts of a national group of 64 experts who participated in the three-day invitational NMDS Conference at the University of Wisconsin–Milwaukee. The NMDS Conference was conducted in the tradition of other conferences that were held to identify the earlier UMHDSs. The participants at the conference included nurse experts in practice, administration, research, and education; health policy spokespersons; information systems, health data, and health record specialists; governmental and proprietary agency personnel; and persons knowledgeable about the development of previous UMHDSs.[50-52]

Purposes of the NMDS

The purposes of the NMDS are these: (*a*) establish comparability of nursing data across clinical populations, settings, geographic areas, and time; (*b*) describe the nursing care of patients or clients and their families in a variety of settings, both institutional and noninstitutional; (*c*) demonstrate or project trends regarding nursing care provided and allocation of nursing resources to patients or clients according to their health problems and nursing diagnoses; (*d*) stimulate nursing research through links to the more detailed data existing in NISs and other health care information systems (HCISs); and (*e*) provide data about nursing care to facilitate and influence clinical, administrative, and health policy decision making.

NMDS elements

The NMDS comprises three broad categories of elements: (1) nursing care, (2) patient or client demo-

ELEMENTS OF THE NURSING MINIMUM DATA SET

Nursing care elements

1. Nursing Diagnosis
2. Nursing Intervention
3. Nursing Outcome
4. Intensity of Nursing Care

Patient or client demographic elements

*5. Personal Identification
*6. Date of Birth
*7. Sex
*8. Race and Ethnicity
*9. Residence

Service elements

*10. Unique Facility or Service Agency Number
11. Unique Health Record Number of Patient or Client
12. Unique Number of Principal Registered Nurse Provider
*13. Episode Admission or Encounter Date
*14. Discharge or Termination Date
*15. Disposition of Patient or Client
*16. Expected Payer for Most of This Bill (Anticipated Financial Guarantor for Services)

*Elements comparable to those in the Uniform Hospital Discharge Data Set.

graphics, and (3) service elements. Ten of the sixteen elements also are included in the previously mentioned UHDDS.[20,33] Those elements presumably would not need to be recollected in hospitals, where they should be available through existing relational database management systems because the federal government has mandated that the UHDDS items be collected on all Medicare patients. The NMDS elements are listed in the box above.

Benefits of the NMDS

There are numerous benefits for nursing if the NMDS were adopted nationwide in ongoing data collection systems. These include: (a) access to comparable, minimum nursing care and resources data at local, regional, national, and international levels; (b) enhanced documentation of nursing care provided; (c) identification of trends related to client problems and nursing diagnoses, as well as to nursing care provided; (d) impetus to improved costing of nursing services; (e) improved data for quality enhancement; (f) impetus to developmentand refinement of nursing information systems; (g) comparative research on nursing care, including research on nursing diagnoses, nursing interventions, nursing intensity, nursing outcomes or resolution status of nursing diagnoses, and referral for further nursing services; as well as (h) contributions toward advancing nursing as a research-based discipline.

PROGRESS TOWARD ADOPTING AND IMPLEMENTING THE NMDS

To realize the full benefits of the NMDS, widespread adoption of the data set must occur. The concept of the NMDS should be taught in all nursing educational settings. Nurse administrators and policy makers must continue to demand and use nursing data-based information in their decision making process. Nurse researchers should learn to use information gained from the NMDS in research programs and participate in the testing and further development of the NMDS. Within the past decade, progress has been made in the adoption of the NMDS. The following are examples of how the NMDS currently is being used in different areas, such as nursing education, clinical practice, administration, health care policy, and research. The NMDS elements must be used in patient care documentation with assurance that these data can be retrieved readily from computerized systems in all practice settings.

Nursing education

The NMDS has become part of course curricula at the graduate and undergraduate levels. Some university professors are using the Werley and Lang[50] book on the NMDS in nursing courses on informatics. Through course assignments designed to teach computer skills and potential uses of a nursing database, the nursing elements of the NMDS have been linked to one another.[12] Presentations on the NMDS have been made nationally and internationally at professional conferences to share information, and the *NMDS Data Collection Manual*[44] has been used widely as a teaching tool.[24,53]

Clinical practice

The NMDS is becoming an inherent part of nursing information systems being developed in many institutions and agencies. Computer vendors are structuring their nursing information systems data to include the NMDS elements (e.g., N-Touch, 3M, Health Data Sciences' Ulticare, and HBO & Co's Health Quest).

Administration

At the Milwaukee County Medical Complex, master staffing plans currently are being determined in part by a patient's individualized plan of care that links nursing interventions to the staff mix and hours of care required. Thus, the intensity of nursing care provided can be measured.[1] Nursing intensity and nursing diagnosis have been shown to be predictors of resource consumption in home health care.[17] Nursing problems, defined according to the Omaha System,[40] have been shown to account for 55% of the variance in determining resource use in home health care when compared with medical diagnoses, which accounted for only 17.2% of the variance.[26]

Health care policy

The American Academy of Ambulatory Nursing Administration (AAANA) reflected its interest in the NMDS by sponsoring a workshop on this topic prior to its annual meeting in 1990. Publication of these proceedings show that the outcomes were considered fruitful.[4]

The ANA has been interested in having nursing included in the World Health International Classification of Diseases (ICD), a system that includes a family of classifications. In preparation for a request to have nursing included in the ICD-10 revision, the North American Nursing Diagnosis Association's (NANDA) nursing diagnoses were coded to be in consonance with the ICD-9 system, and an article on this matter was published in the *American Journal of Nursing*.[15] The request to be included in the ICD-10 revision was not approved, but there is ongoing work being done nationally and internationally at the International Council of Nurses and the World Health levels to bring about a common classification system. The proposed International Classification of Nursing Practice (ICNP) would include nursing diagnoses, interventions, and outcomes.[8] Norma Lang from the United States and representatives from other countries are involved in this work. Several teams other than NANDA (e.g., Omaha, Psychiatric Nursing) also are working on classification systems for nursing diagnoses, and until a single system of nursing diagnoses is agreed upon by the profession, widespread adoption of the NMDS may be difficult.

Research

Research on the NMDS is being approached in a variety of ways. The NMDS is being tested and used by several master's and doctoral students. For example, Tillman[39] completed a master's thesis by testing availability and reliability of the NMDS in a community academic nursing center. His findings were positive, and he encouraged continued research and implementation of the NMDS in independent nursing practice settings. Marek[26] used the Omaha System for classification of nursing problems and patient outcomes in her study of correlates of utilization and outcomes in home health care. Correlates tested included nursing diagnoses, medical diagnoses, nursing interventions, as well as payers and selected demographic variables. In addition, several doctoral students across the country have expressed interest in using the NMDS in their dissertation research and have requested information about it.

To date, Connie Delaney[9] has developed the largest research program on the NMDS. In an abstract published in the Australian Nursing Informatics '91 conference proceedings, Delaney reported on "Research Utility of the Nursing Minimum Data Set." Her research questions for this pilot study pertained to nursing diagnoses validation, incidence of associated etiologies, relationship of nursing diagnoses to diagnostic-related groups (DRGs), length of hospital stay, patient demographic variables, specific patient care outcomes actualized, nursing order sets selected, and intensity and costs of nursing care. Her data were collected on 215 patients and stored in a computerized NIS in a U.S. health care center. Unfortunately, her paper was not included in the proceedings. Delaney is at the University of Iowa College of Nursing and can be contacted there for a list of her publications on the NMDS.

The NMDS was tested initially in a pilot study of availability of data and reliability.[10] Subject records (n = 116) used were from a hospital, nursing home, home health care agency, and two clinics. Overall intercoder agreement was satisfactory (91%). The implications of these results are that the definitions and protocol for coding were generally acceptable. Most of the NMDS elements were available for greater than 90% of the cases. One conclusion that can be drawn from these results is that existing records were an adequate source for most of the elements in the NMDS.

Leske and Werley[24] conducted a questionnaire survey of those who requested the *NMDS Data Collection Manual*. The intended use of the *Manual* was compared with the later actual use, and availability and retrievability of the data also were examined.[53] There was a 44% return before the deadline for submission of the paper for the Australian Nursing Informatics '91 Conference. Analysis of these data showed that the NMDS elements were recorded on an ongoing basis by 86% of the respondents; more than half (63%) could retrieve the data over time, but only 31% could readily retrieve all the elements. In the main, the stated intended uses of the *Manual* were to serve as a guideline or educational tool, library reference, or example for information systems that include the NMDS. The reported actual uses were to educate other nurses (43.5%), to structure collection of the NMDS (39.1%), and for nursing documentation (30.4%). With multiple choices possible, the total percentages may exceed 100%.

Ryan, Coenan, Devine, and Werley from Milwaukee, Wisconsin, currently are conducting descriptive research in which selected elements of the NMDS are being abstracted from the medical records of patients who had been hospitalized in a Midwest hospital during the 1991 calendar year. Data from one site have been obtained, and data from two other sites in different geographic locations are being sought so that comparisons may be made across sites in different geographic locations. The research questions include: (*a*) What are the nursing diagnoses that have been identified in patients with one or more of the most frequently occurring medical diagnoses or surgical procedures? (*b*) What are the nursing interventions, patient outcomes, and intensity of nursing care in patients with one or more of the six most frequently occurring nursing diagnoses, and do these differ by selected patient characteristics (i.e., length of stay, geographic location, medical diagnoses, surgical procedures, age, gender, and race/ethnicity)? and (*c*) Which combination of patient characteristics and nursing interventions in each of the most frequently occurring nursing diagnoses explain variation in patient outcomes, as defined by resolution of the six selected nursing diagnosis?

Preliminary analyses at the Midwest hospital site indicated that the most common nursing diagnoses identified during the first half of 1991 were: pain ($n = 2186$), anxiety ($n = 1260$), potential for injury ($n = 1410$), decreased cardiac output ($n = 887$), potential for infection ($n = 584$), and knowledge deficit ($n = 495$). Final analyses will include descriptive statistics and logistic regression. Nursing diagnoses, interventions, and outcomes will be compared for similarities and differences across sites and settings. This study has significance for nursing practice, education, research, economics, and health policy.

Several professors from the University of Wisconsin–Milwaukee submitted abstracts for presentation at the Nursing Informatics '94 Conference, to be held in San Antonio, Texas. Eileen Shiel and Mary Wierenga are pursuing research questions in the clinical areas of maternity and diabetes, using computer technology to retrieve the data from computerized documentation of patient care, including the NMDS. Judy Diekmann conducted an experimental study and will report on the effect of implementation of a computerized documentation system on nurses' attitudes toward computers and work stress levels.

It is essential that research nurses and others interested in studying nursing practice and documentation data to assess care use the computerized data that are saved for research in various settings. Otherwise, other professionals will exert pressure to have the nonused nursing data purged from the computerized system.

ISSUES RELATED TO IMPLEMENTING AND USING THE NMDS

Nursing is still in its infancy in regard to implementing, testing, and conducting research using the NMDS to pursue research questions. Physicians and hospital administrators have had much support for research and development of their medical information systems (MISs) and hospital information systems (HISs). For years, nurses have been urged to move in the direction of developing NISs. However, in the 1970s, when federal money was available, nurses did not use the opportunity to develop NISs and databases.[49] To a large extent this was due to the fact that the concept of a NMDS was, and still is, ahead of its time for many nurses. Sadly, this is still true for those who should be funding nursing research and development in this area. Because of the lack of support by a major funding agency, it has not been possible to take the second major step in testing the NMDS—a regional study.

A number of major issues concerning the NMDS relate to implementation of this powerful small data set. These include: (*a*) need for *consistent* documentation, computerization, as well as review and assessment of the nursing data; (*b*) recognition that the NMDS is appropriate for use wherever nursing care is provided; (*c*) understand what it means to test the NMDS across settings; and (*d*) acceptance of the NMDS by the nursing profession. These issues are by no means exhaustive, but they are crucial ones. These issues do not deal with roles that nurses in the various functional areas should assume if nursing is to realize the full benefits of widespread use of the NMDS. Some of these nurse roles were mentioned briefly earlier in this chapter.

Documentation, computerization, and review of nursing data

An issue related to implementing the NMDS is the need for standardized, *consistent* documentation of nursing practice and review of these nursing data. Following the definitions for the NMDS elements as presented in the Werley and Lang[50] book chapter in the *NMDS Data Collection Manual*[44] continues to be a major step in insuring standardization. The NMDS draws on the documentation of the nursing process used when nurses provide care to people in any setting. The documentation can be effective only if nurses in practice and administration document fully both the care provided and the nurse resources used to provide that care. It should be remembered that, as early as 1962, at a conference on information systems, cosponsored by the National Center for Health Services Research and Case Western Reserve University School of Nursing, nurses and information systems specialists agreed that frequently some of the same nursing data can be used by both clinicians and the administrators.[37]

Every effort must be made to be certain that mechanisms are developed to insure accurate and complete documentation, or health records will be an inadequate source of the nursing data needed by clinicians, administrators, researchers, and healthy policy makers. However, efforts to increase the quality of documentation must minimize the additional demands made on clinicians, who already are experiencing considerable stress in providing care under growing cost containment measures.

In addition to the documentation of data, the computerization of data is an issue related to the testing and implementation of the NMDS. In certain areas, computerization of nursing information is becoming more common. Nurses must be certain to be involved in the philosophical discussions preceding adoption of an information management system and in the day-to-day decision making about NISs. In addition, nurses must be involved in the research and development of these NISs.

Computerized nursing data do not always mean *retrievable* nursing data; the data must be saved and be available readily for later abstraction and use. The entry of nursing information must be done in such a way that the data are keyed and can be retrieved as needed in order to examine and use nursing's subsystem of data.[54] In the future, these NISs will be computerized and operational at the institutional or agency level where, through relational database management systems, the nursing data can be related to other HCISs. The goal is to include the NMDS elements in the NISs as these systems are being developed and refined, so that the NMDS can be incorporated in *ongoing* data collection systems. Nurses must, however, be able to pull out nursing's information systems data so they can see in actuality just what nursing data are recorded and saved in nursing's own language.

Nursing must be accorded its proportionate share of the total computerization support available in facilities for the development of computerized information systems. Unfortunately, external funding sources, such as those available from the U.S. Agency for Health Care Policy and Research, the National Library of Medicine, and others too frequently are not sought or are not available for nursing administrators, practitioners, and researchers for the support of information systems research, development, and management. As mentioned earlier, this was the situation in the 1970s, when hospital and medical information systems were being developed. Nursing missed out on those millions of dollars that were devoted to the research and development of information systems through the National Center for Health Services Research. Thus, there has been far too much delay in nurses' taking advantage of the resources and technology related to the information management and computerization of nursing services data.

Because the NMDS also is built on the UHDDS, which currently is required for clients under Medicare coverage in hospitals, the cost of implementation may be considerably less in settings currently providing care to this particular patient group. This is a practical and a financial advantage. Only four nursing care elements and two of the service elements are additional; the other 10 elements are comparable to those already being collected in the UHDDS. Nurses should recognize the merits of having built the NMDS on the UHDDS and capitalize on this fact in justifying that the NMDS elements be included in NISs and other HCISs. As Thompson[38] stated during the 1985 NMDS Conference, linkage with the UHDDS "is valuable not only because of information this data set contains, but more importantly as a key to enter other data sets to obtain an almost complete picture of the total period of hospitalization."[37]

The NMDS is appropriate wherever nursing care is provided

It must be understood that the NMDS is not the combination of different minimum data sets currently used in various areas of nursing to make clinical decisions. The use of multiple different data sets would result in a proliferation of data sets having questionable comparability. Instead, the NMDS is a set for retrospective collection of comparable, minimum, essential, common core data across all settings that describes the nursing care provided and the nurse resources used. Elements of the NMDS are consistent from site to site, location to location, and time to time.

It is important that nurses understand that the NMDS is appropriate for use wherever *nursing care* is provided, including hospitals, nursing homes, home health or community health care agencies, and ambulatory clinics. It is agreed by most personnel that wherever nurses practice, a nursing diagnosis is made to direct nursing interventions and outcomes. Hettinger and Brazile[21] recently described a design for community health data using the NANDA nursing diagnosis classification system. They also presented at the ANA convention Computer Application Demonstration Theater that was planned and overseen by the ANA Council on Computer Applications in Nursing. And, due to the high interest in the Hettinger and Brazile content, the presentation was scheduled several additional times to accommodate the participants' desire for this information.

Use of the NMDS would facilitate the evaluation component of the nursing process. As nurses assume more autonomy for their practice, the ability to evaluate adequately and to demonstrate their contribution to health care becomes even more crucial. In addition, increased accountability for the resources used and the client outcomes achieved is required. Access to comparable data related to patient outcomes across settings and populations would enhance greatly the evaluation of nursing care provided.

The philosophy of the UMHDSs allows for the collection of additional data as needed for specific research or evaluation projects by certain groups or specialties, but that does not mean that one alters the basic minimum data set without a reason shown through research. It is, of course, expected that the power of the basic minimum data set is not destroyed.[13] This powerful, small NMDS is appropriate for use in any setting where nursing care is provided and nurses make a nursing diagnosis.

Testing and implementation of the NMDS will be both facilitated by and, in turn, will facilitate the continuing development and refinement of classification systems for nursing practice. For example, a particularly exciting development is the recently published research by the Iowa Intervention Classification Project of McCloskey, Bulechek, and colleagues[22] at the University of Iowa College of Nursing and their related publications.[5-7,25] In addition, further testing of the NMDS will provide considerable data for the continual refinement of classification systems for nursing diagnoses, interventions, and outcomes.[54]

The knowledge that nurses possess and develop is essential for theory building in nursing. Implementing the NMDS can result in readily retrievable data for research focused on a variety of nursing concerns. This research then can serve as a link to develop theories that are based on nursing practice, and in turn, have nursing recognized more readily as a data-based discipline.

What it means to test the NMDS

Testing the NMDS requires a commitment to the elements of the data set and the definitions of these elements.[44,50] That is, the NMDS cannot be modified to meet perceived individual or specialty needs before testing because modification destroys the standardization of the NMDS as a data collection tool. Testing the set means just that. Changes, if needed, should be based only on the research pursued in the testing. The testing should include examination of the availability of the data elements in the nursing practice documentation, reliability with which the data can be collected, and difficulties encountered in regard to data coding and retrieval.

It must be realized that a study or testing of the data set will be useful not only to the nurses doing the testing but also to the practicing nurses, the personnel who oversee the documentation, and the nurse coordinators working with the information management and computer systems personnel. This is a matter of working together, so the data that are documented and saved are the data needed and are in nursing's language. This must include the NMDS elements that can be retrieved readily for use in assessing nursing practice and patient care, conducting research on care, and decision making by clinicians, administrators, as well as health policy makers.

There is confusion among some individuals who want to compare studies across settings where different nursing diagnoses labels and different intervention classification systems are used. Until the profession has adopted a single set of diagnoses and intervention labels, plurality will exist. As a consequence, only NMDS data from settings using similar diagnosis and intervention classification systems may be compared. One must first identify which nursing diagnosis system is used, such as the NANDA or the Omaha System. The classification system for nursing interventions also must be identified, for example, the Omaha System[40] or the Iowa Intervention Project.[22]

Acceptance of the NMDS by the profession

As nurses are working toward implementation of the NMDS, they also should assume a leadership role in the implementation of the *Computer-Based Patient Record* (CPR). Failure by nurses to design and implement NISs that include the NMDS during this period of rapid movement on the CPR will result in nonnurses making decisions that will influence nursing directly for generations. Numerous texts, references, and professional organizations are available to assist in the development of NISs pertinent to the content of the Institute of Medicine book on the *Computer-Based Patient Record,*[11] so that nursing practice data can be included in nursing's terminology.

Many opportunities for involvement exist to advance the testing and further work of the NMDS, to conduct research on this data set across settings, and to try out the information systems where nurses have been entering the NMDS elements as an inherent part of the computerized NISs. Until practicing nurses and research nurses do these things, it will not be known how closely the documentation of care meets nurses' needs, nor will it be known if the data can be retrieved readily from their respective computerized systems. The NMDS was identified by a group of expert individuals, and it should receive more attention from nursing as a scientific discipline. Futuristic thinking also is needed on the part of funding agencies. Unless the decision makers in such agencies can envision the value of futuristic projects, the profession will never be able to shape its future.

In the work on the NMDS, nurses should be mindful of Jacox's discussion on the inclusiveness of scope in nursing diagnoses. She stated, "It may be that a broad organizing framework such as the Nursing Minimum Data Set, which includes nursing diagnoses, nursing interventions, patient outcomes, and nurse intensity is a sufficiently neutral framework with which to organize the language of nursing."[23] Through the use of the NMDS, the essence of nursing practice can be described, and a database can be developed.

SUMMARY

In this chapter, background information about the NMDS has been summarized, including the concept, purposes, elements, and benefits. Specific examples of ongoing research and implementation in education, practice, administration, and healthcare policy have been provided. Finally, several issues pertinent to the implementation and use of the NMDS were discussed. A plea for stronger acceptance and implementation of the NMDS by the profession was set forth, and specific strategies to facilitate this acceptance were identified.

Constructive criticism of these views will be welcomed, as well as suggestions about how nurses and nursing can be helped to move further into the information management and computerization age. This ultimately would benefit nursing practice, administration, research, and education—all of which would help nurses to influence practice and health policy decision making.

REFERENCES

1. Albrecht, C. A. (1987). Hours of direct nursing care. *Computers in Nursing, 5*(2), 46-49.
2. American Nurses Association. (1986). *Development of computerized nursing information systems in nursing services* (Resolution No. 24). Kansas City, Mo: Author.
3. American Nurses Association. (1991). National data bases/sets to support clinical nursing practice. *Report to the Nursing Organization Liaison Forum* (pp. 2-3). (Unpublished).
4. Androwich, I. M., & Phillips, K. *Use of the nursing minimum data set in ambulatory nursing*. Pittman, N.J.: American Academy of Ambulatory Nursing Administration.
5. Bulechek, G. M., & McCloskey, J. C. (Eds.). (1992a). Defining and validating nursing interventions. *Nursing Clinics of North America, 27,* 289-299.
6. Bulechek, G. M., & McCloskey, J. C. (Eds.). (1992b). Nursing interventions. *Nursing Clinics of North America, 27,* 289-598.
7. Bulechek, G. M., & McCloskey, J. C. (1992c). *Nursing interventions: Essential nursing treatments* (2nd ed.). Philadelphia: W. B. Saunders.
8. Clark, J., & Lang, N. (1992). Nursing's next advance: An international classification for nursing practice. *International Nursing Review, 39,* 109-112, 128.
9. Delaney, C. (1991). Research utility of the Nursing Minimum Data Set. In E. J. S. Hovenga, K. J. Hannah, K. A. McCormick, & J. S. Ronald (Eds.), *Nursing informatics '91. Proceedings of the fourth international conference on nursing use of computers and information science* (p. 104). Berlin: Springer-Verlag.

10. Devine, E. C., & Werley, H. H. (1988). Test of the Nursing Minimum Data Set: Availability of data and reliability. *Research in Nursing and Health, 11,* 97-104.

11. Dick, R. S., & Steen, E. B. (Eds.). (1991). *The computer-based patient record: An essential technology for health care.* Washington, D.C.: National Academy Press.

12. Doheny, M. O. B., Eddy, D. M., Black, S. O., Wyper, M. A., Coeling, H. V., & Turkoski, B. B. (1992). Creation and use of a nursing diagnosis data base related to nursing of adults. In J. M. Arnold & G. A. Pearson (Eds.), *Computer applications in nursing education and practice* (pp. 287-295). New York: National League for Nursing (Publication No. 14-1406).

13. Experts push for the Nursing Minimum Data Set. (1991). *Nursing & Technology, 2*(4), 4-5.

14. Felts, W. R. (1989, October). *Need for standardized ambulatory care data: National provider perspective.* (Abstract 3023). Paper presented at the meeting of the American Public Health Association, Chicago.

15. Fitzpatrick, J. J., Kerr, M. E., Saba, V. K., Hoskins, L. M., Hurley, M. E., Mills, W. C., Rottkamp, B. C., Warren, J. J., & Carpenito, L. J. (1989). Translating nursing diagnosis into ICD Code. *American Journal of Nursing, 89,* 493-495.

16. Hawes, C., Morris, J., Phillips, C., Mor, V., & Fries, B. (1992). *The reliability of the minimum data set (MDS) for nursing home resident assessment and care planning and its utility in clinical practice and research.* (Abstract). (From Abstracts, Health Services Research Conference). AHSR and FHSR Ninth Annual Meeting, Chicago. Health Services Research: Implications for Policy, Management, and Clinical Practice. Washington, D.C.: Association for and Foundation for Health Services Research.

17. Hays, B. J. (1992). Nursing care requirements and resource consumption in home health care. *Nursing Research, 41,* 138-143.

18. Health Information Policy Council. (1983). *Background paper: Uniform minimum health data sets.* (Unpublished). Washington, D.C.: Department of Health and Human Services.

19. Health Information Policy Council. (1984). *1984 revision of the uniform hospital discharge data set.* (Unpublished). Washington, D.C.: Department of Health and Human Services.

20. Health Information Policy Council. (1985). 1984 revision of the uniform hospital discharge data set. *Federal Register, 50*(147), 31038-31040.

21. Hettinger, B. J., & Brazile, R. P. (1992). A database design for community health data. *Computers in Nursing, 10,* 109-115.

22. Iowa Intervention Project. (1992). In J. C. McCloskey & G. M. Bulechek (Eds.), *Nursing interventions classifications (NIC).* St Louis: Mosby.

23. Jacox, A. (1992). *Toward inclusiveness of scope in nursing diagnoses.* Paper presented at the meeting of the North American Nurses Diagnosis Association, San Diego, Calif.

24. Leske, J. S., & Werley, H. H. (1992). Use of the NMDS. *Computers in Nursing, 10,* 259-263.

25. Maas, M., Buckwalter, K., & Hardy, M. A. (Eds.). (1991). *Nursing diagnoses and interventions for the elderly.* Redwood City, Calif: Addison-Wesley Nursing.

26. Marek, K. D. (1992). *Analysis of the relationships among nursing diagnosis and other selected patient factors, nursing interventions and other measures of utilization, and outcomes in home health care.* Unpublished doctoral dissertation, University of Wisconsin–Milwaukee.

27. Morris, J. N., Hawes, C., Fries, B. E., Phillips, C. D., Mor, V., Katz, S., Murphy, K., Drugovich, M. L., & Friedlob, A. S. (1990). Designing the national resident assessment instrument for nursing homes. *Gerontologist, 30,* 293-307.

28. Murnaghan, J. H. (Ed.). (1973). Ambulatory care data: Report of the conference on ambulatory medical care records. *Medical Care, 11*(2, Suppl), 1-205.

29. Murnaghan, J. H. (Ed.). (1976). Long-term care data: Report of the conference on long-term health care data. *Medical Care, 14*(5, Suppl), 1-233.

30. Murnaghan, J. H. (1978). Uniform basic data sets for health statistical systems. *International Journal of Epidemiology, 7,* 263-269.

31. Murnaghan, J. H., & White K. L. (Eds.). (1970). Hospital discharge data: Report of conference on hospital discharge abstract system. *Medical Care, 8*(4, Suppl), 1-215.

32. National Committee on Vital and Health Statistics. (1980a). *Long-term health care: Minimum data set.* (DHHS Publication No. PHS 80-1158). Hyattsville, Md: U.S. Department of Health and Human Services, National Center for Health Statistics.

33. National Committee on Vital and Health Statistics. (1980b). *Uniform hospital discharge data: Minimum data set.* (DHEW PUblication No. PHS 80-1157). Hyattsville, Md: U.S. Department of Health, Education, and Welfare, National Center for Health Statistics.

34. National Committee on Vital and Health Statistics. (1981). *Uniform ambulatory medical care: Minimum data set.* (DHHS Publication No. PHS 81-1161). Hyattsville, Md: U.S. Department of Health and Human Services, National Center for Health Statistics.

35. NCVHS Subcommittee on Ambulatory and Hospital Care Statistics. (1992). *Proposed revision to the uniform hospital discharge data set, June 1992.* Hyattsville, Md: U.S. Department of Health and Human Services, National Center for Health Statistics.

36. Shugars, D. A., O'Neil, E. H., & Bader, J. D. (Eds.). (1991). *Healthy America: Practitioners for 2005: An agenda for action for U.S. health professional schools.* Durham, N.C.: The Pew Health Professions Commission.

37. Study Group on Nursing Information Systems. (1983). Special report, computerized nursing information systems: An urgent need. *Research in Nursing & Health, 6,* 101-105.

38. Thompson, J. D. (1988). Introduction (Part Six): Nursing Minimum Data Set and effectiveness of nursing care. In H. H. Werley & N. M. Lang (Eds.), *Identification of the Nursing Minimum Data Set* (pp. 282-288). New York: Springer Publishing.

39. Tillman, H. J. (1990). *Test of the Nursing Minimum Data Set in a nursing center.* Unpublished master's thesis, Marquette University, Milwaukee, Wis.

40. Visiting Nurse Association of Omaha. (1986). *Client management information system.* Washington, D.C.: U.S. Department of Health and Human Services, Health Resources and Services Administration, Division of Nursing.

41. Werley, H. H. (1987). Nursing diagnosis and the Nursing Minimum Data Set. In A. M. McLane (Ed.), *Classification of nursing diagnoses: Proceedings of the seventh conference* (pp. 21-36). St Louis: Mosby.

42. Werley, H. H., & Devine, E. C. (1987). The Nursing Minimum Data Set: Status and implications. In K. J. Hannah, M. Riemer, W. C. Mills, & S. Letourneau (Eds.), *Clinical judgment and decision making: The future with nursing diagnosis* (pp. 540-551). New York: Wiley.

43. Werley, H. H., Devine, E. C., & Zorn, C. R. (1988a). The Nursing Minimum Data Set: Effort to standardize collection of essential data. In J. Ball, K. J. Hannah, U. Gerdin Jelger, & H. E. Peterson (Eds.), *Nursing informatics* (pp. 160-167). New York: Springer-Verlag.

44. Werley, H., Devine, E., & Zorn, C. R. (1988b). *The Nursing Minimum Data Set data collection manual* (reprint ed.). Milwaukee, Wis: University of Wisconsin–Milwaukee, School of Nursing. (Original work published 1988; reprinted 1990, 1992)

45. Werley, H., Devine, E., & Zorn, C. R. (1988c). Nursing needs its own minimum data set. *American Journal of Nursing, 88,* 1651-1653.

46. Werley, H., Devine, E., & Zorn, C. R. (1989). Status of the Nursing Minimum Data Set (NMDS) and its relationship to nursing diagnosis. In R. M. Carroll-Johnson (Ed.), *Classification of nursing diagnoses: Proceedings of the eighth conference* (pp. 89-97). Philadelphia, Pa: J. B. Lippincott.

47. Werley, H. H., Devine, E. C., & Zorn, C. R. (1990). The Nursing Minimum Data Set (NMDS): Issues for the profession. In J. C. McCloskey & H. K. Grace (Eds.), *Current issues in nursing* (3rd ed., pp. 64-70). St Louis: Mosby.

48. Werley, H. H., Devine, E. C., & Zorn, C. R., Ryan, P., & Westra, B. L. (1991). The Nursing Minimum Data Set: Abstraction tool for standardized, comparable, essential data. *American Journal of Public Health, 81,* 421-426.

49. Werley, H. H., & Grier, M. R. (Eds.). (1981). *Nursing information systems.* New York: Springer Publishing.

50. Werley, H. H., & Lang, N. M., (Eds.). (1988). *Identification of the Nursing Minimum Data Set.* New York: Springer Publishing.

51. Werley, H. H., Lang, N. M., & Westlake, S. K. (1986a). Brief summary of the Nursing Minimum Data Set conference. *Nursing Management, 17*(7), 42-45.

52. Werley, H. H., Lang, N. M., & Westlake, S. K. (1986b). The Nursing Minimum Data Set conference—executive summary. *Journal of Professional Nursing, 2,* 117-224.

53. Werley, H. H., & Leske, J. S. (1991). Use and implementation of the Nursing Minimum Data Set. In E. J. S. Hovenga, K. J. Hannah, K. A. McCormick, & J. S. Ronald (Eds.), *Proceedings of the fourth international conference on nursing use of computers and information science* (pp. 91-99). Berlin: Springer-Verlag.

54. Werley, H. H., & Zorn, C. R. (1989). The Nursing Minimum Data Set and its relationship to classification for nursing practice. In *Classifications for nursing practice* (pp. 50-54). Kansas City, Mo: American Nurses Association.

55. Zielstorff, R. D., McHugh, M. L., & Clinton, J. (1988). *Computer design criteria for systems that support the nursing process.* Kansas City, Mo: American Nurses Association.

CHAPTER 16

Nursing diagnosis taxonomy development

Overview and issues

JUDITH J. WARREN

Development of the North American Nursing Diagnosis Association's (NANDA) Nursing Diagnosis Taxonomy during the past 20 years has had great significance for the profession of nursing and the organization of nursing knowledge. The effort and vision of many nurses have created a document that has led to much debate concerning the need for a standardized language, how the diagnoses should be classified, and even what constitutes a nursing diagnosis. The following is a discussion of the benefits of a taxonomy, the development of Taxonomy I, the evolution to Taxonomy II, and the issues concerning NANDA's Nursing Diagnosis Taxonomy.

BENEFITS OF A TAXONOMY

There are four major purposes for constructing a taxonomy regardless of the types of objects being classified. First, a taxonomy describes the structure and relationships of the objects between each other. The relationships are simplified so that general statements can be made about groups of objects. Second, the taxonomy generates hypotheses that describe the relationships among the objects. Third, the taxonomy achieves an economy of memory (the mind can deal with classes of objects, not numerous single cases) and facilitates communication. Without the ability to summarize information and label conveniently, people are unable to communicate. Fourth, the taxonomy eases the manipulations of observations. It makes the retrieval of information easy—a must in the age of computerized records.

Fleischman and Quaintance[10] proposed that taxonomic development has both scientific and practical benefits. The scientific benefit for nursing is the promotion of research and theory development for use in practice. First, the diagnoses may be used as key words for the communication of nursing knowledge and the storage and retrieval of nursing information. Second, similar diagnoses suggest similar databases (variables of concern) that facilitate the comparison of results between studies. This enables previous research results to be generalized or extended to include new diagnoses as they are developed. Third, by studying the relationships between and among the diagnoses in the taxonomy, gaps in nursing knowledge become apparent. Fourth, by naming nursing phenomena, nursing diagnoses assist in nursing theory development.[13,33] Walker and Avant[30] even suggest that well developed nursing diagnoses are mid-range theories.

Some possible practical benefits involve uses of the diagnostic labels and taxonomy for purposes other than labeling patient problems. Fleischman and Quaintance suggest "a number of ostensibly disparate problems are drawn together and can be viewed in a new light by the application of such a taxonomy."[10] Job descriptions contain the responsibility to diagnose patient problems for which the nurse is accountable, while performance criteria include accurate identification and treatment of specific nursing diagnoses. Diagnostic ability could be part of a set of criteria for job placement. Since the taxonomy organizes and explicates part of the domain of nursing practice, nurse-patient system designs must account for nursing diagnoses and their function (the original challenge that led to the development of nursing diagnoses). The taxonomy's coding scheme and relational structure can provide the standardized nomenclature for computerized documentation of nursing's contribution to patient care (the second part of the original challenge).

Finally, the taxonomy provides a convenient structure that clusters groups of diagnoses. These clusters may provide organizing frameworks for educational program designs.[28]

DEVELOPMENT OF TAXONOMY I

In the early 1970s, two nurses were asked to participate in a project that required patient data to be computerized (including retrievability of the data set) and discipline-specific care to be provided in a multidisciplinary setting (each discipline providing unique care). The nurses were frustrated because there was no standardized list of nursing problems that could be used to code patient data for retrievability or to communicate the unique services of nursing. Their efforts to solve this dilemma led to the first meeting of the National Conference Group for the Classification of Nursing Diagnoses in 1973. This group began the formal effort of identifying, developing, and classifying nursing diagnoses.[15]

The national conference group convened invitational meetings again in 1975, 1978, 1980, and 1982 to continue this work.[11,22,23] Nurses were invited to participate in the second through fifth conferences based on clinical experience with nursing diagnoses and expertise in taxonomic development. Diagnoses during this period were accepted and/or rejected by a majority vote of the conference participants. This practice accounted for some diagnoses being added to and deleted from earlier lists. The National Conference Group, unable to agree on a conceptually based classification scheme, decided to organize the diagnoses alphabetically. Since the majority of the diagnoses began with "A" for alteration, a second decision was made to list the basic concept of the diagnosis first, followed by the descriptive modifiers. For example, "alteration in bowel elimination, constipation" was listed alphabetically as "bowel elimination, alteration in: constipation." As the use of nursing diagnoses began to spread, many nurses used the diagnoses as alphabetically listed instead of writing the diagnosis in a grammatically correct format. This made learning and working with nursing diagnosis difficult. The language seemed awkward, and many nurses dismissed nursing diagnosis as a quickly passing fad. It was clear more work on nursing diagnoses and on the classification system was needed.[19,33]

A group of nurse theorists, chaired by Sr. Callista Roy, was invited to the third conference to develop a conceptually based taxonomic structure. Using induc-

tive methods, they identified nine domains or patterns that grouped similar diagnoses.[22] At the fifth conference the nurse theorists presented a proposed model for the development of the taxonomy—the nine "Patterns of Unitary Man."[23] The group, however, only identified and described the patterns. No classification of diagnoses within the patterns was attempted by the theorists. Neither was a detailed report of the inductive process ever published.

Also at the fifth conference, a special interest group interested in taxonomic structures used clustering techniques to explore the relationships between some of the diagnoses. When they encountered different conceptual levels, they used branching networks or "trees" to visually display the relationships. The first branch contained the most abstract diagnoses while the most concrete diagnoses were in the more distant branches. This activity led to the development of the "taxonomic trees" published in several conference proceedings. The clusters of diagnoses were very similar to the patterns proposed by the nurse theorists.[23] This work plus the theorist model was used a basis for the development of the current NANDA taxonomy.

Before the sixth conference, a taxonomy committee was appointed to continue the work begun by the nurse theorists and the special interest group. Furthermore, a formal process for peer review and acceptance of new nursing diagnoses was developed. This process was implemented to improve the quality and to document the validity of each nursing diagnosis. The peer review process began phasing in requirements for validation studies as part of the diagnosis submission process. See the following for diagnosis validation methods: Fehring,[8] Grant, Kinney, & Guzzetta,[14] NANDA.[26]

Valid diagnoses are crucial to developing a valid taxonomy. At the seventh conference, there was a debate about whether or not to use the nine patterns as an organizational structure for the taxonomy. Many participants wanted specific nursing theories or assessment frameworks to guide classification. It was reiterated that the taxonomy was not to be developed to endorse a specific nursing theory or assessment framework. The debate stemmed from a lack of clarity concerning the rules of diagnosis classification and definitions of the nine patterns. The Taxonomy I, as proposed by the taxonomy committee, was finally endorsed for further development by the membership at this conference. The taxonomy committee published the rules used to classify the diagnoses (see the box on page 125) and developed extensive definitions for the

---

RULES FOR CLASSIFICATION[26]

1. There is no inherent order in the numbering of the nine patterns. The patterns and diagnoses were sequentially numbered as they were considered.
2. The level of abstraction determines the level of placement within the taxonomy. Supporting literature from the submitter, expert opinion, and nursing literature assist in making the determination of placement within a pattern.
3. The diagnosis is classified by considering the consistency between the definition of the pattern and the definition of the diagnosis.
4. The placement of the diagnosis must be conceptually consistent with current theoretical views within nursing.
5. Categories in brackets were developed by the committee to clarify why certain diagnoses were placed at a specific level. It is hoped that these bracketed categories or other diagnoses will be submitted for inclusion.
6. The numbering system was developed to facilitate computerization of the taxonomy.

From: The North American Nursing Diagnosis Association. Used with permission.

---

patterns.[20] These were adopted by NANDA in 1990 and published in the introduction to Taxonomy I Revised.[6,27]

During the fifth conference, NANDA became an official nursing organization.[23] Five conferences have been held since 1982, all open to nurses wanting to become involved in the excitement of identifying and classifying nursing diagnoses.[5-7,17,25] During these years, NANDA has collaborated with the American Nurses Association (ANA) and other nursing specialty organizations to further this work (see Table 16-1).

Translation of Taxonomy I Revised into ICD Code. As part of the ongoing collaboration with the ANA, the taxonomy committee translated NANDA's taxonomy into the format used by the World Health Organization (WHO). WHO revises and publishes the International Classification of Disease (ICD), which organizes an international database for health care and is used to standardize the reporting of mortality and morbidity rates. The inclusion of nursing diagnoses facilitates the development of an international nursing database within the ICD framework.[9] Two characteristics of this translation were (1) coding only at two levels of abstraction and (2) using "high risk" instead

Table 16-1 History of nursing diagnosis

Year	Author	Event
1973	American Nurses Association	Published first standards of practice; Standard II specifically recognized nursing diagnosis
1973	Gebbie & Lavin	First conference for the classification of nursing diagnoses
1975	Gebbie	Second conference for the classification of nursing diagnoses
1978	Kim & Moritz	Third conference for the classification of nursing diagnoses; nursing theorists joined the effort
1980	Kim & Moritz	Fourth conference for the classification of nursing diagnoses
1980	American Nurses Association	Published *Social Policy Statement*; defined nursing as diagnosis and treatment of human responses to health problems
1982	Kim, McFarland & McLane	Fifth conference for the classification of nursing diagnoses; NANDA organized; nurse theorists submitted proposed taxonomic structure
1983	Warren	Demonstrated use of nursing diagnosis in establishing accountability measures in nursing
1984	Hurley	Sixth NANDA conference, taxonomy committee met for first time
1986	McLane	Seventh NANDA conference, endorsed Taxonomy I
1987	Hanna, Reimer, Mills & Letourneau	First international nursing diagnosis conference in Canada
1987	American Nurses Association	Endorsed NANDA as responsible for classification of nursing diagnoses
1988	Carroll-Johnson	Eighth NANDA conference
1990	Carroll-Johnson	Ninth NANDA conference, taxonomy committee presented possibilities for Taxonomy II
1992	Carroll-Johnson	Tenth NANDA conference, possible linkages with other databases discussed
1992	American Nurses Association	Revised nursing practice standards still recognize nursing diagnoses

of "potential." The boards of NANDA and ANA approved the final document, which was forwarded to WHO. The list of nursing diagnoses was also submitted to the publishers of the FCD-10 CM (*International Classification of Disease tenth edition–Clinical Modification*). The clinical modification of the ICD provides the major coding scheme used by most third-party payers and reporters of health care resource utilization in the United States. Inclusion of nursing diagnoses in the FCD-10 CM would articulate patient conditions requiring nursing care (this decision has yet to be made). Nursing diagnoses were not included in the ICD-10, but ANA and NANDA were encouraged by WHO to resubmit for the ICD-11.

DEVELOPMENT OF TAXONOMY II

Recent developments of the taxonomy have evolved from the work on the ICD translation and study of issues raised by the NANDA membership. A series of papers was presented at the ninth conference to include the membership in a dialogue about the future of NANDA's taxonomy. The major issues presented were (*a*) the use of axes to facilitate classification, (*b*) the reduction of the number of levels of abstraction from six to two, (*c*) some methods for testing the taxonomic structure and classification rules, (*d*) the use of the taxonomic structure in practice, and (*e*) the deletion of diagnoses that did not meet the criteria specified in the new NANDA definition of a nursing diagnosis. Detailed discussions of these points can be found in the proceedings of the ninth conference and the series of articles by the taxonomy committee.[6,16,19-21]

ISSUES CONCERNING THE NANDA TAXONOMY
Conceptual framework

One of the primary issues concerning the NANDA taxonomy is the conceptual framework, used to organize the taxonomy. This framework, developed by the nurse theorists, was inductively derived by observing similarities and differences between 42 diagnoses—the complete diagnostic list in 1978. The identification of the similarities and differences of the diagnoses is the first step in organizing knowledge about this nursing phenomena. These observations became the basis for the classification of diagnoses and for the formulation of criteria of category inclusion or exclusion.

Fleischman and Quaintance state, "classification is necessary for drawing generalizations across events, one of the important goals of science, and for establishing efficient communication among scientists."[10]

The difficulty is that the identification of the similarities and differences depends on the purpose of the taxonomy. This is best explained using the example of a cookbook. One author may note similarities based on the course of the meal—appetizer, salad, main course, or dessert. Another book may be categorized by type of dish—pasta, crepe, quiche, or casserole. Both classifications are useful, unless the cook wishes to look for a recipe using eggs or beef. Then another cookbook is needed or the cook looks through each recipe in both books.

As with cooks, nursing must keep an open mind as to the development or evolution of nursing diagnosis taxonomies; however, that does not mean that nursing should wait until the perfect classification framework appears. The Omaha VNA system[24] and the home health care system developed by Saba et al.[29] are two systems that also have nursing diagnoses classified, even though diagnostic labels and organizing frameworks are different. These two systems have been developed for specific types of nursing practice, while the NANDA system has been developed to identify and classify all those things that nurses identify or diagnose in patients regardless of setting. Thus, there is no single framework for classifying the phenomena in nursing and nurses need not be sensitive about attaining a single framework for taxonomic development.

Validating Taxonomy I

Validation of Taxonomy I Revised is the second major issue. The lack of taxonomic validation has been a major concern of the proponents and critics of the NANDA taxonomy. Both Kerr[21] and Warren[1,32] have proposed models and methodologies for the process. The biggest roadblock to validation is money. Validating or testing a taxonomy the size and scope of NANDA's requires considerable resources. While the Omaha VNA System[24] and the Home Health Care Classification Project[29] have been able to obtain federal grants to fund their validation projects, NANDA has not had the resources or institutional support to do the same. Validation of this taxonomy is critical for nursing as computerized databases are developing and linking. There must be coded, retrievable data that captures what nurses do for and with patients—the phenomena nurses treat and the patient outcomes that are nurse sensitive.

Collaboration with the American Nurses Association

NANDA has had very positive experiences collaborating with the ANA. The Social Policy Statement defined nursing in terms of diagnosing.[3] Nursing diagnoses have been integral to the Standards of Nursing Practice.[2] The 1992 standards mandate guideline development in nursing based on nursing diagnoses and other care problems. In 1987 ANA agreed that NANDA was the organization responsible for classifying nursing diagnoses. Currently, NANDA has representation on an ANA committee—the Steering Committee on Data Bases to Support Clinical Nursing Practice.[35] This committee has been asked to identify essential data elements and databases necessary to document the services provided by nursing. All current databases and taxonomies are being evaluated (for example, Bulechek & McCloskey,[4] Martin & Scheet,[24] NANDA,[27] Saba et al.,[29] Werley & Lang[34]). These databases will provide nursing with statistics on prevalence rates of nursing diagnoses, frequencies of specific nursing interventions, patient acuity, nurse-sensitive outcomes, and resultant costs. Nursing will be in a much stronger position to lobby for health policy and reimbursement reforms if hard data describing the impact of nursing, instead of stories about individual patient responses, are available. Nursing needs instant access to summaries of large patient information data sets, achievable only through computerized patient records where nursing information is coded and retrievable. While the NANDA taxonomy is not perfect, it is available and it does describe what nurses diagnose. The taxonomy provides a coding scheme and structure for a computerized database—one of the prime reasons for the beginning nursing diagnosis work. Nursing no longer has the luxury to wait until there is one perfect database; in fact, there never will be *one*. Medicine learned that lesson long ago with the development of the ICD, SNOMED (pathology codes), CPT codes (medical procedures code), DSM III (psychiatric diseases), and many other taxonomies that describe medical practices in a variety of settings and for a variety of purposes. The ANA committee supports multiple taxonomies and will be recommending the use of many databases, both nursing and nonnursing, in order to capture the data that supports nursing practice.

The ability to accomplish the goal of accessing and analyzing data across patients, units, hospitals, states, and nations requires a "standard" vocabulary for nursing diagnoses, nursing interventions, and patient outcomes. The standardization of terms does require consensus within the nursing community, but a word of caution: The use of standardized labels for describing patient phenomena does not imply a turning away

from nursing's commitment to individualized patient care. The use of standard databases does imply that nursing will have the tools necessary to identify, describe, and document the current use and future need for resources required for the delivery of individualized patient care.

Communication between databases

The ANA steering committee was also asked to identify other health care databases and whether or not nursing-sensitive issues could be identified within them. The National Library of Medicine (NLM) has developed a program that searches the known, accessible computerized databases, called the Unified Medical Language System and semantic network (UMLS). It is possible, using this system, to search databases such as HCFA (Health Care Finance Administration) claims database, HCFA uniform clinical data set, HCFA minimum data set for nursing facility resident assessment and care schema (in process of development), Medline, COSTAR (a computerized ambulatory medical record), ICD, CPT, and SNOMED to find information on resource utilization, patient conditions, or treatment options. Zielstorff,[35] a member of the steering committee, used the UMLS to query the available databases for evidence of nursing's contribution to patient care. She was not able to retrieve any nursing information because data were not coded for retrieval by nursing vocabulary, even though many of the databases contained information of interest to nursing. ANA has negotiated with the NLM to collaborate on a project that would create the necessary translations for the semantic network feature of the UMLS to access nursing phenomena. One taxonomy to be used will be the NANDA taxonomy. With the ability of the semantic network to link between standard databases, nursing will be free to use multiple taxonomies. All that is required is the translation from one taxonomy to another so that access can be facilitated. The UMLS is the tool nursing has needed to free it from premature closure in choosing THE taxonomy.

SUMMARY

There is still work to be done. Existing nursing diagnoses need to be refined and clinically tested in a variety of settings and with different patient populations. New diagnoses need to be identified, developed, tested, and classified. The role and articulation of nursing diagnoses in other computerized health care databases needs to be developed.[34,35] The need for a standardized language of nursing and measures of accountability are as great now as they were in the early 1970s.[31]

REFERENCES

1. Aden, C., & Warren, J. J. (1991). A validation study of NANDA's Taxonomy I. In R. M. Carroll-Johnson (Ed.), *Classification of nursing diagnoses: Proceedings of the ninth conference* (p. 273). Philadelphia: J. B. Lippincott.

2. American Nurses Association. (1973, 1992). *Standards of nursing practice.* Kansas City, Mo: Author.

3. American Nurses Association. (1980). *Nursing: A social policy statement.* Kansas City, Mo: Author.

4. Bulechek, G. M., & McCloskey, J. C. (1992). *Nursing interventions: Essential nursing treatments.* Philadelphia: W. B. Saunders.

5. Carroll-Johnson, R. M. (Ed.). (1989). *Classification of nursing diagnoses: Proceedings of the eighth conference.* Philadelphia: J. B. Lippincott.

6. Carroll-Johnson, R. M. (Ed.). (1991). *Classification of nursing diagnoses: Proceedings of the ninth conference.* Philadelphia: J. B. Lippincott.

7. Carroll-Johnson, R. M. (Ed.). (in press). *Classification of nursing diagnoses: Proceedings of the tenth conference.* Philadelphia: J. B. Lippincott.

8. Fehring, R. J. (1986). Validating diagnostic labels: Standardized methodology. In M. E. Hurley (Ed.), *Classification of nursing diagnoses: Proceedings of the sixth conference* (pp. 183-190). St Louis: Mosby.

9. Fitzpatrick, J. J., Kerr, M. E., Saba, V. K., Hoskins, L. M., Hurley, M. E., Mills, W. C., Rottkamp, B. C., Warren, J. J., & Carpenito, L. J. (1989). Translating nursing diagnosis into ICD code. *American Journal of Nursing, 89,* 493-495.

10. Fleischman, E. A., & Quaintance, M. K. (1984). *Taxonomies of human performance.* New York: Academic Press.

11. Gebbie, K. M. (Ed.). (1976). *Summary of the second national conference: Classification of nursing diagnoses.* St Louis, Mo: Clearinghouse—National Group for Classification of Nursing Diagnoses.

12. Gebbie, K. M., & Lavin, M. A. (Eds.). (1975). *Classification of nursing diagnoses: Proceedings of the first national conference.* St Louis: Mosby.

13. Gordon, M. (1990). Toward theory-based diagnostic categories. *Nursing Diagnosis, 1*(1), 5-11.

14. Grant, J. S., Kinney, M., & Guzzetta, C. E. (1990). Using magnitude estimation scaling to examine the validity of nursing diagnoses. *Nursing Diagnosis, 1*(2), 64-69.

15. Hannah, K. J., Reimer, M., Mills, W. C. & Letourneau, S. (Eds.). (1987). *Clinical judgement and decision making with nursing diagnosis (Proceedings of the international conference).* New York: John Wiley & Sons.

16. Hoskins, L. M., Kerr, M. E., Fitzpatrick, J. J., Warren, J. J., Avant, K., Carpenito, L. J., Hurley, M. E., Jakob, D., Lunney, M., Mills, W. C., & Rottkamp, B. C. (in press). Axes: Focus of Taxonomy II. *Nursing Diagnosis.*

17. Hurley, M. E. (Ed.). (1986). *Classification of nursing diagnoses: Proceedings of the sixth conference.* St Louis: Mosby.

18. Kerr, M. E. (1991). Validation of taxonomy. In R. M. Carroll-Johnson (Ed.), *Classification of nursing diagnoses: Proceedings of the ninth conference* (pp. 6-13). Philadelphia: J. B. Lippincott.

19. Kerr, M., Hoskins, L., Fitzpatrick, J., Hurley, M., Mills, W., Rottkamp, B., Warren, J., & Carpenito, L. (1991). From Taxonomy I to Taxonomy II. *Nursing Diagnosis, 2*(3), 131-136.

20. Kerr, M. E., Hoskins, L. M., Fitzpatrick, J. J., Warren, J. J., Avant, K. C., Carpenito, L. J., Hurley, M. E., Jakob, D., Lunney, M., Mills, W. C., & Rottkamp, B. C. (1992). Development of definitions for Taxonomy II. *Nursing Diagnosis, 3*(2), 65-71.

21. Kerr, M. E., Hoskins, L. M., Fitzpatrick, J. J., Warren, J. J., Avant, K. C., Carpenito L. J., Hurley, M. E., Jakob, D., Lunney, M., Mills, W. C., & Rottkamp, B. C. (submitted). Taxonomic analysis: An overview. *Nursing Diagnosis.*

22. Kim, M. J., McFarland, G. K., & McLane, A. M. (Eds.). (1984). *Classification of nursing diagnoses: Proceedings of the fifth national conference.* St Louis: Mosby.

23. Kim, M. J., & Moritz, D. A. (Eds.). (1982). *Classification of nursing diagnoses: Proceedings of the third and fourth national conferences.* New York: McGraw-Hill.

24. Martin, K. S., & Scheet, N. J. (1992). *The Omaha system: Applications for community health nursing.* Philadelphia: W. B. Saunders.

25. McLane, A. M. (Ed.). (1987). *Classification of nursing diagnoses: Proceedings of the seventh conference.* St Louis: Mosby.

26. North American Nursing Diagnosis Association. (1989). *Monograph of the invitational conference on research methods for validating nursing diagnoses.* St Louis: Author.

27. North American Nursing Diagnosis Association. (1990). *Taxonomy I Revised with official nursing diagnoses.* St Louis: Author.

28. Pearce, C. W., Gelser, L., Phillips, M., Tyra, P. A., Stecchi, J. M., & Gardner, M. (1990). Nursing diagnosis as content organizer. *Nurse Educator, 15*(1), 31-35.

29. Saba, V. K., O'Hare, P. A. Zuckerman, A. E., Boondas, J., Levine, E., & Oatway, D. M. (1991). A nursing intervention taxonomy for home health care. *Nursing & Health Care, 12*(6), 296-299.

30. Walker, L. O., & Avant, K. C. (1988). *Strategies for theory construction in nursing.* Norwalk, Conn: Appleton-Lange.

31. Warren, J. J. (1983). Accountability and nursing diagnosis. *Journal of Nursing Administration, 13*(10), 34-37.

32. Warren, J. J. (1987). A proposal for testing the Nursing Diagnosis Taxonomy I. In K. J. Hannah, M. Reimer, W. C. Mills, & S. Letourneau (Eds.), *Clinical judgment and decision making: The future with nursing diagnoses* (pp 111-114). New York: John Wiley & Sons.

33. Warren, J. J., & Hoskins, L. M. (1991). The development of NANDA's nursing diagnosis taxonomy. *Nursing Diagnosis, 1*(4), 162-168.

34. Werley, H. H., & Lang, N. M. (Eds.). (1988). *Identification of the Nursing Minimum Data Set.* New York: Springer.

35. Zielstorff, R. (in press). National databases: Nursing's challenge. In R. M. Carroll-Johnson (Ed.), *Classification of nursing diagnoses: Proceedings of the tenth conference.* Philadelphia: J. B. Lippincott.

CHAPTER 17

Nursing interventions classification (NIC)

Defining nursing care

GLORIA M. BULECHEK, JOANNE COMI McCLOSKEY

Classification is . . . at the heart of doing science. For science to operate and for scientists to communicate with one another, it is essential that practitioners share a common way of looking at phenomena and a vocabulary for talking about them.[26]

Although nurses are the largest group of health care professionals, their work is little understood and the impact of nursing care is virtually invisible. While nurses have been doing important work for decades, there is no systematic documentation of the problems they treat or the treatments they perform. In recent years, there has been recognition by the leadership of the nursing profession that classifications of nursing knowledge are needed in the areas of nursing diagnoses, nursing interventions, and patient outcomes. These classifications will enable nurses to communicate to clients and others what it is that they do, to provide a common language for nurses to talk with each other, and to illustrate areas where little is known and more study needs to be done. The efforts to systematize knowledge in the areas of nursing diagnoses and outcomes are described elsewhere in this section. This chapter provides an overview of the work to construct a classification of nursing interventions.

DEVELOPMENT OF NIC*

In May of 1992, the *Nursing Interventions Classification (NIC)* was published.[14] NIC contains a standardized

---

*Much of this section also appears in two other chapters: McCloskey, J. C., & Bulechek, G. M. (forthcoming). Classification of nursing interventions: Implications for nursing research. In J. Fitzpatrick, N. Polis, & J. Stevenson (Eds.), *Proceedings from State of the Science Congress.* New York: Springer Publishing; and McCloskey, J. C. & Bulechek, G. M. (forthcoming). Classification of nursing interventions: Implications for nursing diagnoses. In *Proceedings of the 10th national conference on the classification of nursing diagnoses.* Philadelphia: J. B. Lippincott.

list of 336 direct care nursing interventions, each with a definition, a set of activities that a nurse would do to carry out the intervention, and a short list of background readings. Five chapters overview in detail the ongoing research effort to develop and expand the classification. That effort is briefly outlined here.

The *Nursing Interventions Classification* is the work of a large University of Iowa research team done with the help of nurse experts from many specialties and with input and endorsement by the American Nurses Association. A grant from the National Center for Nursing Research, NIH (RO1-NR02029), as well as other support from the Rockefeller Foundation and the University of Iowa, has facilitated the effort. To make the project more manageable, five steps were identified:

1. Identification and resolution of the conceptual and methodological issues
2. Generation of an initial list of interventions
3. Refinement of the intervention labels and defining activities
4. Arrangement of the interventions in a taxonomic structure
5. Validation of the interventions and taxonomic structure

Each of these steps is explained briefly as follows.

Identification and resolution of the conceptual and methodological issues

During the first step of the research, a number of methodological and conceptual issues were identified and resolved. For example, one major conceptual issue was the question of what sorts of nursing activities should be included in an intervention taxonomy. Nursing interventions represent nurse actions or behaviors. This is different from nursing diagnoses and nursing outcomes, which represent the patient's actions or behaviors. Nurses, in fact, perform many activities to benefit the client. Seven groups of nursing activities were identified:[3]

1. Assessment activities to make a nursing diagnosis
2. Assessment activities to gather information for a physician to make a medical diagnosis
3. Nurse initiated treatments, in response to nursing diagnoses
4. Physician initiated treatments in response to medical diagnoses
5. Daily essential function activities that may not relate to either medical or nursing diagnoses but are done by the nurse for clients who cannot do these for themselves
6. Activities to evaluate the effects of nursing and medical treatments. These are also assessment activities but they are done for purposes of evaluation, not diagnosis
7. Administrative and indirect care activities that support the delivery of nursing care

We determined that the intervention taxonomy should include all direct-care treatment activities (both physician-prescribed and nurse-prescribed) that nurses do on behalf of patients. We expanded our definition of a nursing intervention:

A nursing intervention is any direct-care treatment that a nurse performs on behalf of a client. These treatments include nurse-initiated treatments resulting from nursing diagnoses, physician-initiated treatments resulting from medical diagnoses, and performance of the daily essential functions for the client who cannot do these.[3]

We used this definition to guide the selection of data sources so that we captured the type of activities found in categories 3, 4, and 5. More detail on this list of activities and other background for our research are available in a number of publications.[3,4,14,18,19] (See the box on this page for a summary of terminology related to nursing intervention taxonomy development.)

Generation of an initial list of interventions

We reasoned that nurses have documented their treatments for decades but at a very concrete level of action.

DEFINITION OF INTERVENTION TERMS

Classification of nursing interventions

The ordering or arranging of nursing activities into groups or sets on the basis of their relationships and the assigning of intervention labels to these groups.

Taxonomy of nursing interventions

A systematic organization of the intervention labels into what can be considered a conceptual framework with rules and principles for ordering the labels clearly articulated.

Nursing activities

Those behaviors or actions that nurses do to assist clients to move toward a desired outcome. Nursing activities are at the concrete level of action and examples include: "Raise the head of the bed 30 degrees," and "Explore the need for attention with the patient."

Nursing intervention

Any direct-care treatment that a nurse performs on behalf of a client. Nursing interventions include nurse-initiated treatments and physician-initiated treatments. Nursing intervention labels are at the conceptual level and require a series of actions or activities to carry them out.

Nurse-initiated treatments

Interventions initiated by the nurse in response to a nursing diagnosis: "an autonomous action based on scientific rationale that is executed to benefit the client in a predicted way related to the nursing diagnosis and the stated goals." Examples might include Patient Contracting, Counseling, Reminiscence Therapy, Preparatory Sensory Information, and Oral Health Promotion.

Physician-initiated treatments

Interventions that are initiated by a physician in response to a medical diagnosis but are carried out by a nurse in response to a "doctor's order." Examples might include Medication Administration, Electrolyte Monitoring, and IV Therapy.

From: Iowa Intervention Project. (1992). (*In J. C. McCloskey, & G. M. Bulechek [Eds.] Nursing interventions classification (NIC). St Louis: Mosby.*)

We reviewed nursing textbooks, published care planning guides, and nursing information systems that contain innumerable concrete nursing activities. Typically, textbooks include long lists of nursing actions for each type of patient; the list in one book is not the same as the list in another even though the same patient condition is being discussed. For example, if we compare the suggested nursing interventions for the nursing diagnosis of activity intolerance in several books, we find big differences. For treatment of activity intolerance, Moorhouse, Geissler, and Doenges[21] list 6 independent interventions (e.g., "Check vital signs before and immediately after activity") and 1 collaborative intervention ("Follow graded cardiac rehabilitation and activity program"); McFarland and McFarlane[20] list 3 goals with 24 interventions (e.g., "Assess the patient's past and present activity pattern" and "Engage immobile patient in passive exercise regimen"); and Carpenito[7] lists 8 major categories of interventions and 46 discrete activities (e.g., "Instruct person to practice controlled coughing four times a day" and "Discuss the need for annual immunizations [against flu, bacteria]"). The problem, we figured, was not to ignore these rich sources of data but to organize, categorize, and label the activities at higher levels of abstraction.

We reviewed and rated more than 30 possible data sources. We choose 14 of the highest rated sources for use in 8 content analysis exercises to create an initial list of intervention labels. Each content analysis procedure was done as follows: (1) approximately 250 concrete nursing activities from 2 related sources were randomly selected and entered into a computer file, (2) each activity was printed on a separate slip of paper and the slips distributed to all members of the research team, and (3) each team member independently categorized the activities and gave each category an intervention label. In the beginning, each label had to be generated by the team members based upon their knowledge and experience. As the list of labels grew, members selected a label already identified or added a new label if an appropriate one was not on the list. After eight exercises, the number of new labels being generated was small and the team felt it was time to go on to the next step.

Refinement of the intervention labels and defining activities

Following the literature-based exercises, we had a list of approximately 350 intervention labels each associated with anywhere from one to several hundred activities. Many of these activities were redundant as different sources proposed the same activity but with different wording. The task was the refinement of the labels and activities to begin to establish validity. Two methods were used: expert survey and focus group.

For the expert survey process, a two-round Delphi questionnaire to certified master's prepared nurses in particular specialty areas was used. Groups of related intervention labels were selected, lists of their accompanying activities generated by the computer, and, after some cleaning for face validity, each activity was rated as to the extent it characterized the label. Each survey used a Delphi technique with an adaptation of the Fehring method[10,11] for establishing content validity. Fehring's method adapted for intervention labels consists of the following steps:

1. Nurse experts rate the activity for each intervention on a scale of 1 (activity is not at all characteristic of intervention) to 5 (activity is very characteristic). They are also asked to suggest any missing activities and to comment on the definition.
2. The Delphi technique is used to enhance consensus among experts. Two rounds of questionnaires are used. Round 2 presents a refinement of the first list of activities and interventions based on previous responses by the nurses.
3. Weighted ratios are calculated for each activity. These are obtained by summing the weights assigned to each response and then dividing by the total number of responses. The weights established by Fehring were used: $5 = 1$, $4 = 0.75$, $3 = 0.50$, $2 = 0.25$, and $1 = 0$.
4. Activities with ratios equal to or greater than 0.80 are labeled as critical activities. Activities with ratios less than 0.50 are discarded. These cutoffs were set by Fehring as established conventions.
5. A total intervention content validity (ICV) score is obtained for each intervention by summing the individual activity ratings and averaging the results.

Between June 1989 and March 1991, we validated 138 interventions in 14 surveys to 483 nurse experts. Twelve of the surveys were published in the June 1992 issue of *Nursing Clinics of North America*.[5,6]

The second method, using a focus group, was instituted when it became apparent that the survey process was too time consuming and not appropriate for all labels. We could only include 12 to 15 labels on each survey in order to keep to a reasonable length. It was taking a minimum of six months to prepare questionnaires, obtain mailing lists, mail out, analyze responses and revise, mail again, and analyze and revise a second time. We also learned that interventions that have a known research base and are well-developed in the

---

EXAMPLE OF ONE INTERVENTION FROM NIC

Crisis intervention

Definition: Use of short-term counseling to help the patient cope with a crisis and resume a state of functioning comparable to or better than the pre-crisis state

Activities:

Provide atmosphere of support

Determine whether patient presents safety risk to self or others

Initiate necessary precautions to safeguard the patient or others at risk for physical harm

Encourage expression of feelings in a nondestructive manner

Assist in identification of the precipitants and dynamics of the crisis

Assist in identification of past/present coping skills and their effectiveness

Assist in identification of personal strengths and abilities that can be utilized in resolving the crisis

Assist in development of new coping and problem solving skills as needed

Assist in identification of available support systems

Provide guidance about how to develop and maintain support system(s)

Introduce patient to persons (or groups) who have successfully undergone the same experience

Assist in identification of alternative courses of action to resolve the crisis

Assist in evaluation of the possible consequences of the various courses of action

Assist patient to decide on a particular course of action

Assist in formulating a time frame for implementation of chosen course of action

Evaluate with patient whether crisis has been resolved by chosen course of action

Plan with patient how adaptive coping skills can be utilized to deal with crises in the future

Background readings:

Aguilera, D. C. (1974). *Crisis intervention: Theory and methodology.* St Louis: Mosby.

Chandler, S. C. (1989). Crisis theory and intervention. In B. S. Johnson (Ed.), *Psychiatric-mental health nursing: Adaptation and growth* (pp. 641-656). Philadelphia: J. B. Lippincott.

Kanak, M. F. (1991). Development and validation of selected patient safety nursing interventions. Master's thesis, University of Iowa, Iowa City.

Kanak, M. F. (1992, June). Interventions related to safety. In G. M. Bulechek, & J. C. McCloskey (Eds.), *Symposium on nursing interventions* (pp. 371-395). Nursing Clinics of North America.

Kus, R. J. (1985). Crisis intervention. In G. M. Bulechek, & J. C. McCloskey (Eds.), *Nursing interventions: Treatments for nursing diagnoses* (pp. 277-187). Philadelphia: W. B. Saunders.

Morley, W. E., Messick, J. M., & Aguilera, D. C. (1967). Crisis: Paradigms of intervention. *Journal of Psychiatric Nursing, 5,* 537-540.

From: Iowa Intervention Project. (1992). (*In J. C. McCloskey, & G. M. Bulechek [Eds.]* Nursing interventions classification (NIC). *St Louis: Mosby.*)

literature received few comments from our expert raters. For all of these reasons, we moved to the focus group method. For the focus group method, a team member prepared a draft of the label definition and activities for initial review by a small group of core team members followed by review of the entire team. Each review led to further refinement of the label, definition, and activities. Through the focus group method, 198 labels were prepared in 12 months.

At this point in the research, we published *NIC,* an alphabetical list of 336 interventions. (See the box above for one example.) While the work was by no means finished, we believed it was necessary to get something into the literature so the project would be known and others could use and provide feedback. We have, however, continued the work to identify and standardize interventions and to organize them in a taxonomy.

Arrangement of the interventions in a taxonomic structure

We have been using hierarchical clustering techniques to guide the development of a system of classification, or *taxonomy* of nursing interventions. Hierarchical cluster analysis groups nearby (that is, similar) interventions into clusters of related interventions and the clusters in turn can be grouped into "super-clusters" of similar clusters.[9,24] (See Fig. 17-1.) Now that we have the interventions defined, we need to identify an easy-to-use and clinically meaningful organizing structure.

At this time, we have identified an initial 26 groups of interventions,which we are calling classes, and we have 6 super-groups, which we are calling domains. In the next year, we will validate the groupings and define a three-tiered taxonomic structure for the interventions. The top level consisting of the 6 domains is the

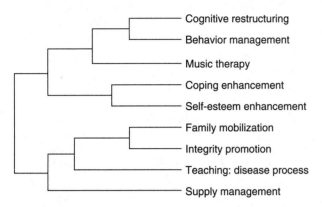

Hierarchical Cluster Analysis

- Cognitive restructuring
- Behavior management
- Music therapy
- Coping enhancement
- Self-esteem enhancement
- Family mobilization
- Integrity promotion
- Teaching: disease process
- Supply management

Fig. 17-1. Example of hierarchical clustering of nursing interventions.

most abstract. The second level consists of the 26 classes; the third level consists of the interventions.

Validation of the interventions and taxonomy

In order for the classification to be used, it needs validation from nurses in practice. In the spring and summer of 1992, we distributed a questionnaire asking for feedback on the interventions from the 45 clinical specialty nursing organizations participating in the American Nurses Association Committee on Nursing Practice Standards and Guidelines joint meetings. A similar questionnaire is also being distributed to a national sample of staff nurses in order to gain the perspective of the nurse in practice. We have also included a review form in the book, *Nursing Interventions Classification*. A questionnaire to assess the meaningfulness of the classes and domains is being constructed at the present time and will be distributed to a national sample of nurse experts in the future.

Future work to be done includes the development of a mechanism to evaluate and incorporate feedback on specific interventions, the development and validation of indirect care interventions, and the translation of the classification into a coding system that can facilitate computerization and can be used for articulation with other classifications and for reimbursement. Depending on continued funding, we will also field test the classification in four agencies. The field testing will be used to construct mechanisms to facilitate future research.

FEATURES OF NIC

NIC includes all direct care interventions that nurses do on behalf of patients, including both independent and collaborative interventions. The classification applies to nurses in all specialties and in all settings. While an individual nurse will have expertise in only a limited number of interventions, the entire classification is meant to capture the expertise of all nurses.

Although NIC was constructed inductively from activities used to document nursing care, we believe that it encompasses the lists of interventions currently in the literature. That is, it covers: Benner's Domains of Nursing Practice,[1] Bulechek and McCloskey's beginning taxonomy,[2] Griffith et al., CPT Routine Nursing Tasks,[12] Henderson's components of basic nursing practice,[13] National Council of State Board's Seventeen Categories of Client Needs,[15] Omaha Intervention Scheme,[16,28] Saba et al., Intervention Taxonomy for Home Health Care,[22] Sigma Theta Tau's Classification of Nursing Knowledge, Nursing Care/Interventions,[23] and Verran's Ambulatory Care Taxonomy.[8,27]

Nurses will use NIC just as they use a list of nursing diagnoses. That is, they will choose from the list the interventions appropriate for their particular patients. The classification does not prescribe interventions for particular diagnoses or populations of patients. The choosing of a nursing intervention for a particular patient is part of the clinical decision making of the nurse. In our book, *Nursing Interventions: Essential Nursing Treatments*, we discuss six factors that a nurse considers when choosing an intervention for a particular patient: (1) desired patient outcomes, (2) characteristics of the nursing diagnosis, (3) research base for the intervention, (4) feasibility for doing the intervention, (5) acceptability to the patient, and (6) capability of the nurse.[5]

NIC has been endorsed by the American Nurses Association as one of the nursing classifications that should be part of a unified nursing language and is one of the few nursing classifications that will be included in the National Library of Medicine's Metathesaurus for the Unified Medical Language System. An initial report indicates that only 15% of the NIC terms match the Metathesaurus medical terminology. This means that the nursing interventions contained in NIC are unique to nursing. NIC and other standardized nursing classifications also need to be included in other national databases concerned with our nation's health care. A number of such databases have been developed under the auspices of the National Committee on Vital and Health Statistics. Nursing needs to become visible in these databases that are used for the determination of national health care policy.[31] The Institute of Medicine is aggressively advocating computer-based patient records. The nursing data elements for an automated patient record will be needed before the end of the century. NIC is a major contribution toward this goal.

Many practice settings are working on the development of nursing and health care information systems. Institutions and vendors have long bemoaned the difficulty of building computerized systems for lack of standardized language representing nursing practice.[30] NIC provides a standardized language that helps to fill this void. It can be used across units within an agency, across health care settings, and across health care disciplines. Nursing information systems should be built with the capability of producing reports from actual patient data[25] that can help nurse executives with the planning for resources needed in nursing practice settings. As information about the most prevalent diagnoses and interventions is provided on a particular unit, there will be clear justification for the type of staff needed, the type of staff development required, and the amounts of equipment to be procured. This new generation of nursing information systems will also provide the data elements to determine the cost of services provided by nurses. New models of determining nursing cost[17] based upon the interventions performed are now possible with NIC. NIC can help in the construction of a reimbursement system for nursing care—a key issue in the reduction of health care cost, and it provides a classification for one of the key nursing care elements in the Nursing Minimum Data Set.[29]

NIC will also be very useful in nursing education. Current nursing textbooks are still based primarily upon medical knowledge, although many new editions have expanded their content to include more on nursing diagnoses. These books, however, are sparse on nursing treatments, and content consists largely of discrete activities at the procedural level. NIC provides the intervention concepts to better describe the work that nurses do and can help faculty determine curriculum sequencing. In the future, some of the more basic interventions will be taught to all students at the undergraduate level; others will be taught in advanced specialty courses at the master's level. Nursing education will also use the databases created in the nursing practice settings to build case scenarios to help students learn decision making through the analysis of actual clinical data.

The construction of NIC advances the state of nursing science by identifying and making possible new avenues of research. As indicated in the quotation at the beginning of this chapter, classification is essential in organizing the knowledge of a discipline. NIC makes explicit what previously has been implicit about nursing treatment. The creation of databases derived from actual patient data containing nursing elements will make possible new kinds of studies. It will be possible to look at the linkages between nursing diagnoses, nursing interventions, and desired outcomes and between nursing interventions and medical diagnoses and the interventions of other providers. Such studies will help to determine the most effective treatments for patients and the costs in providing these treatments.

REFERENCES

1. Benner, P. (1984). *From novice to expert.* Menlo Park, Calif: Addison-Wesley.
2. Bulechek, G. M., & McCloskey, J. C. (1987). Nursing interventions: What they are and how to choose them. *Holistic Nursing Practice, 1*(3), 38.
3. Bulechek, G. M., & McCloskey, J. C. (1989). Nursing interventions: Treatments for potential diagnoses. In R. M. Carroll-Johnson (Ed.), *Proceedings of the eighth conference, NANDA* (pp. 23-30). Philadelphia: J. B. Lippincott.
4. Bulechek, G. M., & McCloskey, J. C. (1990). Nursing intervention taxonomy development. In J. C. McCloskey & H. K. Grace, (Eds.), *Current issues in nursing* (3rd ed., pp. 23-28). St Louis: Mosby.
5. Bulechek, G. M., & McCloskey, J. C. (1992). *Nursing interventions: Essential nursing treatments* (2nd ed). Philadelphia: W. B. Saunders.
6. Bulechek, G. M., & McCloskey, J. C. (Eds.). (1992). Symposium on nursing interventions. In *Nursing clinics of North America.* Philadelphia: W. B. Saunders.
7. Carpenito, L. J. (1989). *Nursing diagnoses: Application to clinical practice* (3rd ed.). New York: McGraw-Hill.
8. Cohen, S. M., Arnold, L., Brown, L., & Brooten, D. (1991). Taxonomic classification of transitional follow-up care nursing interventions with low birthweight infants. *Clinical Nurse Specialist, 5,*(1), 31-36.
9. Everitt, B. (1974). *Cluster analysis.* London: Heinemann.
10. Fehring, R. J. (1986). Validating diagnostic labels: Standardized methodology. In M. E. Hurley (Ed.), *Classification of nursing diagnoses: Proceedings of the sixth conference.* St Louis: Mosby.
11. Fehring, R. J. (1987). Methods to validate nursing diagnoses. *Heart and Lung, 16*(6), 625-629.
12. Griffith, H. M., Thomas, N., & Griffith, L. (1991). MDs bill for these routine nursing tasks. *American Journal of Nursing, 91*(1), 22-25.
13. Henderson, V. (1961). *Basic principles of nursing care.* London: ICN.

14. Iowa Intervention Project (1992). In J. C. McCloskey & G. M. Bulechek (Eds.), *Nursing interventions classification (NIC)*. St Louis: Mosby.

15. Kane, M., Kingsbury, C., Colton, D., & Estes, C. (1986). *A study of nursing practice and role delineation and job analysis of entry-level performance of registered nurses.* Chicago: National Council of State Boards of Nursing.

16. Martin, K. S., & Sheet, N. J. (1992). *The Omaha system: A pocket guide for community health nursing.* Philadelphia: W. B. Saunders.

17. McCloskey, J. C. (1989). Implications of costing out nursing services for reimbursement. *Nursing Management, 20*(1), 44-49.

18. McCloskey, J. C., & Bulechek, G. M. (1992). Defining and classifying nursing interventions. *Proceedings from conference: Patient outcomes research: Examining the effectiveness of nursing practice* (pp. 63-69). Rockville, Md.

19. McCloskey, J. C., Bulechek, G. M., Cohen, M. Z., Craft, M. J., Crossley, J. D., Denehy, J. A., Glick, O. J., Kruckeberg, T., Maas, M., Prophet, C. M., & Tripp-Reimer, T. (1990). Classification of nursing interventions. *Journal of Professional Nursing, 6*(3), 151-215.

20. McFarland, G. K., & McFarlane, E. A. (1989). *Nursing diagnosis and intervention.* St Louis: Mosby.

21. Moorhouse, M. F., Geissler, A. C., & Doenges, M. E. (1987). *Critical care plans: Guidelines for patient care.* Philadelphia: F. A. Davis.

22. Saba, V. K., O'Hare, A., Zuckerman, A. E., Boondas, J., Levine, E. & Oatway, D. M. (1991). A nursing intervention taxonomy for home health care. *Nursing and Health Care, 12*(6), 296-299.

23. Sigma Theta Tau International Honor Society of Nursing. (1987). *Introduction to the international classification of nursing knowledge.* Indianapolis: Author.

24. Sokal, R. R. (1974). Classification: Purposes, principles, progress, prospects. *Science, 185,* 1115-1123.

25. Study Group on Nursing Information Systems. (1983). Computerized nursing information systems: An urgent need. *Research in Nursing and Health, 6*(2), 101-105.

26. Suppe, F. (1989). Classification. *International encyclopedia of communication* (pp. 292-296). New York: Oxford University Press.

27. Verran, J. (1981). Delineation of ambulatory care nursing practice. *Journal of Ambulatory Care Management, 4,*1-13.

28. Visiting Nurse Association of Omaha. (1986). *Client management information system for community health nursing agencies* (Pub. No. HRP-0907023). Washington, D.C.: U.S. Department of Health and Human Services.

29. Werley, H. H., & Lang, N. M. (Eds.) (1988). *Identification of the Nursing Minimum Data Set.* New York: Springer.

30. Zielstorff, R. D. (1984). Why aren't there more significant automated nursing information systems? *Journal of Nursing Administration, 14*(1), 7-10.

31. Zielstorff, R. D. (1992, April). National databases: Nursing's challenges. Presented at NANDA's 10th Conference on Classification of Nursing Diagnosis, San Diego, Calif.

CHAPTER 18

Nursing-focused patient outcomes

Challenge for the nineties

MARION JOHNSON, MERIDEAN MAAS

The current emphasis on the use of patient outcomes for the evaluation of health care effectiveness results from concerns about the cost, quality, and distribution of health care services. Costs can be controlled most efficiently by reducing health care services,[2] but maintaining quality becomes problematic when little is known about the relative effectiveness of health care interventions. As a result, government and private sources who pay the health care bill are putting pressure on physicians and other health care providers to define and justify what they are about.[4] This has created the need for information about the effects of health care interventions and precipitated the interest in patient outcomes.

The political interest in outcomes has produced an influx of money for outcomes research and has created a distinct area of study that Wennberg calls clinical evaluation science.[8] For nursing to become a full participant in this developing discipline, it is essential that patient outcomes influenced primarily by nursing care (nurse-sensitive patient outcomes*) be identified and measured.[16,23,25,26] The importance of outcomes research for nursing is demonstrated by the number of conferences focusing on outcomes assessment and research and the continued emphasis on outcomes in nursing literature.

This chapter will give an overview of the development of outcomes research with an emphasis on the role of nursing, identify conceptual issues in outcomes research, and address the need for standardization of nursing-sensitive patient outcomes.

THE EVOLUTION OF OUTCOMES RESEARCH

The study of patient outcomes is not a new endeavor for health care professionals. It had its beginnings when Florence Nightingale recorded and analyzed health care conditions and patient outcomes during the Crimean War.[20,41] Since that time, the measurement of patient outcomes has been sporadic, often discipline-specific, and frequently focused on medical practice. In the early 1900s, Codman, a Boston surgeon, proposed the use of outcome-based measures as indicators of medical quality. His work is considered the precursor of modern outcomes research.[37] Outcomes research was emphasized again in the mid 1960s when Donabedian[9] proposed a model utilizing structure, process, and outcome to assess medical care quality. This model received wide attention, was adopted by other health care disciplines, and is widely used today to direct the evaluation of health care quality.

Nursing also has a history of using patient outcomes to assess nursing care quality. In 1962, Aydelotte published one of the first studies to use changes in behavioral and physical characteristics of patients as outcomes of nursing care.[3] Since that time a number of nursing studies have used patient outcomes to measure the quality of nursing care and the effects of specific nursing interventions.[19] Considerable effort has been expended on developing outcome measures useful for nursing research and quality assurance and on categorizing these outcomes.[7,14,15,24,30,39,46]

---

*The term *nurse-sensitive patient outcomes* was coined by an expert planning group called together by the National Center for Nursing Research in May 1990 to discuss strategies for nursing outcomes research. NOTE: Some of the ideas presented in this paper are the result of the work of the Nursing Sensitive Patient Outcomes Research Team at the University of Iowa, College of Nursing. The team is co-chaired by Marion Johnson and Meridean Maas.

Despite the use of patient outcomes for medical and nursing research and quality assurance programs, outcomes research was not emphasized and, consequently, poorly funded until health care cost and quality became an economic and political issue. Funding is now available through the federal government and private enterprise, but much of it is targeted for the evaluation of physician practice. Federal funding is channeled through the recently formed Agency for Health Care Policy and Research (AHCPR) as well as through established health research centers and institutes.* Private funding has come from foundations, the Rand Corporation, and other businesses and insurance companies. This infusion of money has served to both stimulate and define outcomes research.

Effectiveness: The current focus

Government and other payers are interested in the appropriateness and effectiveness of interventions, as well as the benefits that can be accrued at a given cost.[34,40] Appropriateness is a measure of the ratio of benefit to risk; that is, does the benefit of an intervention exceed its risk sufficiently to justify its use?[4] Effectiveness is a measure of the relative costs and outcomes of alternative modes of treatment[33] and is determined through the study of linkages between health care structure, process, and outcome. The expectation is that effectiveness research will suggest how services can be eliminated, reduced, or altered to control costs, increase access, and maintain quality.

Outcomes have long been used in clinical research to evaluate the effects of new methodologies for treating disease conditions or controlling symptoms. What is new is the emphasis on research that ties cost to benefits and outcomes to structural and process components of practice. Additionally, the concept of outcomes has been expanded to include measures other than physiological parameters, and efforts are under way to standardize outcomes and facilitate database development. These changes require that health care professionals consider the purpose for which outcomes are assessed.

Efficacy and effectiveness

Historically, health care professionals have used efficacy, the outcomes that can be achieved under ideal conditions, to evaluate health care interventions.[22,40]

---

*For a historical account of the development of the Agency for Health Care Policy and Research, see Rettig.[36]

Studies are designed to control variables, interventions are well-defined, providers are often few and carefully trained in the techniques to be used, and patient populations are carefully selected. This type of clinical research is important to refine knowledge, test new innovations, and describe care modalities that promote positive outcomes. It provides answers to the questions, What is the right thing to do?[50] or What outcomes are possible with a given intervention?

The current focus on effectiveness of medical care and, by implication, the effectiveness of care provided by all health care providers emphasizes the results of health care interventions for normal practice conditions rather than ideal conditions.[22] Studies are designed to compare outcomes associated with interventions provided in multiple practice settings, by multiple health care providers, as part of routine practice, and with cross-sectional populations. Effectiveness answers the question, What outcomes are achieved with varied interventions and providers and at what cost? Ideally, both the efficacy and the effectiveness of an intervention are needed to evaluate quality.[5] Answers to the questions, What *can* be achieved? and What *was* achieved? allow us to ask, Why or why not?

Nursing, like other health disciplines, has focused on studying the efficacy of specific nursing interventions and the quality of nursing care, a concept that after three decades and numerous attempts to study has remained difficult to define and, consequently, to measure.[44] Efficacy studies continue to have an important role in nursing research, particularly in the evaluation of new innovations, but attention must also be given to effectiveness research. Focusing on effectiveness may assist in defining quality and generating new approaches for the identification and measurement of nursing-sensitive patient outcomes. The difficulty is that it also creates conceptual, design, and methodological challenges for nurse researchers. Few conceptual frameworks are available to guide research design and instrument development, and methods and instruments necessary for gathering and anlyzing outcome data are underdeveloped.[40]

A number of recent articles provide excellent discussions of the numerous design and methodological issues pertinent to the measurement of nurse-sensitive patient outcomes.[13,16,22,34,46] The remainder of this chapter will focus on some of the conceptual issues that need to be addressed in nursing outcomes research.

CONCEPTUAL ISSUES IN OUTCOMES RESEARCH

Conceptual issues are related to the complexity inherent in specifying patient outcomes and developing a model that portrays the influence of structural and process variables on patient outcomes. What outcomes are measured and how measures are developed is ultimately determined by the way in which outcomes are defined.

Definitional issues

Patient outcomes are an "immensely complex construct"[22] and the intricacy necessary for measurement has been difficult to capture without creating complex definitions. Definitions have varied from the simple: the end results of medical care[22] to the complex: functional, objective, and measurable changes in the health state of an individual or patient population of interest, upon which nurses have a direct influence and should be held accountable.[14] Despite the differences, most definitions imply that outcomes measure patient states and that the measurement occurs after the implementation of a health care intervention. The way in which the elements of the definition are conceptualized has implications for assessing nursing-sensitive patient outcomes.

Who is the patient? Patient outcomes focus on the recipient of care, but the term *patient* may be too limiting for evaluating nursing interventions. Patient connotes a single individual, but nursing interventions may be directed at a family, a group, or a community. Marek[25] has suggested the use of the term *client* rather than patient as the recipient of nursing care. The measurement issue suggested by this semantic debate is determination of the unit for data collection. In most cases, data will be collected at the individual level and aggregated to provide information about a group of interest; for example, all patients on a designated nursing unit, all patients with a medical diagnosis of acute myocardial infarction, all patients with a nursing diagnosis of urinary incontinence. Some outcomes may, however, require data to be collected at a group level; for example, interaction patterns among family members may not be adequately assessed by collecting individual data.

A second issue related to the definition of patient is the inclusion of significant others in the assessment of outcomes. Nursing has a history of focusing on family members, caregivers, and other individuals significant for the care of the individual patient. When assessing outcomes of nursing care, it would seem imperative to assess pertinent outcomes relative to these individuals to appreciate the full impact of nursing services.

What is patient state? The outcomes traditionally used to measure patient state—mortality, morbidity, laboratory results, and other signs and symptoms[12,22]—are no longer sufficient. Measures of patient state now include health status, quality of life, and patient satisfaction.[12,22,38] Even these expanded measures may not be sufficient to assess the effects of nursing interventions. Other patient states, such as patient behaviors, knowledge, and perceptions, may need to be measured. Specifying the states to be assessed is a prerequisite to the development of data collection tools and instruments.

A second issue in specifying patient state is related to the expectation that interventions will produce a positive change in patient state. This expectation causes confusion when using the terms *outcome, outcome criteria,* and *outcome standard. Outcome criteria* defined as statements of expected changes for a specific patient category—a definition consistent may be with standards—or as a component or aspect of structure, process, or outcome that reflects quality of care.[9] Additionally, the Joint Commission on Accreditation of Healthcare Organizations has introduced the term *indicator* to identify quantitative measures used to evaluate health care quality.[32,35,48]

In contrast, *outcomes* refer to the state of the patient, whether positive or negative, desirable or undesirable,[48] at the time data are collected. This may or may not reflect a change in the patient's condition when compared with previous patient states. McCormick[29] suggests the following states can occur after nursing interventions: improvement, stabilization, deterioration, and death. Because patient state, and thus outcomes, can be described along a continuum, rating scales can be applied to the measurement of client outcomes. The scale can be developed to measure individual outcomes in relation to a described population (norm-referenced) or in relation to objectives of care stated as client outcomes (criterion-referenced).[27] Rating scales developed for use in community settings are illustrated in the box on page 139. Scales of this type can be developed for specific outcomes and used to evaluate individual patient progress as well as the progress of a patient in relation to a larger population.

When to measure? Evaluation of the *changes* produced by a nursing intervention requires the assessment of patient state before and after the intervention.

A PATIENT OUTCOME RATING SCALE USED IN COMMUNITY HEALTH					
Concept	**1**	**2**	**3**	**4**	**5**
Knowledge The ability of the client to remember and interpret information	No knowledge	Minimal knowledge	Basic knowledge	Adequate knowledge	Superior knowledge

From: Martin, K. S., & Scheet, N. J. (1992). *The Omaha system: Applications for community health nursing.* Philadelphia: W. B. Saunders. Used with permission.

Comparison of the *effects* of more than one intervention, as is done in effectiveness research, can be made by contrasting post-intervention outcomes only but requires large sample size. The underlying assumption of either of these measures is that nursing interventions have an effect on patient state, but current nursing research is insufficient to support such a causal link.[25] Thus, the current emphasis on outcomes research provides nursing an unprecedented opportunity to identify and verify relationships between nursing interventions and patient outcomes.[16]

Although there is general agreement that outcomes should be measured following nursing interventions, the timing of data collection is problematic when studying structure-process-outcome-linkages. Data collected too soon after an intervention might not reflect the overall result of treatment while data collected too long after the intervention makes it more difficult to isolate the effects of the intervention from other variables that can influence outcomes. Timing of data collection is further complicated by the fact that outcomes often vary over the course of an illness, which makes it necessary to collect multiple measures of patient states. The advantage is that interval measures, if timing is specified, can provide longitudinal data useful

Activities of daily living (ADL) function level			
25%	**50%**	**75%**	**100%**
Needs total assistance	Needs partial assistance	Needs supervision	Independent

From: Wilson, A. A. (1988). Measurable patient outcomes: Putting theory into practice. *Home Healthcare Nurse, 6*(6), 15-18. Used with permission.

for comparisons and trending[26] and for making associations with structure and process variables. Jennings[16] has suggested the use of short-term, intermediate, and long-term outcomes to capture the relationships between nursing interventions and patient outcomes. The Council on Medical Service (1986) of the American Medical Association has determined that the evaluation of intermediate outcomes is acceptable and often more feasible.

Although agreement about what constitutes a patient outcome (what we are measuring) and how and when we measure needs to be reached, Schroeder[42] cautions that undue amounts of time and money should not be spent on determining correct terminology until outcomes research is developed further. Nursing must also turn its efforts to the development of a conceptual framework that links outcomes with other relevant variables and provides the information necessary to evaluate nursing practice.

Theoretical issues

Conceptual frameworks are needed to facilitate the identification, measurement, classification, and study of patient outcomes. Reviews of research point up the fact that conceptual frameworks are seldom used to support the identification of outcome variables.[19,45] Furthermore, Waltz and Strickland[45] found that studies examining relationships between nursing processes and outcomes frequently have failed to differentiate process and outcome variables and in some cases used the same tool to measure both variables. Development of a theoretical framework requires the resolution of a number of issues germane to the study of patient outcomes.

Outcome models. Patient outcomes have been studied primarily in relation to specific diagnoses—medical or nursing—and specific interventions, but a model of diagnosis --->intervention--->outcome is too simplistic for nursing outcomes research. The model does not account for the multiple patient related variables that can influence patient outcomes: patient characteristics and preferences, environmental and financial conditions, and social and family support. The model also fails to account for the structure and processes used in the delivery of health care; for example, the way in which nursing care is organized and delivered, the characteristics of the health care provider, the amount and type of communication between disciplines. All of these factors have the potential for influencing patient outcomes and need to be recognized in a model of patient outcomes. The question that needs to be addressed in outcomes research is: Can patient outcomes be interpreted to reflect the care delivered and *not* . . . other factors?[12]

The model also does not account for generic measures that do not relate to a specific diagnosis, nor for the fact that a given outcome may be the outcome of more than one diagnosis or intervention. Generic outcomes "measure concepts that are relevant for everyone" with the "focus on such basic human values as emotional well-being and the ability to function in everyday life."[47] With the emphasis nursing places on holistic care and caring, generic outcomes are particularly pertinent for the evaluation of nursing interventions. These outcomes, however, may not be derived if the model is based solely on nursing diagnosis, intervention, and outcome.

A model based on Donabedian's components of structure, process, and outcome was developed for the Medical Outcomes Study (MOS)[43,47] to evaluate the impact of physician practice on patient outcomes. The MOS study and framework has received wide attention among health service researchers and has implications for the development of nursing models. The MOS model might serve as a template for the development of a nursing model that reflects nursing structures, processes, and nursing-sensitive patient outcomes. Outcomes influenced by nursing and other disciplines—general well-being, quality of life, and patient satisfaction—are included in the model. Expansion of the model or the development of a similar model reflecting nursing practice would enhance collaborative studies of patient outcomes and assure that outcomes important for the evaluation of nursing are included in outcomes research.

Organizing nursing-sensitive patient outcomes. Efforts to organize nursing-sensitive patient

---

TWO CATEGORIES OF NURSING-SENSITIVE PATIENT OUTCOMES

Donabedian[10]

Physical health status
Mental health status
Social and physical functioning
Health attitudes/knowledge/behaviors
Utilization of professional health resources
Patient perceptions of the quality of nursing care

Marek[25]

Physiological indicators	Goal attainment
Psychosocial measures	Patient satisfaction
Functional status	Safety
Client behaviors	Frequency of service
Client knowledge	Cost
Symptom control	Rehospitalization
Home maintenance	Resolution of nursing
Well-being	diagnosis

---

outcomes can be traced to the landmark research of Horn and Swain[14] in the 1970s. They conducted extensive research to identify patient outcomes influenced by nursing care, validate outcome measures, and categorize the outcomes. More recently, efforts have focused on identifying and categorizing outcomes used to measure the effects of nursing care. Lang and Clinton[19] based their discussion of outcomes described in nursing literature on the 6 outcome categories identified by Donabedian[10] (see the box above). Marek[25,26] identified the 15 categories shown in this box. The categories used by Lang and Clinton reflect patient state, behaviors, and perceptions—concepts consistent with definitions of patient condition or state. The categories developed by Marek include greater specificity of patient states and also include items such as cost, home maintenance, goal attainment, and resolution of nursing diagnosis that, while important measures of nursing care effectiveness, are not direct measures of patient condition. The use of these elements to evaluate nursing interventions does, however, provide support for the inclusion of variables other than patient state to evaluate nursing care effectiveness.

Nursing or multidisciplinary outcomes? The majority of patient outcomes are not the result of the interventions of one discipline but rather reflect the coordinated efforts and interventions of a multidisciplinary health care team. Within such a context, is there a need to develop nursing-sensitive patient outcomes, or should the focus be on multidisciplinary outcomes only? Given the state of nursing science and the often-unrecognized role of nursing in health care, it behooves nursing to identify those patient outcomes most sensitive to nursing interventions, define the outcomes, and develop measures for these outcomes. Nursing-sensitive patient outcomes can then be included in multidisciplinary studies and other collaborative efforts. Identification of nursing-sensitive outcomes will ensure that a wider range of patient outcomes are assessed and allow the unique contributions of nursing to be recognized. For example, nursing has developed measures for well-being, quality of life, knowledge and compliance behaviors, coping behaviors, and a multiplicity of other patient outcomes that may not be captured by other disciplines. The challenge for nursing is to organize and validate these measures, for without the inclusion of nursing outcomes, "the validity of attempts to measure national health care quality is compromised"[25] and contributions of nursing will continue to be unrecognized.

Resolution of the conceptual and measurement issues in outcomes research is not the only challenge facing nursing in the next decade. To fully participate in outcomes research, nursing needs to standardize outcomes and contribute to data sets used in the evaluation of health care effectiveness.

DATA SET DEVELOPMENT

Computer technology has precipitated the development and use of large data sets for health care evaluation and outcomes research. The Health Care Financing Administration (HCFA) collects data on mortality, morbidity, disability, and cost for Medicare and Medicaid recipients and is currently expanding the database to monitor variations in interventions and outcomes. The government also is instituting the National Practitioner Data Bank to collect information on health care practitioners; the first to be monitored will be physicians and dentists, followed by nurses.[28] Additionally, the government is investigating the feasibility of linking clinical, research, and administrative data.[1] Development and use of data sets will undoubtedly accelerate with technologic advances, and it is imperative that nursing be represented in national data sets.

The current turmoil in the U.S. health care system provides an unprecedented opportunity for nursing to contribute to health care policy and influence system change. As policy makers become disenchanted with the current system, there is growing recognition that physician practice alone does not explain patient outcomes.[31] To seize the opportunity, nursing must establish a unified national database[21,29,33] that reflects the practice and outcomes of nursing.

Database development requires a common language and a standard way to organize data.[16] The essential first step in organizing and standardizing nursing information is to develop meaningful categories of data and establish uniform terminology.[17] Currently, a research team at the University of Iowa is conducting a study to identify, label, define, and classify nursing-sensitive patient outcomes and develop valid, reliable outcome measures. Other efforts are also under way. The American Nurses Association is working toward the establishment of standardized data sets for nursing in conjunction with the AHCPR.[18] Although the need for nursing data sets is immediate, the elements selected must be scientifically sound to assure sound effectiveness research[33] and to capture the impact of nursing interventions and practice.

CONCLUSION

The way in which nursing revolves the issues discussed in this chapter may well influence nursing's future roles in health care as well as the development of nursing science. Identifying and measuring nurse-sensitive patient outcomes is an arduous task, but the rewards will be great for both the profession and the clients we serve.

REFERENCES

1. Agency for Health Care Policy and Research. (1991). *Report to Congress: The feasibility of linking research-related data bases to federal and non-federal medical administrative data bases* (AHCPR Publication No. 91-0003). Rockville, Md: Author.
2. Aiken, L. (1988). Assuring the delivery of quality patient care. *Nursing resources and the delivery of patient care* (NIH Publication No. 89-3008, pp. 3-10). Washington, D.C.: U.S. Government Printing Office.
3. Aydelotte, M. (1962). The use of patient welfare as a criterion measure. *Nursing Research, 11,* 10-14.
4. Brook, H. L. (1989). Practice guidelines and practicing medicine: Are they compatible? *Journal of American Medical Association, 262,* 3027-3030.
5. Bunker, J. P. (1988). Is efficacy the gold standard for quality assessment? *Inquiry, 25*(1), 51-58.
6. Council on Medical Service. (1986). Quality of care [Council Report]. *Journal of American Medical Association, 256,* 1032-1034.

7. Daubert, E. (1979). Patient classification system and outcome criteria. *Nursing Outlook, 27,* 450-454.

8. DeFriese, G. H. (1990). Measuring the effectiveness of medical interventions: New expectations of health services research [Editorial Preface]. *Health Services Research, 25,* 697-708.

9. Donabedian, A. (1966). Evaluating the quality of medical care. *Milbank Memorial Fund Quarterly, 44*(3, Part 2), 166-206.

10. Donabedian, A. (1980). *The definition of quality and approaches to its assessment.* Ann Arbor, Mich: Health Administration Press.

11. Donabedian, A. (1986). Criteria and standards for quality assessment and monitoring. *Quality Review Bulletin, 12*(3), 99-108.

12. Greenfield, S. (1990). What's the next step for outcomes assessment? *The Internist, 31*(1), 6-9.

13. Hegyvary, S. T. (1991). Issues in outcomes research. *Journal of Nursing Quality Assurance, 5*(2), 1-6.

14. Horn, B. J., & Swain, M. A. (1978). *Criterion measures of nursing care* (DHEW Pub. No. PHS78-3187). Hyattsville, Md: National Center for Health Services Research.

15. Hover, J., & Zimmer, M. (1978). Nursing quality assurance: The Wisconsin system. *Nursing Outlook, 26,* 242-248.

16. Jennings, B. M. (1991). Patient outcomes research: Seizing the opportunity. *Advances in Nursing Science, 14*(2), 59-72.

17. Johnson, M., & Maas, M. (1992). Classification of nurse sensitive patient outcomes. Grant submitted to Sigma Theta Tau International.

18. Johnson, M., & McCloskey, J. C. (1992). Quality in the nineties. In M. Johnson (Ed.), *Series on nursing administration, vol. 3, the delivery of quality health care* (pp. 59-68). St Louis: Mosby.

19. Lang, N. M., & Clinton, J. F. (1984). Assessment of quality of nursing care. In H. H. Werley & J. J. Fitzpatrick (Eds.), *Annual review of nursing research* (vol. 2, pp. 135-163). New York: Springer.

20. Lang, N. M., & Marek, K. D. (1990). The classification of patient outcomes. *Journal of Professional Nursing, 6,* 153-163.

21. Lang, N. M., & Marek, K. D. (1991). The policy and politics of patient outcomes. *Journal of Nursing Quality Assurance, 5*(2), 7-12.

22. Lohr, K. N. (1988). Outcome measurement: Concepts and questions. *Inquiry, 25*(1), 37-50.

23. Lower, M. S., & Burton, S. (1989). Measuring the impact of nursing interventions on patient outcomes—the challenge of the 1990s. *Journal of Nursing Quality Assurance, 4*(1), 27-34.

24. Majesky, S. J., Brester, M. H., & Nishio, K. T. (1978). Development of a research tool: Patient indicators of nursing care. *Nursing Research, 27,* 365-371.

25. Marek, K. D. (1989a). Outcome measurement in nursing. *Journal of Nursing Quality Assurance, 4*(1), 1-9.

26. Marek, K. D. (1989b). Classification of outcome measures in nursing care. In American Nurses Association (Ed.), *Classification systems for describing nursing practice* (ANA Publication No. NP-74-500, pp. 37-41). Kansas City, Mo: ANA.

27. Martin, K. S., & Scheet, N. J. (1992). *The Omaha system: Applications for community health nursing* (pp. 90-98). Philadelphia: W. B. Saunders.

28. McClure, M. L. (1991). The uses and abuses of large data sets. *Journal of Professional Nursing, 7,* 72.

29. McCormick, K. A. (1991). Future data needs for quality of care monitoring, DRG considerations, reimbursement and outcome measurement. *Image: The Journal of Nursing Scholarship, 23,* 29-32.

30. McDaniel, C., & Nash, J. (1990). Compendium of instruments measuring patient satisfaction with nursing care. *Quality Review Bulletin, 16,* 182-188.

31. Moritz, P. (1991). Innovative nursing practice models and patient outcomes. *Nursing Outlook, 39,* 111-114.

32. Nadzam, D. M. (1991). The agenda for change: Update on indicator development and possible implications for the nursing profession. *Journal of Nursing Quality Assurance, 5*(2), 18-22.

33. Ozbolt, J. G. (1991). Strategies for building nursing databases for effectiveness research. Abstract for paper presented at Patient Outcomes Research: Examining the Effectiveness of Nursing Practice (September 12, 1991). Rockville, Md.

34. Peters, D. A. (1989). An overview of current research relating to long-term outcomes. *Nursing and Health Care, 10*(3), 133-136.

35. Podgorny, K. L. (1991). Developing nursing-focused quality indicators: A professional challenge. *Journal of Nursing Quality Assurance, 6*(1), 47-52.

36. Rettig, R. (1991). History, development, and importance to nursing of outcomes research. *Journal of Nursing Quality Assurance, 5*(2), 13-17.

37. Reverby, S. (1981). Stealing the golden eggs: Ernest Amory Codman and the science and managment of medicine. *Bulletin of the History of Medicine, 55,* 156-171.

38. Revicki, D. A. (1989). Health related quality of life in the evaluation of medical therapy for chronic illness. *Journal of Family Practice, 19,* 337-380.

39. Rinke, L. (1988). *Outcome measures in homecare* (vol. 3). New York: National League for Nursing.

40. Roper, W. L., Winkenwerder, W., Hackbarth, G. M., & Krakauer, H. (1988). Effectiveness in health care: An initiative to evaluate and improve medical practice. *New England Journal of Medicine, 319,* 1197-1202.

41. Salive, M. E., Mayfield, J. A., & Weissman, N. W. (1990). Patient outcomes research teams and the Agency for Health Care Policy and Research. *Health Services Research, 25,* 697-708.

42. Schroeder, P. (1991). From the editor. *Journal of Nursing Quality Assurance, 6*(1), VIII.

43. Tarlov, A. R., Ware, J. E., Greenfield, S., Nelson, E. C., Perrin, E., & Zubkoff, M. (1989). *Journal of American Medical Association, 262,* 925-930.

44. Taylor, A. G., & Haussmann, G. M. (1988). Meaning and measurement of quality nursing care. *Applied Nursing Research, 1*(2), 84-88.

45. Waltz, C. F., & Strickland, O. L. (1989). Issues and imperatives in instrumentation in nursing research. In I. L. Abraham, D. M. Nadzam, & J. J. Fitzpatrick (Eds.), *Statistics and quantitative methods in nursing* (pp. 202-214). Philadelphia: W. B. Saunders.

46. Waltz, C. F., & Strickland, O. L. (1988). *Measurement of nursing outcomes: Measuring client outcomes* (vol. 1). New York: Springer.

47. Ware, J. E. (1991). Conceptualizing and measuring generic health outcomes. *Cancer, 67* (February supplement), 774-779.

48. Williams, A. D. (1991). Development and application of clinical indicators for nursing. *Journal of Nursing Quality Assurance, 6*(1), 1-5.

49. Wilson, A. A. (1988). Measurable patient outcomes: Putting theory into practice. *Home Healthcare Nurse, 6*(6), 15-18.

50. Wyszewianski, L. (1988). Quality of care: Past achievements and future challenges. *Inquiry, 25*(1), 13-22.

CHAPTER 19

The international classification of nursing

JUNE CLARK

While attending a special meeting of the International Council in Paris, I was naturally at once struck by the fact . . . that the methods and the ways of regarding nursing problems were, in many respects, as foreign to the various delegations as were the actual languages; and the thought occurred to me that if . . . we hoped ever to realize the aims of the International Council, one of which is "to confer upon questions relating to the welfare of their patients," sooner or later we must put ourselves upon a common basis and work out what may be termed a Nursing Esperanto which would, in the course of time, give us a universal nursing language and methods for all our affiliated countries.

E. HAMPTON-ROBB[5]

It seems incredible that 83 years after Hampton-Robb identified a fundamental need to the development of nursing, we still do not have a means of expressing the elements of our practice in terms that mean the same thing to other nurses who are doing exactly the same things elsewhere.

Is there something called "nursing" that has common elements, whether it is being done by a nurse in a modern hospital in New York, in a mission hospital in Uganda, in a primary health care center in Finland, or in a clinic in the Amazon rainforest? The paradox is that until we have terms that ask and answer the question, we will never know.

While we may strongly value that nursing is universal because the human needs that it exists to meet are universal, we have no existing empirical data to describe nursing practice across clinical settings, patient or client populations, geographic areas, or time. There is no precise way to know how, or to what extent, the dimensions and characteristics of clinical practice vary according to these or other factors. We cannot know the incidence or prevalence of the human responses or health problems that are the target of nursing actions, and we cannot describe, let alone measure, the effects of such actions because we do not

have a shared meaning about what it is that we are to measure.

Language can be a barrier to having a shared meaning. Even within the English-speaking world, different words describe the same thing and the same word means different things. The problem is not just about making comparisons. As Lang[7] has pointed out, "If we cannot name it, we cannot control it, finance it, teach it, research it or put it into public policy." American nurses know to their cost (literally, as well as metaphorically) that if they cannot name it, they cannot claim reimbursement for it. Even in countries where claiming reimbursement is not relevant because the health care system is different, the "invisibility" of nursing is a major problem. Experience in many countries has demonstrated the vulnerability to which this exposes nursing, especially in an environment where there is competition for control of resources. How can one argue a case for more nurses, or a different kind of nurse, or even know how many nurses you need, if you have no way of describing what nurses do, in response to what kind of problems, and with what results?

Until we have word labels for the symbols we are trying to articulate, we cannot begin to organize them. It appears to be an intrinsic need of the human mind to organize information systematically by grouping data according to common features and distinguishing one group from another by their commonalities and differences. At an individual level, the process is frequently subconscious, and the criteria for the grouping are rarely made explicit. We use this mental process to make sense of the mass of data that continually bombards our senses, learning the "new" by contrasting and comparing it with the previously known, felt, or experienced. This is how babies learn, and children who are unable to manage the process become defined as having "learning difficulties." The process is, in effect, one of creating "categories" for classification.

This same process is also the basis of science, and recognition of its importance to the development of nursing science is also not new. In 1926, Harmer wrote:

If nursing is ever to make even a remote claim to being a science, or even to being conducted on a scientific basis, it must be built up like all branches of science; that is by the most careful, unbiased observation and recording of often seemingly trivial details from which—by organizing, classifying, analyzing, selecting, inferring, drawing and testing conclusions—a body of knowledge or principles are finally evolved.[6]

If the need was identified so long ago, why has it taken so long for us to respond? The linguistic problem should not be underestimated, but I believe the real problems are conceptual and attitudinal. The conceptual problem has been the slow development of theoretical frameworks for nursing and the apparent resistance of practicing nurses to the relevance of theory to their practice. This attitudinal resistance leads many nurses to dismiss the intellectual activity of conceptualizing and categorizing what they do as "mere theorizing." The tragedy is that practicing nurses themselves fail to recognize the complexity of their practice and the intellectual processes that underpin it; they do not see any need to "fuss" about what Benner has called "the knowledge embedded in clinical practice."[2]

Until now.

Where scientific imperatives failed, financial imperatives and technology are succeeding. Cost constraints and greater emphasis on the efficient (and therefore systematic) development of resources require sound information and management systems. The development of computers has leapt into the breach and spawned a whole new science of informatics. Computers work by sorting, classifying, and manipulating data items and, therefore, require clear rules for defining and categorizing data input.

But in the excitement of the data processing, the significance of defining the data input may be overlooked. The invisibility of nursing in the policy and commercial aspects of health care has led to the assumption that medical nomenclature and classification systems (such as ICD) are adequate for nursing or, worse, that some "common sense" or ad hoc system developed by the system vendors or information experts will do. Nursing must not leave the decision making about nursing's essential data to system vendors or other health care professionals. It is nursing's responsibility to define its own phenomena in ways which are consistent with its own purposes.

Nurses in the United States were the first to recognize the need and to begin the work. Harriet Werley[13] began to develop the concept of the Nursing Minimum Data Set (NMDS), built on the concept of the Uniform Minimum Health Data Sets (UMHDSs) in the late 1960s. The work of the American Nurses Association on the development of standards of practice during the 1970s identified the elements for a nursing practice classification in its delineation of "assessment factors, nursing diagnosis, interventions, and outcomes,"[14] and these ideas were reinforced by their 1980 definition of nursing as "the diagnosis and treatment of human responses to actual or potential health problems."[1] One recommendation in this publication was the pursuit of a classification system for nursing and, in 1982, the ANA Cabinet on Nursing Practice appointed a steering committee on classifications of nursing practice phenomena. Meanwhile, the development of a classification of nursing diagnoses was being pursued through the North American Nursing Diagnosis Association, and McCloskey and Bulechek began their work at Iowa on a classification of nursing interventions.[8] Werley and Zorn note that the work on NMDS spurred further elaboration of intervention classifications and the nursing diagnoses taxonomy and that, similarly, continual testing and implementation of the NMDS are not possible without the development and refinement of the classification of nursing interventions.[14] Many other American nurses are similarly working on a variety of projects, and the American literature is now considerable and rapidly expanding. Significantly, it was the American and the Canadian Nursing Associations who proposed the resolution to ICN that led to the development of the ICNP project.

Unfortunately, however, there is still an intellectual and linguistic resistance in many countries, in Europe and Africa in particular, to what they perceive as the

American predilection for "mere theorizing." In the United Kingdom, for example, nurses are "switched off" by terms such as "nomenclature," "taxonomy," or "interventions" and are distinctly uncomfortable with words such as "diagnosis" or "prescription," which are still perceived as being relevant only to medical practice. One of the key challenges for the ICNP project is to bridge the culture gap by making it simple enough, conceptually and linguistically, to be seen as meaningful a description of the practice by a nurse working in a rural clinic in Africa as for a nurse working in high-tech in New York.

To find out what was happening in other parts of the world, in 1991 the International Council of Nurses undertook a survey of its 105 member National Nursing Associations (NNAs) and of the 21 World Health Organization Collaborating Centers for Nursing and commissioned a pilot literature search. The response rate to the questionnaire was not great (perhaps inevitable when one considers the problems of communicating with 105 countries), but of the 29 responding countries, 14 had a system for describing clinical problems and 9 had a system for describing the effects of care on patients. Of the WHO Collaborating Centers, 6 reported a system for describing activities, 5 a system for describing patient problems, and 5 a system for describing the effects of care. Among the systems identified were the use of DRGs in Australia and Taiwan, the Philippine Nurses Association Patient Classification System, several medical information systems used in Greece, the Classification of Medical Procedures in Finland, the Canadian Classification of Clinical Procedures, the Kenya Format for Medical Officers of Health, the NANDA taxonomy of nursing diagnoses on Spain and the United States, and the Programme de Recherche d'Indication d'Activité in France.[15]

The literature search similarly indicated that naming and classification systems in varying degrees of development exist in nursing around the world. For example, Enfors et al.,[4] described efforts in Sweden to identify key words for documentation across the nursing process. Australia's Community Nursing Minimum Data Set (DNMDS-A) was summarized by Turley.[12] Sermeus[11] indicated that nursing-related groups (NRGs) are part of a hospital data set required by law in Belgium. Several countries have some kind of nursing workload analysis system and/or a system for classifying patients according to their dependency.

In Europe, driven no doubt by the imperatives of computerized information and management systems,

several countries are developing minimum data sets for health care, but nursing has generally not been in the forefront of these initiatives, which are overwhelmingly dominated by medicine. The problems of Europe's linguistic variability are balanced by the political goals of standardization and harmonization within the European Community that already includes 12 countries, soon to be joined by the remaining countries of Western Europe and then Eastern Europe. A European Minimum Data Set initiative was begun in 1976 by the directorate general XIII of the Commission of the European Communities, which is concerned with telecommunications, informationindustries and innovation, and recognition of the need for common action, and has led to a program for advanced informatics in medicine (AIM). Nursing Minimum Data Sets are being developed in Belgium, Denmark, Portugal, Holland, and the United Kingdom.

Meanwhile, the WHO/Euro project "People's Needs for Nursing Care"[15] between 1976 and 1985 brought together nurses from Belgium, Czechoslovakia, Denmark, Finland, France, Greece, Norway, Poland, the United Kingdom, and Yugoslavia in an effort to standardize essential nursing data within the framework of the nursing process. This project was, however, pursued as part of the professional development of nursing and not as part of the development of computerized information systems. As Mortensen[9] has pointed out, European nurses (at least those in Denmark and the United Kingdom) seem to be divided into two groups—one group who is interested in information technology but without any great interest in clinical nursing based on the concept of nursing diagnosis, and another group who is actively interested in identifying nursing diagnoses in clinical practice but less interested in computers. This divide has to be overcome, and Mortensen's own work at the Danish Institute for Health and Nursing Research is designed to bring together the development of nursing diagnoses and the development of nursing informatics.[10] Mortensen, who is a leader in the European work on nursing classification, is now developing a concerted action (a technical term used within the European Community institutions) on a European Nursing Minimum Data Set.

In all these circumstances, the need for an international classification for nursing practice is urgent. All around the world, we are faced with demands for information about health care and the development of systems for providing it, in which the largest component of health care—nursing—is at risk of being invisibly absorbed, its distinctive contribution unseen, undervalued, sunk without trace.

THE ICNP PROJECT

The necessity for an international classification for nursing practice was first proposed to ICN at the Council of National Representatives meeting in Seoul in 1989. Prepared by the American and Canadian Nurses Associations, the resolution expressed nurses' concerns about the effects of nursing's inability to define the problems to which it addressed its activities and the distinctive contribution it makes to solving them. The resolution asked that ICN encourage member nurses' associations (NNAs) to become involved in developing classification systems for nursing care, nursing information management systems, and nursing data sets to provide tools that nurses in all countries could use to describe nursing and its contributions to health.

The resolution was referred by the ICN board of directors to its professional services committee (PSC), which in turn appointed June Clark of the United Kingdom, Norma Lang of the United States and, later, Randi Mortensen of Denmark to work with Margretta Styles (PSC Chairperson) and ICN staff to study the feasibility of such a system and to consider how ICN can best support it.

The specific objectives of an international classification for nursing practice are:

- To establish a common language about nursing practice to improve communication among nurses and between nurses and others
- To describe the nursing care of people (individuals and families) in a variety of settings, both institutional and noninstitutional
- To enable comparison of nursing data across clinical populations, settings, geographic areas, and time
- To demonstrate or project trends in the provision of nursing treatments and care and the allocation of resources to patients according to their nursing needs based on nursing diagnoses
- To stimulate nursing research through links to detailed data available in nursing information systems (NIS) and other health care information systems (HISs)
- To provide data about nursing practice to influence health policy decision making

To be useful and applicable to nurses in all countries, an international classification for nursing practice must be:

- Broad enough to serve the multiple purposes required by different countries
- Simple enough to be seen by the ordinary practitioner of nursing as a meaningful description of practice and a useful means of structuring practice
- Consistent with a clearly defined conceptual framework but not dependent upon a particular theoretical framework or model of nursing
- Based on a central core to which additions can be made through a continuous process of development and refinement
- Sensitive to cultural variability
- Reflective of the common value system of nursing across the world as expressed in the ICN Code for Nurses
- Usable in a complementary way with the family of disease and health–related classifications developed by WHO, the core of which is the WHO International Classification of Diseases (ICD)

A strategic plan outlining the major goals and the means to their achievement has been proposed. The strategies are:

- To develop an ICNP with specified process and product components that is recognized by the national and international nursing communities
- To achieve integration of the ICNP within the ICD and the WHO "family" of classifications
- To achieve utilization of ICNP by nurses at country level for development of databases
- To establish an international database that incorporates the ICNP, a nursing minimum data set, human resource data set, and regulatory information

Work has begun. The ICN has given its support to the submission by the American Nurses Association and NANDA of a classification of nursing diagnoses for inclusion in the ICD 10th Revision. Collaboration has also begun with the WHO Department of Epidemiological and Health Statistical Services, and with the WHO Collaborating Centers for the Classification of Diseases. Norma Lang represented ICN at the WHO workshop on Nursing Informatics held in Washington, D.C. In addition, a review has begun of the ICD-10 and related documents to identify labels already included that are relevant to nursing with view to developing an "application of the ICD and other health-related classifications to nursing."

A preliminary literature search and a survey of ICN's 105 member associations have identified classification systems in use or being developed around the world, from which we have begun to develop exemplar lists.

Publications[3] and conference presentations in several countries are beginning to spread around the world. There will be both a plenary presentation and a workshop on the ICNP at the Quadrennial Congress of the International Council of Nurses in Madrid in June 1993.

CONCLUSION

The ICNP is seen as a useful tool to nursing in all countries in many ways. The task is enormous, but it is fundamental to the continued development and recognition of nursing. It is the kind of project that never ends but for which there is a timely beginning—now. With justification, it has been called "nursing's next advance."

REFERENCES

1. American Nurses Association. (1980). *Nursing: A social policy statement*. Kansas City, Mo: Author.
2. Benner, P. (1984). *From novice to expert: Excellence and power in clinical nursing*. Reading, Mass: Addison-Wesley.
3. Clark, J., & Lang, N. (1992). Nursing's next advance: An international classification for nursing practice. *International Nursing Review, 39,* 4, 109-128.
4. Enfors, M., Thorell-Ekstrand, I., & Ehronberg, A. (1991). Towards basic nursing information in patient records. *Vard I Norden, 21*(11), 12-31.
5. Hampton-Robb, E. (1909). Report of the third regular meeting of the international council of nurses. International Council of Nurses.
6. Harmer, B. (1926). *Methods and principles of teaching the principles and practice of nursing*. New York: Macmillan.
7. Lang, N., & Clark, J. (1991). Nursing's next advance: Development of an international classification for nursing practice: Final Proposal submitted to the Board of Directors. ICN (unpublished).
8. McCloskey, J. C., & Bulechek, G. M. (Eds.) (1992). *Nursing interventions classification*. St Louis: Mosby.
9. Mortensen, R. A. (1991). *Experiences in health care data base development*. Paper presented to the WHO Workshop on Nursing Informatics in Washington, D.C., October 1991. Copenhagen: Danish Institute for Health and Nursing Research.
10. Mortensen, R. A. (1992). *Concerted action of nursing: European action on information requirements for nursing practice. European classification of nursing practice with regard to patient problems, nursing interventions, and patient outcomes, including educational measures*. Unpublished paper. Copenhagen: Danish Institute for Health and Nursing Research.
11. Sermeus, W. K. (1991). Comparing information on medical condition and nursing care for the management of health care. In E. J. S. Hovenga, et al. (Eds.), *Nursing Informatics '91: Proceedings of the fourth international conference on nursing use of computers and information science*. Berlin: Springer-Verlag.
12. Turley, J. P. (1991). Community nursing minimum data set—Australia. In J. P. Turley & S. K. Newbold, (Eds.) *Nursing Informatics '91: Pre-conference proceedings*. Berlin: Springer-Verlag.
13. Werley, H. H., & Lang, N. M. (Eds.). *Identification of the nursing minimum data set*. New York: Springer.
14. Werley, H. H., & Zorn, C. R. (1989). The nursing minimum data set and its relationship to classifications for nursing practice in ANA. Classification Systems for Describing Nursing Practice: Working Papers. Kansas City, Mo: American Nurses Association.
15. World Health Organization. *People's needs for nursing care: A European study*. Copenhagen: Author.

PART THREE

CHANGING EDUCATION

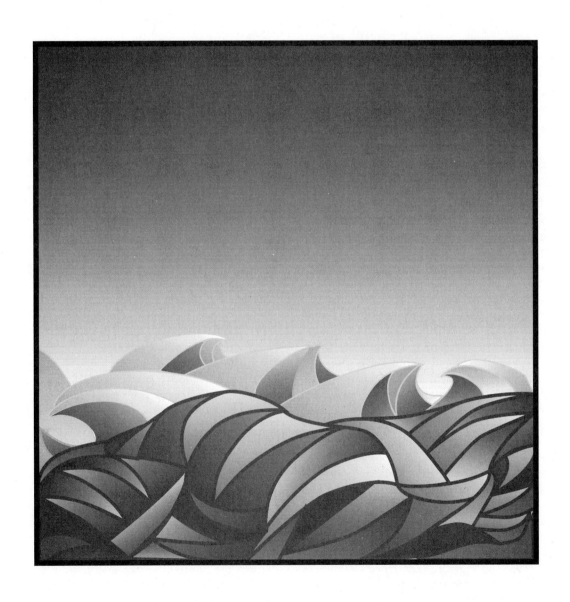

The need for educational reform

JOANNE COMI McCLOSKEY, HELEN KENNEDY GRACE

Placement of this section on nursing education between those on nursing knowledge and nursing practice is not accidental. Nursing education looks in both directions: nursing educators must provide an atmosphere in which nursing knowledge can be generated and refined and also must prepare competent practitioners. Disagreement within nursing about how best to accomplish these goals has led to the proliferation of different types of nursing programs.

The debate chapter is about "entry into practice," but rather than continue the stale argument about professional versus technical education, DeBack focuses on the pros and cons of diversity. The approach is refreshing: she surveys the history of nursing education in the United States and points out that diversity in education existed within 25 years of the establishment of the first nursing schools. She presents both pro and con arguments regarding diversity in nursing education. While nursing programs are opened with relative ease, it is difficult to close them. DeBack says that this is because external pressures on the profession carry more weight than the values and philosophy of nursing leaders. She notes that the recent interest in "differentiated practice" is a way to accept educational diversity while at the same time applying professional control over practice. Is she right? Is this the answer? Should we celebrate rather than denigrate our diversity in education and focus our energies for change on practice applications?

The theme of diversity is continued in the first two viewpoint chapters, which address our student population. Naylor notes that after a severe national nursing shortage in 1988, we began to experience an influx of students into nursing programs. In her chapter she examines two unexpected challenges resulting from the influx: (1) an imbalance in the distribution of new enrollments and (2) slow growth in the number of minority students. Disproportionally, the new students are selecting associate degree rather than baccalaureate programs. This, says Naylor, is due to several things, including the reduced time and expense for completion and the absence of a differentiated practice system.

Naylor outlines several ways in which our higher education systems need to be more responsive to attract a diverse pool that includes new high school graduates, associate degree graduates, older people, and those with degrees in other fields. She also examines the challenge of recruiting minority students. While recent gains have been made in this area, the profession still has too few minority members. She examines the reasons for this situation and outlines several minority recruitment strategies. Retention mechanisms are a part of a recruitment package. While the overall shortage of nurses may have abated at least for the time being, the shortage of baccalaureate and minority nurses is still a problem.

Bednash agrees and points out that, increasingly, nursing students are nontraditional learners. She compares the traditional beginning student (just out of high school, late teens, receiving financial help from parents, studying full time) to the nontraditional student (older, working, supporting a family, and studying part time). The new nontraditional student reflects the changes in American society. A change in society *not* yet reflected in our enrollments is the increasing diversity of the workforce. Bednash, like other authors in the section, makes the plea that nursing recruit more racial and ethnic minorities. She overviews some changes that higher education programs have made to attract the nontraditional student and a more diverse student body. For example, 40 schools have developed accelerated baccalaureate programs and 12 have generic master's programs. Bednash says, however, that associate degree programs still remain more attractive for older students than baccalaureate programs, as evidenced by the average age difference of students. She also makes the point that graduate programs need to rethink the entry requirement that many have for nursing experience after graduation; older students with life experience do not want or need to delay graduate education. Both Naylor's and Bednash's chapters urge nursing educators to examine current practices and revise educational programs to accommodate diverse students.

The need for educational programs to recognize the many changes taking place and to develop ways to adapt is taken up in the next chapter. Rothert, Talarczyk, and Awbrey discuss the mechanism of partnerships as the means to cope with changes in student population characteristics, changes in the health care delivery system, and changes in institutions of higher education. A new diverse student body challenges nursing programs to provide access and to be concerned about retention. The authors review the many ongoing collaborate efforts in nursing. Excellent references are provided for the reader who wants more detail on any one strategy. Partnerships include those with other provider disciplines, with nursing service, with community health care agencies, and between different types of educational programs. The authors say that the needs of the community in the area where the nursing program is located will increasingly be a factor in determining the curriculum and student experiences. Nursing programs will increasingly be challenged to provide nursing students with both high tech and primary care skills. The traditional full-time faculty member who provides clinical supervision in one health care facility may be a thing of the past. This chapter is about change and the responsibility of nursing educators to develop new partnerships to meet the needs of new, different students.

An example of a partnership that has resulted in major curriculum reform is discussed in the next chapter. Until recently, the curricula of our more than 800 associate degree (AD) programs focused on the acute-care hospital setting. The chapter by Sherman and Waters outlines a massive change process to add a focus on long-term care in nursing homes. In 1986, a demonstration project funded by the W. K. Kellogg Foundation was conducted in six associate degree nursing programs located in different parts of the country. Each program developed a partnership with a nursing home to improve nursing care in the homes and to enhance the knowledge and skills of nursing students about long-term care. Continued funding in 1990 helped to

disseminate the results to the associate degree community at large. Today, approximately 300 AD programs have expanded the teaching of gerontological nursing and include practice experience in a nursing home. The project also resulted in a revision of the National League for Nursing's document describing competencies of AD nurses. The authors describe the change process and note that the most successful model was one led by a strong in-house leader. The chapter will interest all those interested in educational reform and change strategies for curriculum revision.

The next three chapters focus on graduate education. First, Poteet, Hodges, and Tate address the concerns of nurses contemplating a return for an advanced degree. Choosing a graduate program, say the authors, is one of the most important career decisions a nurse can make. They begin their chapter by overviewing the history of master's and doctoral education and then discuss professional and personal reasons for returning for a graduate degree. Often, the choice to go back to school is made when one feels a sense of stagnation in the job. Nine essential elements to consider when selecting a program are discussed, including the national standing of the program, its institutional climate, and the availability of assistantships. Future directions in graduate education may include more-focused clinical specializations, more preparation for primary care, and more emphasis on the role of case manager. This helpful chapter is must reading for anyone considering graduate education.

Graduate education is undergoing constant change and faces many challenges. After reviewing the beginnings of graduate education in nursing, Ketefian and Redman discuss issues for both master's and doctoral education. They address three areas of issues for master's education: the role of the master's degree, changing consumer demand, and curricular content. One interesting discussion is about the two differing focuses of master's programs (as stepping stone for a doctorate versus practitioner preparation) and whether a university can afford to do both in an environment of constrained resources. They also point out the growing trend and associated challenges of more international students. They then turn to a discussion of issues in doctoral education in six areas: conceptions, nursing knowledge, scientific integrity, accreditation, students, and faculty. They note the recent trend away from focus on process courses (e.g., nursing methods and statistics) to a focus on substantive courses (e.g., aging or nursing service administration). They issue a challenge that we should reexamine our policy not to admit non-nurses by pointing out that many nurses pursue graduate education and make good contributions in other fields. Perhaps, they say, we should include nonnurses and be enriched by their fresh perspective. They argue for both standardization and flexibility. This is a helpful chapter that provides fruitful ideas for debate and discussion on important issues in U.S. graduate education.

In the next chapter, Conway-Welch continues the case for reform in graduate education. Reviewing a number of recent reports, she predicts that the emphasis of the health care delivery system will shift from curing to caring and that there will be an increased demand for nurses with advanced degrees. New models of graduate education are needed, she says, to prepare these nurse leaders of tomorrow. Our challenge in graduate education is to "create a teaching environment focused on transforming existing power relationships rather than replicating learning relationships based on dominance-submission models." She makes the case that clinical majors also need content on leadership and management skills. Three trends are discussed: the need for content on continuous improvement, acquisition of dual degrees, and the merging of advanced practice roles. Conway-Welch calls for a paradigm shift in graduate nursing education. The traditional focus of professional knowledge on subjects, discipline, and values resulted, she says, in our expensive biobehavioral model, which requires people to get ill before treatment is given. New knowledge is needed about systems, effectiveness of care, and intrinsic motivation to shape a better health care delivery system for tomorrow.

In the last chapter in the section, Fenton makes the case for international exchange as a means to find answers to some of our pressing health problems. She gives many reasons for promoting international exchange in nursing education, including the fact that such exchange is now feasible, that the knowledge learned about other cultures transfers to our own diverse patient population, and that the primary care models of other countries may help us to find cheaper, less-invasive care models for this country. The time has come, she says, to address international exchanges as a method of increasing our ability to meet the needs of our population. She lists many questions that faculty ask when considering the development of an exchange program. The numerous concerns require commitment on the part of faculty and deans, but the benefits, she believes, are well worth it. Nurses who have obtained health care experiences in other countries often are stimulated to create new, less expensive methods of care, become more astute about the role of women in our society, reevaluate the relevance of nursing theories, and become more aware of U.S. health policy abroad. This is a well-reasoned and convincing presentation for promoting educational models of international exchange.

As the chapters in this section demonstrate, nursing educators must both educate future scholars and leaders who will continue to advance the knowledge base of the discipline and must prepare competent practitioners who can manage the increasingly complex challenges of the workplace. They need to permit access while maintaining standards. The many recent changes in the practice setting demand changes in the educational setting. Many educational reforms are suggested by our chapter authors. The challenges are laid out. Despite recent budget cutbacks and other barriers, faculty need to take action and design more accommodating and flexible programs for today's diverse student population.

CHAPTER 20

Debate

Diversity in nursing education

Does it help or hinder the profession?

VIVIEN M. De BACK

Today there are four types of undergraduate, preservice educational programs to prepare for a career in nursing. The graduates of three basic nursing education programs—diploma, associate degree, and baccalaureate degree—are eligible to take the licensure exam for registered nurses (RN). Practical nursing education programs prepare their graduates to take state examinations to become licensed practical nurses (LPN). (See the box on page 154.) These programs were developed by nurses, and each type was initiated to solve specific patient care or nurse supply problems in the nation.

In addition to developing new types of programs, nurse leaders, educators, and practitioners also have attempted to close certain types of nursing education schools. Many excellent, rational reasons have been advanced to support closure recommendations. While a trend toward two types of educational programs, baccalaureate and associate degree, has been apparent for more than 10 years, four types of undergraduate programs remain.

Clearly, the ability or power of a group to open schools is different than the ability or power to close schools as attested to in the nursing profession by its great diversity of educational programs. It is believed by some that such diversity is confusing to potential students, while others suggest that many types of nursing programs offer multiple opportunities for men and women of varying backgrounds to choose nursing as a career. This chapter addresses the questions of diversity: Does it help or hinder the profession?

HOW DID WE GET HERE?

There are many excellent historical accounts of the development of nursing education in this country, some of which are cited here for those wishing to find more in-depth treatment of the subject.[2,7,8,10]

The following overview of the issue is meant to set the stage for the debate regarding the value of educational diversity. By all accounts, nursing education started in the United States in 1873, based on Florence Nightingale's work and the training plan developed for St. Thomas Hospital School of Nursing in London.[4] These hospital-based diploma schools proliferated as demonstrated by the rapid expansion of over 500 schools by 1900, to 1,844 by the early 1930s. Physicians and hospital administrators were strongly supportive of nursing school development because the students and graduate nurses provided the needed care for the growing hospital industry and medical community.

Nurses were educated under an apprenticeship model of education characterized as a training program in which students could learn by working with and being directed by nurses on a clinical unit. The tasks students performed included patient and hospital ward activities and housekeeping chores. Early apprenticeship nursing programs had no formal classes or textbooks. This model of nurses training began to be questioned as early as 1900, with recommendations from the Curriculum Committee of the National League of Nursing Education (NLNE), which proposed guidelines on how to set up actual courses.[2] Curriculum guides for schools of nursing continued to evolve and were revised approximately every 10 years. NLNE published "A Standard Curriculum for Schools of Nursing" in 1917, revised in 1927 and again in 1937. The development of standards signaled an expectation by the nursing community that the preparation of nurses should be an educational rather than an apprentice experience.

UNDERGRADUATE EDUCATIONAL OPPORTUNITIES IN NURSING

Prototype

1. Short-term vocational education
2. Occupational education in multipurpose collegiate institutions
3. Occupational education in noncollegiate single-purpose schools
4. Undergraduate education in senior colleges
   a. Complete programs leading to first professional degree
   b. Provisions for admission with advanced standing

Type of program in nursing

1. Practical nurse program
2. Associate degree programs in junior community colleges
3. Diploma programs in hospital schools or independent noncollegiate schools
4. Baccalaureate degree programs with a major in nursing in senior colleges and universities
   a. Complete programs typically 4 years in length (basic, generic or primary)
   b. Programs for graduate of diploma and associate degree schools

---

The demand for well-trained nurses started early in the development of nursing education programs. Establishing schools was not enough to meet the demand. More well-educated teachers and administrators were needed for schools and hospitals, and, therefore, the universities, particularly those with hospitals, were recognized as the place for educating these new nurse leaders. The first university education for nurses is a subject of some debate. However, it appears from the work of Mary Elizabeth Carnegie that Howard University, a school for black students, was the first to train nurses in theory and practice when it established an 18-month program at the School of Medicine. Seven women graduated from that program in 1895.[6] Teachers College, Columbia University, offered a course for nurses in hospital economics in 1899.[2] In 1908, the University of Minnesota made its School of Nursing a part of the university.

The important point to be made for this discussion is that the diversity in nursing education began within 25 years of the establishment of the first nursing schools in the country. Different nurses prepared in different schools with different expectations for the graduates is a concept almost as old as American nursing education itself.

Baccalaureate schools opened slowly during the early 1900s. By 1940, the external forces of war affected nursing education in another way. During World War II, the Surgeon General recognized the need to increase the pool of nursing personnel for the war effort. The U.S. Cadet Nurse Corps came into being in 1943, supporting student nurses with stipends, tuition,

and books in accelerated education programs, usually two years in length. Some nurse leaders believed that although the original intent was good, the accelerated program was ultimately detrimental to nursing education. Between 1943 and 1945, 179,000 nurses graduated from the Cadet Nurse Corps programs. These nurses were educated differently than their counterparts in traditional diploma programs.[11] Slowly but continuously new baccalaureate programs in nursing opened. Several attempts were made to "differentiate" graduates from diploma and university programs. Dr. Esther Lucille Brown published the Brown Report[5] in 1948, recommending that the term *professional* be applied only to those nurses who graduate from a university program. She also recommended that different levels of nursing be identified, such as professional and technical.

Numerous studies encouraged nursing to take control of education from hospitals and place professional education in schools of higher education. This recommendation, first heard from Annie Goodrich in 1912, was respected for many years without significant response.[9]

The most rapid change in nursing education began in the 1950s. Based on Dr. Mildred Montag's study of the two-year program of nursing education in community colleges,[14] associate degree programs in nursing began to develop. The first program opened at Fairleigh Dickinson College, in New Jersey, in 1952.[18]

Continued pressure to move nursing into schools of higher education began to have an effect on the diploma schools in the country. In 1970, the National

Commission for the Study of Nursing and Nursing Education noted that in the United States between 1958 and 1968, nearly 200 diploma schools closed and 350 associate degree programs were established.[15]

In 1965, the American Nurses Association (ANA) made a historic statement when its Committee on Nursing Education issued a position paper declaring that education for nurses should take place in institutions of higher learning within the general system of education.[1] This formalization of the position that nursing leaders had taken for years was expected to end the debate about nursing education. However, debate and dissension has continued.

Nursing education programs continued to open and close. In 1973, there were 574 associate degree in nursing (ADN) programs, 494 diploma programs, and 305 baccalaureate programs in nursing. Five years later, ADN had 656 programs, diploma, 367 and baccalaureate 349. In 1990, diploma schools represented less than 12% of total programs while more than half of the nursing programs in the country were ADN.

In 1990, there were 489 baccalaureate schools of nursing for entry-level students (basic). It is significant to note that in 1990 there were an additional 139 baccalaureate schools with programs that admitted diploma and associate degree nurses only.[17]

Schools of nursing (basic students)

	1973	**1978**	**1990**
ADN	574	656	829
DIPLOMA	494	367	152
BSN	305	349	489

The graduates from these programs, except those who are RNs already, take the same licensing exam to become registered nurses although the programs have different outcomes and, therefore, different practice expectations.

In spite of many reports, studies, commissions, and recommendations, nursing education continues to have great diversity in its ranks. Although changes continue, with some schools closing and others opening, the diversity remains. The expected movement to two types of nursing education is slower than nurse leaders predicted in 1965, and the potential for nursing to continue to have multiple pathways to enter the profession remains high.

ARGUMENTS AGAINST DIVERSITY

There are many thoughtful arguments against the wide variety of nursing programs available today. For example, it is suggested that many different types of nursing programs serve to confuse the public about nurses. They cannot know what a nurse is or what a nurse does because diverse educational programs graduate nurses with different abilities. Diversity in nursing education makes it difficult for consumers to identify the type of nurses needed for their care or to evaluate the nursing care received. What is really being said here is that different nurses are treated the same in the work setting, and, therefore, the nurse and the public are less able to identify the differences in each nurse's competencies and scope of practice. Thus, the argument against educational diversity could be addressed by workplace differentiation of nursing practice. It will be noted in the following pages that such practice differentiation is given as rationale to *support* the many types of educational programs for nurses.

Another argument against many types of nursing programs is the problem it creates for potential nursing students who must make a decision about what kind of school to enter. Career advisers in high schools often lack the information needed to supply potential nurses with accurate educational materials and comparisons of types of schools. Few counselors can articulate the advantages and disadvantages of each type of program so that informed decision making can occur. Therefore, some argue, diversity continues simply because information about choices is not available.

The trend in changes in nursing education programs has continued slowly but steadily for more than 25 years toward baccalaureate and associate degree nursing programs. This trend suggests a growing consensus in the nursing community on rationalizing the educational system and restructuring the nursing delivery system to include job descriptions based on education and experience. Increasing numbers of diploma schools are translating their educational programs into baccalaureate or associate degree programs.[16] In cooperation with junior or senior colleges, numerous nursing education models, as well as some independent degree-granting institutions, have developed. Practical nurse programs are closing or using their resources to develop associate degree programs in nursing. The organized nursing community has gone on record to support the concept of professional and technical nurses educated in baccalaureate and associate degree programs. The growing body of literature on effective and efficient models of care delivery provides further evidence of "different education equals different role expectations." All this suggests a move toward a reduction in types of nursing education programs.

Finally, it is suggested that diversity in nursing education is antithetical to advancing the profession. Professions, it is argued, have one entry point and a trajectory of practice and research that is well defined in higher education. Without this clear pathway, nursing can be viewed as a technical job (because of lower level education) rather than a practiced profession.

ARGUMENTS FOR DIVERSITY

The Pew Health Professions Commission[19] has described the diversity in nursing education as a tremendous asset. In today's environment, diversity is both a strength and weakness. It is a strength because of the wide variety of programs from which potential nurses may select. The weakness stems from the fact that there is little differentiation in the roles of nurses in the practice setting. The continual growth in interest in different role expectation will support the position of educational diversity as a strength in nursing.

The continued shortage of nurses in many areas of the country has increased the community support for all types of nursing programs.[13] As the population ages and the needs for nursing care escalate, advocates for nursing schools of all kinds will grow. This support is expected to continue as long as the community is unaware of the differences in nurses' abilities.

Many nursing programs are located in the community where the students live. The type of nursing school a potential student selects is often dependent upon what kind of program is in proximity to home. It is argued that diverse programs offer a student an opportunity to enter nursing at a reasonable cost and begin work in one or two or three years.

The recent interest in career progression demonstrated by increasing numbers of nurses in advanced programs strengthens arguments for diverse programs in many communities. Nurses can advance in their education once they have entered the profession at any level, and nurses are financially able to return to school to get their degrees when they are already in the field. Nursing has been a second or delayed career for many women and men, in part, a result of economic depressions in other job markets. The variety of nursing programs attracts the second-career candidates and further supports educational diversity. Career mobility programs available throughout most of the country are appealing to adult students. Defined "step-off points" fit today's lifestyles. Part-time study for advanced degrees has increased in popularity. This supports the diversity argument by appealing to a much broader audience and thus helps to relieve the ongoing nursing shortage.

SUMMARY OF THE ARGUMENTS

The support for and against multiple paths for nursing education are compelling. Unfortunately, the debate seems to be based on the assumption that the nursing profession has control over closure of its schools. Rosalie C. Yeaworth addressed this issue.

I am struck by how nursing education is determined not so much by the philosophy and values of nursing leaders and educators, but by legal, economic and social situations. We believed that if we could just give rational reasons to change and show substantiating data for our beliefs we could convince people and implement the needed changes.

However, we lacked the central control or power to require such a minimum level of education so we continue to have diploma schools. With educational, political, social and economic values favoring accessibility to education and the community college concepts, we soon discovered that the primary educational preparation occurred at the associate degree level.[20]

This lack of control over educational issues has been observed by Baldridge[3] and Matejski,[12] both of whom noted that where professional organizations are well insulated from external pressures, the professionals themselves control the organization, determining its professional norms and defining its tasks and work routines. Such organizations possess a large measure of professional autonomy. However, where there is little isolation between the professional organization and the environment, there is a lessening of professional autonomy, including the profession's ability to determine educational preparation for its future practitioners.

While nursing has achieved a measure of autonomy and professional status, the power associated with these abilities does not extend to the authority to close schools of nursing. The result is educational diversity.

Nursing leaders are cognizant of this dilemma and the problems and divisiveness created during the long "entry into practice" debate. Therefore, a new direction for the goal of increasing professionalism and controlling education and practice has developed. That change of focus is "differentiated practice," which recognizes educational diversity and supports variations in nursing practice based on education, ability, and experience. Differentiated practice sites are characterized by a change in their previous single job description for nurses with various educational backgrounds. Practice competencies form the core of differentiated job descriptions for nurses with different education and experience.

This shift to differentiated practice seems to represent an acceptance of educational diversity while at the same time applying professional control over practice parameters. It is important to note that the concept of differentiated practice has grown in acceptance in recent years but cannot be considered an integrated phenomena throughout the health care industry or the nursing education community. However, differentiation offers the best opportunity for the profession to control and define who nurses are, what educational outcomes can be expected, and what nurses do for clients.

CONCLUSION

The nursing profession continues to grow in status, research-based knowledge, political impact, and leadership. It is difficult to argue that nursing has been hindered by educational diversity when we cannot know what the profession would look like today without that history.

What is clear is that nurse leaders have reiterated for more than 50 years the belief that upgrading nursing education is necessary to meet the complex health needs of this country. Whether nursing does this by redesigning the educational system to provide the community with different types of nurses for different population needs or identifies more clearly what each nurse brings to the practice arena is yet to be seen.

Whether helpful or hindering, educational diversity in nursing is here. What the profession does with that reality is the future challenge.

REFERENCES

1. American Nurses Association. (1965). *Educational preparation for nurse practitioners and assistants to nurses: A position paper.* Kansas City, Mo: Author.
2. Anderson, N. (1981). The historical development of American nursing education. *Journal of Nursing Education, 20*(1), 18-35.
3. Baldridge, J. V. (Ed.). (1971). *Academic governance: Research on institutional politics and decision making.* Berkeley, Calif: McCutcheon Publishing.
4. Bayldon, M. (1973). Diploma schools; the first century. *Registered Nurse, 36*(2), 33.
5. Brown, E. L. (1948). *Nursing for the future.* New York: Russell Sage Foundation.
6. Carnegie, M. E. (1986). *The path we tread: Blacks in nursing, 1854-1984.* Philadelphia: J. B. Lippincott.
7. Fitzpatrick, M. L. (1983). *Prologue to professionalism: A history of nursing.* Bowie, Md: Robert J. Brady.
8. Glass, L. (1985). A dream come true: Richard Olding Beard and the University of Minnesota School for Nurses. *Nursing and Health Care,* 323-325.
9. Goodrich, A. W. (1912). The complete nurse. *American Journal of Nursing, 12,* 777-782.
10. Hanson, K. (1989). The emergence of liberal education in nursing education, 1893 to 1923. *Journal of Professional Nursing, 5*(2), 83-91.
11. Kingsbury, V. (1947). The philosophy of nursing education as influenced by the development of professional nursing education in the United States from 1873 to 1947. Master's thesis, St Louis University.
12. Matejski, M. P. (1977). The influence of selected external forces on medical education at the University of Maryland School of Medicine, 1910-1950. Dissertation, University of Maryland, Baltimore.
13. Miller, N. (1987). *The nursing shortage: Facts, figures and feelings.* Chicago: American Hospital Association.
14. Montag, M. L. (1951, 1971). *The education of modern nursing.* Original publisher: G.P. Putnam's Sons. Reprinted.
15. National Commission for the Study of Nursing and Nursing Education. (1970). Summary report and recommendations. *American Journal of Nursing, 70*(2).
16. National Commission on Nursing Implementation Project. (1987). Work Group I, Education. 1987 invitational conference papers. Milwaukee: Author.
17. National League for Nursing Division of Research. (1991). *Nursing data source: Volume I—Trends in contemporary nursing education.* New York: Author.
18. Oderkirk, W. W. (1985). Setting the record straight: A recount of late nineteenth century training schools. *Journal of Nursing History, 1*(1).
19. Pew Health Professions Commission. (1991). *Healthy America: Practitioners for 2005.* Durham, N.C.: Author.
20. Yeaworth, R. (1991). An educator's response to models of differentiated practice. In *Differentiating nursing practice into the twenty-first century.* Kansas City, Mo: American Academy of Nurses.

CHAPTER 21

Viewpoints

Recruitment of students into nursing

MARY D. NAYLOR

The influx of new students entering nursing programs that began in 1988 points to a brighter future for many of the nation's nursing schools. The remarkable 10% upswing in nursing school enrollments between 1988 and 1990 surpasses that of the nation's colleges, where an increase of 3.4% was found.[7] The findings from the 1990 National League for Nursing annual survey are the first in half a decade to indicate an increase in graduations. As suggested by these admission data, the number of new graduates is expected to grow over the next few years. While increased admissions alone do not suffice to stem the nursing shortage, these new graduates are welcome additions to the profession.

Despite these positive developments, it is premature to abandon the efforts to understand and correct the recent nursing shortage. The recent increase in students entering the nation's nursing schools has unleashed some unexpected issues and challenges. Two trends that warrant further examination are (1) the significant imbalance in the distribution of new enrollments between associate and baccalaureate programs and (2) the relatively slow growth in the recruitment of minority students coupled with continuing problems with their retention.

IMBALANCE IN ENROLLMENTS BETWEEN ADN AND BSN PROGRAMS
An issue of balance

The well-publicized nursing shortage, projected demand for nurses well into the twenty-first century, and major media campaigns designed to change the public's image of nursing have obviously achieved some measure of success. Men and women of all ages and backgrounds have turned to nursing as their career choice. Most of these people, however, have selected the associate degree nursing program (ADN) as the route to begin their life's work. A significant consequence of the unprecedented growth in ADN programs is that greater proportions of new entrants to the nursing supply (64% in 1990) are graduates of this program.[7] This is occurring despite the presence of data that indicate our society has enough ADN graduates through the year 2000. Currently, fewer than one third of registered nurses possess a baccalaureate degree.

In its 1990 Report to the President and Congress, the Department of Health and Human Services forecast that by the year 2000, there would be one half as many baccalaureate-prepared and higher-degree nurses as needed.[11] For the year 2000, these projections represent a deficiency of more than 400,000 nurses. This same report projects an excess of nearly 200,000 nurses prepared at the associate degree level.

For years, the nursing profession has affirmed that minimum preparation for professional nursing practice should be the baccalaureate degree in nursing (BSN), yet the vast majority of new recruits are beginning their socialization in programs designed to prepare technically competent nurses. The arguments in favor of entry through the BSN have focused on the importance of having the professional course of study build on a solid base in the arts and sciences. Baccalaureate education provides the needed breadth and depth for students preparing for a lifelong career. This entry route enables the profession to meet its obligation to prepare safe, competent caregivers in a system that is consistent with the norm for American higher education. Graduates from BSN programs provide a pool from which persons capable of graduate study in nursing can be drawn. If the case for baccalaureate education is so compelling, why are many capable students choosing ADN programs?

Roots of the issue

A range of factors has contributed to the incredible comeback in enrollments in ADN programs. Generally thought to be two years in length with relatively inexpensive tuition, more than 800 associate degree nursing programs are widely distributed throughout the nation in local community and junior colleges and, therefore, very accessible to the students they attract.

Students choosing ADN programs represent a disproportionate share of older students. Many of these students have prior college experience; some possess baccalaureate or graduate degrees in other fields. A few of the reasons why many of these students decide not to enroll in four-year (frequently residential) BSN programs include financial concerns, distance from home to college, and the presence of major family responsibilities. The availability of financial aid is a major factor affecting the choice of educational routes. Students who are college graduates, for example, rely heavily on personal savings, spousal support, and work to fund their nursing education. This group often has accumulated debt and typically does not meet eligibility requirements for the traditional forms of student assistance.[2]

Certainly, a major force driving new recruits in large numbers to ADN programs is the absence of a differentiated practice system.[8] The public recognizes that in most practice environments, graduates from a variety of educational routes will assume the same entry-level positions at the same competitive salaries. Further, these individuals will be able to continue their nursing education while working and having tuition paid by their employers. Numerous educational models emphasizing educational advancement and career mobility have made it relatively easy for ADN graduates to pursue advanced degrees.

A more responsive educational system

Despite dramatic changes in the demographic and social profile of the nursing population, many BSN programs are organized today as they were two or three decades ago. Significant changes in this type of program are needed if nursing is to attract the quality and numbers of students that should be entering the profession through the baccalaureate route. A more responsive and creative nursing education system should be designed so that within each region the following types of baccalaureate programs are available:

- Programs that have established a partnership with two-year liberal arts colleges

- Programs that provide work study options and include cooperative programs for nursing education
- Accelerated pathways or combined degree options (e.g., BSN/MSN) for second-degree students

Some four-year, upper-division nursing programs should consider affiliations with two-year junior or community colleges. Partnerships with high-quality, two-year colleges offer a cost-effective liberal arts education for many students currently not choosing to enter BSN programs. Qualified students could complete their liberal education base in colleges close to their homes and their professional course of study in schools of nursing closely linked with junior colleges.

Within each region of the country, it is desirable to have programs that specialize in cooperative approaches to nursing education. These programs would enable students with family responsibilities and financial concerns to work for periods of time while completing their undergraduate nursing program. Strong partnerships with hospitals and other health care agencies could be developed to facilitate the appropriate placements of these individuals.

At least two categories of educational models that are attractive to students with degrees in other fields have been developed. The first type is an accelerated program that capitalizes on the college graduates' backgrounds and is designed to prepare these students for entry-level positions as staff nurses. The second category of programs combines basic and advanced nursing preparation through submatriculation or direct entry into a MSN or combined BSN/MSN program. Graduates from this latter type are prepared for roles as nurse practitioners, nurse-midwives, or clinical nurse specialists.

Schools of nursing that offer baccalaureate and graduate degrees in nursing need to continue their efforts to design curricular models and restructure their programs so that they are accessible and attractive to students from a variety of backgrounds. Each school should examine how it can best contribute at a local and regional level to an open educational system that encourages entry of most of its recruits at the baccalaureate level.

Financial incentives

In addition to creative curricular options, efforts to increase financial aid for these students should be pursued vigorously. Recently, a number of innovative models of financial aid have been initiated that will benefit students from diverse backgrounds. Individual schools of nursing have collaborated with employers in the design and implementation of work-study or work-grant programs. Private foundations have joined forces with nursing schools to provide scholarship or loan support for undergraduate and graduate nursing students. This experience has been very instructive in demonstrating how valuable even partial funding can be in enabling nontraditional students to enroll in and complete BSN programs. Finally, schools of nursing have joined forces with national nursing organizations to strengthen the financial aid programs available to this student population.

The importance of differentiation

If the profession is to attract the quality and number of new recruits into baccalaureate programs that society needs, a more fundamental change in nursing education and practice is warranted. Distinct levels of nursing education linked to practice and credentialing are necessary. The advantage of linking education to credentials is that prospective students will understand the trade-offs in time and money among the various educational routes to a career in nursing. Additionally, different examinations and credentials would clarify entry-level competencies for employers and encourage pay differentiation on a basis accepted by many other professions. The baccalaureate degree would be a more desirable educational route if the relationships among education, competence, and compensation were more closely associated.

In summary, shifting the balance to BSN entry requires that nursing education and practice respond to those factors that have resulted in the current imbalance. A more coherent, better understood, and fair educational system can be devised that expands access to generic baccalaureate programs. The practice environment can be modified to encourage and reward entry into professional practice through the BSN route. It is important to note that these changes can occur without diminishing the value of ADN programs and their graduates.

RECRUITMENT AND RETENTION OF MINORITY STUDENTS INTO NURSING
Recruitment and retention barriers

The two fastest-growing segments of the U.S. population are blacks and Hispanics. By the end of this decade, one in every three Americans will be a member of an ethnic minority. Recently, important gains in minority recruitment to nursing have been made. In 1990, nonwhites represented 18% of the total admissions to

nursing schools: 11.1% black; 3.2% Hispanic; 3.0% Asian; and 0.6% American Indian.[7]

The relatively recent establishment of baccalaureate nursing programs at historically black colleges and universities (HBCUs) is a phenomenon that has contributed to this growth. According to a 1990 report on the status of minorities in higher education, HBCUs are increasing in popularity and enrolling significantly larger numbers of blacks in recent years.[3] The majority of minority students, however, are attending integrated nursing programs. Despite considerable effort and recent gains, the nursing profession continues to be underrepresented by individuals who are members of minority groups.

The problems encountered by schools of nursing in attracting, retaining, and graduating minority students are shared by many colleges and universities throughout the country. In most academic communities, for example, there is considerable concern and discussion about the declining enrollment and attrition of black students. Studies of both two- and four-year colleges have revealed an alarming gap between the number of black and white students who complete their degree requirements within a reasonable time.

The Allen, Nunly, and Warner[1] study of black students in baccalaureate nursing programs resulted in the identification of six barriers to recruitment and retention: inadequate financial aid, feelings of loneliness and alienation, failure to use available counseling, inadequate secondary school preparation, cultural and racial identity adjustment problems, and problems with social and sexual relationships. Other researchers agree with these findings and identify lack of academic preparedness, racism, social isolation, and alienation as the factors most likely to have the greatest negative impact. Additionally, Orque et al.[9] found that nursing was viewed negatively by black parents. Many parents considered nursing to be a menial job with low prestige; they did not support this profession as a career choice for their children. To attract and graduate the number of minority nurses needed, schools of nursing must devise strategies that address these barriers. Recent efforts to enhance the recruitment and retention of minority nursing students have yielded an important database regarding the effectiveness of selected strategies.

Recruitment strategies

Programs that link minority nursing role models and students in primary and middle schools have been found to be effective.[10] Career theorists suggest that elementary school children should be targeted for career education because by the time they reach junior high, they have formulated attitudes, both positive and negative, toward most careers. A sustained contact between a positive role model and child is needed to assist the child in emulating and incorporating the behaviors associated with a particular career into the child's self-concept. A prenursing club for minority school-age children is a program that could stimulate the interest of these children in a nursing career. Schools of nursing could adopt one or more health careers or prenursing clubs and facilitate minority children's access to excellent role models and relevant experiences.

Other linkages between nursing schools and high schools could assist in the preparation of students for a positive collegiate experience. Examples of successful outreach programs are tutoring for high school students, precollege skill building programs, and intensive summer orientation programs.[6] Summer on-campus programs for middle and high school students have proved to be very beneficial in promoting academic success. Not only can these programs assist students to develop the skills needed to be successful in college, they can also provide participants with a more realistic view of the college experience. Summer programs should include dormitory living, planned academic, sports, and cultural experiences, as well as workshops designed to improve study and test-taking skills. It is very desirable for nursing faculty to actively participate in these offerings to foster the students' exposure to positive role models.

The recruitment of minority students with prior college degrees is an area recently targeted by some nursing schools. Efforts to build linkages with students at HBCUs that do not have schools of nursing, for example, could yield significant returns for the profession. One successful mechanism is to offer summer research or clinical fellowships for minority students attending college. Fellows would be linked with a faculty or clinical preceptor. These fellowships could provide students with challenging learning opportunities and offer excellent exposure to the nature of nurses' work and some of the leaders in the profession.

Institutional commitment

Students who are attracted to a campus will expect to see widespread evidence of the institution's support for diversity.[4] A strong minority faculty presence is an im-

portant indicator of institutional commitment to minority students. Visiting scholars or faculty exchange programs may provide nursing schools with a minority presence until there is adequate representation within the school. Schools of nursing can enlist the help of associations, such as the Black Nurses Association, in their efforts to recruit minority faculty.

A curriculum that is rich in content related to ethnic and racial diversity is another important sign of a commitment to the recruitment and retention of minority students. According to Glock,[5] general education offerings should be structured to give students the skills and resources needed to understand their particular ethnicity, while emphasizing the world shared by other students and their faculty. Offerings in literature, language and civilization, and art and music that expose students to the contributions of diverse groups to American culture are needed to promote a positive ethnic and racial identity.

As a profession concerned with caring for people with compassion and respect, nursing has been a leader in promoting the study of multiculturalism and its impact on health care. At the 1989 National League for Nursing convention, for example, the membership approved a resolution for curriculum innovation that fosters social values that recognize the multicultural, multiracial, and growing diversity of individual and family lifestyles in society. Many schools have begun to offer courses or integrated relevant content in efforts to promote these social values. A multicultural center that offers programs for faculty and culturally diverse learning experiences for students is excellent evidence of an institution's investment in diversity.

In addition to learning opportunities that encourage students to appreciate cultural differences and the unique health needs and problems of various minority groups, nursing schools should expose students to minority nursing organizations and leaders. Minority leaders should be included as speakers for student functions and ceremonies.

Retention mechanisms

Once the student has been recruited, efforts to assure retention must be rigorous. Institutional support, such as an extensive orientation program, academic advising, personal counseling services, and financial aid services, are critical to promoting the retention of minority students.[6] Summer transition programs for incoming freshmen should include testing to determine if any academic deficiencies exist and a thorough orientation to available support services. It is important to encourage students' use of these resources and to alleviate any concerns that using these services will mark the student as deficient. Exposure to both staff and other students who have benefited from these programs is often helpful in minimizing these feelings.

The summer transition program might be designed to simulate the experiences of students during the first few weeks of school. Time could be spent assuring that students both understand the expectations of faculty and believe that faculty are committed to their academic success. If possible, stipends should be provided for students who participate in the transition program. Stipends help to replace lost summer earnings and encourage students to enroll.

Freshman orientation programs should be extended throughout the freshman year to assist with this difficult transition. Formally structured peer support groups should be an integral part of this program. Peer support groups can assist minority students to network with other students and become involved in campus life. Peer tutoring programs or programs that encourage group study are particularly helpful because they provide both academic support and increased peer interactions.

A strong academic advising system is essential to assist the students with academic planning, monitor students' progress, identify problems early and guide students to appropriate services. Programs that help all faculty to explore their attitudes, perceptions, and behaviors toward minority students should be encouraged. The development of close relationships with advisors should be facilitated through opportunities for multiple faculty and student interactions. It is very desirable for students to be assigned to the same advisor throughout the program.

Social connections are very important for all students and may be a challenge for minority students at predominantly white schools. Chi Eta Phi, the black nursing sorority, alumni groups, and local chapters of the National Black Nurses Association can provide support, role models, and mentors. Minority students should also be encouraged to participate in the nursing student organizations and other campus activities.

The recruitment and retention of minority students must continue to be a priority for all nursing schools and the profession. Minority nurses are essential to keep the evolving health care system focused on the unique needs of an increasingly diverse society. The provision of care, the expansion of knowledge, and the establishment of policy related to all underrepresented groups require the involvement of a critical mass of minority nurses.

REFERENCES

1. Allen, M., Nunly, J., & Scott Warner, M. (1988). Recruitment and retention of black students in baccalaureate nursing programs. *Journal of Nursing Education, 27*(4), 107-116.
2. American Association of Colleges of Nursing. (1989). *The economic investment in nursing education: Student, institutional and clinical perspectives.* Washington, D.C.: Author.
3. Carter, D. J., & Wilson, R. (1991). *Ninth annual status report: Minorities in higher education.* Washington, D.C.: American Council on Education.
4. Crawford, L. A., & Olinger, B. H. (1988). Recruitment and retention of nursing students from diverse cultural backgrounds. *Journal of Nursing Education, 27*(8), 379-381.
5. Glock, N. C. (1990). *Rethinking the curriculum to meet the needs of underprepared, underrepresented, and economically disadvantaged students: Majors and courses for the 21st century.* Paper presented at the Annual Conference on Ethnic and Languages Minorities, Sacramento, Calif.
6. Jones, S. H. (1992). Improving retention and graduation rates for black students in nursing education: A developmental model. *Nursing Outlook, 40*(2), 78-85.
7. National League for Nursing Division of Research. (1991). *Nursing datasource: Volume I—Trends in contemporary nursing education.* New York: Author.
8. Naylor, M. (1990). Nursing education and the shortage. *The nursing shortage: Opportunities and solutions.* (Monograph No. 5, AHA No. 154184). American Hospital Association and the American Nurses Association.
9. Orque, M., Bloch, B., & Monrroy, L. (1983). *Ethnic nursing care: A multicultural approach.* (pp. 81-108). St Louis: Mosby.
10. Stearns, S., & Marchione, J. (1989). Pre-nursing club: A recruitment program for minority school age children. *Nurse Educator, 13*(3), 34-36.
11. U.S. Department of Health and Human Services. (1990). *Nursing—Seventh report to the President and Congress on the status of health personnel.* Washington, D.C.: U.S. Public Health Service.

CHAPTER 22

The changing pool of students

GERALDINE POLLY BEDNASH

Students entering or preparing to enter higher education in the 1990s are markedly different from students several decades ago. These differences represent both enormous potential and serious challenges for nurse educators and practitioners. The potential is represented by the increasing diversity that provides new pools from which nursing can draw. The challenges are a result of the need to reformulate how we educate nurses for the future.

Student pools must be defined very broadly. High school students constitute a smaller proportion of new enrollees in higher education; instead, nursing students are increasingly nontraditional learners. Moreover, the changing demographics and economics of the United States have created a rich diversity of potential students with new education and career patterns. These changes mandate that the education options available to future nurses also be more diverse and responsive to these new realities.

SOCIAL, ECONOMIC, AND CULTURAL REALITIES

Hodgkinson's[6] report on shifting demographics in the United States provides an overview of how these shifts have changed and will continue to change the face of student populations. The shifting socioeconomics of American society are represented in changing social structures, population characteristics, and patterns of education.

Today, only 6% of American families have a "traditional" family composed of a working father, a stay-at-home mother, and children.[6] In fact, more than two

This paper was written by Dr. Bednash in her private capacity. No official support or endorsement by the American Association of Colleges of Nursing is intended or should be inferred.

thirds of all husbands and wives between the ages of 20 and 55 both have full-time employment.[11] By some estimates, almost 60% of all children will live in a single-parent household at some time of their life. In addition, the number of married couples with children under the age of 18 declined 1.7% between 1980 and 1990, while the number of single-parent women has increased 21.2% and the number of single-parent men has increased 87.2%.

A recent report of the American Council on Education titled *Financing Nontraditional Students* provides evidence that the changes seen in American social structures highlighted by Hodgkinson are reflected in the markedly different student body of today. In that report, Ross and Hampton[9] analyzed the changes seen in postsecondary student populations as reported in the National Postsecondary Student Aid Study and in data reported to the National Center for Educational Statistics. These researchers brought together diverse data sets to allow them, for the first time, to get an accurate total for the number of individuals now enrolled in postsecondary education programs—almost 18 million individuals—and to more fully describe this extremely large and diverse group.

Traditionally, a college student has been perceived to be immediately out of high school, in her or his late teens, financially dependent upon parents or guardians, enrolled in a course of study full time, and focusing full energies on the higher education experience.

The reality, however, is quite different. Ross and Hampton[9] were able to document that the traditional student is no longer the major force in higher education, but has instead been supplanted by a group of individuals who are older, studying part-time, working, and supporting families. Ross and Hampton define nontraditional students as those over the age of 22, who are no longer financially dependent on their parents or guardians, are most often enrolled on a part-time, hourly basis, live off campus, have full-time or almost full-time employment, and have a greater likelihood of being a member of a racial or ethnic minority group.

Although 6 million individuals meet the earlier definition for "traditional students" and continue to be an important element of higher education today, more than two thirds of all postsecondary students, or more than 12 million individuals, meet Ross and Hampton's definition for "nontraditional" students. This new reality has dramatically changed the nature of higher education and will likely continue to do so for the foreseeable future. Moreover, the clear domination of the nontraditional education patterns has created calls for new terms other than traditional or nontraditional to describe these very distinct groups.

Nontraditional students are more likely to be enrolled in community colleges. In both two-year community colleges and four-year senior colleges and universities, women represent the majority of nontraditional students, but students in community colleges are likely to have a higher average age (30) than those in four-year institutions (27 in public institutions and 29 in private institutions). Almost 40% of nontraditional students are married, in marked contrast to the 2% of traditional students who are married.

Clearly, changing economic and social conditions in the United States today have created a surge in the number of individuals who are returning to college for a new career or reexamining college as an opportunity for enhancing their potential for economic security. And traditional patterns of education will not meet the needs of this new student majority.

A second, more dramatic change—the growth in the number of individuals who are members of a racial or ethnic minority group—is also reshaping the composition of student pools. Currently, almost 25% of the U.S. population is a member of a racial or ethnic minority group. In some areas of the country, minority may be a misnomer. For example, in the elementary and secondary systems in California, New Mexico, Hawaii, and the District of Columbia, more than half of the population under the age of 18 are members of a racial or ethnic minority group. Hodgkinson reports that in 26 cities in California, no single racial or ethnic group made up a majority of the population.[6] At a recent presentation by The College Board, Claire Pelton, director of Educational Services for San Jose, California, reported that in the San Jose population of

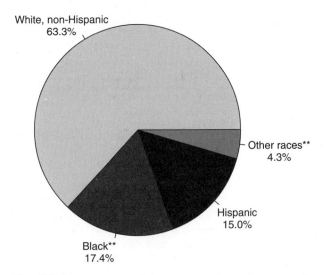

Fig. 22-1 Projections of the U.S. population by race and ethnicity, ages 0-17, 2010. (Source: *National Center for Education Statistics (1991)*. Youth Indicators. *Washington, D.C.: Department of Education.*) **Includes a small number of Hispanics; "other races" are primarily Asian and American Indian.

30,000 elementary and secondary students, 77 languages are spoken (personal communication, April 30, 1992). The U.S. population of elementary and secondary education age represent a much greater diversity than is seen in the total population (see Fig. 22-1). This data suggests that the future composition of students in postsecondary programs will also have a much greater diversity.

Much of the growth in racial and ethnic diversity is a result of the surging growth in immigration to the United States. According to the U.S. Census Bureau, during the decade of the 1980s, almost 7 million legal immigrants entered the United States.[8] An additional untold number of illegal immigrants have also entered the United States, bringing demands for social, health, and educational services. This immigration boom, the largest in the country's history, has and will continue to create a dramatically different workforce. It will also bring a cultural richness, and an additional strain, to the higher education community.

Recent data on enrollments in higher education suggest that a growing number of post–high school students are members of a racial or ethnic minority group. However, racial and ethnic minorities are still underrepresented in higher education (see Fig. 22-2). Moreover, the increase in racial and ethnic diversity

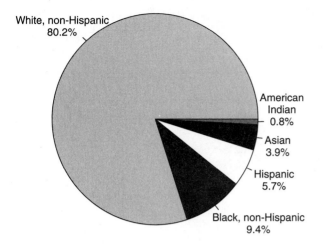

Students Enrolled in All Undergraduate Programs (a)

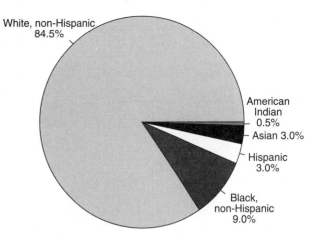

Students Enrolled in Baccalaureate in Nursing Programs (b)

Fig. 22-2 Comparison of all undergraduate and baccalaureate in nursing programs by race and ethnicity. (Source (*a*): *National Center for Education Statistics (1991). Digest of education statistics. Washington, D.C.: Department of Education.* Source (*b*): *American Association of Colleges of Nursing (1992).* Enrollments and graduations in baccalaureate and graduate programs in nursing 1991-1992. *Washington, D.C.: Author.*)

has not produced an increase in the diversity of graduating students. Astone and Nunez-Wormack[1] note that large portions of minority students either fail to complete a secondary school education or a postsecondary education program. Moreover, few of those minority students who do graduate from high school enroll in a higher education institution.

NURSING STUDENTS: REFLECTIONS AND FAILURES

These data provide evidence that diversity is a part of the American mainstream and that it must become a mainstay of nursing education to prepare an adequate number of highly skilled and capable nurses for the future. The growing number of nontraditional students and the increasing racial and ethnic diversity of the U.S. population are the two student pool characteristics that will have the greatest impact on nursing education's ability to do that.

Nontraditional student trends have already affected nursing education. In the most recent report (1988)[7] on the registered nurse population in the United States, the Department of Health and Human Services (DHHS) summarizes trends in nursing education: the average age of a graduate of an associate degree program was 28.7, and the average age of a graduate of a

baccalaureate nursing program was 23.8. The more recent data on enrollment trends in higher education in general presented by Ross and Hampton[9] suggest that the next report on nursing student characteristics will indicate further aging of the beginning nursing student population.

Moreover, if only 6% of all families have a traditional composition, and if 40% of nontraditional students are married, large numbers of nursing students must be maintaining both their studies and their familial responsibilities. The growth in the number of single parents in the general population predicts a high likelihood that a nursing student will also increasingly be the only parent in a home. Nursing students who must juggle school, work, and child care will continue to expand the time required to successfully complete a course of study. Data from the American Association of Colleges of Nursing study of the costs of a nursing education indicated that baccalaureate students took an average of 4.9 years to complete the degree.[3] These data suggest that nontraditional patterns of learning are a common part of nursing education.

Clearly, old ways of educating that require Monday through Friday, daytime class work will not meet the needs of the growing number of nontraditional students. This shift in student populations has already dramatically changed the types of nursing programs

Table 22-1 Enrollments by race and ethnicity in baccalaureate and graduate programs in nursing 1991-92*

	Undergraduate			Graduate			Generic	
	Generic	RN	Total Bacc.†	Master's	Doct	Post Doct	Master's	Gen ND
Number of programs reporting Race/Ethnicity	328	392	431	209	53	3	10	3
Asian or Pacific Islander	1,970	474	2,815	572	67	0	12	6
(%)	(3.1)	(1.8)	(2.9)	(2.5)	(2.5)		(2.6)	(4.5)
Black, non-Hispanic	5,598	1,961	8,448	1,205	112	1	14	9
(%)	(8.8)	(7.4)	(8.8)	(5.2)	(4.3)	(7.1)	(3.0)	(6.7)
American Indian or Alaskan native	337	91	434	77	15	0	5	0
(%)	(0.5)	(0.3)	(0.5)	(0.3)	(0.6)		(1.1)	
Hispanic	1,793	692	2,779	387	45	0	5	5
(%)	(2.8)	(2.6)	(2.9)	(1.7)	(1.7)		(0.4)	(3.7)
White	52,670	21,804	78,883	19,915	2,184	13	423	114
(%)	(83.1)	(82.5)	(81.9)	(86.1)	(83.0)	(92.9)	(92.1)	(85.1)
International student	245	138	413	249	68	0	2	0
(%)	(0.4)	(0.5)	(0.4)	(1.1)	(2.6)		(0.4)	0
Unknown	851	1,284	2,508	731	140	0	2	0
(%)	(1.3)	(4.9)	(2.6)	(3.1)	(5.3)		(0.4)	0
Not reported	3,308	1,873	5,181	684	0	0	120	0

*Institutions that reported estimated data are excluded.
†Twenty-three institutions did not report separate generic and RN baccalaureate race/ethnicity data.
Reprinted by permission: American Association of Colleges of Nursing. (1992). *Enrollment and graduations in baccalaureate and graduate programs in nursing 1991-1992*. Washington, D.C.: Author.

being offered, and many nurse educators have responded to these changing realities with new programs for nonnurse students. These programs have seen marked growth in response to an older, nontraditional population of students. New "accelerated" baccalaureate nursing programs began developing approximately five years ago as an option for individuals with baccalaureates in a field other than nursing to acquire the baccalaureate in nursing. In that short period, over 40 programs have opened and another 17 are in planning stages.[2]

These "accelerated" programs are an evolutionary variation on the generic master's programs for nonnurses begun with great controversy by Yale University. Yale's programs, designed to allow the individual with a baccalaureate degree in a field other than nursing to do entry-level nursing studies at the master's level, were hotly debated as a workable model. Today, however, the number of generic master's in nursing programs is also increasing. A number of institutions have begun these programs in response to a growing interest in nursing by nontraditional, older students

with previous college education. In 1992, 12 of these generic master's programs existed, and another 9 were in planning stages.

Both the accelerated baccalaureate and the generic master's programs are clear indications that nursing education is evolving in response to new pools of students. These variations are a beginning. However, other changes are vitally needed. As the increasingly complex health care delivery system demands more nurses with advanced-level clinical skills, the demand for master's and doctorally prepared nurses will continue to grow. Unfortunately, many graduate programs in nursing require an entering student to have one or more years of experience before entering graduate studies.

The requirement that a newly graduated nurse with a baccalaureate degree wait several years to begin advanced studies seriously elongates the time between entry into a generic nursing education program and the availability of a more highly trained individual to the health care system. Moreover, recent data indicate a serious concern regarding the aging of the nursing population. In 1988, less than 16% of all nurses were

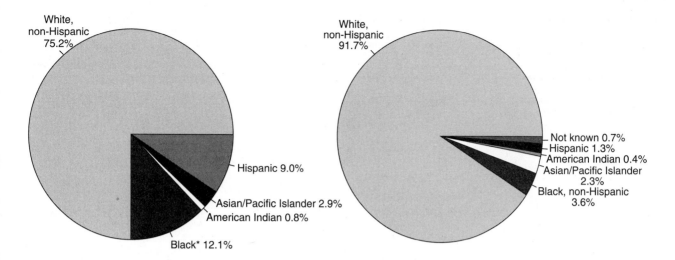

U.S. Population 1990 by Race and Ethnicity (a)   Registered Nurse Population, March 1988, by Race and Ethnicity (b)

Fig. 22-3 Comparison of total U.S. population and registered nurse population by race and ethnicity. (Source (a); *Hodgkinson, H. L. (1992). A demographic look at tomorrow. Washington, D.C.: Institute for Educational Leadership.* Source (b): *Moses, E. B. (1990). The registered nurse population. Washington, D.C.: U.S. Department of Health & Human Services.*) *Includes a small number of Hispanics.

under the age of 30. The growth in nontraditional students in nursing will greatly accelerate the aging of the nursing population. Increasing the time required to complete graduate studies will cut the number of years a nontraditional graduate will be able to practice as an advanced nurse clinician.

As was evident in the AACN study on nursing costs,[3] the majority of graduate students are employed an average of 32 hours per week during their studies, a factor that further elongates the education experience and shortens the time the advanced nurse clinician is available to the health care system. The goal of the educational system should be to facilitate progression to the highest level of practice with the fewest barriers.

The new realities of student pools also creates a need to focus efforts to recruitment of greater numbers of minority students. Although the percentage of nursing students who are members of a racial or ethnic minority group has increased in the last decade, these percentages still fall behind the total population representation. The most recent American Association of Colleges of Nursing report on enrollments and graduations in baccalaureate and graduate nursing education provides evidence that the greatest representation occurs at the undergraduate level (see Table 22-1). Mi-

nority enrollment at the graduate level continues to lag far behind, a result of the very small number of minority registered nurses (see Fig. 22-3). The disparity between enrollments and graduations of minority students gives some indications that the difficulties experienced by minority students as noted above may also be affecting the success of minority nursing students (see Table 22-2).

The realities of the demographics of the future mandate greater attention to recruitment of larger numbers of minority students. Besides issues of equity and representativeness, the reality is that the student body of the twenty-first century is likely to be predominantly composed of minority students. To maintain a stable supply of nursing personnel, a consistent effort must be made to attract students from diverse backgrounds. In addition, Smith[10] notes that by increasing the numbers of nurses and health professionals who are members of a minority group, the professions also increase their ability to address the health care needs of diverse populations.

NEW DIRECTIONS FOR NEW ISSUES

In a recent policy discussion on human resources for health care, Bulger and Osterweis[4] detail some of the

Table 22-2 Graduations by race and ethnicity in baccalaureate and graduate programs in nursing 1990-91*

	Undergraduate			Graduate			Generic	
	Generic	**Total RN**	**Bacc.†**	**Master's**	**Post Doct**	**Doct**	**Master's**	**ND**
Number of programs reporting Race/Ethnicity	334	396	450	185	54	3	5	2
Asian	337	144	544	112	10	0	0	0
(%)	(2.2)	(1.7)	(2.1)	(2.0)	(3.1)			
Black	1,128	613	1,911	260	11	0	0	5
(%)	(7.4)	(7.5)	(7.5)	(4.5)	(3.5)		(21.7)	
Native American	72	31	112	13	0	0	0	0
(%)	(0.5)	(0.4)	(0.5)	(0.2)				
Hispanic	438	178	694	76	3	0	2	0
(%)	(2.9)	(2.2)	(2.7)	(1.3)	(0.9)		(3.3)	
White	12,788	6,770	21,327	5,081	282	2	59	18
(%)	(84.2)	(82.6)	(83.6)	(87.1)	(89.0)	(100)	(96.7)	
International student	40	18	68	49	11	0	0	0
(%)	(0.3)	(0.2)	(0.3)	(0.8)	(3.5)			
Unknown	385	446	853	240	0	0	0	0
(%)	(2.5)	(5.4)	(3.3)	(4.1)				
Not reported	776	534	1,434	310	34	0	1	0

*Institutions reporting estimated data are excluded.
†Twenty-six institutions did not report separate generic and RN baccalaureate race/ethnicity data.
Reprinted by permission: American Association of Colleges of Nursing. (1992). *Enrollment and graduations in baccalaureate and graduate programs in nursing 1991-1992*. Washington, D.C.: Author.

dramatic changes that the system of health care delivery is undergoing. They note that "the number and kinds of health professionals society needs depends on the social choices we make in light of perceived threats to health, demographic shifts, technologic advances, costs, and the value that we place on health care."

Detmer[5] details the steps necessary to fulfill a vision of the future. First, realities must be clearly understood. Second, the goal or vision must be fully articulated. And, third, the infrastructure to achieve the vision must be put in place.

For nursing education, the reality is that new pools are and must continue to be tapped. The vision is to create a wealth of diversity in the nursing profession that is representative of social, economic, and cultural changes in the population at large. The infrastructure is only partially developed. The move to less traditional ways of becoming a professional nurse are a beginning. The challenge is to bring more diverse groups of individuals to these new options.

REFERENCES

1. Astone, B., & Nunez-Wormack, E. (1990). *Pursuing diversity: Recruiting college minority students* (ASHE-ERIC Higher Education Report No. 7). Washington, D.C.: The George Washington University, School of Education and Human Development.
2. Bednash, G., Berlin, L., & Chan, L. (1992). *1991-1992 enrollment and graduations in baccalaureate and graduate programs in nursing*. Washington, D.C.: American Association of Colleges of Nursing.
3. Bednash, G., Redman, B., & Southers, N. (1989). *The economic investment in nursing education: Student, institutional, and clinical perspectives*. Washington, D.C.: American Association of Colleges of Nursing.
4. Bulger, R. J., & Osterweis, M. (1992). Human resources policy and academic health centers. In C. M. Evarts, P. P. Bosomworth, & M. Osterweis (Eds.), *Human resources for health: Defining the future* (pp. 1-12). Washington, D.C.: Association of Academic Health Centers.
5. Detmer, D. (1991). Reducing the discontinuities between vision and practice. In C. Rich, A. Barbato, & J. Griffith (Eds.), *Vision: Leadership and values in academic health centers* (pp. 97-103). Washington, D.C.: Association of Academic Health Centers.
6. Hodgkinson, H. (1992). *A demographic look at tomorrow*. Washington, D.C.: Institute for Educational Leadership.
7. Moses, E. (1990). *The registered nurse population: Findings from the national sample survey of registered nurses, March 1988*. Washington, D.C.: U.S. Department of Health and Human Services.
8. Population-Environment Balance. (1992). *Balance data*. Washington, D.C.

9. Ross, L., & Hampton, D. (1992). "How the nontraditional student finances her education." In J. Eaton (Ed.), *Financing nontraditional students: A seminar report* (pp. 7-32). Washington, D.C.: American Council on Education.

10. Smith, M. (1992). Health personnel in a diverse society. In C. M. Evarts, P. P. Bosomworth, & M. Osterweis (Eds.), *Human resources for health: Defining the future* (pp. 26-33). Washington, D.C.: Association of Academic Health Centers.

11. Snyder, D. P., & Edwards, G. (1992). *America in the 1990s: Strategic insights for associations.* Washington, D.C.: The Foundation of the American Society of Association Executives.

CHAPTER 23

Partnerships in nursing education

Expanding the boundaries

MARILYN L. ROTHERT, GERALDINE J. TALARCZYK, SUSAN M. AWBREY

In today's world, more than ever, nursing education must be considered part of a dynamic system of interrelated components to deal with current needs and issues. To understand issues involving nursing education requires an understanding of population characteristics, students, health care delivery mechanisms, and institutions of higher education. Changes in any one component influence the other components, requiring each area to be both proactive and reactive to address emerging issues and needs. Currently, each one of these components is experiencing and coping with dramatic change, which in turn strongly influences the other parts of the system. Considering the rapid changes taking place and the interrelatedness of the components of the system, *partnerships* are essential to provide quality health care and prepare the nurse of the future.

This chapter provides a brief overview of changes in student population characteristics, health care delivery, and institutions of higher education, followed by a review of current collaborative programs in nursing education. The chapter concludes with a discussion of the major implications for future partnerships in nursing education.

POPULATION SHIFTS

The future of our nation depends on our ability to attract and retain today's educational consumers who are the work force of tomorrow. At the same time that the complexity of health care work settings is increasing, the preparation of students entering our educational institutions is expected to decline. Overall, the U.S. population is undergoing drastic change. As we begin the new century, white males, currently a major group in the workforce, will constitute under 20% of the new labor force entrants.[15] The "vanishing white male" is being replaced with a diversity of new workers.[58] By the year 2000, one in three Americans will be a person of color and 60% of new job entrants are expected to be minorities or immigrants.[59] Women are expected to make up 47% of the work force.[27] More and more of these new workers will be coming from disadvantaged circumstances. One third of the new entrants will be from single-parent homes and one fifth from families below the poverty line.[59] Because our future work force depends on the education of groups once relegated to the margin in our society, what was once deemed desirable because it was fair and ethical has now become a matter of economic survival.

New entrants to nursing practice will also face a dramatically reshaped work environment where the very nature of work has been redefined by the information revolution, where the diversity of co-workers and clients is rapidly increasing, where new models for the integration of home and work life are being seen, and where a growing awareness of international responsibilities, a renewed social agenda, new organizational structures, and new managerial practices exist.[27] Adaptability and flexibility must be primary concepts for the training and education of new nurses. Because many workers will also face the prospect of changing fields multiple times during their lifetimes, new strategies will be needed to educate and upgrade the skills of existing workers who choose nursing as a second career. Seventy-one percent of mothers with children under 18 are already working,[40] and the median age of workers will approach 39 by the year 2000.[57]

Registered nursing ranks second among occupations that will generate the most new jobs between 1988 and

2000. There will be an estimated 613,000 new jobs for registered nurses, an increase of 39%.[57] The annual survey of nursing schools by the National League for Nursing found that overall nursing enrollments increased 7.5% during the 1991-92 academic year. Although nursing educators can currently be encouraged by the success of their efforts to recruit students to meet the projected increase in positions, they still face the challenge of developing programs that will retain this new diverse population of students. Since the greatest enrollment increases are in baccalaureate programs, the challenge will intensify as educators are faced with developing less well-prepared students into the highly trained professionals who can assist in finding solutions to the massive health care problems created by the changes in our overall population.

HEALTH CARE DELIVERY SYSTEM

A second major area influencing nursing education is the health care delivery system. There is a health care crisis in the United States. In 1986, infant mortality (under one year of age) in the United States was 10.4%, behind many other countries in the world.[39] Access to affordable and available health care services stands as a major challenge, and nursing must prepare to address this challenge. The United States is the only industrialized country besides South Africa that does not guarantee health care for its citizens.[48]

There is a disproportionately larger number of providers practicing in the wealthier urban and suburban areas, creating an imbalance in the availability of services. There was actually a decline in use of medical care for all population groups between 1982 and 1986, and this decline is attributed to an increase in persons without a regular source of care, an increase of 65%.[19] To address these needs, nurses must be prepared to deliver care in rural and urban areas, inner city and suburban areas, and primary care and high-tech acute care.

In 1989, approximately 30 to 40 million people were without health insurance, and an additional 65 million were underinsured.[47] Since 1965, spending for health care has grown almost twice as fast as the GNP.[31] Health care costs now constitute about one eighth of the nation's productive effort, and health plan costs for employees continue to rise, reported by a health care benefits survey by A. Foster Higgins & Co. as averaging $1,724 in 1985, and rising to $3,605

in 1991.[12] The Employee Benefits Research Institute reported the number of nonelderly uninsured Americans increased to 35.7 million in 1990, up from 33.6 million in 1988. The rise is attributed to increased unemployment and increased costs of health benefits, causing many to lose their employer-sponsored health coverage. As a percentage of the entire population, 55.2% of the uninsured in the United States in 1990 were working adults.[24] Business is not ready to take on more responsibility to pay for health care, since they already assume a significant portion of health care costs. All indications are that health care costs will continue to escalate, and uncompensated care has become a major health care issue.[42]

With the high cost of health care, reimbursement is a major issue and nursing has a central role in it. Several new initiatives have already been developed. As of January 1, 1991, services delivered by nurse practitioners and clinical nurse specialists in rural areas can be reimbursed under the Medicare program. Beginning in 1992, Medicare payment to physicians is based on a fee schedule as a result of provisions in the Omnibus Budget Reconciliation Act of 1989 (OBRA-89), signed into law (PL101-239) in December 1989. The relative value of each service is now determined by estimates of average time and effort, practice expense, and costs of professional liability insurance. Geographic adjustments will also be made. How the payment formula is determined is a significant issue for nurses, as it is expected to influence insurance reimbursement for all practitioners.

A changing focus on the health care consumer is also evident, and efforts such as Nursing's Agenda for Health Care Reform place the consumer at the center of the issues. There are increased efforts to focus on enhancing patient involvement in decision making. A major portion of chronic illness is recognized as related to individual lifestyle and behavior. In addition, businesses are expecting informed patients involved in decision making to be more likely to act in their best medical and financial interests. Involving the employee, and respecting the employee's autonomy and the right to choose, requires providing the employee the tools to make wise choices and places a renewed emphasis on patient education.[34] Major health care issues such as AIDS, infant mortality, and drug abuse must increasingly be viewed within the context of social, economic, political, and cultural issues and be integrated into the nursing curricula.

INSTITUTIONS OF HIGHER EDUCATION

In addition to shifting demographics and crises in our health care delivery system, changes in institutions of higher education continue to have an impact on nursing education. Alpert[1] noted that economic retrenchment has focused attention on the nation's commitment to its institutions of higher education as well as questioning the responsibilities of universities to society. Retrenchment revealed serious problems related to management and governance, identity and purpose, including faculty morale and recruitment of new faculty. While the university focused inward, it was seen as out of touch with the population and the environment it served.

The confusion of mission has also been reflected in questions regarding the faculty reward system, which no longer matches the full range of academic functions and leads to competing obligations. If institutions of higher education are to meet today's academic and social mandates, their missions must be redefined and the meaning of scholarship creatively reconsidered to give legitimacy to the full scope of academic work.[7] Thus, universities are trying to find ways to be more responsive to society through the generation, application, and dissemination of knowledge. This requires assessing the role of outreach, faculty involvement, and rewards for teaching, research, and service.

Bok has addressed the issue from the perspective of what the community demands. As the economic situation worsens, the United States is faced with a deteriorating quality of life and a serious challenge to revitalize its stance to provide well being for all its citizens. "With 27 million functional illiterates, 33 million in poverty, and many millions addicted to drugs and alcohol, vast sums of money must be spent on programs of welfare, law enforcement, social work, and other services that do not add to productivity."[6] What role will universities play in this scenario?

Traditionally, universities have shied away from practical, social issues. A variety of factors have combined to create this reluctance to act. Although the average person may believe that universities have been less than successful in addressing society's ills because they are isolated ivory tower environments, it would be more accurate to say that "universities are captive to the very social values and priorities that caused these problems in the first place. . . . universities are responsive, but what they respond to is what the society chooses to pay for, not what it most needs."[6] Clearly, much social reform is beyond the mission of the uni-

versity. However, future social well-being and economic strength are inextricably tied to the values of individual citizens. "Nearly half of the population . . . enters our colleges and professional schools. For several formative years, the university is the dominant influence in their lives."[6]

There are many ways that universities can contribute to building a humane, responsible, and responsive citizenry. Perhaps, most basic is a more balanced program of support between the traditional arts and sciences and the practice-based, professional programs such as nursing, social work, education, and other service disciplines that have historically focused on society's needs. Students can be involved in applied research that studies the assumptions imbedded in the actions people take and the decisions they reach.[8] Creating an awareness of cultural diversity and challenging students to think critically about the assumptions they hold will assist them in coping with the changing landscape of the future. Universities can empower students to actively participate in the life of their communities.[20]

COLLABORATIVE EFFORTS IN NURSING EDUCATION

Over the years, nursing education has reached out to form various partnerships and collaborative relationships as a part of the solution to meeting the expanding needs of the times. For example, individual programs—to create a climate for collaboration in the delivery of health care services—have joined with other health care disciplines to promote interdisciplinary educational opportunities for students. Nursing has created these educational partnerships with medicine,[4,22,33,60] pharmacy,[10] nutrition,[5] dentistry,[32] social work,[29] as well as with multidisciplinary groups.[41]

To improve nursing education and the care provided to nursing home patients, nursing education has participated with nursing service in at least two large projects. One was the Robert Wood Johnson Foundation Teaching Nursing Home Program, funded from 1982 to 1987, to evaluate what happens to care of the elderly when nursing homes and nursing schools collaborate. The demonstration project with a three-pronged thrust—education, service, research—was carried out at 11 sites.[23] A second project was the Community College–Nursing Home Partnership: Improving Care Through Education, which was funded by the W. K. Kellogg Foundation. Six demonstration sites engaged in activities to develop nursing potential in long-term settings through in-service education and to influence associate degree education to include educational experiences in long-term care settings.[21]

In another effort, nursing education and nursing service have united in some medical centers to meet common goals. This model exists at Case Western Reserve University,[42] the University of Rochester,[18] and Rush-Presbyterian-St. Luke's Medical Center.[9] Where these models do not exist, other efforts to strengthen the link between nursing education and nursing service have been implemented. In some instances, this has been through joint appointments, i.e., as a faculty member in a nursing program and as a member of nursing service in a health care agency.[16,26,28] In others, it has been through cooperative arrangements in providing continuing education opportunities for service personnel[38] or faculty,[50] or through collaborative research.[36]

Nursing service has supported nursing education programs in a variety of ways. Examples of nursing service support include providing preceptors for nursing students,[13,14,17,25,52] providing tuition reimbursement for employees enrolling in nursing programs, having representatives serve on advisory committees of nursing education programs, and by entering joint venture arrangements with educational programs.[3]

Nursing education and nursing service have also been working together to identify differentiated nursing practice.[51] Several projects sponsored by the Midwest Alliance in Nursing and funded by the W. K. Kellogg Foundation brought together nursing service managers/staff developers and ADN and BSN educators to develop a regional consensus on the differentiated scope of practice for ADN and BSN graduates.[44,53] This understanding could not only provide reasonable employer expectations but could also serve to define an educational articulation model for ADN and BSN programs. In several states, including Minnesota, Maryland, and Colorado, planning between ADN and BSN programs has provided statewide articulation plans for nurses.[11,45,61]

In 1989, the W. K. Kellogg Foundation initiated its Community Partnerships program to establish models of academic, community-based, primary health centers. The goal of the initiative is to significantly change the way health professionals are educated by assisting a few institutions in creating new organizational structures in partnership with communities. The program is built on the concepts that the nature of health profes-

sions education, including research and teaching, is a function of the clinical settings where academic health centers provide their services. The initiative intends to demonstrate that communities are willing and able to join in partnership with academic institutions to address important local health care issues. The initiative requires medicine and nursing to work together with the community in both education and service.[46] Nurses in expanded practice are a major component of the seven projects funded across the country.

IMPLICATIONS FOR NURSING EDUCATION

Changes and shifts in populations, health care delivery, and institutions of higher education will push nursing education to expand its collaborative efforts. Changes in population characteristics of our students will challenge nursing programs to provide greater access and to retain students whose cultures, lifestyles, and age may vary markedly from traditional students of the past. To meet this challenge will require university-based nursing educators to form linkages not only with secondary education to recruit students but also with community colleges and public/private sector retraining programs for returning adult students. Assisting this diverse pool of students to remain in school will require close partnerships with other on-campus units and community agencies to provide tutoring, counseling, financial aid, and flexible community-based and distance education programs.

Population shifts and cost control efforts have also impacted the nature of our client population. Cost control efforts such as DRGs have resulted in early discharge from acute health care settings and a patient population that is less accessible to health professional students or more widely distributed in the health care system as they return to local health care provider settings. The increase in the population of uninsured and underinsured has also decreased the number of persons in the health care system, thereby again, decreasing the number of learning opportunities for health professional students. The shift from acute care to primary care with an emphasis on disease prevention and health promotion has also shifted student learning opportunities from the acute-care setting to a broad-based community setting of clinics and health care provider offices. To have access to learning opportunities in this changing health care environment, nursing education programs will have to work closely with these less centralized systems. It will mean not only working together to access clients/patients but to also develop a teaching-learning relationship. Nursing programs will become increasingly dependent on practitioners other than traditional full-time faculty to supervise student learning as students are spread throughout the community rather than concentrated in a single health care agency such as the hospital.

The shift to a community-based health care delivery system will place an increasing emphasis on community assessment, utilization of community resources, interdisciplinary team health care, and client/patient education in nursing curricula. In addition, there will be a focus on the use of the political system to initiate and bring about change within the health care system itself and within local, state, and federal government health care policy-making bodies. The problems of cost, access, and quality of health care for all populations will bring a renewed interest in the ethical dilemmas resulting from various proposed policies and solutions. Rationing of health care, choosing the decision makers in the health care system, and other issues will continue to be debated.

Perhaps the biggest challenge for nursing educators will be assisting students to develop the skills necessary to actively participate in and provide leadership for addressing the nation's health care problems, including skills such as creatively adapting to change, being sensitive to individual differences and multicultural issues, having respect for and working in concert with other professions, and, most importantly, thinking critically[8] to identify and challenge assumptions, to examine the contexts for decisions, and to explore alternatives. With such skills, future nurses can facilitate community partnerships that empower people to find creative health care solutions.

As universities struggle to identify strategies useful to meet the expanding educational needs of society in a time of serious economic constraint, new partnerships are emerging. With citizens funding institutions of higher education, both through taxes and tuition, the lack of practical application and dissemination of knowledge to address major social problems is highly visible and highly criticized. Nursing education has focused on application of knowledge as a service profession, yet the practice of nursing and the preparation of new nursing professionals has not reached its potential to address the societal issues related to access, quality, and cost of health care.

Nursing education must enhance its partnership with communities and service institutions to produce community-based education. This means that nursing students will be practicing their clinical skills and meeting their educational objectives in community hospitals, agencies, clinics, and offices; the needs of the community will be a factor in determining the curriculum and educational experiences. Students will not only be expected to function in a high-tech academic health care center but also to have the skills to practice community-based primary care for underserved populations. This shift, to meet the health care needs of our citizens, will require different and expanded skills from our students and will require a partnership with our state licensing and our professional accrediting bodies. These partnerships will be needed to align approval and accreditation criteria of our educational programs and credentialing of new professionals with our values in education and service.

The changes will require new skills of our faculty, and collaboration between universities and colleges/schools of nursing to expand the skills and credentials required and valued in an academic setting. Ongoing continuing education will be an essential ingredient for faculty and service providers. Research, teaching, and service will become redefined as generation, application, and dissemination of knowledge, and outreach will become an integral part of the mission of the university.

Changes in institutions of higher education will also require a redefinition of the educational site and the geographical boundaries of the university. If we are to prepare nursing professionals to address the health care needs of citizens in underserved areas, we must educate students in underserved areas such as inner cities and rural communities. This will require new partnerships between the community and university to develop community-based educational experiences drawing on faculty who are integrated into the community setting.

The health care issues facing society today require multifaceted approaches. Future health care professionals must learn in an interdisciplinary environment to understand their separate roles and shared goals across disciplines. Nursing is challenged along with other health care professions to develop the educational experiences that will prepare students for interdisciplinary practice. To achieve the goal, faculty with skills in collaborative practice and experience in community settings will be needed.

The financial constraints facing universities are also breaking down barriers to alliances among educational institutions. Universities are assessing opportunities to collaborate which will provide broader opportunities for students. Community colleges and universities are expanding linkages and diminishing barriers for students moving from the community college to a four-year institution. These alliances will not only reduce cost and expand educational opportunities but also better prepare students to respond to societal needs.

In summary, the educational system, health care delivery system, and consumers of these services are rapidly changing, both individually and collectively. Those responsible for educating the new nursing professional must recognize the interrelatedness of education, health, and community, and develop new partnerships to meet the expanding educational and service needs.

REFERENCES

1. Alpert, D. (1985). Performance and paralysis: The organizational context of the American research university. *Journal of Higher Education, 56*, 241-281.
2. Andrews, M. M. (1992). Cultural perspectives on nursing in the 21st century. *Journal of Professional Nursing, 8*(1), 7.
3. Bargagliotti, L. A., Jones, D. L., Trygstad, L., Hayward, M., Crow, G., & Bowe, F. L. (1991). Joint venture arrangement for RN to BSN: A model of synergy between academia and service. *Nursing and Health Care, 12*(7), 380.
4. Barnum, B. J. (1990). At New York University, the Division of Nursing develops a model for nursing and medical school collaboration. *Nursing and Health Care, 11*(2), 89.
5. Baumslag, N., Gatins, K., Watson, D. R., & England, A. (1976). Interdisciplinary nutrition education. *Journal of Medical Education, 51*(1), 64.
6. Bok, D. (1990). *Universities and the future of America.* Durham, N.C.: Duke University Press.
7. Boyer, E. L. (1990). *Scholarship reconsidered: Priorities of the professoriate.* Princeton, N.J.: The Carnegie Foundation for the Advancement of Teaching.
8. Brookfield, S. D. (1991). *Developing critical thinkers: Challenging adults to explore alternative ways of thinking and acting.* San Francisco: Jossey-Bass.
9. Christman, L. (1979). The division of nursing and the college of nursing: An overview. *Nursing Administration Quarterly, 3*(3), 7.
10. Collier, I. M. (1981). Educational cooperation among nursing, medicine and pharmacy: A success story. *Journal of Nursing Education, 20*(7), 23.
11. Colorado Council on Nursing Education. (1990). *The Colorado nursing articulation model.* Denver: Author.
12. Data watch. (1992). *Business and Health, 10*(3), 18.
13. Davis, L. L., & Barham, P. D. (1989). Get the most from your preceptorship program. *Nursing Outlook, 37*(4), 167.
14. Donius, M. A. H. (1988). The Columbia precepting program: Building a bridge with clinical faculty. *Journal of Professional Nursing, 4*(1), 17.
15. Doyle, F. P. (1989). Who will be? Challenges and opportunities of U.S. population change. In *Proceedings of the new America: Prospects for population and policy in the 21st century* (pp. 1-6). Washington, D.C.: Committee for Economic Development.
16. Fasano, N. (1981). Joint appointments: Challenge for nursing. *Nursing Forum, 22*(1), 72.
17. Ferguson, M., & Hauf, B. (1973). The preceptor role: Implementing student experience in community nursing. *Journal of Continuing Education in Nursing, 4*(1), 12.
18. Ford, L. C. (1980). Unification of nursing practice, education and research. *International Nursing Review, 27*(6), 178.
19. Freeman, H., Blendon R., Aiken, L., Sudman, S., Mullinix, C. F., & Corey, C. R. (1987). Americans report on their access to health care. *Health Affairs, 6*(1), 6-8.
20. Grace, H. K. (1990). Building community: A conceptual perspective. *W. K. Kellogg Foundation International Journal, 20-22.*
21. Hanson, H. A., & Waters, V. (1991). The sequence of curriculum change in gerontology. *Nursing and Health Care, 516.*
22. Harding, E. H., Fowler, M., & Gordon, N. (1975). A nursing course for medical students. *Nursing Outlook, 23*(4), 240.
23. Huey, F. (1985). What teaching nursing homes are teaching us. *American Journal of Nursing, 85*(6), 678.
24. Issues and trends. (1992). *Business and Health, 10*(3), 22.
25. Joel, L. (1985). The Rutgers experience: One perspective on service-education collaboration. *Nursing Outlook, 33*(5), 220.
26. Kelly, K., Gardner, D., Johnson, M., Maas, M., McCloskey, J. C., Bowers, M., Maske, J., Mathis, S., Specht, J., & Watson, C. (1990). Adjunct executive appointments for faculty. *Journal of Nursing Administration, 20*(10), 35.
27. Kreitner, R., & Kinicki, A. (1992). *Organizational behavior* (2nd ed.). Homewood, Ill: Irwin.
28. Kruger, S. (1985). The demonstration of a joint faculty/practice position. *Journal of Nursing Education, 24*(8), 350-352.
29. LaMonica, G., & Schmidt, M. G. (1986). Teamwork training polishes students' home care skills. *Nursing & Health Care, 7*(8), 451.
30. Lindquist, G. J. (1986). Programs that internationalize nursing curricula in baccalaureate schools of nursing in the United States. *Journal of Professional Nursing, 2*(1), 143.
31. Levit, K., Freeland, M., & Waldo, D. (1989). Health spending and ability to pay: Business, individuals and government. *Health Care Financial Review, 10*(3), 1-11.
32. Lough, M. A., Weinstein, L., & Abrams, R. A. (1986). Pre-school screening: An interdisciplinary training experience for nursing and dental students. *Journal of Nursing Education, 25*(4), 170.
33. Luginbill, C. (1978). Nurse-instructors for medical students. *American Journal of Nursing, 78*(5), 869.
34. Making the patient a partner. (1991). *Business and Health Special Report: Integrating Managed Care,* 25.
35. Meleis, A. I. (1987). International nursing research. In J. J. Fitzpatrick & R. L. Tauton (Eds.), *Annual review of nursing research, vol. 5.* New York: Springer.
36. Minckley, B. B., Anderson, R., & Sands, D. (1989). Collaborative research: The Arizona experience. *The Journal of Continuing Education in Nursing, 20*(5), 228.
37. Mooneyhan, E. L., McElmurray, B. J., Sofranko, M. S., & Campos, A. B. (1986). International dimensions of nursing and health care in baccalaureate and higher degree nursing programs in the United States. *Journal of Professional Nursing, 2*(2), 82.

38. Moore, P., Beckman-Pace, K., & Rapacz, K. (1987). Collaborative model for continuing education for home health nurses. *The Journal of Continuing Education in Nursing, 22*(2), 67.

39. *Nursing's vital signs: Shaping the profession for the 1990s.* (1990). A Design for Nursing's Future from the National Commission on Nursing Implementation Project. Battle Creek, Mich: W. K. Kellogg Foundation.

40. Offermann, L. R., & Gowing, M. K. (1990). Organizations of the future changes and challenges. *American Psychologist,* 95-108.

41. Oishi, N., Oki, G., Itano, J., Stringfellow, L., & Kurren, O. (1986). Professional schools team students to improve oncology care. *Nursing and Health Care, 7*(8), 446.

42. Perkins, C. B., & Perkins, K. C. (1992). Uncompensated care: The millstone around the neck of U.S. health care. *Nursing and Health Care, 13*(1), 20.

43. Pierek, M. (1973). Joint appointments: Collaboration for better patient care. *Nursing Outlook, 21*(9), 576.

44. Primm, P. L. (1986). Entry into practice: Competency statements for BSNs and ADNs. *Nursing Outlook, 34*(3), 135.

45. Rapson, M. F. (1987). *Collaboration for articulation: RN to BSN.* New York: National League for Nursing.

46. Richards, R. W., Grace, H. K., & Henry, R. C. (1991). *Community partnerships: A Kellogg initiative in health professions education.* Battle Creek, Mich: W. K. Kellogg Foundation.

47. Short, P., Cornelius, L., & Goldstone, D. (1990). Health insurance of minorities in the United States. *Journal of Health Care for the Poor, 1,* 9-24.

48. Shugars, D. A., O'Neill, E. H., & Bader, J. D. (1991). *Healthy America: Practitioners for 2005: An agenda for action for U.S. health professional schools.* Durham, N.C.: The Pew Health Professions Commission.

49. Siciliano, R. C. (1989). Introduction. In *Proceedings of the new America: Prospects for population and policy in the 21st century* (pp. i-ii). Washington, D.C.: Committee for Economic Development.

50. Smith, C. E., Baasch, L., & Hoffman, S. E. (1984). Back to the bedside. *The Journal of Continuing Education in Nursing, 15*(2), 45.

51. Stevens, B. J. (1981). Program articulation: What is and what it is not. *Nursing Outlook, 29*(12), 700.

52. Stuart-Siddall, & Haberliln, J. M. (1983). *Preceptors in nursing education.* Rockville, Md: Aspen.

53. Stull, M. K. (1986). Entry skills for BSNs. *Nursing Outlook, 34*(3), 138.

54. Tesch, R. (1992). *Qualitative research: Analysis types and software tools.* New York: Falmer Press.

55. Toffler, A. (1991). *Powershift: Knowledge, wealth, and violence at the edge of the 21st century.* New York: Bantam.

56. Tripp-Reimer, T., & Dougherty, M. C. (1985). Cross-cultural nursing research. In H. H. Werley & J. J. Fitzpatrick (Eds.), *Annual review of nursing research, vol. 3.* New York: Springer.

57. U.S. Bureau of the Census. (1990). *Statistical abstract of the United States* (110th ed., Table no. 646, p. 392.) Washington, D.C.: U.S. Government Printing Office.

58. Weber, A. R. (1989). Shaping a competitive work force. In *Proceedings of the new America: Prospects for population and policy in the 21st century* (pp. 14-24). Washington, D.C.: Committee for Economic Development.

59. Wharton, C. R. (1989). The new diversity—special needs, special challenges. In *Proceedings of the new America: Prospects for population and policy in the 21st century* (pp. 7-13). Washington, D.C.: Committee for Economic Development.

60. Wheeler, L. A., Burke, M. M., & Ling, F. W. (1981). Nurse-midwife involvement in medical student education: The pelvic examination. *Journal of Nurse-Midwifery, 26*(1): 34.

61. Zusy, M. L. (1986). RN to BSN: Fitting the pieces together. *American Journal of Nursing, 86*(4), 394.

CHAPTER 24

Community college–nursing home partnerships

Successful strategies for change in nursing education

SUSAN SHERMAN, VERLE WATERS

It has been said that changing the curriculum is like moving a graveyard: there are all those buried bodies, all that sacred ground, and all those hallowed icons of yesteryear. This discussion will present an account of successful curriculum change in associate degree education in the space of a few years, notable because the change meant confronting personal and professional biases about old people and nursing homes. Initiated in 1986, the W. K. Kellogg-funded project The Community College–Nursing Home Partnership: Improving Care Through Education had, as of 1992, significantly increased curriculum emphasis on gerontologic nursing in associate degree education and fostered new clinical affiliations with nursing homes in more than a third of the nation's 830 associate degree nursing programs. Strategies and factors associated with this remarkable success story will be described. While cause-and-effect relationships cannot be clearly established, the ingredients of successful change will be identified and described in this account of project activities and outcomes.

Over the past decade, nursing educators have grown increasingly conscious of the need to provide more instruction in the knowledge and skill of caring for older clients. Gunter and Estes[3] and Brower[1,2] recommended essential undergraduate content. Yet despite the evidence of need for more instruction on nursing care for the elderly, academic leaders and faculty have been reluctant to alter the curriculum to provide substantially different learning experiences.[2]

The history of associate degree nursing demonstrates the ability of these programs to produce significant numbers of nurses to meet the nursing needs of society. From the establishment of the associate degree nursing program in 1952, the curriculum has focused on the knowledge and job skills essential for the registered nurse who works in an acute-care hospital. Demography and shifting patterns of health care delivery prompted a reexamination of this focus through the activities of the Community College–Nursing Home Project.

The proposal funded by the W. K. Kellogg Foundation in 1986 had two purposes: to improve care in nursing homes through staff development and affiliation with nursing students and to substantially alter the associate degree curriculum such that graduates were prepared for practice roles in long-term care and acute-care organizations. The structure of the four-year project specified demonstration sites in six associate degree nursing programs in different parts of the country, each of whom would, in partnership with nursing homes, develop site-specific activities to meet project goals. At least four assumptions or beliefs about conditions necessary to successfully bring about change underlay the project structure and calendar of project activities:

1. Change is more likely if the oligarchy advocates it. With this assumption in mind, demonstration sites were selected where the nursing program held National League for Nursing (NLN) accreditation, a positive local reputation, and a director seen as a national leader. Within the demonstration sites, the oligarchy principle argued for the recruitment of tenured, full-time, well-regarded faculty to coordinate project activities. Not all six sites found it

possible to place full-time faculty in project leadership positions. A fuller discussion of leadership occurs later in this paper.

2. Campaigns for change are made more effective by combining ideology and conceptual arguments with compelling demonstrations of how-to-do-it. To achieve such a campaign, the project provided an "umbrella" structure identifying objectives and activities relating to a national perspective. A national advisory committee assisted in planning, analyzing, and synthesizing experiences from the six demonstrations. The six demonstration sites, on the other hand, built advisory committees that suited local needs and characteristics.

3. Change agents need support. For the period of the project, principals from all six sites met and worked together. At least two times per year, key people from each site gathered to collaborate, share, and plan.

4. Systematic formative evaluation and feedback fosters successful change. An evaluation specialist assisted both the national project and each demonstration site to develop evaluation protocols and analyze data.

The demonstration phase of the project began in 1986 and ended in 1990. Continued funding was provided by the W. K. Kellogg Foundation for the 1990-93 period to disseminate the results and achievements of the demonstration phase to the associate degree nursing community at large. Following successful curriculum change, the six demonstration sites assisted other ADN programs to commit to similar curriculum activities. Approximately 300 second-generation associate degree nursing programs have expanded the teaching of gerontologic nursing to increase classroom content and to provide clinical laboratory experience in a nursing home in the second year of their program. The journey from 1986 to 1992 has been eventful, enlightening, and rewarding. There have been false starts and dead ends, but an undeniably real change has occurred in associate degree nursing. An account of the experiences of those years yields valuable insights for others contemplating curriculum change.

The first step toward curriculum change is faculty development.[4] The traditional emphasis in the associate degree nursing curriculum has been on acute care. Faculty interests, loyalties, and specialized knowledge rests there. Reluctance to endorse substantive curriculum alterations and particularly to place students in nursing homes for clinical education was expressed in

several ways. Common expressions of resistance in a nursing faculty included:

- Since most hospital patients are over 65, gerontology is adequately taught without further change.
- Since only 5% of the over-65 population is in a nursing home, added learning experiences with that age group should focus on the majority of the elderly, those who are healthy and active.
- The idea has some merit, but there is no time left in the curriculum.
- The idea has merit, but the students will resist.
- There are no good role models in the nursing home, and it is a deprived learning environment.
- Affiliating ADN programs with the low-valued nursing home will refuel the "entry into practice" agenda.

LEADERSHIP

Two different models of leadership emerged. At three project sites, tenured faculty were released from teaching assignments to provide in-house leadership. At the other three sites, a grant coordinator was employed. Each model has strengths and weaknesses.

Every faculty group has a history, values, and established patterns and norms. An in-house leader understands this and has a sensitivity to timing that an outsider may not have. In this project, change was observed to occur more rapidly with in-house leaders. A strong inside leader, supported by a strong, committed administrator, can manage resources and time more effectively, particularly if that person has a history of leadership in the faculty organization.

New individuals, regardless of their credentials, always need to "pay their dues" to the group to gain acceptance. On the other hand, a new leader can stimulate and energize faculty. Without a personal history in the faculty or nursing program, the new leader can concentrate on project activity with a fresh perspective. The outside leader, however, is vulnerable to predictable pitfalls and their position is interim in nature. Interim leaders may lead a faculty to interim short-term change. This leader must understand faculty values, goals, and priorities to avoid pitfalls.

New ideas take time to work their way into faculty norms, need nurturing, and may require faculty modeling. Participation in project activities by the most respected members of the faculty should not be underestimated. Respected faculty who take the risk of getting involved in project activities stimulate recalcitrant faculty to participate. Soon, "joining in" becomes the group norm. The power of group norms is one of the leader's most important tools, whether the leader is an insider or an outsider.

FACULTY DEVELOPMENT

Three models of initiating and sustaining faculty development emerged. We call these the "we're all in this together" model, the "carrots to individuals" model, and "the credible in-house leadership" model.

The project leaders on campuses electing the "we're all in this together" model held the belief that the desired changes called for all full-time faculty to receive the same treatment and opportunity. These leaders assumed that faculty would support each other during the linear movement of the curriculum toward the desired goal. Faculty in this model were required to attend retreats with outside experts and to work cohesively to bring about program changes regardless of where their individual interests were at the time. In the programs electing this approach, "the grant" was for the common good and the mandate was to reeducate all members of the faculty.

In the second model, "carrots to individuals," leaders approached grant objectives with a more laissez-faire attitude. Grant objectives were shared with faculty who volunteered to pursue one or more areas within the umbrella of the overall goals. In these programs, faculty dropped in and out of project activities as time, energy, and interest permitted.

The third model, "credible in-house leadership," emerged as the structure most conducive to creating change. In this model a highly respected, tenured faculty member assumed leadership in achieving project goals. Endorsement of change by a strong faculty leader moderates the inevitable criticisms of the disbelievers, and risk taking is elevated to an acceptable, even desirable, faculty activity. Stepping out of a secure faculty position is a risk. At one site, the in-house coordinator quickly built a support group of interested faculty, known as "the gang of six," who supported and learned from each other. They developed resources for other faculty and advanced the idea that integration of gerontology is supplemental to, rather than different from, faculty's traditional nursing expertise.

CURRICULUM CHANGE

As project schools developed grant activities, changes began to show up in all nursing courses in the curriculum. All faculty, not only those carrying project assignments, gained knowledge and sensitivity to the needs of the elderly client. As nursing textbooks and journals were searched for information and perspective, faculty slowly realized that the literature is thus far inadequate to support faculty or student mastery of this field. This discovery sparked debate: Is there too little to know or is the area untapped? A positive outcome of this debate was that faculty concluded that available resources, activities, and references were needed. Over time a number of publications and contributions to the literature were developed. In some schools, change began slowly and developed its own momentum, in others, it occurred more rapidly.

In all cases curriculum change was fostered by the opportunity provided by the Kellogg grant for faculty leaders in the six schools to meet together. At various points in time, different project schools emerged as leaders in curriculum discussions. Ideas were exchanged, challenges taken up, and successes and disappointments shared fully.

In the dissemination project phase, workshop plans for the second generation schools were based on this model. The networking of faculty, so successful in the demonstration site experience, became a powerful tool for faculty development. The recognition that if desired outcomes are clearly stated, pathways for their achievement can differ, has enriched the project and its participants. Two key curriculum outcomes, a well-elder experience in the first year of the curriculum and a second-year nursing home clinical experience were common to all sites. But, as described in *Teaching Gerontology*,[8] the specific design of these activities varies among all project schools.

Faculty with clinical teaching assignments in the nursing home found themselves unprepared for the role changes they experienced. Accustomed to teaching in acute care, faculty felt outside their comfort zone as they confronted long-established patterns and traditions associated with hospital-based teaching. New patterns, traditions, and relationships among teachers, agency staff, and students emerged. The concept of participatory clinical education, described by Tagliareni et al.,[7] evolved as project faculty struggled to resolve their discomfort while providing successful learning experiences for students. Faculty who embrace a collaborative, participatory role as clinical teachers in the nursing home have found their teaching behaviors in acute-care settings are transformed as well.

Operational objectives derived from the two project goals served as the evaluation criteria for all project activities and provided the framework for the project implementation and evaluation plans developed at each of the six project sites.

Evaluative findings support the conclusion that the project achieved its intended outcomes regarding faculty knowledge about and attitudes toward aging, curriculum emphasis on gerontological nursing, and student knowledge about aging and interest in working in long-term care facilities. The findings indicate that planned faculty development activities, especially those that lead to gerontological nursing credentials, have a positive effect on faculty knowledge of and attitudes toward care of elderly people.[4]

INSTITUTIONALIZING CHANGE

The dissemination phase of the Community College–Nursing Home Partnership included collaborative activities with regulatory and accrediting bodies to support increased curricular attention to gerontological nursing. A collaborative relationship developed between the dissemination project staff and the committee assigned to revise and update the 1978 NLN-CADP "Competencies of the Associate Degree Nurse on Entry into Practice." The NLN committee was charged to revise the competencies and to develop the broadest possible understanding of the current and future practice patterns of associate degree nurses. The committee studied detailed reports for the Partnership Project along with other contemporary data. The resultant document, *Education Outcomes of Associate Degree Nursing Programs: Roles and Competencies,*[6] addresses the nursing needs of an aging population in emphasizing knowledge and skills required to serve the elderly population, to manage client care resources, to think critically, and to embrace values and practice ethically. These NLN-CADP competencies specifically address the preparation of registered nurses to provide direct care to clients across the life span, with an emphasis on adults. Three roles are identified as basic to associate degree nursing practice and within each role, concern for the older client is emphasized, as is the need for the development of practice patterns unique to both acute and long-term care settings.

Curricular emphasis represented in the 1990 NLN-CADP competency document reflects not only the value of practice roles in long term care settings, but the deemphasis of the traditional specialty areas of nursing practice. While advocacy for such a shift in the ADN curriculum arises from other sources as well, project faculty concluded that a change of this nature was warranted by work patterns of new graduates, as reported by Kane et al.,[5] and national demographic shifts. Emphasizing the necessity of preparing nurses for a work world where they will spend 75% of their work lives caring for people over the age of 65 became an early mission of project principals; it is a message that accrediting and regulatory agencies along with other audiences have heard.

SUMMARY

One purpose of nursing education is to serve society. Nursing education approaches the new millenium with challenges to adapt curricula to new care delivery systems, to rapidly expanding technology, and to dramatically different populations. Managing curriculum change is central in the work life of every nurse educator.

It is usually easy to note whether a change has been accomplished. Explaining how it occurred, or accounting for why it was possible is considerably more difficult. Yet we seek to know how and why to become better at managing it. The W. K. Kellogg-funded project, The Community College–Nursing Home Partnership, has successfully accomplished an intended change in at least one third of the nation's associate degree nursing programs; the effect is believed to be considerably broader. Factors related to the success of this change include the organizational structure of the project, the enlistment and training of capable leaders, the stability of leadership at all levels over the life span of the project, the timely evaluative feedback during the change process, and a conscious effort to institutionalize the change wherever possible.

REFERENCES

1. Brower, H. T. (1983). The nursing curriculum for long-term institutional care. In *Creating a career choice for nurses: Long-term care* (pp. 45-64). New York: National League for Nursing.
2. Brower, H. T. (1985). Knowledge competencies in gerontological nursing. In *Overcoming the bias of ageism in long-term care* (pp. 55-82). New York: National League for Nursing.
3. Gunter, L. M., & Estes, C. A. (1979). *Education for gerontic nursing.* New York: Springer.
4. Hanson, H. A., & Waters, V. (1991). The sequence of curriculum change in gerontology: Faculty first. *Nursing and Health Care, 12,* 10.
5. Kane, M., Kingsburg, C., Colton, D., & Estes, C. (1986). *A study of nursing practice and role delineation and job analysis of entry-*

level performance of registered nurses. Chicago: National Council of State Boards of Nursing.

6. National League for Nursing Council of Associate Degree Programs. (1990). *Educational outcomes of associate degree nursing programs: Role and competencies.* New York: Author.

7. Tagliareni, E., Sherman, S., Waters, V., & Mengel, A. (1991). Participatory clinical education: Reconceptualizing the clinical learning environment. *Nursing and Health Care, 12,* 5.

8. Waters, V. (Ed.). (1991). *Teaching gerontology.* New York: National League for Nursing.

CHAPTER 25

Graduate education
Making the right choice

GAYE W. POTEET, LINDA C. HODGES, SHARLA TATE

One of the most critical decisions a nurse will make is whether or not to attend graduate school. The second most important decision is where to attend graduate school. No matter whether a master's program or a doctoral program, a commitment to graduate education represents a high investment of time, energy, and financial resources. In most instances, it also involves personal sacrifice on the part of the individual and his or her significant others. The choice one makes about graduate education determines in large part the course of career development over a lifetime. At the same time that one considers personal factors, one needs to consider marketplace forces that will provide a fit between current and future employment opportunities and educational preparation.[9]

Downs[7] pointed out that graduate education is preparation for scholarship and that demonstration of scholarship occurs through a consistent pattern of productivity. Therefore, the choice of a program in which to acquire the knowledge and skill during the preparation phase is crucial.

HISTORY

The first master's degree in nursing was awarded in 1916 by Teachers College, Columbia University, Department of Nursing Education, New York, New York.[3] Graduate education has really developed along the lines of role preparation in three phrases. Early programs were designed to prepare administrators and teachers to serve as directors of nursing services and nursing education programs.

Frances Richter coined the term *clinical nurse specialist* in the early 1940s.[8] This nurse was viewed as a specialist with advanced knowledge and expertise in a specialized area of clinical practice. Preparation for this role had the improvement of patient care as its primary focus. Since that time, more than 231 schools of nursing have developed programs leading to a master's degree with 78% accredited by the National League for Nursing.[12] These programs range in areas of broad specialization, such as community health nursing, to narrow fields such as adult oncology. Three functional areas of study represent approximately 98% of all students enrolled in master's programs. These include teaching (9.3%), administration and management (18.4%), and advanced clinical practice (70.9%). In the area of advanced clinical practice, the four areas representing greatest enrollment are medical-surgical (30.9%), maternal-child (28.2%), psychiatric mental health (10%), and community nursing.[12]

The first program to award a doctoral degree in nursing was Teachers College, Columbia University, New York, New York. This program was designed to prepare nursing educators and was based upon the EdD model. The second doctoral degree program in nursing was New York University's nursing science program that awarded the PhD. Like the program at Teachers College, the degree was also modeled on the PhD from the College of Education. In 1960, the first doctoral program with a practice discipline focus was developed at Boston University.[18] Graduates of these programs were awarded the DNSc.[14] In 1960, nurses choosing to attend doctoral programs in nursing had only four choices; by 1992, the number of programs had grown to fifty-four.[1]

Graduate nursing education grew rapidly during the next three decades. This growth occurred at both the master's and doctoral levels. In addition, the opportunities for specialization multiplied, and a variety of degrees were chosen to be awarded for completion of the various programs. In 1988, 22,259 students were pursuing graduate nursing degrees, 20,182 master's, with the remaining 2,077 in doctoral nursing programs.[18]

TYPES OF DEGREES

The proliferation of graduate degrees has created less confusion at the master's level than at the doctoral. Whether the master's degree is a master of science in nursing (MSN), master of science (MS), master in nursing (MN), or master of arts (MA) is a practical matter. At this level, it is commonly understood and accepted that the end result is preparation for practice whether it be administration, education, or advanced clinical practice.

Degrees at the doctoral level are usually classified within two categories, academic and professional. Academic degrees are generally designed to prepare the individual for knowledge development. The professional degree is awarded following a program designed for the preparation of practitioners. According to Marriner-Tomey,[10] nurses had the following options for doctoral education in the 1960s:

(1) The EdD, the professional degree in education, which was the degree most commonly held by the few nurses with doctorates at that time; (2) the PhD in a cognate discipline, which was encouraged by the Nurse-Scientist Graduate Training Program; (3) a professional degree exclusively for nursing [DNS, DNSc, DSN]; and (4) the PhD in nursing.[10]

As a matter of choice, the majority of nurses completing doctoral degrees emerged from one of these programs well into the 1970s. Since that time, the number of doctoral nursing programs has increased and presently numbers 50.[12] For the nurse in the nineties, the same options exist. In some instances, the choice of the degree for a nursing doctorate rests more on the choices open to nursing faculty on individual campuses than on the actual differences in the curriculum plan for the various programs leading to a nursing doctorate. Because of the necessity for advanced clinical knowledge and the attention of nursing faculty to research skills, nursing doctoral programs are largely indistinguishable from each other by doctoral degree awarded.

The preparation of researchers in any discipline takes place at the doctoral level, and the doctor of philosophy degree is recognized as the "mark of highest achievement in preparation for active scholarship and research" by the Council of Graduate Schools in the United States:

The doctoral program is designed to prepare a student for a lifetime of intellectual inquiry that manifests itself in creative scholarship and research, often leading to careers in social, governmental, business, and industrial organizations as well as the more traditional careers in university and college teaching.[6]

CONTINUING YOUR EDUCATION: WHY GRADUATE SCHOOL?

Professional practice implies a commitment to lifelong learning. With the rapid growth of knowledge and the predicted almost-instant obsolescence of knowledge, continuation in a career demands continued updating and development of new skills and knowledge. This can be done either through formal degree granting institutions or informal continuing education. The choice is not whether one continues to learn but rather by what method one chooses to learn.

There are many career advantages to acquiring advanced degrees through formal education programs for those committed to a career. Nursing has developed a professional model of practice that, in many instances, requires a master's degree in nursing for attainment of positions such as head nurse or advancement via a career ladder. Holding the formal credential provides access to advanced positions, increased salary, key positions on institutional committees, and increased status in the organization.

Most often the people who advance in professional organizations are those who hold advanced degrees. Attending a formal advanced degree program puts one in touch with potential leaders in nursing, i.e., classmates who can form a close personal and professional network and who, in later years, are in a position to assist in career development. Additionally, formal degree-granting programs bring the student in contact with mature professionals who are committed to the advancement of bright and eager graduate students. Most likely, it is in the master's program that the student acquires the skill for formal presentation and scholarly writing so necessary for overall career success.[15]

Perhaps the best reason for returning to graduate school is personal fulfillment and professional commitment. When one is motivated to acquire an advanced degree only to qualify for a job, the goal becomes paramount often to the exclusion of enjoying the journey. The student with limited motivation often fails to become immersed in a field of study, its literature, and the scholarly inquiry process. For these persons, the goals of graduate education become a series of checkoffs—products produced and designated hurdles jumped—rather than the acquisition of knowledge for professional enhancement and personal fulfillment. The learning that occurs from being a participant in the academic community under these circumstances is lost.

Many educators in practice disciplines support the position that a period of time as an active practitioner is needed to internalize the theories and skills learned so that practice and clinical decision making become automatic.[2] In the past, nurses seeking degrees have tended to complete doctoral programs at a later age as compared to women completing doctorates in other fields.

Potential candidates often arrive at the decision to commit to graduate study when they feel capable of handling the challenges of their present position and begin to experience a sense of stagnation. Potential applicants verbalize this sense of frustration and boredom with statements such as the following examples:

- I have learned all I can in this job.
- The mold is beginning to grow.
- Is this all there is?

Formal educational programs offer the opportunity and challenge for personal and professional development needed for those committed to career growth.

CHOOSING A PROGRAM

Many variables need to be considered when making a commitment to a program of graduate studies. The most critical factor is to have formulated a clear idea of one's individual career goals. One cannot prepare for all areas or roles in nursing in a single program. The danger in choosing too broad a field of study is that one may end up being unemployable because one lacks expertise in a particular area. This pitfall is seen more commonly at the master's level.

Once a definable career goal is in mind, then the next step is identifying graduate programs that offer the chosen area of study. These programs must be accessible, given individual constraints such as personal responsibilities, finances, family responsibilities, distance, and the need for job continuance. One's previous academic record and general academic ability should also be considered.

When shopping for the ideal graduate program, there are nine factors that should be considered. Indi-

---

ASSESSING ESSENTIAL ELEMENTS IN GRADUATE NURSING EDUCATION

1. Accreditation status
2. National standing
3. Admission requirements
4. Faculty qualifications
5. Institutional climate
6. Resources
7. Clinical facilities
8. Assistantships
9. Program requirements

---

vidual needs and interests will serve to modify and refine this list; however, every potential student should address each of the items shown in the box above.

One of the first elements to be determined when selecting a quality graduate program is the program's accreditation status. Brochures and catalogs should list National League for Nursing Accreditation and regional accreditation status. Speciality accreditation, such as that granted by the American College of Nurse Midwifery for graduate nurse-midwifery programs, is a prerequisite for writing for certification upon graduation.

Another dimension to be considered is the national standing of the school and the university. Those schools that hold national prominence generally have attained that standing through demonstration of outstanding facilities, faculty qualifications and scholarship, the presence of outstanding students, and a cadre of alumni with nationally recognized achievements. Information about the national standing of schools of nursing can be found in the Gorman Report, although some individuals have questioned its authenticity. Recent nursing research studies have also addressed the relative status of schools of nursing.[4,17]

Admission standards not only tell you whether or not you are likely to be accepted or rejected; they also provide information about the type of classmates you are likely to have. Potential applicants should pay particular attention to such aspects as the minimum grade point average and the minimum scores required on the Graduate Record Examination.

Underlying the belief system of graduate education, especially at the doctoral level, is the premise that the student has the opportunity to be guided or mentored by an active scholar. Thus, nonproductive faculty whose only qualification is a doctoral degree and a completed dissertation do not meet the qualification for teaching at the graduate level. A graduate faculty composed primarily of junior faculty members is not likely to meet the needs of doctoral students for a rich academic climate.

An aggregate of senior faculty with a recognized record of scholarly productivity is essential if doctoral students are to realize their full potential.[11] Unfortunately for some, career potential may well be limited as a result of lack of attention to this factor when selecting a program.

One determines the caliber of faculty available by first inspecting the catalog to establish a sufficient number of faculty with appropriate credentials. Many schools of nursing also publish lists of faculty research interest and expertise. Additionally, the more recent National League of Nursing (NLN) self-study report provides detailed information about faculty experience and scholarly accomplishments. For schools where the NLN accreditation may be several years old, this source may be outdated. In that case, an author search would provide insight into the faculty's commitment to and productivity in the area of scholarship.

The student who has previously identified an area of study should determine whether or not faculty with similar interests and the requisite expertise are available to direct student research. This is particularly important at the doctoral level.

To assess the climate that prevails in an individual institution, the best source of information is other students or alumni. Key questions should include:

1. Are relationships characterized by supervisor/subordinate roles or by patterns of mentoring?
2. Are opportunities available for students to work with faculty on research projects?
3. How accessible are faculty for advisement?
4. To what extent are faculty involved in classroom teaching versus the use of research assistants and guest lecturers?
5. Does the right to challenge existing opinions exist without fear of retribution?

Adequacy of institutional resources to support the program of study is best demonstrated by the presence of statistical consultation, computer services, facilities to support presentation, i.e., instructional aids development, and the availability of student study space and lounges. A simple walk through the library to assess the nursing and related holdings is advisable.

An environment rich in clinical facilities provides the learning laboratory for master's programs whose purpose is the education of the advanced practitioner. At the doctoral level, opportunities to access populations for clinical research can be essential to the development of the dissertation and the identification of a career-long focus for research. While contractual arrangements offer many successful affiliations, the availability of the university hospital and associated clinical services generally provides opportunities and advantages not always found in patient-care oriented institutions. For example, a primary mission of the university hospital is the conduct of research. Faculty and students in associated health professional schools are involved in research and can serve to facilitate, and often times collaborate, on nursing student and faculty projects.

When assistantships are available, it is advisable to explore the responsibilities and opportunities the position provides before making a commitment. Generally, assistantships are available in two areas—teaching and research. Graduate teaching assistantships usually require a designated number of hours of classroom or clinical teaching, primarily in undergraduate programs. Research assistant responsibilities may vary according to both institutional policy and the needs and preferences of individual faculty to whom the assignment is made. Traditionally, these positions are considered opportunities for the development of abilities not normally available in classroom work. Unfortunately, in some instances, faculty take advantage of teaching and research assistants, and students find that, instead of enjoying a unique opportunity to acquire additional skills outside of the formal program, they are merely used as gofers in the system. If holding a teaching or research assistantship is required to financially support one's education or desire for personal growth, then it is advisable to assess the nature of these positions within the school of nursing before agreeing to serve.

The last element to be considered when selecting a graduate program is the program requirements. At the master's level, the number of hours required, the existence of a thesis option, and requirements for comprehensives are key factors often considered. Potential candidates are wise to validate time requirements and curriculum organization along with the flexibility of practicum requirements before enrolling. Of paramount importance is determining the average length of time it takes full-time and part-time students to complete the program requirements. For example, some programs are advertised as a year in length for full-time study, but in actuality few are able to complete them in one year.

At the doctoral level, special attention should be given to determining the number of hours required for the degree and whether or not hours earned at the master's level can be counted. The qualifying process should also be explained to determine the nature of comprehensives within the graduate school. Other requirements to determine include demonstrated competencies in computers, statistics, and foreign languages. Just as with the master's level, the prospective student is advised to investigate the usual length of time it takes to complete program requirements.

PERSONAL CONSIDERATIONS

Depending upon preference, other factors to be considered include the availability of social and cultural events and student organizations in keeping with student university life. While these opportunities are of differing importance to more mature students, return for graduate education provides the opportunity for further leadership development and expands the growth achieved through earlier education in the liberal arts. Involvement in graduate student organizations and on university committees provides additional experience in leadership roles that are the foundation of career development.

Other factors that many students must consider when choosing a graduate program are a match between family and employment responsibilities, the scheduling of classes, and commuting requirements. Increasingly, students returning for master's degrees and doctorates require flexible programs that allow part-time study and evening or back-to-back classes. For students who must retain employment, ease in scheduling is essential.

FUTURE DIRECTIONS IN GRADUATE NURSING EDUCATION

Opportunities for different specializations at the master's level and innovative dual double degrees, such as the MBA-PhD, are now available. More than 10 universities have developed joint master's in business and in nursing (MBA-MSN) graduate degree programs. Start-up funding for many of these programs was provided by The Commonwealth Fund.[13] Numerous programs across the country have developed RN to master's pro-

grams to facilitate graduate studies for bright returning nurses educated in diploma and associate degree programs in earlier times.[5] As market demands for specialization change, innovative programs, such as the University of Maryland's master's degree in nursing informatics, which features a multidisciplinary approach, have been developed. Upgrading of credentials required by ANA and speciality organizations, such as American College of Nurse Midwifery and the American Association of Nurse Anesthetists, are moving preparation for these roles into the mainstream of graduate nursing education. For example, effective December 1991, ANA requires the master's degree for certification as a nurse practitioner.

Other specializations at the graduate level can be anticipated as graduate education in nursing moves away from the medical model to a nursing model. Conceivably in the future, concentrations will be developed in areas such as specialization in pain and incontinence management. For example, in the area of incontinence, the cost to the country in health care dollars runs into millions and is the single most important factor that prompts institutionalization of the elderly person. Incontinence and the restoration to normal functioning is nursing's domain. As the population ages, clearly this area of specialization is likely to be in increased demand.

In response to major policy statements regarding health care in the twenty-first century (the Healthy People 2000 Agenda, ANA Statement on Health Care Reform, and Pew Commission Report), graduate nursing education is challenged to place a greater emphasis on preparation for primary care. This emphasis will no doubt address underserved populations throughout the country. It is anticipated that federal and foundational support for nurse practitioners, nurse-midwives, and nurse anesthetists will grow in response to this need.

With the advent of prospective payment and the move by third-party payers to ensure cost effectiveness, the role of case manager has emerged. The nurse is more appropriately prepared to handle the comprehensive nature of this role than social workers or physicians. The ranks of staff nurses are being depleted by employment in the insurance companies and industries to manage patients' holdings, disability claims, and patients with chronic health care problems. Graduate nursing education has not responded to the need to clearly define and prepare nurses for this advanced role. Within the next few years, it can be anticipated that role development in case management will take its place alongside clinical specialization, administration, and education.

Doctoral education in nursing can also be expected to change. The past few years has witnessed an increased emphasis on the PhD degree in nursing to meet market demands for faculty who can achieve promotion and tenure in research universities. More and more advertisements appearing in *The Chronicle of Higher Education* call for candidates holding the PhD in nursing. It seems likely this preference will continue. Additionally, the increasing complexity in the health care environment will require innovation in programming to meet the need for nurse executives prepared to manage multifocused health care corporations. One such program is the University of Pennsylvania/Wharton School of Business PhD/MBA program.

Research priorities at the National Center for Nursing Research have recently focused on the need for more nurses with research preparation in the biological and biomolecular sciences. The aging population, AIDS, and rising patient acuity levels are examples of the need to refocus on the biophysical aspects of patient care. In the future, it can be anticipated that funding opportunities will be increased for doctoral and postdoctoral study to support this agenda.

It is anticipated that as the acuity of care merges with advanced technology, there will be a need for the preparation of a clinician researcher who will be capable of dealing with clinical problems in the highly complex health care setting. Because of the emerging preference for the PhD, it is anticipated that this preparation will also award the PhD.

SUMMARY

The critical matter of choosing a graduate program has emerged as the most important career decision a nurse who is committed to lifelong work in the field can make. Graduate studies represent huge investments of time, energy, and money. As with other major investments made in life, the wise professional should assess carefully the human resources and the climate the school has to offer before making a commitment. A program of studies is greater than the curriculum outlined in the catalog. It also includes the learning that occurs in the relationship between student and teacher and activities occurring in the environment. The quality and standards of excellence vary among graduate programs. The wise professional will gather data and base a decision on the fit between professional and personal needs and the many parameters of the school chosen.

REFERENCES

1. Bednash, G. D., Berlin, L. E., & Alsheimer, D. (1993). *1992-1993 enrollment and graduations in baccalaureate and graduate programs in nursing* (Publication No. 92-93-1). Washington, D.C.: American Association of Colleges of Nursing.
2. Benner, P. (1984). *From novice to expert: Excellence and power in clinical nursing practice.* Menlo Park, Calif: Addison-Wesley.
3. Brown, J. M. (1979). *History of master's education in nursing in the United States, 1945-1969.* New York: Teachers College, Columbia University.
4. Chamings, P. A. (1984). Ranking the nursing schools. *Nursing Outlook, 32*(5), 238-239.
5. Conway-Welch, C. (1990). Vanderbilt University School of Nursing's "bridge" to the future. In M. A. Wandelt & B. J. Thomas (Eds.), *Innovations in nursing education administration* (pp. 81-82). New York: National League for Nursing.
6. Council of Graduate Schools of United States. (1977). *The doctor of philosophy degree.* (ERIC Document No. ED 153 546). Washington, D.C.: Council of Graduate Schools.
7. Downs, F. S. (1978). Doctoral education in nursing: Future directions. *Nursing Outlook, 26*(1), 56-61.
8. Edlund, B. J., & Hodges, L. C. (1983). Preparing and using the clinical nurse specialist: Shared responsibility. *Nursing Clinics of North America, 18*(3) 499-507.
9. Kelley, E., Morris, G. W., & Duffy, M. E. (1990). Returning to school: Guide for the RN consumer. *Imprint, 36*(5) 43,45,47.
10. Marriner-Tomey, A. (1990) Historical development of doctoral programs from the Middle Ages to nursing education today. *Nursing and Health Care, 11*(3) 132-137.
11. Murphy, R. F. (1990). Motivation of postgraduate students: Transatlantic comparisons. *Biochemical Society Transactions, 18*(2) 160-161.
12. National League for Nursing. (1991). *Nursing datasource 1991, volume III. Leaders in the making: Graduate education in nursing* (Pub. No. 19-2422). New York: Author.
13. News, notes, and tips. (1990, May/June). *Nurse Educator, 35,* 39.
14. Parietti, E. (1979). *Development of doctoral education for nurses: A historical survey.* New York: Teachers College, Columbia University.
15. Poteet, G. W., Edlund, B. J., & Hodges, L. C. (1987). Consider this . . . Support scholarship in the health care system. *Journal of Nursing Administration, 17*(9), 4, 8.
16. Report on enrollment and graduations in baccalaureate and graduate programs in nursing, 1983-1988.
17. Wandelt, M. A., Duffy, M. E., & Pollock, S. E. (1985). *Profile of a top-ranked school of nursing* (Pub. No. 41-1990). New York: National League for Nursing.
18. Werley, H. H., & Leske, J. S. (1988). Pinning down the tracks to doctoral degrees. *Nursing and Health Care, 9*(5), 238-243.

CHAPTER 26

The changing face of graduate education

SHAKÉ KETEFIAN, RICHARD W. REDMAN

Rapid change characterizes society today. Reform of the health care system has emerged at the forefront of public discourse and in recent political elections as a pressing domestic issue. The health professions both lead and follow changes in health care delivery. Rapid social and technologic change also presents challenges in the education of health professionals, especially in the graduate education of nurses.

A number of trends in society and health care, summarized by participants in the Future of the Health Professions Project of the Pew Charitable Trusts,[21] influence health professional education. Among them are: the change in focus of health care from acute-care settings addressing individual needs to ambulatory settings concerned with broader populations and chronic conditions; the rising cost of health care, its impact on the economy, and its affordability; specialization in the professions while the need for primary care has become greater; the need to incorporate quality measures into the assessment of outcomes; a broader definition of health that transcends the traditional conception; changing expectations of "consumers," including patients and students; demographic trends in the population, including a rise in the number of elderly and in the number of minority groups; and expansion of knowledge.

These trends, and others unfolding with each passing day, demand a degree of unprecedented vigilance on the part of health professional schools if they are to prepare effective practitioners. In this chapter, we aim to present selected issues and challenges in graduate education in nursing, including postdoctoral study, from the perspective of current and evolving social, technologic, professional, and clinical practice needs and to suggest evolving trends.

To accomplish this aim, we begin with a historical overview of the development of graduate education in nursing. We then examine a number of critical issues in contemporary graduate nursing education at the master's, doctoral, and postdoctoral levels.

GRADUATE EDUCATION – HISTORICAL OVERVIEW

The vision of the American graduate school was to train scholars for the creation and transmission of knowledge. The master's degree has been associated with pedagogy.[22] First granted by Harvard University in 1642, it was a rigorous degree, involving three years of study beyond the bachelor's. This degree later diminished in importance. According to M. J. Pelczar, Jr., the University of Michigan is credited with reviving the master's degree. Adopted through regents' action in 1858, it involved a course of study and a thesis. This model was adopted by other institutions and variations of it obtained throughout the country. The master's degree achieved its identity, as distinct from the doctoral degree, when offerings expanded in education, and institutions began admitting women to graduate study. The majority of the master's degrees were earned by public school teachers, a situation that continued through the late 1950s.[22]

Graduate education received its impetus in 1867 by the opening of Johns Hopkins University, devoted exclusively to graduate study. The German model of education was adopted, emphasizing generation of new knowledge.[4] Following the German model, basic sciences gained ascendency in the late nineteenth century, and the scientific model became the prototype for emerging disciplines. Thus was born the American

PhD degree, which was quickly adopted by major universities; the graduate school became the producer of the American scholar. The first part of the twentieth century saw great expansion in graduate education and doctoral training. New knowledge generated gave rise to even more specialties and professional fields of study.

Rapid expansion in higher education occurred following World War II. Many returning veterans sought college and graduate degrees. Government and foundations invested heavily in university research, students, and buildings.[4] Soviet scientific and space achievements in the late 1950s gave further impetus to graduate education. New national objectives were set for scientific training, and fellowships were made available, though they tended to support doctoral rather than master's education.[22]

Graduate education in nursing

Graduate education in nursing began at Teachers College, Columbia University, in the early 1920s and was designed to prepare educators and administrators. This model remained until 1954 when Rutgers University initiated a graduate program at the master's level to educate clinical nurse specialists in psychiatric nursing.

During the 1950s and 1960s, the master's degree in nursing was viewed as a terminal degree,[14] and role preparation continued to be its focus. In the early 1970s, clinical specialist and nurse practitioner preparation emerged and continued to hold sway. By the late 1970s, role preparation made a comeback. Such pendulum swings as to program focus and the development of new specialties and degrees reflected the discipline's readiness to evolve in response to changes in society and in nursing and the need to incorporate the new knowledge that was becoming available at a rapid rate within nursing and related fields.

Forni[8] has reported 11 master's degree titles being offered by nationally accredited master's programs in 1984. In 1983, Williamson's analysis of nationally accredited programs revealed 130 combinations of available areas of study by 109 programs then accredited.[28] By 1986, Starck reported 247 different program titles/specialties being offered by 143 accredited master's programs.[27]

Doctoral education was first initiated at Teachers College, Columbia University (1933), and at New York University (1934). These programs offered the doctor of education degree. In the next 25 years, only 2 more doctoral programs were established. Since then, their growth has been exponential. At last count, 55 institutions were offering doctoral degrees. Grace[11] and Murphy[19] have described the development of doctoral programs in phases: Phase I—education *for* nurses for functional roles (inception to 1959); Phase II—education *for* nurses in a second discipline, referred to as nurse scientist training (1960-69); Phase III—education *in* and *of* nursing (1970 to present). Seven degree titles are currently offered, each claiming a distinctive purpose and goals.[16,17] The majority of the programs (72%) offer the PhD degree, which is the research doctorate and has wide acceptance and recognition in higher education.

ISSUES IN GRADUATE EDUCATION

Graduate education in all disciplines has evolved to the present day in response to several driving forces. Graduate education parallels forces such as social values, priorities in the public sector, technologic capabilities, knowledge development, maturity in the professions, and changing student demographics. These forces in turn shape curricular content, program requirements, and issues in higher education.[14]

Graduate education in nursing is no exception. The rapid social and technologic change experienced during the past 20 years in American society has interacted with the evolution of professional nursing. During this time, there has been a rapid growth in graduate nursing education. A number of issues have presented both challenges and opportunities for nursing education. While these issues vary somewhat, depending on the level of graduate education, they present themes that are common to many professional disciplines.

Issues in master's education

At the master's degree level, the issues closely reflect the rapid changes in the profession and in clinical practice. In addition, they reflect the social, cultural, and technological transformations under way in society. Out of a wide range of issues that could be examined, three critical ones have been selected to portray the types of challenges that master's education in nursing is facing today. They are meant to be illustrative, rather than comprehensive.

1. Role of master's degree. The focus of master's degree education in many disciplines has evolved over time, reflecting both the maturity of higher education in the United States and changing social forces and values. Before 1900, the master's served primarily as a scholarly degree for college teachers. Between 1900 and 1945, the master's degree began to serve multiple purposes, ranging from a terminal degree to a stepping stone to the doctorate. From 1945 to 1970, master's education underwent rapid expansion, diversification, and professionalization. Since 1970, change and innovation have been the hallmark of master's education. Rapid change in consumer demand has resulted in new formats, such as external degree programs and interdisciplinary degrees.[6]

In many academic settings, particularly the research university, master's degree education has been assigned second-class citizenship. It is viewed primarily as a screening device or stepping stone to the doctorate. In response to this designation, a study on master's education was commissioned by the Council of Graduate Schools to examine the role that master's degree education currently serves and the issues related to that role in American education. Data reveal that over 300,000 master's degrees are awarded annually in the United States, with 52% going to women and 12% to racial and ethnic minorities. Master's degrees constitute about one fourth of all academic degrees awarded. Nearly 85% are in professional fields. The overall conclusion of this study is that master's education has made a far greater impact than either doctoral or baccalaureate education in the lives of students and society. This impact is described as a "silent success" because of the major social benefits derived within various professions and across communities from master's-prepared individuals.[6]

Of particular interest in the Conrad study is the typology of master's degree programs developed from their findings. Four major types of educational programs were described; these are presented in the box on this page. Many of the issues in master's degree education in nursing parallel this typology.

One issue facing master's education is the type of educational program that will best address the pressing social and disciplinary issues that nursing faces. In graduate nursing programs, this issue is often described in terms of "research versus professional" degrees. In graduate programs where the research doctorate is offered, the issue is particularly acute. Whether one graduate program can offer two types of master's degrees, i.e., an ancillary and a career advancement or apprenticeship program, in a time of constrained resources is a dilemma that will be faced with increasing frequency. While it is clear that more than one type of master's degree is needed in nursing,

---

TYPOLOGY OF MASTER'S DEGREE PROGRAMS IN THE UNITED STATES

Ancillary program

Program is a stepping stone, screening device and subordinate to the doctoral degree; learning takes place primarily through faculty-directed scholarly training; practical work experience is tacked on to degree requirements but not cherished.

Career advancement program

Program is career-oriented training which provides terminal credential; heavy emphasis on preparing experts in a field with theory-to-practice focus.

Apprenticeship program

Program follows model used heavily in the biologic sciences with heavy emphasis on "doing" and strong foundation in theory; faculty serve as master practitioners who facilitate student apprenticeships into a profession.

Community-centered program

Program is a dialogical learning community wherein faculty and students are collegial participants; heavy emphasis on social stewardship and critically informed thoughtful action.

Adapted from: Conrad, C., Haworth, J., & Millar, S. (1993). *A silent success: Master's education in the United States.* Baltimore, Md: Johns Hopkins University Press. Used with permission.

---

it is not certain where these educational programs should be based.

Another issue deals with the rapid clinical specialization developing in nursing and the concomitant need for more apprentice-type programs where graduate students in nursing are involved with expert practitioners in clinical settings. This is an ongoing challenge for faculty, especially in university-based programs, who are pressed with the need to maintain clinical proficiency along with demands for scholarly productivity. It also raises curricular issues concerning the balance between theory versus practice content at the master's degree level.

The rapid transformations taking place in master's degree education in general and in nursing education, in particular, will continue in these times of rapid social change. It is also clear that nursing is not the only academic discipline grappling with these issues.

2. Changing consumer demand. The graduate student population in nursing has undergone tremendous change. In fact, the typical graduate student is often characterized as "nontraditional." The vast majority of nursing graduate students today are women with multiple professional and personal responsibilities. Often they are full-time employees seeking part-time graduate study in programs that are flexible and designed to fit their demanding schedules. Typically, students are not only place-bound and unable to relocate to attend graduate school but also are dependent on the income that full-time employment provides. This transformation in graduate student demography has created several concerns in graduate nursing education.

One change, generated from student demand, has been in program structure and format. Several nontraditional approaches have been attempted, including a range of models from external degree programs to off-campus, satellite, outreach formats and include a blend of on-campus, off-campus offerings. Technologic developments have enabled distance learning through video and electronic communications. Consortiums between existing programs also have been experimented with. Several successful models for these new approaches exist.[13,24]

Many concerns have been generated by these non-traditional approaches to graduate education. When educational offerings are delivered off-campus, maintenance of program quality and integrity is always an issue. Another issue is the extent to which socialization toward role behaviors and values of the profession can occur when students are not in residence and do not have regular, ongoing interactions with nursing faculty. In addition, nonresidential students often have limited access to liberal arts course offerings and the wide range of learning resources available on campus. Program resources often are strained when both residential and nonresidential programs are offered within the same unit. Finally, the need for educating students in many advanced specialty practice areas must be balanced with the opportunities for learning experiences available off-campus.

We cannot anticipate that simply increasing the flexibility in educational programs will cause these barriers for those seeking graduate education in nursing to diminish sufficiently. It is clear that these issues will continue to challenge educational institutions and their faculty.

3. Curricular content. The rapid changes in undergraduate nursing education and in clinical practice roles have resulted in many challenges to the content in master's degree programs. The tensions between generalist versus specialist content and standardization versus diversity and flexibility have resulted in a wide variation among approaches. The diversity in master's education in nursing has been well documented and suggests a lack of consensus regarding the structure of master's degree programs. The content in many programs more typically reflects faculty philosophy than consensus within the discipline. In turn, this has resulted in role confusion across practice settings.[27] The need for standardization in educational programs with a more uniform approach to preparation for advanced practice roles presents a major challenge to nursing education.

As we rapidly become a global community, program standardization becomes a challenge from another perspective. Major variation exists in the health care and educational systems in the world community,[10] and the need to consider standards beyond the United States must be dealt with as more international students seek education in American programs.

The rapid changes that undergraduate nursing programs are experiencing also produces a problem of standardization. As these programs change and include content in areas such as conceptual models of nursing practice and research methodology, there is need for adjustment in graduate curricula. In addition, these changes affect the learning requirements of graduate students who have completed their undergraduate education at different points in time and at different institutions.

In response to the rapid specialization in clinical practice, new issues have arisen about certification and regulation. Various specialties within nursing are rapidly moving to the requirement of advanced degrees for certification in a specialty. To date, certification has generally been on a voluntary basis, and within the control of the profession. The lack of standardization of curriculum content takes on a new dimension in this realm. One proposal is to consider licensure for advanced practice roles and thus regulate through governmental authority the requirements for entry into specialty practice roles.[20]

Another challenge in graduate education is related to rapid technological changes and their impact on both process and content of graduate education. Certainly, information technology continues to change the way we carry out our personal and professional responsibilities. One result, however, has been ongoing debate about how it should be incorporated into graduate learning experiences. The same challenges exist with all the enabling technologies available in the patient care environment. It presents major challenges in terms of curriculum content, faculty proficiency, and program resources.

Issues in doctoral education

At the doctoral level, the issues reflect both the evolving trends in society and the field as a whole, especially the changes in the discipline and science of nursing. It is impossible to delineate an exhaustive list of these issues. Those identified will give readers a sense of what doctoral programs and educators are grappling with, and stimulate them to further explore this area.

Conceptions of doctoral education. The broad goals of doctoral education are to prepare nurses who will: (*a*) expand the scientific knowledge base for the field through research and scholarly activities and (*b*) serve in leadership capacities in a variety of arenas within society and nursing.[7] A longstanding debate has taken place within nursing about the nature of each of the seven types of degree designations, and about which should be the standard or the ideal. On the one hand, the proponents of the professional doctorate (DNS/DNSc) have contended that, as a practice discipline, all intellectual endeavors should be connected to the practice concerns of nursing. On the other hand, the proponents of the PhD degree hold that the academic/research degree is needed to strengthen the scientific base of nursing.[16] Christman[5] has advocated even a narrower conception, focusing on a clinical doctorate; Schlotfeldt[25] and others hold that there is sufficient flexibility inherent in the nature of the PhD to accommodate various types of pursuits; while Peplau[23] has argued for the need for both professional and academic doctorates as being of value to the discipline. Many authors have reviewed and elaborated on these issues, and discussed the varying conceptions and justifications regarding doctoral preparation.[4,9,11,17,18] (A clarification is needed regarding the ND or doctor of nursing degree: this is offered by two institutions and prepares individuals for basic practice in nursing, and represents neither an advanced degree nor an investigative one.)

While these descriptions regarding differentiation of major degree types are ostensibly clear, it is the case that in practice such differentiation is not clear in program goals or in program execution. Nor is there any evidence that prospective students make a deliberate choice of program on the basis of type of degree offered. It is rather the case that the more important elements in program differentiation have to do with type of faculty expertise and their research, the nature of the substantive content being offered, and institutional support and resources available to the program, among others.

Substantive nursing knowledge. Historically, the majority of doctoral programs have focused on teaching "process" courses, such as research methods, statistics, and theory development. More recently, a distinct move is evident toward focusing on substantive courses in the discipline of nursing. This movement has received impetus as a result of the efforts of groups such as the American Association of Colleges of Nursing and the National Forum on Doctoral Education in Nursing. It has been motivated by the expansion of the research base of nursing and the number of nurses engaged in knowledge generation. There is great variation across programs in the focus of nursing knowledge and phenomena being taught and investigated and how that knowledge is organized.[15] The consensus within the field at present is to endorse this diversity of theoretical and research approaches, as it is deemed premature at this juncture to dictate a uniform approach. It is felt that such diversity makes for richness and enhances the discipline.

Scientific integrity. The recent spate of cases in the media involving various forms of scientific misconduct threatens to undermine the credibility of the scientific community at large. These cases also highlight an important oversight in the training process of scholars. Various governmental agencies have established offices and panels to deal with cases brought to their attention. In the main, this development is the result of inability or unwillingness of institutions themselves to set appropriate standards and monitor the integrity of science on their campuses.

An important ingredient of education during doctoral training is a systematic approach to dealing with issues such as fabrication and falsification of data, plagiarism, and the murkier issues related to access to data, allocation of authorship credit, what constitutes exploitation of subordinates, and the like.

Some of these are clearly ethical and integrity concerns, while others relate to norms and conventions. Disciplines vary in the way in which they socialize their scholars about these matters. At present, nursing does not have its own guidelines about research integrity. The result is a situation whereby doctoral mentors aim to socialize their own students according to the tenets of their particular discipline and according to the tenets of their own best judgment. It is typically the case that doctoral program faculties have individuals with doctorates from many disciplines, each bringing different norms and expectations on matters of scientific integrity. To rectify this rather chaotic situation, it is imperative for nursing to develop its own guidelines and set forth disciplinary norms related to scientific integrity. Research universities need to develop their own standards as well, and have monitoring mechanisms in place.

Monitoring program quality. Following extensive discussions within nursing, it is now the case that doctoral programs are not accredited by either the National League for Nursing, the specialized accrediting agency for baccalaureate and master's degree programs, or any other agency. It is the contention that such accreditation is not necessary, since quality monitoring is provided by the parent institution.[26] The American Association of Colleges of Nursing has developed quality indicators in order to provide guidance with regard to various indicators of quality and program functioning.[1] These indicators have been widely used by programs themselves; however, there are no data available at present to suggest the extent to which institutions do in fact monitor quality, whether for the PhD degree—which is typically administered under the aegis of the "graduate school"—or for the professional degrees, and what type of variations might exist across institutions in this regard.

Students. Who are the students in doctoral study and what is their composition? Currently, 9.1% of doctoral students are members of underrepresented minority groups;[2] these are broken down as follows: 4.3% Black, 2.5% Asian or Pacific Islander, 1.7% Hispanic, 0.6% American Indian or Alaskan Native.[2] The current climate in higher education unequivocally emphasizes diversity in its broader meaning. The population trends are changing, and it is expected that the proportion of previously underrepresented minority groups will be high in the twenty-first century. Efforts to recruit a diverse student body need to be stepped up by doctoral programs. With regard to the matter of intellectual diversity, it is now the case that nonnurse potential applicants are not eligible for admission into nursing doctoral programs. While many nurses hold doctoral degrees in another discipline and are making important contributions both to nursing and that discipline, nursing excludes nonnurses from becoming scholars of nursing. Inclusion of such individuals could imbue nursing with fresh perspective and enrich the field.

Faculty. The majority of doctorally prepared nurses are employed in colleges and universities as faculty and/or academic administrators, and a small percentage are engaged by health care institutions, government agencies, and other enterprises. According to AACN data, in 1978, AACN member schools reported 15% of their faculties as having doctoral preparation (944 faculty); by 1991-92, the figure had risen to 48% (3690 faculty). Despite this growth, which has paralleled the growth in doctoral programs, demand appears to be rising faster than the supply, with some schools reporting inability to locate individuals to fill vacant faculty positions.[3] Faculty salaries are not competitive with those within the service sector. This is a concern within the field; were this trend to continue, some educators fear that prospective students may not be motivated to seek doctoral degrees or will choose employment in settings other than higher education.

POSTDOCTORAL TRAINING

Postdoctoral training is relatively recent within nursing. As nursing science has developed and the number of nurse scholars has increased, efforts to develop postdoctoral opportunities for nurses and in nursing have been stepped up. Historically, small numbers of nurses have sought postdoctoral training in a variety of disciplines through individual initiative. The impetus for postdoctoral training came following the establishment of the National Center for Nursing Research (NCNR) within the National Institutes of Health in 1985 (now the National Institute of Nursing Research). The purpose of postdoctoral training is "to provide time, space, an intellectual and colleague support system, as well as a safe, risk-taking environment for becoming an independent researcher;"[12] this level of training is intended to enable nurses to "position [themselves] so that we can shape the cutting edge of science."[12]

Under the aegis of the NCNR, a career trajectory has been developed whereby scientific development is viewed as a lifetime commitment; under center programs, opportunities are provided for nurse scholars to pursue postdoctoral training at different career phases. This conception is unique in nursing and is designed to be responsive to the unique career patterns of nurses and the needs of the discipline for science development. In most disciplines, the typical pattern is for an individual to move into a postdoctoral fellowship immediately following the completion of the doctorate.

This level of study is now recommended more and more for individuals who expect to pursue research and teaching careers in research universities. At the present time only a small number of nurses pursue postdoctoral training, mostly due to limited funding opportunities. Eighteen institutions currently offer postdoctoral and/or predoctoral training under funding from the NCNR, the agency responsible for a large portion of funding for postdoctoral training. In addition, 13 postdoctoral fellows are individually funded through NCNR. Other sources of funding are also available; for example, the National Science Foundation, the Robert Wood Johnson Foundation, and the American Nurses Association Minority Fellowship Program/W. K. Kellogg Foundation provide support for postdoctoral training.

It is expected that postdoctoral training will be a more common feature in the training of nurse scholars in the years to come.

CONCLUSION

At this moment graduate education in nursing is like a kaleidoscope and is in a dynamic state of change. To what extent can graduate education in nursing be standardized? What are the tensions between standardization and flexibility? The NLN sets standards for master's education and accreditation of these programs; the AACN has quality indicators that guide doctoral programs. While quality monitoring is crucial, flexibility needs to be maintained in order to make these programs responsive to the needs of society and those of students. Nursing has been criticized for developing an ethnocentric science applicable to white, middle-class populations. Meleis[18] calls for nursing to develop a world view of phenomena so that an awareness of issues faced by minority groups and by other nations can be an integral part of its science and instruction. She recommends that this criterion become an indicator of quality of doctoral programs.

Within the past few years, a number of new specialties have developed in nursing, such as space nursing, AIDS, addictions, and the like. A constraint to be mentioned relates to the fiscal picture across the nation that has affected graduate education. Many institutions are cutting budgets and are emphasizing the concept of "innovation by substitution," rather than by addition. In the 1970s and 1980s, programs expanded offerings without much concern for cost. Now they are being challenged to be responsive to consumer demands and high quality, and be cost efficient at the same time.

At the time of this writing, there are no data about how nursing programs are dealing with the constraints imposed on them and whether the addition of a new specialty means the elimination of defunct specialties/subspecialties. This is a matter of urgent concern for educational administrators because they are accountable for balancing the budget and for delivering high-quality programs. The environment in which we find ourselves is dynamic and the challenges are many.

While it is impossible to say what graduate education will look like in the twenty-first century, one thing is certain: it will be different from what it is today. If the past is prologue, we have reason to believe that it will be stronger for the challenges and will be even more central to the health care delivery system of the twenty-first century than it is today.

REFERENCES

1. American Association of Colleges of Nursing. (1987). Indicators of quality in doctoral programs in nursing. *Journal of Professional Nursing, 3*(1), 72-74.
2. American Association of Colleges of Nursing. (1992a). *1991-1992 enrollment and graduations in baccalaureate and graduate programs in nursing* (Pub. No. 91-92-1, pp. 14-15). Washington, D.C.: Author.
3. American Association of Colleges of Nursing. (1992b, June). *AACN Issue Bulletin, 3.*
4. Brodie, B. (1986). Impact of doctoral programs on nursing education. *Journal of Professional Nursing, 2*(6), 350-357.
5. Christman, L. (1977). *Clinical doctorates—A means of increasing the clinical competence of nurses.* Unpublished manuscript.
6. Conrad, C., Haworth, J., & Millar, S. (1993). *A silent success: Master's education in the United States.* Baltimore, Md: Johns Hopkins University Press.
7. Crowley, D. M. (1977). Theoretical and pragmatic issues related to the goals of doctoral education in nursing. In *Proceedings of the first national conference on doctoral education in nursing* (pp. 25-29). Philadelphia, Pa: The University of Pennsylvania School of Nursing.
8. Forni, P. R. (1987a). Nursing's diverse master's programs: The state of the art. *Nursing and Health Care, 8*(2), 70-75.
9. Forni, P. R. (1987b). Models for doctoral programs: First professional degree or terminal degree? In S. E. Hart (Ed.), *Issues in graduate nursing education* (Pub. No. 18-2196, pp. 45-73). New York: National League for Nursing.
10. Glittenberg, J. (1987). The scope and trends of international nursing education. In J. Roode (Ed.), *Changing patterns in nursing education* (Pub. No. 14-2203, pp. 133-142). New York: National League for Nursing.
11. Grace, H. (1978). The development of doctoral education in nursing: An historical perspective. *Journal of Nursing Education, 17*(4), 17-27.
12. Hinshaw, A. S. (1991). The federal imperative in funding postdoctoral education: Indices of quality. In *Proceedings for the 1991 forum on doctoral education in nursing. Postdoctoral education in nursing science: Purpose, process, outcome* (pp. 81-108). Amelia Island, Fla: The University of Florida.

13. Holden-Lund, C. (1991). Consortium model for master's education in nursing. *Nurse Educator, 16*(5), 13-17.

14. Jolly, M. L., & Hart, S. E. (1987). Master's prepared nurses: Societal needs and educational realities. In S. E. Hart (Ed.), *Issues in graduate nursing education* (Pub. No. 18-2196, pp. 25-31). New York: National League for Nursing.

15. Ketefian, S. (1993). Moving beyond traditional boundaries: Diverse models for structuring knowledge and funding doctoral education. *Journal of Professional Nursing, 9*(5).

16. Lash, A. A. (1987a). The nature of the doctor of philosophy degree: Evolving conceptions. *Journal of Professional Nursing, 3*(2), 92-101.

17. Lash, A. A. (1987b). Rival conceptions in doctoral education in nursing and their outcomes: An update. *Journal of Nursing Education, 26*(6), 221-227.

18. Meleis, A. I. (1988). Doctoral education in nursing: Its present and its future. *Journal of Professional Nursing, 4*(6), 436-446.

19. Murphy, J. F. (1981). Doctoral education in, of, and for nursing: An historical analysis. *Nursing Outlook, 29*(11), 645-649.

20. National Council of State Boards of Nursing. (1992). Position paper on the licensure of advanced nursing practice. Revised March 5th.

21. O'Neil, E. H., & Hare, D. M. (Eds.). (1990). *Perspectives on the health professions.* Durham, N.C.: Duke University Press.

22. Pelczar, M. J., Jr. (1980). *The value and future of graduate education leading to a master's degree: A national perspective.* Washington, D.C.: American Association of Colleges of Nursing.

23. Peplau, H. E. (1966). Nursing's two routes to doctoral degrees. *Nursing Forum, 5*(2), 57-67.

24. Reilly, D. E. (1990). *Graduate professional education through outreach: A nursing case study* (Pub. No. 15-2340). New York: National League for Nursing.

25. Schlotfeldt, R. M. (1966). Doctoral study in basic disciplines—A choice for nursing. *Nursing Forum, 5*(2), 68-74.

26. Spero, J. R. (1987). Specialized accreditation of doctoral programs in nursing: To be or not to be. In S. E. Hart (Ed.), *Issues in graduate nursing education* (Pub. No. 18-2196, pp. 75-88). New York: National League for Nursing.

27. Starck, P. L. (1987). The master's-prepared nurse in the marketplace: What do master's-prepared nurses do? What should they do? In S. E. Hart (Ed.), *Issues in graduate nursing education* (Pub. No. 18-2196, pp. 3-23). New York: National League for Nursing.

28. Williamson, J. A. (1983). Master's education: A need for nomenclature. *Image: The Journal of Nursing Scholarship, 15*(4), 99-101.

CHAPTER 27

National initiatives for change

COLLEEN CONWAY-WELCH

While 1988 was considered a benchmark year for the publication of agenda for change in nursing,[7] reports and articles in the 1990s may have surpassed this agenda in terms of urgency for change in the way we prepare nurses on the master's level for advanced practice. To paraphrase an old seer—we have met the enemy and he is us.[22] Recent reports and publications add fuel to this fire. They are forcing nursing educators to examine the relevance of where they are going, who and what they are preparing, and how they are preparing them.

The Pew Foundation Report[31] suggests that "education and training of health professionals is out of step with the evolving health needs of the American people. Simultaneous improvements in the education and training of health professionals are required." Professionals of every health discipline need to understand better why people behave the way they do, particularly in distress. The Pew Report listed the following competencies needed by practitioners in the year 2005:

expand health access to effective care; provide contemporary clinical care; emphasize primary care; participate in coordinated care; ensure cost-effective and appropriate care; practice prevention; involve patients and families in the decision-making process; promote healthy lifestyles; assess and use technology appropriately; improve the health care system; manage information; understand the role of the physical environment; provide counseling on ethical issues; accommodate expanded accountability; participate in a racially and culturally diverse society and continue to learn.[31]

The report also suggested that schools must redesign their educational core regarding: "(1) the disciplines represented in the core; (2) the setting in which clinical education occurs; (3) the teaching-learning process; (4) health care teamwork; (5) curricular effectiveness; and (6) educational flexibility."[31]

The Secretary's Commission on Nursing points to the twofold nature of the solution for the cyclical nursing shortage/turnovers: to increase nurse productivity and to increase the attractiveness of a nursing career. Recommendations were developed from both demand and supply sides of the nursing shortage issue: better nurse compensation, better health care financing, improved nurse decision making, and better development, maintenance, and utilization of nursing resources.

Healthy People 2000[37] outlines the health goals for the nation for the next 10 years: to increase the average span of healthy life, to reduce disparities in health among our citizens, and to provide access to health maintenance activities for all Americans. It addresses 22 priority areas of our nation's health and establishes specific and attainable goals for each. These priorities areas cover physical activity, nutrition, tobacco use, the use of alcohol and other drugs, family planning, mental health and mental disorders, violent and abusive behavior, educational and community-based programs, unintentional injuries, occupational safety and health, food and drug safety, oral health, maternal and infant health, heart disease and stroke, cancer, diabetes and chronic disabling conditions, human immunodeficiency virus infection, sexually transmitted diseases, immunization and infectious diseases, and clinical preventive services. An even cursory review of these areas suggests the critical role that nurses—particularly nurses in advanced practice—can and must play.

Several of the recommendations of the Public Health Service Task Force on Women's Health Issues[40] focus on the need to provide services for the prevention and treatment of disease and conduct biomedical and behavioral research emphasizing conditions and diseases unique to or more prevalent in women in all age groups, particularly in the areas of acceptable contraceptive methods and debilitating, chronic diseases.

"Nursing's Agenda for Health Care Reform" was developed by the American Nurses Association (ANA), the National League for Nursing (NLN), and 40 other nursing organizations representing almost 1 million nurses to propose a nursing perspective on the health care debate.[2] It calls for a basic "core" of essential health care services to be available to everyone and restructures the health care system to deliver services to consumers in convenient sites such as schools, workplaces, and homes. It also calls for a shift from the predominant focus on illness and cure to an orientation toward wellness and care. Nursing's plan represents a fundamental shift in focus to the need to decrease costly hospital stays and unnecessary procedures while placing a stronger emphasis on prevention, primary care, and long-term care. In addition, the plan suggests that "incentives be put in place to select nurse-managed care centers in the community to provide basic health services to groups such as mothers and infants, businesses seeking lower health costs, and children in schools."[30] There are approximately 250 nursing centers in operation nationwide.

The 1990 Report to Congress on the Study of the Need for Nurse Advanced Trained Specialties, by the Health Resources and Services Administration, documented that, in 1990, 84 schools of nursing offered nurse practitioner programs. "Increasing interest in nurse practitioners, nurse anesthetists and nurse-midwives is evidenced by the growing demand for these cost-effective and patient-focused primary care givers and by the federal government's ongoing research in the area."[39]

The National Center for Nursing Research State-of-the-Science Invitational Conference in 1991 identified new roles for nurses in advanced practice, including infection control, risk management, quality assurance, information systems, and case management.

The report of Lewis–ICS and the National Committee for Quality Healthcare, titled "Tracking the System: American Healthcare 1992,"[23] explored four indices that measured the demographic, technological, and economic demands placed on our healthcare system and provided fertile ground for demonstrating the need for nurses in advanced practice. The facilities and personnel index shows a steady growth and demand for health care personnel of all types and an expansion of the need for nursing homes and ambulatory facilities. The utilization index illustrates the focus of patient care shifting from in-patient to the out-patient sector, a trend driven by the new medical technology, changing physician patterns, and increased hospital efficiency. The demographics/environment index shows that the increase in demand due to the aging of the population may be offset by the expansion of managed care and other cost-saving activities. The population/outcomes index suggests that there may have been some improvement in health outcomes including reduced infant mortality and heart disease, but these were offset by the increase in AIDS deaths and no change in life expectancy.

STIMULUS FOR CHANGE WITHIN GRADUATE NURSING EDUCATION

The acute care health system, built on rescuing people from an unpredictable disease process, will be replaced by a system focused on early intervention and chronic disease processes as disease becomes more predictable. "Changes in the next 50 years will demolish what remains of the acute-care system and force our health insurance system and society to confront the increased predictability of disease risk. This revolution will be fueled by developments in pharmaceuticals, genetics, and immunology. The traditional approach of diagnosis and treatment will be replaced by the prediction and early management of illness."[15] The emphasis of the health care delivery system will shift from curing to caring and focus on personal, community, and environmental health. The development of outcome measures will lead to improved therapies.[13]

The NLN *Nursing Data Source*[29] reports that 231 master's programs and 50 doctoral programs in nursing were in operation in 1990-91. However, government projections estimate significant shortfalls in the supply of RNs with advanced degrees.[32] This is coupled with an impending faculty shortage caused by the increased demand for RNs with advanced degrees in "nonacademic" settings, such as research, administration, and advanced practice.

The American Association of Colleges of Nursing's draft *Position Statement on Differentiated Practice*[1] defines differentiated practice as practice based on education, experience, and demonstrated competence. The draft also emphasizes the need for students to acquire mastery at collaboration, independent decision making, and evaluation of health care.

The Sample Survey of Registered Nurses, conducted by the Division of Nursing, Bureau of Health Professions, Department of Health and Human Services, and most recently performed in 1988, reports that 40% of the 2 million nurses in the United States hold diplomas as their highest earned credential.[36] Associate degrees and baccalaureate degrees account for 25% each. Under 5% of RNs have earned master's degrees in nursing, and an additional 2% have obtained master's in other disciplines. Fewer than one half of 1% hold doctorates in nursing or a related field. Approximately 124,000 nurses held master's degrees in 1988, and almost half were employed in hospitals. The majority of master's-educated RNs were prepared to hold positions characterized as advanced clinical practice (52%). Another 24% are educators and 20% are in administrative positions.[36] This gives one pause for thought in that our clinical specialties focus on practice to the virtual exclusion of administration, process variation, and team-building and delegation skills, yet these skills are essential to success in the clinical area.

The biomedical perspective of health care is forcing us to change our focus from requiring patients to become ill before receiving attention to assisting patients in remaining healthy and to be knowledgeable about major societal conditions that lead to disease such as poverty, homelessness, pollution, poor nutrition, and chemical abuse:

A different approach is needed to meet the needs of a vulnerable population suffering from chronic health problems. This must emphasize continuity of care and shift the locus of care to the community. . . . The highly bureaucratic, specialized, territorial, fragmented, and rigid model for acute care has long dominated the nursing curriculum.[12]

A curriculum revolution in nursing began in 1986 and is continuing to gather momentum. The 1987 National Conference on Nursing Education was devoted to "Curriculum Revolution: A Mandate for Change" and led to additional national conferences and meetings to focus on major themes and values of the revolution. "There is a growing sense of malfunction in the continued use of a behavioral model of education for nursing.[35] This model led to a slavish generation of objectives to meet predetermined behavioral goals with the expectation that all students will meet all objectives."[12]

The major themes of the revolution that must be integrated into nursing curricula at every level are:

1. Our social responsibility to transform the health care delivery system because health promotion depends very little on access to care but rather on healthier living conditions
2. Our commitment to caring that allows the nurse or teacher to understand and act on the broader concerns and issues of patients or students
3. Our need to unveil, understand, and criticize beliefs and assumptions that guide practice and teaching
4. Our rejection of the behavioral model (rational-technology model or Tyler model) or reductionism
5. Our renewal of the primacy of the teacher-student relationship and student-student relationship as interactional and transactional where the relationship *is* the curriculum and learning occurs through meaningful dialogue[14,35]

EMERGING MODELS

Our challenge in graduate education is to create a teaching environment focused on transforming existing power relationships rather than replicating learning relationships based on dominance-submission models.[5,25,26,43] Our student-teacher partnership must be flexible and knowledgeable about individual differences in learning styles.

I have documented earlier my concern that nursing education must abandon the BSN in favor of an AD/MSN (or ND) model similar to all other health disciplines. The information summarized in this paper underlines the obvious fact that the professional nurse of tomorrow will need a strong liberal arts background to manage the knowledge base needed for practice.[7]

The NLN *Nursing Data Source Vol. 1: Trends in Contemporary Nursing Education*[30] validates the influx of older students, the increase in the number of part-time students, and the increase in academic and cultural diversity. "Their rich diversity includes differing life experiences and values. A singular manner of organizing learning experiences can no longer effectively serve the complex demands of [these] students."[12] The median age of a 1990 graduate was 31, compared to 1982s age of 25; 21% of our students are part time, and Hodgkinson[18] prophesied that, by the turn of the century, one third of the American population would be minority. His predictions are rapidly becoming reality.

Some schools of nursing are adjusting their master's programs to respond to this older, goal-oriented student who is pursuing a second degree and comes with either an undergraduate degree in another discipline or the equivalent of three years of liberal arts/sciences courses. The schools recognized by the NLN as having point-of-entry master's programs for these students are Vanderbilt University, University of Texas at Austin, University of Tennessee at Knoxville, Case Western Reserve, Massachusetts General Hospital Institute of

Health Professions, Yale University, University of San Francisco, and Syracuse University.

Hill[16] asked 47 Indiana nurse administrators and educators to make predictions and provide judgments about content both critical to survival in practice and best learned at the master's level. She organized their recommendations into a 42-semester credit program covering the four areas of care, options, specialty, and practicum. "Care" included seven 3-credit-hour courses—counseling, legal and government issues, personnel, leadership, ethical decision making, research, and statistics. "Options" included two 3-credit-hour courses selected from staff development, economics, organizational behavior, communication, and wellness/preventive care. The "specialty" included two 5-credit-hour courses, including nursing theory and gerontological nursing. The practical courses included 6 credit hours. While the study was small, it suggests that there are several content areas critical to survival that most of our master's programs do not address in their clinical majors. The acquisition of these skills will cause us to look at knowledge for practice in dramatically different ways.

We are also seeing several trends in graduate nursing programs suggesting that some nurse educators are forging ahead in the curriculum revolution to the incorporation of the "continuous improvement" process, joint degrees with other disciplines, and a merging of the nurse practitioner and clinical nurse specialist roles into one role of advanced practice.

CONTINUOUS IMPROVEMENT

The gaps in our discipline-focused educational efforts on the master's level are nowhere more evident than in the lack of content relative to total quality management (TQM), total quality improvement (TQI), and continuous improvement (CI) efforts that are sweeping our agencies under the rubric of work restructuring. Today's graduates are virtually clueless as to what this will mean to their practice and how they will need to incorporate this nondiscipline-specific knowledge into their activities.

The pioneers of quality improvement—Shewhart,[33] Crosby,[8] Juran,[19,20] Deming,[9,10,11] and Wadsworth, Stephens, and Godfrey,[41] among others—left a "rich heritage of theory and technique by which to analyze and improve complex production processes."[4]

The paradigm of delivery of traditional nursing care and traditional nursing education has changed to pro-

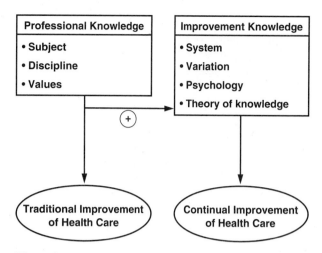

Fig. 27-1. Underlying knowledge. *(Reprinted from Batalden, P. B., & Nolan, T. W. [1994]. Knowledge for the leadership of continued improvement in health care. The AUPHA Manual of Health Services Management [p. 71]. Reprinted with permission of Aspen Publishers Inc. © 1994.)*

ducing products (services and graduates) that meet patient/customer expectations, provide true value for the money, and do not require the system to engage in rework.[44] As nurses become familiar with TQM/TQI as customer-driven, value-added, process-focused and statistically, analytically measured through quality improvement tools, they will become more and more interested in basing curricula strategies and design on "continuous improvement" theory where "as the discipline-specific knowledge domain for nursing has continued to grow, the curricula has become filled to capacity. We need to step back and look at a different set of knowledge needed for tomorrow's nurse."[44]

The underlying knowledge we need as nurses has changed. The traditional focus of professional knowledge (on subjects, discipline, and values) led to improvement in health care but has left us with an expensive biobehavioral model that requires people to become ill before the treatment/reward system kicks in. An improved and new core of knowledge must be added to traditional knowledge to build a health care delivery system for tomorrow (see Fig. 27-1). Those new knowledges that are linked and will improve the effectiveness of our actions are: (1) Knowledge of systems as interlinked processes, each with its five elements of (*a*) suppliers who provide, (*b*) inputs on which an (*c*) action produces (*d*) outputs for (*e*) customers. For example:

Process: Design an exam.
Supplier: Nurse faculty.
Inputs: Content taught.
Action: Questions generated.
Output: Exam.
Customer: Student.

Knowledge of the system allows sharpening of vision and mission and suggests a set of measures that show an improvement. (2) Knowledge of variation—"a statistical, analytical way of thinking that sees variation as a natural part of every process and that, to understand the variation and be able to take appropriate action, should be measured over time."[10,42] (3) Knowledge of psychology and intrinsic motivation to improve. (4) New theory of knowledge regarding implementation which allows us to "predict and gather data by developing knowledge about variation, make an improvement, and collect information to know the effect of the change and the new level and variability of output that the process has achieved."[3] Viewing work in terms of a system can assist people to better understand how their efforts are part of a greater whole and makes them aware of their suppliers and customers.

DUAL DEGREES

The Commonwealth Fund's report on the nursing shortage[6] discusses changes in medical practices and changes in patient demographics. It includes the professional beliefs of leaders of organized nursing, who have advocated for a better-educated nurse workforce to provide adequate patient care in light of the growing needs and complexity of medical technology and the rising acuity of hospitalized patients. A few members of this educated workforce will increasingly be prepared in two disciplines. Even a few years ago, if a nurse acquired a nonnursing graduate degree, she was in danger of "being drummed out of the corps." The board of directors of the Commonwealth Fund, concerned that nurse executives lacked the language of business and were, therefore, merely observers at the policy table, initiated a courageous program—the Nurse Executive Fellowship Program—to support master's-prepared nurses pursuing an MBA. Several years later, they "seeded" 10 universities to develop joint master's in nursing/master's in business administration programs. Today, there are more than 35 joint master's in nursing/master's in business administration programs in major universities.

ADVANCED PRACTICE ROLES

The roles of the nurse practitioner (NP) and the clinical nurse specialist (CNS) are merging. The American Nurses Association recently combined its two separate councils into one Council for Advanced Nursing Practice. With so much patient care moving out of acute-care settings and into the community, NPs need many acute care skills; while CNSs are redefining and broadening their role in the hospital and need the NP assessment skills.

Language and lines blur. We now have neonatal critical care nurse practitioners and adult acute care nurse practitioners. The challenge to educators is to review, refine, and distill educational content, avoid the temptation to keep adding more, and distill the essential elements of critical thinking, delegation, business, and quality improvement skills into the education of the nurse prepared on the master's level for advanced practice.

REFERENCES

1. American Association of Colleges of Nursing. (1992). *AACN position statement on differentiated practice* (draft). Washington, D.C.: Author.
2. American Nurses Association & National League for Nursing. (1991). *Nursing's agenda for health care reform*. Washington, D.C.: American Nurses Association.
3. Bataldon, P., & Buchanan. (1989). Industrial models of quality improvement. In N. Goldfield & D. Nash (Eds.), *Providing quality care: The challenge to clinicians* (pp. 133-155). Philadelphia: American College of Physicians.
4. Berwick, D. (1989). Continuous improvement as an ideal in health care. *New England Journal of Medicine, 320*(1), 53-56.
5. Bevis, E., & Watson, J. (1989). *Toward a caring curriculum. A new pedagogy for nursing*. New York: National League for Nursing.
6. Commonwealth Fund. (1989). *What to do about the nursing shortage?* New York: Author.
7. Conway-Welch, C. (1990). Emerging models of post-baccalaureate nursing education. In J. McCloskey and H. Grace (Eds.), *Current issues in nursing* (3rd ed., pp. 137-141). St Louis: Mosby.
8. Crosby, P. B. (1979). *Quality is free: The art of making quality certain*. New York: McGraw-Hill.
9. Deming, E. (1982). *Quality, productivity, and competitive position*. Cambridge, Mass: Massachusetts Institute of Technology, Center for Advanced Engineering Study.
10. Deming, W. E. (1986). *Out of the crisis*. Cambridge, Mass: Massachusetts Institute of Technology, Center for Advanced Engineering Study.
11. Deming, W. E. (1992). TQM/TQI in business and healthcare: an overview. *American Association of Occupational Health Nursing Journal, 40*(7), 319-325.
12. de Tornyay, R. (1990). The curriculum revolution. *Journal of Nursing Education, 29*(7), 292-294.

13. Dezold, C. (1992). Five futures. *Healthcare Forum Journal, 35* (3), 29-42.
14. Diekelmann, N., Allen, D., & Tanner, C. (1989). *The National League for Nursing criteria for appraisal of baccalaureate programs: A critical hermeneutical analysis.* New York: National League for Nursing.
15. Goldsmith, J. (1992). The reshaping of health care. *Healthcare Forum Journal, 35*(3), 19-27.
16. Hill, B. (1989). Development of a master's degree program based on perceived future practice needs. *Journal of Nursing Education, 28*(7), 307-313.
17. Hodgkinson, H. L. (1931). *Economic control of quality of a manufactured product.* New York: D. Van Nostrand.
18. Hodgkinson, H. L. (1985). *All one system: Demographics of education, kindergarten through graduate school.* Washington, D.C.: Institute for Educational Leadership, Inc.
19. Juran, J. M. (1964). *Managerial breakthrough.* New York: McGraw-Hill.
20. Juran, J. M., Gryna, F. M., Jr., & Bingham, R. S. (Eds.). (1979). *Quality control handbook.* New York: McGraw-Hill.
21. Kacker, R. N. (1985). Off-line quality control parameter design and the Taguchi method. *Journal of Quality Technology, 17,* 176-88.
22. Kelley, W. (1977). Pogo comic strip.
23. Lewis-ICS and the National Committee for Quality Healthcare. (1992). *Tracking the system: American healthcare.* Washington, D.C.: National Committee for Quality Healthcare.
24. Meyer, J., Silow, C., & Sullivan, S. (1990). Critical choices: Confronting the cost of American health care. *A report to the National Committee for Quality Healthcare.* Washington, D.C.: U.S. Government Printing Office.
25. Moccia, P. (1989). Curriculum revolution: Integrating the voices of revolution. *Curriculum revolution: Reconceptualizing nursing education.* New York: National League for Nursing.
26. Moccia, P. (1990). No sire, it's a revolution. *Journal of Nursing Education, 29*(7), 307-311.
27. Moccia, P. (1992). A nurse in every school. *Nursing and Health Care, 13*(1), 14-18.
28. National Center for Nursing Research. (1988). *State of the Science Invitational Conference: Nursing resources and the delivery of patient care* (NIH Pub. No. 89-3008). Washington, D.C.: U.S. Department of Health and Human Services.
29. National League for Nursing Division of Research. (1992). *Nursing data source 1991. Volume 3: Leaders in the making: Graduate education in nursing.* New York: Author.
30. National League for Nursing. (1992). *NLN Division of Research, nursing data source 1992. Vol. 1: Trends in contemporary nursing education.* New York: Author.
31. Pew Foundation. (1991). *Healthy America: Practitioners for 2005, an agenda for action for U.S. health professional schools.* Philadelphia: The Pew Health Professions Commission.
32. *Seventh Report to the President and Congress on the status of health personnel in the United States.* (1990, March). Washington, D.C.: U.S. Department of Health and Human Services.
33. Shewhart, W. A. (1925). The application of statistics as an aid in maintaining quality of a manufactured product. *Journal of American Statistical Association, 20,* 546-8.
34. Sullivan, Louis. (1990). Sounding board: Healthy People 2000. *New England Journal of Medicine, 223*(15), 1065-1067.
35. Tanner, C. (1990). Reflections of the curriculum revolution. *Journal of Nursing Education, 29*(7), 295-299.
36. U.S. Department of Health and Human Services. (1988). *Secretary's Commission on Nursing* (Volumes I & II). Washington, D.C.: Author.
37. U.S. Department of Health and Human Services. (1990). *Healthy people 2000: National health promotion and disease prevention objectives.* Washington, D.C.: Author.
38. U.S. Department of Health and Human Services. (1992). *The national primary care conference: Executive summary.* (March 29-31). Washington, D.C.: Author.
39. U.S. Health Resources and Services Administration, Public Health Service. (1990). *Report to Congress on the study of the need for nurse advanced trained specialties.* Washington, D.C.: Author.
40. United States Public Health Service. (1991). *Action plan for women's health.* Washington, D.C.: Office of Women's Health.
41. Wadsworth, H. M., Stephens, K. S., & Godfrey, A. B. (1986). *Modern methods for quality control and improvement.* New York: John Wiley.
42. Walton, M. (1986). *The Deming Management Method* (pp. 40-51). New York: Doss, Mead & Co.
43. Wheeler, C., & Chinn, P. (1989). *Peace and power: A handbook of feminist process* (2nd ed.). New York: National League for Nursing.
44. Widtfeldt, J., & Widtfeldt, J. (1992). Total quality management in American industry. *American Association of Occupational Health Nursing Journal, 70*(7), 311-318.

CHAPTER 28

Development of models of international exchange to upgrade nursing education

MARY V. FENTON

WHY INTERNATIONAL EXCHANGE?

Although international exchange has occurred between schools of nursing for many years, it is now becoming a reality for many schools and colleges that would not have considered it 5 or 10 years ago. The rapid changes in our world are not only facilitating more international exchange but almost demanding it. Barriers have fallen, borders have changed almost overnight, and many countries, including the United States, are placing a greater priority on nursing as an underutilized health care resource. Because of more international conferences and the availability of international travel, nurses from all over the world are meeting colleagues in other countries and, even more important, discovering that nursing speaks a common language regardless of the country, native language, or culture. This has led to an increase in interest in learning about other countries' health care systems and nursing education programs. In addition, many of the foreign nursing students who came to the United States for nursing master's and doctorate degrees in the 1970s and 1980s have returned to their countries to provide nursing leadership. Therefore, in developing an exchange program with a foreign university or ministry of health, it is usually possible to find a nurse administrator or faculty member who has studied in the United States through whom an initial contact can be made.

However, there are more pressing reasons for international exchange in nursing education today. First, the increase in immigration and travel has greatly increased the ethnic diversity of our population, and U.S. nurses are providing care for patients with a wide variety of customs, beliefs, and health practices. This diversity often leads to frustration and values conflicts, so there is a tremendous need for students and nurses to have the kinds of multicultural experiences that can be provided through international exchange programs. Second, the last decade alone has brought about an explosion of knowledge in the biomedical sciences, resulting in an ever-expanding system based on delivery of high-tech health care. Because of this, today's nursing students face a far more complex environment requiring advanced high-tech clinical skills. Third, while the high-tech explosion has emerged in many countries, a tremendous need still exists to provide primary health care. In many countries, both developing and developed, people do not have access to basic health care, including disease prevention and health promotion. International exchange can directly address this problem by making possible the sharing of models and concepts for the development and implementation of community-based primary health programs.

Access to basic health care has become a major issue at both the consumer level and the political level. For example, the United States no longer ranks at the top for common health statistics, such as infant mortality. In 1918 with an infant mortality rate (IMR) of 77 per 1000 live births, the United States ranked 6th in the world for the lowest death rates. By 1991, the IMR had been reduced to 9.1 per 1000—a vast improvement but a rate that now places the United States 24th internationally. This may be more of a reflection of our increased ability to save sick babies than to produce healthier ones.[5] The overall IMR, too, is misleading for if specific ethnic minorities are studied—for example, blacks—the infant mortality rate is 18.6 compared to 8.1 for whites.[6] These statistics become even more significant if we accept Assistant Secretary for Health Dr. James Mason's assertion that "a nation's infant mortality rate is a measure of its success in combating poverty, ignorance, and disease."[5]

Dr. Mason's assertion raises the question of why the United States, with its vast resources and health care expenditures, has health indices worse than many developing countries. One answer can be found by looking at the deteriorating infrastructure of our health care system. For the past 10 to 15 years, many basic public health disease prevention and health promotion programs have been cut at the federal, state, and local levels and literally made unavailable to much of the population. This policy was carried out in the United States at the same time that many developing countries were developing programs that focused less on high tech and more on the provision of basic primary health care to the population. These programs had to be cost-effective because of the lack of available resources. Therefore, you will find developing countries with immunization rates for children that exceed those of the United States. For example, in the United States vaccination rates for children ages 1 to 4 for measles, rubella, DTP, polio, and mumps range from 58.9% through 64.9%, though technically speaking 90% of all children "have access" to immunization. And even with higher rates of immunization, reported cases of measles alone have more than doubled since 1970.[6] In rural areas in Texas, the state health department estimates that 20% of all preschoolers have received no immunizations whatsoever.[2]

With its emphasis on acute and high-tech care, the United States has been slow to adopt the World Health Organization's goal of "Health for All by the year 2000" through primary health care, and it only recently has become part of discussions among health care providers, educators, and policy makers. The United States has gone from being the world model for public health policy and structure in the early and mid-twentieth century to one of "disarray" that must be redefined and restructured if we are to assume that a healthy population will move into the twenty-first century. A focus on primary health care is critical to addressing problems here in the United States and worldwide. Alternative models of health care with appropriate technology are needed to demonstrate that in many situations more can be done with less.

THE ROLE OF NURSING AND HIGHER EDUCATION

With the U.S. system of health care no longer affordable or accessible to large segments of the population, nurses functioning in both traditional and advanced practice roles are being utilized in more and more diverse ways. They cost less than physicians and can perform a wider range of responsibilities appropriate to meet primary care needs. Thus, nurses prepared for advanced clinical nursing roles are in higher demand than ever before, and many past legal barriers to advanced nursing practice are disappearing, primarily for economic reasons. The situation is right for nurses to move toward more active participation in shaping a system that will be effective in meeting the needs of the population. This fact, however, is not a sufficient base for a "newer, better, more efficient" system. Serious deficiencies and the focus of our delivery system are difficult issues for a country that has always considered its health care system as the "biggest and best."

Since the end of World War II, world politics and health care have undergone a radical transformation, and the late 1980s and early 1990s will perhaps go down in history as a time when the world did not ask for change, but demanded it. And, as might be expected, one of the most difficult aspects of rapid evolution is general confusion as to which direction to go and who should lead. As early as 1983, Earl Backman asserted in *Approaches to International Education* that if Americans are to be able to understand and cope with the changing environment, "the higher education community should—in fact, must—take the lead in developing international education programs."[1] However, in the United States as elsewhere, funding is scarce for development and sustenance of such programs, and the bulk of the burden for development and implementation of programs will fall directly upon institutional leaders and participating faculty.[1] If we are going to utilize some of the successful experiences of our colleagues in other countries in developing cost-effective and accessible systems of health care to restructure our own system, we will need to research, evaluate, present, and publish these ideas and systems in order to promote change. Higher education institutions, including schools of nursing, are logical choices.

In summary, as we near the century mark, we have as a nation reached a crisis in health care, and the lack of access to care has become one of our country's primary focuses. Having fallen behind in meeting many basic health needs of the population, we are increasingly forced to look internationally for health care models. Nurses have a vital role to play in primary health care in both developing and developed countries. The time has come to address international exchange as a viable method of increasing our ability to meet the needs of our population and to educate nurses prepared to deal with life and nursing practice in the future.

DEVELOPMENT OF MODELS OF INTERNATIONAL EXCHANGE

There is a wide range of models of international exchange in schools of nursing today, ranging from individual, informal contacts by faculty to more highly formalized models with university agreements and contracts spelling out specific objectives and missions. Activities may include faculty exchange and/or consultation, project and research collaboration on common problems, joint publication, sharing of ideas and resources, student exchange, and sharing of courses, materials, and resources.

Many concerns are encountered in the development and implementation of an international educational exchange program. Some key questions include: How does a school of nursing committed to development of an international educational exchange program identify resources for funding and planning and use them most efficiently? How can the use of scarce resources for international exchange be justified? Is it possible to work within the existing academic system? How do faculty and students become involved and committed to such a program? Should the program stand alone in the nursing school or be integrated into the overall university program, if one exists? How should institutional goals and objectives be designed? How could a program be designed to meet the needs of the institution, faculty, administration, and students?[1] In addition to these general questions, schools of nursing have additional concerns: First, it is a time of diminishing budget support for higher education and a time of competition for available funds. Finding funding is often difficult and may require creative financing ideas. Second, the nursing discipline requires complex licensing and registration procedures in order for graduates to practice; therefore, to bring foreign students and visitors to the United States to gain educational and clinical experience often requires special policies that either show compliance with local licensing requirements through demonstration of equivalence or waive local requirements under proper conditions.

To deal with the concerns expressed above, great commitment on the part of faculty and nursing school deans is required. Numerous models have been developed and implemented for international exchange in schools of nursing with various degrees of success. The most important concept is that the model be feasible, for no two institutions or schools will or should have identical programs, if only because no two institutions can or will have the same needs or population. Some schools have been able to integrate international health concepts into their general international programs and other activities; others have treated them as a separate entity.

International faculty exchange

An international faculty exchange program between schools of nursing is a two-way street. Although the transfer of high-tech acute-care knowledge may be seen as flowing primarily one way from the United States, the transfer of knowledge about using less invasive, less expensive, and less intense methods may be primarily in the opposite direction. It is often surprising to U.S. nurses to discover that many less technology-based methods get equivalent results when compared with outcomes of health care in the United States. Therefore, visits and discussions with colleagues from other countries often stimulate thinking about more creative and less expensive ways to provide health care.

Often faculty return from an international consulting visit and begin to ask more questions about our current health care system. At the same time, they often become more politically astute about the role of women in society and the role of nursing in health care, coming to the realization that until those inequities are addressed, "Health for All" will probably only remain a slogan and unattainable goal. Faculty are exposed to a wealth of information relating to health such as the World Health Organization publications and, by incorporating this information into their curriculum, are able to create a more common language for working with schools in other countries. Because of the more centralized governmental-controlled system of health care in countries other than the United States, nurses from other countries have been more exposed to the World Health Organization's goals, policies, and information than U.S. nurses.

U.S. faculty also come face-to-face with the influence that U.S. nursing has had on nursing education abroad. Because the United States has been seen as the leader in nursing education, many countries have adopted U.S. curriculum models. If you ask to see their curriculum, you will be handed, in some situations, a model U.S. curriculum that may or may not have relevance for nursing in that country. One also may see either outdated or even brand new equipment and technology sitting in rooms with no one trained to use it, or no repair or parts available, or, in the case of computers, no software to run on it or no printer. The problems of exporting inappropriate technology without knowing the setting or needs of the country or situation become evident. As a result, faculty begin to question the appropriateness of their own curriculum and teaching methodologies not only for the United States, but for other countries as well.

One example of this is the export of U.S. nursing theory as the basis for conceptualization of nursing school curricula and research. In most cases, U.S. nursing theorists did not expect their theories to be used as the basis for developing curricula. However, during the 1970s and early 1980s many schools of nursing in the United States adopted developing nursing theories as the basis for their curricula. This use of theory sometimes resulted in disjointed, awkward, and confusing curriculum design. When international graduate students and visiting faculty returned from U.S. schools to their countries, they attempted to use the theories, often with similar results. The result was that in many cases the curriculum stayed on the shelf and was only shown to visiting dignitaries, and the old curriculum continued to be taught.

International students

Educational exchanges must be carefully planned. The first step after committing to develop an international exchange program is to assess the needs of the student, faculty, the school, and the institution and to identify the available resources. In 1992, more than 407,000 foreign students were enrolled in U.S. schools, the largest foreign population in the world.[4] Many of these students are sponsored by their governments or home institutions in the hope that the education they gain will provide them with the professional, social, and personal skills required to play meaningful leadership roles in their societies. Many of these programs are successful, but when they are not, it is often because of students' difficulty in adaptation to U.S. culture.[3]

Providing an international exchange program for students can range from accepting foreign students into the program, to taking and accepting students on exchange visits either for short or long term, to arranging for preceptorships for students in other countries. All of these experiences will broaden and enrich the knowledge and understanding of students. For example, in collaboration with faculty from the University of Nuevo Leon School of Nursing in Monterrey, Mexico, the University of Texas Medical Branch School of Nursing conducted a community health elective for undergraduate students in Mexico. The program consisted of intensive preparation classes, including information on culture, customs, and simple Spanish phrases, before leaving the United States and then classes and community health clinical experiences with faculty and students from Nuevo Leon.

The majority of students who took the elective were RN-BSN students, most of whom had considerable nursing experience in the United States. For many of them it was an experience in culture shock but also a turning point in their careers. They came home convinced they could do a better job of providing health care even with fewer resources. They also had a better appreciation of the origins and experiences of many of their patients from Mexico and the border areas of Texas. They were proud of their ability to cope with all the situations they encountered although, at the time, they were not sure they would be able to. If you ask them today what was one of the most significant learning experiences they had while earning their BSN, they would all say their elective in Mexico. The fact is that even though faculty may try to create experiences to challenge students and to make them critically evaluate our health care system, an international experience makes that happen.

An international exchange program brings a nursing school faculty and students face-to-face with the policies of the U.S. government. For many faculty and students, it is often the first time they have been exposed to any viewpoint other than that of the United States. In many cases the experience is positive, but in other situations it may be negative. It often results in the development of more political awareness and interest in the U.S. role in world politics. For example, faculty and students have become aware of U.S. policy that does not discourage U.S. companies who are aggressively developing new markets for cigarettes in developing countries with the principal targets being young people and women. This has happened concurrently with the outlawing of most cigarette advertising in the United States and more stringent control over secondhand smoke. A second example is U.S. policy that allows the exportation of pesticides banned in the United States because of their harmful effects on the people and environment. Awareness of such policies can raise faculty and students' awareness of the connection between politics, economics, and health care policy in their own community and state.

Funding of international exchange

Over the past 30 years, many state and private universities have implemented international education programs with the assistance of the federal government and private foundations, such as Carnegie, Kellogg, Rockefeller, and, before 1970, the Ford Foundation.[1] The emphasis on international affairs in the 1940s resulted in the development of international assistance programs in the early 1950s, particularly through the Federal Operations Administration, which awarded contracts to several large universities to develop and implement programs. After 1960, the United States Agency for International Development continued this unique role.

However, many successful international programs are not the result of large grants from private foundations and U.S. governmental agencies. Many programs are supported on an individual project-by-project plan by the schools themselves. For example, a successful short-term faculty exchange program can be conducted by simple agreements between the two schools involved. In many situations, the institution sending the faculty member continues to pay the salary and also for airfare and travel expenses while the host school provides housing and transportation. The faculty member is responsible for paying for food and incidentals. This does not put a great drain on either institution to find large amounts of new money and yet can result in a very successful exchange.

Longer-term exchange programs may require the assistance of private foundations and government agencies. Another way to fund a successful program is to write grants jointly to fund programs that benefit both schools. This can be especially effective when U.S. schools can provide technical and writing assistance for international schools applying to U.S. foundations.

SUMMARY

The effect of international exchange on schools of nursing both in the United States and in other countries is just beginning to be realized. International exchange programs have exposed students and faculty to other cultures' beliefs and health care models. They are having a major impact on developing a more culturally sensitive approach to health care around the world. Although in the beginning there was more of a one-way exchange, this is beginning to change as we become more exposed to different ways of providing health care developed in other countries and as we learn to do more with less. International exchange is contributing to the development of more relevant nursing curricula and research as we search for better ways to meet the health care needs of our societies. It also contributes to better educated nurses who are more willing to participate in the development of health policy for their communities, states, and countries due to their increased awareness of the effect of policy on health care. International exchanges also result in better understanding of the differences and similarities of nursing around the world and, most important, build confidence that nurses can make a significant impact on the health of the people.

REFERENCES

1. Backman, E. L. (Ed.). (1984). *Approaches to international education.* New York: American Council on Education/Macmillan.
2. Crider, R. (1992). Texas immunization levels rank below Third World. *Rural Health Reporter, 6.*
3. Lee, M. Y., Abd-Ella, M., & Burks, L. A. (1981). In S. C. Dunnett (Ed.), *Needs of foreign students from developing nations at U.S. colleges and universities.* Washington D.C.: National Association for Foreign Students Affairs.
4. Institute of International Education. (1992). *Open doors, 1990-91.* New York: Author.
5. Mason, J. O. (1991). Today's challenges to the public health service and to the nation. *Public Health Reports, 106*(5), 473-477.
6. National Center for Health Statistics. (1992). *Prevention profile. Health, United States, 1991.* Hyattsville, Md: U.S. Public Health Service.

PART FOUR

CHANGING PRACTICE

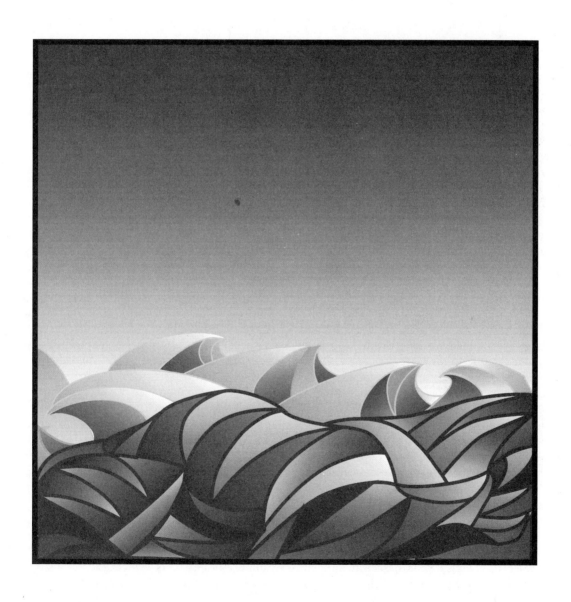

Change creates opportunities

JOANNE COMI McCLOSKEY, HELEN KENNEDY GRACE

The practice of nursing is challenged by the dramatic changes occurring in health care. Pressures to reduce the costs of care result in patients being kept out of acute-care hospitals to a later stage in illness. Patients who are hospitalized are more acutely ill, and their treatment involves a high level of technological care that requires counterbalancing by "high touch" on the part of nursing staff. With patients being discharged into the community at an earlier point in their illnesses, families are increasingly providing care for family members in home settings. Fragmentation of services and funding sources creates demands for coordination if individuals and their families are to receive adequate and accessible health care services. The health care delivery system is experimenting with new modes of delivery to speed up services and reduce costs. The challenge to nursing in the face of many changes is to bring coherence to a chaotic and fragmented system. This requires a greater degree of autonomy and leadership than has been customary in the recent past of nursing practice. At the same time, it requires the ability to work as part of a collaborative team. This section discusses some of the dilemmas of nursing practice as viewed from various perspectives.

The debate chapter addresses an important and growing concern—the increasing use of unlicensed assistants. In 1991, the American Nurses Association (ANA) created a task force to study the issue and make recommendations. Dietz discusses the ongoing work of the task force and the progress made to date. Just coming to some agreement on definition of terms for this emotionally laden, complex issue has been difficult. The task force has come up with four helpful decision criteria that can be used to judge whether something should be delegated. The criteria relate to the complexity of the task, the repetitiveness of the task, the condition of the patient, and the requirements of the environment. Dietz presents arguments for and against use of unlicensed assistants in four areas: practice, training, utilization, and regulation. Nurses are using many kinds of assistants, but issues related to control and training are problematic. Dietz makes it clear that nursing needs to come to terms with the issues involved with using unlicensed personnel, and soon—before others make decisions for us. Our decisions need to be made carefully because they may lead to the creation of yet another level of nurse provider.

Increased use of assistants and many other changes are evident in hospitals. Noting the effects of changed reimbursement systems on the composition of the patient population in hospitals, Joel succinctly describes nursing in today's hospitals. Enumerating the differences made by skillful nursing in the clinical management of acutely ill patients, particularly the elderly, Joel notes that "hospitals were blind to the inherent value of nursing as they first began to consider approaches to cost-effectiveness." The change in payment systems has increased the importance of nurses in moving patients in and out of hospitals quickly. The ability to move patients through the system quickly is largely contingent on the capabilities of nurses to provide expert clinical care. Joel says that the large numbers of unlicensed assistive personnel now used in hospitals have resulted in unsafe staff-mix ratios. Assistive personnel, she says, should never be assigned directly to the patient, but to the nurse. She outlines the vicious cycle in nursing: A shortage results in higher nursing salaries; higher salaries prompt a more efficient use of nurses and use of assistants, which leads to a surplus; salary gains are slowed until nurses are cheap again and another shortage created. The future for nursing in hospitals, she says, may include admitting privileges for nurses and full practice partnerships *if* we are prepared to take advantage of emerging opportunities.

The next two chapters address changes in the community. First, Farley addresses needed change in the community. She says that when health care agencies, such as hospitals, place their outreach programs in the community, they are not really creating community centers. They are expanding themselves and are not willing to share their power. Instead of these programs, what is needed, she says, are real partnerships with communities where decision making is shared and the community is empowered. An example of a real community partnership is the Rural Elderly Enhancement Program (REEP) in Alabama. The goal of the project is to develop community leadership so that project staff are no longer needed. The structure and activities of REEP are explained and a case study is used to illustrate how the partnership between health professionals and citizens can make a difference in patient care. Farley also discusses several factors critical to success and gives many helpful tips based on her experience. To be successful in communities, nurses must form partnerships with citizens and share power and decision making.

Next, Salmon continues the discussion of the critical leadership role of nurses in community health. Leadership interventions are needed in the following domains: (1) social—for example, in shifting the focus away from the treatment of disease to health promotion and disease prevention; (2) medical, technological, and organizational, ensuring that adequate care is provided by a system driven by financial concerns; (3) environmental, in light of needs for an adequate knowledge base and for interdisciplinary, collaborative approaches to addressing environmental concerns; and (4) human and biological challenges, such as those posed by AIDS and the potential of genetic engineering. The chapter addresses multiple challenges, including the changed family structure, the effective use of appropriate technology, and environmental pollution. Community health nurses need to play leadership roles in addressing these and other issues, requiring vision, conviction, the courage to act, and the willingness to work with others.

The next two chapters shift to a focus on particular specialty areas within nursing: nurse-midwifery and long-term care nursing. Ernst notes that although nurse-midwives have demonstrated an ability to deliver low-cost, high-quality health services, nurse-midwifery has never really taken hold in the United States, as reflected by problems in maternity care. The momentum of the natural childbirth movement has created a

void in maternity services that poses a particular challenge for nurse-midwifery. Producing adequate numbers of appropriately prepared nurse-midwives is one problem. A second problem is that of constraint of practice and the malpractice insurance crisis. Birth centers are seen as an essential component of low-cost, high-quality maternity care, and as they develop, they provide opportunities for expanded practice and also serve as training sites for future nurse-midwives. Noting that it took half a century to move maternity care into hospitals, Ernst projects that the third-party reimbursement system will be the force that moves maternity care out of hospitals and into birthing centers. During this time of change and opportunity, she challenges nursing to take responsibility for developing ambulatory maternity care services.

Turning to the other end of the age continuum, Strumpf and Kaufmann argue for greater attention to the health care needs of the elderly. The chapter demonstrates three things: that reforms in long-term care are urgently needed, that nursing is a potentially powerful force in the care of older people, and that the aging of America is an opportunity for nursing as a profession to demonstrate value. After presenting demographic data regarding the aging U.S. population, the authors outline the problems of long-term care. The United States will soon be home to one of the oldest populations in the world. Temporary and inadequate funding, funding from multiple sources, and the focus on funding for illness care rather than for a spectrum of services all contribute to fragmentation of care for the elderly. Nursing has a vital role to play in improving care for the elderly. Important reforms include making gerontological nursing a viable and desirable career choice, increasing the emphasis on long-term care in the educational process, conducting research on the contributions of nursing to an improved quality of life for the elderly, and improving care in nursing homes.

A strategy to improve care and decrease costs that crosses setting boundaries and is useful to many populations is managed care. In her chapter, Zander urges nurses to be more collaborative in their development and use of the tools of managed care. She sounds the warning bell that nurses who are too controlling of critical paths and case management policies may encounter resentment from the larger system. Nurses, she says, must enter the multidisciplinary arena with more than lip service. The nurse who is in charge of implementing case management in an agency must make "allegiance to nursing secondary to the goal of cost/quality outcomes for patients." Zander gives many concrete examples and strategies that will facilitate the design of true collaborative practice. Nurses, she says, must not assume that physicians will not participate and must not assume the role of policeman/woman for physician practice. She stresses repeatedly that no one owns case management—it is *not* another *nursing* model. Critical paths need a common language, but to get to a common interdisciplinary language, nurses need to be able to articulate their own practice. Zander's chapter points out the complexities and high-level skills needed for interdisciplinary collaboration.

One high-level skill is decision making. Nurses who are working collaboratively with other providers and are meeting the expectations of today's practice environment also desire control over their own work schedules. As a result, many clinical settings have introduced the use of flextime and self-scheduling. Wulff says that these strategies meet the needs of an increasingly diverse workforce. Flextime is a system of scheduling work that allows each employee to select a starting and quitting time. This is a difficult challenge in most nursing situations where patients require continuous coverage. Self-scheduling is the process whereby nursing staff on a unit decide and implement the monthly work schedule. Each of these practices has been adopted in attempts to increase nurses' job satisfaction and reduce turnover. Each has benefits and difficulties discussed thoroughly by Wulff. In particular, self-scheduling is not easy to implement and requires time, communication, and interpersonal skills for discussion and negotiation. Anyone interested in trying these management practices in her or his work environment will find this a helpful chapter.

The many changes in practice are also changing the nature of the care plan. The current controversy about the nursing care plan stems from the Joint Commission on Accreditation of Healthcare Organizations' (JCAHO) 1991 change in standards. The requirement for an individualized plan was deleted in the Accreditation Manual and replaced with a requirement for demonstrating planned care "consistent with the therapies of other disciplines." Tucker gives an overview of the nature of the traditional nursing care plan, the JCAHO requirements relating to patient care since 1946, and health care agencies responses to the requirements. Care plan books and computer software programs have been used to reduce the time of writing care plans. The current JCAHO standard encourages interdisciplinary planning, and timeline care plans or critical paths are increasingly being used to demonstrate this process. Tucker concludes that the traditional nursing plan as "a provider-driven, single-discipline tool is moribund." The new care plan, she says, is flexible and multidisciplinary and includes the patient as a partner.

While practice has seen many recent changes, more are coming. According to Simpson, the most significant change in nursing practice in the next decade will result from the computer-based patient record. Simpson outlines the history, from the narrowly focused electronic medical record, to the automated patient chart, to the electronic medical record, and now to the computer-based patient record. He says that the ambitious goal set by the Institute of Medicine to have the computer-based patient record by the year 2000 will require close collaboration between nurses and vendors. He takes nurses to task for their pervasive distrust of vendors. He points out that the presence of inadequate nursing information systems is more the fault of nurses who buy these systems than the vendors who sell them. Simpson outlines the many changes he predicts will happen at the bedside and in the nursing profession as a result of the computer-based patient record. Simpson urges nursing leaders to get involved and to make sure that nursing has an active and central part in the implementation of the computer-based patient record.

The international chapter in this section discusses primary health care in developing countries. Robertson says that the concept of primary health care has many interpretations and at least three models of implementation. She says that effective primary health care requires a paradigm shift away from the "biological-health-provider-knows-best" approach to the empowerment of communities to handle their own health problems. Health care workers need to develop partnerships with the community and to be accountable to the communities they work in. In South Africa and elsewhere, members of the community are being trained as health workers, but they need education, support, and help from health care workers to be successful. A proliferation of community health workers has caused fragmentation in care and conflicting messages. Unfortunately, nurses delivering primary care in South Africa have received mixed reviews from community members. Robertson explores the reasons for this and discusses the skills nurses need to be effective community change agents. She challenges academic institutions to develop curricular models that will both prepare primary health providers and undertake the needed research. While the focus of the chapter is on primary health care in developing countries, the chapter's content and message are relevant to nurses everywhere.

As the chapters in this section demonstrate, nursing practice is challenged to keep up with many health care system changes. As we attempt to streamline our care to save unnecessary steps and cost, we must also continue to provide enough time to attend to the people tasks. The change in health care attitudes and practice are creating enormous opportunities for nurses and nursing if we have the leadership skills and the courage to act.

CHAPTER 29

Debate

Should nurses use assistants?

ELIZABETH O. DIETZ

Few nursing issues spark as heated debate as the employment of unlicensed assistive personnel (UAP) in providing nursing care. Lines are immediately drawn between administrative nurses and the general bedside staff nurses. In many instances, it is like a pitched battle with nurses fighting nurses. Administrative nurses are continually trying to simultaneously provide better patient care with less resources. Staff nurses are often ill-prepared to function within the changing nursing care delivery system and the transition from primary nursing to team nursing. These staff nurses are being asked to care for more patients at a higher acuity level and provide the care with less professional support. Patients are caught in the middle, trying to obtain the best possible care with even less knowledge of the new system than they had of the traditional one.

At first glance, the title of this chapter seems an easy question to answer. After all, we all subscribe to the tenets of primary nursing that registered nurses can do and will do all of the care themselves. However, do we all subscribe to the nursing delivery system of primary nursing? Are we sure that we can do it all, and do we really believe that we want to do all of the nursing care ourselves?

Recent statistics from the American Nurses Association (ANA) indicate that most of us were educated during the period of nursing when "team nursing" was appropriate. Why are we having questions now? Why can we not accept help and why do we even wonder if we should or should not use assistants?

In 1991, the ANA created the Task Force for Unlicensed Assistive Personnel (TFUAP) to look at this very question. The task force has not answered the question yet but is still gathering data to help the membership of the ANA assess the issues. What seemed like a simple choice of yes or no is not. The issue has grown and evolved into a maze in which we are lost and unable to see the big picture from above.

Nursing is also not aware of the extent of the usage of unlicensed assistive personnel. In a national study, Blegen, Gardner, and McCloskey[2] found that 80% of registered nurses in acute-care institutions and 98% of registered nurses working in long-term care are involved in some capacity with the assignment/delegations and supervision of UAPs in the delivery of their nursing care.

As we contemplate and research this issue, we further refine our definition of the problem, look at the issues, and try to clarify our terms. However, the deciphering of semantics to distinguish among these terms, such as *nursing assistant, nursing aide,* or *assistant to the nurse,* fosters as much confusion as the topic itself. What are the necessary categories, terms, and definitions? What is the extent of the problem? Is it even a nursing problem? What can we, or should we do about assistive personnel? As ANA and other organizations began to look at the issues, they quickly realized that there is no agreement on terms or issues.

Nurses do not see clear lines of demarcation but a mosaic of intertwining issues and more questions. No one agrees on the definitions of terms for assistive personnel. State boards of nursing and state nurses' associations (SNAs) do not agree upon definitions of terms or titles. The North Dakota Nurses Association looked at the very same question of assistive personnel in health care and determined there were over 250 titles of assistive personnel.[4] A further review of the state nurse practice acts yields numerous lists of titles for unlicensed assistive personnel that may or may not be under the supervision and direction of registered nurses.

The task force created by ANA to study the unlicensed assistive personnel was to comprehensively look at the subject and its diverse issues. The task force was created as an outgrowth of concern about lack of empowerment by nurses in some areas of the country and in some nursing specialties. Other reasons for the creation of the task force was the perception that there was encroachment into nursing practice by other professions. There was also a concern that there is a realignment and reassignment of registered nurses with unlicensed assistive personnel and other mixes of personnel in some agencies and specialties to the detriment of the registered nurse staffing.

The task force did not work in isolation and used the first meeting to speak with representatives of five major nursing groups. These representatives come to the task force from the Nursing Organization Liaison Forum (NOLF), American Organization of Nurse Executives, American Association of Critical Care Nurses, Emergency Nurses Association, and the American Association of Operating Room Nurses. They believe that together they can achieve a better outcome. During the prior year (1991-1992), there were five face to face meetings and numerous conference calls to work on this subject. After many months of deliberation, definitions and two position statements were drafted (see the box on page 214).

To ensure a global professional consensus, the ANA task force, during its first year, communicated extensively with 53 state and territorial nurses associations and other nursing organizations. The task force developed and implemented two state nurse association surveys regarding specific states' positions on the utilization of unlicensed assistive personnel and their organizations' views and definitions of regulations of unlicensed assistive personnel. At the same time, the state nurse practice acts were reviewed and analyzed by the nursing practice lawyer within the ANA to inject the legal perspective of the key definitions of nursing, delegation, supervision, and assignment. Legal interpretations were also elicited from other leading nurse attorneys.

The specific results during this first year have been a compilation of ANA and other state nurses association policy statements. Now there is a generally agreed-upon list of definitions, but not all states support one set of definitions. For example, the definitions of assignment and delegation are reversed in the California Nurse Practice Act. California defines delegation as RN to RN while assignment is from RN to UAP. The ANA definition has delegation as RN to UAP and assignment as RN to RN. Two position statements have been created and disseminated on (a) registered nurse utilization of unlicensed assistive personnel, and (b) registered nurse education relating to the utilization of unlicensed assistive personnel. A state nurses' association advisory concerning the pros and cons of UAP regulation has been disseminated. Finally, a listing of questions and answers on the topic has also been printed.[1]

The decisions to use unlicensed assistive personnel or not use them should not be on a blanket yes or no basis, but rather on four factors. First, is the complete nursing process or are the more complex portions of the nursing process to be utilized? If the task is simple and the needs of the nursing process are data gathering or assessment, a unlicensed assistive personnel might be an appropriate delegate. If complex, multiple dimensions or complex areas of nursing process are needed, then the assistive personnel are not a choice to be utilized at that time.

Second, is the task or service involved of a repetitive nature? If so, an unlicensed assistive person might be useful in completing the task.

Third, what is the patient's condition and has the task or procedure already been performed on the patient by a licensed provider? If the task has been performed once and the patient is stable, then the UAP might be the appropriate person to perform the task. If the task is complex, multidimensional, and it is the patient's first time for the task, then a UAP might not be appropriate.

Fourth, does the environment specifically mandate a particular level of task implementation; e.g., ICU, CCU, ER? Here again, the UAP might not be the appropriate person. If there are no environmental mandates, then the UAP might be the appropriate person to deliver the patient care.

The statements that a UAP might be appropriate or might not be appropriate are very vague and indefinite, and this lack of clarity has caused poor communication and distrust between and among nurses and administrators.

Regardless of setting or acuity level of the patients, the UAP is not the appropriate person to be delivering complex patient teaching, intubation, complex portions of the nursing process, and all areas of intravenous therapy.

A decision to use a UAP should be made based on the following criteria:

AMERICAN NURSES ASSOCIATION DEFINITIONS RELATED TO ANA POSITION STATEMENTS ON UNLICENSED ASSISTIVE PERSONNEL 1992

The ANA Task Force on Unlicensed Assistive Personnel developed the following definitions to clarify the ANA position statements on the role of the registered nurse working with unlicensed assistive personnel. These definitions reflect a review of current regulatory, legal, practice, and professional terminology and are intended to be used only in the context of these position statements.

1. Unlicensed assistive personnel (UAP)

An unlicensed individual who is trained to function in an assistive role to the licensed registered nurse in the provision of patient/client care activities as delegated by the nurse. The term includes, but is not limited to, nurses aides, orderlies, assistants, attendants, or technicians.

2. Technician

A technician is a skilled worker who has specialized training or education in a specific area, preferably with a technological interface. If the role provides direct care or supports the provision of direct care (Monitor tech, ER tech, GI tech), it should be under the supervision of a registered nurse.

3. Direct patient care activities

Direct patient care activities assist the patient/client in meeting basic human needs within the institution, at home, or other health care settings. This includes activities such as assisting the patient with feeding, drinking, ambulating, grooming, toileting, dressing, and socializing. It may involve the collecting, reporting, and documentation of data related to the above activities. These data are reported to the RN who uses the information to make a clinical judgment about patient care. Delegated activities to the UAP do not include health counseling, teaching or require independent, specialized nursing knowledge, skill or judgment.

4. Indirect patient care activities

Indirect patient care activities are necessary to support the patient and their environment, and only incidentally involve direct patient contact. These activities assist in providing a clean, efficient, and safe patient care milieu, and typically encompass chore services, companion care, housekeeping, transporting, clerical, supply stocking, and maintenance tasks.

5. Delegation

The transfer of responsibility for the performance of an activity from one individual to another while retaining accountability for the outcome. Example: the registered nurse, in delegating an activity to an unlicensed individual, transfers the responsibility for the performance of the activity but retains professional accountability for the overall care.

6. Assignment

The downward or lateral transfer of both the responsibility and accountability of an activity from one individual to another. The lateral or downward transfer of skill, knowledge, or judgment must be made to an individual, within the individual's scope of practice.

7. Supervision

The activity process of directing, guiding, and influencing the outcome of an individual's performance of an activity. Supervision is generally categorized as on-site (the nurse being physically present or immediately available while the activity is being performed) or off-site (the nurse has the ability to provide direction through various means of written and verbal communications).

NOTE: Judgment as it relates to the above definition is defined as the intellectual process that a nurse exercises in forming an opinion and reaching a clinical decision based upon analysis of the evidence or data.[1]

- First, the delegated skills must consist of highly proscribed activities that do not require nursing judgment. There should be no room for independent nursing judgment by the UAP.
- Second, the UAP must have the specific competency or certification and have received the appropriate training for the implementation of the delegated tasks.
- Third, there must be a process in place for evaluating and monitoring the implementation of the task.
- Fourth, the registered nurse must consider the severity of the patient care task and the overall physical and psychological stability of the patient.

Not all situations are appropriate for performance by a UAP, and a licensed provider should carry out the task. The "four rights" of delegation were identified in an article in the *American Journal of Nursing*: (1) the right task, (2) the right person, (3) the right communication, and (4) the right feedback.[3] The specific task should be done by the most appropriate person qualified to do that task. This person needs a clear description of the instructions and objectives and verbal and written feedback on his or her performance. The registered nurse must consider all of these rights in relationship to the clinical setting, patient acuity, and staffing within the unit.

BASIC PROBLEM

The central debate concerning whether or not registered nurses should use UAPs presents many issues, but the strongest issue deals with the dichotomy of views between the staff nurse, who is delivering the bedside patient care, and the nurse manager or nurse administrator, trying to direct the patient's care with an allegiance to the functioning of the hospital administration (see Fig. 29-1). The basic challenge is seeing the problem through different eyes, yet both wanting the same outcome of patient care. The state nurses' associations (SNAs) of the American Nurses Association view nursing as a collective whole but have a strong allegiance for workplace advocacy issues and respond to the philosophy of the staff nurse. The staff nurse views the agency structure from his or her level up the chain of command to the chief nursing administrator. The staff nurse rarely communicates directly to this chief nurse administrator and feels a sense of frustration having to work through the many levels of organization, and not directly with the administrator.

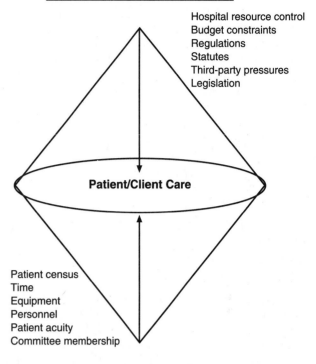

ADMINISTRATIVE NURSING VIEW

Hospital resource control
Budget constraints
Regulations
Statutes
Third-party pressures
Legislation

Patient/Client Care

Patient census
Time
Equipment
Personnel
Patient acuity
Committee membership

STAFF NURSING VIEW

Fig. 29-1. Perspectives on the issue of UAP.

The chief nurse administrator, on the other hand, has divided loyalties, caught between allegiance to the institution, on the one hand, and special insight with the problems and needs of direct patient care, on the other hand. There is a basic conflict between duty to the hospital (and or employer), the staff nurses, and the patient. The nurse administrator rarely communicates directly to the staff nurse but relies on the infrastructure of the organization. The staff nurse in turn rarely communicates directly to the nurse administrator because of the many layers of administration between the two individuals.

We must remember that the chief goal of our nursing care is to deliver competent patient care. One of the ways that we can do that is by having full, clear, open, and honest communication among all of the parties involved in this issue. Nurse administrators and staff nurses want the same things. Staff nurses have responsibility to provide care in a fiscally sound manner. Staff nurses must also pay attention to the costs of care for equipment and supplies and promote the viability of the organization. Nurse administrators must assure that the nursing care provided is fiscally sound, and that it provides comfort, knowledge, and skills to patients.

The Executive Boards of the California Nurses Association (CNA) and the Organization of Nurse Executives-California (ONE-C) have been meeting to discuss the issues of the UAP and nursing in general. It is one of the few times when these two diverse groups have tried to obtain unification. Both groups have had to compromise in their ability to reach consensus. Both realize that the final objective of care is to the patient.

The debate these two groups and others have concerning registered nurse use of unlicensed assistive nursing personnel centers around four areas: (1) practice, (2) training, (3) utilization, and (4) regulation.

PRACTICE
Pro argument

UAPs can be a viable part of our health care delivery system now and can help nurses advance their real role in patient care by eliminating unimportant, repetitive, routine tasks from the registered nurse practice. UAPs provide care of value and can make contributions to patient care. The purpose of using the UAP in direct and indirect patient situations should be to free the RN from needless tasks and assignments. Registered nurses must first define their own total patient practice and not just focus on specific simple patient care tasks. Through proper utilization of UAPs, the registered nurse is able to provide nursing care with appropriate personnel. The registered nurse must be the individual who defines the assignment, work, and tasks of the unlicensed assistive personnel. The delivery of professional nursing care can be facilitated by the proper use of UAPs.

Con argument

UAPs will replace the registered nurse and will become a cheaper alternative for delivering basic bedside nursing care. Fewer registered nurses will be needed per shift, thereby utilizing more UAPs and encroaching into professional nursing care. Patient care will suffer as less-qualified individuals provide the required patient care. Registered nurses will be responsible for larger numbers of patients who will be served by increasing numbers of UAPs. The image of the registered nurse as a direct provider of care will be eroded because of their being only seen as a "director" or "administrator" of the necessary care and not the real provider of the direct patient care.

TRAINING
Pro argument

The specific training program for the UAP involved in patient care (either direct or indirect patient care) should be under the guidance and direction of the registered nurse. Nursing should control nursing practice. The RNs must be responsible for the planning, implementing, and evaluating of all of the UAP curriculum and instruction. The programs created for training UAPs should be designed to meet the needs of the students. The training programs should be economically based and soundly developed programs that will meet in convenient locations providing day, evening, and weekend classes. They will provide both the depth and breadth of knowledge to allow for flexibility and growth of the students. Opportunities should be provided for UAP graduates to entry professional nursing programs at a later date if they desire to expand their skills and mastery levels.

Registered nurse education programs in the undergraduate and graduate level need to provide information about the proper use and training of UAPs. Continuing education and staff development personnel must also provide programs to teach their participants the proper use of UAPs. Part of this material might also be appropriate for the basic NCLEX-RN examination.

Con argument

It is impossible for all nurses to be all things to all people especially when there are 53 different state and territorial nurse practice acts and over 250 job classifications or categories for UAPs. The idea is too great a task. We have neither the resources, time, or allocation of money to handle the training. No two patient care agencies can agree on the one way to provide skills training for their respective agencies. With multiple entry points to nursing, how can we believe that we can create the proper entry for UAPs? Since people move from institution to institution and state to state, how do we know that one program is equal to another? How do we validate skills and abilities? The patient care needs of acute care vary so greatly from home health and community-based care needs that we would then have to create different programs for all different settings. With resources being so tight, how do we create all of these levels of programs for people we do not know have equal entry-level skills?

UTILIZATION
Pro argument

The assistive personnel that are involved in patient care (either indirect or direct patient care) should be supervised and guided by the registered nurse. This necessitates that the nursing department of the agency will define the job descriptions, set the criteria and methods for the utilization of the UAP, and evaluate the performance of the UAP. Registered nurses in each facility need to have the right to choose to use UAPs or not. With appropriate education, nurses will know how to use unlicensed assistive personnel.

Con argument

Since there are many identified categories of UAPs, some that provide low-skill nursing care and others that provide nonpatient care, how do registered nurses have the knowledge base and authority to train and utilize the patient care UAPs? We have failed to identify lists of appropriate tasks and skills. We continue to function state-by-state with individual nurse practice acts that do not transfer state to state. Even within one acute-care institution, the needs vary from department to department because of the acuity of the patient, technological knowledge base, and other patient care needs. Nursing is not the only important cornerstone of patient care; there are other providers who are licensed and covered by his or her own professional health care acts, and each has his or her own practice and utilization standards. How can we, as nurses, say that we can control all of the utilization of UAPs for patient care?

REGULATION
Pro argument

It is the responsibility of the profession of nursing to protect our patients and the public in general. We must create appropriate mechanisms to control the practice of unlicensed personnel by registered nurses. With standardized training programs for the different categories of unlicensed assistive personnel these nonlicensed personnel would have the necessary check off system to move from agency to agency and state to state. The state boards of nursing must control regulation of all individuals who provide nursing care within the scope of that practice in the state. Since nursing is responsible for the training and utilization of the UAP, it is best that the nursing profession regulate the practice of UAP. Most nurse practice acts determine that the RN is accountable and legally responsible for all tasks and assignments that are delegated to less-skilled individuals and for improperly delegated assignments. It is only a logical step for nursing to control the practice of its assistants by regulating these individuals.

Regulation is not a singular category but, in fact, has three levels or forms of established regulation programs: (1) licensure, (2) certification, and (3) registry or registration.

Licensure. Permission is given to an individual by a granting authority, by virtue of its legal standing, to engage in activities or provide care that would be illegal without the licensure. Licensure is granted on basis of credentials, education, and examination.

Certification. A voluntary granting by a nongovernmental authority of certain privileges or standards to an individual. Certification is a manner to prove minimum competency of a particular specialty or of acquired skills and knowledge. The process may be created by proof of completion of an approved education or training program and or completion of skills testing.

Registry or registration. A listing of names and demographic data of individuals who have completed prescribed training or education programs. The individual documents in this process can list past and current competency and achievements of the individuals who are thus listed. The listing can be maintained by an independent nongovernmental or governmental authority or board.

Con argument

By virtue of using any level or form of the regulation process, we are legitimizing and accepting the responsibility for another separate group of individuals to practice in the health arena. Once a registry has been established, it would be possible to then certify these individuals and, within another period of time, legitimize and codify these unlicensed assistive personnel into licensed personnel. Since this group costs less to educate and is paid a lower salary or wage, there would be justification to replace RNs with the newly licensed assistive individuals. RNs would now be held completely liable for all individuals to whom they have delegated their authority in an assignment.

SUMMARY OF PRO AND CON ARGUMENTS

It is time for change, and registered nurses must not participate in the repetitive, nonessential patient care tasks that can be reassigned to others. It is time to assess reallocation of registered nurse time to perform appropriate nursing tasks. Primary nursing as a delivery model is no longer financially feasible, and we do not have adequate resources and personnel at all levels. (Some individuals might think this a short-term view, once the financial difficulties of the health care system were dealt with we could go back to primary nursing. This chapter does not deal with the revamping of the health care delivery system in the future and is the topic of other chapters or papers in the future.) We must look at different staff blends and other nursing delivery systems. All nurses, regardless of whether they are bedside staff or administrative nurses, must communicate directly, assertively, and together. The misunderstanding of the registered nurses is due to failure to communicate. Communication must improve between and among registered nurses throughout their own institutions and between the various professional nursing organizations.

The concept of regulation for unlicensed assistive personnel has caused the greatest discomfort for all nurses, whether they are assigned as staff or administrators. This issue is so complex and difficult, that the ANA Task Force For Unlicensed Assistive Personnel could not provide adequate information for or against regulation. There is no agreement on regulation of unlicensed assistive personnel. Further, this disagreement extends to the questions of regulation. Should the control of unlicensed assistive personnel be internal to nursing or external from a governmental regulating body? No one can agree on appropriate staff mix, RN to RN, RN to LVN, and RN to UAP. In many states, there are no specific numbers or ratios within the statutes and ordinances. Finally, if regulation by a statutory body is not the answer, should one of the other less stringent regulatory processes be implemented such as certification or registration? We must answer our own questions, or someone else will.

Additional meetings and concept papers are needed before definite consensus can be achieved. The tasks and questions are not fully answered and the debate still rages. During the 1992 ANA House of Delegates Convention in Las Vegas, Nevada, a resolution was passed that continued the quest for answers regarding UAPs. The resolution indicated four statements of action:

1. A request that the association assess the issues and make recommendations related to the utilization of UAPs and delegation of tasks by RNs to UAPs
2. That every effort be made for the recommendations to be developed in such a fashion as to permit critique by the SNAs before the December 1992 Constituent Assembly
3. That the recommendations shall be submitted to the 1993 House of Delegates as an Action Report
4. That the ANA Board of Directors make funding available to continue the work of the task force for the urgent work that needs to be completed on this issue within the next biennium

These issues need to be further investigated before nursing can make the important decisions.[1]

The legal responsibility to perform licensed professional nursing functions rests on the registered nurse. When the registered nurse appropriately delegates tasks to the appropriate person the liability is attenuated. The nurse must make sure that the person delegated to has the proper training and is the appropriate person to be delegated to. However the RN is, in fact, at risk and liable when the nurse delegates tasks that are beyond the bounds of the legal statutes. The risk continues if the task involves a substantial risk or harm to the patient.

If the registered nurse does not provide the appropriate supervision for unlicensed assistive personnel and if the registered nurse delegates a patient care task to a UAP who has not had the appropriate training or orientation for the task, liability remains with the registered nurse. More in-depth investigation and interpretation are needed by the entire nursing community to analyze the legal consequences of this issue.

There is a continued need for further nursing research in the area of nursing care delivery systems. Health care agencies and schools of nursing need to work together to look into this important area. Across the country, there are initial investigations involving the appropriate use of UAPs, how to mix staff and how to delegate patient and nonpatient care assignments to them. One example is a continuing project by Susan Neidlinger and Patricia Sparacino titled "The effect of supplemental staffing with permanent unit-based nurses' aides on patient outcomes and cost," involving the University of California, San Francisco School of Nursing and the Nursing Services Department at the University of California, San Francisco Hospital Center. Initially in the project, nursing assistants were assigned to patients, but now the nursing assistants are assigned to the staff nurses on the units. This particular project is an excellent example of the continued cooperation needed between schools of nursing and the nursing departments of health care agencies.

The work of the ANA task force is not completed and the remainder of the issues must be investigated. A final American Nurses Association monograph or position paper is needed to try to gain consensus on the topic of regulation of unlicensed assistive personnel. Discussion papers must be developed on the following topics:

1. Medication administration aides
2. Nursing students
3. Community health–home health aides
4. School system aides
5. Emergency medical technician paramedics
6. Multipurpose personnel/cross-training aides

At this time, nurses must document, in their best judgment, occasions when they believe that there have been inappropriate delegation to unlicensed assistive personnel. Many hospitals with workplace advocacy programs or collective bargaining contracts specify forms that can be utilized to report problems in nursing care and staffing problems. The many levels within the agencies must be made aware of these issues. Staff mix and ratios of RN to UAP, RN to LVN, and RN to RN must be investigated.

The one issue throughout this entire subject that is clear is that nursing must commit itself to investigate these dilemmas. If not, other professions and the judicial/legislative offices within the local and national government will investigate and make decisions for us. Nurses must take and keep control of practice in this area as in others.

REFERENCES

1. American Nurses Association. (1992). Progress report on unlicensed assistive personnel: Informational report. Report: CNP-CNE-B. Washington, D.C.: Author.
2. Blegen, M. A., Gardner, D. L., & McCloskey, J. C. (1991). Who helps you with your work? *American Journal of Nursing, 92*(1), 26-31.
3. Hansten, R., & Washburn, M. (1992). How to plan what to delegate. *American Journal of Nursing, 92*(4), 71-72.
4. North Dakota Nurses Association, Congress of Education and Professional Nursing Practice. (1989). *Study of unlicensed personnel who provide assistance to the nurse.* Bismarck, N.D.: Author.

CHAPTER 30

Viewpoints

Changes in the hospital as a place of practice

LUCILLE A. JOEL

Burgeoning technology, advances in medical science, shifts in demography, and the economics of health care have dramatically changed hospitals and hospital nursing practice. This chapter establishes a historical perspective to allow a better understanding of nursing practice in contemporary hospitals. Given an idea of what exists and why it has come to be, the reader will be able to distinguish current trends and what nurses can expect under a variety of circumstances.

THE ORIGINS OF CHANGE

The conquest of infectious disease and advances in the treatment of traumatic injury and acute illness have created a world where chronic conditions are common. Medical science and technology, coupled with reimbursable services to the elderly through Medicare, have caused a dramatic shift in demographics. We are confronted with a population that is older and more characterized by chronic disease and disability. By the year 2030, 20% of Americans will be over the age of 65, and many will be over 75 years old. In 1900, 4% of the elderly were 85 years or older; by 2050 that figure will be 25%.[11]

Where health care coverage is provided through the workplace, reimbursement has begun to favor treatment in community settings; however, public entitlement programs such as Medicare continue to be biased toward traditional hospital- and physician-based models of service. Given these factors, it is no surprise that 40% of hospital admissions are Medicare recipients and 60% of hospital days are Medicare days.[10] The elderly predominate among hospital patients, and unstable or acute exacerbations of chronic illness are the most frequent clinical situations. Ready access to state-of-the-art technology and an extremely litigious environment create circumstances in which aggressive therapy has become more the rule than the exception.

The changes attributable to medical science, an aging and more chronically ill population, and expanded access to services pale next to the manner in which hospitals have been reshaped by economics in the last decade. By end of the 1970s, the federal government began to feel uneasy about the magnitude of its financial obligation to Medicare and Medicaid recipients. By 1980, cost effectiveness in health care reimbursed through public entitlement programs was mandated by the government. Hospitals, the most costly element in the delivery system, were targeted for cost containment.

In a sequence of events from 1980 through 1983, hospital rates and fees for inpatient ancillary services paid by the Medicare program were negotiated downward, and related expenses, such as capital improvements, interest payments, and the cost of care to the indigent, were disallowed. In October 1983, the Medicare prospective pricing system (PPS) was instituted for hospitals. This system awarded a fixed-dollar amount for an episode of illness based on a cluster of variables found to be highly predictive of hospital resource use (diagnosis, complications, surgery, age). The taxonomy of diagnostic-related groups (DRGs) provided the reimbursement categories for PPS.

To ensure fiscal solvency, hospitals were obliged to influence the prescriptive practices of physicians. Reducing the length of stay and the use of ancillary services became critical. The use of proprietary as opposed to generic drugs and defensive diagnostic testing for protection in a litigious milieu both create serious financial liability for hospitals. From another perspective, physicians construed the need to be judicious in their ordering practices as administrative intrusion into clinical management. The reaction has been for physicians to favor treatment of patients in the community and to choose hospitalization only as a last resort.

PPS has been described as the ultimate in both regulation and deregulation. Cost-benefit decisions were decentralized to the facility level, and the hospital was able to predict the dollar amount of Medicare revenue based on its historic case mix. Further, by striking reimbursement rates according to the average cost of treatment in a category, PPS intended hospitals to assume some risk for patients who consume resources in excess of the usual. The industry's response has been less humanistic, often denying admission to patients who appear to be a financial liability. Such cases often become the charge of public sector facilities.

The efficiencies imposed by Medicare and, in most instances, state Medicaid programs shifted some of the costs of doing business to patients who paid out-of-pocket or were reimbursed by private sector insurers, predominantly through the workplace. It is important to note that this common practice of cost shifting has been recently declared unconstitutional by the New Jersey Supreme Court. To safeguard their premium payments, insurance intermediaries and employers began to limit reimbursable treatment options and to monitor clinical management practices. In other words, it has been many years since most Americans have had total freedom of choice in health care. Community care is favored over hospitalization except in the most serious instances. The effect of these complementary private and public sector trends has been the unprecedented severity of illness of hospitalized patients and aggressive treatment both to speed discharge and to serve as a therapeutic response to acutely ill patients. Clinical intensity is also affected by the need to maintain high patient volume and maximum occupancy rates. In today's reimbursement environment, three patients each hospitalized for 10 days generate more revenue than one patient hospitalized for 30 days. Each new admission requires assessment, development of a plan of care, and subsequent implementation and integration of a therapeutic regimen. The increased demands on nursing are obvious.

NURSING IN TODAY'S HOSPITALS

In the midst of a hospital environment where the physician continues to be the gatekeeper and reimbursement focuses on medical management, nursing has become the single, most essential service. There are few, if any, medical conditions that cannot be treated in the community. An increasing number of surgical procedures are appropriate to freestanding surgical centers or day-of-admission programs. Patients come to hospitals for nursing because of the need for monitoring and surveillance on a continuous basis, because of self-care deficits and compromised functional statuses and because of the need for teaching, counseling, coordination of services, development of community support systems, and preparation of the family to cope with an individual's changed health status. Consumers have begun to distinguish the roles that hospitals and physicians play in promoting return to health. Consumers are more judicious in selecting their hospitals and their physicians. This choice is often based, either consciously or unconsciously, on the perceived quality of nursing.

Competent nursing is also critical to the financial integrity of hospitals. Skillful clinical management of the acutely ill elderly can minimize functional deficits and avoid costly disposition problems. Advancing the patient's diet on a meal-to-meal basis, furthering self-care as motivation appears, and seizing the opportunity to teach and counsel at the moment of receptiveness all contribute to reducing the length of stay, and shortened lengths of stay contribute to the financial well-being of the hospital. Documenting complications at the first detectable clinical signs and immediately instituting a corrective regimen may increase short-term costs but may avert the need for a protracted hospital stay and, even ultimately, create a higher level of reimbursement. Skillful clinical observation can reduce the need for testing. Careful coordination of hospital services can speed diagnosis, treatment, and stabilization of the medical regimen.

Cash flow concerns and maximizing reimbursement demand thorough documentation executed with a cost-conscious eye. Chart completion and the establishment of a principal diagnosis are critical for reimbursement. Nurses' notes often provide information overlooked by physicians. Given the potential clinical and financial benefits of sophisticated nursing, regionalization and organization of clinical services based on nursing specialties is more prudent than consolidation reflecting the medical model.

Hospitals were blind to the inherent value of nursing when they first began to consider approaches to cost-effectiveness. In the early days of cost containment, nursing departments—as labor-intensive centers—were targeted for downsizing. The hospital budget was often balanced on the back of nursing, most notably by reducing the numbers of registered nurses. Those nurse executives who had the foresight to document increased resource consumption by patients were the most successful in maintaining their staffs. As hospital patients became more acutely ill, the wisdom of decreasing the number of registered nurses became suspect. Instead, hospitals began to cut back on the support services available to nursing and to thin the ranks of other provider professionals in such areas as pharmacy, physical therapy, and respiratory therapy, in favor of increasing the number of nurses on staff. Registered nurses were recognized as versatile, ready, and able to assume the duties of a wide variety of skilled and unskilled work and an extremely good value since sometimes only a few dollars an hour separated them from technical or assistive personnel. Nursing practice in hospitals began to be characterized by all-registered nurse (RN) staffs.[1] In truth, there was a lack of appreciation for what nurses could contribute as nurses. There are two hidden issues here: (1) the use of nurses to perform nonnursing activities and (2) nurses performing clinical duties below their skill levels. The latter situation, at least, has been well documented.

Management studies have found that up to 40% of a nurse's time may be invested in nonnursing functions.[9] Research in New Jersey in the 1980s indicated that 23% to 48% of the nurse's time is invested in work inappropriate to the role.[12] Great variation exists in the creation of support systems for nurses that allocate more professional nursing time to the bedside. The "unit assistant" created at Rush-Presbyterian-St. Luke's Medical Center in Chicago is one example. The unit assistant takes on a variety of nonnursing tasks rather than operating exclusively as a messenger, a transporter, or a clerical worker. This approach is based on the fact that because the needs of each hospital unit are different, it is unwise to create specific categories of supportive workers or to detail their tasks. The essential role that nurses play in coordinating and integrating the hospital routine makes it prudent to place support workers under the control of nursing. Ideally, the money for these positions should come from the nursing budget and the support worker should be assigned consistently to one registered nurse. This arrangement creates the best environment for shaping the support role and allows the nursing philosophy of care and work ethic to be clearly communicated and modeled by the responsible superior.

Similar nonclinical, nursing-designed, unit-based models have been reported at Providence Medical Center in Seattle and at Miami's Children's Hospital.[2] In a 1988 survey of hospitals conducted by the American Nurses Association (ANA) and the Association of Nurse Executives (AONE), 84% of the respondents reported creating support personnel to perform nonnursing duties.[4] The result is an increase in the amount of time nurses can devote to patient care.

The question remains: Is there a role in hospitals for personnel who can assist nurses with direct care? Until the nursing shortage of the mid 1980s, there was an observable decline in the number of both assistive and technical nursing personnel in hospitals because of increased use of registered nurses. However, by the end of the decade, staff composition was characterized by nursing care providers with a variety of skill levels and capabilities and a decreasing ratio of registered nurses to unlicensed assistive personnel (UAP). At this writing, more than half of the state nurses' associations have reported instances in which staff mix ratios (RNs to UAPs) are unsafe.[6] The clinical condition of the hospital patient should be the critical element in this debate. While it is impossible to deny the need for assistive workers who have direct care functions in long-term and home care, there is no ability to generalize for acute care. The American Nurses Association has given significant attention to this issue and offers some initial guidance. Decisions on the need for clinical or direct care support personnel and their level of training are best made by the nursing staff at the facility level. Assistive personnel should never be directly assigned to a patient; they should be assigned to the registered nurse. It then becomes the professional nurse's responsibility to use that human resource wisely, assigning or delegating activities while maintaining personal accountability for the quality and safety of care. Finally, credentialing assistive personnel holds a substantial element of risk. Human nature being what it is, there will be inevitable movement towards independence and recognition.[5,6]

The reader is cautioned about the danger of moving too quickly to embrace direct care support systems for nursing before adequately assessing the nonnursing duties that have become part of the nurse's role. It is also necessary to lobby for hospital policies that allow nurses to control the introduction of support personnel and that establish the nurses' authority over their work. In recent years, nurses have accepted new categories of clinical workers in specialty areas with little protest, viewing each incident as an isolated occurrence. Specific examples can be cited in dialysis, critical care, emergency services, anesthesia, and the operating room. This trend gained little attention until the American Medical Association proposed a new class of caregiver, the registered care technologist (RCT), as its response to the nursing shortage.

Both personnel utilization patterns and compensation were positively influenced by the nursing shortage of the 1980s. The market for nursing responded to supply and demand. Nurses' salaries increased significantly in some geographic areas. Hospital nurses, as the most visible group, profited the most. Starting salaries have often been increased at the expense of economic growth within existing nursing positions. The AONE suggests a 100% range between beginning and maximum salaries. Establishing unrealistic entry salaries creates future problems in the attempt to solve present ones. Salary compression creates a serious obstacle to nurse recruitment and retention.

The tendency to pay more for personnel during a shortage has always been the first step in a vicious cycle. Nursing salaries have always been increased in times of shortage. The high cost of nursing then prompts a more cost-efficient use of nurses and the introduction of support systems to take over nonnursing duties and those less-skilled activities commonly delegated to nurses. A nursing surplus gradually develops and salary gains are slowed, at which point it becomes feasible to hire nurses rather than less-skilled workers. This returns us full circle to a demand-driven shortage.[1]

Benefits have also been reshaped by the nursing shortage to address personal and professional needs. More than 93% of the respondents in a 1988 ANA/AONE survey of 1065 hospitals offer flexible work schedules for nurses seeking degree education. More than 81% of these hospitals provide financial assistance to licensed practical nurses (LPNs) and licensed vocational nurses (LVNs) enrolled in RN-educational programs, and almost 81% subsidize baccalaureate and graduate courses for registered nurses. Nurses who take on less desirable work schedules are rewarded financially by 63% of the hospitals. Clinical excellence and productivity are identified as the basis for promotion by 52.4% of the respondents.[4]

On another note, there is a positive correlation between more flexible and creative professional employee policies and the degree of nursing shortage experienced by the hospital. Where there is little or no shortage, there is little openness to change.[4] This is unfortunate and demonstrates the need for progressive hospitals to publicize their incentive and practice programs to attract nurses. Market competition may be the most effective tactic to restructure hospital nursing.

OUR PREFERRED FUTURE

I have already offered examples of how hospital nursing is being restructured to promote professionalism. The nursing shortage has been the catalyst. Moving beyond salary and benefits, it will be the practice programs and role relationships in hospitals that provide status and prestige. Hospital nursing can only flourish in an environment of status and prestige. The elements critical to a preferred future have been thoroughly described by organized nursing.[3,13,14]

A preferred future must include the ability to distinguish nurses according to education, seniority, experience, supervisory and peer evaluations, and certification, as well as any other appropriate variables. Job descriptions, clinical ladders, or both may be the vehicles to formalize these distinctions. It is critical that roles and responsibilities change as a nurse advances within a system and that salary and benefits are tailored to recognize these levels of personal growth and accomplishment. Ideally, there is a hierarchy of clinical competencies that complements the variations in patient complexity seen in the hospital. A staff hierarchy also accommodates variable expectations in the areas of research, mentoring, and institutional involvement.

Dissatisfaction with hospital nursing is closely associated with the growing fragmentation of practice and the consequent loss of control over plans of patient care. The intimacy and holism that lie at the core of nursing have been seriously compromised by attempts to accommodate more profoundly ill patients, technology, specialization, and rapid discharge. Hospitals that successfully retain their nurses organize service delivery to reinstitute continuity, comprehensiveness, and control of the clinical nursing regimen. The principles are the same whether we talk about primary nursing, case management, district nursing, or a variety of other models. The role of the nurse as patient advocate, systems coordinator, and integrator of the total hospital experience is logical and cost effective.

The decentralization of clinical authority and the establishment of systems of reward based on competence demand that nurses be accountable to and for one another. A practice council becomes the forum in which interdisciplinary clinical management can be discussed. Practice councils allow the resolution of problems between groups of provider professionals; this resolution is achieved without administrative intrusion but with administration serving in an advisory capacity and offering a broader perspective on operations. A nursing staff organization provides the self-governance structure to develop and institute a program of peer review.

The roles and relationships that have been described can only flourish in an environment where the chief nursing executive has the status of other major department heads. This individual must be secure enough in status and ability to recognize that one cannot be an expert in all areas. One must have the self-assurance to allow people to fail, to delegate authority, as well as responsibility, and to give people some latitude in approaching their responsibilities.

There is no single best structural and functional design for hospital nursing services. Modeling must be done at the facility level within a system of participatory management. Individuals invest highly in systems that they help to develop and by which they will have to live. A tertiary provider institution with high levels of clinical intensity and well-developed specialization will require a different organization and mix of resources than a community hospital with a simpler patient population.

In effect, the test of any system is to look at outcomes. Are patients discharged in fewer days? Is recidivism lower? Are iatrogenic occurrences less frequent? What about drug errors and accidents? Is staff turnover lower? Is research a part of everyday life? Is the facility a desirable place for students? Do faculty from affiliated schools participate readily in staff development activities? This is not an exhaustive list, but it does begin to identify critical indicators against which to measure our preferred future. Moving beyond guild issues, hospital nursing will flourish only to the extent that it makes a difference to patients and to the well-being of the institution.

THE INEVITABLE FUTURE

The years between the first writing of this chapter and the current revision have been the occasion of intense debate around health care reform. The debate is gradually revealing consensus on select aspects of a preferred infrastructure. These observations hold implications for hospitals and nursing.

There is predictable movement towards a "seamless fabric," or integrated system, of health services, allowing the client to move fluidly between levels of care. Artificial barriers between acute, long-term, and community care will be minimized or eliminated. The trend for hospitals to establish long-term care beds, home care agencies, and community-based satellites is good business and socially sensitive. The challenge is, wherever possible, to expand nursing practice to address the entire episode of illness.[7]

The presence of a case manager for those clients who are intense users of services is an additional requisite included in most pending public policy.[8] This role goes beyond the nursing care manager models that have become visible in nursing circles. The case manager in the former context advocates to maximize the client's resources for an entire episode of illness. Brokering and procuring services are essential skills. Where such case manager roles exist, they are usually open to either nurses or social workers. In reality, nurses have been less than eager to assume this responsibility.

Both an integrated system and case management allow hospital nurses to expand their practice beyond the institutional walls. Given an adventurous spirit, there is the promise of exciting practice, clinical gain for the patient, and the opportunity to directly contribute to the fiscal integrity of the system.

The over-bedding that persists in many areas of this country and the fragile nature of the elderly, the chronically ill, and the disabled have given rebirth to some old hospital practice models. Strong nursing leadership has seized this opportunity to establish "progressive nursing units" or "short-term, long-term care." This concept, harkening back to the model first executed at Loeb Center of Montefiore Hospital in the Bronx, requires admission by a nurse in advanced practice, and the physician becomes consultative to the attending nurse. Patients are only admitted if they conform to stringent criteria that predict a return to some degree of independence and self-care within a reasonable period. These units are not a place to house disposition problems, but an intense nursing program to avoid them.

This revival of a pioneering spirit also adds credibility to nursing's demands for practice privileges in hospitals. Membership of nurses on the professional staff is consistent with Joint Commission and Medicare criteria. Institutional policies create obstacles and disallow nurses from being recognized as full-fledged professional colleagues. These limitations and stereotypes have to be challenged immediately, consistently, and continually to position nursing strategically for a future with profound demands for accountability.

A growing outcry for accountability to the public is directed towards provider professionals and the health care industry in general, but hospitals in particular. In repeated public opinion surveys, respondents identify greed and waste as the major culprit in creating our mean-spirited, inadequate health care delivery system. This consumer sentiment has been the impetus for the federal medical effectiveness initiative. Through an amendment to the Omnibus Budget Reconciliation Act of 1990(OBRA90), the 101st Congress established the Agency for Health Care Policy and Research (AHCPR). This agency is to work with the professional community towards consensus, in the form of guidelines, on the clinical management of conditions that are costly to Medicare, differ significantly in treatment depending on the provider, yet have an identifiable body of research. Three sets of guidelines for nursing-friendly conditions have already been authored: postoperative pain, decubiti prevention, and urinary incontinence. The content is important, but not the most critical point here. These federal guidelines have established a new legal standard. In turn, there are new demands for staff development, and an outcry for research-based practice as opposed to care based on intuition or outdated information. And the value of a provider will depend both on how it impacts the bottom line and how it contributes to quality outcomes. An awareness of the cost of nursing and nursing's role in revenue generation has been slow to develop among members of the profession.

In conclusion, recent years have held dramatic changes in hospital practice. Where we were once limited to accommodating change that was upon us, we can now anticipate the next frontier. If we are ill-prepared for a new reality, it will be because we have chosen to close our eyes.

REFERENCES

1. Aiken, L., & Mullinex, C. (1987). The nursing shortage: Myth or reality. *The New England Journal of Medicine, 317*(10), 641-646.
2. American Hospital Association. (1989). *Restructuring the work load: Methods and models to address the nursing shortage.* Chicago: Author.
3. American Nurses Association. (1983). *Magnet hospitals: Attraction and retention of professional nurses.* Kansas City, Mo: American Academy of Nursing.
4. American Nurses Association. (1988). *Nursing practice update.* Kansas City, Mo: Author.
5. American Nurses Association. (1991). *Resource packet on unlicensed assistive personnel to the registered nurse.* Kansas City, Mo: Author.
6. American Nurses Association. (1992). *Progress report on unlicensed assistive personnel.* Report to the House of Delegates. Washington, D.C.: Author.
7. American Nurses Association. (1992). *Nursing's agenda for health care reform.* Washington, D.C.: Author.
8. Bowers, K. (1991). *Case management by nurses.* Kansas City, Mo: American Nurses Association.
9. Ernst & Whinney. (June, 1988). Personal communication to the American Nurses Association.
10. Joel, L. (1984). Geriatric imperative: The acutely ill elderly. *Journal of the Medical Society of New Jersey, 81*(8), 655.
11. Koop, E. E. (1985). The strengths and needs of the elderly. In *Issues and strategies in geriatric education* (pp. 59-63). McLean, Va: The Circle.
12. New Jersey Department of Health. (1978). *A prospective reimbursement system based on patient case mix for New Jersey hospitals, 1976-1983* (2nd annual rep, vol. 1). Trenton, N.J.: State of New Jersey Department of Health.
13. Nursing summit statement on short-term strategies to address the nursing shortage. May, 1988. Washington, D.C.
14. Secretary's Commission on Nursing. (1988). *Interim report.* Washington, D.C.: U.S. Department of Health and Human Services.

CHAPTER 31

Developing community partnerships

Shifting power from health professionals to citizens

SHARON FARLEY

Community-based primary health care is like motherhood and apple pie; everyone praises it. And yet there are various interpretations of how community-based programs should be implemented. Also, in spite of public rhetoric, some health professionals may be ambivalent toward the concepts of community partnerships and citizen empowerment that must accompany successful community-based primary health care.

Some public and private agencies physically place community health centers, mental health centers, nursing care centers, and the like in the community but keep them responsible to the system instead of to the citizens they serve. McKnight[6] believes that outreach programs are a way for systems to expand themselves and diminish communities. In these programs, health and social service providers view people as clients instead of citizens. The clients are people who are defined by their needs and are dependent on the programs to fix their problems.[3]

Sometimes these systems promise partnerships with the community to identify needs and design programs to fill the gaps in services. However, these powerful outside groups and bureaucracies are not willing to share power with their citizen partners or to give up the supervisory role. These "partnerships" perpetuate the paternalistic health and social service delivery system and, consequently, the community-based programs often are not successful.

Many social and health reformers are advocating that citizens become genuinely involved in making decisions about programs and policies that affect their health and quality of life.[2,6,9] This community empowerment is a process of increasing control by groups over consequences that are important to their members.[4] Research by McKnight[6] indicates that it is impossible to produce health among the powerless but that it is possible to allow health by transferring tools, authority, budgets, and income to those with the malady of powerlessness.

The health status of those with the least power, minorities and the poor, remain unconscionably low. The *Report of the Secretary's Task Force on Black and Minority Health*[8] noted that minorities experienced approximately 60,000 "excess deaths" annually. Signs of the health costs of powerlessness among the poor and disenfranchised are interpersonal violence, dangerous housing, drug overdoses, alcoholism, teenage pregnancy, etc. Powerlessness and poverty of the spirit and of resources are the antecedent risk factors of preventable disease.[2]

Nurses and other health professionals need new actions and allies to solve the health problems of the 1990s and beyond. Communities have an abundant capacity for caring about their citizens. When people are enabled to work with professionals in real partnerships where decision making is shared, changes will occur that improve health and quality of life. Nurses, traditionally committed to involving individuals in decision making, can play a key role in empowering citizens for participation in community-based health care programs.

BUILDING COMMUNITY-BASED PARTNERSHIPS

The Rural Elderly Enhancement Program (REEP)* in Alabama is a nurse-initiated project developed on a

*The Rural Elderly Enhancement Project is partially funded by the W. K. Kellogg Foundation.

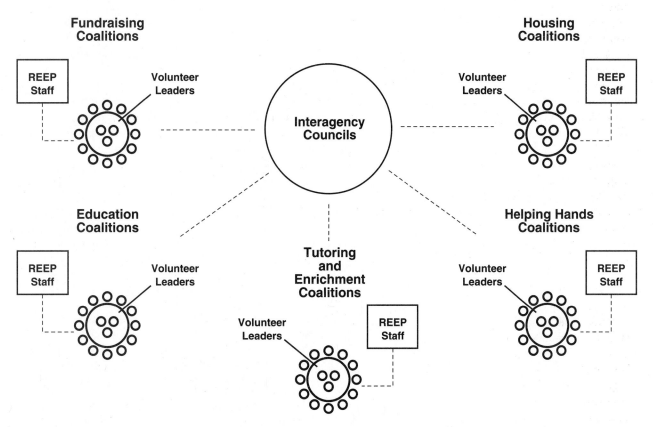

Fig. 31-1. Organizational structure of community coalitions.

model of community empowerment. REEP's initial goal was to maintain the health and independence of the elderly, but in response to citizens' demand, it was expanded to an intergenerational focus with a strong commitment to youth. The majority of the target population in the two Alabama counties is black, poor, and medically underserved.

The project views health according to the World Health Organization's definition, which is: (1) adequate food, shelter, and clothing; (2) access to medical care when needed; (3) an opportunity to participate; and (4) a safe, healthful environment. Therefore, nurses work with other health and human service professionals, local and state government units, agencies, volunteer coalitions, and schools to: (1) stimulate rural development involving community volunteer coalitions, leadership training, intergenerational programs, and public education; (2) provide accessible and potable water and improved housing and transportation; and (3) conduct assessments of the elderly and school-age children and respond to their needs with linkage to services, education, and appropriate volunteer coalitions.

The organizational structure for the Rural Elderly Enhancement Program supports its philosophy of community participation and empowerment. Fig. 31-1 depicts the organization structure. The project staff and members of the interagency councils build partnerships with each other and with the community volunteer coalitions but do not function in a supervisory role. Leadership and decision making reside with each coalition.

Project staff roles

Project staff, which includes three nurses and two social workers, provide educational and leadership training activities for the coalitions. These activities develop citizens' organizational, technical, and human relations skills necessary to identify issues, set goals, and implement programs that will improve their health and quality of life. The project's goal is to develop community leadership so that coalitions will not need the staff to sustain activities. One of the nurses said, "My goal is to work myself out of a job."

Interagency council roles

In each county there is an interagency council with representatives from health, service, and education agencies. The councils serve four purposes: (1) to plan and implement cooperative programs with the volunteer coalitions that assist the communities; (2) to assist with volunteer training; (3) to play an advisory role to the coalitions and provide linkages between community initiatives and available services and resources; and (4) to communicate with each other and decrease duplication of services. Project staff provide leadership and educational activities for council members which enable them to implement a community empowerment model and to assume an advisory instead of a supervisory role for community-based programs.

Community volunteer coalitions

Volunteer coalitions are the heart of the REEP project. Although the needs are great and the resources are few, volunteers are giving 800 hours of free services to assist their neighbors and friends. The tradition of "neighbor helping neighbor," long recognized as a hallmark of rural life, forms the value base for these volunteer coalitions. These citizens, many impoverished themselves, recognize their interconnectedness and responsibility for the well-being of each other, and believe in their capacity to act to solve their communities' problems.

Both counties have housing, fund raising, education, and helping-hand coalitions that assist the elderly and tutoring and enrichment coalitions that assist school-age children. Each coalition has one to three coordinators who are elected by its members. The housing coalitions improve the access and safety of older persons' homes by building steps, ramps, and porches and replacing roofs, windows, and floors. The high school vocational students improve their carpentry skills by participating in these activities under the supervision of retired teachers. The fund-raising coalitions assist the elderly to buy medication, obtain transportation, and get public water to their homes. Registered nurses from the REEP staff train volunteers in the education coalition who then provide health education for residents of their communities. The helping-hand coalitions provide friendly visiting, homemaking, personal care, and respite for the elderly and their families. Volunteers in these coalitions are graduates of the home health aide training classes taught by nurses in the project. These volunteers also assist the project nurses with assessments, case finding, and referral as well as helping the elderly gain access to the fragmented health care system. Sixty percent of the home health aide graduates, many of whom were on welfare, are employed by home health agencies.

The tutoring and enrichment coalitions assist school-age children with mathematics, reading, and science in after-school and summer programs. Also, they implement programs in the arts and humanities. Retired school teachers and other older residents use story telling to connect children to their history, culture, and values.

Partnership case study

The following case study illustrates how health professional–citizen partnerships can make a difference in community-based programs:

A member of the helping hand coalition called the project nurse because she was worried about a neighbor who was a diabetic and a stroke victim. The client was 64 years old and was not Medicare or Medicaid eligible. Therefore, she "fell through the cracks" of the system. The client needed help with activities of daily living. When the nurse went to the house to do an assessment, she found the entrance to the trailer had narrow, steep steps. There was a rickety wooden rail on one side, and she wondered if the old boards could support her weight. The house needed cleaning.

The nurse contacted the helping hand coalition member, who provided housekeeping, personal care, and friendly visiting. The vocational students built new front steps for the trailer. Six months after the initial assessment, a helping hand volunteer again called the project nurse because the woman was refusing insulin and was not eating. Since the woman was now 65 years old, the nurse called the home health agency to inquire if she was eligible for nursing services. A nurse from home health began visiting the client for diabetic teaching and blood sugar monitoring. Volunteers continued providing services on days when home health did not see her. Through efforts of citizens working in partnership with health professionals, the woman was able to remain safely in her home.

FACTORS CRITICAL TO SUCCESS

Cooperative goals, trusting relationships, and commitment are the foundation for coalition building and partnerships. Increasingly, collaboration becomes a necessity as individuals and groups seek to develop individual competencies, solve problems, and respond to a rapidly changing world. Some factors are critical to building successful coalitions and partnerships for community-based primary health care programs.

Respect for individual and community values

The underlying goal of successful coalitions is to improve the quality of life, and the underlying value is to maintain the dignity of every individual. Health professionals who respect the dignity of people emphasize the concept of possible change created by local leaders and volunteers versus the fantasy of "saviors." The issues, solutions, and programs flow from the people. Alinsky[1] said, "Denial of the opportunity for participation is the denial of human dignity and democracy."

The community's sense of dignity and confidence in directing its own efforts is an essential element in developing community-based programs. The community existed long before the community organizer came into it, and it will exist long after the community organizer is gone. Time in rural communities is measured not in days or weeks but in decades and centuries; time in rural communities is a smooth, ever-flowing big river. From this perspective, community-based programs become mere ripples in the stream—they come and they go.

Many rural communities, having seen community-based programs come and go, have little faith in the longevity of projects, and this is an obstacle to overcome. Since the underlying purpose in developing volunteer coalitions is to create both an organized approach to the community's problems and a leadership group that will survive or evolve into another group when the project's goals are completed, the issue of time and making lasting changes is a major concern. REEP chose to address this concern by selecting staff community development coordinators who were natives of the counties. These coordinators gave the project credibility with the local population. Their commitment to their communities, their sterling character, and their willingness to listen and learn enhanced the possibility of lasting changes.

Focus on issues that matter most

The place to begin is with what matters most, that is, what matters most to the people in the community. Of course, this must be tempered with rational thought and the probability of success, for it is important that the first projects be achievable. Given that consideration, the choice of types of coalitions and the projects they undertake should be left to the discretion of the group. The guidance and advice of the project staff can prevent the selection of first projects that will be difficult to complete or that will not allow the group to experience an early success.

It is essential to remember that communities have many problems and that it is very likely that they will always have problems. The goal is not to eliminate all problems; the goal is to focus the community's energies toward those problems that they are willing to work together to solve. These problems then become issues, which should be grouped in related categories, around which volunteer coalitions can be developed. The development of successful coalitions and the selection of successful projects will depend on these factors: the selection and grouping of issues into possible projects for the different volunteer coalitions and the concentration on developing only two or three coalitions at first.

The first community meeting of REEP was a joint meeting of community leaders from both counties. Before this meeting, the project staff had listed opportunities for volunteer involvement related to each project goal and grouped these opportunities into fields of interest such as transportation, housing rehabilitation, water, health education, fund-raising, nutrition, recreation, chore services for the elderly, and clerical support for the project staff. The project staff envisioned that each field of interest would be the basis for a possible volunteer coalition, and they developed job descriptions for each possible coalition. The project staff also had definite opinions about those coalitions they felt were most needed in the two counties and were definitely surprised when their opinions were not shared by those present at the meeting. The additional surprise came when these two counties, very similar in demographic profiles, also had differing opinions concerning the coalitions they wanted to form. From the outset, the project staff learned a valuable lesson: Never assume that you know what the community needs and is willing to work together to achieve; always ask them what their needs are and what they want to work to achieve.

Continuous leadership development

Leadership development for local community leaders often consists of an organized program of meetings, seminars, and workshops that last one or two days, one week or several weeks. Leadership development is seldom viewed as a continuous need. When one-shot leadership training is the mode of instruction, several problems occur. If the leadership program is not relevant to the leader's current situation, the knowledge and skills gained in the training will suffer from a lack of application and often be forgotten. Leadership development, for both community leaders and coalition members, should be ongoing, and the topics of the development programs should meet the participants' current needs.

Oftentimes, one training session on a particular topic will not be sufficient. For the REEP project, planning workshops were held in both counties, and project staff *assumed* (that deadly word) that all coalition members understood both the elements of the planning process and methods used in developing strategic and long-range plans. During the training, all coalition members received instruction in the use of Gantt and PERT charts. The coalition's use of these planning tools in subsequent meetings convinced the project staff that they understood the planning process. Only 9 months later did they realize that the coalition members may have understood how to use some planning tools but had not completely internalized what they knew about the planning process. Following a second planning workshop, one participant said, "I attended the first workshop you did on this, but I didn't realize that we were going to have to keep doing this. I was used to our getting together to help someone when their house burned. I didn't realize that we were going to have to continuously develop plans to reach all the people who are in need." The cyclical nature of planning as it related to their coalition and their county was slowly becoming an accepted fact of life, but it was not the result of one-shot leadership training and development.

Experiential learning is the most effective learning. It is only in repetition that one gains confidence and belief in newly gained skills. Learning reinforced with positive experiences is also most successful. All leadership training should focus only on the skills the coalition members need to develop at that time, and it should allow for the successful practice of newly gained skills. Allowing the coalition members to determine the projects they want to undertake, helping them to set realistic goals, and giving them the training they need to accomplish these goals is essential to the long-term success of any volunteer community development project.

Leadership development should also be open to everyone; it is not the blessing given to a few. All members of the coalitions should participate in the leadership development events, which should be scheduled with their attendance in mind. Essential topics for all leaders and members of volunteer coalitions include group management skills, including conflict resolution, methods of encouraging participation, and group dynamics; organizational skills including planning, delegation, fund raising, and budgeting; problem resolution skills including problem identification and analysis, setting goals, and group decision making; evaluation skills, including assessment of results and revision of approaches. In addition, all leadership programs should include a reiteration of basic values: the improvement of the quality of life and the maintenance of the dignity of every individual.

Natural leaders have emerged in most of the REEP coalitions, but in some, leadership is sporadic. Lack of strong local leaders is a problem facing many communities, and the causes of this problem are often similar. Many communities have lost their strong leaders of the past, and the opportunities for leadership development have not been readily available to the young. Many communities have "risen to the bait" only to be disappointed, and they are reluctant to rise again. Many have seen daily life situations remain unchanged while being hailed as great changes. It will require much time and patience to develop the leadership strength needed by communities, and it is a problem that, at times, seems unresponsive to outside intervention. Yet leadership training is the key—leadership training that provides opportunities for practice and success with newly learned skills, that does not push the coalitions into efforts they are unready or unwilling to undertake, and that constantly reaffirms the possibility of actual change is essential. At the same time, be aware that communities have not reached the state they are in overnight and that state will not be changed overnight.

Remember to celebrate

A fringe benefit of working with REEP is the experience of participating in community celebrations. Rural people constantly incorporate parties and social events in their activities. Every REEP coalition meeting begins with social chatter and food and ends with more food. McKnight[7] believes, "You will know that you are in a community if you often hear laughter and singing. You will know you are in an institution, corporation, or bureaucracy if you hear the silence of long halls and reasoned meetings."

Social events and celebrations are effective tools for building trust between health professionals and citizens and for recruiting volunteers and motivating community participation. REEP staff sponsor two or three community parties each year to thank volunteers, to celebrate progress, and to laugh and play together. One of the most successful events was a Christmas parade and party organized by a helping hand coalition for the elderly they served. Ten 80 and 90 year-olds, some in wheelchairs, rode on floats blowing kisses and throwing candy to the children.

BARRIERS TO SUCCESS

When REEP was implemented in the counties, many health and social service providers were skeptical about its chance for success. One health provider's comments illustrate this attitude: "These people don't care, and they really don't want any change. They won't volunteer. We are giving them plenty of services and welfare. You are really spinning your wheels." So, the first barrier encountered was professionals who did not trust the capacity of community people to work as equal partners. McKnight[7] says that they see communities as collections of "parochial, inexpert, uninformed, and biased people."

Another barrier is the resistance of hierarchial social service institutions to share power and decision making with citizens. They do not want to lose control and supervisory power over community-based programs. A social service professional was willing to support "using" REEP volunteers to support the agency's programs, but was not willing to "include" volunteers in planning and establishing priorities for those programs.

The interagency councils are assisting to breakdown barriers. Members participate in the leadership training with the coalition members as well as participating as advisors and partners in the coalition's programs. They experience the capacity of the volunteers to make a difference when citizens become empowered. When they embrace the concepts of partnerships and empowerment, they spread the word to their colleagues in the agencies. Slowly, agencies are asking to participate as partners in REEP's community-based programs.

PHILOSOPHICAL ADMONITIONS

Health professionals should enter communities with the purpose of mobilizing the capacities of people to respond to issues. However, communities are not managed, orderly environments, and disenfranchised people are sometimes the least organized, and their voices the most angry or despondent.[3] So, some philosophical admonitions are offered as a foundation for developing community-based primary health care programs that empower citizens.

Community development is a process, not an event

Evolutionary change is not an event that happens one day like Christmas. All evolutionary change takes time, but more often results in a stable organization. Revolutionary change will create an organization that exists only a short time for a purpose that, when achieved, leads to the dissolving of the organization.

Avoid developing a "Messiah complex"

Community empowerment is a process that enables, but does not impose. For community members to recognize and meet the needs of their community may require the intervention of persons or institutions outside the community. This intervention may be teaching the methodology of problem resolution, but the specific solutions to specific problems must be decided by the citizens. Professionals do not simply provide communities with set "answers."

Maintain a policy of inclusion

Respecting the dignity of the individual and community means opening the door to all "stakeholders" who want to participate. Have a policy of inclusion, not exclusion. During leadership training, choose words carefully and constantly repeat key ideas:

- "Working together we can do wonderful things."
- "Involve others, not use others."
- "Who else should we involve in this?"
- "Develop resources, develop people, build communities."
- "When you help to build a cathedral, you may not see it completed in your lifetime."

Go beyond promises

Universities as well as government and private agencies have started many community-based programs to improve citizens' health and quality of life. Some have been very successful, but many have failed. At an organizational meeting for REEP an old woman said, "Other universities have promised to help us. They have used statistics from our county to get funding for themselves. We've been studied and written up. People have created charts and figures and told us that we'll hear from them later. We've never heard from them again. All we want is water, better houses, and jobs. We don't need any more studies. Don't promise if you can't help us."

Nurses can assist communities to organize successful programs that improve health and quality of life. To go beyond promises and to build programs that flourish, nurses must form partnerships with citizens and share power and decision making. George[5] writes, "Successful organizers are those willing to enjoy the reflected glow of others' successes, those who find satisfaction, not in their own production, but in the production of others. We can starve ourselves and others with promises or we can feast together."

REFERENCES

1. Alinsky, S. D. (1971). *Rules for radicals.* New York: Vintage.
2. Braithwaite, R., & Lythcott, N. (1989). Community empowerment as a strategy for health promotion for black and other minority populations. *Journal of the American Medical Association, 261*(2), 282.
3. Dewar, T. (1990). 'Systems' talk turns off citizens. *Metro Monitor, 21*(7), 3.
4. Fuchs, V. R. (1983). *Who shall live.* New York: Basic Books.
5. George, I. R. (1983). *Beyond promises: A guide for rural volunteer program development* (p. 42). Montgomery, Ala: Alabama Office of Voluntary Citizen Participation, State of Alabama Commission on Aging.
6. McKnight, J. L. (1985). Health and empowerment. *Canadian Journal of Public Health, 73,* 37.
7. McKnight, J. L. (1987). Regenerating community. *Social Policy,* 54.
8. U.S. Department of Health and Human Services. (1986). *Report of the secretary's task force on black and minority health.* Washington, D.C.: Author.
9. Williams, D. M. (1991). Policy at the grassroots: Community-based participation in health care policy. *Journal of Professional Nursing, 7*(5), 271.

CHAPTER 32

Leadership for change in public and community health nursing

MARLA E. SALMON

The focus of this chapter* is on leadership as an essential intervention for change in the practice of public and community health nursing. Leadership has come to mean many things in our society and has numerous definitions. For the purposes of this chapter, *leadership* is defined as the ability to envision and communicate a changed future and to foster a dynamic that mobilizes and catalyzes the efforts of many toward that end. In this definition the dynamic between leader and follower is "leadership"; it is not simply what the leader does.

Leadership is viewed as the hallmark of professional nurses. For nurse administrators and supervisors, it is an integral component of the managerial and administrative strategies used to optimize clinical practice. For the overall profession, leadership is seen as a means of advancing the professionalization of nursing; but it has not been viewed as a key intervention strategy for the direct practice of nursing. Nursing care plans or other documentation of the nursing process generally do not include leadership as an intervention; its inclusion would be viewed as highly unconventional. With one critical exception, the clinical practice of individual nurses can proceed on a day-to-day basis without any consideration or utilization of leadership as an intervention strategy. The exception is the practice of public and community health nursing.

Public and community health nursing practice differs from all other nursing practices in a number of significant ways. The departure point for practice, particularly for public health nurses, is public mandate

and responsibility for the health of the public. This mandate translates into a focus on the prevention of premature death and disability and the preservation of health. The client is the public or community; advocacy is for the public and community good. This form of advocacy and focus of practice demand that interventions involve both the formal and informal structures of society and communities. In other words, the policies, organizations, institutions, and other components of the community infrastructure are the focuses for action; the community is the client. The tangible, reassuring, here-and-now character of other types of clinical nursing practice is not a constant dimension of public and community health nursing. While the practice for the entry-level practitioner of public health and community health nursing may involve predominantly hands-on nursing care, the *raison d'être* is the well-being of the community and public. Advanced practice, which may appear indirect relative to other forms of nursing, is quite direct in the domain of moving the health status of communities and populations.[13] To accomplish this, nurses must effectively use leadership as an applied clinical strategy.

THE CLIENT'S CURRENT CONDITION

The nature of leadership as an essential strategy for public and community health nurses is best emphasized by examining the condition of the client. Currently, there are some key factors or determinants of health in communities and American society in general that seriously affect the health of their members. These determinants constitute the domain of public health and community health nursing practice and require that interventions address them directly, rather than

---

*The views expressed in this chapter are solely those of the author and not necessarily those of the Department of Health and Human Services.

focusing only on the person whose health is affected. The determinants are classified in four general categories: (1) social, (2) medical/technological/organizational, (3) environmental, and (4) human or biological.[20] The common theme in all these determinants is that the ability of individuals to affect them on behalf of communities and society is greatly enhanced by the leadership in public policy and social institutions. For public and community health nurses to play a role in these arenas, leadership must also be their key intervention.

SOCIAL DETERMINANTS OF HEALTH

The concept of society is frequently viewed as the backdrop for public health nursing interventions. Most of us have a general understanding that individuals and families exist in a social context and that there is some relationship between their health and that of the broader society. However, what is frequently not operationalized is the understanding that the well-being of individuals and families is, in large measure, a direct consequence of social forces. For public health nurses to be effective, these social forces must be altered. Part of the challenge of leadership in public health nursing is to move the social backdrop of health into the forefront as a target of intervention. To do this, one must also know both in broad and highly specific terms the forces with which they should relate. Some of these are discussed here.

One significant social trend affecting the health of people today has been the emergence of concern for health promotion and disease prevention. In 1979, the federal government published "Healthy People: The Surgeon General's Report on Health Promotion and Disease Prevention."[18] It was the first report of its type and clearly outlined a national agenda for health promotion and disease prevention in the United States. This report and its successor, "Healthy People 2000: National Health Promotion and Disease Prevention Objectives,"[19] reflect two major social phenomena: Americans' realization that lifestyle is a major determinant of health and the burgeoning cost of health care.

While recognition of the importance of health promotion and disease prevention (HPDP) and concern for rising costs of health care are important, they do not alone describe the social forces requiring the leadership of public health nurses. In fact, they cannot be viewed in isolation from the larger social picture in which they exist. To have any impact on either the expansion of HPDP or reduction of health care costs, this larger context must be understood.

As we approach the twenty-first century, we are facing challenges the magnitude of which make them unlike any we have faced previously. There are emerging social trends that call for major shifts in both what individuals and institutions do if they are to have any positive impact. Perhaps the most significant of these trends fall into the category of "demographics."

To preface this discussion of demographics, or measures of different aspects of society, it is important to understand two simple facts: culture changes over time and variations among groups. What this means for this discussion is that the diversity that is created by both the changes in the "aging" of our society and those that come with changes in our ethnic and racial makeup, is the central challenge in all of the demographics trends described here.

Let us begin by considering the family. We are no longer a society in which the nuclear, dual-parent, married family constitutes the largest proportion of households. While this was the case in 1970, it is not the case today. Traditional family households have decreased and have been offset most significantly by nontraditional households, including those with only one individual, single parent, and married households without children.[17] While many conclusions can be drawn from this, perhaps the most important is that our operating assumptions about our society and how to provide services to "families" need to change dramatically and that our clients' understandings of "family," dependent upon age group, will be very different.

Taking a closer look at those people who make up our households, we find that the age profile has shifted. By the year 2020, we will have a society in which almost 1 of every 5 persons is beyond retirement age. We have been successful in expansion of the overall lifespan,[16] but with it has come the complex problems of prolonged illness, disability, and emerging new chronic diseases.

Demographics are also changing for children. For example, the annual increase in the white population between 1980 and 1989 was about 0.8%, approximately half of the increase among blacks, which was 1.5%. The growth in the Hispanic population, which was about 3.7%, was more than 4 times the rate of increase of the white population.[16] With these difference in population growth rates come many opportunities and challenges. One specific challenge is that of making our health promotion and disease prevention efforts truly relevant to children whose color, culture, and language at home may be totally different from the public health nurses and institutions who serve them.

Our children are really a mirror for our overall society. Their demographics are both created by and a reflection of those of their parents and the larger social context. Children are leading the trend that is becoming known as "the emerging majority." What this means, quite simply, is that our basic assumptions about the majority/minority makeup of our society are rapidly becoming obsolete. The current white, "mainstream," majority population is increasingly being replaced by the current ethnic and racial minority populations. With the growth of these minority populations comes a wealth of different cultures, languages, and traditions—as well as new challenges relating to the disparate risk for health problems among some of these peoples. Consider the challenge represented in the simple projection that by the year 2000, the majority of school children will come from ethnic and racial minority groups. The challenges of the year 2000 are not far away; for some areas of the country, they are here. "Ethnicity is a challenge itself. Nearly 100 languages are spoken in state schools. In San Francisco, classes may well be taught in Chinese, Japanese, Spanish, Tagalog, Korean, Polish, Russian, and Armenian."[9]

The demographics of household composition and diversity do not capture the totality of social conditions impacting health. Intertwined with these are some major social trends impacting all groups. Among these are increasing poverty and violence. It is important that these be considered relative to each group and their impact assessed. For the purposes of discussion here, let us look briefly at how these affect the well-being of children. A sobering glimpse of this impact was presented in a *Washington Post* interview with Marion Wright Edelman:

Every 39 seconds in the United States an infant is born into poverty; every 14 minutes an infant dies; every 117 seconds an infant is born too small to be healthy; every 2 minutes an infant is born to a mother who received late or no prenatal care; every 31 seconds an infant is born to an unmarried mother; every 64 seconds an infant is born to a teenage mother; and every 3 hours another child is murdered.[4]

We also know that the children of today are increasingly a part of our homeless population. Women and children are among the fastest growing group of homeless people in our country, and the majority of homeless children in shelters are in their pre-school years.

Other major social trends impacting on the health of all people in our society are those relating to the breakdown of national barriers in a variety of areas. Among these the most important is the emergence of a global economy in which the United States is but one of a number of major players. The impact of emerging nationalism in many parts of the world, including the former Soviet Union and the related warfare, all have an effect on our society as well. We are no longer isolated, nor will we ever be again.

The well-being of all people in our society is clearly related to those social factors briefly discussed in this section. To impact the health of these people, the origins of their conditions must be altered. What this means for public health nursing is that we must also alter our assumptions and paradigms; we cannot operate individually or organizationally as if society is or will be the same as it was yesterday. We must also operate in concert with others. Social forces are simply not amenable to the actions of one discipline alone. Interdisciplinary strategies are the only ones that have promise for success.[7] The implications for public health nursing practice are simple: leadership is required to create this type of change.

MEDICAL/TECHNICAL/ORGANIZATIONAL DETERMINANTS OF HEALTH

The nature of medical technology and services and how they are organized and financed reflect and also affect the values, resources, and nature of society in general. Too often, however, these factors are not viewed by health professionals as key determinants of the health of communities and their members for which they are responsible.

We are currently experiencing a wide-scale recognition that health care costs are too high, too many people are uninsured, and the way we currently provide services is inadequate to meet the health care needs of this country. This recognition is now so pervasive that it is a part of almost every national political campaign. The debate is on, but where we go as a country is quite unclear. This discussion will specifically address some key themes that are or will impact on health.

"Health care reform" is the catch-all phrase that reflects two major areas of the ongoing debate. How we should organize the delivery of health care and how/who should pay for it? The underlying concerns are increasing access to care while decreasing or controlling cost. Public health nurses should become conversant in the key proposals that are or will be put forth in the coming years. Among these is one which specifically incorporates the potential contributions of nursing: "Nursing's Agenda for Health Care Reform."[11]

Some crucial tensions in the debate about health care reform have not been resolved. Perhaps the most important from a public health perspective is how to assure that public health services are not omitted from the frequently narrow concepts of what constitutes adequate services. Because of the highly medical "nature" of the health care system and fairly widespread lack of appreciation for the role of primary prevention and interventions beyond the "patient" and his or her provider, public health may be inadequately addressed in this emerging system. Many of the discussions have focused on the need to move the trend toward specialization in medicine back to generalization.[10] The need for expanding primary care services has also been addressed.

Another tension is between whole scale reform of financing and modification of the current methods, including expansion of reimbursement to encompass some health promotion and disease prevention activities, as well as those provided by nurse practitioners, certified nurse-midwives, and others.[3] Because financing of services, particularly since the advent of Medicare and medical assistance, has had a tremendous impact on the delivery of public health nursing services, this current debate is one in which public health nurses should play a major part.

The "access to care" discussion is a major part of the current debate. Managed care, case management, and cost containment are dimensions of access that should be of particular interest to public health nurses. Managed care may well be a future domain for health departments; case management should already be part of the practice of public health nurses. The fact that public health nurses have done case management for as long as the profession has existed carries little weight in the discussions today of who should do case management. The leadership of public health nurses is needed in this area of debate.

What is frequently not recognized in other areas of discussion of access is that access to services is not assured simply by enabling payment for services. The serious health care questions of today transcend payment for services to individuals and are systems-level questions that need to be asked by public health nurses and others. Among these is, How can we assure that there are appropriate providers available to those who need them? This includes concerns for well-prepared, culturally competent providers who not only are there when care is sought, but are also seeking those who should receive services. There is an operant premise in many of today's debates that services begin when a person "presents" to the system for care. This premise is woefully inadequate when considering those problems that most impact the health of our society. It is frequently those who do not recognize the need for services, preventive or otherwise, who need those services most.

Another dimension to the question of assuring that appropriate providers are available is that of assuring that they are permitted to practice.[12] In the cases of nurse-midwives and nurse practitioners, there is a long history of situations in which they have been prepared and available to practice but not able to do so because of unreasonably restrictive laws or policies relating to scope of practice or prescriptive authority and reimbursement. Unless progress is made in these domains, the promise of expanded access will not be fulfilled.

Another important question addresses how we can support and further develop a public health infrastructure that "assures" the health of the public and deal with those health problems not addressed in the primary care domain.[5] Most proposals for reform of our systems focus on making people well; few focus on the importance of protecting their health. If ignored, this failure can have serious consequences.[2]

To enhance the health of people in this country, it is essential that we have adequate surveillance and the ability to employ targeted responses to health problems in a timely manner. AIDS, multidrug resistant TB, and infant mortality are all nationwide examples of problems dependant on this type of infrastructure at national, state, and local levels if they are to be addressed or prevented.

The public health infrastructure question is particularly important for public health nurses—and one not often understood. Public health nurses cannot be effective in health promotion and disease prevention activities in systems that are unable to identify "need" and impact. All too frequently, public health nurses grow to assume that the services they provide (often clinic based) are meeting the health needs of the public. Unfortunately, they are at best only meeting the needs of those who "show up." Unless there is system that can tell us whom we miss and what we do, public health nurses cannot be effective.

Finally, whether direct or indirect services are the focal point of health care reform, one must question how we can assure that quality is as much a driving force as cost containment. Establishing and maintaining quality assurance mechanisms at all levels of service are essential. Part of these quality assurance mechanisms should be ways of assuring adequate educational preparation. We know that there is a significant gap already in what PHNs are prepared to do and what they actually do.[6,14] This gap could, in part, be addressed through appropriate quality assurance mechanisms. Although they should be addressed, it is fairly certain that they will not be adequately addressed without the leadership of public health nurses.

Although health care reform is the centerpiece of current activity in the medical/technical/organizational domain, the technology and state of "medical" arts should not be ignored. We are clearly a society in which technology is viewed as an answer to almost every problem, particularly in health care. The cost of both the development technology and its use/misuse have become part of much of the discussion about health care today. What technology should we develop and use? Which should be avoided? Public health nurses and their work is generally "low tech" in nature and, sometimes, technology preventing. What this means is that if the health promotion and disease prevention efforts of PHNs are successful, then the later need for technology dependent treatments can be avoided. This does not mean, however, that the practice of public health nursing cannot be enhanced through technology.

Public health nurses are scarce resources who should look to technology as a means for decreasing their unnecessary work and enhancing the services they provide. PHNs should be on the forefront of exploring ways in which technology might better enable them to reach their clients. The telephone is a technology that we use on a daily basis without giving it a second thought. We use it to communicate and observe or receive observations. We should be looking at other ways of doing these simple actions. For example, the promise of fiber optics might offer PHNs ways of interacting with their clients visually. To be able to teach or answer a client's question through visual demonstration would be of tremendous assistance and would allow the PHN to observe the client. We could also transfer data through this mechanism, including monitoring blood pressures or other physiologic measures.

We should also be expanding our use of computers and the roles that we play in developing and using data. Modem-linked, miniature computers could allow PHNs to link up with information needed from almost anywhere. Again, this is an example of technology enhancing practice.

The interface of public health nursing and health-related technology is practically unlimited. As genetic solutions to health problems become increasingly incorporated in preventive strategies, PHNs will need to become better informed and able to combine their "high-touch" skills with the high-tech solutions.

The effective use of appropriate technology, as well as the development of mechanisms to decrease misuse of technology, should all be viewed as within the domain of public health nurses. Quite simply, technology can and does either enhance or harm the health of people.

ENVIRONMENTAL DETERMINANTS OF HEALTH

In terms of impact, the environment may be the single most important determinant of health in the very near future. It is also the determinant about which nurses perhaps know the least. The nursing literature on environmental health and the role of public and community health nurses is alarmingly sparse. Most content is found in the area of occupational health nursing, particularly in the industrial context. Environmental problems of concern to public health nurses include the disposal of hazardous waste (including toxic industrial waste and radioactive-contaminated materials), acid rain, urban lead poisoning, air pollution, and water pollution. Global concerns include the depletion of the ozone layer, with its accompanying weather changes and warming of oceans. We also face environmental threats relating to thermonuclear and chemical arms proliferation and warfare.

Part of the leadership required of public and community health nurses relates to the task of educating ourselves and others about what environmental health issues are and how to intervene effectively. Clearly all of the environmental issues relate to the state of environmental policy and regulation, but nurses must learn to insert themselves into the debates surrounding these issues, while, at the same time becoming involved in the specifics of potential and actual exposures of their clientele. Macinick and Macinick[8] suggest some action guidelines for nurses to begin to solve the problems of our environment, including the following: being willing to admit to the idea of asymptomatic, subclinical toxicity and the multiple-effects disease model; being aware that environmental toxicology is a politically charged issue involving the world of high finance and corporate egos; being able to accept disbelief and even anger toward the messenger; and being aware that almost no research on the synergistic effects of low-level toxins has been done, leading to downplaying of their importance. They suggest that nurses' most helpful tool is knowledge, which will also enable the nurse to begin educating the community about the effects of low levels of pollution. Macinick and Macinick's suggestions are particularly useful to public health nurses, whose practice frequently include some types of hazard communication.

Another aspect of the environment not often considered as part of public health nursing is the weather and its health effects. The increase in malignant melanoma is but one aspect of this factor. Another aspect is the effect of violent weather, as was recently evidence in the hurricanes Andrew and Iniki. Both the direct impact, such as injury and destruction, as well as those from water contamination, lack of safe food, psychological trauma, and inadequate health services are all within the domain of public health nursing. In areas where violent weather is fairly common, PHNs should be involved in the development of community education to minimize the human impact and to maximize emergency preparedness.

Finally, a whole category of environmental hazards relates to physical safety, including vehicle safety, workplace safety, household, school, and day care safety. These hazards can include everything from asbestos to poorly lit stairways and many times are amenable to simple interventions, such as protective devices (seatbelt and helmets); preventive strategies, including regulation (equipment shields, inspections, smoke alarms, etc.); and educational strategies. Given the tremendous impact of these hazards on morbidity and mortality[11] and, frequently, the ease with which they can be addressed, public health nurses have a major role to play.

Leadership strategies for public health nurses that relate to these and other environmental determinants must again cross disciplines and include the community, particularly in the area of environmental determinants. Nurses generally do not possess the technical sophistication and specialized knowledge required to assess and monitor hazards. They do, however, have the general leadership and health knowledge required to bring together the many people needed to address these issues.

HUMAN AND BIOLOGICAL DETERMINANTS OF HEALTH

The human and biological health determinant, probably the most familiar and comfortable to nurses, is one in which significant public health issues have emerged in this last decade. We have observed the appearance of devastating and exotic infectious diseases such as AIDS, toxic shock syndrome, herpes, and Legionnaires' disease. More than any other disease, AIDS, coupled with the reemergence of new strains and epidemics of diseases formerly thought to be under control, such as tuberculosis (now multi-drug resistant TB), syphilis, gonorrhea, mumps, measles, diphtheria, and flu, has radically altered the course of public health in this nation. The global eradication of smallpox in the 1970s signaled a new era in public health in which there was great optimism that the age of infectious disease was coming to an end, but this hope has been erased. Not only has there been a resurgence in infectious diseases, public health practitioners are also faced with challenges of chronic disease associated with growing numbers of the elderly. The increasingly grave and diverse disease picture in public and community health has not been accompanied by an increase in resources or systems to address these problems. The development of effective strategies, including those relating to resources, must involve the leadership of public and community health nurses to be appropriately responsive.

Public health practitioners are also confronted with the promises and threats to society inherent in the reality of genetic engineering. The ethical, moral, legal, social, and economic questions surrounding developments in this area fall squarely in the domain of public health. Society will confront these issues in all arenas: individual, family, community, state, and national. How these issues are resolved depends greatly on who provides the leadership. The inclusion of public and community health nurses in these debates is essential to an outcome sensitive to and respectful of the public good and the public health.

A final concern relating to human biology and overall well-being is the challenge of enabling people to optimize their own health. Although the lifestyle movement certainly provides answers for the middle and upper classes, which have options associated with their financial resources, it does not address the needs of less fortunate people. Questions of how to ensure that all people are equipped with the advantages of a healthy fetal and early childhood experience, adequate nutrition, immunizations, exercise, and the skills of self-development are not easily answered through most of the current lifestyle programs. Children are still bearing children and are destroying themselves and others through drug abuse, suicide, and other forms of violence. These questions clearly cannot be addressed solely at the one-to-one level. They require the leadership of those close to the problems, committed to the good of the community, and skilled in understanding the relationship between the health of the individual and the broader society.

THE NEXT STEPS

Although the condition of the client—our communities and society—is clearly grave, it is not without hope or an agenda for action. "Healthy People 2000" provides a clear sense of national direction.[19] What is perplexing, however, is that for many of the problems that we face today, we already know many of the answers. Never before have we known as much about health as we do now; what we do not seem to know is how to put this knowledge into action. Again, this requires leadership.

The July 4, 1988, issue of *Newsweek* published a special report that portrayed a number of "unsung heroes."[15] This classic article is noteworthy because it highlighted the accomplishments of "everyday" people who had made a major positive impact on the well-being of others. These stories are really lessons in leadership. Each of these "heroes" was unwilling to accept the status quo; he or she took action and effected change. Although not trained to accomplish what they undertook, they had a vision of a better situation and pursued this vision with personal commitment, courage, and involvement with the community. Of all of the attributes of leadership, these are perhaps the most important. Another noteworthy theme in this report was that for each of these individuals, *people* were the primary means for achieving change. These leaders relied on themselves and others as the means for effecting change; they did not wait for technical or economic answers.

The message here for public and community health nurses is that leadership is necessary and attainable. The lessons from the unsung heroes—vision, conviction, and the courage to act—are an excellent departure point. Another worthwhile lesson was their willingness to work with others. Finally, the reason that these heroes are "unsung" is that they did things in their own backyards and communities; their actions were local, beginning at home.

The next step for public and community health nursing is to focus on nursing's leadership interventions. Understanding the condition of the client and the factors creating this condition is only the beginning. The future health of the client—our communities and society—relies greatly on the development of leadership as the key strategy for public and community health nursing. The challenge is perhaps best stated by a memorable aphorism from the 1960s: If you are not part of the solution, you are part of the problem. If public and community health nurses are not part of the leadership required to enhance the health of society, then we are, in fact, contributing to its decline.

REFERENCES

1. American Nurses Association. (1991). Nursing's agenda for health care reform. *American Nurse,* Supp. PR-3, 220M.
2. Braunstein, J. (1991). National health care: Necessary but not sufficient. *Nursing Outlook, 39*(2), 54-55.
3. Brecht, M. C. (1990). Nursing's role in assuring access to care. *Nursing Outlook, 38*(1), 6-7.
4. French, M. (1992, May 10). The measure of her success, Marian Wright Edelman's lessons on raising kids, and on raising consciousness. *The Washington Post,* Sec. F1.
5. The future of public health. (1981). *Report of the Institute of Medicine Committee for the study of public health.* Washington, D.C.: National Academy Press.
6. Jones, D. C., Davis, J. A., & Davis, M. D. (1987). *Public health nursing education and practice.* Springfield, Va: National Technical Information Service.
7. Lindsey, A. M. (1988). Editorial, strengths and challenges: Nursing in the 21st century. *Journal of Professional Nursing, 4* (2), 71-72.
8. Macinick, C. G., & Macinick, J. W. (1987). Toxic New World: What nurses can do to cope with a polluted environment. *International Nursing Review, 34*(2), 40.
9. Michael, M. (1992, May 4). Society education, Another lost generation. *Newsweek,* pp. 70-72.
10. Mullan, F. (1992). Missing: A national medical manpower policy. *The Milbank Quarterly, 70*(2).
11. The National Committee for Injury Prevention and Control. (1989). Injury prevention: meeting the challenge. *Oxford University Press, 5*(3).
12. Safriet, B. J. (1992). Health care dollars and regulatory sense: The role of advanced practice nursing. *The Yale Journal on Regulation, 9, 2.*
13. Salmon, M. E. (1989, Sept/Oct). Public health nursing: The neglected specialty. *Nursing Outlook, 37*(5), 226-229.
14. Salmon, M. E., Selby, M. L., & Muller, R. (1989). Master's-level community/public health nursing needs: A national survey of leaders in service and education. *Research Report to the National League for Nursing.* New York: National League for Nursing.

15. Special report: A holiday for heroes. (1988, July 4). *Newsweek,* p. 34.
16. U.S. Bureau of the Census. (1988). *Projections of the population of the United States by age, sex, and race: 1988-2080.* (Pub. No. 1018). Washington, D.C.: U.S. Government Printing Office.
17. U.S. Department of Commerce, Bureau of the Census. (1992). *How we're changing, demographic state of the nation: 1992.* (Pub. No. 177). Washington, D.C.: U.S. Government Printing Office.
18. U.S. Department of Health, Education, and Welfare. (1979). *Healthy people: The Surgeon General's report on health promotion and disease prevention.* Washington, D.C.: Author.
19. U.S. Department of Health and Human Services, Public Health Service. (1990). *Healthy people 2000: National health promotion and disease prevention objectives.* (Pub. No. PHS 91-50213). Washington, D.C.: Author.
20. White, M. S. (1982). Construct for public health nursing. *Nursing Outlook, 30*(9), 527.

CHAPTER 33

Nurse-midwifery

A nursing challenge

EUNICE K. M. ERNST

Nurse-midwifery in the United States was founded by Mary Breckinridge at the Frontier Nursing Service in the Appalachian Mountains of southeastern Kentucky in 1925. Although the service was established primarily to address the needs of children, the underlying principle was that if one cared for the mother, the mother would care for the child. Thus flows the logic that the care of children begins with the care of the mother and family. This comprehensive view sent Mary Breckinridge in search of a provider to meet the needs of the people to be served. After careful study of nursing in the United States and midwifery in Europe and Britain, she determined that the needs of rural families would be served best by combining the talents of the public health nurse and the midwife as seen in the highlands of Scotland.

The Maternity Center Association (MCA) in New York City came to much the same conclusion after an independent investigation of British and European education for midwifery. In 1931, MCA opened the first school of midwifery for registered nurses in affiliation with its urban nurse-midwifery clinic and home birth service for poor and new immigrant women. The outstanding records of these two pioneering services are well documented and legendary.[2,7,10,22,24]

Similar demonstrations of the effectiveness of midwifery care, of nurse-midwives and physicians working together in a common commitment to improve care for childbearing families, have been replicated in a variety of settings in the United States over the past 60 years. In large medical centers, small community hospitals, and freestanding birth centers, nurse-midwives have shown that they can provide safe and satisfying care to women. In both rural and urban areas, medically underserved and overserved areas, in public service and private practice, nurse-midwives provide high-quality, cost-effective care.* Yet, nurse-midwifery has never really been embraced by the health care delivery system, and the problems of maternity care in the United States give evidence to this. Our rates of infant mortality, cesarean sections, teen pregnancy, and access to care is well below other industrialized nations, while our costs are the highest in the world. The wealthiest nation in the world seems unable to guarantee even the simplest care to all women who have willingly or unwittingly embarked on bringing forth and nurturing a new generation.

Only in the past decade have health policy makers on national and state levels begun to recognize the potential of nurse-midwifery care and have recommended expansion of nurse-midwifery services. Former Surgeon General Dr. Julius Richmond, in a symposium on nurse-midwifery in 1986, exhorted nurse-midwives to stand firm in the face of barriers to their profession and to recognize their invaluable contributions to improving the health status of women and infants, especially minority women, saying, "To a large degree it lies in your power to realign the national and local debate to include issues of social justice, equity and compassion. Perhaps more than any other health profession, midwifery has been able to inject human values into the provision of health care."[18]

This is a broad challenge to nurse-midwifery and nursing. Decisions on how to meet this challenge raise issues about nurse-midwifery and its role in the evolving system for health care delivery.

---

*References 3, 5, 6, 8, 12, 18, 20, 23.

BACKGROUND

Significant changes began in the late 1940s when the postwar demand for greater access to medical care spawned publicly funded expansion of medical education and construction of community hospitals. Third-party reimbursement, which paid only for physician and hospital services, became available through employer benefit programs. In the 1960s, the poor gained access to medical and hospital care through tax-supported Medicaid programs. The place of birth became the acute-care hospital and the sole care provider the physician. Birth was removed from the bosom of the family and became a fragmented medical care event. Home birth and midwives became almost extinct.

All of this was done without studying the potential impact on families or society. Hospitalization is often credited with the improved outcomes of pregnancy and birth, which is true for the minority of women who have complications. However, subsidized nutrition and women's ability to exercise control over their reproduction also had a significant impact on outcomes for the majority of women. In 1982, the Institute of Medicine reviewed all research on birth settings and reported that the place of birth had never been adequately studied.[6]

In 1959, the Maternity Center Association, struggling to keep midwifery education alive and in keeping with the shift to university-based nursing education, accepted the invitation of Dr. Louis Hellman to move the School of Midwifery into the Downstate Medical Center of the State University of New York, Kings County Hospital. The home birth service was closed. At Kings County Hospital, nurse-midwives demonstrated their ability to work closely with the resident medical staff in the acute-care setting. In the 1960s and 1970s, 24 educational programs opened in affiliation with universities across the country, and nurse-midwives began to be recruited for employment by public hospitals and clinics to supplement physician care to low-income women.

As nurse-midwives demonstrated their abilities to care for the poor, the natural childbirth movement gained momentum among informed and insured middle-class women. They began to ask for more than what was offered by the physician/hospital acute-care system. In response, two studied demonstrations were mounted to meet their needs:

- In Philadelphia in 1971, a childbirth educator, an obstetrician, and a nurse-midwife proposed to the Salvation Army that its underutilized hospital for unwed mothers be converted into a family-centered, one-class care facility staffed by an obstetrician/nurse-midwife team. Philadelphia is a city with five medical schools providing ample access to medical care, yet Booth Maternity Center, supported by the Maternity Center Association and the Salvation Army, conducted a highly successful demonstration of the readiness of middle-class American women for family-centered, nurse-midwifery care that crossed all class barriers.[4]

- In New York in 1975, the Maternity Center Association established the demonstration of the freestanding birth center for women seeking more control over their childbirth experience. The freestanding birth center, a concept primarily developed by nurse-midwives and sometimes owned and operated by nurse-midwives and nurses, became licensed health care facilities and eligible for third-party reimbursement.[9]

These demonstrations of organized obstetrician/nurse-midwife collaboration in the private sector raised new issues about third-party reimbursement for both nurse-midwives and birth centers and about hospital practice privileges for nurse-midwives. Private nurse-midwifery practices grew. The relationship of nurse-midwives to physicians and hospitals had begun to change. A new joint statement between organized obstetric and organized nurse-midwifery was drafted.

THE CONSTRAINTS AND THE CHALLENGE

It has taken 60 years to bring nurse-midwifery near to the mainstream of health care in the United States. One nursing leader describes nurse-midwifery as "the flying wedge for nursing."[16] Those who have worked to document the contribution that nurse-midwifery could make to the health and welfare of childbearing families will tell you that it has been an uphill climb all the way and that medicine and nursing sometimes present the most formidable constraints.

Constraints on education

The most effective constraint on the expansion of nurse-midwifery in the first four to five decades was at the point of entry: the education programs. When nurse-midwifery education moved into the university teaching centers, the clinical teaching sites came under the control of medicine. Student nurse-midwives, who had made a career commitment to serve childbearing women, stood at the end of a long line for clinical teaching experience. Medical students and interns, who might never again care for a woman in childbirth, were given priority. This single factor, more than any other, limited the number of nurses admitted to nurse-midwifery education programs and therefore the number of nurse-midwives in practice.

By the mid-1980s, in spite of the increase in the numbers of education programs and federal funding for education through the division of nursing, the profession failed to produce the numbers needed to meet a growing demand for its services. As practice opportunities expanded and service salaries increased, it became more and more difficult to recruit faculty for education programs. This limited student admissions and made it difficult for new programs to be established. Nurse-midwifery was in a catch-22. A resurgence of lay midwifery emerged to fill the void.

Over the past decade major medical centers across the nation have begun to include nurse-midwives on the perinatal care teams, and a concerted effort has been made to establish new education programs. Community hospitals and private obstetricians are employing or contracting with nurse-midwives to provide care to clients at all income levels. As reimbursement for services became available, freestanding birth centers and private nurse-midwifery practices have grown.[1,13,15,19] The increased variety and volume of practice sites is making it possible to place increasing numbers of students, thereby reducing the barrier of competing with medical students and residents for clinical learning opportunities.

A major breakthrough in education was realized in 1989 by a pilot program of community-based nurse-midwifery education (CNEP). Nurses often express a desire to become a nurse-midwife. Many nurses report that they entered nursing to become a midwife but they married, had children, and were unable to leave children and employment to pursue an on-campus education. The CNEP removed these barriers to education for these nurses. This program alone admitted 110 students in 1992.

Constraints to practice

Initially the primary constraints to the practice of nurse-midwifery were the myths about the safety of midwifery care and the view that it was second-class care. This has been refuted by research showing that nurse-midwives can reduce rates of neonatal mortality and cesarean sections, reduce or contain costs, and increase client satisfaction.

Barriers to the development of nurse-midwifery practice today vary from state to state and community to community. They have included the temporary loss of the profession's liability insurance coverage, which in turn caused a temporary but serious reduction of applications to education programs in the mid-1980s; denial of hospital and prescription-writing privileges; rulings by state nursing boards permitting nurses to take orders only from physicians; inability to obtain agreements from physicians for obstetrical consultation and referral for midwifery clients who develop problems; a liability insurance surcharge on physicians working with nurse-midwives; and, most recently, denial of liability insurance for nurse-midwives attending women giving birth at home.

Underlying these visible barriers is the physician's fear of competition from nurse-midwives for the private patient. The opportunities for gatekeeping are found at many levels in the delivery of health care services. The gatekeepers of most barriers to nurse-midwifery practice in the health care system, if not physicians, are usually indoctrinated to the premise that health care is medical care and that the physician is the only eligible provider. This premise is supported by the negative reference to all other providers as "non-physician providers." One nurse-midwife observes that, like a nondairy creamer, the reference acknowledges what you are not rather than what you are.

Nurse-midwifery practice opportunities have grown in spite of these conflicts and constraints because of the growing need for providers in underserved areas and consumer demand for midwifery care in the private sector and, yet to be fully appreciated, the cost benefits of matching the numbers of primary health care providers and specialist medical care providers to the needs of the population being served.

NURSING PREREQUISITE CHALLENGED

Over the past two decades, also in response to women seeking alternatives to physician-hospital services, there has been a rebirth of the "lay midwife," the empirically trained midwife. She is usually a mother who learned by apprenticing to another lay midwife and is responding primarily to women who seek to give birth at home. Unlike the "granny midwife" of old, today's lay midwife is usually middle class, well educated, articulate, and well paid for her services. As she has gained experience and confidence, she questions the need for the prerequisite of nursing for midwifery education. Serious criticism is leveled at nursing by these new midwives. They allege that nursing education promulgates the medical model of pregnancy as an illness and birth as a medical event. They further allege that nursing education teaches subservience to medical doctrine even when that doctrine is not supported by scientific research.

There has not been a serious study of nurse-midwifery versus direct-entry midwifery education in the United States. The graduate program at Yale University offers direct entry to midwifery in a three-year program that includes nursing. The Seattle School of Midwifery offers direct entry to a three-year midwifery program. The views of individual nurse-midwives are divided and the profession has avoided taking a stand on whether it is essential to be a nurse before becoming a midwife. However, most agree that, if not a prerequisite, the inclusion of aspects of nursing education are desirable.

Efforts to separate midwifery from nursing have been taken into the political arena in state legislatures. As this publication goes to press, proposed legislation on midwifery in New York State has brought to the public forum the conflicting interests of organized obstetrics to retain control over the practice of midwifery, lay midwives to establish a profession independent of nursing, nursing to retain the broad base of nursing education as a prerequisite for midwifery, and the conflicted views of the nurse-midwives caught in the middle.

Empirically trained midwives have succeeded in legitimizing their practice in a number of states. Although there are one or two recognized formal education programs for direct entry to midwifery (Washington and California), apprentice programs are offered by groups in several states including Texas, New Mexico, California, and Colorado. Some feel that the emergence of this new midwife is a clear sign that there are voids in the present system of care that nurse-midwives and physicians are either unable or unwilling to fill.

Other countries, in exploring more efficient and effective models for delivery of maternity care services, have also looked at issues of midwifery education and practice. The Ministry of Health in the province of Ontario, Canada, reacting to consumer pressure for midwifery care and intense lobbying by articulate women's groups and lay midwives, conducted an exhaustive study of midwifery education in Britain, Europe, and the United States.[11] Upon review of the information collected, a decision was made to open a four-year, university-based, direct-entry midwifery education program. Also in response to consumer demand the Ministry of Health established four hospital-based birthing centers and recently authorized three free-standing birth centers. In 1993 the provinces of Quebec and British Columbia are following the path taken by Ontario.

These events notwithstanding, it remains that most of the hard evidence on midwifery care available in the United States has been generated by nurse-midwives. It is this evidence that has caused policy makers to look at nurse-midwifery as a viable adjunct to improving our system of health care to childbearing families. This 60-year record of nurse-midwives educated in an organized program of study of theory and practice has sometimes been transposed to make a case for midwives trained only by apprenticeship without an organized curriculum or standards for practice. Midwives trained in the apprentice system without a sound theoretical base need to apply the same rigorous evaluation of their education and practice. Only then can these two approaches be objectively appraised. A university-based, formal program for "direct entry" to midwifery education, as proposed in Canada, would be a new model of education for the United States.

The challenge to nursing on the issue of whether or not nursing is an essential requirement for entry to midwifery education is that there is evidence of a vacuum in the system for providing maternity care services that must be filled. If nurses do not move to fill the vacuum, it will be filled by others. How important is midwifery to the profession of nursing? How important is nursing to the profession of midwifery? Will nurse-midwifery expand or will a new midwife evolve?

These questions are unsettling in a time when American nurse-midwives appear to be on the verge of overcoming major barriers to expanding practice opportunities and educational programs. It is clearly a time for nursing to look carefully at the leadership nurse-midwifery has provided for nursing over the past six decades in establishing practice models. It is also a time for obstetrical nurses to examine their role in meeting the challenges posed by women, parents, government, business, and industry for affordable solutions to the delivery of health care. Judith Rooks has described this time as a "window of opportunity" for nurse-midwives.[17]

Prudence almost dictates that nurses and nurse-midwives come together in a concentrated effort to build on the foundation for growth that has been carefully laid down over the past 60 years. Other routes of entry to midwifery education are certainly an option that may be explored, but it should not impede the development of nurse-midwifery and the nursing contribution it can make at this critical time.

THE BIRTH CENTER: A PLACE FOR MIDWIFERY
The birth center

The freestanding birth center is defined by the National Association of Childbearing Centers as a primary care service, "a place for the practice of midwifery." It is based on principles that propose a view of pregnancy and birth as normal until proven otherwise and that care of women anticipating normal progress in pregnancy and birth does not require admission to the acute-care setting until indicated. This represents a major change in the restructuring of the delivery of maternity and women's health care delivery services. It challenges us to match the providers and services to the people we serve. If 75% to 80% of women in pregnancy and birth do not require the medical/surgical intervention of an obstetrician in the acute-care setting, it is logical to begin to educate women to the primary care of the nurse-midwife in the birth center setting. This will necessitate a significant increase in midwifery providers and a reeducation of the public and of medical specialists to the benefits of collaboration and cooperation in the delivery of services.

The Maternity Center Association (MCA) is a 70-year-old voluntary health agency with a commitment to demonstration of innovative care that is sensitive to the needs of childbearing families. In 1975, perceiving the ferment brewing in the delivery of maternity care services, MCA opened the Childbearing Center, a demonstration of a freestanding birth center with a program of care directed at healthy women and families seeking more control, more responsibility, and more participation in their childbirth experience. The Childbearing Center is one of the earliest demonstrations of a community nursing center.

Program. The clinical aspects of the program pivot on careful and continuous screening for problems that may require medical specialist consultation or confinement in the acute-care setting, an emphasis on self-care and self-help education in pregnancy, close home followup after discharge at 6 to 12-hour postpartum. The social and emotional aspects of the program focus on encouraging and preparing family or friends of the woman's choice to participate in supporting the expectant and new mother throughout the childbearing year. The nurse-midwives and physicians work together in a team staff arrangement, each bringing their special expertise to the childbearing woman and her family.

Safety. After more than two decades of careful evaluation, the freestanding birth center has emerged as a safe, cost-effective place for birth.[1,13,14,19] The outcomes for mothers and infants in centers participating in the National Birth Center Study reported by Rooks, in the *New England Journal of Medicine* concluded that "few innovations in health service promise lower cost, greater availability, and a high degree of satisfaction with a comparable degree of safety. The results of this study suggest modern birth centers can identify women who are at low risk for obstetrical complications and can care for them in a way that provides these benefits."[19]

Cost. Maternity is currently the most frequent reason for admission to hospital and is costing business, industry, and taxpayers upwards of $15 billion annually. It is estimated that approximately 75% of American women do not need acute care during childbirth. Birth centers participating in the National Association of Childbearing Centers (NACC) annual survey have consistently reported charges for total care that are up to 50% less than regular hospital stays for normal birth and 30% less than short hospital stays. In 1991, the NACC estimated that if only 50% of the 4 million births in the United States were attended in freestanding birth centers, not only would access to care be greatly improved, savings would be almost $4 billion annually. This figure does not include the savings that would accrue from a 50% reduction in cesarean sections and other routine medical interventions in the low risk births.[15]

Potential. Birth centers, like nurse-midwifery, present a compelling argument for major changes in the delivery of care to childbearing families. Birth center programs fit the current focus of third-party payers for a greater emphasis on prevention of disease and education for healthier lifestyles. The birth center removes a major constraint to the education of nurse-midwives by providing clinical teaching sites dedicated to the practice of midwifery. It is a place where students witness the uninhibited role of the midwife and the practice of midwifery.

The freestanding birth center has the potential to greatly improve access and availability of maternity care services in geographical areas where they are presently lacking or inadequate. Small community hospitals would do well to look at converting their small obstetrical units to autonomous (freestanding) birth centers and triaging the women with complications. The difference between meeting the national standards for a primary care facility and an acute-care facility represents significant savings in the cost of construction and operation.

The birth center has been identified as a major catalyst in bringing about changes in hospital maternity care and for opening up hospital privileges for nurse-midwives. In almost every community where a freestanding birth center has been established, hospitals have established birthing suites or adopted a short-stay option. In some communities, competition from freestanding birth centers have persuaded hospital medical staffs to put aside their concerns about competition and open practice privileges to nurse-midwives.

The most important consideration for nursing posed by the freestanding birth center is that it provides an unprecedented opportunity for nurses and nurse-midwives to take more responsibility and control (they are inseparable) in accepting the challenge to improve care for *all* women and childbearing families. It holds the potential for being a nursing part of the solution to today's problems in providing maternity care services.

THE CAVEAT: ENOUGH MIDWIVES

The expanded opportunities for practice are creating an increased demand to educate nurse-midwives. It is clear that professionals trained exclusively in medical centers experience discomfort practicing in the birth center setting. Therefore, if nurse-midwives are to be the primary care providers for childbearing families, and the birth center a place for the practice of midwifery, a new approach to the education and training of all practitioners is called for.

In 1984 a consortium comprised of the Maternity Center Association, the Frontier School of Midwifery and Family Nursing, the Frances Payne Bolton School of Nursing of Case Western Reserve University, and the National Association of Childbearing Centers came together to design a community-based education program that would allow students who accepted the role of an adult learner to take a large portion of their credits for graduate study in a community-based study program. In other words, the community of the individual student becomes her classroom. She communicates

with faculty on her coursework through a computer network and bulletin board, fax, telephone, and mail. In addition to the standard for curriculum required for accreditation by the American College of Nurse-midwives, the program includes course and field work on an assessment of the needs of the student's community and its readiness for nurse-midwives and/or birth centers. Students contract with approved nurse-midwifery services in or near their communities for clinical practicum. Part of their clinical practicum is planned in a freestanding birth center.

While all nurse-midwifery education programs have reported an increase in the numbers of students enrolled in the past three years, none compare with the 150 students admitted to the Frontier School of Midwifery and Family Nursing CNEP class in 1993. To date, more than 8,000 nurses have requested information or applications for admission. The program is tuition driven and plans to admit all students who meet the admission criteria for graduate study in nursing at Case Western Reserve University and have approved clinical sites.

THE FUTURE

It took more than half a century to move all births into the acute-care setting of the hospital, and it was accomplished largely by a third-party system that paid only for hospital and physician services. It is reasonable to expect that the driving force to take normal birth out of the acute care setting will also be the third-party payers presently struggling to contain costs in a health care system that some feel is out of control. How long it will take depends upon how well we are able to overcome barriers and to evaluate and report to the public the advantages of a shift of this magnitude.

As we move into an era of more careful evaluation of the benefits, hazards, and costs for hospital acute care for all women versus health-oriented primary care, we can expect to see a contraction and consolidation of expensive acute care services and expansion of lower cost, preventive, primary care services. Both nurse-midwifery and birth centers are in line for this expansion.

The current issues for nursing presented here pose three questions. Will we, as individual nurses and as one of the largest blocks of professionals voting in the nation, organize to take responsibility for expanding nurse-midwifery? Will we take responsibility for developing ambulatory maternity care services? Will we take responsibility for containing costs and maintaining quality?

If we do not take responsibility, we cannot expect to have control. The ball is in our court.

REFERENCES

1. Bennetts, A. B., Lubic, R. W. (1982, Feb. 13). The freestanding birth centre. *The Lancet, 1,* 378-80.
2. Browne, H., & Isaacs, G. (1976). The frontier nursing service. *American Journal of Obstetrics and Gynecology, 124,* 14-17.
3. Ernst, E. K. M. (1979) The evolving practice of nurse-midwifery. *Health Law Project Library Bulletin, 4*(a), 289-294.
4. Ernst, E. K. M., & Forde M. (1975). Maternity care: An attempt at an alternative. *Nursing Clinics of North America, 10*(2).
5. General Accounting Office. (1979). Better management and more resources needed to strengthen federal efforts to improve pregnancy outcome. *GAO,* Washington, D.C.
6. Institute of Medicine. (1982). *Research issues in the assessment of birth settings.* Washington, D.C.: National Academy Press.
7. Laird, M. (1955). Report on the maternity center association, NY, 1931-1951. *American Journal of Obstetrics and Gynecology, 69,* 178-184.
8. Levy, B., Wilkinson, F., & Marine, W. (1971). Reducing neonatal mortality rate with nurse-midwives. *American Journal of Obstetrics and Gynecology, 109,* 50-58.
9. Lubic, R. W. (1983, July). Birthing centers: Delivering more for less. *American Journal of Nursing,* 1054-1056.
10. Metropolitan Life Insurance Company. *Report on the FNS of Hyden, KY,* May 9, 1932.
11. Ministry of Health. (1987). *Report of the task force on the implementation of midwifery in Ontario.* Toronto: Author.
12. Montgomery, T. (1969). A case for nurse-midwives. *American Journal of Obstetrics and Gynecology, 105,* 3.
13. Murdaugh, A. (1976). Experiences of a new migrant health clinic. *Women and Health, 1*(6), 25-28.
14. National Association of Childbearing Centers. (1990). *Report of the 1990 NACC official survey of birth center experience 1987-1989.* Perkiomenville, Pa: Author.
15. National Association of Childbearing Centers. (1991). *Report of the 1991 NACC official survey of birth center experience 1990.* Perkiomenville, Pa: Author.
16. Personal conversation with Mary Mallison, RN, Editor, *American Journal of Nursing.*
17. Rooks, J. (1990). Nurse-midwifery: The window is wide open. *American Journal of Nursing, 90*(12), 30-6.
18. Rooks, J., Haas. J. E. (1986). *Nurse-midwifery in America—A report of the American College of Nurse-Midwives Foundation.* Washington, D.C.
19. Rooks, J., Weatherby, N., Ernst, E., Stapleton, S., Rosen, D., & Rosenfield, A. (1989, Dec. 28). The national birth center study. *New England Journal of Medicine, 321,* 1804-1811.
20. Sharp, E. (1984). A decade of nurse-midwifery practice in a tertiary university affiliated hospital. *Journal of Nurse-Midwifery, 29*(6), 353-364.
21. Slone, C., Wetherbee, H., Daly, M., Christensen, K., Meglen, M., & Theide, H. (1976). Effectiveness of certified nurse-midwives. *American Journal of Obstetrics and Gynecology, 124,* 177-182.
22. Stewart, D. (1981). *The five standards for safe childbearing* (p. 118). Marble Hill, Mo: NAPSAC Publications.
23. Stewart, R., & Clark, L. (1982). Nurse-midwifery practice in a hospital birthing center: 2050 births. *Journal of Nurse-Midwifery, 27*(3), 21-26.
24. Summary of first 10,000 confinement records of the frontier nursing service. (1958). *Quarterly Bulletin of Frontier Nursing Service, 33,* 45-55.

CHAPTER 34

Long-term care

Meeting obligations to the elderly

NEVILLE E. STRUMPF, KAREN SUE KAUFFMAN

Three statements continue to summarize the situation for nursing and long-term care:

1. Nursing remains a potentially powerful force in the planning and humane execution of care for older people.
2. Reform of, and alternatives to, the existing system of long-term care are urgently needed.
3. The presence of a growing number of older persons needing care is an opportunity for nursing to demonstrate its political and social maturity as a profession.

As has been the case for the past decade, a number of critical issues are affecting services for the elderly, including widening national concern for the costs of care, genuine limitations in material and human resources, changing priorities about the use and distribution of technology and sophisticated interventions in health care, a growing proportion of older people who are quite vulnerable because of their frailty and meager financial circumstances, and a shortage of health care workers (professional and nonprofessional) trained in geriatrics. Nevertheless, the character of a society and of the professions it generates and rewards is mirrored in the response to persons in need. The *Social Policy Statement* formulated by the American Nurses Association states that nursing is "owned by society" and "must be perceived as serving the interests of the larger whole of which it is a part."[3] Meeting that obligation and fulfilling that promise as it pertains to the old among us are the central challenges of long-term care.

Wholehearted acceptance of biomedical strategies as the framework for the health professions has left "little place for the chronically ill, the marginally dysfunctional, or the aged. . . . the siren song of cure sounds sweeter to Americans than the gentler refrain of comfort and care,"[28] helping to create the pressing problem of care for the very old, especially those most dependent and in need of institutional care or other support. This reality also carries with it the growing burden of technological and moral choices likely to shape the availability and the quality of health services well into the twenty-first century.

For our purposes here, long-term care refers to a range of health and support services carried out over an extended period of time in a variety of community or institutional settings for individuals lacking some or all ability to care for themselves. This chapter provides background essential to understanding long-term care: changing demographics, a fragmented system of health care, needed reforms, and the role that must be assumed if nursing is "to take hold of aging the way medicine took hold of disease."[27]

DEMOGRAPHY AND OLD AGE
Statistical data

At this writing, results of the 1990 census are still being analyzed, although data compiled by the U.S. Administration on Aging[41] and the American Association of Retired Persons[1] are excellent sources of information. More than 30 million persons, or approximately 12.6% of Americans, are 65 years of age or older. By 2040 about 20% of the population will be 65 or older; 13 million of these will be over the age of 85. Among the rapidly enlarging group over 85, approximately 20% are in institutions and most of the rest live alone.

These shifts are the result of increased life expectancies along with recent declines in the birth rate. On average, females can expect to live longer than males, with white females having the longest life expectancy

(79.6 years), followed by black females (75.0), white males (72.7), and black males (67.7). The black elderly are the fastest growing segment of the African-American population.[5] Currently, about 7% of the black population is 65 and over; by 2030 it will increase to just above 17%. Overall, older women outnumber older men 3 to 2, and the disparity is even greater at age 85-plus: There are only 40 men for every 100 women.

Despite an ongoing debate concerning the economic status of elders in the United States, the Census Bureau's latest figures show that 12.4% of Americans over 65 live in poverty.[40] Many of these persons are women and minorities and rely solely on social security for support.

Most older persons describe their health as "good" or "excellent" and are able to manage their daily needs. Not until the 80s do older persons show greater signs of dependency, throwing into question a young "sandwich generation" in their 40s or early 50s who are faced with caring for them.[11] Increasingly, informal caregivers are getting older themselves and are often in their 60s.

Most older people report at least one chronic health problem, and multiple conditions are commonplace. In addition, mental health problems, although they often go unrecognized, are significantly more frequent in later life and can influence the course of physical illness. Alzheimer's disease may affect as many as 42% of persons over the age of 85,[17] and cognitive impairment, whether from Alzheimer's or other causes, is one of the principal reasons for institutionalization. Suicide is a more frequent cause of death among older adults than among any other age group. However, the majority eventually die from heart disease, cancer, or stroke, with heart disease being the major cause of death.

The risk of needing some nursing home care over a lifetime may be as great as 43% for those 65 and over.[22] These alarming projections notwithstanding, the number of available beds for persons aged 65 and over has recently been declining, probably the result of efforts by the states to control costs.[19] Of the approximately 5% of aging persons who do reside in nursing homes, most are very old, female, white, markedly impaired physically and mentally, and without a spouse, family member, or significant other to provide care and support.

Almost half of the older population lives in eight states: California, New York, Florida, Pennsylvania, Texas, Illinois, Ohio, and Michigan. A little-appreciated exodus of young people from the farm states, such as Iowa and North and South Dakota, however, is leaving these states with a relatively high percentage of the "oldest old," people age 85-plus.[11] In a few decades, the United States will be home to one of the oldest populations in the world. What remains unknown about this large group of future older Americans is the nature of their unique health problems and the results of changing environmental and social conditions and risk factors over time.

Implications of statistical data

Shifts in age structure are already having profound effects on the delivery of services and are a major consideration in plans for the future. The significant increase in numbers of older persons means a greater incidence of functional disability or debilitating illness and greater use of acute and long-term care services. That most of the very old are women who have faced structural inequities intensifying their disadvantaged economic and health situation also cannot be ignored.[7]

The chance of developing one or more chronic conditions or disabilities increases with age. About one fourth of the noninstitutionalized older population have functional limitations in one or more of several areas, including personal care and home management.[15] The ability of older people to get help with activities is an important factor in determining whether they can continue to reside in the community or must move to a long-term setting. The significant personal cost for at-home care, little of it covered by insurance, entitlement, or welfare, is yet another risk factor for institutionalization.

Americans spent over $666 billion on health care in 1990, 12.2% of the gross national product.[39] Of this amount, a very substantial portion (33%) was spent for care of the elderly.[2] Rates of hospitalization and lengths of stay are greater for the elderly when compared to younger persons. Average annual Medicare costs per person rise substantially with age, from $2017 for individuals aged 65 to 74 years, to $3215 for those aged 85 years and above.[42] Total expenditures for in-home aging services grew from $67 million in 1984 to $80 million in 1990.[37] Care in nursing homes went from 20 billion dollars annually in 1980 to 53 billion dollars in 1990, an increase of 165%.[24] The latter figure represents $30,000 to $40,000 annually for each of more than 1.6 million residents. About half of this is paid by Medicaid, the rest by residents or their families. Once individuals have spent down any personal resources that could be used for nursing home care, they are eligible for Medicaid, which over the years has become the major third-party payer for long-term care. For those persons whose incomes are too high to obtain eligibility for Medicaid yet too low to cover the cost of nursing home care as private pay patients, their primary caregivers face tremendous financial and emotional burdens with little hope of relief.[31]

The proportion of money spent to care for older people is large relative to their proportion in the population, and that money comes mainly from public funds. This focuses considerable attention on the aging population in any discussion of the cost of care, especially as general consumer and political interest shifts from long-term care needs of the elderly to the millions of younger persons without any health protection whatsoever. At the same time, aging members of society must not be made scapegoats for consuming what appears to be a disproportionate share of available resources. Although the average amount spent on health care for those 65 and older is greater than that spent for people under 65, expenditures vary with health status, and older people usually have modest expenditures during most years. For those older persons who do experience hospitalization, poor health, or institutionalization, however, the expenditures are significant, whether paid for with personal or public funds. Thus, the need is obvious for maintenance of functional ability and independence for as long as possible through community-based and institutional supports that are high quality, economically feasible, and equally accessible. The current system of long-term care, unfortunately, falls far short of these ideals.

THE SYSTEM OF LONG-TERM CARE
Current problems

A comprehensive care system for older people must offer a full range of integrated services, including "primary care, preventive and maintenance care, acute hospital care, extended care, home support services, and long-term care services, tailor-made for each individual."[44] In general, we have failed to appreciate the fact that the chronic impairments of older people are often more complex than the problems experienced by other age groups. The current approaches to care by both providers and the health system itself have not been entirely responsive or sensitive to this important point. The persistent efforts of many health providers, agencies, family members, and advocacy groups are often required to find even the most basic services or to coordinate these services for one individual. The present system, or more accurately nonsystem, satisfies no one.

The central problem facing long-term care in the United States is its peculiar financing. Existing mechanisms for eligibility and reimbursement for health care continue to emphasize an institutional model of care with its related biomedical and technological "solutions." Dealing with acute illness is favored over more comprehensive approaches to care, with the result that short-term hospitalization or nursing home placement are virtually the only choices available to older people and their families. In a thorough examination of care for the disabled elderly, Rivlin and Wiener[32] summarize the major problems in long-term care: (1) the burden falls heavily on persons unlucky enough to need extensive care and on their families; (2) public costs are rising rapidly, primarily in Medicaid, leaving poor families with children and the frail elderly to compete with one another for limited funding; (3) a two-class system of long-term care, especially in the case of nursing homes, is perpetuated by dependence on individual out-of-pocket spending or Medicaid as the chief means of reimbursement; (4) access to care is often limited, with patients capable of paying privately preferred over those who must rely on public funds; and (5) reimbursement for home care services is limited, and financing those home care services that are available is extremely fragmented.

Long-term care depends heavily on public funding, although expansion in private long-term care insurance has occurred in recent years, and on multiple agencies, each with their own eligibility and service provision requirements. The "unresolved catastrophe," to use Brody's[9] apt phrase, is the need, despite a maze of funding sources and agencies, to achieve continuity of care for the multiproblem client. Brody describes continuity of care as moving through three stages: (1) acute care, usually representing a hospital stay; (2) short-term/long-term care, which is the brief time period, often less than 90 days, following a hospital stay that allows for transition to community living; and (3) long-term/long-term care, which may be intermittent, of varying intensity and locations, but continuous.

Several highlights of the current system of financing health services for older people are essential to understanding why gaps in continuity of care are so great. Medicare, a federal entitlement program for all persons aged 65 and older, mainly covers acute care. Little coverage is available as part of Medicare for home care or for care in a nursing home.

Since 1983, Medicare has paid for hospital care with essentially a fixed rate per discharge, depending on the diagnostic-related group (DRG) in which the patient is classified. Prospective payment, intended to curb soaring medical costs, substantially changed the structure and function of the long-term care system because reduction in length of hospital stay dramatically increased the practice of discharging patients "quicker and sicker."[33] As a consequence of the early discharge of many older patients, home care services are unusually burdened, and nursing homes are being forced to accept a heavier care case mix to accommodate those needing post-hospital extended care.[35] Increased reliance by hospitals on nursing home care following early discharge may be contributing, however inadvertently, to unnecessary or even permanent institutional placement. Hospitals also continue to have few incentives for establishing specialized geriatric evaluation or consultation units or services, although these have been shown to improve functional outcomes, lessen readmission after discharge from the hospital, and decrease institutionalization.[6,8,20,29,34,38]

Unlike Medicare, Medicaid is a means-tested welfare program for the poor financed by individual states and the federal government. It now accounts for about half of all nursing home reimbursement, usually at a fixed daily rate per resident that varies greatly among the states. Rarely does it provide funding sufficient to meet all of the costs of care, a major reason why most nursing homes strive to have as many private-pay residents as possible. In several states, case-mix adjustment, which allows for reimbursement according to characteristics and resulting care needs of residents, has been attempted in an effort to improve access and quality and to lower costs. Findings to date are inconclusive on the benefits of such systems.[43]

What should be obvious from the above description of the two primary sources of reimbursement for health services for older people is the lack of organization among the five essential components of a long-term care system: (1) the client, (2) informal support services, (3) formal direct services, (4) linkages, and (5) the financing mechanism itself.[25] Along with insufficient reimbursement mechanisms for the health care of older people, some additional reasons for suboptimal conditions in the existing set of long-term care services include poor public and provider attitudes toward aging persons, inadequate education about the clinical problems of older people, perceived lack of stature and attractiveness of careers in gerontology and geriatrics, and a low level of expectations from both recipients of services and society regarding the therapeutic potential of older adults.[36]

Although provision of health care for older people inevitably must span a continuum of services from home to hospital to long-stay institution, the nursing home dominates and symbolizes many problems and dilemmas in long-term care. Placed in the ambivalent position of being "second-class hospitals,"[21] they are increasingly called upon to provide services for a heterogeneous clientele, among them a growing number of persons with AIDS or other terminal illnesses, a range of psychosocial and behavioral problems, head injuries and developmental disabilities, individuals needing a period of convalescence or intensive rehabilitation, and frail older people too impaired physically and mentally to remain at home.[26]

Directions for reform

The cry to reform health care, including long-term care, has hardly been louder since enactment of Medicare-Medicaid legislation in 1965. The presidential stance since 1980 has clearly favored "maintaining the integrity of the private-public partnership,"[39] but demands from the political opposition, many consumer groups, professional organizations, policy analysts, and average citizens are urging a stronger initiative from the public sector.[30] No one denies that health care costs are increasing at unsustainable rates and that Americans are worried about obtaining necessary health care coverage.[13]

Of course, there have indeed been favorable developments in the delivery of comprehensive long-term care in the past two decades, with and without government support, including among them the Chelsea Village Program of home care services, a component of the Department of Community Medicine at St. Vincent's Hospital and Medical Center in New York; the Continuing Care Retirement Communities and Life Care at Home; the On Lok Community Care Organization for Dependent Adults in San Francisco; and a variety of other experimental and innovative approaches to community-based services. Although scattered throughout the country, and clearly not available to all, these programs demonstrate the positive outcomes so desired in any system providing long-term care services to the elderly. On the other hand, their successes stand in such sharp relief because of a growing national trend toward decentralization "away from a primary concern for community and access to care, in the name of containment and cost effectiveness."[16] It will thus challenge us politically, socially, and morally to devise a system that allows for access and quality of life in a fiscally responsible and ethical manner.

According to Rivlin and Wiener,[32] the objectives of any reform of long-term care are to (1) reduce the uncertainty and anxiety that now surround paying for long-term care, (2) enable older people to remain at home for as long as possible, and (3) improve the quality of care and the flexibility and efficiency of the delivery system. To do this, Somers and Livingood[37] argue that we must profit from what has been learned during the past decade and devise systems, with federal support, that, as their goal, maximize functional independence, utilize an interdisciplinary approach, provide for coordination of services (increasingly referred to as "managed care"), have effective quality controls and incentives to contain costs, promote patient responsibility and autonomy, and are firmly rooted in the local community.

As changes in the delivery of long-term care are considered, the allocation of resources to older people is likely to be debated further. Two arguments for the rationing of health care by age have been put forward by Daniels[14] and Callahan.[10] If their proposals are not entirely tenable, we must still accept the fact that a form of rationing does exist in the United States, namely access to care based on ability to pay. Churchill[12] lucidly argues for overcoming misguided commitments to very expensive, high-technology interventions in favor of universal recognition of the collective vulnerability to disease, disability, and death. Perhaps the clinical dialogue necessitated by passage in 1990 of the Patient Self-Determination Act[23] can guide that complex task. Difficult decisions about allocation of societal resources in general and health care dollars in particular will have to be made. In that intersection between the competing forces of ethical care and cost containment, nursing is presented with the challenge and the opportunity to help reshape long-term care.

THE ROLE OF NURSING IN LONG-TERM CARE

Demographics, reimbursement structures, the need for a more comprehensive approach to the care of older people, and a growing concern for a reformed, morally just, and efficient system of long-term care form both background and context for the role of the nurse in gerontology.

The framework for gerontological nursing practice is delineated in a statement on standards and scope prepared by the American Nurses Association.[4] The standards call for quality care at a level beyond that required by minimal regulatory criteria and serve as a model for basic and advanced professional practice in the areas of organization of services, generation and testing of theory as a basis for clinical decisions, data collection, health assessment, planning and continuity of care, intervention, evaluation, interdisciplinary collaboration, research, ethics, and professional development. Emphasis is placed on maximizing functional ability in activities of daily living; promoting, maintaining, and restoring health, including mental health; preventing and minimizing the disabilities of acute and chronic illness; and maintaining life in dignity and comfort until death.

Given the existing state of long-term care, nursing can make its most significant contributions by:

1. Increasing the pool of baccalaureate, master's, and doctorally prepared nurses in gerontology
2. Participating actively in the delivery of health services aimed at the enhancement of accessibility, management, and continuity of long-term care for older people
3. Improving care in nursing homes
4. Conducting research documenting impact by the nurse on clinical outcomes and quality of care for older people

An ideal community ensures the personal liberties of older people, protects their individuality and enhances the integrity of the aging experience.[18] The nurse who chooses long-term care will be expected, above all, to contribute to the preservation of these values. At the same time, this nurse will also be living in a nation with a growing percentage of older people, a fragmented system of health care, and a finite supply of resources. Nonetheless, it is possible for gerontological nurses to influence the care older people will receive through their advocacy of a reformed and more equitable system of services, participation in assessment and management of the health care problems of aging persons in the community and institutions, and conduct of part of the research essential to understanding the needs of older people. In fulfilling these obligations of a caring community to the old among us, we fulfill, as well, these same obligations to ourselves.

REFERENCES

1. American Association of Retired Persons. (1991). *A profile of older Americans: 1991.* Washington, D.C.: Author.
2. American Medical Association. (1990). White paper on elderly health. *Journal of the American Medical Association, 150*(12), 2459-2472.

3. American Nurses Association. (1980). *Nursing: A social policy statement*. Kansas City, Mo: Author.

4. American Nurses Association. (1987). *Standards and scope of gerontological nursing practice*. Kansas City, Mo: Author.

5. Angel, J., & Hogan, D. (1991). *Minority elders: Longevity, economics, and health*. Washington, D.C.: Gerontological Society of America.

6. Applegate, W., Miller, S., Graney, M., Elam, J., Burns, R., & Akins, D. (1990). A randomized controlled trial of a geriatric assessment unit in a community rehabilitation hospital. *New England Journal of Medicine, 322*(22), 1572-1578.

7. Arendell, T., & Estes, C. (1991). Older women in the post-Reagan era. *International Journal of Health Services, 21*(1), 59-73.

8. Barker, W., Williams, T., Zimmer, J., Van Buren, C., Vincent, S., & Pickerel, S. (1985). Geriatric consultation teams in acute hospitals: Impact on back-up of elderly patients. *Journal of the American Geriatrics Society, 33*(6), 422-428.

9. Brody, S. (1987). Strategic planning: The catastrophic approach. *The Gerontologist, 27*(2), 131-138.

10. Callahan, D. (1987). *Setting limits*. New York: Simon & Shuster.

11. Carlson, E. (1992). Redrawing America. *Bulletin of the American Association of Retired Persons, 33*(6), 1,11-12.

12. Churchill, L. (1988). Should we ration health care by age? *Journal of the American Geriatrics Society, 36*(7), 644-647.

13. Clinton, B. (1992). The Clinton health care plan. *New England Journal of Medicine, 327*(11), 804-807.

14. Daniels, N. (1985). *Just health care*. Cambridge, England: Cambridge University Press.

15. Dawson, D., Hendershot, G., & Fulton, J. (1987). *Aging in the eighties, functional limitations of individuals age 65 years and over*. (Pub. No. 87-1250). Hyattsville, Md: U.S. Public Health Service National Center for Health Statistics.

16. Estes, C., & Wood, J. (1986). The nonprofit sector and community-based care for elderly in the U.S.: A disappearing resource? *Social Science and Medicine, 23*(12), 1261-1266.

17. Evans, D., Funkenstein, H., Albert, M., Scherr, P., Cook, N., Chown, M., Hebert, L., Hennekens, C., & Taylor, J. (1989). Prevalence of Alzheimer's disease in a community population of older persons. *Journal of the American Medical Association, 262*(11), 2551-2556.

18. Gadow, S. (1984). Humanities teaching and aging: Issues and approaches in medical education. In S. Spicker & S. Ingman (Eds.), *Vitalizing long term care, the teaching nursing home and other perspectives, Part III*. New York: Springer.

19. Harrington, C., Preston, S., Grant, L., & Swan, J. (1992). Revised trends in states' nursing home capacity. *Health Affairs, 11*(2), 170-180.

20. Hogan, D., & Fox, R. (1990). A prospective trial of a geriatric consultation team in an acute-care hospital. *Age and Aging, 19*(2), 107-113.

21. Kane, R., & Kane, R. (1980). Long term care: Can our society meet the needs of its elderly? *Annual Review of Public Health, 1*, 227-253.

22. Kemper, P., & Murtaugh, C. (1991). Lifetime use of nursing home care. *New England Journal of Medicine, 324*(9), 595-600.

23. LaPuma, J., Orentlicher, D., & Moss, R. (1991). Advance directives on admission. *Journal of the American Medical Association, 266*(3), 402-405.

24. Levit, K., Lazenby, H., Cowan, C., & Letsch, S. (1991). National health expenditures, 1990. *Health Care Financing Review, 13*(3), 29-54.

25. Lubben, J. (1987). Models for delivering long term care. *Home Health Services Quarterly, 8*(2), 5-21.

26. Lusk, P. (1990). Who's knocking now? New clientele for nursing homes. *Journal of Gerontological Nursing, 16*(6), 8-11.

27. Lynaugh, J. (1983). *Care of the aged: Society's mandate to nursing*. Paper presented at Nursing Research Conference on Gerontology, Mid-Atlantic Regional Nursing Association, Hershey, Pa, September 30.

28. Lynaugh, J. (1990). Is there anything new about this nursing shortage? In J. McCloskey & H. Grace (Eds.), *Current issues in nursing* (3rd ed.) St Louis: Mosby.

29. McVey, L., Becker, P., Saltz, C., Feussner, J., & Cohen, H. (1989). Effect of a geriatric consultation team on functional status of elderly hospitalized patients. *Annals of Internal Medicine, 110*(1), 79-84.

30. Moon, M. (1989). Taking the plunge—The arguments for a comprehensive long term care system. *Journal of the American Geriatrics Society, 37*(12), 1165-1170.

31. Quadagno, J., Meyer, M., & Turner, J. (1991). Falling into the Medicaid gap: The hidden long term care dilemma. *The Gerontologist, 31*(4), 521-526.

32. Rivlin, A., & Wiener, J. (1988). *Caring for the disabled elderly*. Washington, D.C.: Brookings Institute.

33. Rogers, W., Draper, D., Kahn, K., Keeler, E., Rubenstein, L., Kosecoff, J., & Brook, R. (1990). Quality of care before and after implementation of the DRG-based prospective payment system. *Journal of the American Medical Association, 264*(15), 1989-1994.

34. Rubenstein, L., Josephson, K., Wieland, G., English, P., Sayre, J., & Kane, R. (1984). Effectiveness of a geriatric evaluation unit: A randomized clinical trial. *New England Journal of Medicine, 311*(26), 1664-1670.

35. Shaughnessy, P., & Kramer, A. (1990). The increased needs of patients in nursing homes and patients receiving home health care. *New England Journal of Medicine, 332*(1), 21-27.

36. Siu, A. (1987). The quality of medical care received by older persons. *Journal of the American Geriatrics Society, 35*(12), 1084-1091.

37. Somers, A., & Livengood, W. (1992). Long term care for the elderly: Major developments in the last ten years. *Pride Institute Journal, 11*(1), 6-18.

38. Sullivan, E., Wanich, C., & Kurlowicz L. (1991). Nursing assessment, management of delirium in the elderly. *American Operating Room Nurses Journal, 53*(3), 820-828.

39. Sullivan, L. (1992). The Bush administration's health care plan. *New England Journal of Medicine, 327*(11), 801-804.

40. The far-reaching human toll of the sour economy. (1992). *Philadelphia Inquirer*, September 6, Section F, p. 2.

41. U.S. Administration on Aging. (1991). *Aging in America: Trends and projections*. Washington, D.C.: Office of Management and Policy.

42. Waldo, D., Sonnefeld, S., McKusick, D., & Arnett, R. (1989). Health expenditures by age group, 1977 and 1987. *Health Care Financing Review, 10*(1), 111-120.

43. Weissert, W., & Musliner, M. (1992). *Access, quality, and cost consequences of case-mix adjusted reimbursement for nursing homes: A critical review of the evidence*. Washington, D.C.: American Association of Retired Persons.

44. Williams, T. (1987). Extended care: A physician's perspective. In B. Vladeck & G. Alfano (Eds.), *Medicare and extended care: Issues, problems, and prospects*. Owings Mills, Md: Rand Communications.

CHAPTER 35

Nurses and case management

To control or to collaborate?

KAREN ZANDER

Nurses are having a difficult time changing their habits. Accustomed to taking on the pressures in institutions and accommodating to added responsibilities, nurses are creating potential longer-term problems for the profession and themselves by making managed care and case management just one more nursing model. Critical paths or their next generation, CareMaps,* managed care, and case management are powerful clinical systems that will backfire on nurses if they do not allow and expect the ownership of them to be held throughout all levels of the institution.

By "backfire," I mean that nurses may invest their hearts and time in a managed care/case management project only to discover there is resentment, acting-out, and lack of consistent support from the larger organization. Certain design factors will add only to nursing's responsibilities rather than address responsibility and accountability from other key sectors of the institution. If the project works too well, there will be competition as well as threatened departments and people— including some within nursing. At risk is valuable time, people's morale and confidence in attempting any future innovations, administrations' credibility, and, most important, the spirit of collaboratively investing in raising standards to achieve patient outcomes.

How do you know if you are "at risk"? Symptoms include frequent use of the word *buy-in*, nurses perfecting CareMap tools before they include any other discipline in a discussion, only nursing diagnoses and nursing signoffs on CareMap documents, absence of a multidisciplinary steering committee, CareMap pro-

cesses taught only to nursing rather than to all clinicians, a board that has not heard that the hospital is using a CareMap system, and physicians calling CareMap tools "that nursing thing." Similarly, case management policies, procedures, structures, and roles determined solely by nursing will not gain interest or instill ownership. Within each of these insular scenarios, nurses and others will perceive that manpower resources have decreased rather than increased.

To conserve itself, nursing must enter the multidisciplinary arena with more than lip service. This necessitates changing our own behavior to have people respond differently to us. Only then will there be enough total resources for patient care.

BACKGROUND

Managed care and case management in acute care are often construed as nursing models because they were originally developed by nurses[7] and because the coordination of the volume of details written on a CareMap tool is a responsibility that other professions are usually satisfied to give to nurses. This trend is a credit to the capability of professional nurses and has taken the form of diverse and exciting models that are inextricably tied to nursing staffing issues.[2]

There will never be enough nurses to do everything we would like done for our patients. There will also never be enough time for each individual nurse to establish meaningful, continuous relationships with every acutely ill patient because the patients are moving through each care area more rapidly as length of stay decreases. In addition, the intensity of care increases as length of stay goes down, so patients often receive more interventions (i.e., tests and treatments) from

*CareMap is a trademark and concept of The Center for Case Management, South Natick, Massachusetts.

various departments per day.[3] Therefore, both patients and staff are more stressed and have less time and energy to process events. Furthermore, Dr. Donald Berwick, renowned for his leadership in quality improvement in health care, states that because of increased service fragmentation patients need a system but get "events."[1]

All these trends speak to the need for methods that assure cost and quality outcomes. Six years after their inception, multidisciplinary CareMap tools are generally accepted as a method for the providers of care to maintain control over their own practices.[5]

Institutionally controlled managed care entails the use of CareMap tools 24 hours a day. Case management is a generic process that may encompass the use of CareMap tools and extends across care areas. Case managers are clinicians who, as individuals or part of collaborative groups, are overseeing the management of case-type-based care (i.e., DRG, etc.) and are usually held accountable to some standard of cost effectiveness and quality. The actual model in each institution is a combination of at least two of these three elements: (1) Critical Path/CareMap documents (see Fig. 35-1); (2) managed care; and (3) role changes establishing case managers and/or formal collaborative practices.

At issue in this chapter is the way nurses, in their eagerness to assist health care agencies in addressing the impact of prospective payment and related crises, have defined, or "concretized," the three elements too narrowly and not collaboratively enough. This chapter gives suggestions on how nurses can become more system savvy.

ESTABLISHING GOALS AND INFRASTRUCTURE

To stay focused throughout a managed care/case management project and evaluate its results fairly, goals must be determined and disseminated from the executive level outwards through the organization. This group will need up-to-date information to make its decisions and should meet monthly over at least two years for adequate implementation.

Goals tend to cluster around cost, quality, and collaboration. One, *cost* goals become defined as length of stay and technical resources. Managed care/case management should be implemented with a budget-neutral stance in terms of manpower resources. Two, *quality* goals become clarified as meeting measurable intermediate and discharge or transfer outcome criteria per

case type. (There is a built-in assumption that the staff of all disciplines already use quality clinical processes.) Additionally, organizations are realizing how the CareMap tools link continuous quality improvement (CQI) tangibly to the patient. "CareMapping is a way to assure that we're constantly and continually applying a high standard of quality care," says St. Elizabeth's of Boston president Theodore Druhot. "When we do that, efficiency results, and the patient will get what the patient needs when the patient needs it—no more, no less, no sooner, no later."[9] Three, *collaboration* goals become clarified as not only discussions between physicians, nurses, and others in crises but also the setting, managing, and evaluation of the clinical outcomes that are the institution's best practice.

Other goals that are currently important to most institutions are patient satisfaction, the ability to contract/market, streamlining documentation, restructuring nursing roles, and meeting JCAHO and other regulatory agencies' requirements. All of these goals can be accomplished within one to two years, but none of them should be set by nursing or any other department in isolation from the larger group.

The infrastructure for a CareMap system should be designed to neutralize territory and turf issues, while simultaneously creating continued active involvement. The CEO should appoint a steering committee that should interview and appoint a project manager. Fig. 35-2 gives a rudimentary diagram of infrastructure. Even if nursing suggested the project, nursing should not begin any activity except gathering information until there is a set avenue for processing decisions.

The project manager is usually a nurse who takes the position for at least two years. He or she must instantly become a person without a country in order to help the organization look at itself and make change. To be effective, the project manager must make any allegiance to nursing secondary to the goal of cost/quality outcomes for patients. He or she will be privy to information from every sector of the organization and will be expected to resolve age-old discrepancies in the way things work. Initially, managed care/case management might open Pandora's box—a necessary step for improvement. The project manager has to allow disclosure without exposing any one person or group to blame. Inquiry rather than blame is indeed very different behavior than what health care professionals are accustomed to. If the project manager cannot rise above the overt and covert vested interests in the organization, diverse groups within the organization will not be

CHF CareMap ™	1-Feb	1-Feb	2-Feb	3-Feb	4-Feb	5-Feb	6-Feb
	Benchmark Quality Criteria:						
Location-Day: **Problem:**	ER 1 - 6 hours	Floor Telemetry or CCU 6 - 24 hours Day 1	Floor Day 2	Floor Day 3	Floor Day 4	Floor Day 5	Floor Day 6
1) Alteration in gas exchange/perfusion & fluid balance due to decreased cardiac output, excess fluid volume	Reduced pain from admission or pain tree Uses pain scale O2 sat. Improved over admission baseline on O2 therapy	Respirations equal to or less than on admission	O2 sat = 90 Resp 20-22 Vital signs stable Crackles at lung bases Mild shortness of breath with activity	Does not require O2 Vital signs stable Crackles at base Respirations 20 - 22 Mild shortness of breath with activity	Does not require O2 (O2 sat. on room air 90%) Vital signs stable Crackles at base Respirations 20 - 22 Completes activities with no increase respirations. No edema.	Can lie in bed at baseline position Chest X-ray clear or at baseline	No dyspnea
2) Potential for shock	No signs & symptoms of shock	No signs/symptoms of shock No signs/symptoms of MI	No signs/symptoms of shock	No signs/symptoms of shock Normal lab values	No signs/symptoms of shock	No signs/symptoms of shock	No signs/symptoms of shock
3) Potential for consequences of immobility & decreased activity: skin breakdown, DVT, constipation, injury	No redness at pressure points No falls	No redness at pressure points No falls	Tolerates chair, washing, eating and toileting	Has bowel movement Up in room and bathroom with assist	Up ad lib for short periods	Activity increased to level used at home without shortness of breath	Activity increased to level used at home without shortness of breath
4) Alteration in nutritional intake due to: nausea & vomiting, labored breathing		No c/o nausea No vomiting Taking liquids as offered	Eating solids Takes in 50% each meal	Taking 50% each meal	Taking 50% each meal Weight - 2 lbs from patient's normal baseline	Taking 75% each meal	Taking 75% each meal
5) Potential for arrhythmias due to decreased cardiac output: decreased irritable foci. valve problems, decreased gas exchange	No evidence of life-threatening dysrhythmias	Normal sinus rhythm with benign ectopy	K(WNL) Benign or no arrhythmias	Digoxin level WNL Benign or no arrhythmias	Digoxin level WNL Benign or no arrhythmias	Digoxin level WNL Benign or no arrhythmias	Digoxin level WNL Benign or no arrhythmias
6) Patient/Family response to future treatment & hospitalization	Patient/Family expressing concerns Following directions of staff	Patient/Family expressing concerns Following directions of staff	Patient/Family and staff discussing degree of CHF and its causes	States reasons for and cooperates with rest periods Patient begins to assess own knowledge and ability to care for CHF at home (meds, diet, activity, other)	Patient decides whether he/she wants discussion with physician about advanced directives	States plans for 1-2 days post discharge as to : meds, diet, activity, follow-up appointments Expresses reaction to having CHF	Repeats plans States signs and symptoms to notify physician/ER Signs discharge consent
7) Individual problem:							
Staff Tasks	Staff Tasks: ER	Staff Tasks: 6-24 hr. Day 1	Staff Tasks: Day 2	Staff Tasks: Day 3	Staff Tasks: Day 4	Staff Tasks: Day 5	Staff Tasks: Day 6
Assessments/Consults	Vital signs q 15 min Nursing assessments focus: lung sounds, edema, color, skin integrity, jugular vein distention Cardiac monitor Arterial line if needed Swan Ganz Intake & Output	Vital signs q 15 min - 1 hr Repeat nursing assessments Cardiac monitor Arterial line Swan Ganz Daily weight Intake and Output	Vital signs q 4 hr. Repeat nursing assessments D/C cardiac monitor 24 hr D/C arterial and Swan Ganz Daily weight Intake and Output	Vital signs q 8 hr. Repeat nursing assessments Intake and Output Daily weight	Vital signs q 8 hr. Repeat nursing assessments Intake and Output Daily weight Nutrition consult	Vital signs q 8 hr. Repeat nursing assessments Intake and Output Daily weight	Vital signs q 8 hr. Repeat nursing assessments Intake and Output Daily weight
Specimens/Tests	Consider TSH studies Chest x-ray EKG CPK q 8 hr X 3 ABG if Pulse Ox: (range) Lytes, Na, K, Cl, CO2, Glucose, BUN, Creatinine, Digoxin: (range)	EKG	Evaluate for ECHO Lytes, BUN, Creatinine			Chest X-ray Lytes, BUN, Creatinine	
Treatments	O2 or intubate IV or Heparin lock	O2 IV or Heparin lock	IV or Heparin lock	DC pulse Ox if stable D/C IV or Heparin lock			
Medications	Evaluate for Digoxin Nitrodrip or paste Diuretics IV Evaluate for antiemetics Evaluate for antiarrythmics	Evaluate for Digoxin Nitrodrip or paste Diuretics IV Evaluate for pre-load/after-load reducers K supplements Stool softeners if indicated	D/C Nitrodrip or paste Diuretics IV or PO K supplements Stool softeners Evaluate for Nicotine Patch	Change to PO Digoxin PO diuretics K supplements Stool softeners Nicotine patch if consent	PO diuretics K supplement Stool softeners Nicotine patch if consent	PO diuretics K supplement Stool softeners Nicotine patch if consent	PO diuretics K supplement Stool softeners Nicotine patch if consent
Nutrition	None	Clear liquids	Cardiac, low salt diet	Cardiac, low salt diet	Cardiac, low salt diet	Cardiac, low salt diet	Cardiac, low salt diet
Safety/Activity	Commode Bedrest with head elevated Reposition patient q 2 hr. Bedrails up Call light available	Commode Bedrest with head elevated Dangle Reposition q 2 hr. Enforce rest periods Bedrails up Call light available	Commode Enforce rest periods Chair with assist 1/2 hr. with feet elevated Bedrails up Call light available	Bathroom privileges Chair X 3 Bedrails up Call light available	Ambulate in hall X 2 Up ad lib between rest periods Bedrails up Call light available	Encourage ADLs which approximate activities at home Bedrails up Call light available	Encourage ADLs which approximate activities at home Bedrails up Call light available
Teaching	Explain procedures Teach chest pain scale & importance of reporting	Explain course, need for energy conservation Orient to unit & routine	Clarify CHF Dx and future teaching needs. Orient to unit and routine. Schedule rest periods Begin medication teaching	Importance of weighing self every day Provide smoking cessation information Review energy conservation schedule	Cardiac rehab level as indicated by consult Provide smoking cessation support Dietary teaching	Review CHF education material with patient	Reinforce CHF teaching
Transfer/Discharge Coordination	Asses home situation; Notify significant other if no arrythmias or chest pain, transfer to floor. Otherwise transfer to ICU	Screen for discharge needs Transfer to floor	Consider Home Health Care referral		Evaluate needs for diet and anti-smoking classes Physician offers discussion opportunities for advanced directives	Appointment and arrangement for follow-up care with home health care nurse Contact VNA	Reinforce follow-up appointments

Fig. 35-1. Congestive heart failure CareMap.

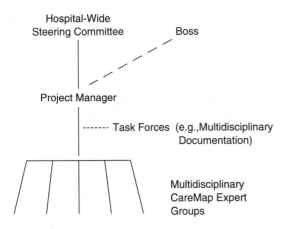

Fig. 35-2. CareMap system infrastructure.

able to engage in the new behaviors of continuous quality improvement.

These new behaviors can be understood in light of the three central questions which must be answered to begin managed care and/or case management. They are:

1. What is the work required to get patients within certain case-types to desired outcomes?
2. What is the best way to produce the work? i.e., the clinical decision-making process and the structure (people for care-giving, their responsibilities, relationships, and documentation)
3. Who is accountable for the results?

Nursing's tendency is to answer the second question first and then to not really address the third question. A better and new behavior is to spend a few hours in dialogue with a multidisciplinary team of clinical experts sharing practice beliefs and patterns to define the work, as the first question suggests. The answers to the second question involve a very prolonged design phase, which will then point the way to answering the third question.

CAREMAP DEVELOPMENT

Nurses must be ready to bend paradigms and develop a common language for the CareMap tools. For instance, in one multidisciplinary discussion about patients undergoing colectomies, the physician described the experience of the patient waiting (5 days) for a pathology report as "dread." The nurses transcribed the discussion and changed the problem statement to "anxiety related to unknown diagnosis," even though "dread" was agreed upon by the group. Such behavior unravels collaborative endeavors.

In similar CareMap sessions, mainstream nurses do not have a language yet to articulate their own practice and are tentative when discussing practice with physicians. Nurses need to find words for what they are trying to achieve with their interventions. For example, a nurse in a neonatal ICU spoke of the potential for an intercranial bleed in neonates of a certain gestational age on "Day 2." The problem statement was obviously "potential for intercranial bleed," but she had no words to measure an outcome. Responding to a series of questions, she was able to say that "no evidence of seizures" was a good realistic outcome, stating that the interventions of nursing and other professionals would appropriately monitor blood pressure, pulse, and other signs and symptoms. Once the nurse acknowledges this criteria as genuine, it needs to be presented for multidisciplinary validation. This is a golden opportunity for nurses to advocate for both patients and nursing.

All the work nurses have done on nursing standards must be woven into a CareMap tool, which means that they must be discussed and explained within a multidisciplinary arena. This is a healthy but uncomfortable step for nurses to take, having tried to perfect their standards. The problem is that nursing should have standards, but those standards will not be actualized unless there is consensus about them from professionals of other disciplines and unless they are operationalized by the entire institution. Otherwise, nurses will continue to feel burdened, angry, and depleted.

Nurses are experts in coordinating most and delivering much of the detailed interventions suggested on the CareMap tools. However, little progress has been made in true collaborative practice until there is:

1. Agreement about the expected clinical outcomes of interventions (which should be added to Critical Paths to make CareMaps) and
2. Determination made as to which clinical departments have the authority to validate outcomes achievement

How "multidisciplinary" should be nursing be? *Totally!* The ultimate goal is that professionals of each discipline who give direct care evaluate the patient and/or family against the intermediate outcomes every day, shift, hour, or visit. When used for documentation, CareMap tools have the potential of replacing progress notes for all disciplines unless there are variances, in which case a progress note is required by the discipline(s) determined best qualified to evaluate that outcome. Otherwise, the professionals authorized to sign off outcomes can put their initials on the actual CareMap document and enter a signature log on the back. Use the following checklist to evaluate the extent of multidisciplinary design of your CareMap System. Have all related disciplines and departments been actively involved/represented in:

- Steering committee
- Determining case types
- Creation of CareMaps
- Validity/reliability from literature review
- Meeting professional/state standards
- Setting thresholds for variance
- Orienting peers to CareMap process
- Signing-off tasks and/or outcomes
- Variance coding
- Concurrent revisions of CareMap
- Progress notes
- CQI by "expert" groups
- Developing and teaching case-type management
- Research[9]

NURSES AND PHYSICIANS

Another common behavior of nurses as they enter the CareMap arena is the self-defeating assumption that physicians will not participate, not like, and not use a CareMap system. In actuality, CareMap tools are a written algorithm of clinical progressions and are based on the scientific method. If structured for individual preference, physicians will consider how CareMap tools can benefit them.

Nurses need to present themselves as allies of physicians in the cost/quality challenge. There are at least 30 ways to involve physicians in CareMapping, all which require a nonbiased spirit of clinical inquiry and desire to really learn from, as well as teach, physicians.[8] The most important behavior is to never let the CareMap system or Case Management be designed as a policing system of physician practice. That is definitely not a collegial role for professional nurses.

DOCUMENTATION AND RESPONSIBILITIES

The CareMap tool should ultimately be the core of the medical record. Nurses should think of each new ver-

sion of the tool as a revised improvement rather than the final format. In other words, the format must keep changing to accommodate new demands, such as when the clergy want to be acknowledged on a "consult" category or utilization review staff request a new piece of data. In a typical dilemma, staff nurses may want nonduplication variance entry forms, while quality assurance will want lots of variance information. The answer?

Nurses should never solve the dilemma through the nursing department alone. Take the issues to various multidepartmental task forces and find mutual solutions. Keep returning to the organization's goal for the project. It is highly possible that professionals other than nurses have too much documentation as well, and have similar needs and goals. It is equally possible that nonnursing departments do not share equal pressures or goals. Either way, problem solving in isolation from other professionals will, by definition, be the wrong solution.

Another behavior that is adaptive to today's environment is a readiness to try new interventions and learn new skills. For example, open heart surgical patients are being sedated and vented for shorter periods of time postoperatively. This creates the need for heightened levels of assessments at different treatment junctures. Similarly, staff nurses have to be more proactive in moving patients' care along through a weekend and in making very timely use of discharge planning resources. CareMap tools will reflect current "best practice" but will continue to evolve their content as practice evolves.

New clinical management skills for staff nurses and other direct-care professionals are using case consultation and participating in health care team meetings when patients are at variance. Other new behaviors are inclusion rather than delegation, principled negotiation as a basis collaboration, and followup/follow-through.[4]

As far as nurse managers (and all department heads for that matter) new behaviors are also needed because "status quo management is obsolete."[6] In their book, *Health Care Managers in Transition,* Leebov and Scott offer a useful list of the attitudes and behaviors that health care managers must undergo to make a necessary transition. Some are highlighted below:

1. From tradition and safety to experimentation and risk
2. From busyness to results

3. From turf protection to teamwork across lines
4. From "we-they" thinking to organizational perspective
5. Gaining organizational support for making role changes[6]

WHO OWNS CASE MANAGEMENT?

No one owns case management. It is a process in which all care givers can partake. However, the issue of whether an organization wants or needs case managers, and who should have a case manager role, is complex.

Nurses make excellent case managers and the literature grows monthly with their documented successes. However, at issue in this chapter is the process used to determine the role and accountabilities—not necessarily the final decision itself.

The steering committee, not the nursing department, should survey case management design choices and their consequences. Figures 35-3 and 35-4 display

basic choices. Some institutions are wisely avoiding confusion and conflict with the belief that all patients should be managed by CareMap documents, but perhaps only certain case-types/patient populations need the extra continuity of case managers. Other institutions have decided, wisely again, to consider each CareMap development team clinical experts, the collaborative embodiment of case management, and avoided the term *case manager*. These formal, defined, long-term collaborative groups are authorized to review aggregate variance and are held accountable for the cost/quality results of their patients.

Nurses will need to be comfortable with diversity to be creative in the design and redesign of work. There may even be different managed care or case management programs within the same institution. For instance, stroke patients may need long-term case managers, orthopedic patients may need home visits by physical therapist case managers, and prostatectomy patients may require simply a CareMap tool

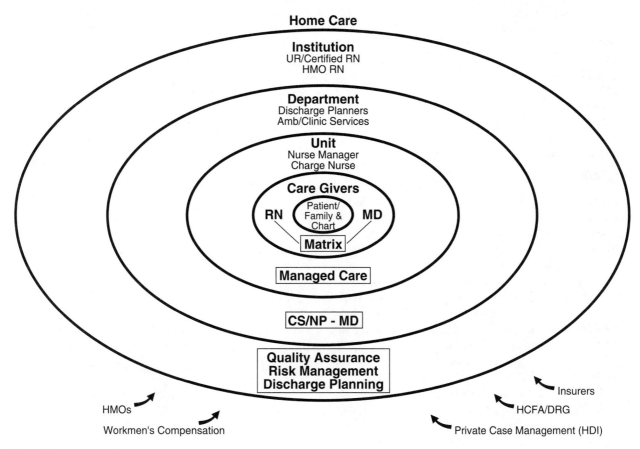

Fig. 35-3. Locus of control options.

Locus of Control	Reports to	Span of Authority	Time Solely Spent on CM	Reimbursement
1. Staff nurse as CM				
a. Direct care	NM	a. Solo or group practice with other RNs, MDs	a. 3 hrs/wk	Clinical ladders
b. Indirect care, charge nurse	NM	b. Line control	b. 40 hrs/wk	Differential, salary, etc.
2. Clin. spec. /NP as CM				
a. Clinical, direct care	NM and/or MD	a. Solo or member of cross-hospital group	40 hrs/wk	Flexibility of time
b. Administrative, consultative	NM and/or MD	b. Facilitate group practice	1 to 2 hrs/wk	Flexibility
3. Administrative CM (non-direct care)	Internal MC/CM Department	Across departments	1 to 2 hrs/wk unless 40 hrs week as product line manager	Salary
4. External case managers	HMO, PPO, Insurer, Private, etc.	All patients under contract	40 hrs/wk	Salary

Fig. 35-4. Case management design choices.

and a followup phone call from their staff primary nurse. All this variety is confusing but exciting.

SUMMARY

In conclusion, form should follow function. In other words, if a proposed structure promises to meet a goal, try it temporarily and evaluate the fit to that goal. Pilot projects should be short-term, with a true beginning, end, and official evaluation.

The habits that keep nursing insular will soon be dysfunctional. The behaviors that stem from true pride in nursing practice will need to be stretched to include other disciplines in the commitment and skills needed for outcome-based practice. Let everyone "own" quality, and expect everyone to "own" the responsibilities inherent in producing quality. Behaviors that grow from security in nursing knowledge and nurses' unequaled ability to operationalize anything from new

equipment to new concepts will serve well in establishing CareMap systems and case management.

REFERENCES

1. Berwick, D. (1992, March/April). Seeking systemness. *Healthcare Forum Journal,* 23.
2. Bower, K. (1988). Nursing case management: The strategic management of cost and quality outcomes. *Journal of Nursing Administration, 18*(5).
3. Cohen, E. (1991). Nursing case management: Does it pay? *Journal of Nursing Administration, 21*(4).
4. Fisher, R., & Ury, W. (1988). *Getting to yes.* New York: Penguin.
5. Health Care Advisory Board. (1990). *Superlative Clinical Quality, 1.*
6. Leebov, W., & Scott, G. (1990). *Health care managers in transition.* San Francisco: The Jossey-Bass Health Series.
7. Zander, K. (1988). Nursing case management: The strategic management of cost and quality outcomes. *Journal of Nursing Administration, 18*(5).
8. Zander, K. (1992). Physicians, CareMaps and collaboration. *The New Definition, 7*(1).
9. Zander, K. (1992). Quantifying, managing, and improving quality, Part II. *The New Definition, 7*(3).

CHAPTER 36

Flextime and self-scheduling

Benefits and difficulties

KAREN S. WULFF

An increasing level of knowledge and education and a greater mix of professionals among American workers has resulted in a heightened demand for worker involvement in decisions and for management flexibility. Flextime requires increased organizational or management flexibility. Self-scheduling represents a complex form of worker participation in decision making.

BACKGROUND

Jamieson and O'Mara describe a workforce that is more diverse in six perspectives: age, gender, culture, education, disabilities, and values.[7] They go on to prescribe flexible management to meet the needs of this more diverse workforce. Flexible management requires a shift in focus from the worker being expected to conform to the organization's norms, or one way of doing things, to the employer being expected to make adjustments to meet the individualized needs of a more varied workforce. Management practices are based on accepting individual differences, valuing people, and providing choices. Policies are minimal and expectations are focused on outcomes rather than constraints and rules on how to do things.[7]

Higher levels of education, along with more leisure time and greater affluence of American workers, have shifted workers' values, priorities, and expectations of work to greater autonomy, respect from superiors, open communication, and opportunities to participate in decision making.[12] Based on Maslow's theory of motivation, the lower needs of food, shelter, and security are met, and workers now desire conditions that provide for increased esteem (recognition from superiors and others they respect) and self-actualization (challenge, learning, and achievement).[3]

In the past decade, three separate national studies have been commissioned to focus on recruitment and retention issues of the nursing profession. The values and expectations of nurses for their work (as documented in these studies) were similar to those described for the general workforce. As partial solutions to the issues of recruitment and retention, all three studies recommended that nurses be given more involvement in decision making and be provided a work environment conducive to professional growth and autonomy.

The National Commission on Nursing, formed in 1980 with 31 leaders from the fields of nursing, hospital administration, medicine, government, academia, business, and hospital trustees, made 18 recommendations aimed at improving recruitment and retention in nursing. Three recommendations specifically relevant to flextime and self-scheduling include: (1) nurses should be involved in policy development and decision making throughout the organizations in which they work; (2) nursing should be recognized as a clinical practice discipline with authority over its management process; and (3) nurses should be provided a work environment that fosters professional growth and development with approaches such as flexible scheduling, appropriate staffing patterns, and career advancement and recognition programs.[9]

The Task Force on Nursing Practice in Hospitals of the American Academy of Nursing (1981-1983) studied the characteristics of hospitals that attracted and retained nurses (magnet hospitals). This study revealed that the great majority of magnet hospitals had heavy nurse involvement in the hospital committee structure and decentralized nursing department structures. This decentralization resulted in staff nurses reporting a sense of control over their immediate work environments, greater autonomy in individual nurse practice, and more flexible work schedules.[1]

The most recent study, which was conducted by a 25-member advisory panel to the Secretary of the Department of Health and Human Services, concluded that "failure on the part of health care delivery organizations, physicians, and health policy-making bodies to fully recognize the decision-making abilities of registered nurses has contributed to problems in recruiting and retaining nurses, hindered the development of a cancer orientation in professional nursing, and limited the efficiency and effectiveness of patient care delivery."[5] This study also called for increased participation of nurses in decision making and an improved work environment that promoted flexibility and professional autonomy.

Thus, the realization that nurses "love their work, but hate their jobs"[11] has led health care administrators to adopt more flexible management practices and to restructure to provide nurses more involvement in the organizations in which they work. Flextime and self-scheduling are two management practices adopted in an attempt to increase registered nurses' job satisfaction and to reduce nurse turnover.

FLEXTIME

Flextime is a system of scheduling work that allows each employee to select a starting and quitting time that best meets personal needs and preference while still meeting work responsibilities.[3] In some work situations, employees may have the discretion to report to work at varying times daily within some established parameters. This generally is only possible within management and leadership roles or where the work done by the individual is independent and does not interface directly with other work.[6] Work that requires continuous coverage, is interdependent to work performed by other employees, or interfaces with other work within or outside the company generally requires a predictable schedule and is incongruent with daily employee discretion regarding work hours.

While nurses in administrative, management, consultation, academic, and research roles have some discretion in selecting daily work hours, most staff nurses—because of the nature of their work, which requires continuous coverage—do not have this discretion. Staff nurses either work as a member of a group practice in a hospital setting, where continuous nursing coverage is required, or within an outpatient setting, where nursing care is administered by appointment. Because of the continuous coverage required within staff nursing, flextime is accomplished by providing variable prescheduled shift start times, shift lengths, and percentages of work.

Because the numbers of patients requiring care and because care requirements are not evenly spread over the hours in a shift or day, the number of nurses needed differs from time to time. This provides an opportunity for both the organization and individual nurses to implement and benefit from variable prescheduled start times and shift lengths. Nurses in many hospital settings now can find work schedules that vary from the traditional shift start times of 7:00 A.M., 3:00 P.M., and 11:00 P.M. These variations from the traditional shifts may start at 1:00 A.M., 3:00 A.M., 5:00 A.M., 6:00 A.M., 9:00 A.M., 11:00 A.M., 1:00 P.M., 5:00 P.M., 7:00 P.M., 9:00 P.M., 10:00 P.M., and 12 M.N. These variable start times are usually associated with either shorter or longer shift lengths than the traditional 8-hour shift. Some nursing units offer shorter 4-hour, 5-hour, or 6-hour shifts to meet peaks in workload that occur in the middle of the traditional shifts, or to match the gap between two 10-hour shifts that other nurses on the unit are working. These shorter shifts with variable start times allow nurses the capability of matching their work schedules with children's school schedules, with spouse's availability for care of children or other family members, or with other social, job, or school commitments.

Many nursing units are offering longer work shifts to accommodate nurses' desires to consolidate their work time into fewer days and to provide longer stretches away from work while maintaining full-time work status. These longer shifts include 9-hour, 10-hour, 12-hour, a mix of 12-hour and 8-hour shifts, or 16-hour shifts. The 9- and 10-hour shifts usually start an hour or two before the traditional shifts or extend an hour or two beyond them. Sixteen-hour shifts are usually just two consecutive traditional shifts. Although 12-hour shifts could start at any time of the day provided the nurses were paired and assumed each other's patient care assignments, they are usually restricted to just a few start times within any unit to minimize confusion and disruption to the unit group process. Extensive use of 12-hour shifts is most easily done in critical care settings, where the number of nurses required for patient care remains about the same during the 24-hour period. Where this is not the case, the number of 12-hour shifts that can be accommodated is restricted by the number of staff required to cover the evening and night shifts. Popular start times for 12-hour shifts include 7:00 A.M. and 7:00 P.M., 9:00 A.M. and 9:00 P.M., 11:00 A.M. and 11:00 P.M., and 1:00 A.M. and 1:00 P.M. The two shifts must be equally attractive and tolerable for staff in order for the combination to work.

Factors contributing to the use of variable percentages of work or job sharing in nursing include the continuous coverage required from staff nurses to meet patient care needs, the repeated shortages of nurses, and the predominance of women in nursing. Without the flexibility of working part-time, the lifestyle demands of managing a household, raising children, or attending graduate school, would force many nurses to quit work. Given the ongoing demand for nurses and the short supply, organizations adapted to these lifestyle needs of nurses by offering them part-time work, job sharing opportunities, and flexible schedules. This benefit lessens the impact of the nursing shortage for organizations, retains nurses in the profession, and offers nurses options to increase and decrease the amount that they work at different times in their careers as their personal lifestyle demands change.

Benefits

Flextime in the forms of variable prescheduled shift start times, shift lengths, and percentages of work required offer benefits to both the organization and individual nurses. For the organization, being able to increase the number of nurses at peak workload times and to decrease the number at low workload times results in more efficient and cost-effective patient care. For example, having some predictability of when a surgical patient will be admitted postoperatively to the unit, surgical units can schedule nurses to begin their shifts at those peak times rather than staffing up for the whole shift in anticipation of the surgical patient admittances.

Reported research has shown flextime to increase productivity and job satisfaction and to improve employee morale and motivation.[2] Flextime is most successful when implemented in a culture that fosters independence and self-motivation, which in turn contributes to increased nurse satisfaction and retention. Increased nurse satisfaction and retention help organizations meet the increased demands for nurses in the face of repeated nursing shortages. Moreover, decreased turnover resulting from flextime reduces ori-

entation costs and contributes to more cost-effective patient care.

For nurses, prescheduled variable shift start times, variable shift lengths, and the ability to share jobs or work part-time offer more choices for balancing work responsibilities and personal lifestyle priorities. For example, the ability to work part-time while children are young or to match children's school hours or the ability to work evening or night shift or only weekends so spouses are available to relieve for child care or elder care are all advantages of the flextime variations offered in nursing. Flextime contributes positively to nurses' perceptions of increased control, increased involvement in decision making, and an enhanced feeling of being valued as an individual. Negativism and burnout are less likely to result with flextime benefits because of a decreased sense of being trapped without choices for balancing lifestyle.

When attempting to recruit individuals into the profession, nurses have not effectively marketed flextime options as one of the unique, positive features of nursing. Given the priorities of the workforce for balancing work and lifestyle, these abilities to work variable schedules to match changing lifestyle needs throughout a career should be publicized.

Difficulties

Flextime can also present difficulties for both individual nurses and for the organization. Because successful implementation requires a balance between meeting nursing care needs of patients and nurses' work scheduling preferences, not all nurses will be able to always work the flextime option which they desire. Thus, it is important that nurses agree with the expectations for required coverage and that they feel scheduling decisions are made fairly. Ease of transfer to other nursing units within the organization where the preferred scheduling options are available also should be facilitated.

Introducing a new role for involvement in work unit decisions and for negotiation of scheduling options with peers will result in staff difficulties unless needed education and skill development are provided. Any change in scheduling patterns can initially be disruptive and require time for staff adjustment. Thus, flexible schedules should be initiated as a trial both for the unit and the individual.

Without careful planning and evaluation, flextime schedules can result in disruptions to the unit routines and nursing practice and result in decreased continuity of care for patients. Initially, the number of different shifts tried on a single unit should be limited to determine the effects on nursing unit routines and to make appropriate adjustments to prevent any negative impacts on nursing practice, patient care, and individual staff. Patient assignments, communications between nursing staff, and physician rounds are examples of unit routines that might need adjustments with flextime schedules. For example, if primary nursing was accomplished by the full-time staff because of its frequency of being at work when 12-hour shifts are initiated, adjustments may be needed to assure nurse accountability for coordination and continuity of patient care and for patient outcomes via multiple nurses rather than a consistent nurse.

One of the consequences of job sharing and increased use of part-time staff is a net increase in numbers of staff a manager supervises. This may necessitate an adjustment in management communication methods. It also increases the numbers of staff requiring feedback, orientation and education, goal setting, scheduling, and performance evaluations. Depending on organizational benefit policies, the increased numbers of staff may result in increased benefits being paid. Hopefully, these increased benefit costs are offset by the decreased orientation expenses of reduced turnover and the increased productivity gains associated with flextime.

SELF-SCHEDULING

Self-scheduling is the process by which nurses and other staff on a nursing unit collectively decide and implement the monthly work schedule.[8,10] Self-scheduling requires staff involvement to develop rules and guidelines for staffing and scheduling that seem fair and equitable to each staff member. Staff also set parameters for minimum numbers and mix of staff required to deliver care to the average number and acuity of patients on each shift and each day of the week. These parameters must also meet budget. The guidelines include procedures for scheduling, requirements for weekend and shift rotations, and rules for handling requests, vacations, and holidays. They also may define consequences for staff members who do not follow the guidelines set for self-scheduling.

Successful implementation of self-scheduling requires staff commitment to the concept and participation in its development on the individual nursing unit. Adequate time must be allowed initially for staff to learn needed concepts about scheduling, to increase interpersonal and negotiation skills, and to adequately participate in every aspect of self-scheduling. The actual scheduling process usually involves staff initially sharing their ideal schedule and then making changes and negotiating with each other until a schedule is produced that optimizes staff desires while still meeting the staffing parameters required for patient care.[4,8,10] Evaluation of the success of this process is based on each staff member feeling that the scheduling process and outcome were fair and that the patient care staffing parameters were met.

Self-scheduling represents a complex form of nurse involvement in unit-level decision making. The goals for self-scheduling include increased nurse recognition, increased perceived autonomy and involvement in decision making, and increased sense of control over the work environment by nurses. As with flextime, self-scheduling is one management practice aimed at increasing nurse satisfaction, improving recruitment into the profession, and decreasing nurse turnover.

Benefits

Self-scheduling offers benefits to both individual nurses and the organizations for which they work. Miller studied the effects of implementation of self-scheduling on a 62-bed medical unit and reported a 55% reduction in turnover rate on the unit, increased awareness of nursing staff for the unit's need for nursing care, a new team spirit among staff, and a more cooperative attitude between staff nurses and nursing administration.[8] Cooperrider reported that participatory scheduling reinforced the beliefs that each staff member is important to the unit and that their ideas are respected and needed in the group process.[4]

Self-scheduling offers the nurse increased individualization and creativity in scheduling, increased sense of control and involvement in unit decisions, and an overall sense of increased autonomy. The individual nurse also benefits from the required change in style of the unit manager because of the self-scheduling process from a negative controlling style of supervisor to a facilitating style of coach. This style change promotes a professional, participatory environment of mutual respect.

The organization benefits from increased nurse satisfaction and retention as a result of the self-scheduling process. Another benefit is increased staff awareness of the difficulties of balancing individual staff scheduling desires with nursing care requirements of patients.

This increased awareness results in increased nurse acceptance of accountability for not only meeting the scheduling needs required for patient care but also for other professional contributions toward the success of the nursing unit and the speciality patient program. Self-scheduling refocuses the nurse manager from schedule development to individualized mentoring of staff toward increased professionalism and accountability.

Difficulties

Self-scheduling is not an easy concept to implement. Success depends on the nurse manager's strong support, patience, and perseverance with implementation. Success also requires staff acceptance of the concept and participation in every aspect of the change to self-scheduling. As stated earlier, adequate time must be allowed for discussion and negotiation at every stage of the process to facilitate staff taking ownership for the schedule. Management must be flexible and allow staff to learn and to be creative with the schedule. The time spent initially in getting ready to implement self-scheduling will be saved later with a smoother implementation.

Self-scheduling is easier to implement with a stable staff where team efforts, trust, and participation are already established norms than with a staff that is experiencing turnover and not yet functioning as a team. Because extensive staff participation, discussion, and negotiation are required to successfully implement self-scheduling, implementation is more easily accomplished with small staffs than with large staffs. If extensive shift rotation is not required for coverage, large staffs might be more successful in implementing self-scheduling among the staff on each shift rather than among the whole staff. Because of the complex communication and interpersonal skills required to implement self-scheduling, this should not be the first participatory concept attempted in any work area. Self-scheduling is more likely to be successful in an already-established high-involvement, professional environment where participatory leadership, open communication, trust, and peer support are norms.

CONCLUSION

Flextime and self-scheduling are being implemented within organizations employing nurses in response to ongoing recruitment and retention issues that contribute to a nursing shortage. In the past decade, three national studies have recommended that health care organizations provide nurses with increased participation in decisions throughout the organizations in which they work and improved work environments that foster professional autonomy and promote flexibility. Flextime and self-scheduling are two management practices that increase nurse involvement in unit-level decisions, promote autonomy, and enhance flexibility and nurse control of the work environment. Implementation of these concepts has proven to increase nurse satisfaction and reduce nurse turnover.

Health care is experiencing a rapid succession of changes spurred by concern for escalating health care costs and compromised health care access. Nurse practice models are changing and patient care is being planned and administered as a continuum of care rather than a hospital episode. These rapid changes and others yet to be defined will result not only in altered nursing practice models, but also in further changes in nurse work patterns and in nurse-employer relationships. The key to effective leadership to meet the future needs of nurses is flexibility. Nurse leaders need to encourage flexible management with a primary focus on the needs of patients and staff nurses and with anticipation because of an awareness of ongoing changes in the health care environment.

While flextime and self-scheduling are congruent with increased nurse involvement in decision making and with an environment conducive to professional practice and autonomy, these are only two management practices. The challenge of nurse leaders is to provide vision and, through flexible management, to provide a culture that promotes positive patient care outcomes and meets individualized needs of professional nurses.

REFERENCES

1. American Academy of Nursing. (1983). *Magnet hospitals: Attraction and retention of professional nurses* (Report of Task Force on Nursing Practice in Hospitals). Kansas City, Mo: American Nurses Association.
2. Buckley, M. R., Fedor, D. B., & Kicza, D. C. (1988). Work patterns altered by new lifestyles. *Personnel Administrator, 33*(12), 40-43.
3. Callahan, R. E., & Fleenor, C. P. (1988). *Managing human relations: Concepts and practices.* Columbus, Ohio: Merrill.
4. Cooperrider, F. (1980). Staff input in scheduling boosts morale. *Hospitals, 54,* 59-61.
5. Department of Health & Human Services. (1988). *Secretary's Commission on Nursing: Final report.* (Vol. 1). Washington, D.C.: Author.
6. Huse, E. R., & Cummings, T. G. (1985). *Organization development and change* (3rd ed.). St Paul: West.

7. Jamieson, D., & O'Mara, J. (1991). *Managing workforce 2000: Gaining the diversity advantage.* San Francisco: Jossey-Bass.

8. Miller, M. L. (1984). Implementing self-scheduling. *Journal of Nursing Administration, 14*(3), 33-36.

9. National Commission on Nursing. (1983). *Summary report and recommendations* (Trust Catalog No. 654200). Chicago: Hospital Research and Education Trust.

10. Ringl, K. K., & Dotson, K. (1989). Self-scheduling for professional nurses. *Nursing Management, 20*(2), 42-44.

11. Wyatt Company. (1989). *I love my work. I hate my job: The nursing crisis in America. A report.* Atlanta: Wyatt Asset Services.

12. Yankelovitch, D. (1982). The work ethic is underemployed. *Psychology Today, 16*(5), 5-8.

CHAPTER 37

Death of the care plan

SUSAN M. TUCKER

Some say the nursing care plan is dead; others say it is alive and well. Why the conflict? The nursing care plan has been around for a long time. Most of us were educated in nursing programs wherein the nursing care plan was the vehicle upon which the student learner's synthesis of theory or course content was applied to a single patient. Patient problems or needs and appropriate interventions and an evaluation were identified. The format followed what is now referred to as the nursing process (assessment, planning, intervention, and evaluation). In recent years, the addition of another step to the process was the making of the nursing diagnosis as the second step of the process. According to Henderson,[4] the nursing process is an analytical process that should be used by all health care providers who are problem solving. The process of care is currently referred to as clinical decision making, which is based on clinical knowledge.

In addition to the nursing process or clinical decision-making framework, many institutions have required nursing care plans to be based on a theoretical model, such as those of Orem,[8] Johnson,[5] Roy,[12] Rogers,[11] Peplau,[10] or others. The application of these theories to the planning of care ranges from its concepts applied to policies and procedures, to the use of verbiage from the model in the care plan or on the patient's record.

The requirement for the use of the nursing care plan has been written into the regulations of some states through the nursing practice acts and hospital licensing regulations. The Joint Commission on Accreditation of Healthcare Organizations (JCAHO) in the Nursing Services chapter of the *Accreditation Manual for Hospitals* has had a standard on the nursing care plan for several years (Table 37-1). Although there has not been an official requirement for a nursing care plan by JCAHO since the early 1980s, the interpretation of the

standards, supported by surveyors, was to have a nursing care plan on all patients who were not exempted from a plan by local hospital policy.

During the 1980s, the nursing staff at several acute care hospitals did, in fact, exempt certain patient populations from the individual nursing care plan requirement of the JCAHO. The exemption often included patients with a length of stay of less than 24 hours and patients undergoing diagnostic or therapeutic procedures. A few creative facilities exempted all or the majority of their inpatients from having individual care plans and referred to reference texts as their source of care planning guides. This practice was congruent with JCAHO standards providing there was evidence of application of the guidelines of care to patients as individuals. For example, the 10-year-old patient undergoing an appendectomy had different needs than a 70-year-old person having the same procedure, and the documentation in the patient's record needed to reflect the individuality of the patient.

Care plan reference books, used to demonstrate compliance with JCAHO standards, varied in format. Some contained guidelines or plans of care based on the medical admitting diagnosis and simply listed the anticipated routine care in a sequential format. Others were divided by body system and admitting medical diagnosis, and contained the most expected nursing diagnoses for the condition and related care and teaching. These references most frequently reflected dependent, independent, and interdependent components of patient centered care. Dependent care is based on the physician's orders, while independent care is based on nursing orders or directives. Interdependent functions are based on the merging of nursing, medicine, and other disciplines to achieve a patient centered (as opposed to a provider centered) quality outcome of care. Other reference books were based on the independent

Table 37-1 Developmental sequence of Joint Commission standards relating to patient care from 1946 to 1980

1946	Due care shall be exercised at all times to ensure safe and efficient nursing care of the patient.
1953	Bedside nursing for all patients is a primary responsibility of the nursing department.
1964	It is axiomatic that adequate nursing service to patients is essential if a hospital is to be accredited. It is expected that there be written nursing care plans for patients. The principle is that thoughtful planning has been done to make sure that the patient received the nursing care he needs.
1969	There shall be evidence established that the nursing service provides safe, efficient, and therapeutically effective nursing care through the planning of each patient's care and the effective implementation of the plans.
1980	The nursing department/service shall be organized to meet the nursing care needs of patients and to maintain established standards of nursing practice. Individualized, goal-directed nursing care shall be provided to patients through the use of the nursing process.

practice of nursing as reflected by nursing diagnoses, sometimes with the addition of a dependent intervention such as to administer medication as ordered (by the physician) for pain control.

Hospitals using reference books as a source of care plans reflected this approach in nursing department policies and procedures. The intent was to provide consistency in care, continuity in care, standardization, and a decrease in the repetitive activity of writing an individual plan of care for patients undergoing the same surgical procedure. This activity also tended to decrease the amount of time spent in documentation by referring to the care planning/guideline reference in the patient's medical record.

In addition, in an effort to reduce the time of writing care plans, promote increased direct nursing time, and demonstrate compliance with JCAHO standards, a plethora of computer software programs have been made available to hospitals. Most of these programs have a variable component in which the using nurse can alter the contents of the plan of care to best reflect the individual needs of the patient.

When a team of nursing experts were convened in 1989 and 1990 to revise the nursing care standards in the *Accreditation Manual for Hospitals*,[6] the requirement for an individualized nursing care plan was

clearly deleted in the 1991 edition of the manual. However, a requirement was specified for planning care "based on identified nursing diagnoses and/or patient care needs, and patient care standards that are consistent with the therapies of other disciplines." The methodology is left up to each institution. Many facilities that have finally perfected their approach to providing individual care plans—whether through a preprinted form, use of reference books, or use of computer programs—are reluctant to give them up. As the average length of stay decreases, acuity mix increases; and as staff mix changes with an increase in the use of nurse extenders, there is and will be less time for registered nurses to do that which is exclusively in their domain of practice. With limited resources, it becomes much more important to reexamine existing practices with regard to the planning of patient care in collaboration with other disciplines and to decrease inappropriate tasks that are labor intensive, time consuming, and extraordinarily costly when there are more efficient methods of achieving similar quality outcomes.

The response to the revised JCAHO nursing care standards that were published in the 1991 *Accreditation Manual for Hospitals* was overwhelmingly positive with regard to the clarity of the omission of a requirement for a nursing care plan. Brider[2] interviewed many of the task force members about the revision and its significance to nursing. The responses were unanimous about the need to lay to rest a tool that is useful for the student nurse or novice but unwieldy and impractical for the majority of practicing nurses.

It continues to be interesting to ask a nurse what is good about a care plan regardless of its type. Nurses may say that a particular plan provides continuity, consistency, and direction; drives professional practice; is convenient; gives a picture of the patient; and shows progress, when and if it is updated. They may also tell us what can be bad about a care plan. It can be repetitive; time consuming; boring; outdated; have subjective goals; have unmeasurable outcomes; create needless paperwork; not always be patient centered; and be wordy, nondescript, and too detailed.

Sovie[13] pointed out that "practicing nurses have been demonstrating with their overwhelming lack of enthusiasm for compliance to the nursing care plan standard [of the JCAHO] that written care plans are not essential to quality patient care." This has been supported in studies by Ferguson, Hildman, and Nichols,[3] where no significant differences were found on any of the outcome variables of three types of nursing care planning systems. These were the (1) printed Kardex with physicians' orders and a list of nursing tasks, (2) standardized nursing care plans with the provision for individualizing them on the chart and (3) a Kardex that was a permanent part of the chart with inclusion of nursing diagnoses and orders as well as physicians' orders.

Benner[1] has described how five different levels of nurses approach their patients and how they perceive clinical situations. These levels are the novice nurse, advanced beginner, competent, proficient, and expert. The change of shift report tells the expert nurse the status, the goals, and the needs of the patient. The expert nurse synthesizes data from multiple sources, makes a nursing diagnosis, and then initiates or appropriately delegates those interventions required to remediate the patient care problem. The relevance of the nursing process was studied by McHugh[7] using Benner's five levels of skill proficiency. The conclusion of this study was that the nursing care plan or the documented nursing process served the novice or advanced beginner, while the advanced practitioner and expert could do very well without the written nursing care plan.

The revised Joint Commission standards are very specific that nursing care should be consistent with the therapies of other disciplines. To ensure this, some hospitals have begun to use multidisciplinary timeline care plans that spread the expected care and expected outcomes across the course of time. Some of these are done by days and others by periods. The prototype for the time line type of care plan is the "critical path" described by Zander, Etheredge, and Bower,[17] and Zander,[15] which is now referred to as a "clinical path" or CareMap.[16] These types of multidisciplinary plans seem to hold the hope for those concerned with providing consistency, continuity, and quality within an expeditious time frame.

The good news is that there is neither a right nor a wrong as to how the planning for care is demonstrated. There are many acceptable alternatives, and that is good for all of us. The Joint Commission has become less prescriptive and seems to welcome the creative approaches of nurses and other clinical leaders in the creation of a multidisciplinary/interdisciplinary plan of care.

With regard to the differences between the traditional nursing care plan and the multidisciplinary plan of care, we can all take a lesson from Florence Nightingale[14] about being flexible: "Everything which succeeds is not the production of a scheme, of rules and regulations made beforehand, but of a mind observing and adapting itself to wants and events." The nursing care plan in its historical sense as a provider-driven, single-discipline tool is moribund. We must be flexible adapting to "wants and events." The multidisciplinary/interdisciplinary planning for patient-centered care is very much alive; with the patient as a partner in establishing outcome goals, the needs of our patient populations will be better served in the future.

REFERENCES

1. Benner, P. (1984). *From novice to expert.* Menlo Park, Calif: Addison-Wesley.
2. Brider, P. Who killed the nursing care plan? *American Journal of Nursing, 91*(5), 35-38.
3. Ferguson, G. H., Hildman, T., & Nichols, B. (1987). The effect of nursing care planning systems on patient outcomes. *Journal of Nursing Administration, 17*(9), 30-36.
4. Henderson, V. (1982). The nursing process—is the title right? *Journal of Advanced Nursing, 7,* 103-109.
5. Johnson, D. E. (1980). The behavioral system model for nursing. In J. P. Riehl & C. Roy (Eds.), *Conceptual models for nursing practice.* New York: Appleton-Century-Crofts.
6. Joint Commission on Accreditation of Healthcare Organizations. (1991). *Accreditation manual for hospitals.* Chicago: Author.
7. McHugh, M. (1986). Nursing process: Musings on the method. *Holistic Nursing Practice, 1*(1), 21-28.
8. Orem, D. E. (1991). *Nursing: Concepts of practice* (4th ed). St Louis: Mosby.
9. Parsek, J. D. (1989). Memorandum to the Nursing Standards Task Force from the Joint Commission on Accreditation of Healthcare Organizations Department of Standards.
10. Peplau, H. E. (1952). *Interpersonal relations in nursing.* New York: G.P. Putnam's Sons.
11. Rogers, M. E. (1970). *An introduction to the theoretical basis of nursing.* Philadelphia: F. A. Davis.
12. Roy, C. (1976). *Introduction to nursing: An adaptation model.* Englewood Cliffs, N.J.: Prentice-Hall.
13. Sovie, M. D. (1989). Clinical nursing practices and patient outcomes: Evaluation, evolution, and revolution. *Nursing Economic$, 7*(2), 79-85.
14. Ulrich, B. (1992). *Leadership and management according to Florence Nightingale.* Norwalk, Conn: Appleton and Lange.
15. Zander, K. (1988). Nursing case management: Strategic management of cost and quality outcomes. *Journal of Nursing Administration, 18*(5), 23-30.
16. Zander, K. (1992). Nursing care delivery methods and quality. *The Delivery of Quality Health Care: Series on Nursing Administration, 3,* 86-104.
17. Zander, K., Etheredge, M., & Bower, K. A. (1987). *Nursing case management: Blueprints for transformation.* Boston: New England Medical Center Hospitals.

CHAPTER 38

The computer-based patient record and how it will affect the nurse's practice

ROY L. SIMPSON

Imagine charting without pen or paper. Imagine being able to organize the information in a patient's medical record to reflect how a nurse thinks. "Decouple the idea from its physical medium and all sorts of possibilities emerge."[1] The purpose of this chapter is to explore the possibilities for nursing that emerge from the decoupling of the medical record from its physical medium. In particular, the chapter will examine the impact that the computer-based patient record (CPR) will have on the nurse's practice.

The chapter opens with a primer on technology. In discussions about technology, terminology can often be troublesome. To avoid such problems, relevant concepts are defined, and a brief history of the computer-based patient record is presented. The recent report from the Institute of Medicine represents a significant moment in the development of the CPR, and for this reason the strategic vision elaborated in this report is briefly discussed.[2]

Vendors play a critical role in the development of the computer-based patient record. Even so, nurses continue to misunderstand what vendors do, often displaying an appalling lack of information about the inner workings of capitalism. This incomplete knowledge base means that nurses are unable to negotiate effectively in the marketplace, leaving the critical information systems development and selection processes to others. To address this disparity, the "business point of view" is described briefly. The bottom line is: A meaningful partnership between the nursing profession and health care computer companies must be de-

veloped to produce a product line fully supportive of the computer-based patient record.

Once these general ideas are discussed, the specific issues to do with nursing and the CPR are approached. The computer-based patient record is expected to impact the nurse's practice in two fundamental ways. First, the nurse's actual day-to-day practice will be changed in significant ways by the presence of the computer-driven record. Second, the nursing profession as a whole will be affected more globally, which, in turn, will impact the nurse's practice. Both types of change are discussed.

Two additional items should be remembered when considering these points. First, how other, more universal health care issues, such as those of cost, access and quality, play out will affect profoundly the development of the computer-based patient record. For example, if the U.S. health care system is nationalized, reimbursement will no longer be a problem, and as a result, the critical security issues surrounding preexisting conditions, such as HIV status, will no longer require debate. Second, knowledge is power, and as nurses grapple for a stake in the future of health care, the structure and nature of nursing knowledge increasingly becomes a point of dispute.[6,9] If computerization is knowledge engineering,[7] then the "knowledge is power" struggle of this decade and the next will most likely be played out in the information systems arena. Under these circumstances, computerization clearly becomes a central, if not fundamental, concern for nursing. In fact, it may well be *the* issue—and must be appreciated as such—so that nurses can learn to maneuver and establish their practice domain. The first step in recognizing the importance of computers to the future of nursing is to develop a basic understanding of technology in general and the CPR in particular.

The author would like to thank June B. Somers, RN, PhD, for her scholarly assistance in preparing this chapter.

A TECHNOLOGY PRIMER

Background information is especially important in discussions that focus on technology. First, important points can often be obscured by acronyms and jargon. Second, common terms and concepts frequently change meaning from vendor to vendor, further complicating discussion. The section that follows is intended to set the stage for future discussion by defining terms and identifying basic concepts.

Donald Englebart, a remarkably talented engineer at Stanford Research Institute, identified that his early work with computer technology had one goal, namely, to develop systems "to augment human intellect."[3] By defining technology as tools to augment human intellect, the proper focus is brought to bear on the idea of technology. First, the definition emphasizes that technology assists people and supplements their basic capabilities. The individual remains accountable and responsible. Second, in this definition, the "making of technology" remains grounded in thinking and intellect, regardless of mechanistic appearances. Bringing this definition to a discussion on the computer-based patient record elevates the idea of electronic documentation to its proper place. That is, a computer-based patient record is more than a way of storing data or recording data; it represents a way of thinking and acting that will have far-reaching implications for the practice of nursing.

Electronic documentation[10] began as the narrowly focused *electronic medical chart* (EMC). The generic process of electronic charting began with isolated vendors or computer companies providing "quick-and-dirty system upgrades" for individual client hospitals. The focus was the episodically based hospital chart. With the EMC, system functions were limited to support for one episode per patient and one provider. The next step in the evolution of electronic documentation was the *automated patient chart* (APC) or the *electronic patient chart* (EPC). The use of one term over the other was a matter of vendor preference, and vendor marketing collateral reflected these decisions. Basically, the APC and the EPC were one and the same, and the focus of the record remained the same as for the EMC; that is, the patient's chart for one stay or one visit established the boundaries for the data. The progression was seen in the behavior of computer companies in that vendors began to write software in a more orderly fashion and provide the same product line to a number of clients or providers. Vendors were motivated to improve software to maintain their market share.

The next step in the development of electronic documentation was represented by a product called the *electronic medical record* (EMR). Vendors expanded the software away from the one-episode, chart-by-chart focus to include all episodes of care for a patient. The electronic document remained tied to a particular provider but was expanded to include all activities in all sectors, whether inpatient or outpatient.

The final and last step is represented by the computer-based patient record, which represents the culmination of efforts in electronic documentation. This type of electronic record includes all visits or stays for all providers for the lifetime of the patient, from birth to death. In their report on the patient record of the future, the Institute of Medicine (IOM) defined the CPR as follows:

[The computer-based patient record is]. . . an electronic patient record that resides in a system specifically designed to support users through availability of complete and accurate data, practitioner reminders and alerts, clinical decision support systems, links to bodies of medical knowledge, and other aids. This definition encompasses a broader view of the patient record than is current today, moving from the notion of a location or device for keeping track of patient care events to a resource with much enhanced utility in patient care (including the ability to provide an accurate longitudinal account of care), in management of the health care system, and in extension of knowledge.[2]

The Committee on Improving the Patient Record, Division of Health Care Services, Institute of Medicine, concluded that *"no current system, however, is capable of supporting the complete CPR."*[2] Prototypes of systems that approach the concept of the CPR are found primarily in teaching hospitals. They include the Summary Time-Oriented Record (STOR) system at the University of California at San Francisco; the HELP model from Utah's Latter-Day Saints Hospital; the THERESA system at Grady Hospital in Atlanta; and The Medical Record developed at Duke University in North Carolina.[10]

In their report, the committee opened the section on "User Need and System Requirements" by emphasizing that "direct providers of care will remain the users of highest priority in design considerations."[2] The objectives for the CPR include: supporting patient care and improving the quality of that care; enhancing administrative control; supporting health services research; accommodating future developments in technology, policy, management and finance; and maintaining patient confidentiality.[2] While the committee concluded that most technological barriers to the creation and implementation of the CPR have disappeared or are about to disappear, nontechnological barriers remain. These include a lack of understanding of the nature of the task and a lack of infrastructure to support the CPR. Adequate funding and effective organization were identified as necessary for overcoming these barriers.[2] Even though most patient records today are paper records, the committee set the year 2000 as the year for achieving a computer-based patient record.[11]

Reaching the ambitious goal of having a CPR by the year 2000 will require close collaboration between nurses and vendors. Before this can happen, nurses need to develop an understanding of the role of the vendor as a capitalist, a subject explored in the next section.

THE REALITY OF THE MARKET

Repeated questioning by nurses of vendors' intentions suggests that nurses have a pervasive distrust of computer professionals in the private sector. This is not a personal issue but a professional one. This is an issue of great importance to nurses because vendors make technology, and, as indicated above, the making of technology is pivotal to the future viability of nursing as a profession. In 1990, Woolery stated "Nurse administrators should question the ethics of computer vendors who are obviously in the business to sell systems."[17] This statement reflects a profound misunderstanding of the capitalist system. Of course, vendors are in the business of selling systems—that is what capitalism is all about. Certainly there are unethical salespersons, but this statement suggests that one of the basic activities of capitalism is unethical itself. How can nurses who have this viewpoint collaborate with vendors on product development? What kind of products will nursing have on hand, if their input is not forthcoming? Where does this leave the computer-based patient record? In an effort to begin the building of bridges, the following points are offered to assist nurses in understanding and appreciating what it means to be a vendor.

Basically, understanding where technology makers are coming from means understanding the business point of view because most of today's technology is made in the private sector or in partnership with the private sector. The business point of view is made up of six primary aspects.

Aspect one is capitalism. In technology, the market economy rules. Capitalism defines the rules of the game. This may be an undesirable state of affairs. Nevertheless, this is the way it is, at least for now.

Aspect two is entrepreneurism and intrapreneurism. The nature of technology development is innovation and product development. By definition, entrepreneurs and intrapreneurs assume a risk for the sake of profit. They innovate to make money. A person who does so within an organization is called an intrapreneur. Persons who have their own organizations are called entrepreneurs. Both entrepreneurs and intrapreneurs are needed in nursing, so that the profession can thrive in the world of computers.

Aspect three is the market, which is the guiding light in all technology-design decisions. Technology makers design what sells. Research and development for new product lines is driven by what makes money. As long as nurses continue to buy inadequate nursing systems, new and better nursing systems will not be developed. This is a crucial point for nurses to understand, particularly with regard to the CPR. It is encouraging to note that a recent survey of nursing leaders indicated that 93% of those surveyed think that a form of the CPR is either absolutely essential or important.[12]

Aspect four is the clinical financial tension. All nurses need to realize that this tension, prevalent in most health care organizations, is also present in the private firms that make technology. Nurses need to work together and support each other to improve the balance toward clinical systems. It would be ironic if the CPR were developed because finance supported it as a means to improve revenue.

Aspect five can be described as the "facts of nursing." With regard to computer systems specifically, nurses need to appreciate the task of automating nursing, most particularly the enormity of automating documentation. For example, a single nurse creates 106,000 data points in just *one* hour. Imagine the data points generated in one day! Imagine automating the entry of that amount of data, not to mention dealing with the problems of quality, storage, and retrieval. These issues have to be confronted with the bottom line of the organization in mind.

And finally, there is aspect six, system development. Beyond the simple function of storing and retrieving massive amounts of information, the question is how do you make data systematic so that it can be automated in the first place? Tasks must also be made systematic. The work of the nurse must be "translatable" to become a technical product. This means vendors need nurses to develop their products. Maintaining a hands-off attitude with regard to vendors only hurts nursing. Successful vendors usually appreciate what nurses have to contribute, and they appreciate the honesty of a what's-in-it-for-nursing attitude.

Even though technology is, for the most part, made in the private sector, in the end the responsibility for the quality of nursing systems rests with the nursing profession.[13] Allowing the design process, particularly for a product as important as the computer-based patient record, to default to computer professionals in the private sector because the rules of the game *appear* distasteful is not acceptable. In effect, blaming others, such as vendors, is strategically lethal and pragmatically short-sighted.

NURSING PRACTICE AND THE CPR

The computer-based patient record will affect the nurse's practice profoundly. First, the real work of nursing, the actual hands-on patient care, will be impacted directly. Second, the nursing profession as a whole will be changed, which, in turn, will influence the day-to-day practice of nursing. Both of these types of change are considered.

It is fairly obvious that the real work of nursing will be impacted significantly by the presence of the computer-based patient record. First, the nurse's workplace will be affected. The nurse's workplace encompasses more than the hospital bedside, and includes, among other areas, patients' homes, outpatient clinics, homeless clinics, "the street," and group therapy settings. As nurses move into expanded roles and develop advanced practice models, the nurse's workplace will expand further. Wherever a nurse is practicing, a workplace exists. Primarily, nurses will be more productive. Not only is electronic documentation thought to be faster than manual documentation, but the nurse with a CPR is also expected to work "smarter." Technological "helps," which are part of the CPR, will promote these "smart" work habits. Technological helps include links to secondary, informational databases, image processing and storage, and the presence of fully configured workstations. In fact, a consensus is developing among nursing leaders that computer technology, most particularly bedside terminals, and the resulting improvements in productivity will be one of the best ways to deal with the ever-present nursing shortage.[15,16]

Second, the computer-based patient record will increase accountability and responsibility. It will provide an extremely clear projection of what is to be done for the patient and who should do it, as well as an indisputable record of what was actually done for the patient and who was responsible for carrying out the activity. "Technology promises to provide the tools to restructure the business of nursing by providing the means for accountability and thus, revenue responsibility."[14] The computer-based patient record is a splendid example of the family of technological tools that promotes accountability and responsibility by establishing detailed and accurate audit trails.

The third impact on the nurse's practice that results from the implementation of the computer-based patient record has to do with the type of thinking inherent in the practice of nursing. The fact is that the computer-based patient record will force the nurse to move into the realm of critical thinking. Critical thinking is "thinking that is purposeful, reasoned and goal directed. It is the kind of thinking involved in solving problems, formulating inferences, calculating likelihoods, and making decisions."[4] Components of the computer-based patient record, which include data integration, tools for focusing attention such as alarms and tickler files, decision-support features, access to data analysis software, and online help functions, will encourage and support critical thinking at one level and require it for effective system usage at another level. The use of critical thinking will, in turn, focus the nurse more directly on the patient, rather than on rote tasks. As a result, patient care will become more individualized, which should improve patient outcomes and patient satisfaction.

The fourth impact on the practice of nursing has to do with roles. The computer-based patient record will require two distinct data processing roles, data collector and data manager. The presence of these two roles will facilitate the emergence of clinical role differentiation in nursing, resulting in two levels of nursing, the associate degree (AD) nurse and the master's-prepared nurse. The AD nurse will function in the role of data collector, and the master's-prepared nurse will function as the researcher or the data manager.

The fifth impact, the computer-based patient record, will promote collaboration and consultation among nurses. Nurses will move beyond the boundaries of cities and states, and even countries to consult with each other about the care of particular patients. Instead of moving physically, these nurses will travel along the "national (and international) transportation system for patient data."[2] Colleagueship will be enhanced to include practitioners, educators, and researchers, all of whom will work together to advance and improve individual and collective patient care.

And finally, the presence of the computer-based patient record in the clinical setting is projected to improve the quality of care being delivered. Nurses are estimated to spend up to 44% of their clinical practice time on manual documentation and communication tasks.[10] The computer-based patient record is expected to reduce the time spent on such activities, which should allow for more direct, quality-promoting, patient contact. Also, the CPR will enhance and improve the quality of patient data, that is, the amount, timeliness, content, etc., of the data. Improved patient databases, in turn, should enhance the quality of patient care decisions that should result in improved patient care. Further, because of built-in system features, required data will be controlled and nurses will not be allowed to leave the system until all data entry is complete. These features will reduce critical omissions from the patient database, further improving the quality of the data and the quality of the care.[10]

The computer-based patient record is also expected to affect the nurse's practice indirectly. These changes are more global in nature. The computer-based patient record is expected to change the focus of the practice of nursing. The focus will be expanded to include patient outcomes, particularly with regard to reimbursement protocols. The CPR will encourage this shift, and a balance between outcome and process is expected to be achieved for the first time in the history of nursing.

The change in focus to outcome, which is encouraged by the CPR, will promote a refocusing of the nurse's practice from an emphasis on illness to include a more balanced view which includes wellness. Still allowing for activities to do with practice patterns centered on restoration and cure, the CPR will encourage education and prevention. With the CPR, the patient record will be from birth to death, and it will include all health care encounters. The view of the patient will be broader and longer, and the CPR will present more of an in-depth view of the patient. The picture of the patient will be such that a wellness orientation emerges naturally as a by-product of the system.

Nursing researchers often promote theory to the exclusion of experience.[5] The computer-based patient record will support both theory and practice because it places equal emphasis on data collection and data manipulation. In fact, the computer-based patient record may be revolutionary because it will provide a bridge to link the inductive world of the clinical practitioner with the deductive world of the researcher. The knowledge developed from this collaboration will be complete in a sense never experienced before in the history of nursing.

One of the most fascinating changes projected to develop from implementation of the computer-based patient record has to do with the law. The CPR is projected to push the boundaries of the present law and require additional judicial and legislative support to accommodate the expanded medical record suggested by the CPR. Issues, such as signatures, identification of practitioners, data access, and date ownership, will require thoughtful attention.

The computer-based patient record will require a redefinition of system security. A "public airways" focus may be required, and the possibility of more stringent sanctions for computer-related white collar crime will have to be considered.[8] Tightened security will make system access more difficult for all users, which, in turn, will cause implementation problems for the computer-based patient record. Further, health care professionals may see a licensure procedure that includes a security clearance, leading to the day when provincial interests of state boards of nursing will be forced to give way to a federally supported and nationally focused board of nursing. The clear implication for this change is one license and one number for each nurse.

Nursing administration functions such as staffing and scheduling should be enhanced by having the computer-based patient record in place. One of the goals of the CPR is the support of administration and management.[2] The ability to access aggregate patient data will support and enhance an endless list of activities for managing health care systems such as developing staffing plans, costing-out nursing, designing real-time acuity systems, and measuring the quality of the care being delivered by practitioners.

The impact of the CPR on nursing practice will be massive and far-reaching. Actual day-to-day practice will be affected directly and indirectly as the national health care system moves to expand the medical record to include the features embodied in a computer-based patient record.

CONCLUSION

A future that includes the computer-based patient record holds great promise for the practice of nursing. Health care traditionally spends only 2% to 3% of its total gross dollars on information systems, as compared to almost 8% for industry as a whole.[12] Nurses, and in particular nursing leaders, need to focus their energy on the goal set by the Institute of Medicine, that is, to achieve a computer-based patient record by the year 2000.[2] Specific actions are necessary before change can take place. Nurses need to act. They need to: (1) support the development of taxonomies and nomenclatures which define the practice of nursing; (2) assist in efforts to develop a minimum data set for nursing; (3) get involved in information system activities in current practice settings and encourage development of the CPR; and (4) work within current nursing organizations to address the controversial changes identified as projected outcomes of the CPR. The Institute of Medicine set in motion a plan for achieving the computer-based patient record. It is now up to nurses and other health care professionals to see to it that this plan is implemented.

REFERENCES

1. Belsie, L. (1992, March 26). Publishing without paper or ink. *The Christian Science Monitor,* p. 12.
2. Dick, R. S., & Stein, E. B. (Eds.). (1991). *The computer-based patient record: An essential technology for health care.* Washington, D.C.: National Academy Press.
3. Dunlop, C., & Kling, R. (Eds.). (1991). *Computerization and controversy.* Boston: Academic Press.
4. Halpern, D. F. (1989). *Thought and knowledge.* Hillsdale: Lawrence Erlbaum Associates.
5. Mitchell, G. J. (1991). Diagnosis: Clarifying or obscuring the nature of nursing. *Nursing Science Quarterly, 4*(2), 52.
6. Parse, R. R. (1991). Editorial: Growing the discipline of nursing. *Nursing Science Quarterly, 4*(4), 139.
7. Perrolle, J. A. (1991). Intellectual assembly lines: The rationalization of managerial, professional, and technical work. In C. Dunlop & R. Kling (Eds.), *Computerization and controversy* (pp. 221-235). Boston: Academic Press.
8. Salerno, L. M. (1991). What happened to the computer revolution? In C. Dunlop & R. Kling (Eds.), *Computerization and controversy* (pp. 118-130). Boston: Academic Press.
9. Schlotfeldt, R. M. (1988). Structuring nursing knowledge: A priority for creating nursing's future. *Nursing Science Quarterly, 1*(1), 35-38.
10. Simpson, R. L. (1991). Electronic patient charts: Beware of the hype. *Nursing Management, 22*(4), 13-14.
11. Simpson, R. L. (1991). Computer-based patient records, Part I: The Institute of Medicine's vision. *Nursing Management, 22*(10), 24-26.
12. Simpson, R. L. (1992). What nursing leaders are saying about technology. *Nursing Management, 22*(7), 20-21.
13. Simpson, R. L., & Somers, J. B. (1991). The role of the clinical nurse specialist in information systems selection. *Clinical Nurse Specialist, 5*(3), 159-163.
14. Simpson, R. L., & Waite, R. (1989). NCNIP's system of the future: A call for accountability, revenue control and national data sets. *Nursing Administration Quarterly, 14*(1), 72-77.
15. Sorrentino, E. A. (1991). Overcoming barriers to automation. *Nursing Forum, 26*(3), 21-23.
16. Weisfeld, N. E., & Amor, G. E. (1991). Toward a national policy for nursing. *Nursing Outlook, 39*(2), 73-76.
17. Woolery, L. K. (1990). Professional standards and ethical dilemmas in nursing information systems. *Journal of Nursing Administration, 20*(10), 50-53.

CHAPTER 39

Primary health care in developing countries

BARBARA ROBERTSON

Primary public health care (PHC) is probably one of the most widely used concepts in current health care and has been the topic of numerous debates, articles, and books. Its meaning is variously interpreted by different groups of health workers and, therefore, the implications for practice in a health care system are seldom spelled out clearly. PHC may be interpreted as a second-class service to the poor in rural areas or in institutions as a base for a framework on which to build the more important secondary and tertiary health services. To many nurses, it may be simplistically viewed as any service outside the hospital.

Because of this confusion, it is important to understand some of the factors that led to the development of the primary public health care approach. Walt and Vaughan[9] highlight the issues that linked health status to other sectors outside of the traditional health ministry. They point out that food production and the supply of drinking water, housing, and roads are all under the control of other departments; thus the need for a multidisciplinary intersectoral approach to health. With the increasing world population, there was a realization that food and other resources were not limitless. Thus, emphasis had to be placed on mother and child care to control the birth rate, and to try to break the cycle of poverty and high infant and maternal mortality rates. The reliance of Western medicine on sophisticated technology with its attendant high cost made it available to fewer people. This led to dissatisfaction with the medical approach as it overlooked the social, political, and economic aspects of health. In countries where communities become involved in their own health care, people were empowered to take control of their lives and their health. This led to the training of community health workers.

It has become evident that PHC is more than a level of care; it requires a paradigm shift away from the traditional way in which health care is provided, where the biological model with superspecialization takes precedence over all other types of care. The philosophy of PHC is based on a different set of principles, and requires physicians and nurses to be trained for community-based practice. Important aspects for consideration should include:

- The interdependence of health and socioeconomic development. Poor health means low productivity and a decline in economic growth.
- A multisectoral approach, in which the provision of water, basic sanitation, and adequate nutrition are key elements. This requires health workers to work with many other disciplines and to use appropriate technology.
- A comprehensive approach that is more holistic than the medical approach. In line with many Western nations, developing countries have largely adopted the curative model of health care, which allows physicians to dominate.
- The need for health workers to reach out to provide care for high-risk and vulnerable groups, e.g., the under-5 group, women, the aged, and those who, for a variety of reasons, cannot provide for their own health needs.
- Services that are accessible to the community. Services in both the urban and rural areas tend to be out of reach to the majority of the population. Infrastructure is inadequate; e.g., roads and transport are not available. Informal settlements around most big cities in developing countries are at a distance from the nearest health service and are underserved.
- Community participation in health services where community members are in partnership with the health care providers. Alma Ata, article iv, states: People have the right and the duty to participate in-

dividually and collectively in the planning and implementation of their health care.[1]

- Equity of distribution of services across the communities (both urban and rural) in a country. The best services are often based in the urban areas.[9]

The danger is that these PHC principles may be so broad, so politically noncontentious, and so comprehensive as to be difficult to implement.

CURRENT MODELS OF PHC

Different models have been developed for the implementation of the PHC concept. Kaseje[4] describes three.

The top-down approach

PHC is provided by medical and nursing personnel based on their perceptions of the community's health needs; after all, they have the knowledge and know best. There is little or no consultation with the community residents or regard for their views. This system is managed in a top-down fashion and is little more than an extension of the hospital's outpatient department. It tends to be largely curative rather than comprehensive. The motives of those carrying out such an approach are based on their institutional training perspectives on health care. Communities tend to passively accept this approach but may feel abused and dissatisfied with the often impersonal manner in which they are treated. Frequent changes in medical staff and their lack of interest in services outside the institution further bedevil the effectiveness of the approach. The indicators used to measure success are medical and inappropriate to the needs of the community. Because it is added onto an existing institutional service, the budgetary provision is usually inadequate. Bureaucracy, with its authoritarian, self-perpetuating, traditional, and rigid hierachy, makes change difficult and results in discord, anger, and bullying of patients.

The selective approach

This approach has been used by many to try to meet the needs of the community, usually by seeking to improve the health status of certain target groups through the use of technological means. The Growth monitoring, Oral rehydration, Breast feeding, Immunization, Family planning, Food supplements and Female literary (GOBIFFF) Program is an example of this method. Nurses are taught to control dehydration in diarrhea using oral rehydration therapy but are impotent to help mothers and families to handle the social and environmental problems that have caused the diarrhea.

Newell[7] states that selective PHC tends to preserve the status quo by keeping decision making and control in the hands of professional workers. Consultation, because of budgetary and logistic reasons, is with the health authorities and local leaders, not with the people. The community thus retains its powerless position and its socioeconomic needs are not met.

In the above two approaches, health care is understood and interpreted in medical terms.

The community-based approach

Kaseje[4] states that "health is not a commodity to be delivered but a quality of life to be cared for." For this reason, it is essential for communities to take responsibility for their health status. The community-based approach uses a broad approach to empower communities to handle health issues. The focus is on the disadvantaged majority and seeks to address the socioeconomic and political problems that hinder the health of the poor. The communities identify and analyze their needs, seek solutions, and take the necessary action. Health workers act as resource persons, give support, and participate in the program in a manner accepted by the people. In this process of self-discovery, families and communities gain knowledge on the issues affecting their lives and develop confidence in seeking and implementing solutions. In the partnership, each group shares its strengths, and weaknesses are minimized.

Rifkin[8] states that "it is not possible or even useful to have a universally accepted definition of community participation." She outlines three main approaches similar to those of Kaseje, which she calls, first, the medical approach, which has as its objective the medication of individual illness; second, the health service approach in which the community takes an active role in the delivery of health care services; and, third, the community development approach in which the community members are actively involved in the decision on how to improve conditions. These models vary from a top-down to a bottom-up approach.

In many countries, the development of PHC care is still in its infancy. Glatthaar[2] states that "In South Africa, very largely a developing country, it has taken 10 years to discover the importance of PHC. It is further estimated that it will take another 10 years before a network of effective PHC services will be available to all."

Reasons put forward for the delays in implementing PHC are:

- Politics
- Vested interests
- A stubborn unwillingness to cooperate and share
- The stranglehold of bureaucracy
- Territorialism
- Ad hoc decision making
- Uncoordinated planning and decision making
- Marginal support

The existing PHC and the curative services are fragmented and are carried out on an ad hoc basis by a wide variety of government and nongovernment organizations. Models follow the top-down approach.

COMMUNITY-BASED PHC WITH COMMUNITY PARTNERSHIP

There are no quick fixes in moving to a community-based PHC approach as the concept is foreign to health workers, decision makers, and academics. However, no change can take place until the implications of the community-based model are identified and confronted.

A community-based approach involves community partnerships and community empowerment. McMurray[6] says this can only occur "when a community is able to choose strategies for health based on appropriate information, local resources, accessible support, institutional organization, and social approval."

Community partnerships are built on honesty between groups, trust relationships, and a free exchange of ideas. There must be commitment to each other, the service, the community, and, if applicable, the teaching institution. There must be a tolerance of different viewpoints and a willingness to share strengths and weaknesses. Each must take responsibility and handle the relationship with sensitivity and enthusiasm for the cause.

The level of education of the people is immaterial; uneducated people should not be viewed as ignorant but rather as mature people with much life experience. Health committees should be democratically elected, and members should be representative of the community organizations, the disadvantaged groups (e.g., the elderly, women's groups), and individual community members. Realistic and attainable goals need to be agreed upon. In addition, there must be a sensitive regard for political and other differing views between the groups. One of the real dangers in this type of service is to make promises that cannot be fulfilled and, in doing so, to raise unrealistic expectations.

Partnerships should take place in a noncompetitive and nonexploitative atmosphere where participants have faith in the process and are flexible in their approach. There must be ongoing sharing of information because each needs knowledge from the other—one on community norms and the other on health. Health workers need to be accountable to the community. They need to take time and leave their offices to go to the community and earn their acceptance. Working and building partnerships in the community is challenging and demanding because community partnerships can be fragile and should never be taken for granted. It should be born in mind that communities are not necessarily harmonious groups. Community divisions—political, ethnic, religious, social, or factional— can bedevil the formation of partnerships. Apathy, confused leadership, and unresponsiveness further affect the situation. The rewards of such a partnership are far reaching and exciting. It is thrilling to see community groups starting to take responsibility for what is happening to them and to question the standards and type of health care provided for them. This may not always be comfortable for the nurse as his or her methods of care come under scrutiny. This stage must be gone through, and, if necessary, apologies should be given for mistakes made and for insensitive attitudes towards the community. This type of action will build trust.

COMMUNITY NEEDS FOR SERVICES AND HEALTH TEACHING

Community health needs do not necessarily relate only to disease issues. In many rural areas and informal settlements, the overriding needs are for houses, infrastructure, such as roads, drinking water, sewage, refuse disposal, and food production. In recent visits to 13 PHC projects, I learned from a number of communities that "improved nurse attitudes" was their next most important need. This was followed by the need for clinic services with a resident doctor if possible.

The communities were not only asking for help with basic infrastructure that in a developed country is taken for granted but were also asking to be taught leadership, management, teaching, and empowerment skills, including simple bookkeeping, signing checks, keeping a bank account, chairing meetings, and taking minutes. How to talk to authorities from a position of knowledge and strength was a special need.

Community health workers

Because of the failure of the health services to promote community development and because the nurse was seen as inadequately trained to work in partnership in the community, there has been a move to train community health workers (CHWs). These health workers are chosen by the community and are members of the community. It was felt that they would understand the needs of the community better and would be able to educate them in a more acceptable way. The concept has merit and has resulted in some remarkable success stories. On the other hand, the literature abounds with accounts of projects using CHWs that have failed. While not negating the need for such categories, there are lessons to be learned:

- Health services cannot be totally carried out by community health workers. They do play a major role in empowering communities, in providing health education, and in providing basic health services.
- Nurses can provide clinical care for up to 80% of the medical needs of the community. A good referral system with community and regional hospitals are needed for the acutely ill.
- CHWs should be remunerated for their services and be accountable to the community. However, if they are incorporated into the health service, they lose their ability to do what the community sees as a priority. Their loyalty will lie with their employing body. Because they mix with other health workers in the course of their duties, the need for a career ladder and promotion opportunities will become evident.
- CHWs need a support system, ongoing education, and acceptance by other health workers. If they are being trained by nonhealth professionals, the content of what is being taught needs to be checked.
- There appears to be a proliferation of CHWs in many community-related programs without proper planning and consultation with the community. I have come across 9 to 10 different types of CHW categories, including environmentalists, various categories of rehabilitation workers, development workers, care group women, tuberculosis and AIDS assistants, family planning assistants, village health workers, and so on. The proliferation causes fragmentation in care, and the community is being bombarded by these and other workers who might all be giving them different and sometimes conflicting messages. Is this a cost-effective system? Might this system not also be used by professionals to justify their unwillingness to meet real health needs and to remain in the comfort of their institutions. The interrelationship of the community health worker and the professional worker needs to be sorted out.

Community perspectives of nurses

When visiting many communities in and around southern Africa, I listened to community members express some of their views on nursing. These are by no means all negative, and many have high praise for the sacrifices made by them and for the level of medical care given. However, these are some of the aspects that concern them:

- The arrogance of nurses and the way in which they distance themselves from the community.
- Their resentfulness towards suggestions that are made by the community for improvements and their criticism of community ways.
- The general lack of trust that exists between the community members and the nurses. This is largely because of suspicion created because neither party understands what the other is doing. Each has its own agenda, which it pursues with little or no communication between them.
- Community members do not feel that the service is of benefit to them. They are not comfortable with what happens to them, but they do not have the knowledge or resolve to take action.
- The nurses seem to think they have all the health knowledge and speak down to the community in a patronizing manner. This is especially so when they are giving health education talks: "You have to listen to them before you are attended to at the clinic. You feel you are being abused."
- Students come into the area to do "their thing." "You are never introduced to them and do not know why they have come. They use our resources and then go away again without even expressing their thanks."

A colleague of mine was very surprised by the communities' reactions. She had not realized that the nurses have such a poor image in the community. She said, "It was a shock to realize how much we as professional people take the community for granted."

On the other hand, nurses are frustrated and complain about the lack of transport, the absence of a proper communication system, and inadequate supplies and equipment. There is an apathy among nurses towards community work. Most rural nurses questioned would like to go back to the urban areas as soon as they can get a post or as soon as their spouse can get a transfer back to town.

THE NURSE'S ROLE

Nurses are the largest category of health worker in many countries and have the opportunity of playing a major role in PHC if they are willing to change their attitudes, learn new skills, and make major changes to their curriculums so that there are future generations of appropriately trained nurses. Change from a curative hospital-oriented approach will not be without pain, and many nurses will be tempted to perpetuate the present system or at best patch it.

In this new role, nurses should be resource people for the community. Mahler[5] says, "Millions of nurses throughout the world hold the key to an acceptance and expansion of PHC because they work closely with people." He would like to see them become resources to the community rather than to the physicians. There is a need for the nurse to be a generalist with relevant training in PHC. There are many new skills that will have to be learned apart from the nursing, management, and teaching skills. Nurses need good communication skills, with decision-making and problem-solving ability. Harnar[3] says that "it is perhaps most crucial that the nurse be able to trust people, to learn from them, to share leadership with them when it is appropriate and to plan with them." In addition, the nurse needs to be able to network, negotiate, use simple jargon-free language, teach self-help skills, know how to empower people, have knowledge of community procedures, and be able to negotiate expertise across the disciplines, community structures, and government bodies.

CURRICULUM CHANGE

PHC has not had much acceptance in academic institutions. It is necessary that models of excellence be developed in which the students spend 30% to 40% of their time in the community. This will mean that the staff should be rendering care to the underserved, as well as teaching students in the health facility. No existing curriculum can be patched; a new philosophy will have to be developed and community needs will have to be researched. As the focus of education moves to the community, clinical experience in the community will have to be provided at an early stage with suitable reduction of time spent in the tertiary institu-

tion. Course content and learning experiences will have to be constantly checked with the principles of PHC and the needs of the community. It would be wise to have selected community representatives on the curriculum committee.

Didactic teaching should be kept to a minimum and a problem-based approach used, with lots of time for discussion and exploring issues and problems. Where possible, students should live in the community during their community experience in order to understand the community problems. Students who work and live in a rural area are most likely to come back and serve there.[3]

THE WAY FORWARD

The challenge facing nurses is to turn talk into action. If nurses cannot change and work with the community and in a multidisciplinary team, they will be exchanged for other workers. Academic institutions need to meet the example and develop models for comprehensive community-based PHC and to undertake research that has credibility and relevance to PHC.

Nursing is underrated in most countries, and I believe it is time that nurses begin to take part in the planning of health services. The WHO Director General states that many governments do not recognize the demands made on nursing in the community. He says that "it is still rare for nurses to participate in policy making bodies such as national health committees for primary health care. . . ." This is in spite of their well-grounded education and management ability.[10,11,12] The way forward is in the hands of today's nurses. Change is a must.

REFERENCES

1. Alma Ata. (October, 1978). Declaration of Alma-Ata.
2. Glattharr, E. (1992). The slow agonizing birth of primary health care services, Nursing RSA. *Verpleging, 7*(10), 22.
3. Harnar, R. (1985). Nurses: A resource to the community. *Contact, 87,* 1-15.
4. Kaseje, D. (1991). *Community empowerment: The key to health for all.* Keynote address to the Namibian National Primary Health Care Workshop.
5. Mahler, H. (1985, July). Nurses lead the way. *World Health, 85,* 28.
6. McMurray, A. (1991). Advocacy for community self-empowerment. *International Nursing Review, 38*(1), 19-22.
7. Newell, K. W. (1987). Selective primary health care: The counter revolution. *Social Science and Medicine, 24,* 1-4.
8. Rifkin, S. B. (1986). Lessons from community participation in health programmes. *Health Policy and Planning, 1*(3), 240-249.

9. Walt, G., & Vaughan, P. (1991). *An introduction to the primary health care approach in developing countries. A review with selected annotated references* (Pub. No. 13). London: Ross Institute of Tropical Hygiene.

10. WHO. (1982). World health day 1981: Health for all by the year 2000. *WHO Chronicle, 35*(3), 79-85.

11. WHO. (1985). *A guide to curriculum review for basic nursing education. Orientation to primary health care and community health.* Geneva, Switzerland: Author.

12. WHO. (1991). *Strengthening nursing and midwifery in support of strategies for health for all.* Report by the Director General to the Executive Board at the eighty-ninth session. 20 November 1991.

PART FIVE

QUALITY IMPROVEMENT

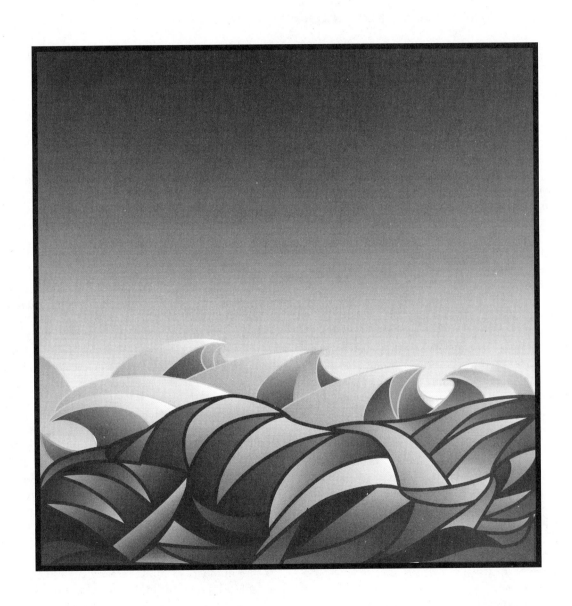

Multifaceted approaches to quality improvement

JOANNE COMI McCLOSKEY, HELEN KENNEDY GRACE

In the changing health care environment, concerns over quality of care are receiving greater attention than ever before. As consumers become more knowledgeable as a result of increased information available to them, much of the mystique surrounding health care is being dissipated. No longer are hospitals, physicians, and, indeed, nurses seen solely as benevolent providers with the patient's welfare central to their concerns. Increases in malpractice suits and dissatisfaction of consumers are indications that all is not well. While quality of nursing in the past has largely been subsumed within the institutional context of the hospital as one of many services, increased emphasis is now being placed upon measurement of quality of nursing care with standards for such care being established by nurses. The focus of efforts to measure quality has also expanded from inside the boundaries of hospitals to community and long-term care settings. This section provides a comprehensive overview of the multifaceted approaches to measuring quality that are developing within nursing.

In the opening chapter of the section, Mitchell challenges the conventional approaches to quality control through governmental regulation and through accreditation processes and proposes that an alternative that involves consumers with providers in establishing agreed-upon standards of care is a more productive approach. Noting that "governmental regulation, emphasizing deficiencies and enforcement philosophies, can actually have an adverse effect on quality," the author states that the alternative of drawing upon components of quality management developed in industrial settings is much more likely to have positive results. The crisis in health care, particularly the high costs and the relatively low returns on the medical model of care and reliance on high-technology tertiary care, is resulting in a redirection of care back to the community. With this change, consumer involvement in health care is increasing. In the past, efforts to define quality have primarily been driven by the providers' definitions. Continuous quality improvement, based on an understanding of individual needs and expectations of consumers, is offered as a promising alternative approach. Voluntary accreditation programs are offered as a promising alternative to governmental regulation and to "closed systems" accreditation approaches.

Drawing on evidence from the business sector and the increasing emphasis on quality, on a more highly knowledgeable consumer population, and on concerns of health professionals and insurers, Hodges et al. argue that measuring the quality of nursing care may be one of the single most important issues of the decade. Quality of health care has traditionally been measured along three dimensions: structure, process, and outcome. Within this framework, the questions of what to measure and at what point in time are posed as critical in measuring the quality of nursing care. Outcome measures at the time of discharge from a health care setting are proposed as critical in appraising quality of nursing care. From these outcome measures, the antecedents of structure and process can be assessed and conclusions reached regarding the quality of nursing care. Challenging nursing to avail itself of the expertise now available in the numbers of nurse researchers and the capability of computer technology to capture and analyze data, the authors conclude by challenging nursing to use an integrative approach in measuring outcome, structure, and process to document cost-effective quality care.

Measurement of quality of care in long-term care facilities poses a separate set of challenges, as Gamroth and Smith note. Most quality assurance standards have been based on a medical model, which does not necessarily apply in long-term care facilities. First, a nursing home is a combination home/care facility, and the measures of quality need to capture both facets. Second, care of patients with chronic conditions where the outcome is most likely that of eventual death poses a different set of challenges in viewing care from the perspective of structure, process, and outcome. A critical question in determining quality of long-term care is, Who determines desirable or appropriate interventions or outcomes? The perspectives of external reviewers and those of the consumers of care (patients and families) may diverge. Tracing the history of review of quality of care in nursing homes, driven primarily from the need to regulate practice, the authors note a change in direction with an increased understanding of the need for greater flexibility in reflecting the patient's perspective in setting criteria for quality care. Concluding that quality is not something that can be regulated, this article concludes by reinforcing the importance of a caring philosophy that is pervasive in long-term care facilities as the ultimate measure.

Many of the problems in establishing quality of care standards in long-term care are also problematic in the home health care field. Colling discusses the issues of care in the home. Although the characteristics of home health care have changed markedly in recent years, with the numbers of patients discharged at earlier points in time from acute care facilities now being cared for in home care settings, the majority of patients cared for in home settings are the elderly with multiple chronic conditions. Contextual factors, the multidiscipline nature of home health care, individual preferences, and difficulty in measuring quality are noted as complicating factors in the home health care field. A promising development in the field is a multisite effort to develop quality indicators that can be used to assess the quality of home health care.

Another approach to standard setting in nursing is that of establishing guidelines for nursing practice by professional organizations. Dean-Baar outlines the framework for nursing practice being developed collaboratively between the American Nurses Association (ANA) and more than 30 specialty groups. This process of standard setting establishes the minimum levels for competent care. In response to the different approaches to establishment of standards for nursing

practice, lack of consistency in the development of standards, and the limited usefulness to nursing of a fragmented system, the ANA has initiated a process to develop guidelines for nursing practice and for professional behavior that would extend across the field. By establishing general guidelines, specialty groups can adapt these to unique characteristics of their area. This approach is serving as a unifying force within nursing to bring together the specialty groups in unifying them around a common concern for establishing measures of quality.

In the business community, total quality management (TQM) has been adopted as a way to increase competitiveness while assuring quality control. With the ever-increasing concerns over quality of care and control of costs, Triolo builds an argument for extending TQM concepts to health care. TQM is a structured system for involving an entire organization in a continuous quality improvement process targeted to meet and exceed customer expectations. After presenting the basic components of TQM and applying them to health care institutions, Triolo summarizes results of application of TQM to 21 health care organizations. The lessons learned are that top management must be totally committed, physicians need to be included from the beginning, and the process must be customized to the organizations. Significant cost savings alone have been realized while quality of care is improved. Cautions offered are that it is a long-term process, that it is possible to become "process" burdened, and that an infrastructure may develop that in effect becomes a "shadow" organization.

Yet another approach to quality control within the profession is that of the certification process to ensure that professionals are qualified to provide specialized services. While certification may be done by a variety of bodies, Bulechek and Maas argue that for nursing specialty practice, it is most appropriately done by specialty organizations. Professional organizations have the responsibility of self-regulation of their membership. The goals of nursing certification are to assure the consumer of the quality of services provided, protect the consumer from substandard practice, and ensure high-quality care at reasonable cost. With this as a framework, the current situation regarding certification of nursing speciality practice is reviewed. The certification field in nursing is divided among the professional organization, the ANA, and certification by speciality groups. Some states certify nursing specialties, while yet another approach is institutional certification. Each of these approaches is analyzed and the conclusion advanced that the preferable model is that of certification by the professional organization.

Testing of knowledge and skills alone is a limited approach to determining competence. Demonstrations in actual practice situations of clinical judgment and decision-making skills are also needed. Yocum summarizes the current approaches used to measure degree of clinical competence. Performance testing involves the use of skill inventories, peer evaluation, and chart/record audits. This approach is open to a high probability of measurement errors. Objective testing involves the use of standardized objective questions developed by panels of experts and taken in the form of paper and pencil tests. While this approach may be valid and reliable in measuring knowledge and ability to analyze and synthesize, it is questionable that it measures clinical judgment and decision making. Development of patient management problems has been an approach to addressing this concern. With the advent of computer technology, computerized clinical simulation testing holds promise of more accurately measuring the ability of nurses to make sound clinical judgments and decisions.

While there may be general approaches to measuring competence of nurses and quality of care, it is important that care-providing organizations build within their structures ongoing processes for monitoring quality of nursing practice. One comprehensive system that has been developed is that for the Visiting Nurse Service of Omaha described by Martin. The Omaha system is a comprehensive, multifaceted approach to measuring quality of nursing care. Seven measurement approaches are included within this system: (1) practice, documentation, and data-management orientation; (2) case conferences, where nurses describe their patient encounters to supervisors; (3) shared evaluation visits and observations in which supervisors visit families with the nurse and evaluate the encounters with standardized approaches; (4) practice-based in-service education; (5) record audit, peer review, and utilization review; (6) accreditation and external audit; and (7) client satisfaction surveys. While this approach has been developed within a home health care agency, the same model could be used profitably in other settings.

An international perspective brings yet another dimension toward measuring quality of patient care. In the concluding article of this section, Lange and Jaimovich points out that perhaps the ultimate measure of quality of care lies in how successful we are in increasing the capacity of the individual to care for him or herself and his or her families. When the person becomes a patient, the tendency is for the "professionals" to take over responsibilities that prior to this time have been under the control of the person and his or her families. Linking self-care concepts with qualitative measures of health care results in reformulation of some of the central issues. For example, patients may be much more satisfied with taking a pill for hypertension than modifying their behavior to increase exercise and change their diets. This section concludes with an argument for a need to shift to a self-care model in which the individual assuming greater responsibility for his or her own health and that of his or her families. Within this framework, the measures of quality for patient care are those that indicate change in the behavior of the patient as reflective of the interpersonal and educative skills of the provider.

In this section, approaches to measuring quality are multifaceted. The ultimate measure is that of improving the quality of life for those we serve. Whether it be through a framework of minimal standards necessary for acceptable practice or through the ability to "empower" individuals to apply knowledge to better care for themselves and their families (a measure requiring a high level of interpersonal skills), the ultimate test of a health profession is its faithfulness to its societal mission to contribute to the improvement of health for people.

CHAPTER 40

Debate

How can we assure health care quality?

MARIA MITCHELL

The U.S. health care system is facing a growing crisis in quality. Reports of substandard care in various sectors of the system have raised alarm among consumers, who are becoming more sophisticated in negotiating the health care system and have simultaneously developed greater expectations about the quality of care they receive. Concerns about quality, fueled by consumer vigilance, have stimulated policy makers across the nation to enter the debate about (1) the components of quality and (2) appropriate strategies for measuring and improving quality. There is growing evidence that governmental regulation, emphasizing deficiencies and enforcement philosophies, can actually have an adverse effect on quality, and alternate approaches are being explored. At the same time, a growing body of research is demonstrating that the components of quality management, first developed in industrial settings, are relevant to the management of health care organizations and ought to be integral to evaluative processes.

Improving the value of the health care system has become the primary goal of policy makers in the 1990s. This movement follows a decade of crisis marked by the inexorable decline of key indicators of cost, access, and quality. The nation as a whole has expressed considerable dissatisfaction with the status quo and distrust of the provider and insurance community they hold largely responsible for the failure of the health care system. Consumers have begun to demand better quality in terms of the processes and outcomes of care and better information to make informed choices among providers. The groundswell of support for the new imperative of consumer value has been acknowledged among businesses, insurers, and other purchasers of health care as they begin to view themselves as consumers and suppliers or brokers of health care services.

At the federal level, the Department of Health and Human Services is supporting both legislative and regulatory approaches to assure quality, as well as strengthen private sector approaches, such as accreditation. But it is the private sector that holds the greatest promise in terms of innovation and flexible approaches to quality management since private initiative and commitment on the part of industry managers is essential to the process of continuous quality improvement. Regulation will always play an important adjunct role in the imposition of sanctions, such as fines and penalties. This chapter discusses the current crisis in the health care system and how the consumer clamor for quality can be met through a regulatory approach that utilizes the benefits and advantages of a private/public partnership.

THE CRISIS IN HEALTH CARE

For many years, the health care system has been in a state of sustained crisis. The picture remains bleak for the future, barring significant changes in the way health care services are planned and financed. Municipalities across the country are beginning to function like Third World nations. The problems they face are the result of the convergence of a host of medical, socioeconomic, and demographic realities that highlight the inadequacies of the present configuration of the health care delivery system. In cities and states across the nation, the health care system is struggling to address an endless litany of problems—the twin scourges of AIDS and drug addiction, the reemergence of TB, the weakening of childhood immunization programs, overflowing emergency rooms, rising poverty especially among children, homelessness, and the growth of the uninsured and the underinsured.

To make matters worse, we are in the middle of a demographic revolution: the ranks of the elderly are growing rapidly. The over-65 population is expected to increase 15% between 1990 and 2010. Most dramatically, the number of people over 85 has grown from 300,000 in 1930 to about 3.3 million today—and a projected 18.7 million in the year 2080. New projections from researchers at the National Institute on Aging place this number at 72 million, after considering declines in the death rate of the adult population.[15] With family size shrinking, there will be fewer and fewer caregivers. Instead, we face a future scenario of the old caring for the very old. Exacerbating this is the fact that the people who are living longer are impaired by the debilitating, chronic physical and mental ailments of old age that require greater service input. Medicare recipients older than 85 use about four times as many services as do those between 65 and 69—the very conditions that our health care delivery systems do not address well.

While the demographic changes were foreseen long ago, as a nation we have failed to make the necessary systemwide adjustments. Chronic care services to enhance independent functioning and improve the quality of life are sorely underfunded. The financing and delivery of health care remains centered on the huge medical industrial complex of acute care hospitals. This biomedical enterprise grew out of the infectious disease era where the task was to diagnose and treat acute illness through intensive, high-technology services. The flaws in this system are increasingly apparent as consumers and purchasers discover that the full continuum of their needs is going unmet. Rather than addressing these needs, the provider-driven system asserts the prerogatives of science and determines which needs can be met by science.

HEALTH CARE FINANCING ISSUES

Financial considerations limit the availability and access to health care services. Health care expenditures have risen dramatically since 1980—from $250 billion to $820 billion today and a projected $1 trillion by 1995. At present rates of growth, we will need another trillion dollars by the year 2000, which, according to economist Eli Ginzberg, translates into an outlay of $30,000 for health care for a family of four—more than

that family will have to spend on food, clothing, housing, and transportation *combined* in 1990.[10]

Health care expenditures are rising two and a half times as fast as the gross national product (GNP). Federal expenditures for health care can currently consume about a third of all federal spending[20] and have increased at a slightly greater rate of growth than private expenditures, including third-party reimbursement.[12] The federal government, faced with a growing deficit, has cut Medicare and Medicaid benefits and increased Medicare premiums.

Economic decline and changing workforce patterns have also led to an increase in the number of uninsured individuals. In fact, since 1975, the proportion of the population without health insurance increased 25%—close to 40 million people. The uninsured are putting greater pressure on providers in terms of charity care and bad debt and on state Medicaid programs struggling to fill coverage gaps caused, in part, by unanticipated federal mandates in whose cost the states must share.

Rising costs have led insurers to look closely at cost-cutting mechanisms and to reduce coverage where necessary. Private insurers have increased deductibles and charged higher premiums. Businesses are also being devastated by competitive pressure and rising employee health care costs, which are eating away a large portion of net earnings. Between 1970 and 1989, spending per full-time employee for health benefits increased 163%.[16] Employers currently pay two thirds of employee's health bills. To reduce expenses, they are forcing providers to lower prices and requiring employees to share the cost burden through increased out-of-pocket expenditures, which have gone up as much as 45%.[9] Some companies are placing caps on the coverage of certain catastrophic illnesses like AIDS and cancer, a practice that has survived legal scrutiny in spite of its disastrous consequences for health policy. Rationing is being avidly discussed among policy makers, and this is inevitable if the factors that fuel rising costs are not adequately addressed. Two thirds of Americans report that they fail to receive the health care they need because of financial constraints. The average person simply cannot afford to be sick.

THE LIMITS OF MEDICAL SCIENCE

The most difficult problems we face, however, are not cost related. Rather, they have to do with the inadequacy of the medical model in meeting our health needs and socioeconomic imperatives and the poor quality of care historically offered through the medical model. The inadequacy of the medical model is everywhere in evidence:

- The United States has the highest infant mortality rate in the industrialized world.
- Children represent more than half of Americans living in poverty without access to health care at all.
- Half of what the elderly spend for their health care is out of pocket.
- Men living in the Harlem section of New York City have a life expectancy worse than that of men living in Bangladesh–a Third World country.
- Half the coronary bypasses, most cesarean sections, and a significant proportion of many other procedures, such as pacemaker implants and hysterectomies, are unnecessary.[4]
- Half of the 1 million coronary angiograms performed each year at $5,000 a test are unnecessary.[1]
- The majority of Medicare dollars are spent on life-sustaining technology in the last year of life in individuals over 80 years of age.
- The leading causes of death are preventable, yet only 1% of the health care dollar is spent on prevention.
- Over 81% of the strides we have made in decreasing the incidence of heart disease are attributable to dietary and lifestyle changes. The other 19% has to do with cardiovascular drugs and surgery, not a very substantial return on our investment.
- One fourth of hospital days, one fourth of procedures, and two fifths of medications could be eliminated, according to Dr. Robert Brock, Rand Corporation fellow.
- Only 21% of the people who incur hospital charges and 29% of those covered by insurance plans feel they have received good value for the money they spent.[5]

During the past decade, key policy makers have questioned the configuration of the current health care system and looked to redirecting the locus of care away from the acute care hospital and toward the home and community. In defining strategic goals for the health care system, they have belatedly recognized a fundamental imbalance in the way resources are allocated, with acute care resources and life-sustaining technologies that arrive late in the patient's stage of illness consuming an inordinate share of the limited health care dollar.

To correct the imbalance between provider-determined need and consumer-based need requires a fundamental and unprecedented redirection of resources toward a coordinated system of community-based care—a system that reaches out to people in their homes, neighborhoods, schools, and community nursing centers and provides essential preventive and primary care services and long-term care services. With this as a clear direction and focus of financial and planning activity, much can be accomplished in terms of improving the responsiveness of the health care system, lowering costs, and meeting payer and patient expectations for an adequate quality of care return on their substantial investment.

GROWING CONSUMER ROLE IN HEALTH CARE

Consumers are playing a key role in reshaping the health care system in defining a set of reasonable expectations in terms of the kinds and availability of services. What is the source of this new-found shift in power to the health care consumer? There has been a major change in consumers' view of their role in health care and their responsibility for taking a more active part in shaping the health care system to meet their expectations.

Ronald Inglehart at the University of Michigan has done a study on culture shift that basically addresses this change in what people expect and value.[13] During the past 20 years, Inglehart argues, American culture in particular, and most Western cultures in general, have moved away from an obsession with economic growth and are becoming increasingly interested in the quality of life. Coupled with this change in what people want out of life is a significant shift in the distribution of political skills. More than ever before, people are taking an active interest in and developing an understanding of the workings of the political system. The educational level attained by the public has never been so high. This educated public has demonstrated a strong desire to participate in decision making and policy making and to actively influence improvements in the quality of their own lives and the lives of the people around them. These developments offer constructive insight into the growing consumer participation in health care. The consumer role will only become stronger in its advocacy for quality of life and will play an increasingly active role in policy making and decision making.

A clear example of where future consumer activism will play an extraordinary role is in long-term care. At present, a younger generation asserts rights on behalf of an older generation. Very soon, however, an older, vocal generation with educational credentials, political savvy, and a clearly articulated notion of quality will be fighting for themselves and on behalf of their spouses and peers.

In *Power Shift,* Alvin Toffler argues that "it is the purchaser of care—insurers and industry groups—not traditional providers of care, doctors, and hospitals, who now control health care in America."[18] Toffler attributes the diminished power of physicians and traditional providers to the advent of the knowledgable society. In the past, purchasers and consumers did not have access to information about the performance of health care providers and, therefore, lacked the ability to identify whose services were worth buying and at what price. This information gap has been an important factor in the relentless escalation of health care costs.

According to Toffler, we are now in an age of information technology that makes it possible to track the results of health care treatments and compare them across providers. Outcomes analysis is fast becoming the consumer's tool for gauging the value, efficiency, and quality of an investment in health care. A half-dozen states are using outcome measurement systems as are numerous corporations, coalitions of businesses, medical providers, insurers, and surveyors. Armed with actual performance data, consumers are gaining leverage over their health care providers.

The search for quality outcomes has empowered consumers to challenge the status quo and to begin to demand information and government-enforced standards of care. In 1987, consumer organizations were successful in pressuring federal regulatory officials to release hospital mortality data that had been collected for internal use. Now, every year comparative data on hospital mortality in selected diagnoses is publicly released, making available to consumers information that can influence the selection of a hospital provider.

Consumer activism around the issue of health care quality also resulted in the exposure of serious deficiencies in the nation's long-term-care system. In home care, for example, the American Bar Association conducted a study entitled "The Black Box of Home Care Quality" that uncovered widespread abuses in the delivery of home health care. The report recommended a number of legislative and regulatory changes that eventually found their way into public law as a part of the Omnibus Budget Reconciliation Act of 1987. New

Medicare conditions of participation for home care providers included significant quality reform, including an unannounced annual survey process using a uniform assessment tool that includes information on outcomes of care, stringent training and competency testing requirements for home health aides, and a patient bill of rights incorporating concepts of self-determination and autonomy. Nursing home reform was also spearheaded by consumer advocacy groups that formed the National Citizen's Coalition for Nursing Home Reform (NCCNHR) in 1975 to improve the long-term-care system and the quality of life for nursing home residents. The NCCNHR successfully coordinated a national effort to achieve the most comprehensive federal nursing home reform in over a decade through the Nursing Home Reform Act of 1987 (P.L. 100-203).

MEASURING QUALITY—INVOLVING THE CONSUMER

The mechanisms that represent the current consensus on how to define and measure quality in health care include regulations, licensing laws, and private accreditation programs. The presumption is that compliance with the standards set forth by these groups results in quality care for the client; however, these systems are not without their shortcomings. Most of the standards are structure and process standards with little or beginning emphasis on the outcome of care. The outcome models in use today are client centered but have been defined and proposed by professionals and payers. This reflects a traditional viewpoint that situates quality of care in the exclusive domain of professionals, yet outcome measures in health care focus on the results of service delivery and determine how a service affects the consumer's well-being. It makes sense, then, that outcomes should include what, for the most part, these models ignore: the preferences and expectations of the consumer regarding the quality of health care services and the concerns about quality of life as a criteria for judging the quality of health care. The innovative "In Search of Excellence in Home Care" research project described in greater detail later in this chapter is addressing this gap by incorporating consumer expectations into the definition of home care quality.

The traditional means of involving the consumer in health care quality has been through the use of patient satisfaction surveys, and indeed, more research is being done on patient satisfaction stimulated by the more sophisticated consumer and intensification of competition for patients. However, in spite of the growing numbers of studies, the inconsistency and problems with methodology currently make it difficult to incorporate satisfaction assessments into evaluations of quality of care.

Another way consumer involvement has been recognized has been through consumers' own definition of quality of life. It is, in fact, the consumer's definition of quality of life that determines the values that are associated with different outcomes. Quality of life is a concept that includes many nonmedical elements such as psychological, socioeconomic, and environmental factors. If measurement of a patient's quality of life is required, it should be done by the patients themselves and not their doctors and nurses. Therefore, it would seem the consumer must have a role in developing any outcome criteria if these criteria are to be useful and meaningful in determining quality.

The professional model of quality has led us to standards that measure quality accurately. The real issue, however, may be greater than measuring quality. It may involve redefining quality to premise it more on client's perception of their condition and the personal nature of services because the thread or theme that keeps emerging is the differing perspectives of the consumer and the health professional.

The challenge of developing a meaningful measure for health care quality is the opportunity to examine the real purpose of health care and to discover how well we currently support clients in their readjustment to altered lifestyles. By including the consumer in the challenge, we can be successful.

CONTINUOUS QUALITY IMPROVEMENT PRINCIPLES – AN OVERVIEW

A customer-centered approach to quality is the essence of total quality management (TQM) or continuous quality improvement (CQI) theories, originally developed for industrial settings but more recently finding practical application in health care settings. This approach focuses on continuous and relentless improvement in the total process that provides care and has demonstrated considerable success in industry in reducing long-range operating expense and improving the overall quality of products and services.

Based on a review of the literature, the following key principles form the core of CQI:[6,7,8,14,19]

- The organization as a whole must be committed to pursuing a long-term mission that is clearly articulated and understood by all the people within the organization.
- The organization must be committed to understanding the individual needs and expectations of its customers, both internal and external, and to designing programs and services that meet those needs.
- There must be a continuous effort to improve the process. The focus is on systems errors rather than on the individual role in quality assurance. J. M. Juran suggests that 85% of the problems in organizations can be attributed to process weaknesses, while only 15% is attributed to the workers.[14] Yet, as Donald Berwick stated, "In modern America health care [we find] the theory of bad apples. Those who subscribe to it believe that quality is best achieved by discovering the bad apples and removing them from the lot."[2]
- Employees must have the authority, the training, and the resources necessary to improve the process. This is the concept of empowerment.
- The organization must be committed to providing high-quality services and products.
- Information and data collection must be viewed as integral to the improvement of processes. Data are used to support the application of judgment in decision making by confirming the existence of problems, identifying opportunities for improvement, and evaluating and monitoring the effectiveness of improvements.
- The organization's top management must be committed to and take responsibility for quality.
- The organization must be committed to learning from the best practices that lead to superior performance and searching for new ideas that go beyond the boundaries of the organization. This is the concept known as "benchmarking."
- The organization should form long-term relationships with a few suppliers who can deliver a quality product and share the same commitment to continuous improvement. This reduces waste, delays, and other costs associated with poor-quality workmanship.

In health care settings, CQI represents a paradigm shift and leads to a number of basic management conflicts. Most notable is the shift from provider values toward customer-based need. The traditional unquestioned professional bureaucracy is replaced with a systemwide, multidisciplinary framework for quality improvement driven by managerial leadership and focused on accountability for both outcomes and process. In the dynamic environment of continuous improvement, the traditional approach in health care of meeting a fixed goal or objective no longer suffices. The role of top management will change dramatically as it focuses on defining the corporate culture and ensuring the adequacy of resources necessary to support the change process. Managers will also need to empower their staffs to solve problems and to be accountable for performance in meeting their own quality objectives. This will require an emphasis on team-building strategies, new reward systems, and structural flexibility. Most importantly, top management will need to drive the benchmarking process—assessing the outside environment, identifying the best of the competition, inside and outside of the health care industry, and comparing these with internal operations.

While CQI presents some basic conflicts, it also presents the best opportunity to improve quality of care and the system designed to provide quality of care.

IMPROVING QUALITY THROUGH STANDARD SETTING

The most striking lessons from the research in quality management is the requirement of an organization's commitment to the process of continuous improvement. A formal quality improvement process is also necessary if the desired organizational transformation is to occur.[17] Other approaches that rely on the extraordinary talents of individuals, trial and error, exhortation or quality reports that gather dust on the bookshelf do not offer the proper framework for sustained growth. A formal process does not focus on a particular problem but provides a system for addressing all problems and reducing the impact of these problems throughout the organization.

Problems cut across organizations, and every member of the organization brings a different perspective on what the problems are, the causes of the problems identified, and the solutions. Resistance to process changes on the part of the staff is alleviated when a formal system is in place. Most importantly, quality improvement efforts will require resources, including time to analyze problems and budgets for training, data collection, and process changes.

The question arises: Can a standard setting process force the kind of organizational transformation neces-

sary to achieve a lasting positive impact on the quality of health care? Currently, standard setting in health care occurs in three ways: Medicare and Medicaid regulations, state licensure of individuals or providers, and private accreditation.

Federal and state regulatory standards operate under a number of constraints that hamper their ability to incorporate CQI principles. First, government regulatory standards are minimum safety standards. Government has rarely taken responsibility for ensuring more than a minimum standard of care and finds support for this among many governmental theorists. Second, assuring a minimum standard requires a framework of sanctions and penalties linked to reimbursement that casts a punitive shadow across the entire regulatory apparatus. A punitive approach, as opposed to a consultative approach, does not create an environment conducive to process change. Third, surveyors bring to the external review process the regulatory habits, biases, and skills of a policing perspective rather than a consultative approach. To change this would require the kind of resource allocations necessary to support extensive education, central office support, and management leadership that is largely unavailable to large governmental bureaucracies. One of the most important aspects of a consultative CQI process, if it is to effect change and process improvement, is the quality of the surveyor's understanding of the management of the organization and the industry in which it operates. The surveyor's expertise and background adds legitimacy to the findings and engenders a mutuality of understanding that permits a consultative approach.

Some attempts have been made to incorporate CQI principles into external regulatory reviews, but none to date have met with success. An evaluation of one such project involving a state's long-term-care quality assurance program found that the concepts of CQI applied to a regulatory effort resulted in the identification of more problems, more severe problems, and more resident-centered problems but that extensive education, support, and management were needed to achieve a role change from policing to consultation. The evaluation also found that government-imposed sanctions remain important motivators for improvement.[11]

PRIVATE ACCREDITATION: THE SEARCH FOR EXCELLENCE

Voluntary accreditation programs offer another source for standard setting in the health care system. Traditionally, accreditation has been a closed system with providers setting standards for themselves and keeping a dark veil of secrecy over the findings. Consumers have long criticized this "fox guarding the hen house" approach to accreditation, and the results in terms of quality assurance have been negligible. One of the most famous reports in the annals of health care quality was a 1988 *Wall Street Journal* article subtitled "Bloody Tables and Maggots," which highlighted the fact that hospital accreditation by the Joint Commission on Accreditation of Healthcare Organizations (JCAHO) often masked sloppy, substandard, and dangerous patient care practices.[3]

Ideally, however, an accreditation program can fulfill an important role in assuring quality and, at the same time, address patient concerns about quality. A member of the Institute of Medicine Committee who developed a plan for assessing and assuring quality in the 1990s stated, "It is always preferable to inspire people to do good, to create an atmosphere where people want to strive to do their best, rather than to depend on an external body to threaten punishment and impose sanctions." The committee report advocated the concept of deemed status or delegation of the responsibility for achieving a higher caliber of care and meeting that standard to private sector organizations.

One organization that has accomplished an incorporation of CQI principles in a consumer-oriented, external evaluative program is the Community Health Accreditation Program (CHAP). A sister organization to the National League for Nursing, CHAP represents nursing's voice in the search for quality health care reform. Recently, CHAP received deemed status recognition from the federal government for its home care accreditation program. In doing so, the federal government acknowledges that CHAP will, in the words of Secretary of Health and Human Services Louis Sullivan, "enhance our efforts to ensure that Medicare beneficiaries are provided only the highest quality care."

What CHAP offers the federal home care certification process is something very different from a traditional accrediting program. CHAP has standards of excellence, not minimum safety standards, and an open system incorporating consumer values, annual unannounced surveys, and a policy of full public disclosure of site-visit reports. An integral part of CHAP's approach is to utilize the accreditation process to address consumer concerns and fears about the quality of home care services and to become a standard bearer of quality for health care reform. CHAP accreditation offers the opportunity to achieve excellence through standards—standards that reflect a total commitment to consumer values and identify the key attributes of organizations providing high quality care. The emphasis is on client outcomes and management.

Consumers are involved throughout the process, from input into the development of standards to participation as purchasers and users of home care services on the CHAP Board of Governors, which sets broad policy, and the Board of Review, which makes the actual accreditation decision.

The CHAP program is ultimately a systematic evaluation of an agency's performance from top to bottom—starting with the agency's mission statement and including a review of the resources available to fulfill that mission. The review also focuses on the agency's total quality management systems and the strategies developed to address long-range viability. CHAP believes that fiscal viability is inextricably linked to the ability to provide high-quality services.

Four key principles form the framework of the standards and CHAP's concept of quality management:

1. The organization's structure and function consistently supports its consumer-oriented philosophy and purpose.
2. The organization consistently provides high-quality services and products.
3. The organization has adequate human, financial, and physical resources effectively organized to accomplish its stated purpose.
4. The organization is positioned for long-term viability.

The program's specific standards emphasize individual client outcomes and program planning and evaluation. All in all, CHAP accreditation is a comprehensive independent management audit covering clinical areas, management, and finances. Akin to the outside financial audits relied upon by corporate boards to assure financial accountability, CHAP accreditation offers an internal assurance that systems are in place that will lead the organization to high-quality, cost-effective service delivery that external customers are more and more looking to find. CHAP offers a consultative process that involves a partnership approach—a dynamic relationship subject to continuing levels of improvement and strengthening the home care industry in the process.

CHAP's expert-site visitors are experienced home care managers with a minimum of 5 years upper-level management experience and at least master's-level educational qualifications. They are capable of providing an organization with a detailed analysis of its administrative and operating strengths and weaknesses together with expert advice regarding these findings.

CHAP's standards development is supported by innovative, consumer-based research. In August 1989, CHAP was awarded $1.2 million by the W. K. Kellogg Foundation to develop standards for measuring the quality of home care services. The purpose of the grant is to strengthen the home care industry by defining quality outcomes in this field: (1) utilizing consumer input as a fundamental source of data, (2) developing a system to assess quality utilizing these outcomes, and (3) incorporating this process into the CHAP standards. The project is significant because it is one of the first endeavors to actually determine quality through valid, reliable outcome measures in the home care industry. Previous approaches have relied upon each provider facility to set its own standards. Utilizing client-centered outcomes, the industry can be held to objective universal criteria that will include clients' assessment of the care they have received.

CHAP represents a model public/private partnership that shows great promise for future arrangements involving consumer-oriented approaches to quality assurance. The federal government will retain oversight and evaluation responsibilities and will have available complete and regular access to site-visit information for purposes of applying federal sanctions, where necessary. The incorporation of standards of excellence within a federal regulatory framework is an explicit acknowledgment on the part of regulatory authorities that the private sector can play a crucial role in improving the quality of health care services, where there is a commitment to consumer values, a conceptual model incorporating principles of continuous quality improvement, and an open system of shared expertise. CHAP demonstrates a powerful role for the nursing community in the development of systems for ensuring the quality of health care in the future. The perspective of the nursing community and its unique ability to bridge the gap between consumer values and provider needs offers multiple, untapped opportunities for creative and innovative approaches to evolving concepts of health care quality.

REFERENCES

1. Altman, L. (1992, November 3). Study sees excess in x-rays of heart. *New York Times*.
2. Berwick, D. M. (1989). Who pays? *New England Journal of Medicine, 1,* 320.
3. Bogdanich, W. (1988, October 12). Small comfort—Prized by hospitals, accreditation hides perils patients face. *Wall Street Journal*.
4. Chambliss, L., & Reier, S. (1990 January 9). How doctors have ruined health care. *Financial World*.
5. The Conference Board, Consumer Research Center, February, 1990.
6. Crosby, P. B. (1979). *Quality is free*. New York: Penguin.
7. Crosby, P. B. (1988). *The eternally successful organization*. New York: McGraw-Hill.
8. Deming, W. E. (1986). *Out of the crisis*. Cambridge, Mass: MIT Press.
9. Freudenheim, M. (1991, January 29). Health care a growing burden. *New York Times*.
10. Ginzberg, E. (1992, November 12). The health swamp. *New York Times*.
11. Gustafson, D. H. (1992, October). *QI implementation in home care programs*. Presentation at CHAP Institute for Quality Leadership.
12. Health Care Financing Administration. (1991). *1991 HCFA statistics* (HCFA Pub. No. 03325). Washington, D.C.: U.S. Government Printing Office.
13. Inglehart, R. (1989). *Culture shift in advanced industrial society*. Princeton, N.J.: Princeton University Press.
14. Juran, J. M. (1989). *Juran on leadership for quality*. New York: The Free Press.
15. Kolata, G. (1992, November 16). New vision on life spans alter forecasts on elderly. *New York Times*.
16. Piacenti, J. S., & Anzick, M. A. (1991, February). Employee benefits in total compensation. *Employee Benefits Research Institute Issue Brief*.
17. Plsek, P. (1992, October). *Total quality management: The key to successfully sustaining growth?* Presentation at CHAP Institute for Quality Leadership.
18. Toffler, A. (1990). *POWERSHIFT: Knowledge, wealth, and violence at the edge of the 21st century*. New York: Bantam Doubleday Dell.
19. Townsend, P. L. (1990). *Commit to quality*. New York: John Wiley & Sons.
20. U.S. Dept. of Health and Human Services. (1992, March). *Report and recommendation to the Congress*. Healthcare Financing Administration, Office of the Actuary.

CHAPTER 41

Viewpoints

Measuring quality

A systematic integrative approach

LINDA C. HODGES, MARY LOUISE ICENHOUR, STARLA TATE

The measurement of the quality of nursing care may be the single most important goal of the nursing profession in this decade. Certainly, all indicators point to the fact that quality will be the new buzzword in health care as we face the beginning of a new century. A renewed emphasis on the measurement of quality in contemporary health care can be attributed to a focus on quality directives instituted by the American business community. This interest, reflected in best seller nonfiction titles on quality measurement from the corporate world, illustrates a new appreciation for the economic power of quality in the market place both in this country, Japan, and the European Community.

Like other sectors of the business community, the health care industry has also shown an increased interest in quality measurement. Now that the shock of DRGs in the 1980s has worn thin and health care professionals have successfully responded to that particular system of reimbursement, efforts to measure the quality of care—particularly as it relates to cost— has reemerged as a major component of health care reform. Other factors have also contributed to a renewed interest in quality health care. Principle among these are consumer demands, health professionals' concern about the impact of shorter hospital stays on patient outcomes, and third-party payer demands for a greater return on dollars spent for health care services delivered.

Consumer demand for quality health care can be attributed to an increase in knowledge of services that meet a degree of excellence. The increased cost for health care has also affected consumer interest in quality services. As more Americans graduate from high schools and universities requiring health education for diploma/degree requirements, and as the public in general becomes more informed about health care delivery through the media, the mystique of medicine disappears. Patients are asking questions about professional credentials and hospital ratings. Increased numbers are also seeking second and third opinions. As third-party payers increase consumer co-payments, the cost of health care is felt on a personal level. Like all goods and services, the consumer is now approaching health care with similar demands for quality at a reasonable price.

The quality of care is also a major concern for health professionals. As a result of DRGs, patients are in the hospital less time and often return to their homes in need of nursing care. The quality of discharge planning as a component of hospital nursing care has received increased emphasis as professional nurses attempt to bridge the gap between the care received while in hospital and the care needed in the home. For example, the stay on maternal infant units is now so short that the notion of waiting to teach the new mother to care for her baby during the "taking-in-phase" has become passé. The concept of quality nursing care, as we knew it before DRGs and the current nursing shortage, has had to be reconceptualized to fit with the rapidly changing health care delivery system.

Third-party payers are also demanding and reemphasizing quality health care services. The cost of health care during the 1980s escalated at an unprecedented rate. At the present time, 12% of the gross national product is spent on health care. Projected expenditure percentages of the gross national product toward health care for 1995 is 14.7% and is 16.4% for 2000.[18] Businesses are finding a greater portion of profits must be allocated to employee health insurance plans, and insurance companies are experiencing difficulty in meeting payment schedules while at the same time increasing insurance premiums. The largest third-party payers, federal and state governments, continue to struggle with increasing demands for Medicare- and Medicaid-funded health care programs in the wake of an exploding federal deficit. As health care costs continue to rise with no ceiling in sight, consumers, businesses, insurance companies, and federal and state governments will increasingly put pressure on providers to deliver quality health care services at an affordable price. Methods for measuring quality care as it relates to cost must be established to answer cost accounting questions of major third-party payers. Since the nursing budget represents a major cost center, there is an urgent need to develop measurement tools/systems to demonstrate the cost-effectiveness of quality nursing care as related to positive patient outcomes, the product line of hospitals.

Although the business community led the way in the 1980s toward quality measurement, the concern for quality care at an affordable price has become the central focus of health care management as the century comes to a close. Beckham[1] states, "the 1980s will go down in history as the decade when quality comes out of the closet." In the 1990s, consumers, health care providers, and third-party payers will demand a full accounting of dollars spent for care received.

CYCLICAL NATURE OF THE HEALTH CARE SYSTEM

Quality is one of four basic concepts underlying any health care system. These four factors include cost containment, equity, access, and quality. Usually, one of these factors tends to dominate the health care system and, thus, health care policy at any one time. For example, equity and access to health care were the dominate themes in the 1960s and 1970s during the Johnson era, when more health care legislature was passed than at any other time in history.[23] The advent of Medicare and Medicaid programs provided for access to the system and increased the use of health care services. As services expanded and demand increased, so did cost. With rising cost, the focus shifted from access and equity to cost containment in the late 1970s and early 1980s as pressure grew to reduce the price tag for health care.

The passage of Public Law 98-21, which instituted the system for prospective payment, was an outcome of the public's growing concern about health care costs.[10] This system of payment, based on time-limited utilization of services for specific medical diagnoses, rewards hospitals for discharging patients early. The move to early discharge has helped to refocus the health care system on the issue of quality health care delivery.

There is a growing concern among all segments of the health care industry that quality may be sacrificed in an effort to contain costs. The quality theme is expected to extend well into the twenty-first century as health policymakers strive to meet the nation's health care needs based on the belief that quality care as an expectation is possible. The ability to deliver quality care at a reasonable cost will be the measure of success in the future.

QUALITY DEFINED

The concept of quality is viewed by different people in different ways. The dictionary defines *quality* as "a degree of excellence; a peculiar and essential character."[5] As applied to quality of care, several definitions are found in the literature. Lang and Clinton[22] suggest that quality assessment is the identification and measurement of a certain level of quality of care. Quality assurance in nursing implies that a level of quality can be defined and measured, and that the public can be assured of that level of care.

In Donabedian's[11] seminal work on quality measurement, quality of care is regarded as "the management by a physician or any other health care practitioner of a clearly definable episode of illness for any given patient." DeGeynt[8] argues that quality is defined primarily as the "degree of conformity with present standards" and is focused on patient care as opposed to medical or health care. Consumer satisfaction as an inherent component of quality of health care is viewed by McMillan[24] as an essential element in the measurement of quality of health care. Universally, the measurement of quality examines the attainment of predetermined norms and standards of health care.

QUALITY CARE MEASUREMENT MODELS

Several authors have proposed models for the measurement of quality of care.[12,19] The most well known was developed by Donabedian and remains the framework for most research in quality measurement. Donabedian suggests that quality of health care can be measured in three ways: structure, process, and outcome. The major structural aspects of health care delivery include institutional characteristics, such as facilities and equipment, health care programs, and health care providers. The level of quality is said to be determined by relating the number of all resources to any and all of the patient/client's or community's health needs. A predetermined standard of numbers and attributes of structural components are needed in order for quality to be judged as present. DeGeynt[8] argues that using the structured method alone to measure quality considerably narrows the meaning of the concept and the extent to which it can be measured.

The process method is the broad view of all activities that go on between health care providers and clients/patients. A judgment of the quality of these activities may be made by either direct observation or an overview of recorded information that allows the evaluator to reconstruct activities occurring between the client/patient and the practitioner. In hospitals, a review of the patient's chart is the measure most commonly used in quality assurance programs. Coyne and Killien[7] state that quality assurance is a process that involves evaluating the quality of patient care provided in a particular setting through establishing standards for care and implementing mechanisms for ensuring that the standards are met. The process method allows for evaluation of quality measures of not only nursing care but care given by other health care practitioners as well.

The third approach to quality measurement receiving the greatest emphasis is the measurement of outcomes. Donabedian refers to outcome as that part of quality measurement indicating a change in the patient/client's current or future health status that can be attributed to antecedent health care. In his definition, *outcome* in its broadest sense means the improvement of social, psychological, and physical health status. He suggests that outcome measures can also measure various patient/client attributes of health care, including satisfaction, the knowledge of health care regimens, and health care behavioral changes. In this approach, the possibility exists to measure the exact outcomes of nursing care—the effectiveness, quality, and time allocated for care.

Interest in the outcome method for quality measurement was apparent in the 1970s. Williamson[29] suggested this method had the greatest potential to measure implications of health care and the patient's/client's health status after care was given. Starfield[28] developed an outcome model of quality measurement that addressed the levels of a patient's health status after discharge. She used a health status profile of 7 categories of patient functioning to indicate the effectiveness of previous care. Brook et. al.[4] also believed that measurement of quality using the process model alone was too narrow and did not adequately measure the care delivered as effectively as outcome measures. More recently, nurse researchers have focused their research on outcomes and have considered the qualitative and quantitative aspects of care.[6,14]

RESEARCH IN QUALITY OUTCOMES

Donabedian[13] reviewed the past 20 years of studies on quality and suggested two new directions in research studying quality outcomes of care. The first group of studies focused on "favorable adverse outcomes," or mortality and case fatality, as quality judgments in and of themselves. An example of such a study would be one conducted at a large university medical center in which institutional differences were noted in the risk of postsurgical fatality. The second grouping of outcome studies identified adverse outcomes as a tool to assess the antecedent process of care. Williamson's[29] studies illustrate this approach. These studies consist of specifying criteria one expects to achieve and whether or not the outcomes have actually been met. If they have not, the antecedent process and structure of care are carefully examined, especially for those group of patients who appear to be more vulnerable to substandard care.

The identification of representative criteria of quality remains difficult to determine since frequently they are value based. It is suggested that all quality criteria are derived from patient/clients' and providers' sets of values and perceptions of quality. An accepted model of quality frequently is developed in which these values are integrated with the organization's realities: what and how care should be delivered. Goals of care based on both patient/client and provider expectations of quality are advantageous since critical components of care are integrated, e.g., health education, patient individuality, and staffing needs.[25]

Hemenway[19] analyzed the use of outcomes measures from an economic perspective. He posited that although measuring process methods of care would be measuring levels of performance, process attributes are not "proxy" measures of outcomes. He quoted Feldstein: "although outcome measures are difficult to determine, it would allow more flexibility for the health care professional to achieve outcomes rather than identifying those process measures that may or may not bring about desired outcomes."

The fact that process measures cannot be used to predict outcome is well illustrated in Icenhour's[20] research findings. When studying quality of care outcomes in ambulatory surgery, it was found that although all surgical patients were taught either at the time of discharge or during their ambulatory surgical stay, few patients achieved learning outcomes as established in the outcome quality criteria.

The following patient examples from Icenhour's study[20] illustrate the difference in measuring process vs. outcome criteria of quality.

John W., a 37-year-old employed postal worker, is discharged after a tumor on his back was excised. It was documented [process measures] that both the patient and his wife received instructions on dressing changes. No determination was made at the time of discharge from ambulatory surgery that they knew or understood sterile dressing changes [outcome measures]. During a one-week postoperative interview, it was found that his dressings were never changed and that he was being treated for a staphylococcal wound infection.

Mary P. is a 57-year-old housewife who had surgery on her foot and required crutches to walk after discharge from ambulatory surgery. Documentation only included that the patient was issued crutches at the time of discharge [process measures]. After discharge, she fell while incorrectly using her crutches, injuring her right wrist. Both the physician's office and the surgery center believed the other had taught her crutch walking. No attempt had been made by either to determine her knowledge proficiency in the use of crutches [outcome measure].

In this study, process methods alone determined that the patients received quality patient teaching; however, when outcome quality criteria were implemented, few patients were found to have achieved the level of patient learning that would have enabled them to carry out compliant, safe, postsurgical care on their own after discharge. Therefore, measuring outcomes of care according to predetermined quality criteria has a greater potential to more accurately identify the areas of nonquality health care interventions.

Although individual writers suggest slightly different views about quality, several commonalities emerge when reviewing their approaches:

1. Quality can be measured.
2. Quality measures a standard or a degree of excellence.
3. Excellence needs to be determined by validating standards of care or by measuring professional conduct when caring for patients.

These statements represent a beginning point in the consideration of quality measurement in health care. The debatable issue—one that will encompass our viewpoints—is the question of what to measure and more importantly at which point in the health care delivery system should quality be measured. The underlying question for professional nursing is when in the nursing management of patients will measurement be most effective and most accurate and assess patient satisfaction? This question must be addressed at the same time nursing interventions that are the most cost effective and provide the greatest opportunity to deliver quality nursing care are determined.[21]

It is our view that the outcomes of nursing care should be the primary focus of quality measurement in nursing practice and should be measured at the conclusion of care in any setting or health care institution. It is believed that measurement of antecedent care is the most informative and has the greatest potential to influence future nursing care and accountability for professional practice and is consistent with new quality measurement directives from such accreditation bodies as the Joint Commission on Accreditation of Healthcare Organizations.[16] Additionally, measurement of nursing care outcomes as related to cost are needed to firmly establish the value of nursing care in the health care delivery system. These data can be used to establish desired staff mix, justify the use of advanced nursing role practitioners—such as clinical nurse specialists, nurse-midwives and nurse anesthetists—and support the nursing service administration operating budget.

The major thrust of quality measurement in nursing in the past has been a measurement of process or an analysis of the degree of compliance with nursing care standards delivered during a specific episode of patient care. In this model, most institutions have developed standards of nursing practice as related to diagnostic-related groups (DRGs) and/or standards related to frequently performed nursing activities, i.e., medication administration, postoperative care, etc.[17] A system for monitoring compliance with the standards, usually through randomized chart audits, is the most commonly used method in quality assurance programs. In this model, a standard for patient education regarding self-medication administration might indicate the question, Was the patient taught the nature of the medication and how to properly self-administer? If the documentation of patient teaching was appropriate, the assumption is that quality nursing care has been delivered. If there is no follow-up on self-

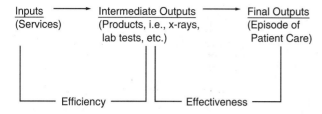

Fig. 41-1. Quality as a measure between efficiency of resource utilization (cost) and outcome effectiveness (benefits).

medication in the home following discharge, one cannot determine whether the time spent teaching the patient (cost of nursing service) indeed resulted in a patient who could appropriately administer his or her own drugs. Therefore, measuring only the structural and process aspects of quality of care, when outcomes can only be determined after discharge, falls far short as a measurement of quality. In other words, efficiency does not always guarantee effectiveness.

MEASURING QUALITY CARE

In 1988, at a meeting of the American Associations of Colleges of Nursing, Diers[9] described a model for quality care measurement (Fig. 41-1). In this model,[15] services rendered in the health care delivery system result in products such as x-rays, lab test results, hours of patient care delivered, meals served, etc. These products or intermediate outputs delivered over a given episode of patient care result in a final output or outcome. When comparing the cost of producing products to final outcomes, a measure of quality of care can be determined based on cost. Diers maintains that data-based arguments in nursing are necessary to relate efficiency to effectiveness and that a comparison of these will be the basis for determining quality in the future. Therefore, unlike past measures of quality that emphasized one component of Donabedian's model (Fig.

41-2) over another, the future of quality measurement will seek an integrative approach that incorporates the cost of nursing care.

This model of measurement of quality of nursing care views nursing services of a specific type (staff mix and model, i.e., case management, primary care, modular care) as an input that results in a product (patient care hours delivered in compliance with predetermined standards). For a specific patient during a given hospital stay, it provides a means for analyzing the efficiency or productivity of the nursing unit. If one stops here with measurement, as do many quality assurance programs, the most critical question, Did efficient utilization of services delivered according to standards result in quality patient outcomes? remains unanswered. By focusing on outcomes as compared to inputs (structure and process), the questions become:

1. How effective is the utilization of services delivered according to standards?
2. Comparing the quality of outcome, was the cost efficiency of services within an acceptable range?

An integrative model has the potential to address all pertinent issues of nursing care while simultaneously using new aspects of measurement, e.g., computers and cost accounting.

A SYSTEMATIC MEASURE OF QUALITY NURSING CARE

With the aid of new computer technology, nursing has a golden opportunity to demonstrate to the consumer the cost effectiveness of the quality of nursing care delivered by professional nurses. In an effort to establish cost for health care services, pressure is being brought to bear on the health care industry to design systems for costing out nursing services. In conjunction with this push from the consumer sector, the Joint Commission on Accreditation of Healthcare Organiza-

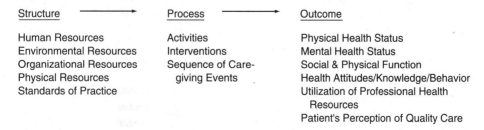

Fig. 41-2. Donabedian's model for quality care measurement. (*From Donabedian, A. [1980]. The definition of quality and approaches to its assessment. Ann Arbor, Mich: Health Administration Press.*) Used with permission.

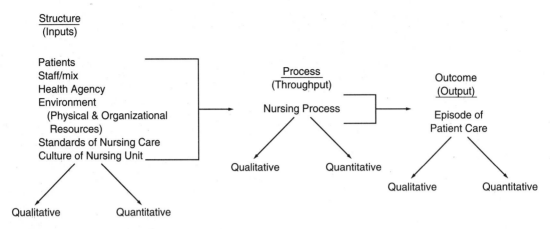

Fig. 41-3. A systematic integrative approach to quality nursing care management.

tions (JCAHO) has refocused accreditation criteria from a primary emphasis on management and equipment, to determining if patient outcomes meet established standards. Effective quality assurance programs in successful health care institutions of the future must be designed to include comprehensive database systems that not only incorporate structure and process variables but also relate these to measurable patient/client outcomes. To survive in the competitive era of today's health care delivery system, these outcomes must be analyzed for cost effectiveness.

A systematic integrative model for quality care measurement, such as delineated in Fig. 41-3, will determine quality of outcomes based on antecedents (structural elements and process). In such a model, structural inputs into the nursing care system would include those elements in the setting in which nursing care is given. Examples include available equipment and supplies, staff mix, standards set for patient care, characteristics of the patients themselves, and cultural norms of the nursing unit. According to Donabedian,[11] the culture within an organization is the most crucial factor associated with quality care. Therefore, the professionalism of the nursing staff should be a consideration in research designs to measure structure.

The process elements measured in such a systemic approach would address the interactions between the nurse, the patient/client, and the patient's/client's environment. Timely nursing interventions must be determined for identified nursing diagnoses. Here, consideration of the complexity of interventions delivered at an appropriate time in the episode of care delivery must be addressed as well as the way the care is delivered (the art of nursing). Standards of care developed today are written to elicit objective data. The more subtle subjective aspects of the nursing process are equally important; however, they are more difficult to determine. These aspects relate to judgments made and attitudes underpinning nursing actions.[3] To date, the most comprehensive nursing study that exemplifies research into this arena of the nursing process is Benner's[2] seminal work on the expert practitioner.

The third component is a systematic model for quality care measurement, and the primary focus is outcome. This aspect of quality of care is highly valued by the consumer but in the past has often been neglected as a major measure in quality assurance programs. Arguments in the past related to difficulty of equating outcomes with care delivered, given the limited control of variables such as genetic makeup, social and environmental factors, and attitudes such as adherence to prescribed self-care regimens. Also research methodologies used to determine outcomes following discharge, such as longitudinal studies that often included time-consuming interviews and content analysis, are costly to conduct.

When considering past nursing research on the assessment and assurance of quality nursing care, Lang and Clinton[22] found many studies that could be categorized as either fitting with the concept of structure, process, or outcome. The number of studies that approach the measurement of quality from a comprehensive perspective relating outcome to structure and process remain relatively few. Clearly, the methodology for research in the field is as yet not well defined. Consideration of quantitative measures alone is too narrow.

Identification of the number of professional nurses on a given unit does not provide information about the qualitative aspects such as attitude and commitment to excellence in patient care delivery. There is a need to design research methods that include both quantitative and qualitative dimensions. These methods must cut across all aspects of quality care measurement: structure, process, and outcome. Additionally, studies must be designed to determine the cost-effectiveness of the measure of the quality determined. Therefore, a model as described by Diers (Fig. 41-1) would fit the requirements of measurement using the relative components of health care.

MEANS TO A METHOD

As we face the task of defining an acceptable measure of quality of nursing care that can be delivered in a cost-effective manner, the development of technology and professional standards will serve the profession well. In addition, a greater number of doctorally prepared nurses are now available with skill both in quantitative and qualitative research methodology. These researchers will provide the designs needed to integrate structure, process, and outcome with appropriate quantitative and qualitative research methods.

The developments in information processing as applied to the health care field now allows comprehensive documentation of nursing care delivery. New software packages are being developed to integrate data on patient/client care outcomes with those of process and structure. The cost aspects are also being programmed into the directives for analysis. Research projects designed by nursing PhDs employed in hospital settings are addressing the efficiency of staff mix and other resource inputs against compliance of nursing standards and patient care outcomes. The profession is on the threshold of a new era in the development of quality assurance programs with dollar signs attached.

SUMMARY

The decade of the 1990s will require the nursing profession to make a strong commitment to the measurement of the quality of nursing care.[26,27] Indeed, nursing's future as a profession may depend upon the ability to statistically demonstrate professional nursing's value to society. This will mean that nursing education and service must work together to address the issue by educating those nurse researchers who have the knowledge and skill to design measurement tools capable of delineating the comprehensive nature of quality nursing care faced by the practitioner in the field. The use of an integrative model focused on outcome has the potential to prove the cost benefit of professional nursing care. Patients/clients recover with fewer complications, need less pain medication, and are better satisfied with their health care when they are cared for by professional nurses. For the first time, the technology is available for quantifying patient/client outcomes based on a rigorous research-based model. Now is the time to make research into the cost effectiveness of quality nursing care a national priority.

REFERENCES

1. Beckham, D. J. (1987, November). *The quality revolution: How to meet the challenge.* Presented at Health Care Competition Week.
2. Benner, P. (1984). *From novice to expert.* Menlo Park, Calif: Addison-Wesley.
3. Boyd-Monk, H. (1991). Quality: A Disney concern. *Journal of Ophthalmic Nursing & Technology, 10*(5), 191-192.
4. Brook, K. R., & others. (1976). *Quality of medical care assessment using outcome measures: An overview of the method.* Santa Monica, Calif: Rand Corporation.
5. Buralnick, D. B. (Ed.). (1980). *Webster's new world dictionary* (2nd ed.). New York: Simon & Schuster.
6. Clark, C. C., Cross, J. R., Deane, D. M., & Lowry, L. W. (1991). Spirituality: Integral to quality care. *Holistic Nursing Practice, 5*(3), 67-76.
7. Coyne, C., & Killien, M. (1987). A system for unit based management of quality of nursing care. *Journal of Nursing Administration, 17*(1), 26-32.
8. DeGeynt, W. (1970). Five approaches for assessing the quality of care. *Hospital Administration, 15*(1), 21-41.
9. Diers, D. (1988, Summer). *Examining options for leadership: How we should respond.* Proceedings from the American Colleges of Nursing Summer Seminar.
10. Dobson, A., Langenbrunner, J., Pelovitz, S., & Willis, J. (1986). The future of medicine policy reform: Priority for research and determination. *Health Care Financing Review,* (Supplement) 1-7.
11. Donabedian, A. (1978). The quality of medical care. *Science, 200*(4344), 856-863.
12. Donabedian, A. (1980). *The definition of quality and approaches to its assessment.* Ann Arbor, Mich: Health Administration Press.
13. Donabedian, A. (1988). The epidemiology of quality. *Inquiry, 22,* 282-292.
14. Erwin-Toth, P., & Spencer, M. (1991). A survey of patient perception of quality of care. *Journal of ET Nursing, 18,* 122-125.
15. Fetter, R. B., & Frieman, J. L. (1986). Product line management in hospitals. *Academy of Management Review, 11*(12), 41-54.
16. Gillette, B., & Jenko, M. (1991). Major clinical functions: A unifying framework for measuring outcomes. *Journal of Nursing Care Quality, 6*(1), 20-24.
17. Harrington, P., & Kaniecki, N. (1988). Standards and 2A—A common sense approach. *Nursing Management, 19*(1), 24-27.

18. Health Care Financing Administration Bureau of Data Management and Strategy. (1991). *1991 HCFA statistics* (HCFA Pub. No. 03325). Washington, D.C.: U.S. Government Printing Office.

19. Hemenway, D. (1983). Quality assessment from an economic perspective. *Evaluation and Health Professions, 6*(4), 379-396.

20. Icenhour, M. L. (1988). Quality interpersonal care: A study of ambulatory surgery, patients' perspectives. *AORN Journal, 47*(6), 1414-1419.

21. Jones, K. R. (1991). Maintaining quality in a changing environment. *Nursing Economic$, 9*(3), 159-164.

22. Lang, N. M., & Clinton, J. F. (1983). Assessment and the assurance of the quality of nursing care. *Evaluation and the Health Professions, 6*(2), 211-231.

23. Litman, T. (1984). Government and health: The political aspects of health care—a sociopolitical overview. In T. Litman & L. S. Robins (Eds.), *Health politics and policy*. New York: John Wiley & Sons.

24. McMillan, J. R. (1987). Measuring consumers' satisfaction to improve quality of care. *Health Progress, 3,* 54-87.

25. O'Brian, N., Lowe, C., & Rennebohm, H. (1987, May). A managerial perspective: In controlling the quality of patient care. *Dimensions,* 22-28.

26. Peter, D. A. (1991). Measuring quality: Inspection or opportunity. *Holistic Nursing Practice, 5*(3), 1-7.

27. Shiber, S., & Larson, E. (1991). Evaluating the quality of caring: Structure, process, and outcome. *Holistic Nursing Practice, 5*(3), 57-66.

28. Starfield, B. H. (1974). Measurement of options: A proposed scheme. *Milbank Memorial Fund Quarterly, 52,* 39-50.

29. Williamson, J. W. (1978). *Assessing and improving health care outcomes: The Health Accounting approach to quality assurance.* New York: Ballinger Publishing Co.

CHAPTER 42

Quality assurance in long-term care

LUCIA GAMROTH, JOY SMITH

Does quality assurance in long-term care (LTC) differ from quality assurance in any other segment of the health care system? This chapter will explore answers to that question, look at different quality assurance efforts, and draw some conclusions about the essence of a quality program. Although LTC covers a whole spectrum of services across settings, this discussion will focus on long-term care facilities licensed and certified as nursing facilities.

Sliefert[11] defines the basic elements of quality assurance as "standard setting, comparison of standard to actual practice, analysis and interpretation of the data, selection and implementation of actions to change practice, and feedback on the results of the action." Continuous quality improvement, a model of quality improvement adapted from the manufacturing field, is a "set of techniques for continuous study and improvement of the processes of delivering health care services and products to meet the needs and expectations of the customers of those services and products."[6] Regardless of the model used, the basic elements in the review process are the same. The process of quality assurance in LTC incorporates those elements and is essentially the same as in any other organization. The differences and difficulties that exist lie within particular elements of the process.

Antecedent to the measurement and assurance of quality is the definition of quality. *Quality of LTC* has been defined as patient/resident satisfaction, safety, prevention of poor outcomes, communication and coordination of care, and/or medical and nursing services that meet recognized standards of care. The Institute of Medicine[6] committee on quality assurance defines *quality of care* as "the degree to which health services for individuals and populations increase the likelihood of desired health outcomes and are consistent with current professional knowledge." Residents in nursing fa-

cilities have defined the elements of quality as ability to make choices, exercise control over their lives, and be treated with dignity by staff with positive, caring attitudes.[12] According to Kurowski and Shaughnessy,[8] "The many definitions (and resulting measures) of the quality of long-term care demonstrate its complexity and multidimensionality."

Several phenomena contribute to the complexity of LTC quality assurance, including the fact that a LTC facility is a home and a treatment center; the nature of chronic illness and disability; confusion about who the consumer is; the development of public policy and the regulatory process for LTC; and the failure of nursing homes to assure adequate quality.

HOME ENVIRONMENT

LTC facilities in general are both treatment and living situations in which health care and social support are provided to persons for a period of months or years. In a survey of nursing home residents, Spalding[12] found that the ability to make choices and to exercise control over such things as food, diet, sleeping and rising times, activities, and visits with friends were considered critical to quality care. These are quite different expectations from those in acute care facilities.

The predominance of the medical model in nursing facilities often prohibits a homelike environment; for example, one cannot have personal towels in the bathroom if the bathroom is shared with any other person because it is then considered a multi-use towel and not allowed under current regulation. Furthermore, personal care items must be labeled with a person's name for proper identification. One would hardly find such practices in a home. Many of the values of a homelike environment are in direct conflict with the acceptable standards of a medical model and, unless a facility is designed with private rooms for residents, it is difficult to personalize or create a homelike living space.

Yet "many aspects of nursing home life that affect a resident's perceptions of quality of life—and, therefore, sense of well-being—are intimately intertwined with quality of care,"[5] and the distinction between quality of life and quality of care thus becomes blurred. An institution can assure quality of care, but how does one assure quality of life? Even assuring quality of care is difficult.

THE NATURE OF CHRONIC ILLNESS

LTC residents typically have multiple diagnoses and interacting conditions for which there are no easy classification schemes or predictable outcomes. For example, if a patient is admitted with a hip pinning, the treatment is fairly predictable. However, the hip wound may be infected and draining, and the person may be a diabetic and have a cardiac condition, greatly complicating the situation.

Chronic conditions generally require restorative or maintenance services, with emphasis on attaining small improvements or preventing undue decline—unlike the intensive efforts of acute medicine that usually aim for cures, remissions, or other substantial improvements.[5]

A look at structure, process, and outcome criteria as defined by Donabedian[2] shows some of the difficulties in determining the criteria for quality assurance in LTC.

Structural criteria

Structural criteria refer to the capacity of the facility to provide good quality care. They include human, organizational, and supply resources. Structural criteria are easily measured and consequently provided the basis for regulatory review until very recently. The problem with structural criteria is that they measure the capacity to provide quality care but do not measure the care actually given or the outcomes of the care. Consequently, facilities may be in compliance with all the structural criteria yet have very poor resident outcomes. Conversely, a facility may demonstrate excellent resident outcomes yet be cited for paperwork deficiencies. Providers have objected to this approach for years, but only recently have regulatory agencies shifted to a process and outcome approach to evaluating quality of care.

Process criteria

Process criteria refer to the procedures or interventions that constitute the services provided. The difficulty in determining process criteria can be illustrated by the treatment of skin conditions. There are many approaches to treating skin conditions, and what works for one patient does not necessarily work for another. The variation is due to many factors, such as nutritional, mobility, and cardiac status, in addition to the individual's immune response and/or cooperation with the treatment protocol. Thus, while process criteria are important, they are very difficult to agree upon and measure with any validity. More work needs to be done to describe effective interventions and to document the relationship of interventions to outcomes.

Outcome criteria

Outcome evaluation in patient care has received a great deal of attention recently; many now consider this the most appropriate way to approach the concept of quality. Kane and Kane,[7] however, note the difficulty of using death, disability, and discharge as outcome criteria in LTC. Death rates in LTC are not good outcome indicators since many people spend their last days in LTC facilities and many come there for terminal care. Disability as an indicator is also problematic since many residents are disabled on admission. Discharge for the short-term resident is a realistic goal but may be inappropriate for the long-term resident.

Kane and Kane[7] also discuss the varied needs for emotional well-being and social interaction of the heterogeneous LTC population. While it is reasonable for staff to address some needs that are short term or related to the residents' condition, staff cannot provide for deficits that have been of life-long duration. Also, for cognitively impaired residents, who represent approximately 60% of the population in nursing homes, there are questions about what are reasonable outcomes and how individual goals affect other residents and staff. Kurowski and Shaughnessy[8] conclude: "Conceptually, attaining appropriate outcome represents the ultimate validation of the effectiveness of the care process. However, it is extremely difficult to specify appropriate outcomes of care and to empirically demonstrate their relationship to the process of care."

WHO DECIDES?

While process and outcome criteria may be the best indicators of quality, a critical question remains: Who determines the desirable and appropriate intervention or outcome? Is it the resident, the family, the professional staff or the regulatory agency? In other words, who is the consumer? Is the consumer the person who receives the care, the one who is responsible for the one who receives the care, or the one who pays the bill? Or are all of these the consumer? The following are examples of dilemmas that occur because of divergent views on this question:

1. The facility dining room seats approximately 50 residents and guests for dinner. Knowing when dinner is served, residents come to the dining room when they wish. Many come early to enjoy a glass of wine with their salad, sitting at the table they have chosen to sit at for many months or years. The entree is then served individually, followed by a dessert and beverage of their choice. The surveyor cites deficiencies in the following areas: (1) the time between the first and main course is too long; (2) salt and sugar are readily available to persons at the table; and (3) the entree is not served *on a tray*.

   In this instance, residents know when the hot food will be served, and many choose to come to the dining room a little early. The presence of salt and sugar is appropriate to the persons sitting at the table, and the entree is served individually as a part of a homelike atmosphere. The surveyor is afraid, however, that someone may get salt and sugar who should not have it. Further, the surveyor is afraid that, without a tray, there may be improper identification of residents and the kind of diet they are to have.

   It seems clear to most persons that the situation allows appropriate choices by residents and staff. The surveyor, however, feels bound to cite this facility in a survey for a "potential hazard to residents," even though *no adverse patient outcomes* were found on the survey. Who has made the quality decision?

2. In another situation, a facility was cited for having a sign on the wall near the bed of a resident describing the procedure for toileting the resident. Information of this kind is generally included in the bedside information sheet, which is protected from public view but accessible to the staff. Because of the concern expressed by the survey team, the director of nursing visited the resident and began to take the information sheet down from the wall. The resident objected, saying that "it is very important that information is there where everyone sees it so

that when I use the commode I am assisted correctly." The nurse talked with the resident about possibly placing the information sheet in the bathroom and the resident refused.

In this situation, the surveyor was concerned about a violation of the dignity and rights of the resident. And at face value, it would appear that putting the information on toileting in full view was a violation of such rights. However, on further exploration, it became clear that it was the resident's wish to have the information sheet where everyone would see and use it. That might not be what staff, family, or a surveyor would choose. Who has made the quality decision?

3. Another example concerns the use of physical restraints in a facility. Over the past two years, this facility reduced the percentage of residents using physical restraints from 25% to 4% ($n=5$). In a quality review of those currently using restraints, 2 of the 5 residents were found to be using them because of family request. Both of these residents were cognitively impaired, so the professional staff met with the two families to discuss alternative ways of dealing with the residents' needs. Both families remained adamant; in their view, restraints were the treatment of choice. The interpretation of the surveyor, however, was that the facility was deficient in meeting professional standards of care. Who decides?

There are many examples of these dilemmas. The point is that values and interpretations of situations differ depending on one's particular perspective. Quality decisions often require balancing conflicting goals and values—e.g., patient safety and patient independence—and those goals must then be evaluated "in the light of each other." The residents and staff deal with these situations every day and are in the best position to evaluate what is appropriate. The surveyor, coming in as an outsider, certainly needs to raise questions, but he or she must have the capability to decide what is reasonable and logical without fear of reprisal from some other regulatory body.

Quality assurance in LTC is in its infancy. A great deal more study is needed to determine appropriate process and outcome criteria. Balancing a homelike atmosphere and personal choices with quality nursing care for individual patients and the total group requires ongoing evaluation.

To summarize, LTC differs from other types of care in three ways: (1) the home environment, (2) the difficulties in defining and measuring appropriate structural, process, and outcome criteria for LTC quality assurance, and (3) divergent perspectives on who is the consumer. In spite of these difficulties, significant efforts have been made to measure and assure quality.

QUALITY ASSURANCE EFFORTS
Peer review

In 1985, the Joint Commission on Accreditation of Healthcare Organizations (JCAHO) published a guide to quality assurance in LTC, and JCAHO has sponsored several workshops on the topic. The commission's LTC standards manual[13] includes revised standards for quality assurance. In 1992, the commission published *Quality Improvement in Long-Term Care,*[14] a guide to how quality improvement can help long-term care facilities comply with the new federal certification requirements. JCAHO is currently working on the development of process and outcome measures as a part of the "Agenda for Change" initiative.

Association efforts

In 1982, the American Health Care Association published *Quest for Quality,*[1] which was one of the first overall descriptions of quality assurance purposes and tools specific to nursing homes. Since 1982, the manual has been revised, but the program continues to target 29 aspects of services for the long-term care population in four categories: resident services, clinical activities, special needs of the frail elderly, and management.[15] *Quest for Quality* provides the basis for QA programs in many homes across the country.

Incentive programs

Several states have developed quality measurement programs based on outcomes. New York State, for example, developed a program to meet the state review requirements, titled Sentinel Health Events (SHE), which identified undesirable or unexpected outcomes.[10] If the incidence of a particular outcome exceeded the norm of the facilities in the state, a second level of review was triggered to look at process in relation to a given outcome. The purpose of the second-level review was to determine whether or not the poor outcome was related to poor care. This program was further developed, broadening the outcome categories, and the state of New York developed the first outcome-oriented resident-based survey process. The New York

survey process served as a model for the development of the new federal survey process.

Illinois initiated a program called the Quality Incentive Program (QUIP). The QUIP program identified standards of quality in specific areas of care and provided a financial incentive to facilities if they showed improvement in these areas.[4] The quality incentive standards were designed to be higher than those for the licensure and certification surveys and, according to proponents of the program, were targeted at those aspects of a facility's care and services that can have the greatest impact on a resident's health, sense of well-being, and quality of life. Geron,[3] however, in an evaluation of the program notes, said "It is impossible to determine whether the program succeeds in improving resident care, or simply represents the ability of providers to meet standards that may not have anything to do with resident care quality." Because of inadequate state funding, the program was discontinued in June 1992.

Regulatory efforts

Regulatory efforts to assure quality have been relatively ineffective for reasons best understood within the context of history. Vladeck[16] in his book *Unloving Care,* and the Institute of Medicine[5] study on quality of care in nursing homes provide excellent historical accounts of the development of LTC public policy and regulatory changes. The growth of nursing homes in this country resulted from the authorization in 1935 of social security, with the Old Age Assistance program. In 1950, amendments to the Social Security Act specified a requirement for state licensure of participating facilities but did not set any standards for care.

It was nearly 30 years after the program began that the Public Health Service issued the Nursing Home Standards Guide, which represented the combined efforts of the Public Health Service, states, and providers of care. Medicare and Medicaid were enacted in 1965, and amendments passed in 1967 authorized the Department of Health, Education, and Welfare (HEW) to develop standards of care and withhold payments from skilled nursing homes not meeting these standards.

Throughout the 1960s, the U.S. Senate's Special Committee on Aging held congressional hearings on nursing home problems. These congressional hearings resulted in a series of reports on the deficiencies of the federal regulatory efforts.

Then, in 1972, Congress passed legislation that federally funded state surveys and certification activities and directed HEW to develop a single set of standards for Medicare/Medicaid participating providers. In 1974, the final rules were promulgated for the certification of skilled and intermediate care facilities; these were titled in 1988 as the Skilled Nursing Facility (SNF) Conditions of Participation and Intermediate Care Facility (ICF) Standards.

Several unsuccessful attempts have been made to revise the 1974 conditions and standards. Continuous opposition to proposed changes in the regulations finally led HCFA and Congress to postpone making virtually any change in the regulations until a committee appointed by the Institute of Medicine studied the issues and reported its recommendations.

Concurrently, the Health Care Financing Administration (HCFA) developed a modified survey instrument, called Patient Care and Services (PaCS), based primarily on direct patient assessments and outcome-oriented indicators of care. Even with the PaCS survey process, however, the pressure on regulatory agencies at the federal and state level during the past 10 years has swung the pendulum to the end of overenforcement or safety at all costs, a phenomenon that has created nightmares for facilities that have given good patient care, whose employees describe "respect for others" as the principle of their practice, and have a record of remarkable outcomes for their residents. The annual survey often cites such facilities for violations like "salt and sugar freely accessible to the residents at their dinner table" or "dinners served without trays."

The Nursing Home Reform Act, often referred to as OBRA '87 because it was incorporated into the Omnibus Reconciliation Act of 1987,[9] has the potential for making the greatest impact yet on the quality of care in nursing facilities in this country.

The new regulations in this act require nursing facilities to provide services that "maintain the highest practicable functioning level"[9] of the resident. Facilities are now required to annually complete a comprehensive assessment on each resident and develop a treatment plan based on the assessment and input from the resident. The Minimum Data Set (MDS) is the primary assessment tool, and the resident assessment protocols (RAPs) include trigger conditions that identify potential problem areas and guidelines for further assessment. Assessments are updated on a quarterly basis for each resident. This database provides longitudinal data on each resident so that key indicators of quality can be tracked over time. In addition to comprehensive assessment and treatment to assure quality of care, OBRA '87 addresses resident rights and quality of life issues, such as autonomy and restraint-free environments.

The focus of the review process for LTC facilities is now on outcomes of care and related processes. In other words: Do the identified processes indicated on the treatment plan relate to the outcomes identified on the treatment plan, the quarterly assessments, and observations of the residents? From the provider's viewpoint, this is certainly a step in the right direction. However, a great deal of discretion is still given to the survey team in determining whether a given situation constitutes a deficiency for a particular facility because it is much easier to determine the presence or absence of decubiti or weight loss than it is to determine whether appropriate care has been provided that honored the wishes and values of the resident. The objective existence of the former does not always constitute poor or deficient care.

Because of inconsistencies among surveyors in applying the guidelines, Congress mandated a program that would measure and reduce inconsistencies among surveyors in the application of the guidelines to individual facilities.[9] The contract to evaluate the new OBRA survey and certification process was awarded to Abt Associates Inc., and the evaluation is currently under way.

In spite of continued problems with the survey process, OBRA '87 calls for a "new mindset" about life within institutions. It is challenging caregivers, families, and residents to reevaluate the age-old beliefs that providers know what is best for the resident. If we really believe in resident rights and consequent responsibilities, we must find new ways to conceptualize quality in long-term care.

Because of this challenge, new ideas are emerging. Two examples may serve to illustrate the new approaches to old problems. A project was recently undertaken by the Benedictine Nursing Center in Mt. Angel, Oregon, to create a model for resident-centered care. The impetus for this change came from a staff RN at the center who died of cancer. During her last days of life, staff from the center volunteered time to care for her in her own home. During that time, she helped them to see that what they wanted for her (as professionals) and what she wanted (as the patient) were quite different. For example, it was not important to her to be turned every two hours to prevent skin breakdown. It was more important for her to be pain free, to sleep through the night, and to be alert enough to spend quality time with her family. This experience made several nurses reevaluate their expectations for resident care and develop a new model of planning care.

The model begins with input from the resident about his or her wishes for care, routines, and goals. If the resident cannot provide that information, the staff seek the family's perceptions of what the resident would choose. This is done only if the resident cannot provide that information firsthand. Then, information from the comprehensive assessment is considered and interpreted in the light of the resident's wishes. A treatment plan is written in the first person, which, in effect, puts the resident "in charge." This approach is difficult for some professional staff—for example, one occupational therapist questioned, "How can I state it in the first person if it isn't the resident's choice?" Good question!

The answer is that this approach requires a different way of thinking than simply "inviting the resident to participate" in the care-planning conference. It goes beyond the requirement in OBRA that residents be included in planning care to the real spirit or intent of the OBRA legislation. The center is now getting requests from other states for information on the project. While in its infancy, the project has the potential to change the standards of what constitutes quality in the care planning process.

The Benedictine Institute for Long Term Care, jointly sponsored by the Benedictine Nursing Center and the Oregon Health Sciences University School of Nursing, now has funding from the Robert Wood Johnson Foundation to demonstrate the effectiveness of a model to assist nursing homes to implement the new federal regulations. The Benedictine Nursing Center has developed a successful process for reducing the use of physical and chemical restraints and, with foundation support, the Benedictine Institute is formalizing the process for nursing homes throughout the state of Oregon.

The Institute is working with other providers, state regulators, and consumers of nursing home care to develop uniform criteria for the use of restraints and policies by which providers can modify their practice. A monitoring system is also being developed to assure that the agreed-upon standards of care are being met. Both providers and state regulators receive training, educational materials, and consultation regarding the criteria for use of restraints.

These efforts have reduced the use of physical and chemical restraints in participating nursing homes in Oregon. The project has also developed a model for bringing providers, regulators, and consumers together to improve nursing home care. Although the initial focus is on reducing the use of physical and chemical restraints, the ultimate intent is to produce a model that can be used for implementing other policy changes in the state of Oregon and adapted for use in other states. The positive response of all participants in the first year of use of the model points to the strong potential for other states to adopt the criteria, monitoring system, and guidelines for modifying practice.

Anecdotal reports of professionals actively working to reduce the use of restraints in facilities across the country indicate that the current use rates in participating facilities are less than 10%, compared with a 40% national average in 1988. Similar reports indicate that chemical restraint use rates are less than 15%, compared to a 50% national rate before these efforts. The professional staff in these LTC facilities have, in effect, set a new standard of care for the appropriate use of physical and chemical restraints, and as staff skills continue to develop, further reduction in these rates is expected. Another by-product of these efforts is that HCFA officials are consulting with these practitioners as the new interpretive guidelines are written and promulgated.

While OBRA '87 set the stage for a new approach to external review of quality, the survey process remains fraught with old attitudes, an orientation toward problems to the exclusion of positive feedback, and, generally, a "policing and enforcement" rather than an "assistance and empowerment" attitude toward providers of care. Negativism and fear will never provide a quality product.

QUALITY SERVICE

Quality of care in LTC has improved over the years. Many changes have taken place as a result of new information about the care needs and illnesses of the older population. Medical and nursing advances in the care of older persons have brought about many changes in both the medical treatment and nursing care of these persons.

In spite of all the advances and the improvements in regulation and training, however, there remain the horror stories of abuse, neglect, and understaffing and a certain proportion of poor quality homes. Why?

The reason is that quality cannot be regulated. Quality relates to excellence, and a belief in and commitment to excellence does not grow out of regulations and laws. It grows out of a philosophy of caring that pervades the staff at every level and is evidenced in interactions between and among the staff, staff and residents, and the facility and community. Quality reflects a pride in who we are as long-term-care providers and an appreciation for the richness of elderly persons' lives and what they have to contribute to our society and our personal lives.

Striving for excellence requires certain basic administrative components. It requires good management and communication. It requires educated, properly prepared staff who keep abreast of new discoveries in their practice fields. It requires an honest, open approach to new ideas, to challenges from within and without. It requires shared responsibility for quality on the part of every single staff person and the board of directors. The responsibility for quality grows out of a respect for the dignity of the people we serve, the people we work with and the community we represent, and it is a positive, creative, forward movement.

The characteristics described here are the characteristics of the facilities that excel in their services to the elderly in our society, facilities that already meet the quality standards of good nursing, and are demonstrating new models of care to improve the quality of care and life for all residents in nursing facilities.

REFERENCES

1. American Health Care Association. (1982). *Quest for quality.* Washington, D.C.: Author.
2. Donabedian, A. (1980). *Explorations in quality assessment and monitoring* (Vols. 1-2). Ann Arbor, Mich: Health Administration Press.
3. Geron, S. M. (1991). Regulating the behavior of nursing homes through positive incentives: An analysis of Illinois' quality incentive program (QUIP). *The Gerontologist, 31,* 292-301.
4. Illinois Register Section 140.525 - .528. (1985). *Quality incentive program.*
5. Institute of Medicine. (1986). *Improving the quality of care in nursing homes.* Washington, D.C.: National Academy Press.
6. Institute of Medicine. Division of Health Care Services. (1990). *Medicare: A strategy for quality assurance* (Vol. I). Washington, D.C.: National Academy Press.
7. Kane, R. A., & Kane, R. L. (1987). *Long-term care: Principles, programs and policies.* New York: Springer.
8. Kurowski, B. D., & Shaughnessy, P. W. (1985). The measurement and assurance of quality. In R. J. Vogel & H. C. Palmer (Eds.), *Long-term care: Perspectives from research and demonstrations.* Rockville, Md: Aspen.
9. Omnibus Budget Reconciliation Act of 1987, Subtitle C, Nursing Home Reform Act, PL 100-203.
10. Schneider, D. *Sentinel health events: A process and outcome-based quality assurance system.* Unpublished manuscript.
11. Sliefert, M. K. (1990). Quality control: Professional or institutional responsibility. In J. C. McCloskey & H. K. Grace (Eds.), *Current issues in nursing* (3rd ed.). St Louis: Mosby.
12. Spalding, J. (1986). *A consumer perspective on quality care: The resident's point of view.* Washington, D.C.: National Citizen's Coalition for Nursing Home Reform.
13. The Joint Commission on Accreditation of Healthcare Organizations. (1988). *Long-term care standards.* Chicago: Author.
14. The Joint Commission on Accreditation of Healthcare Organizations. (1992). *Quality improvement in long-term care.* Oakbrook Terrace, Ill: Author.
15. Trocchio, J., & Holloway, K. (1990, January/February). Quest for quality: Here's a program to help you grade your facility. *Geriatric Nursing.*
16. Vladeck, B. C. (1980). *Unloving care: The nursing home tragedy.* New York: Basic Books.

CHAPTER 43

The status of quality assurance in home health care

JOYCE COLLING

Quality assurance programs are less developed in home health care than in other areas of health care. Although quality assurance programs in some other settings are well accepted and effective, the unique characteristics of providers, services, and recipients of home care create difficulties in adapting quality assurance programs from other settings or in designing comprehensive quality assurance specifically for home care. The pressure for quality assurance programs in home health care, however, has intensified during the past several years because consumers demand high-quality care, fiscal constraints have increased, the home care services are vulnerable to fraud and abuse, and services provided in the home have become increasingly sophisticated.

This chapter reviews recent changes in health care that have had a profound effect on home health care and on the development of quality assurance in home health. It also presents issues to consider in designing quality assurance programs in home health care or in applying knowledge on quality assurance from other settings and for other populations. Finally, a multisite project that proposes to overcome deficiencies of previous quality assurance programs in home health care is described.

HEALTH CARE SYSTEM CHANGES THAT HAVE INFLUENCED HOME HEALTH CARE AND QUALITY ASSURANCE

Several recent social and legislative changes have had a significant effect on the health care system in general. First, there is an ever-increasing number of people aged 65 and older. Those 85 years and older are the fastest-growing segment of society and are the most likely to need frequent, episodic or continuing care for multiple chronic conditions and functional disabilities.

Second, recent Medicare legislation has created the incentive for the proliferation of home health agencies because it provides limited reimbursement for eligible posthospital Medicare-certified patients. Home health agencies now number over 6000, and in the past decade there has been an 800% increase in the number of proprietary agencies that are Medicare certified.[21] In addition, the limit on the number of home health and skilled nursing visits that can be provided was lifted in 1981 for eligible Medicare beneficiaries. At the same time, Congress authorized the Health Care Financing Administration (HCFA) to permit states to waive eligibility requirements for Medicaid coverage of home health care if the care is a substitute for nursing home care. However, a review of some of these programs suggests that they are not a substitute for nursing home care, but instead are reaching persons who would otherwise receive no care.[31] Both of these actions increased the demand as well as the intensity of home care services.

A third factor that has had a profound influence on health care delivery has been legislation mandating a prospective payment system for medical care. This has decreased the length of hospital stays still further and has shifted a greater number of acute and chronically ill patients into home health care agencies.

The rising demand for high-quality health care by numerous consumer groups in the past two decades is a fourth factor that has affected health care delivery. Consumers want high-quality technical care that also is accessible and provided in a manner that conveys respect and dignity for the individual.[13] They are becoming increasingly vocal and sophisticated in stating what they want and are demanding a role in policy-making groups where decisions are made about the future of health care. Initial efforts in response to these demands for quality control have occurred mainly through regulation, certification, and licensure at both the institutional and individual levels for various categories of health care workers.[17] These actions, however, fall far short of achieving the current objectives of active consumer groups.

Fifth, the Omnibus Budget Reconciliation Acts of 1986 and 1990 (OBRA) included mandatory discharge planning and a uniform needs assessment. Further, Congress ordered the Department of Health and Human Services to develop general criteria to establish priorities for the allocation of funds and personnel and for reviewing and assuring quality of care.

Sixth, during this same period of time nursing has experienced dramatic changes that have had an impact on home health care. These changes include a rapid decline in the number of graduates from diploma-granting programs, a large increase in graduates prepared at the associate degree (AD) level and relatively little change in the percentage of graduates from four-year baccalaureate programs. Traditionally, baccalaureate nurses were the only nurses specifically prepared to function in nonhospital settings. Now, however, many diploma and AD nurses are employed in home health where an increasing amount of high-technology nursing is carried out with considerable independent judgment expected of the nurse.

Finally, the Joint Commission on Accreditation of Healthcare Organizations (JCAHO) has shifted its monitoring and evaluation standards for quality assurance to a continuous quality improvement (CQI) approach. This shift was reflected in the 1992 Joint Commission's quality assurance (QA) standards and will be fully implemented in the 1994 standards. CQI emphasizes continual improvement of care by establishing an ongoing, comprehensive self-assessment system that involves all levels of personnel rather than a single QA department. In the CQI approach, there is a focus on the processes of care and service that takes into account the contextual variables influencing quality care rather than the performance of individuals.

STATUS OF QUALITY ASSURANCE IN HOME HEALTH CARE

The structure-process-outcome framework for determining quality proposed by Donabedian more than a decade ago has been widely applied in different areas of health care.[23] Early efforts at measuring quality relied mainly on structural resources, which are relatively easy and inexpensive to measure. Unfortunately, although adequate resources are necessary ingredients for quality care, they are not sufficient to ensure quality. That is, they do not guarantee that the resources will be used to achieve quality care. More recently process variables—procedures, activities, and services carried out on behalf of clients—have been widely used as measures of quality, but again procedures or activities alone cannot predict that the client will progress satisfactorily and certainly predict nothing about client satisfaction with the care received.

The final aspect of the quality triad proposed by Donabedian is outcome measures. They focus on the consequences of care activities. Outcomes are particularly difficult to measure reliably because they can be influenced by many factors, including contextual differences, individual differences (genetic, physical, social, economic, and psychological), and the specific and interactive contributions of all health care professionals engaged in the client's care.[12]

Building on the less-than-satisfactory results of previous attempts to measure quality, the most recent quality assurance programs have recognized that the combined components of structure, process, and outcome are all important measures of quality. The American Nurses Association's Standards of Home Health Nursing Practice has recognized this combined approach to measuring quality. They define quality assurance as the "estimation of the degree of excellence in the alteration of the health status of consumers, attained through provider's performance or diagnostic, therapeutic, prognostic or other health care activities."[2] This definition places considerable emphasis on the skills used by the practitioner to work toward a positive health outcome, and recognizes that the outcome of a positive alteration in the recipient's health status is the goal of therapeutic activity. It also recognizes that quality assurance is broader in scope than what nursing alone contributes. Other factors include fiscal constraints and deficiencies in a comprehensive social policy for home care services.

Table 43-1 describes a number of individually focused quality assurance programs in home health care. As the table shows, few of the early programs were developed with outside funding to support the time-consuming pilot testing and evaluation necessary to ensure reliability and validity. There is remarkable

Table 43-1 Summary reports on quality assurance programs in home health care

Year	Author/source	Agency	Key aspects of program
1977	Vincent & Price[28]	Cleveland VNA	Focused on mental health patients; social behavior, employment, medication compliance, and hospital readmission used as outcome measures
1977	Daubert[8]	New Haven, Conn, VNA	Developed patient classification system by prognosis; focused on process and outcome measures
1979	Decker & others[9]	Minnesota Dept. of Health	Based on medical diagnoses with functional and other criteria as subsets of outcome criteria
1980	Legge & Reilly[19]	Altanta VNA	Focused on cancer patients, using functional status as one outcome measure
1983	Visiting Nurse & Home Care, Inc.[29]	Hartford, Conn, VNA and Home Care	Multidimensional outcome-oriented instrument; focused on self-management
1984	Ansak & Zawadski[3]	San Francisco	Focused on elderly clients; functional and cognitive status, institutionalization, health, and cost were outcome measures
1985	Gould[11]	Philadelphia, United Home Health Services	Used nursing diagnoses as focus of outcome criteria
1985	Miller & others[20]	—	Focused on elderly clients; ADL, IADL,* mental status, number of nursing home days and hospital days were measured
1986	Brouton & others[6]	—	Focused on low birth weight infants; standardized physical and mental growth outcome measures were used
1986	Kline & others[15]	Georgia Dept. of Human Resources	Focused on process measures
1986	Lalonde[18]	Home Care Assn. of Washington	Federally funded study in progress; developing a number of outcome-oriented scales
1986	Simmons[26]	Omaha Visiting Nurse Association	Federally funded project; outcome criteria developed based on nursing diagnoses
1986	Sorgen[27]	Alberta, Canada	Funded study completed in 1988; focused on key structural, process and outcome criteria; a classification system was developed
1988	Applebaum & Christianson[4]	—	Funded National Channeling Demonstration projects to monitor quality of services with case management
1988	Wilson[32]	Hudson Valley VNA	Four functional assessment instruments were developed as outcome measures
1990	Kramer & others[16]	University of Colorado Health Science Center	Robert Wood Johnson and HCFA funded project to develop a comprehensive system of outcome and process measures of quality of care
1991	Saba & others[22]	Georgetown University	Funded study which focused on a method for classifying nursing actions provided to home health Medicare patients to predict resource requirements and measure outcomes
1992	Goodwin[10]	Family Home Care, Spokane, Wash	Study focused on identifying a process for developing critical pathways for achieving a specific outcome of care for particular DRGs**

*ADL, activities of daily living; IADL, instrumental activities of daily living.
**DRG, diagnostic-related groups.

dedication and creativity involved in developing these early models of quality assurance in home care. They serve as guides for future development. The more recent examples cited in the table are federally funded programs that are more likely to achieve the goals of reliable and valid measures of quality. The most extensive project by Kramer et al.[16] proposes a comprehensive quality assurance system and is described in more detail in this chapter.

ISSUES OF QUALITY ASSURANCE IN HOME HEALTH CARE

Four major issues to resolve or consider in developing quality assurance programs for home care are contextual factors, multidisciplinary care delivery models, individual differences, and the measurement of quality care. It is unlikely that small independent efforts, no matter how dedicated and creative, can effectively untangle the interrelationships among these areas. Well-designed, well-funded, multisite studies are needed that combine the best thinking of informed consumers, methodological experts, and expert clinicians from diverse health care disciplines.

Multiple contextual factors

Developing useful quality assurance measures in home care is complicated by the fact that each home in which the care is delivered poses differing and multiple contextual factors that can have a bearing on the outcomes of client care. For instance, treating an elderly client's stasis ulcers in a home environment in which the hygiene, nutritional conditions, and opportunities for adequate rest and sleep are poor may yield a different outcome than if the home environment is optimal for healing to occur. In addition, a number of other factors about the client's family situation may have a negative or positive bearing on how well the client responds to care provided by agency personnel. These factors include how supportive the family is in allowing the client to assume the sick role and what competing psychological or physical stressors may be present among other family members.

Multidisciplinary care delivery models

It is estimated that 70% to 80% of all home care services are delivered by paraprofessionals such as aides who provide homemaker and personal care services. Other therapies can include physical therapy, occupational therapy, social work, medicine, and specialized nursing. Nurses are often responsible for coordinating, supervising, and evaluating the overall plan of care. Thus, process measures may be a major component of a quality assurance program where the contribution of each health care worker is measured. The client's satisfaction, however, is not assessed using this perspective, nor does it take into account the interaction and coordination among the several health care workers and family members who may be crucial in determining the overall outcomes of care in a comprehensive quality assurance program.

Accounting for individual differences among clients

One of the most difficult problems to overcome in developing reliable and valid quality assurance measures for home care is that of accounting for individual differences. Although there is some homogeneity among children and younger adult clients, one of the most distinctive characteristics of elderly persons is their *heterogeneity*. As people age, they tend to become less like others who are the same chronological age, which makes the development and testing of measurement instruments difficult to standardize. This problem is an important consideration because the majority of home care clients are elderly. Further, about two thirds of the elderly population have multiple chronic diseases or disability problems. Although these problems may not be the cause of the home care referral, they must be taken into account when developing a plan of care and in assessing the potential for a specified outcome. Knowledge about gerontology and geriatrics is clearly essential to accurately assess and evaluate care. Unfortunately many disciplines, nursing included, do not currently include this content in their curricula.[1]

Measurement limitations

A number of quality assurance projects have developed and tested instruments for use in institutional settings such as hospitals and nursing homes. However, use of these instruments without careful testing for modifications needed to account for the unique characteristics of home care is questionable. Specific areas of knowledge gleaned from previous research on quality assurance model development that can be useful in the development of home care quality assurance programs include the following:

- Measures that capture relationships, particularly among process, outcome, and even structural components, are necessary to yield useful quality measures.

- Given the cost constraints on health care services and the potential for rationing of care, it may be necessary to determine points at which increases in services result in diminishing outcomes of patient status.
- Knowledge from gerontology and geriatrics is needed to define positive outcomes of maintaining current levels of functioning, rather than recognizing only improvement in function or cure.
- Multivariate techniques should be used that allow one to evaluate all criteria and to determine what combinations of criteria best predict quality of care.
- Providers' qualifications and skills should be included.
- Computerization of systems of care monitoring allows easier manipulation of variables.

A proposed comprehensive quality assurance system

A multiproject agenda between 1988 and 1993, funded by HCFA and the Robert Wood Johnson Foundation, has undertaken a research program to develop a broad-based quality assurance system for home health care.[16,24,25] The quality assurance system is based on two premises: (1) it is necessary to measure outcome, process, and structural measures to assess quality home care; and (2) home health patients should be classified into homogeneous quality indicator groups (QUIGs) to assess home health care quality. The researchers use the term *quality indicator* to denote "constructs, patient characteristics or service attributes that can be used to assess quality home health care."[16] Further, they divide QUIGs into focused measures and global measures. This classification approach began by listing quality indicators and specifying the types of patients for whom each indicator was appropriate. These small lists then grouped similar patient types according to the constellations of appropriate quality indicators. The classification system was then field tested on 300 Medicare patients to determine that all patients could be classified adequately. In addition, a Delphi process was conducted using interdisciplinary panels to determine face validity of the classification scheme.

At present, 26 QUIGs of patient conditions have been identified to measure quality, and approximately 100 outcomes have been established. Work is also under way to identify key process components of assessment, planning, intervention, and care coordination that are essential to achieve a positive outcome for each of the 100 outcomes identified. Currently, 45 home health agencies are involved in data collection and testing the proposed system. The goal of the project is to identify a set of uniform items for home health care that can be used to measure key outcomes and form the basis for a broader set useful for care planning at the agency level and for administrative purposes at the agency and regulatory levels. Thus, this multiproject is an effort to empirically associate process and outcomes of care and holds promise to provide a comprehensive system to measure quality in home care services.

CONCLUSIONS

Quality assurance (QA) in home care is currently less developed than in other settings, and few programs have been tested for reliability and validity. Because of the unique characteristics of home care, QA measures developed for other settings and populations cannot readily be adopted for the home setting. Finally, the need to develop effective QA in home care is increasing as a greater number of clients receive a wide variety of complex health care services in the privacy of their homes that in the past were carried out in institutions. This creates the potential for less-than-optimal outcomes if quality is not monitored carefully. The need is even more urgent because QA and reimbursement are likely to be linked in some way in the near future.

REFERENCES

1. American Nurses Association. (1986). *Gerontological nursing curriculum: Survey analysis and recommendations.* Kansas City, Mo: Author.
2. American Nurses Association. (1986). *Standards of home health nursing practice.* Kansas City, Mo: Author.
3. Ansak, M., & Zawadski, R. T. (1984). On-lok CCODDA: A consolidated model. In R. T. Zawadski (Ed.), *Community-based systems of long-term care.* Philadelphia: Haworth Press.
4. Applebaum, R., & Christianson, J. (1988). Using case management to monitor community-based long-term care. *Quality Review Bulletin, 14,* 227-231.
5. Barkauskas, V. H. (1983). Effectiveness of public health home visits to primiparous mothers and their infants. *American Journal of Public Health, 73*(5), 573.
6. Brouton, D., et al. (1986). A randomized clinical trial of early hospital discharge and home follow-up of very low–birth weight infants. *New England Journal of Medicine, 15,* 934.
7. Cox, C. L., Wood, J. E., Montgomery, A. C., & Smith, P. C. (1990). Patient classification in home health care: Are we ready? *Public Health Nursing, 7*(3), 130-137.
8. Daubert, E. A. (1979). Patient classification system and outcome criteria. *Nursing Outlook, 27,* 450.
9. Decker, F., et al. (1979). Using patient outcomes to evaluate community health nursing. *Nursing Outlook, 27*(4), 278.

10. Goodwin, D. R. (1992). Critical pathways in home health care. *Journal of Nursing Administration, 22*(2), 35-40.

11. Gould, E. J. (1985). Standardized home health nursing plans: A quality assurance tool. *Quarterly Research Bulletin, 11,* 334.

12. Horn, B. J., & Swain, M. A. (1976). An approach to development of criterion measures for quality patient care. In *Issues in evaluation research.* Kansas City, Mo: American Nurses Association.

13. Kelman, H. R. (1976). Evaluation of health care quality by consumers. *International Journal of Health Services, 6*(3), 431.

14. Kenney, G. M., & Dubay, L. C. (1992). Explaining area variation in the use of Medicare home health services. *Medical Care, 30*(1), 43-57.

15. Kline, M. M., Tracy, M. L., & Davis, S. L. (1986) Quality assurance in public health. *Nursing and Health Care, 1*(4), 192.

16. Kramer, A. M., Shaughnessy, P. W., Bauman, M. K., & Crisler, K. S. (1990). Assessing and assuring the quality of home care: A conceptual framework. *The Milbank Quarterly, 68*(3), 413-443.

17. Kurowski, B. D., & Shaughnessy, P. W. (1985). The measurement and assurance of quality. In R. J. Vogel & H. C. Palmer (Eds.), *Long-term care: Perspectives from research and demonstrations.* Rockville, Md: Aspen.

18. Lalonde, B. (1986). *Quality assurance manual of the home care association of Washington.* Edmonds, Wash: Home Care Association of Washington.

19. Legge, J. S., & Reilly, B. J. (1980). Assessing the outcomes of cancer patients in a home nursing program. *Cancer Nursing, 3*(5), 357.

20. Miller, L. S., Clark, M. L., & Clark, W. F. (1985). The comparative evaluation of California's multi-purpose senior services project. *Home Health Care Services Quarterly, 6*(3), 49.

21. Mor, V., & Spector, W. (1988). Achieving continuity of care. *Generations, 4*(3), 47.

22. Saba, V. K., O'Hare, P. A., Zuckerman, A. E., Boondas, J., Levine, E., & Oateway, D. M. (1991). A nursing intervention taxomony for home health care. *Nursing and Health Care, 12*(6), 296-299.

23. Schneider, D. (1986, May). *Sentinel health events: A process- and outcome-based quality assurance system.* Paper presented at Oregon Health Sciences University, Portland.

24. Shaughnessy, P. W., Crisler, K. S., Schlenker, R. E., Bauman, M. K., & Kramer, A. M. (1992). Developing a quality assurance system for home care. *Caring, 11,* 44-48.

25. Shaughnessy, P. W., & Kramer, A. M. (1990). The increased needs of patients in nursing homes and patients receiving home health care. *The New England Journal of Medicine, 322*(1), 21-25.

26. Simmons, D. A. (1986). Implementation of nursing diagnosis in a community health setting. In M. E. Hurley (Ed.), *Classification of nursing diagnosis: Proceedings of the sixth conference.* St Louis: Mosby.

27. Sorgen, L. M. (1986). The development of a home care quality assurance program in Alberta. *Home Health Services Quarterly, 7,* 13.

28. Vincent, P., & Price, J. R. (1977). Evaluation of a VNA mental health project. *Nursing Resident, 26*(5), 361.

29. Visiting Nurse and Home Care, Inc. (1983). *Guidelines: Self-management outcome criteria.* Plainville, Conn: Author.

30. Visiting Nurse Association of Metropolitan Detroit. (1984). *Guide for the development of the nursing care plan.* Detroit: Author.

31. Waldo, D. R., Levit, K. R., & Lazenby, H. (1986). National health expenditures. *Health Care Financing Review, 9*(1), 1.

32. Wilson, A. A. (1988). Measurable patient outcomes: Putting theory into practice. *Home Health Care Nurse, 6,* 15-18.

CHAPTER 44

Standards and guidelines

How do they assure quality?

SUSAN L. DEAN-BAAR

The purpose of this chapter is to outline the new framework for standards and guidelines for nursing practice developed by the American Nurses Association in conjunction with more than 30 specialty nursing organizations. This framework for standards and guidelines for practice has the potential to serve as a unifying framework to evaluate the quality of nursing in a variety of practice settings and areas. Schroeder[8] provides a comprehensive review of other approaches to standards in nursing.

A component of the American Nurses Association's (ANA) core mission is its responsibility for defining nursing, establishing the scope of nursing practice, and for setting standards of nursing practice. ANA has been involved in setting standards of practice for many years. In 1952, ANA established functions, standards, and qualification committees that serve as the roots of today's current standards of practice.

The development of standards is an important step toward assuring quality of nursing care. Next in importance to the development of nursing standards is the application of the standards to actual nursing practice. Standards of nursing practice provide a means for determining quality of care as well as accountability of the practitioner.

In 1973, ANA's Congress for Nursing Practice published the generic *Standards of Nursing Practice,* which laid the foundation for professional nursing practice. They were based on the nursing process and provided a systematic approach to nursing practice in any setting and in any specialty area. Following the publication of the generic standards, many of the ANA practice councils collaborated with specialty nursing organizations to develop and publish standards of practice for their particular areas of practice. Over the years, there has

been an evolution in nursing standards of practice. From 1975 until 1990, standards published by ANA used a structure, process, and outcome format that reflected the ANA model for quality assurance.[4] In 1982, some standards documents began to include standards in areas other than the nursing process.

The range of definitions for standards resulted in some standards referring to a baseline for practice or minimum expectations and others referring to a goal for practice or level of excellence. This diversity in definitions and frameworks has resulted in a fragmented approach and understanding of the purpose of standards for nursing practice.

McGuffin and Mariani[6] analyzed the content of 27 clinical standards developed and published by the American Nurses Association from 1973 to 1989. Many of these were developed in conjunction with specialty nursing organizations. Twenty-two of the publications reviewed included a nursing process format. They also identified four specialty areas that had published criteria for selected nursing diagnoses in the specialty area.

In addition to standards related to the nursing process, they found that nine other standards were frequently included. These were theory, organizations, continuity of care, collaboration, professional development/continuing education, quality assurance/peer review, research, community systems, and ethics. McGuffin and Mariani's analysis found repetition and also little difference under the theory, organizations, continuity of care, collaboration, research, community systems, and ethics standards, and an apparent confusion between the concepts of professional development/continuing education and quality assurance/peer review. They recommended that those aspects of practice that consistently appear in or affect practice be shared among areas of nursing to avoid duplication and that agreement be reached on the broad category headings. In addition, they concluded that clarification and consistency are needed in several areas, including how the categories of professional practice and professional performance standards are defined, and whether standards indicate a minimum or maximum level of practice.

In 1988, ANA began a process of reevaluating the nature and purpose of standards of nursing practice because the evolution of standards had raised several concerns. These concerns included the lack of utility in the profession's standards to measure the effectiveness of health care, the lack of consistency in the process whereby the profession developed standards, the proliferation of standards of nursing practice, and the wide range in the intent, format, and scope of current standards. The divergent and numerous approaches used in standards limited their usefulness to nurses, other health care providers, payers, policy makers, and consumers for use in a variety of activities such as quality assurance, clinical decision making, and reimbursement schemes.[2]

This reevaluation process was guided by an ANA Task Force on Nursing Practice Standards and Guidelines, whose original charge was "in view of current health care quality assurance activities, define the nature and purpose of standards of practice for nursing and the relationship of quality assurance activities and standards of practice to specialization in nursing practice, credentialing, and implications for nursing information systems."[2] As a result of other activities within the health care arena, including some of the work being done by the Agency for Health Care Policy and Research, the charge to the task force was expanded to include the purpose and format of guidelines for practice.

The development of the framework for nursing standards of practice and practice guidelines described here began with a critical analysis of the environment internal and external to nursing. This included discussion representing the perspectives of nurses in a variety of practice roles and settings with input from numerous nursing specialty groups, state nurses' associations, and ANA structural units.

This framework is substantially different from previous standards work done by the American Nurses Association. The framework is innovative and brings nursing to a new stage in its development. The framework has the potential to provide unity and a common point of reference regarding the use of standards and guidelines for all of nursing.

STANDARDS OF CLINICAL NURSING PRACTICE

Standards of Care	Standards of Professional Performance
Assessment	Quality of Care
Diagnosis	Performance Appraisal
Outcome Identification	Education
Planning	Collegiality
Implementation	Ethics
Evaluation	Collaboration
	Research
	Resource Utilization

The combined framework for standards of nursing practice and practice guidelines is designed so that it can provide direction for nursing practice, a means to evaluate practice, and a way in which the profession can be accountable to the public. Each of these is important to building a foundation to assure quality.

Within the framework, standards and guidelines primarily differ in their scope and intent. The purpose of standards is to provide broad direction for the overall practice of nursing, including the provision of care and professional role activities. Standards are authoritative statements that describe a level of care or performance common to the profession of nursing by which the quality of nursing practice can be judged. Standards define professional practice and reflect the values of the profession. Standards of clinical nursing practice are divided into two categories: standards of care and standards of professional performance. The intent of standards of care is to describe an acceptable level of patient care; the intent of standards of professional performance is to describe an acceptable level of behavior in the professional nurse's role.

Standards of care describe a competent level of care as demonstrated by the nursing process involving assessment, diagnosis, outcome identification, planning, implementation, and evaluation. Standards of professional performance describe a competent level of behavior in the professional role, including activities related to quality of care, performance appraisal, education, collegiality, ethics, collaboration, research, and resource utilization[3] (see the box above).

These definitions of standards clearly delineate the role of standards as setting a competent level of care or performance. This is a significant change from previous standards, which have been designed to describe excellence and were not intended to define minimum levels of nursing care or legal parameters for measuring the quality of care. This framework provides for the inclusion of components of the professional nursing role in addition to the provision of care. The need for the inclusion and delineation of these two components of professional nursing activity has become clear.

Standards of nursing practice will include general criteria that will allow them to be measured. Criteria will be variables known to be relevant, measurable indicators of the standard. Although standards are anticipated to remain relatively stable over time, criteria may change over time due to advancements in knowledge and technology.

Specialty areas of nursing practice will be able to define themselves by developing criteria by which each standard is measured. These criteria will be specific to the specialty area. Thus, the standards would not change, but the criteria will change to reflect the specialty area of practice, in essence creating standards of practice for that specialty area.

In contrast, the purpose of guidelines for nursing practice is to guide practice by providing linkage among diagnoses, treatments, and outcomes, to describe alternatives available to each patient/client or patient/client population, and to provide a basis for evaluation of care and allocation of resources. The goal of guidelines is to describe a recommended course of action to address a specific nursing diagnosis, clinical condition, or the needs of a particular patient/client population. Guidelines will describe a process of patient/client care management that has the potential of improving the quality of clinical and consumer decision making. A guideline includes a diagnosis, intervention(s), and expected patient/client outcome(s).

This approach to guidelines has similarities with previous work done within nursing and that frequently was labeled standards. This is most commonly reflected in the standardized care plan approach to planning and providing nursing care. Both approaches described a course of action to address a specific need or diagnosis.

However there are some significant differences in the approaches. One of the major differences is in the change in terminology from standards to guidelines. Standards are intended to be applied rigidly and to be followed in virtually all cases. Exceptions to following the standards would be rare and difficult to justify. In addition, standards are considered to be the foundation for safe health provider practices and not following

them would indicate unsafe and incompetent practice (W. Carson, personal communication, 1992). Guidelines are recommendations for patient management and may include a range of interventions or strategies and, as such, would not meet the characteristics just described. Another difference is the intent of guidelines to describe alternatives and to assist in decision making. One of the difficulties frequently encountered in practice is the inability to use standardized care plans because of the individual characteristics of the patient or client situation. Standardized care plans do not account for the complexity and comorbidity frequently present in individuals. The intent of guidelines is to identify those circumstances when it is known that the guideline would not be appropriate or would need modification in either interventions or expected outcomes.

It is important to remember that guidelines will reflect only recommended actions. Not every guideline will be appropriate for every individual within a patient/client population. In addition, not every intervention within a guideline will always be appropriate.

Guidelines convert science-based knowledge into clinical action in a form accessible to practitioners. They reflect knowledge generated through research and/or professional consensus by practitioners regarding preferred interventions for a particular problem or select group of patients/clients.

In the development of practice guidelines, certain characteristics should be taken into consideration to maximize their usefulness. First, they should be reasonable in view of the state of the art. Interventions and outcomes within a practice guideline should be possible and not developed in a way that makes them unreasonable to implement or achieve. They should be comprehensible or able to be understood by nurses, other health care providers, and consumers. They should be consistent in format across practice specialties. They must be measurable or able to be evaluated, and they must be validated by research or professional consensus. The process for reviewing and updating guidelines will need to be a dynamic one so that guidelines can reflect changes in knowledge and technological capabilities.

The development of guidelines is occurring in many arenas. Specialty nursing organizations are working on revising documents previously described as standards. These publications were intended to be used to assist with clinical decision making and thus, with appropriate revisions, are more appropriately identified as guidelines. In addition, multidisciplinary guidelines are being developed. The Agency for Health Care Policy and Research (AHCPR) has devoted considerable resources to developing guidelines.[1] The overall purpose of the AHCPR is to enhance the quality, appropriateness, and effectiveness of health care services and to improve access to that care. There are numerous panels of experts working on guidelines for AHCPR. The first three guidelines released by AHCPR (acute pain management, urinary incontinence, and prediction and prevention of pressure ulcers) were on clinical conditions where nursing makes a significant contribution to the care and outcomes of individuals experiencing those problems.

The new framework developed by ANA makes clear distinctions between standards and guidelines for practice. These distinctions in intent and definition are important in determining the appropriate use of standards and guidelines. However, they are both equally important in evaluating nursing practice and the quality of care provided. Standards of clinical nursing practice provide a framework to evaluate the individual professional nurse. Guidelines provide a means to evaluate the quality of the nursing care provided to a specific patient or patient population. Components of the standards of care should be embedded within guidelines. Within a guideline should be information about assessment, diagnosis, outcome identification, planning, implementation, and evaluation of that specific diagnosis or clinical condition.

It is believed that standards of nursing practice and practice guidelines can serve as the basis for many activities within nursing aimed at assuring quality. They can serve as the basis for quality improvement systems by identifying important aspects of care within either the standards or a specific guideline. These can be used to identify indicators of quality nursing care that are then monitored. The data collected can be used to improve the quality of care provided. Guidelines can serve as the basis for institution or agency specific policies and procedures. The standards of clinical nursing practice can be used to develop job descriptions and performance appraisals systems that support quality professional practice. In those institutions with clinical or career ladders, the standards can serve as the framework for the initial stage of the ladder with additional stages reflecting increased expectations for practice.

The components of standards and guidelines can be used in conjunction with the Nursing Minimum Data Set[9] to develop database systems that can provide valuable information on the quality of nursing care.

Standards and guidelines can be used in planning, organizing, and evaluating nursing service delivery systems and organizational structures. For example, guidelines could be used to evaluate selected nursing interventions in terms of quality patient outcomes and cost-effectiveness.

In addition, the standards of clinical nursing practice and content of guidelines for practice can be incorporated into certification activities. Particularly those guidelines developed by national agencies or organizations will be the focus of educational offerings aimed at disseminating the information to practitioners so that the quality of care can be improved.

It is hoped that standards of nursing practice and practice guidelines will be used not only by nursing but also by other health care providers, regulatory agencies, consumers, and health care financiers in understanding the scope of nursing and the contribution of nurses and nursing towards the goal of quality health care. Specifically, they could be used to serve as the basis for including relevant nursing information in large database systems, such as the Health Care Finance Administration or insurance companies. The inclusion of nursing components in databases can assist in positioning nursing to be included in health care reimbursement and financing systems. Guidelines can also be used to promote patient/client participation in health care decision making by clarifying health care choices (including choice of practitioner) and their consequences for the patient/client.

The ANA framework modifies the use of the structure, process, and outcome format previously used by deleting the inclusion of structure, process, and outcome criteria in standards. This does not negate the importance of structure, process, and outcome attributes.[5] Structure attributes are those related to the setting in which the care occurs. What had previously been labeled as structure criteria appears to be more appropriate as separate standards related to the administrative domain. Process reflects what is done in giving and receiving care, and thus, in this new framework are reflected both in the standards and within guidelines. Outcomes reflect the effects of care and are patient/client focused. The outcome criteria are more appropriately included as part of the guidelines for practice.

This framework has the potential to be used to develop the patient/client care component of useful and meaningful quality assurance or management programs. These standards and guidelines can be used to develop an institution-, agency-, or unit-based program that demonstrates that the organization is delivering safe, effective, and appropriate care. Written, meaningful standards and guidelines are essential to developing quality assurance programs. Because of the framework's ability to include general and specialty areas of practice, an institution or agency with specialty areas could utilize the same approach as the framework in developing its program. A organization could use the standards of practice and the criteria for each standard to develop their own indicators and make decisions about how and what data should be collected to determine the degree to which the standard is being met.

This approach provides for many possibilities. It provides for the ability to evaluate practice not only within an institution but also across institutions. If nursing organizations utilized the standards of clinical nursing practice and practice guidelines to develop quality assurance programs, the potential of being able to clearly demonstrate the contribution of nursing in providing quality care within that setting would be considerable. As health care becomes increasingly competitive, information on quality becomes even more valuable than in the past.

As the new standards of clinical nursing practice are implemented and work continues on the development and implementation of practice guidelines, all nurses need to think about how this work could be translated in a way that would assist in developing meaningful ways to articulate the importance of quality nursing care. Programs are needed that would allow the evaluation of the quality and cost effectiveness of the nursing care provided in a variety of practice areas and settings.

Mark Phippen, while president of the Association of Operating Room Nurses, wrote "Nursing is at a crossroad. One of the pathways provides an opportunity to move toward professional unity. . . . Acceptance of the proposed ANA model means that AORN will have to rethink its approach to standards of practice. . . ."[7]

This challenge is one for all of nursing; we are at crossroads in the development of standards and guidelines, and this crossroad has the potential to have an enormous impact on nursing practice. There are many different ways for this framework to be adapted for implementation in institutions and agencies where nursing is a part of the health care services provided. A common definition of standard and guideline can only help to clearly articulate the critical role that nursing plays in the planning and delivering of quality, appropriate, and effective health care. This new model is congruent with other work being done in the larger health care arena and has the potential to continue to position nursing in the forefront of activities to evaluate the effectiveness of health care.

REFERENCES

1. Agency for Health Care Policy and Research. (1990). *Clinical guideline development.* Rockville, Md: Author.
2. American Nurses Association. (1991a). Task force on nursing practice standards and guidelines: Working paper. *Journal of Nursing Quality Assurance, 5*(3), 1-17.
3. American Nurses Association. (1991b). *Standards of clinical nursing practice.* Washington, D.C.: Author.
4. American Nurses Association. (1975). *A plan for implementation of standards of nursing practice.* Kansas City, Mo: Author.
5. Donabedian, A. (1988). The quality of care: How can it be assessed? *Journal of the American Medical Association, 260*(12), 1743-1748.
6. McGuffin, B., & Mariani, M. (1990). Clinical nursing standards: Toward a synthesis. *Journal of Nursing Quality Assurance, 4*(3), 35-45.
7. Phippen, M. (1990). President's message. *AORN Journal, 52*(2), 212, 214.
8. Schroeder, P. (1991). *Approaches to nursing standards.* Gaithersburg, Md: Aspen.
9. Werley, H., & Lang, N. (Eds.). (1988). *Identification of the Nursing Minimum Data Set.* New York: Springer.

CHAPTER 45

TQM/CQI

What is it? Does it work?

PAMELA KLAUER TRIOLO

TQM, the new tack in health care quality improvement, has sometimes been called a "semantic nightmare." What is this new focus? *Is* it new? What does it mean for health care, and does it work? This chapter will address these questions. For the purpose of clarity, the term *total quality management* (TQM) will be used throughout this chapter.

To explore the possibility that TQM is not a passing fad or the latest flavor of the month, like management by objectives (MBO) or guest relations, it is important to look at the origins of this expanded emphasis on quality in American business. After World War II, global competition became an issue for almost every manufacturing firm in the United States. By the 1970s, American businesses began losing market share to foreign competitors, like Japan. For example, American manufacturers held 90% of the market share for color television sets in the 1970s. By 1987, that market share had dwindled to 10%.

The Japanese started applying quality principles in their high technology manufacturing areas as early as the 1950s. Early quality efforts were very narrowly focused on quality control, and the main focus was inspection. Rarely was attention paid to the process that created the errors in the product or services. The focus was on inspecting the product after it came off the line and saving the customer from receiving a poorer quality product by pulling it off the line before it left the plant and reached the customer. This early piecemeal approach was later replaced in the 1980s by total quality management.

American companies started addressing these quality issues just one decade ago. In the past 10 years, American companies such as Xerox, Motorola, IBM, Corning, and others began to capitalize on TQM principles and problem-solving approaches and began to pull ahead of their American competitors. The organized quality movement in health care lagged behind that of American businesses.

In the health care arena 10 years ago, patients had limited choices. They were hospitalized at their community hospital or the hospital recommended by their physician. But during the past 5 years, circumstances have changed. Today, patients have many choices, and they hold higher expectations about health care delivery. Not only do they expect the finest technical quality, but they expect that the services surrounding health care be delivered in a courteous, convenient, and efficient manner.

Another force heralding the need for change in health care is the burgeoning cost. In 1992, health care costs in the United States are expected to reach $800 billion, 14% of the gross national product. Industrial research reports that in the production of health care delivery, there is waste. That waste, found in rework, unnecessary lab tests, turnover, errors, waiting time, patient complaints, variation in practice, and litigation, to name a few, is estimated to add up to 25 cents out of every dollar of health care operating expense. And waste is the single most important cause of customer dissatisfaction.[3]

Employers in the search for the best value for the dollar in covering health care expenses are demanding that hospitals provide service at competitive cost. Through selective contracting, employers are choosing to send their employees to the hospital that provides the best quality at the most competitive price.

Most economists agree that the decade of the 1990s in health care begins the era of doing more with either less or the same amount of resources, both human and financial. It will not be possible to purchase improvements, such as MRIs, CAT scans, etc., to compete for the health care customer, since the community hospital down the street has one, or the tertiary care center in another state sends out its mobile unit to your community. The key to success is making the most out of the resources currently available and directing the efforts of all staff, not just managers and clinical staff, toward enhancing quality. A fundamental view in TQM is that quality health care does not cost more; in fact, it costs less. Efforts to date indicate that initiatives designed to enhance the quality of service reduce costs.[1]

These driving forces of competition among hospitals, including competition for staff, rising health care costs, and increasing expectations of regulators and of those that are served by health care, have combined to produce a critical level of interest and momentum in health care focused on continuous quality improvement. In the late 1980s, this heightened interest led to the interest and implementation of TQM in hospitals. And in 1990, in its "Agenda for Change," the Joint Commission on Accreditation of Healthcare Organizations (JCAHO) defined its target as moving from one of meeting standards to evaluating hospitals on continuous quality improvement. The quality improvement journey in health care was officially launched for even those who remained skeptical about this new emphasis.

FOUNDATIONS OF TQM

Simply defined, total quality management is a structured system for involving an entire organization in a continuous quality improvement process targeted to meet and exceed customer expectations. TQM is not a program. It is a process and a philosophy of doing business.

How is TQM different from "TGM," traditional good management? In total quality management, accountability for quality is shifted from management to the entire organization. Staff empowerment is one of the cornerstones, and all staff are encouraged to identify and solve problems. Also, the hierarchy of problem solving is reduced. In other words, staff members are encouraged to solve problems, layering is reduced, and individuals need not ask permission to problem solve. Health care delivery is viewed as a series of processes, and since staff are the closest to the process, their involvement is critical to the solution of problems.

The environment in most health care organizations is characterized by turf battles and fiefdoms, since areas have had to compete for sometimes scarce resources. Professional models of autonomy have also occasionally obstructed the concept of team so essential to providing comprehensive, multidisciplinary care to patients. In TQM, relationships between departments are viewed as a series of customer-supplier relationships. Patients and others served by health care constantly move among departments. Collaboration between departments, for example, between pharmacy staff, the patient, and the unit nursing staff, is essential to providing effective and efficient care.

Another distinction between TQM and traditional management styles is that quality management uses a scientific problem-solving process and a set of data-driven, statistical quality control tools. The problem-solving process is diagnostic in approach, and health care professionals will recognize the similarity to the scientific method and clinical diagnosis (see Fig. 45-1). Although each organization develops its own version of this process, the fundamental steps remain the same. The first step is identification of the problem and its extent. The second step involves identifying the underlying causes of the problem, and the third step developing solutions. The final step is one of monitoring to determine that what was implemented actually works.

Skeptics may ask, how is this different from what managers traditionally do? Managers have fallen into the cycle of identifying a problem and solving it. Rarely do managers explore the extent of a problem to clarify where it occurs, and even more rarely do the solutions identified address the underlying causes of the problem. Finally, managers do not usually continuously monitor a solution to determine if it works.

Though clinicians would never prescribe an antibiotic for a sore throat without a series of assessment and diagnostic steps, managers consistently go for the "quick fix." That is why problems come back on routine cycles, and why if you ask a group of managers from the same area what problems they were dealing with 10 years ago and what problems they were dealing with today, there will be many that are the same.

In the course of working through a problem, this process uses seven statistical quality control tools (Fig. 45-2) and seven management and planning tools. These tools are both investigative, like the fishbone diagram, which looks at cause and effect, and diagnostic, such as the Pareto chart, which exhibits the extent of the problem and assists in prioritizing in what area to concentrate. Although all tools are not used, they eliminate the fatal flaw of jumping to solutions and

① PROJECT ORGANIZATION & DEFINITION	② DIAGNOSTIC JOURNEY
Goal: Develop a problem statement that describes the problem in specific terms, where it occurs, when it happens and its extent.	Goal: Develop a complete picture of all the possible causes of the problem; then agree on basic causes.
③ REMEDIAL JOURNEY	④ CONTINUOUS IMPROVEMENT CYCLE
Goal: Develop an effective and implementable solution and action plan.	Goal: Implement the solution and establish needed monitoring procedures and measures.

Fig. 45-1 The University of Iowa Hospitals and Clinics total quality management/quality improvement storyboard. Used with permission.

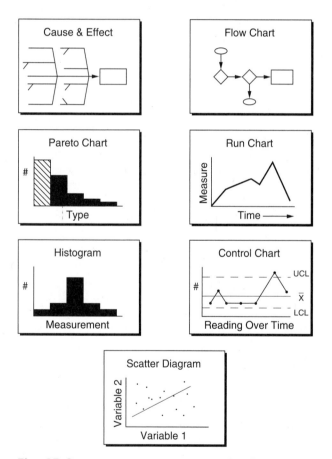

Fig. 45-2 The seven basic quality control tools.

reduce management by instinct or gut feeling. In group process, they are the ultimate equalizer since they facilitate creative thinking and guide teams to make collective decisions based on data, versus forcing teams to succumb to who speaks loudest or may have the greatest political clout.

A final difference in TQM is that the focus in health care is returned to its origin, the patient. Yet health care organizations serve more than patients. The term *customer* is defined as any person or organization that has expectations or makes judgments about the quality of service provided. Some of these customers, beyond patients, include referring physicians, staff, governing bodies, students, faculty, etc. TQM is highly customer focused.

For many years, health care providers managed with the "crystal ball" approach, believing they knew what customers expected. Total quality management actively pursues and identifies the expectations of those served through surveys, interviews, focus groups, and other strategies. Then improvements are targeted to meet and exceed those expectations. Since the philosophy of "if we build it, they will come" no longer applies in the competitive health care arena, new services are developed with the goal of meeting perceived and documented needs of those served by the organization.

RESULTS IN HEALTH CARE: NATIONAL DEMONSTRATION PROJECT

In the fall of 1987, 21 health care organizations met to launch the National Demonstration Project (NDP) on Quality Improvement in Health Care funded by the John A. Hartford Foundation. Hosted by the Harvard Community Health Plan, these organizations were united in an experiment to explore whether the tools of modern quality improvement, which have achieved breakthroughs in performance in other industries, would be applicable in health care.

In the five years since its inception, there have been many lessons learned and results achieved.[5] TQM is not magic. It is hard work, and demands dramatic organizational and personal changes. The following discussion details some of the lessons learned by the health care organizations united in the NDP.

Committed leadership, at the top, is the sine qua non of effective TQM. TQM involves changes in culture, strategic priorities, and organizational structure. Although these can be facilitated by the quality leader, they must be driven from the top. High-level, visible commitment is essential. Skeptics within the organization are quick to point out when senior leadership does not talk the talk or continues to practice autocratic leadership. The most valuable and intrinsic change with TQM comes when each individual changes to be more customer focused, strives to foster relationships between departments, and uses the data-driven problem-solving process to prevent problems, as well as fix them.

Physician involvement is another key component to the success of this new paradigm. Early on, several of the NDP organizations discussed their intentions to involve physicians at a later date. Their first effort would be geared toward improvement of purely administrative processes. This has resulted in a formula for re-work.

The lesson is that any health care organization that begins a comprehensive TQM initiative without the involvement of physicians and physician leaders, a key customer group, does so at its peril. Although it takes time and energy to involve physicians, they are intrinsic to health care delivery, and by involving them early, they serve as some of the greatest champions. Physicians can easily see the merit of both involvement and the diagnostic, problem-solving process.

Although there is no specific recipe for TQM implementation, and each initiative must be customized to the culture of the organization, there are some common structural essentials. Some of these key components are having a clear, shared vision, a quality director, a quality council, a strategic planning process, trained facilitators, a process for nomination and selection of quality projects, and a database of customer expectations.

The vision of continuous quality improvement is one that must be articulated and shared by all staff within the organization. The quality director, in partnership with the CEO and other senior leadership, serves as the designer of organizational change and development, coach for senior managers, trainer, role model, and internal consultant for all staff. Quality directors who report directly to the CEO have been proven to be the most effective. The quality council serves as the policy and decision-making focus for organization-wide enhancements.

Facilitators provide training and support for teams. Facilitators assist teams through the problem-solving process, guide group dynamics, and serve as internal consultants. Facilitators and leadership help each member of the organization see how his or her work clearly supports the long-term vision.

Another key lesson learned is that quality improvement is much more than just teams. Although teams are a component of TQM, this strategy involves a fundamental change in business strategy of which only one element is teams. Organizational change requires systematic review and alteration of management systems, such as human resources, information, leadership behavior, design methods, customer information systems, benchmarking methods, as well as strategic quality planning that sets the organization's priorities.

Unless quality improvement projects are formed and guided by priorities, they tend to be self-serving. They may focus on meeting the needs of internal customers versus developing new processes designed to encompass all those served. Quality improvement projects are an essential part of TQM, but they are not TQM itself.

Another lesson is that training alone is not enough. Early on, organizations seemed to assume that training would produce change. Many organizations launched premature mass training efforts that often left a lag time between application of learning and before top management had laid the groundwork. Training should be for immediate use or as close to the event as possible. Some organizations have adapted the concept of "just-in-time" in their training efforts; where a problem is identified, a team is formed and trained as they work through the TQM problem-solving process.

It is important that training, like teams and benchmarking, not be mistaken for TQM. Training is critical to organizational change, but it should not be mistaken for the whole.

Another lesson is that health care organizations have discovered that they cannot manage what they do not measure. Mining data sources, like patient satisfaction surveys, cultural analysis, Delphi studies of staff priorities, results in the database for improvement. For example, simple measurement of transport time led to an easy rearrangement of equipment, eliminating 15% of transports; measurement of patient admission times led to major changes in admission processes; and measure of medication billing errors led to dramatic improvements in medication charting. These data sources matched with improvement initiatives have resulted in useful measures of internal customer satisfaction and operational efficiency. The payoff is improved care, happier patients, and reduced costs.

A final lesson learned is that health care projects save money. Dozens of hospitals have launched thousands of quality improvement efforts. Although the dollar amount saved has never been quantified, results reported consistently demonstrate financial returns of 400% to 500% or more for specific quality improvement projects. One hospital reduced two full-time equivalents by a simple change in transport procedures. Another cut X-ray retakes to a third, saving tens of thousands of dollars. Another organization saved hundreds of thousands of dollars in unnecessary mailings. Targeted to improve effectiveness, efficiency, and appropriateness, improvement projects have removed anywhere from 10% to 80% of the work in a process.

The University of Michigan Hospitals estimate quality improvement implementation costs at $2.5 million, but the organization has realized a minimum financial gain of $17.8 million. These figures count only the first two years of cost and benefit for each specific project; many benefits will continue for years to come.

THE DARK SIDE OF QUALITY

A discussion of contemporary quality improvement efforts would not be complete without a look at the potential downside of quality. Organizations highly committed to quality improvement require caution in three major areas.

First, organization-wide emphasis on quality improvement is a long-term process. Planning and implementation of TQM in an organization is a long-term process. Transition is not overnight, and administrators who rush for the quick fix will be short-changing their success. Focusing on cost cutting as a way to improve quality results in closed-looped thinking. All efforts to improve quality should address process enhancements, not cost reduction. Cost reduction, through the reduction of waste, will follow process improvement. Reducing costs, without improving the

process, is a Band-aid approach and does not increase the quality of service.

A second obstacle is to become process burdened. In their zeal to foster the new paradigms, teams often proliferate and may be driven to use every tool and every step to problem solve. Teams are not necessary to prevent problems. In fact, teams are not always necessary to solve problems. All tools need not be used for each problem, only those that fit the situation and data. Staff become so preoccupied with following the steps and using the tools that they can be led away from the primary work purpose. Becoming process burdened can slow down TQM in an organization, result in customers not being served, and result in high levels of frustration that can derail even the finest initiatives.

A final threat to TQM was identified by Florida Power and Light, the only American company to win the coveted Deming Prize.[2] In its efforts to improve quality, a tremendous infrastructure had developed to support quality improvement. This infrastructure, which has developed in a number of organizations committed to quality improvement, has sometimes served as a parallel or "shadow" organization. Quality is not integrated into daily responsibilities of all staff but either delegated or supported by a infrastructure that is so far removed from the processes of the company that the customer focus is lost. The managers within the infrastructure also reduce the number of persons allocated to the actual work of the business.

CONCLUSION

The quality improvement journey in health care through the organized process of TQM has just begun. And it will never end. Expectations of those served will continue to evolve. Health care providers will be challenged to provide fine services with decreasing human and financial resources.

Many organizations adopt the philosophy of continuous quality improvement as a reactive response to the JCAHO. Some organizations will launch rapidly into teams without laying the groundwork and structure for success. Many organizations will not undergo the fundamental philosophical change of empowerment but will talk the talk. TQM will fail in these organizations.

Just implementing TQM does not mean an organization will more clearly focus its efforts on the customer, improve its processes, or provide its greater value for the health care dollar. To be successful in continuously improving quality requires tremendous organizational commitment driven from the top. It requires that all staff be customer focused and use a scientific, data-driven problem-solving process. All staff will need to view themselves as a link in the customer-supplier service. And management will need to reward involvement and role model the new behavior.

Without organization-wide change and without organizations moving from a performance to a learning mode,[4] TQM will not grow in the health care delivery system. And TQM will fade and be viewed as just another "flavor of the month," just another fad, like the many that have come before.

REFERENCES

1. Anderson, C. A., & Daigh, R. D. (1991, February). Quality mindset overcomes barriers to success. *Healthcare Financial Management,* 21-31.
2. Broadhead, J. L. (1991, February). The post-Deming diet: Dismantling a quality bureaucracy. *Training,* 41-43.
3. Conway, W. E. (1992, May). Quality management in an economic downturn. *Quality Progress,* 27-29.
4. Fritz, R. (1992). *Creating.* New York: Fawcett-Columbine, Ballantine.
5. Godfrey, A. B., Berwick, D. M., & Roessner, J. (1992). Can quality management really work in health care? *Quality Progress,* 25(4), 23-27.

CHAPTER 46

Nursing certification

A matter for the professional organization

GLORIA M. BULECHEK, MERIDEAN L. MAAS

How to grant credentials to professionals to assure that they are qualified to provide specialized services to consumers is a subject fraught with misunderstanding and vested interests. The controversy has produced a number of views of how professionals should be awarded credentials for specialized practice and who should do it. The nursing profession has experienced this conflict. Several models have evolved for granting credentials to nurses who practice a nursing specialty.

The dominant models for certification of registered nurses for specialty practice are: (1) certification by the professional organization—a statement issued by a professional organization declaring that a nurse has met predetermined qualifications to practice a specialty; (2) certification by the state—a legal endorsement by a state board of nursing certifying that a nurse has met the legal requirements for specialty practice; and (3) certification by an institution—a statement issued by an academic or health service agency recognizing that a nurse has completed the requirements of a program of study for specialty practice.[10] The ambiguous status of nursing certification is confusing both to nurses and to the public.

The American Nurses Association (ANA) and a number of specialty nursing organizations have developed national programs of certification. State certification of the nursing specialties has been a trend in nursing practice law since the mid-1970s.[7] Many nurses are recognized as specialists on the basis of local certification by an academic or service institution. Debate has continued among members of the nursing profession and other interested parties over which of these models best serves the profession's and the public's interests. Certification for entry into specialty practice was one component of *The Study of Credentialing in Nursing: A*

New Approach[1] and *On Specialization in Nursing: Toward a New Empowerment.*[24]

The purpose of this chapter is to clarify the status and functions of nursing certification. A rationale is presented for the view that certification for specialty nursing practice best serves the interests of the public and the profession when it is conducted by the profession. The rationale is based on the concept of a profession, the norms for autonomy and accountability of a profession, and the expectation that professions serve the best interests of their clients. Goals of certification for the profession and the public are discussed. The current status of certification in nursing is described, and the advantages and disadvantages of each of the dominant models for meeting the goals are weighed.

SELF-REGULATION OF THE PROFESSION

Professions evolve in society because their knowledge and services function to meet societal needs.[16] Autonomy is given to professionals so that important work will be done effectively by experts who are competent judges of the needed expertise.[17] It is because of specialized knowledge that professionals are judged competent to define the standards used to assure safe and effective practice. However, society demands accountability of a profession to assure that the profession and its members use authority in the client's best interest. In 1980, ANA outlined in *Nursing: A Social Policy Statement* the specific mechanisms of the nursing profession's "social contract" with society whereby nursing's responsibility for self-regulation is met and the authority for nursing practice is gained. There are a number of ways that professions demonstrate accountability. The definitions of standards for entry into the profession, codes of ethical conduct, standards for practice, and standards for research to define and expand the knowledge base of the profession are some of these mechanisms. Professional peers collectively establish standards for safe and effective practice and use them to evaluate the qualifications and practice of members to hold them accountable.[16]

Accountability for the knowledge possessed and used by members to deliver quality services to clients is a critical obligation of a profession. Changes in the society, in technology, in the values and demands of consumers, and in the growth of knowledge require that the profession develop systems to assure that appropriate knowledge is held by members to deliver specific services. With rapid social change, the threat of obsolescence increases. Universal competence by members of a profession is not possible. To an increasing degree, the knowledge base of professions is highly complex and specialized. The professional's commitment is to a lifetime of learning.[18]

Certification by a professional organization is the model that has been used most commonly to inform the public of the truth of claims to the possession of knowledge for specialized practice. Certification by the professional organization is the process used by the medical profession and most health professions. A number of sociopolitical, economic, educational, and health care trends have influenced the development of certification for specialty nursing practice in such a way that there is little consensus about which model of certification best serves the profession's and public's interests.[20,24] However, there appears to be agreement about the goals that a certification model should strive to meet.

GOALS OF NURSING CERTIFICATION

The appropriate model for certification to practice a nursing specialty must be based on the assumption that both the status of the nurse specialist and the public will be enhanced.[23] More specifically, the goals of a model for certification are to enhance (1) consumer access to quality health care, (2) consumer and provider protection, and (3) consumer and provider benefit over cost.

Consumer access to quality health care

Certification of nursing specialists offers an alternative to consumers for quality health care. Specialization in maternal-child care, gerontology, primary health care, and other areas of nursing is the result of societal pressures for an expanded nurse role in health care and of advances in health care technology and knowledge. To assure that consumers have access to this alternative for health care, a stable, standardized, and credible system for nursing certification must be established. The system should define the appropriate specialty areas of nursing practice, determine the number of specialties, and define the standards and educational qualifications for each area of practice. The system also should provide for orderly translation of new nursing knowledge into the practice of qualified specialists and clearly communicate these credentials to consumers.

Consumer and provider protection

The public needs to be protected from the possible effects of nurses' self-interests and from the vested interests of other organizations and groups. Restriction of qualified individuals from specialty practice, standard setting by persons who lack nursing expertise, and nonuniversally applied standards are some of the possible adverse effects on consumers. Nursing certification procedures should include mechanisms for public input within a structure that can respond quickly to rapid changes in healthcare knowledge, technology, and values. Conversely, nurses need to be assured that they will have autonomy and legal sanction to practice their specialties.

Consumer and provider benefit over cost

There are a number of economic concerns about the appropriate model for nursing certification. The system for certification should minimize costs to both the consumer and provider while maximizing benefits. To minimize costs, overlapping certification processes, limited geographic mobility of practitioners, and inflexible certification processes should be avoided.

CURRENT SITUATION

A description of the current situation for each of the dominant models and a discussion of the advantages and disadvantages of each model for attaining the desired goals will clarify the direction of certification for specialty practice.

Certification by professional organizations

Certification in nursing by professional organizations was begun in 1945 by the American Association of

Table 46-1 Certification programs for nurses

Specialty	Certification Board	Designation
Addictions Nursing	National League for Nursing	CARN
Critical Care Nursing	AACN Certification Corporation	CCRN
Diabetes Educators	National Certification Board for Diabetes Educators*†	CDE
Emergency Nursing	Board of Certification for Emergency Nursing	CEN
Enterostomol Therapy	Enterostomal Therapy Nursing Certification Board	GETN
Gastroenterology	Certifying Council for Gastroenterology Clinicians	CGC
Infection Control	Certification Board for Infection Control*	CIC
Intravenous Nursing	INS Certification Corporation	CRNI
Lactation Consultant	International Board of Lactation Consultant Examiners*	IBCLC
Nephrology Nursing	Board of Nephrology Examiners Nursing and Technology	
Hemodialysis		CHN
Peritoneal Dialysis		CPDN
Neuroscience Nursing	American Board of Neuroscience Nursing	CNRN
Nurse Anesthetists	Council on Certification of Nurse Anesthetists	CRNA
Nurse Midwifery	American College of Nurse-Midwives	CNM
Nursing Administration	Center for Credentialing	C
Long Term Care	Services NADONA/LTC	
Nutritional Support Nurse	National Board of Nutrition Support Certification*	CNSN
Occupational Health Nursing	National Board for Occupational Health Nurses	COHN
Oncology Nursing	Oncology Nursing Certification Corporation	OCN
Ophthalmic Nursing	National Certifying Board for Ophthalmic Registered Nurses	CRNO
Orthopedic Nursing	Orthopedic Nurses Certification Board	ONC
Pain Management	American Academy of Pain Management*	Diplomate, Fellow, or Clinical Associate
Perioperative Nursing	National Certification Board of Perioperative Nursing	CNOR
Plastic and Recontructive Surgical Nursing	Plastic Surgical Nursing Certification Board	CPSN
Post-Anesthesia Nursing	American Board of Post-Anesthesia Nursing Certification	CPAN
Rehabilitation Nursing	Association of Rehabilitation Nurses Certification Board	CRRN
School Nursing	National Board for Certification School Nurses	CSN
Urology Nursing	American Board of Urologic Allied Health Professionals	CURN

Continued

Nurse Anesthetists. The explosion of knowledge and technology during the past two decades have been accompanied by a proliferation of specialty organizations, many of whom offer certification. The purpose of certification by professional organizations is (1) protection of the public and (2) recognition of the expert practitioners. Table 46-1 lists the majority of the professional organizations that conduct certification programs for registered nurses. The two major eligibility requirements are experience and education. The educational requirement varies from a short-term continuing education program to a formal academic program granting a master's degree. The dominant process of certification is for a finite period of time, and a renewal process is designated. Renewal requirements include work experience and continuing education requirements. Each organization awards a specific title of certification, designated by the initials indicated in Table 46-1. The nurse adds the initials to her name and RN designation.

The American Nurses Credentialing Center (ANCC) assumed responsibility for the ANA certification programs in 1989. It is the national program that leads organized nursing in both the number and scope of certification examinations. Of the 225,000 nurses certified in the United States, more than 100,000 are certified through ANCC.[3,8] The ANCC programs are grouped into the four areas indicated in Table 46-1. The largest proportion of certificates are awarded in the nurse generalist program. The five nurse specialist programs, advanced nursing administration program, as well as the nurse practitioner programs, require a master's degree. The other programs will require the BSN by 1998.[5]

Table 46-1 — cont'd Certification programs for nurses

Specialty	Certification Board	Designation
Pediatric Nursing	National Board of Pediatric Nurse Practitioners and Associates	
General Pediatric Nursing		CPN
Pediatric Nurse Practitioner		CPNP
Maternal/Child Nursing	NAACOG Certification Corporation	
OB/GYN Nurse Practitioner		C
Inpatient Obstetric Nurse		C
Neonatal Intensive Care Nurse		C
Neonatal Nurse Clinician/Practitioner		C
Low-Risk Neonatal Nurse		C
Reproductive Endocrinology/ Infertility Nurse		C
American Nurses Association	American Nurses Credentialing Center	
A. Nurse Generalist		
General Nursing Practice		C
Perinatal Nurse		C
Pediatric Nurse		C
School Nurse		C
Medical-Surgical Nurse		C
Continuing Education/Staff Development Nurse		C
Gerontological Nurse		C
Psychiatric and Mental Health Nurse		C
College Health Nurse		C
Community Health Nurse		C
B. Nurse Practitioner		
Family Nurse Practitioner†		CS
Adult Nurse Practitioner†		CS
Pediatric Nurse Practitioner†		CS
School Nurse Practitioner†		CS
Gerontological Nurse Practitioner†		CS
C. Nurse Specialist		
CNS in Community Health Nursing†		CS
CNS in Gerontological Nursing†		CS
CNS in Medical-Surgical Nursing†		CS
CNS in Adult Psychiatric & Mental Health Nursing†		CS
CNS in Child & Adolescent & Mental Health Nursing		CS
D. Nurse Administrator		
Nursing Administration		CNA
Nursing Administration, Advanced†		CNAA

Table constructed from the following sources: Fickeissen, J. L. (1990). 56 ways to get certified. *American Journal of Nursing, 90*(3), 50-57; and American Nurses Credentialing Center. (1992). *Certification catalog.*
*Interdisciplinary program
†Requires a master's degree

Another sizable program is conducted by the American Association of Critical Care Nurses with more than 31,000 CCRNs. Eligibility requirements include RN licensure and one year of experience in critical care. The Council on Certification of Nurse Anesthetists has certified more than 24,000 nurses. Candidates must have a current RN license and be a graduate of an approved nurse-anesthetist program. Certification for nurse-anesthetists and nurse-midwives is necessary for entry into practice in the specialty. Certification of midwives is conducted by the American College of Nurse-Midwives, which has certified approximately 4,200 specialists.

The professional organization model of certification offers many advantages. It fosters responsibility in demonstrating professional accountability. The model enables the profession to use its expertise to determine universal standards, evaluate those competent to practice a specialty, and communicate an orderly, credible, and standardized system of certification to consumers. The profession is best equipped to identify the appropriate areas of specialization and set the qualification for entry into specialty practice. Furthermore, the professional model is more flexible, as opposed to the governmental model, and can respond to new knowledge and changes in practice without the need to revise statutes or governmental rules. This model is less subject to the influence of powerful vested interest groups, such as those supporting medicine and hospitals. The system of granting credentials is supported by the practitioners and professional organization and thus is less costly to taxpayers and consumers. Because the system is voluntary rather than mandatory for the practitioner, geographic mobility of the practitioner is facilitated.

The disadvantages of the professional organization model include public distrust of professional use of autonomy and accountability. There is increasing concern about the restriction of free trade by professional organizations involved in certification. There is also concern about lack of control of economic return and status because of vested self-interest. Raymond and Ketchum[22] illustrate through a task analysis study that the areas of specialty practice in nursing are not currently defined according to knowledge and skills performed but appear to be designated by the social, economic, and political context within which nursing is practiced. There are multiple routes for entry into specialty practice. Educational requirements vary from RN preparation (ADN, Diploma, or BSN) to master's preparation. Required experience varies from completion of an accredited program to two years of supervised practice. Raymond[21] has determined that there is a positive relationship between amount of education and performance on nursing certification exams.

The current major problem of certification by professional organizations is duplication and lack of coordination of criteria and process. Some specialists, including pediatric nurse-practitioners and maternal-child health nurses, could seek certification from more than one professional organization. It is unlikely that an individual would do this because of eligibility requirements and costs. Fees for professional certification are in the $100 to $300 range. Some of the organizations have reduced fees for members and other organizations open certification to members only. In essence, many individual nurses are forced to choose a professional organization to support. Some nurses, believing that ANA is the one professional organization that represents all nurses, seek certification there. Others find that a specialty organization is more responsive to their continuing education needs and brings them together with other health professionals who have similar interests and concerns. Another cadre of nurses takes the "why bother at all" position in view of the current certification situation. A 1979 survey by Edari[11] of certified nurses revealed that little employer support was given for seeking certification and that few nurses received salary increases, job security, or promotion after achieving certification. In 1987, Collins[9] reported that for the most part employers still do not recognize certification, although some hospitals demand certification of nurses in critical care or emergency care so that the institution can be accredited as a trauma center.

Styles[24] is convinced that specialty development and credentialing is an important frontier for the advancement of the profession. The National Federation of Specialty Nursing Organizations and the National Organization Liaison Forum are two organizations that represent nursing specialty groups. A new group, the Committee for the National Board for Nursing Specialties, was convened in 1988. Proposed functions include the establishment of standards for certifications and the promotion of certification to consumers.[6]

Certification by the state

State certification for nursing specialty groups appeared around 1975. Nurse-midwives and nurse anesthetists, as well as other nurse practitioners, began seeking legal endorsement for specialty practice, in addition to the basic license as a registered nurse. These nurses were leading the way with the expanded role of nursing and were encountering opposition to the practice of their specialties. The scope of function for these specialists has been incorporated into a state certification movement that had resulted in legal endorsement for advanced nursing practice in 47 states and territories by 1991.[19] The rules and regulations for state certification are promulgated in each state. La Bar[15] and Styles[24] review these state regulations, noting that they are frequently revised. Several states have mandated that national certification (by professional organization) is required for state certification. In other states, national certification is one option for demonstrating competence in the field. Other options include an education program, a continuing education requirement, or a state examination. The states vary as to whether advanced registered nurse practitioner (ARNP) is mandatory or permissive. In 1992, the National Council of State Boards of Nursing drafted a position paper advocating licensure for advanced nursing practice. The proposal is currently being debated by various audiences.

The trend toward an additional license for specialty practice is not supported by the ANA. ANA's historical position has been that the purpose of state licensure is to protect the health and welfare of the public through legal standards recognized as minimum standards to provide safe and effective nursing practice. Principle 6 in the ANA publication *The Nursing Practice Act: Suggested State Legislation* relates to the question of legal regulation of advanced practice:

The nursing practice act should provide for the legal regulation of nursing without reference to a specialized area of practice. It is the function of the professional associations to establish the scope and desirable qualifications required for each area of practice, and to certify individuals as competent to engage in specific areas of nursing practice above the minimum standards set by law. The law should not provide for identifying clinical specialists in nursing or require certification or other recognition for practice beyond the minimum qualifications established for the legal regulation of nursing.[2]

In summary, ANA's position has been that specialty practice should be recognized through voluntary national mechanisms rather than state statute. This position was reaffirmed by the House of Delegates at the 1992 convention. Two ANA groups, the Task Force to Revise *Nursing: A Social Policy Statement* and the Ad-Hoc Committee on Credentialing in Advance Practice, are collecting information on issues surrounding the definition and regulation of advanced practice.[4]

The advantages of the state model are public recognition of specialty practice and public sanction of those who are certified. There is control of those who identify themselves as qualified to perform specialist activities. Consumers and practitioners tend to recognize certification by a governmental body as indicating superior position and as providing tighter controls on performance. Nurse practitioners see state certification as a way to gain legal sanction for the expansion of their scope of practice, especially in areas of diagnosis and prescription writing. The advantages of obtaining additional legal recognition are related to several areas of concern: (1) establishing requirements that only persons holding such additional recognition be allowed to practice in the given area; (2) reimbursement by third-party payers; and (3) the availability and cost of malpractice insurance.[26]

State certification for specialty practice presents several disadvantages. The intent to give nurse/practitioners legal authority to practice in what has traditionally been medical diagnosis, treatment, and prescription writing can end in limitations to nursing practice, if legal regulations that are promulgated give the physician authority over that practice.[14] The policy of mandating or recognizing certification is, in effect, surrender of the state's authority for establishing standards for protecting the health and welfare of the public to a professional organization. When that professional organization restricts its certification mechanism only to members, the state is in effect requiring membership in a specific organization in order to practice a profession.[26]

The rules and regulations regarding specialty practice are difficult to amend and are subject to powerful lobbies. Employers often resist new licensure attempts. A state agency, typically the board of nursing, must regulate the certification process, and traditionally these agencies have had few economic resources. Overseeing of individual practice typically does not occur unless a complaint is filed. Finally, there is a great deal of diversity among states in the naming of specialties and the qualifications for specialty practice.

Certification by institutions

Many nurses have been awarded certificates to practice a specialty by institutions after the successful completion of advanced educational programs. Nurses enroll in specialty programs sponsored by schools of nursing, medicine, or health science colleges and universities, independent commercial groups, and hospitals. These programs focus on specific content defined according to the needs and structure of the age groups (e.g., child, adult, elderly), diseases (e.g., cardiac, renal, pulmonary), or special skills (e.g., midwifery, anesthesia, critical care).[13] The programs vary in length from a few weeks to two years, and there is little state or professional control over methods and content.

The nurse practitioner movement was launched in the 1970s largely through certificate programs and the support of the Division of Nursing, Department of Health, Education, and Welfare. A three-part series of articles in *Nursing Outlook* in 1983 traced the evolution of this movement. The distinguishing criterion for inclusion in the survey as a nurse practitioner program was because the program prepared nurses for expanded roles in the provision of primary care. In 1973, there were 86 certificate programs and 45 master's programs preparing nurse practitioners; by 1977, there were 117 certificate and 61 master's programs; in 1980, there were 83 certificate programs and 112 master's programs. Thus, during the 1970s, certificate programs were the predominant type of education preparation for nurse practitioners. However, by 1980, the number of master's programs exceeded the number of certificate programs. During the decade the total estimated number of graduates from certificate programs was 12,568, and the estimated number of graduates from the master's programs was 5,586. By 1981, however, the number of graduates from the two types of programs was almost equal.[25] Thus, the trend in nurse practitioner education is toward master's preparation and away from certificate preparation.

Hospitals have become increasingly concerned about the specialty knowledge and skill performance of their nurses. This concern is greatest in complex tertiary care centers where each new specialty unit and each new piece of equipment require additional technological skills in monitoring and intervention. Orientation and continuing education needs in these situations have taken the form of competency-based testing. In essence, the institution is certifying that a nurse is competent to perform certain activities. The standards for this type of certification are unique to each institution although the Joint Commission for Accreditation of Healthcare Organizations (JCAHO) reviews these activities during an accreditation visit.

The advantages of the institutional model of nursing certification arise primarily from the solutions of immediate problems. Nurses who practice in specific organizations or who attend a practitioner program in an educational institution find institutional certification convenient in the short term. Likewise, health care organizations are assured of a supply of nurse specialists to provide needed services. Consumers tend to view academic and health care agencies as organizations that have the expertise and resources required to prepare nursing specialists and to provide surveillance over their practice.

The wide variability in standards among these certification programs is a major disadvantage of the institutional model. Programs appear to be shaped by local needs and resources and are fragmented. Furthermore, institutional certification programs are vulnerable to the competing vested interests of powerful lobbies. Nonuniversally applied standards, the lack of control by professionals with the needed expertise, and lack of interorganizational and interstate practitioner mobility promote satisfaction with lower standards. Clearly, these are weak controls to assure accountability. Self-regulation and colleague control by professionals are inhibited, and governmental regulation is diluted, if not absent altogether. In addition to these disadvantages, the cost-benefit ratio for the institutional model of certification is questionable. The duplication of expensive structures and processes places stress on institutional costs that are already burdensome. Another cost that is often overlooked is the increased liability of institutions for litigations brought by former students who have not been certified for specialty practice by the professional organization. These costs are likely to be passed on to the consumer. Finally, the institutional model is further weakened by the generally accepted belief that education that does not lead to a recognized academic degree lacks credibility and status among consumers and professionals because it may not meet universally recognized standards.

VIEWPOINT

The advantages and disadvantages of the three models of certification for specialty nursing practice are summarized in Table 46-2 according to the desired goals of certification. The preference for a specific model is a matter of judgment. We believe that the advantages associated with the professional organization model hold high value for both the public and the profession, and thus we prefer this model. Attainment of the desired goals of certification is enhanced through professional expertise, development of a standardized system, and geographic mobility of practitioners. The profession is aware of the major problem with this model— the duplication of service and lack of standardization—and is working to correct the situation. We believe that it is essential for the profession to assume responsibility for self-regulation of specialized nursing practice.

The advantage of public recognition of specialty practice associated with the state model holds high value for many nurses. We believe that this is a time-limited advantage that has great potential for creating

Table 46-2 Advantages and disadvantages of models according to goals of certification

	Professional		State		Institution	
Goals/Model	Advantages	Disadvantages	Advantages	Disadvantages	Advantages	Disadvantages
Access to health care	possess needed expertise to define standards standardized specialty areas standardized qualifications national standards established	potential restriction of trade to those qualified	public recognition and sanction	nonstandardized specialty areas nonstandardized qualifications restrict development of new methods, skills	public views/academic health care institutions as experts supply of specialists	public disenchantment with academe fragmented, confusion to public nonstandardized specialty areas nonstandardized qualifications
Consumer and provider protection	combat vested interests of powerful competing groups universal standards responsive to new knowledge/values	potentially self-serving public distrust of professional autonomy	legal control	restricts title—not practice discipline not communicated to other states nonuniversally applied standards difficult to amend subject to powerful lobbies lack expertise dependent on professional organizations need for repeated costly update cost of maintaining boards lack of practitioner mobility	surveillance of practitioners	may make do with lower standards subject to competing vested interests fewer controls nonuniversally applied standards inhibits professional self-regulation
Consumer and provider benefit over cost	interstate and interagency mobile practitioners self-supported by practitioners voluntary rather than mandatory	current duplication of certification by organizations			convenient for practitioner	redundant costs of system passed on to consumer lack of practitioner mobility

problems for both the public and the practitioner. It is forcing edification of rules and regulations for specialized practice that are likely to be outdated in a few years. Each time the rules are updated, the specialty will be subject to the influence of vested interest groups that have traditionally tried to control nursing practice. Even the names of areas of specialization are likely to change as nursing theory develops. What is a prudent direction for the future now that a majority of states have adopted this model? We believe that it would be best to proceed with all due speed to implement the ANA entry-into-practice recommendations and then move to incorporate the expanded role of the nurse into the state practice acts, eliminating the need for state certification. It should also be recognized that state certification is dependent upon certification by the professional organization for establishing competence in the field. It is time for nurses to end the division of loyalties for these two models and unite in developing a certification system that will both enhance the public's access to specialized nursing care and recognize the practitioner.

The usefulness of the third model, institutional certification, also appears to be time limited. The educational trend for specialty practice is clearly toward the master's degree program. This is in keeping with the definition of specialization in the ANA's *Nursing: A Social Policy Statement*. This document establishes two criteria for the specialist: (1) a master's degree, and (2) certification by the professional organization. We lend our support to this definition in the belief that this direction is in the best interest of both the public and the profession.

REFERENCES

1. American Nurses Association. (1979). *The study of credentialing in nursing: A new approach.* (Vol. 7). Kansas City, Mo: Author.
2. American Nurses Association. (1981). *The nursing practice act: Suggested state legislation.* Kansas City, Mo: Author.
3. American Nurses Credentialing Center. (1992). *Certification catalog.*
4. ANA meets with NCSBN on advanced practice. (1992, September). *The American Nurse,* 25.
5. ANCC approves new certification in home health. (1992, September). *The American Nurse,* 20.
6. Beecroft, P. C., & Papenhausen, J. L. (1989). Certification for specialty practice? *Clinical Nurse Specialist, 3*(4), 161-63.
7. Bullough, B. (1982). State certification of the nursing specialties: A new trend in nursing practice law. *Pediatric Nursing, 8*(3), 121.
8. Certification helps RNs achieve their goal. (1991, February). *The American Nurse,* 28-29.
9. Collins, H. L. (1987, July). Certification: Is the payoff worth the price? *RN,* 36-44.
10. Dunkley, P. H. (1974). The ANA certification program. *Nursing Clinics of North America, 9*(3), 485.
11. Edari, R. S. (1979). A profile of the certified nurse. In *The study of credentialing in nursing: A new approach* (Vol. 2). Kansas City, Mo: American Nurses Association.
12. Fickeissen, J. L. (1990). 56 ways to get certified. *American Journal of Nursing, 90*(3), 50-57.
13. Hinsvark, I. G. (1979). Educational preparation for the changed role of the nurse. In *The study of credentialing in nursing: A new approach* (Vol. 2). Kansas City, Mo: American Nurses Association.
14. Kelly, L. S. (1982). Licensure laws in transition. *Nursing Outlook, 30*(6), 375.
15. LaBar, C. (1983). *The regulation of advanced nursing practice as provided for in nursing practice acts and administrative rules.* Kansas City, Mo: American Nurses Association.
16. Maas, M., & Jacox, A. (1977). *Guidelines for nurse autonomy/patient welfare.* New York: Appleton-Century-Croft.
17. Merton, R. (1960). The search for professional status. *American Journal of Nursing, 60*(662).
18. Moore, W. E. (1970). *The professional: Roles and rules.* New York: Russell Sage Foundation.
19. National Council of State Boards of Nursing. (1992). Position paper (working draft) on the licensure of advanced nursing practice.
20. Passarelli, A. (1979). Credentialing in nursing: Background issues. In *The study of credentialing in nursing: A new approach,* (Vol. 2). Kansas City, Mo: American Nurses Association.
21. Raymond, M. R. (1988). The relationship between educational preparation and performance on nursing certification examinations. *Journal of Nursing Education, 27*(1), 6.
22. Raymond, M. R., & Ketchum, E. L. (1988, April). *Certification of nursing.* Paper presented at the annual meeting of the American Educational Research Association, New Orleans.
23. Sammons, L. N. (1983). Control of credentialing for advanced practice analysis using a Lewinian model. *Advanced Nurse Science, 5*(4), 13.
24. Styles, M. M. (1989). *On specialization in nursing: Toward a new empowerment.* Kansas City, Mo: American Nurses Foundation.
25. Sultz, H. A., Henry, O. M., & Kinyon, L. J. (1983). A decade of change for nurse practitioners. *Nursing Outlook, 31* (Parts 1-3), 137-142, 216-219, 266-269.
26. Waddle, F. (1979). Licensure: Achievements and limitations. In *The study of credentialing in nursing: A new approach* (Vol. 2). Kansas City, Mo: American Nurses Association.

CHAPTER 47

Validating clinical competence

Old and new approaches

CAROLYN J. YOCOM

Concern about and recognition of a nurse's level of clinical competence is not of recent origin within the history of nursing in the United States. Initially, in the late 1800s, hospital schools of nursing established registries to assist the public in identifying individuals who had completed a specific nursing education program. However, because educational standards varied greatly, the public continued to experience great difficulty distinguishing between safe and unsafe practitioners.[20] Subsequently, the efforts of early nursing leaders, including Isabel Hampton Robb, Sophia Palmer, and Lavinia Dock, were instrumental to the introduction and passage of legislation establishing state boards of nursing.[8,18] The first boards were established in 1903 in New York, New Jersey, North Carolina, and Virginia.[8,15,18] A primary function of the boards was (and continues to be) to protect the public from unsafe practitioners through the establishment of standards for nursing education programs and maintenance of a registry of nurses who met specified criteria, including graduation from a state-approved school of nursing and passage of a state-recognized examination.[8,18,20]

A nurse's ability to provide competent care to clients continues to be of great importance in today's health care environment. The professional nurse has major accountability for the delivery of safe and effective care to clients in a wide variety of health care settings. Given the increasing acuity levels of clients' health problems within a complex and highly technical health care system, it is crucial to the maintenance of the public's health, safety, and welfare that appropriate mechanisms are available to assess, or measure, the clinical competence of licensed professional nurses and candidates for licensure.

PURPOSE

The purposes of this chapter are to describe approaches currently used to determine a nurse's level of clinical competence and to describe a new, emerging approach that may enhance our ability to accurately assess this trait.

The measurement approaches described are applicable to the assessment of clinical competence of candidates for nurse licensure and those already licensed to practice. They are also applicable to all levels of practice, from the entry-level, professional nurse who is, at the least, minimally competent, to the experienced nurse who is licensed and/or certified as an advanced practitioner. Therefore, intertwined throughout the discussion are references to the assessment of individuals to determine if they are minimally competent to provide safe and effective nursing care, which is the focus of boards of nursing, and the assessment of individuals to determine if they possess characteristics indicative of having reached a higher level of expertise, as exemplified by the certification process.

DEFINITION OF CLINICAL COMPETENCE

As with the measurement of any abstract concept, an identification of its attributes is critical. A competency can be described as a single, observable or definable skill that can be further classified as consisting of knowledge, skills, aptitudes, attitudes, and intellectual strategies, such as problem solving and the ability to deal with ambiguity.[5] Furthermore, a definition of pro-

---

The opinions expressed herein are those of the author and are not those of the National Council of State Boards of Nursing.

fessional competence, introduced by Kane[10] and based on the work of LaDuca, Engel, Risley,[11] Benner,[2] and McGaghie[12] is also relevant. Kane defines an individual's level of competence in an area of practice as ". . . the degree to which the individual can use the knowledge, skills, and judgment associated with the profession to perform effectively in the domain of possible encounters defining the scope of professional practice."

The key phrase in this definition is, "use the knowledge, skills, and judgment associated with the profession to perform effectively. . . ." An individual can possess specific knowledge and/or be able to demonstrate the ability to perform certain psychomotor, communication, or other skills pertinent to a specific domain. However, for an individual's practice to typify that of a clinically competent practitioner, the exercise of appropriate levels of clinical judgment and decision-making skills that incorporate the use and application of knowledge and skills to meet a client's specific needs must be demonstrated.

It is also important to recognize that demonstration of competence within a profession is not, and should not be, a one-time-only endeavor but, rather, an ongoing process. In 1985, the National Council of State Boards of Nursing's position paper on continued competence stated, "Continued competence is the ability to continue to demonstrate competence throughout one's career. In nursing, it encompasses the ongoing ability to render direct nursing care or the ongoing ability to make sound judgments upon which nursing care is based."[15]

MEASUREMENT CONCEPTS

A naive approach used to judge whether or not an individual or object possesses a specific attribute is to fall back on the old adage, "I know one (it) when I see it." This approach is commonly used when shopping for art work or antiques (Is it a "good" piece?). It could also be applied to informal evaluations of members of the nursing profession (Is he or she a competent nurse?). In either case, arriving at a conclusion is based on a personal, internal set of criteria generated and used as a basis for comparing the characteristics of the object or person to be evaluated.

In situations exemplified by the above examples, the reasonableness of the criteria and the generalizability of the evaluation outcomes can be open to question because of the degree of abstractness of the concept being measured, the individual preferences of the evaluator, and the consistency in which the criteria are applied. It is therefore obvious that a more formal, standardized approach is required to obtain consistent, valid judgments about the presence of a trait such as clinical competence.

Within nursing, the development of standardized measurement tools to assess the knowledge, skills, and abilities of professional nurses are exemplified by both licensure and certification examinations. In both cases, empirically grounded indicators (e.g., an examinee's responses to a series of test questions) are compared to predetermined criteria indicative of the desired trait (e.g., clinical competence). The psychometric soundness of the measurement device (e.g., paper-and-pencil or performance examinations) must be supported by evidence of two desirable qualities: reliability and validity.

Reliability concerns the extent to which a measuring procedure yields the same results on repeated trials; there is consistency across repeated measurements.[6] In evaluating the suitability of an examination, its validity is of primary concern. "*Validity* refers to the appropriateness, meaningfulness, and usefulness of the specific inferences made from test scores. Test validation is the process of accumulating evidence to support such inferences."[1]

As Kane[10] points out, "[t]he validity of an assessment of professional competence depends on the evidence supporting inferences from an examinee's score to conclusions about the examinee's expected performance over the domain of encounters defining the area of practice." Three primary inferences are inherent in this process: (1) determining the quality of the examinee's performance—*evaluation*; (2) drawing conclusion about general behavior from the observed behavior—*generalization*; and (3) drawing conclusions about performance in the "real world" from results on the type of assessment performed—*extrapolation*.[10]

CURRENT MEASUREMENT APPROACHES

Methods used to assess the degree of clinical competence possessed by a professional nurse can be grouped within two different types of approaches: performance testing and objective testing.

Performance testing

Examples of performance testing include the use of skill inventories (checklists), peer evaluations, and chart/record audits. Following a brief description of each approach, their advantages and disadvantages will be discussed.

Skill inventories are commonly used in basic nursing education programs and in specialty courses/programs (e.g., nurse-midwifery) to determine whether or not the examinee can demonstrate acceptable levels of performance while interacting with real clients. However, they are not used in professional licensure and certification tests in the United States because of the amount of personnel and fiscal resources necessary to perform performance evaluations on large numbers of examinees.

Peer evaluations of practicing nurses are used in some jurisdictions (states) to validate the continued competence of advanced practitioners. This involves observation of the targeted nurse by a recognized "expert" colleague during the course of regular work assignments and the use of rating forms and/or checklists. This approach also requires extensive personnel and fiscal resources if it is to be used in a large-scale testing/evaluation program.

A chart/record audit entails a systematic review of clients' charts for the purpose of documenting a nurse's accuracy and the thoroughness of client assessments and management. It also is used, on a limited basis, to validate the continued competence of advanced practitioners. A common concern raised in relation to the use of this approach involves claims that a client's written record does not include complete documentation of the processes used by the practitioner and/or all of the activities in which nurses engaged.

Evaluation of the performance of a specific skill (checklist/inventory) and/or a sample of activities commonly used in client interactions (peer evaluations) have a major advantage over objective testing formats because they involve the use of "real" versus contrived or simulated situations. The examinee's ability to provide competent care can be directly observed and evaluated. To a lessor extent, the same also can be said for chart/record audits.

As mentioned above, these approaches currently have limited use in large-scale testing situations because of the need for an extensive number of trained raters and the availability of sufficient fiscal resources to carry out the evaluations in a timely manner. In addition, several other disadvantages of these approaches contribute to their nonuse.[10,19] Because of the use of real clients and a lack of examiner control over (1) client health problems being manifested and (2) the testing environment, standardization of the testing situation across examinees is difficult, at best. In addition, the probability of measurement errors occurring is high and contributes to an unacceptable level of reliability in reported scores. This is related to a lack of specificity in evaluation criteria, which is necessary because of the potential for wide variations in client conditions, the use of multiple raters, and therefore, the potential for interrater reliability problems.

Objective testing

An objective test is usually composed of multiple-choice questions (MCQ) but may also contain true-false, and/or matching type questions. Standardized MCQ examinations are commonly used in high-volume licensure and certification testing because of their relative ease of construction and administration, the use of objective scoring mechanisms, and, through the use of optical mark scanners, short turnaround times for score reporting. The test items on these examinations are developed by content experts who have received instruction in item construction and are recognized by peers as "expert" item writers. Items are developed according to specifications that include the following parameters: specific knowledge, skill, or ability to be measured; degree of difficulty; and level of competency expected (e.g., entry level, expert, etc.). Content validation of newly constructed items can be strengthened through documentation of the correct response in reference materials commonly available to prospective examinees, review by a second panel of experts, and pre-testing of the item.

The *Standards of Educational and Psychological Testing*[1] identifies specific standards for the compilation of a valid examination from available test items. Included is a standard stating that the content domain to be covered is defined clearly and explained in terms of the importance of the content for competent performance in an occupation (Standard 11.1).

Adherence to the *Standards* during the process of examination development results in a valid and reliable evaluation of clinical competence to the extent that one believes that an objective-type test question (e.g., MCQ, true-false, etc.) can test the knowledge, skills, and abilities inherent in the domain of nursing practice. A carefully constructed MCQ-based examination can evaluate knowledge and the ability to analyze and synthesize selected clinical and theoretical facts, or, for example, knowledge of the procedural steps involved in the performance of psychomotor skills. However, it is difficult to make a strong argument that such an examination can effectively measure competence in the areas of clinical decision making and clinical judgment.[16] This is partly due to the level of artificiality imposed by a written test and partly due to the "cuing" effect of item response options. (When was the last time you walked into a client's room and found four options for dealing with the client's problem painted on the wall behind the bed?)

Alternatives to the use of an MCQ examination for the purpose of evaluating clinical decision making and judgment have been explored in both nursing and medicine during the past two decades. One such alternative, the use of paper-and-pencil-based simulations as an examination technique, was pioneered by McQuire and her associates at the University of Illinois.[13] This approach, referred to as a Patient Management Problem (PMP), is characterized by the use of a latent image, branched simulation of a clinical situation in which the examinee is presented with a brief client situation. Patient management skills are demonstrated by making judgments about what types of data to obtain and what nursing actions to undertake. Options for data collection and nursing actions are included in long lists of possibilities. Upon selection of the desired option(s), pertinent client information is revealed by revealing the latent, printed material associated with each option. Progression through the PMP is dependent upon examinee choices.

Within nursing, Holzemer and his colleagues developed and evaluated a series of PMPs designed to evaluate the performance of graduate students in a nurse practitioner program.[7,9,17] Subsequently, these investigators and others (e.g., Noricini et al.[16]) reported continuing concerns regarding the validity of using PMPs for measuring competence in clinical decision making and judgment. Among these were the artificiality imposed by the written format and the linear pathway imposed on the examinee. One further disadvantage of the PMP was the cuing effect imposed by the use of long lists of response options.[21] Therefore, some of the same problems identified with the use of MCQ examinations were not eliminated by PMPs.

FUTURE MEASUREMENT APPROACHES

The advent of major advances in computer technology, including interactive videodisk enhancements, has been instrumental in facilitating exploration of an alternative approach to the evaluation of clinical compe-

tence. The use of computer and interactive videodisk technology opens new horizons in attempts to overcome the disadvantages associated with the use of paper-and-pencil based MCQ examinations and PMPs.

In 1988, the National Council of State Boards of Nursing was the recipient of a major grant from the W. K. Kellogg Foundation for a study to explore the feasibility of developing computerized clinical simulation testing (CST) for evaluating clinical decision-making skills/competencies of entry-level nurses.[3,4,22] The project, conducted in collaboration with the National Board of Medical Examiners (NBME), was designed to address the following areas: (1) adapt technology and software developed by the NBME for the delivery of computer-based clinical simulations for initial nurse licensure; (2) initiate development of 20 computerized simulations in nursing; and (3) examine the validity and reliability of computerized clinical simulation tests as a basis for making nursing licensure decisions.

Computerized clinical simulation testing permits examinees to realistically simulate the problem-solving and decision-making skills used in the management of client needs. In CST, each case begins with a brief description of a client situation, presented on an introductory screen, along with the client's location, the day of care, and the time. The examinee is then free to collect client data through assessment activities and review of client records, and to specify nursing interventions through free keyboard entry. At any point in the case, the examinee may advance the clock in simulated time to evaluate the client at a later point in time and/or to specify further interventions. Originally, the client assessment function consisted of a list of 22 options from which any or all could be selected. This approach is currently being converted to free keyboard entry format to eliminate cuing. No intervention questions or answer options are presented to the examinee.

The simulations are dynamic in that the client's condition changes over time and in response to nursing actions. This permits examinees to evaluate the effectiveness of nursing actions and to provide followup care. In response to a request for assessment data (e.g., vital signs), these are reported in a manner and time frame consistent with current practice. The specification of a nursing intervention (e.g., administer Demerol) results in the provision of a printed message reporting that the medication has been given. To evaluate the client's response to the medication, the examinee must (1) move the simulated "clock" ahead to the desired time and (2) assess the client's comfort level.

As an examinee proceeds through the case, a permanent record of his or her actions is recorded. This is then compared to the case's scoring key by a computer program. The case scoring keys, developed by a committee of expert nurses, specify performance criteria with items defined as benefits (is an appropriate action), neutrals (no positive or negative client impact), or as inappropriates, risks, and flags (cause harm to the client). A feature of the CST scoring system enables the application of procedures which can award credit for different but equally valid nursing actions. It can also award different amounts of credit depending on the timing, sequencing, and level of correctness of nursing actions.

During the course of the project, 27 nursing simulation cases were developed. Of these, 25 were programmed and had scoring keys developed. In addition, audiovisual augmentation, via videodisk, was developed for two cases. A 2500 plus term default nursing intervention database was developed to enable CST to function as a unique uncued examination since it is programmed to recognize a full range of nursing activities specified by examinees through free keyboard entry. A comparable assessment database is currently being developed to support the aforementioned change in format.

The results of a pilot study using diploma, associate degree, and baccalaureate degree graduates who were candidates for RN licensure provided preliminary evidence that a valid and reliable CST examination can be constructed to evaluate clinical decision-making competence in nursing. Statistical evidence supported the hypothesis that CST is measuring something different than that measured by multiple-choice questions. While there was no clear documentation of construct validity, examinee comments strongly suggest that they were able to demonstrate use of clinical decision-making skills. The use of videodisk augmentation had no statistically significant effect on overall examinee performance on two cases. However, there were differences in how examinees performed on different items within these cases, depending on whether or not the cases were augmented with videodisk material.

The findings of this study provide a basis for continued research on CST. Primary issues to be addressed include additional investigation of evidence supporting its validity and reliability as a testing mechanism. Future plans also include an investigation of the feasibility of expanding the use of CST beyond the originally conceived view that it could be used as an adjunct to the computerized adaptive testing licensure examination that uses MCQs (CAT-NCLEX). Current thinking is that CST could potentially be used to test both licensed nurses returning to practice after a period of inactivity in the profession and licensed nurses who are currently practicing in order to determine their continued ability to apply nursing knowledge to the complex health care needs of clients.

The use of CST as a diagnostic assessment tool also has great potential value. One such application would involve its use in those jurisdictions where nursing boards mandate licensees meet specific continuing education requirements. A second application would involve the use of CST to evaluate licensees who have had disciplinary action taken against their licenses. In both of these applications, reeducation could be targeted to identified areas of weakness.

SUMMARY

The ability of a nurse to provide competent care to clients is of primary concern to the profession and to members of the regulatory profession. Several approaches currently used to evaluate clinical competence have been described. These include the use of skill inventories, peer evaluations, chart audits, and standardized, objective tests. With respect to their validity, each approach has contrasting strengths and weaknesses in terms of the reliability of the data provided, and the ability to arrive at valid judgments about the quality of an examinee's performance, to draw conclusions about general behavior based on observed behavior, and to draw conclusions about projected performance in the "real" world based on results on the type of assessment performed. The advent of advances in computer technology has opened up a new avenue of exploration in the attempt to identify a testing methodology that can surmount the disadvantages of using currently available performance and objective testing formats. Preliminary results of research exploring the feasibility of using computerized clinical simulation testing (CST) are promising. If strong evidence can be gathered supporting the validity and reliability of CST, it is possible that CST could be used alone or as an adjunct to other testing methodologies to evaluate the clinical decision-making and judgment components of clinical competence.

REFERENCES

1. American Education Research Association, American Psychological Association, & National Council on Measurement in

Education. (1985). *Standards for educational and psychological testing*. Washington, D.C.: American Psychological Association.

2. Benner, P. (1984). *From novice to expert: Excellence and power in clinical nursing practice*. Menlo Park, Calif: Addison-Wesley.

3. Bersky, A. (1991). The measurement characteristics of computerized clinical simulation tests (CST). In M. Garbin (Ed.), *Assessing educational outcomes* (pp. 107-112). New York: National League for Nursing.

4. Bersky, A., & Yocom, C. (1991). *Computerized clinical simulation testing project: Year three report*. Chicago: National Council of State Boards of Nursing.

5. Callahan, L. (1988). Competence models: From theory to practical application. *Journal of the American Association of Nurse Anesthetists, 56,* 387-389.

6. Carmines, E., & Zeller, R. (1979). *Reliability and validity assessment*. Beverly Hills, Calif: Sage Publications.

7. Farrand, L., Holzemer, W., & Schleutermann, J. (1982). A study of construct validity: Simulations as a measure of a nurse practitioner's problem-solving skills. *Nursing Research, 31,* 37-42.

8. Goodnow, M. (1929). *Outlines of nursing history*. Philadelphia: W. B. Saunders.

9. Holzemer, W., Schleutermann, J., Farrand, L., & Miller, A. (1981). A validation study: Simulations as a measure of nurse practitioner's problem-solving skills. *Nursing Research, 30,* 139-144.

10. Kane, M. (1992). The assessment of professional competence. *Evaluation & the Health Professions, 15,* 163-182.

11. LaDuca, A., Engel, J. D., & Risley, M. E. (1978). Progress toward development of a general model for competence definition in health professions. *Journal of Allied Health, 7,* 149-155.

12. McGaghie, W. C. (1991). Professional competence evaluation. *Educational Researcher, 20*(1), 3-9.

13. McGuire, C., Solomon, L., & Bashook, P. (1976). *Construction and use of written simulations*. New York: The Psychological Corporation.

14. National Council of State Boards of Nursing. (1990). *Member board profiles: 1990*. Chicago: Author.

15. National Council of State Boards of Nursing. (1985). *Position paper on continued competence*. Chicago: Author.

16. Noricini, J., Swanson, D., Grosso, L., & Webster, G. (1985). Reliability, validity and efficiency of multiple-choice question and patient management problem item formats in assessment of clinical competence. *Medical Education, 19,* 238-247.

17. Schleuterman, J., Albano, E., Miller, A., Farrand, L., & Holzemer, W. (1979). *Mr. Ellis, a 48 year old man complaining of chest pain and difficulty breathing*. Chicago: University of Illinois at Chicago, Health Sciences Center.

18. Shannon, M. L. (1975). Nurses in American history. Our first four licensure laws. *American Journal of Nursing, 79,* 1327-1329.

19. Swanson, D. (1990). Issues in assessment of practice skills in medicine. *Professions Education Research, 12,* 3-6.

20. Waddle, F. (1979). Licensure achievements and limitations. In *The study of credentialing in nursing: A new approach. Volume II. Staff working papers* (pp. 126–64). Kansas City, Mo: American Nurses Association.

21. Yocom, C. (1985). *Influence of initial nursing educational preparation on patient assessment*. Unpublished doctoral dissertation, University of Illinois at Chicago.

22. Yocom, C., & Bersky, A. (1992). *The relationship of critical thinking ability and NCLEX-RN performance to performance on computerized clinical simulation tests*. Paper presented at the Tenth Anniversary Conference, Council for the Society for Research in Nursing Education, San Francisco, Calif, February 12-14, 1992.

CHAPTER 48

How can the quality of nursing practice be measured?

KAREN MARTIN

The title question is not a new issue. Nurses in practice, education, and research have asked the question repeatedly, especially since 1961 when Freeman wrote, "There is no problem in public health practice today as important, as haunting, and as frustrating as that of measuring the effectiveness of services afforded the public."[9] Freeman also noted the potential for errors when measurement approaches that are too general or specific are selected. A decade later, the dilemma of "Quantifying the Unquantifiable" was described by Lewis in her 1976 *Nursing Outlook* editorial.[16] Wooley wrote about "The Long and Tortured History of Clinical Evaluation" in 1977.[34]

As we approach the twenty-first century, the question about how to measure quality has not been answered. However, the authors of Part Five describe exciting progress and promising research. They clearly identify the increasing demands of regulatory and reimbursement groups and the potential for linking payment to client outcomes or cost effectiveness. These authors are among the nursing leaders who recognize that, as a profession, nurses must develop skills and research-based, valid and reliable instruments to identify, describe, count, and cost their practice and the quality of that practice.

MEASUREMENT BARRIERS

A variety of factors contribute to the difficulties that practitioners and nursing administrators experience as they attempt to measure the effectiveness of nursing practice. One of those factors involves definitions. To measure is to estimate or appraise by a criterion; quality is a degree of excellence applicable to any trait or characteristic whether individual or general.[33] Freeman defined the effectiveness of nursing services as "the relationship between goals and achievement; it is a measure of the degree to which the service accomplishes the job it sets out to do."[9] Quality of care was defined and adopted as part of the highly publicized Institute of Medicine's Medicare study: "Quality of care is the degree to which health services for individuals and populations increase the likelihood of desired health outcomes and are consistent with current professional knowledge."[13] The previous definitions are well written, understandable, and seem specific. Nurses, however, especially those in the practice setting, are likely to have difficulty operationalizing them.

Conceptual issues are closely related to definitions and represent another difficulty for measuring nursing practice. Donabedian[4] constructed a cubical structure to describe the complex nature of quality. Central to the structure are the client's physiological, psychological, and social functions. The structure also depicts the client and the health care provider on a continuum ranging from the individual client and practitioner to the global community and institution. The literature suggests a shift in emphasis from structure and process to outcomes: a shift from assessing nurses' activities to direct assessment of results or client outcomes.[11,12,25] The practicing nurse is again faced with an overwhelming task of translating a global theoretic perspective into a pragmatic action plan.

Issues related to methods are the third barrier to measuring practice. "Measurable variables include behavioral changes that occur following participation in educational programs or an intervention, as well as general responses (how a person reacts or feels) to different problem areas."[21] Some nursing educators and researchers indicate that measurement of the nurse-client relationship should approach the precision of the chemist in the laboratory or the postal quality inspector calculating the time between pickup and delivery of a box. The methods and procedures these nurses offer are often very complex and consume extensive professional and support staff resources. Designs selected for most measurement research involve a small number of outcome variables that have a narrow focus or limited applicability within acute care and community-based settings.

In contrast, other nursing leaders focus on the art and caring of practice and suggest that actual measurement can only be global or is impossible. They emphasize the unique, human aspect of the nurse-client relationship. The results of global outcome research studies offer practitioners conflicting implications that would be difficult to implement. Therefore, both narrow and global approaches have led to diverse research and produced equally diverse methods which may not be relevant for practice settings.[1,2,5,31]

The complex definitional, conceptional, and methodologic issues offer dilemmas to the practicing nurse and agency or institution as they ask how to measure the effectiveness of practice in their setting. The decision to ignore the entire issue and wait until the "experts" have developed a solution is tempting but dangerous. If the profession does not energetically address client outcomes and quality assurance-improvement issues, nonnurses are likely to impose their own regulations. Because nursing is a complex phenomenon and a practice discipline, practitioners not only can contribute extensively to the developing art and science of measurement but also have a vested interest in ensuring that developments are congruent with the realities of practice and the practice setting.

ADAPTING MEASUREMENT TO PRACTICE

Simultaneously, nurses and their agencies or institutions should make a firm commitment to five recommendations. First, they should appreciate nursing's history and commitment to quality issues; other health care professions such as medicine are experiencing comparable struggles and progress.[10,29] Second, they should contribute to agency-institutional models that are practical and valuable. Third, they should acknowledge that the existing models are commendable, but extensive work remains. Fourth, they should become informed about current efforts to increase the science for measuring nursing practice. Fifth, they should collaborate with educators and researchers to advance scientific rigor.

Many home care and public health agencies, hospitals, and nursing homes use appropriate approaches or models for measuring the quality of nursing practice. These models are multifaceted and involve formative or ongoing evaluation. Some are comprehensive. Many combine quantitative and qualitative measurement techniques. Such an eclectic approach for all health care professionals is strongly endorsed in the conclusions of the Institute of Medicine study.[13]

An important goal for service setting providers is to incorporate the developing science of measurement and research into their models. Another goal is to use the approaches consistently, especially since practice settings often report inconsistent application. Measuring the quality of practice must combine aspects of Donabedian's structure, process, and outcome concepts. Such approaches should reflect inherent assumptions, realities, and constraints of the practice setting:

1. Health care providers and clients desire consistent, high-quality service delivery.
2. Multifaceted, formative approaches strengthen the evaluation of clinical practice since no adequate, single method exists.
3. Discrepancies exist between ideal services and available resources.
4. Providers and clients make occasional errors.

MODELS FOR PRACTICE

Interest in outcome measurement models which are useful in practice settings continues to increase.[18] The benefits of traditional and emerging outcomes for measuring the effectiveness of nursing care were outlined recently.[22] The authors identified mortality, morbidity, and length of hospital stay as traditional indicators. They suggested that functional status, mental status, stress level, satisfaction with care, burden of care, and cost of care were significant emerging measures.

Outcomes of care, such as the traditional and emerging measures, have been of great concern to nurses in home care and public health agencies. Examples of recent, significant home care nursing studies and projects incorporated some of these measures and have been published. A two-volume *National League for Nursing* anthology includes a historical review of quality assurance and outcome standards and various home care outcome research studies, and addresses basic issues in evaluating quality.[26,27] Feldman and Richard[7] developed an episode coding form based on the Omaha Problem Classification Scheme to evaluate nursing outcomes in home health agencies. Peters[24] used the Omaha Problem Classification Scheme as the basis for developing a community health intensity rating scale. Jacobs and dela Cruz[14] developed an instrument to measure the clinical judgment of home health care nurses using simulated client care situations. Eustis and Fischer[6] conducted interviews with home care clients, their home health aides, and personal care attendants. They concluded that the quality of relationships affects quality of care. Martin and Scheet[19] described the Visiting Nurse Association (VNA) of Omaha efforts to develop and refine an outcome rating scale to measure clients' problem-specific knowledge, behavior, and status.

Many important public health studies have been conducted. Oda[23] investigated the effects of telephone contacts and home visits in a preventive child health program. Vahldieck, Reeves, and Schmelzer[30] designed a model to help public health nurses throughout Wisconsin estimate the number and types of client services required. During a recent Indian Health Service study,[8] physical and psychosocial status, health knowledge, and functional behavior outcome achievements were analyzed for clients who received prenatal, postpartum, well child, adult immunization, sexually transmitted disease, and diabetic services. In addition, extensive outcome projects are now being conducted at the National League for Nursing (NLN) and the Joint Commission on Accreditation of Healthcare Organizations (JCAHO).

In order for traditional and emerging measures to be useful to practitioners, the measures must address comprehensive practice, documentation, and data management issues. Seven specific approaches will be described in this viewpoint as will examples of application in the service setting. The approaches are based on practice, documentation, and data management experiences at the VNA of Omaha. The extensiveness and precision incorporated in the approaches vary considerably. The approaches are intended to be introductory and, therefore, do not include the details necessary for actual application and measurement. The VNA approaches reflect current realities and constraints; they do not represent the ultimate solution for measuring the quality of nursing practice in all community-based agencies or other practice settings.

The Omaha System is mentioned in many of the seven approaches. The system consists of nursing diagnosis, nursing intervention, and client outcome terminology and codes. The research-based Omaha System is used consistently as the foundation of professional practice, documentation, and data management throughout the VNA's home care and public health programs.[19,20]

The Omaha System was developed and refined during four research projects conducted between 1975 and 1992. The purpose of the research was to increase the effectiveness and efficiency of nursing practice. The Problem Classification Scheme offers the nurse a holistic, standardized method for client assessment and nursing diagnosis/problem identification. The Intervention Scheme provides a framework for documenting plans and interventions in the client record. It is also the basis of the Supervisory Shared Visit Tool, an evaluation instrument used when supervisors accompany staff members on shared visits. The outcome portion of the Omaha System, referred to as the Problem Rating Scale for Outcomes, is used to document client progress in the record and during the case conferences of hospice staff as they evaluate client change. The Problem Rating Scale was constructed as a relatively simple, criterion-referenced instrument to assist the practitioner with the complex task of measuring client progress. Specifically, it comprises three, 5-point, Likert-type subscales that address the client's problem-specific knowledge, behavior, and status.

The VNA measurement approaches are identified in Fig. 48-1. Included are: (1) practice, documentation, and data management orientation; (2) case conferences; (3) shared evaluation visits and observations; (4) practice-based inservice education; (5) record audit, peer review, and utilization review; (6) accreditation and external audit; and (7) client satisfaction surveys. While they include various aspects of traditional and emerging indicators, the approaches emphasize process indicators, client knowledge-behavior-status outcome measures, and satisfaction with care.

Practice, documentation, and data management orientation

The process of providing orientation for new employees is an important cornerstone in the effort to assure and measure the quality of nursing practice. The new employee needs oral and written information about assignments and client caseload, client-nurse relationships, procedures, equipment, productivity, agency and

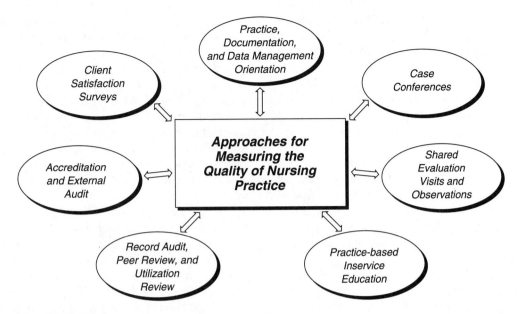

Fig. 48-1 VNA of Omaha measurement approaches.

community resources, and service fees and reimbursement. To meet those needs, employers describe policies and expectations related to practice, documentation, and data management during scheduled sessions. The goal of a competency-based orientation program, such as the VNA's, is to provide essential information that enables the new employee to function effectively, efficiently, and quickly.

Orientees are introduced to the Omaha System while they are learning about the VNA's client record. The system is used throughout the client record and the VNA's quality assurance-improvement program. After the Omaha System is described, new employees view a videotape of a simulated home visit. Working independently, they use the Omaha System to select nursing diagnoses/client problems, nursing interventions, and client outcome ratings depicted in the videotape. Then they discuss their decisions with peers and the presenter to evaluate their diagnostic skills. The speed with which new employees acquire competence applying the Omaha System varies considerably. For many, the idea of documenting outcome measures is a new, and even uncomfortable, experience.

Information about reimbursement is another critical portion of orientation. Community health nurses provide eligibility and cost of service information as they begin visiting newly admitted clients, answer clients' questions throughout the length of service, and assist clients and their families who are confused by the reimbursement process. In addition, nurses must obtain and update physician orders, communicate with third-party providers, and document services appropriately to ensure that services will be reimbursed.

A post-test is administered after the reimbursement orientation to evaluate nurses' knowledge. Developed by the National Association of Home Care, the test includes information frequently misinterpreted when staff members visit clients and complete required forms. As with client record orientation, reinforcement or correction occurs in the groups and/or individually.

Establishing a preceptor program is a recent, important means to increase the quality of practice and documentation and to measure the impact of the VNA orientation process. The VNA goal is to assign each newly employed staff member to one preceptor who has extensive home care experience and demonstrated expertise. Preceptors evaluate clinical, documentation, and communication skills of new employees in comparison to agency standards of competence for a period of several months.

Case conferences

Both new and experienced staff need opportunities to evaluate the clients they are visiting and identify ways to improve their own interventions. Case conferences offer one such method. Conferences can be structured or unstructured, oral or written, brief or long, and involve one staff nurse and supervisor or a multidisciplinary group. Case conferences should be designed to provide positive reinforcement to the direct delivery staff and constructive suggestions for improvement.

The health care professional reviews the client record while preparing for a case conference. The practitioner uses the Omaha System to focus on the client's health-related problems; the client's knowledge, behavior, and status; and the interventions already used. This process alone may help the practitioner gain new ideas about promising interventions and a renewed sense of accomplishment. Publishing case studies in the literature is yet another method for nurses to share expertise and to obtain feedback about the quality of their professional practice.[3,17]

Various methods of conducting case conferences have been used at the VNA. Each method includes inherent advantages and disadvantages. At present, case conferences are most often unstructured, oral, brief, and involve one staff nurse and supervisor. Although these opportunities for communication and problem-solving may not involve formal methods of measuring the quality of nursing practice, they are no less valuable.

Group case conferences are also conducted by the VNA's hospice team. Nurse, social worker, minister, physician, home health aide, pharmacist, and volunteer representatives participate. About every two weeks, case managers describe current data about each client. Other team members contribute the information they have obtained. As part of the conference, the hospice team members review the client's record. They discuss the client's health-related problems, the previous knowledge-behavior-status ratings, and the interventions selected since the last review. The interdisciplinary group discusses the current problem-specific ratings until they reach consensus and record that decision in the client record. They analyze the merits of selected interventions and plan for future interventions. A similar, interdisciplinary approach to case conferences that includes the Omaha System will be used by other groups of home visit staff in the near future.

Shared evaluation visits and observations

Shared staff-supervisory visits and observations offer an important way to measure the quality of nursing practice. Because nursing is a practice discipline, it is logical to evaluate the application of orientation information, principles of nursing practice, and professional development at the time service is provided.

Shared visits and observations are especially valuable because of feedback opportunities. Nurses' abilities to apply the nursing process and their interpersonal and technical skills are relatively easy to evaluate during the nurse-client interaction. Positive reinforcement and constructive suggestions can be offered soon after service is provided. In addition, when supervisors observe nurse-client interaction, they should be able to evaluate documentation in the client record more accurately.

The goal at the VNA of Omaha is for immediate supervisors to accompany each practitioner on home, clinic, or school visits two times a year. To facilitate communication and enhance measurement during shared visits, Jorgensen and Young[15] developed a Supervisory Home Visit Tool. The tool reflects standards of practice familiar to the practitioner and expected at the VNA of Omaha; comparable standards of practice are expected nationally.

The Supervisory Home Visit Tool consists of 34 simple, brief criteria. "This checklist provides consistency in the way supervisors carry out and document supervisory shared home visits, and it affords tabulation of data for both evaluation and quality assurance purposes."[19]

The tool is divided into five major sections: format of home visit; safety factors; health teaching, guidance, and counseling; treatments and procedures/surveillance; and case management/surveillance. In the first two sections, the practitioner is evaluated on criteria such as "carried out home visit in organized, logical manner" and "handwashing done according to policy." The titles of the three remaining sections represent the primary categories of the Omaha System's Intervention Scheme. Examples of criteria on these sections include "gave simple, brief explanations," "demonstrated sufficient technical skills," and "involved client/family in care."

Practice-based inservice education

Principles and procedures pertinent to orientation are also pertinent to practice-based inservice education. Nurses need opportunities to renew existing skills and develop new skills. Ideally, inservice offerings should be part of a logical, annual plan developed as a joint effort by the staff and administrators. Participants' needs should be identified and prioritized based on findings obtained from the other six approaches described in this viewpoint.

Beginning in 1988, data obtained during the supervisory shared visits indicated the need to improve bag technique and infection control procedures. As a result, signs about bag technique were posted throughout the offices and an infection control program was conducted for all staff and supervisors.

During 1988, another educational program was initiated. An agency-based certification program was initiated for a newly-formed VNA infusion therapy team. It included: (1) a self-study packet that includes a self-test, (2) a skills practice and test session with a variety of supplies and equipment and, (3) a 50-item examination that requires an 85% score for passing. As the number of referrals increased, generalized staff completed the same session. More recently, all new home care nurses attend a venipuncture session that includes theory, observation, and practice. The session is designed for the nurses to gain competence with venipuncture, drawing blood from central lines for laboratory specimens, and changing dressings. Similar, competency-based sessions are designed for diabetic and wound care. Nurses who are members of the agency's infusion therapy team establish competence with various pumps, PICC lines, and the administration of blood and blood products.

Record audit, peer review, and utilization review

Efforts to develop client record audit systems were an integral part of early efforts to measure nursing practice. Nursing leaders such as Roberts and Hudson[28] and Wandelt and Phaneuf[32] recognized that excellence in practice should be reflected by excellence in documentation. Instruments developed and tested by such leaders were used in a variety of practice, education, and research settings. That trend is definitely continuing. As a result of an Indian Health Service study,[8] staff nurses became more skillful in discussing and measuring outcomes with their clients and more knowledgeable about standards of documentation excellence.

Peer review can serve as one method of auditing client records. The purpose is to involve those who are documenting service in the evaluation process. As was described in relation to orientation, active participation enhances learning. Thus, staff nurses who critique client records completed by their peers will be more likely to internalize sound documentation practices. Hopefully, they will increase the accuracy and precision of their own client records and decrease unnecessary, confusing, and illegible entries.

Utilization review is a condition of participation required by Medicare legislation. Home health agencies providing Medicare services must conduct a clinical record review of open and closed cases on a quarterly basis.

Record audit, peer review, and utilization review activities occur regularly at the VNA of Omaha. Evaluating client outcomes of care is emphasized. Because the practitioner uses the Omaha System throughout the client record, the practitioner identifies, describes, and counts client data, progress, and service delivery data. A basic assumption when using the Omaha System is that the client record represents a comprehensive photograph of the client or family and home environment. This photograph should provide the reader with *pertinent* details about the client's knowledge, behavior, and status in relation to health-related problems and the provider's plans and interventions for those problems.

During each quarter, a 10% random sample of open and closed records is selected for review. All case managers and supervisors use an audit form to review one record of a client they never visited and discuss their findings with their peers. Recommendations are shared with the case manager responsible for the client and the client's record.

The VNA's quality assurance-improvement team reviews a 100% sample of records for completeness of physician orders and Medicare compliance. In addition, selected records are reviewed in a comprehensive manner to evaluate the quality of service and documentation. Using an audit form, the referral form, demographic data, consent forms, physician's orders, database, medication profile, care plans, problem-specific knowledge-behavior-status ratings, progress notes, and dismissal summary are critiqued. Recommendations and compliments are communicated to staff members and their supervisors.

Accreditation and external audit

In contrast to the first five approaches for measuring the quality of care, accreditation and external audits are conducted by persons not employed by the host agency or institution. Home care and public health agencies can seek accreditation from the Community Health Accreditation Program (CHAP), a subsidiary of the National League for Nursing (NLN), or the Joint Commission on Accreditation of Healthcare Organizations (JCAHO).

Both organizations provide an opportunity for participating agencies to engage in self-review and peer review. CHAP accredits about 350 home care organizations, while JCAHO accredits 2500 organizations. CHAP received deemed status in 1992; the JCAHO application is still pending.

Third-party payers schedule a variety of surveys and site visits, as well as client record and financial audits. Medicare regulations have created standards and procedures that Medicaid, health maintenance organizations, preferred provider organizations, and private insurance companies often follow. As a CHAP-accredited and a Medicare/Medicaid–certified agency, the VNA of Omaha hosts site visitors and auditors and submits client record data and financial statements regularly. Although reviewers still require structure and process data, the focus on client progress and outcomes has definitely increased.

Client satisfaction surveys

Client satisfaction surveys are another method of gathering data to evaluate the quality of services. Data are usually gathered through telephone interviews, mailed questionnaires, or home visits. Questions may relate to the types of services and attitudes about the service and health care providers. McNeese (1988) identified three benefits to the agency and its clients: (1) use of the research process in evaluating the quality and appropriateness of services, (2) provision of a scientific basis for evaluating and modifying health care delivery systems or models, and (3) identification and integration of individual clients and family concerns into quality improvement activities.

Within one or two weeks of the start of care date, VNA of Omaha home care clients receive a telephone call from a volunteer. Three attempts are made to call and ask a series of seven questions. Included are, "Was the VNA service explained to you?" and "Do you know how to reach your nurse?" Data from the telephone surveys are screened by a staff nurse from the agency's information and referral department. Most comments vary from positive to very positive. When negative comments are received, the nurse contacts the appropriate administrator or supervisor for immediate action. Data are compiled each quarter and discussed during the quarterly quality assurance meetings.

After clients are dismissed from service, a survey which consists of 19 items and a 5-point, Likert-type scale are mailed to their homes. Statements include, "The VNA staff explained things in words I could understand" and "The VNA staff saw me as often as I wanted them to." As with the previous surveys, nega-

tive responses are reviewed and corrected as soon as possible. Responses are tabulated each quarter, presented to the quality assurance committee, and shared with agency personnel.

SUMMARY

Seven approaches for measuring the quality of nursing practice have been adopted at the VNA of Omaha. These or similar approaches are used in many other community-based agencies, nursing homes, and acute care facilities. The approaches are congruent with resources, regulations, and contracts of the practice setting. Some are relatively simple while others are complex. They include quantitative and qualitative characteristics and vary greatly in their research foundation. When considered collectively, the approaches contain aspects of traditional and emerging indicators including process indicators, client knowledge-behavior-status outcome measures, and satisfaction with care.

The profession is making remarkable progress toward the goal of measuring the quality of nursing practice. Considerable time and commitment will be required, however, before nurses consistently use scientifically rigorous, practical, client-focused approaches. It is possible that not all nurses will use such ideal approaches. That possibility, however, should not diminish our collective effort. "The task ahead is arduous; the benefits are far reaching."[30]

REFERENCES

1. Abraham, I., Nadzam, D., & Fitzpatrick, J. (1989). *Statistics and quantitative methods in nursing.* Philadelphia: W. B. Saunders.
2. Barkauskas, V. (1990). Home health care: Responding to need, growth, and cost containment. In N. Chaska (Ed.), *The nursing profession: Turning points* (pp. 394-404). St Louis: Mosby.
3. Chapman, C. (1988, June). Of mice and Merle. *American Journal of Nursing, 88,* 938.
4. Donabedian, A. (1976). Some basic ideas in evaluating the quality of health care. In *Issues in evaluation research* (pp. 3-28). Kansas City, Mo: American Nurses Association.
5. Donabedian, A. (1988, September). The quality of care: How can it be assessed? *Journal of American Medical Association, 260,* 1743-1748.
6. Eustis, N., & Fischer, L. (1991, August). Relationships between home care clients and their workers: Implications for quality of care. *The Gerontologist, 31,* 447-456.
7. Feldman, J., & Richard, R. (1988). A measure of nursing outcomes for home health care. In C. Waltz & O. Strickland (Eds.), *Measurement of nursing outcomes, Vol. 1: Measuring client outcomes* (pp. 475-495). New York: Springer.
8. Fish, C. (1989). *Evaluation of a quality assurance model for public health nursing: Final report* (Contract No. BOA-240-88-0007). Washington, D.C.: Native American Consultants, Inc.

9. Freeman, R. (1961, October). Measuring the effectiveness of public health nursing service. *Nursing Outlook, 9,* 605-607.

10. Geigle, R., & Jones, S. (1990, Spring). Outcomes measurement: A report from the front. *Inquiry, 27,* 7-13.

11. Hinshaw, A., & Atwood, J. (1982). A patient satisfaction instrument: Precision by replication. *Nursing Research, 31,* 170-175, 191.

12. Horn, B., & Swain, M. (1977). *Development of criterion measures of nursing care, Vol. I.* Ann Arbor, Mich: University of Michigan.

13. Institute of Medicine. (1990). *Medicare: A strategy for quality assurance, Vol. 1.* Washington, D.C.: National Academy Press.

14. Jacobs, A., & dela Cruz, F. (1990). Measuring clinical judgment in home health nursing. In C. Waltz & O. Strickland (Eds.), *Measurement of nursing outcomes, Vol. 3: Measuring clinical skills and professional development in education and practice* (pp. 125-141). New York: Springer.

15. Jorgensen, C., & Young, B. (1989, May/June). The supervisory shared home visit tool. *Home Healthcare Nurse, 7,* 33-36.

16. Lewis, E. (1976, March). Quantifying the unquantifiable. *Nursing Outlook, 24,* 147.

17. Magnan, M. (1989, February). Listening with care. *American Journal of Nursing, 89,* 219-221.

18. Marek, K. (1988). Classification of outcome measures in nursing care. In *Classification systems for describing nursing practice* (pp. 37-42). Kansas City, Mo: American Nurses Association.

19. Martin, K., & Scheet, N. (1992). *The Omaha System: Applications for community health nursing.* Philadelphia: W. B. Saunders.

20. Martin, K., & Scheet, N. (1988, May/June). The Omaha System: Providing a framework for assuring quality of home care. *Home Healthcare Nurse, 6,* 24-28.

21. Mateo, M., & Kirchhoff, K. (1991). *Conducting and using nursing research in the clinical setting.* Baltimore: Williams & Wilkins.

22. Naylor, M., Munro, B., & Brooten, D. (1991). Measuring the effectiveness of nursing practice. *Clinical Nurse Specialist, 5,* 210-215.

23. Oda, D. (1988, December). The outcome of public health nursing service in a preventive child health program: Phase 1, health assessment. *Public Health Nursing, 5,* 209-213.

24. Peters, D. (1989, March). An overview of current research relating to long-term outcomes. *Nursing & Health Care, 10,* 133-136.

25. Remington, M. (1990). Measuring the quality of nursing care among critical care nurses. In C. Waltz & O. Strickland (Eds.), *Measurement of nursing outcomes, Vol. 3: Measuring clinical skills and professional development in education and practice* (pp. 69-84). New York: Springer.

26. Rinke, L. (Ed.). (1987). *Outcome measures in home care, Vol. I: Research.* New York: National League for Nursing.

27. Rinke, L., & Wilson, A. (Eds.). (1987). *Outcome measures in home care, Vol. II: Service.* New York: National League for Nursing.

28. Roberts, D., & Hudson, H. (1964, April). *How to study patient progress* (Pub. No. 1169). Bethesda, Md: U.S. Department of Health, Education, and Welfare, Public Health Service, National Institutes of Health.

29. Tarlov, A., Ware, Jr., J., Greenfield, S., Nelson, E., Perrin, E., & Zubkoff, M. (1989, August 18). The medical outcomes study: An application of methods for monitoring the results of medical care. *Journal of American Medical Association, 262,* 925-930.

30. Vahldieck, R., Reeves, S., & Schmelzer, M. (1989, June). A framework for planning public health nursing services to families. *Public Health Nursing, 6,* 102-107.

31. Waltz, C., & Sylvia, B. (1991). Accountability and outcome measurement: Where do we go from here? *Clinical Nurse Specialist, 5,* 202-203.

32. Wandelt, M., & Phaneuf, M. (1972, August). Three instruments for measuring the quality of nursing care. *Hospital Topics, 50,* 20-23, 29.

33. *Webster's College Dictionary.* (1991). New York: Random House.

34. Wooley, A. (1977, May). The long and tortured history of clinical evaluation. *Nursing Outlook, 25,* 308-315.

CHAPTER 49

Self-care as a concept to guide quality nursing practice in Latin American countries

ILTA LANGE, SONIA JAIMOVICH

In developing countries, high rates of population growth have generated rural labor surpluses that cannot be fully absorbed under current conditions related to the level of development of agricultural technology and social organization. As a result of inadequate resources in rural areas, migration rates to urban settings have been high. Although a proportion of the migration is among rural areas, the number of people moving to the cities has significantly increased urban growth rates. Most migrants to urban areas find income-earning opportunities that offer a higher standard of welfare than does life in rural areas; nevertheless, governments face great difficulties in meeting the public service requirements to respond to the needs of a rapidly growing population. The governments of some countries have adopted policies to retain population in rural areas, but this strategy has encountered certain difficulties. Rural income and welfare levels remain low, and a high proportion of the rural population in many Latin American countries live in extreme poverty.[7]

The developing countries, as they progress, are confronted with many of the problems of the industrialized world; as they become urbanized, they also begin to share their morbidity patterns.[10] At the same time they are also challenged to deal with the traditional problems of developing countries. The main causes of death in the Latin American adult population, just as in the industrialized world, are cardiovascular diseases, cancer, and accidents. However, in regard to infant mortality, the first cause of death in many developing countries still is infectious diseases, especially diarrhea; 45% of the world's population still has infant mortality rates higher than 50 per 1000 live births. Life expectancy is bordering 70 years in several Latin American countries

(1985 to 1990), such as Argentina, Chile, Uruguay, Costa Rica, Cuba, and Puerto Rico. However, other countries, such as Bolivia, Guatemala, Honduras, Nicaragua, and Haiti, are still bordering 60 years or less. In most developing countries, crude birth rates vary between 20 to 40 per 1000 inhabitants. The great difference between birth and death rates in these countries produces a high growth rate and, consequently, a high proportion of young population. Mexico, for example, has a crude birth rate of 40 per 1000 inhabitants and a crude death rate of 10 per 1000, thus being the Latin American country with the highest growth rate.[16]

We can conclude then, that the biggest health care concerns in Latin America are still related to the maternal child group; however, as life expectancy is rapidly increasing, the problems related to the adult and elderly population are having a greater relative importance each day. In fact, the main challenge of health care in the twenty-first century will be the prevention and management of chronic diseases in the adult population.[20]

CHARACTERISTICS OF THE HEALTH SERVICES IN LATIN AMERICA

The implementation of primary health care strategy has been a preoccupation in Latin America since the WHO conference in Alma Ata in 1979. Efforts have been made to improve access to health care through the organization of primary, secondary, and tertiary levels of care in the health system. The primary level of care is defined as the level closest to where the people are and is responsible for offering basic health services through the implementation of health programs that strengthen basic sanitation, foster maternal/child health, improve nutrition, prevent infectious diseases, and treat minor illness. Nevertheless, health services are still failing to reach out to those who need them most.[11]

In Latin America, people are used to receiving health care, treatments, and medicines without participating in the decision-making process. Hospitals have been oriented traditionally to offer curative care to individuals, ignoring the importance of incorporating family members into the health care delivery process. In this system, professionals make health decisions for the patients, focusing on a specific disease (typhoid fever, hepatitis, liver cirrhosis, etc.) or health problem and the treatment of symptoms without taking into consideration the patient's psychological, social, and spiritual needs or their self-care practices. The patient's compliance to treatment is very low, especially in those who suffer from chronic diseases.

Usually a Latin American person who has a health problem will adopt self-care behaviors according to what he has learned from his mother, neighbors, or friends. Formal education has minor influence on these self-care activities. When the individual feels that he cannot solve his health problem by himself, he will search for professional help. In the health institutions, this person—who was independent up to this moment—will be made very dependent upon the health care providers (professionals and nurse's aides). He will be called and treated as a "patient" who has only minor possibilities of participating in the decisions that affect his own health and well-being. His self-care behaviors are usually ignored by the health care providers and the participation of his family is limited (Fig. 49-1).

In this traditional health care model, health professionals are considered by the public and by themselves as the owners of the truth, wisdom, experience, and knowledge to improve health. The patient is considered a "health consumer" with scarce knowledge or experience in health matters. The professional/patient relationship is a hierarchical one in which the health care provider decides what is best.[9]

SELF-CARE NURSING: A CONCEPTUAL APPROACH

Health can be defined as a dynamic state of biopsychosocial well-being in which individuals are able to perform those functions deemed necessary and desirable to maintain existence in their environment.

Self-care seems upon first consideration to be a straightforward and simple topic. People have always assumed responsibility for their personal safety and for the well-being of the group or family with whom they live. Moreover, they have taken measures, however primitive they might seem to us, to deal with illness.

We can define self-care as all voluntary actions or activities in which individuals, families, and communities engage to promote and maintain their health and prevent and/or cure diseases.

Woods defines self-care as an attempt to promote optimal health, prevent illness, detect symptoms at an early date, and manage chronic illness. Self-care also includes processes of self-monitoring and assessment; symptom perception and labeling; evaluation of severity; and evaluation and selection of treatment alternatives such as self-help, lay-helping resources, or formal health services.[22]

Self-care nursing is a particular approach of nursing practice in which special emphasis is given to the clients' capacity to attain and maintain their health. Self-care nursing incorporates strategies, methodologies, and activities into nursing care geared towards helping individuals, families, and community learn how to care for themselves and when to search for professional help.[6]

Self-care nursing is considered a philosophy of care as well as a specific professional intervention. "It is a perspective that permeates all aspects of care, guiding nurses to consider all the ways clients can care for themselves in illness and in health.[19] One of the consequences of this health approach is that the clients learn to make better health-related decisions and to use the health services more efficiently, thus reducing their health costs.

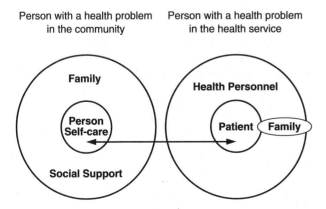

Fig. 49-1 Traditional health care model.

If we review nursing history, we can recognize that nurses have always been concerned about teaching patients self-care practices. Florence Nightingale believed that every woman is a nurse because, at some point in time, each woman has been in charge of the health care of somebody: a child, an elderly person, etc.[19]

Dorothea Orem has been undoubtedly the person most commonly associated with the incorporation of the self-care concept into nursing practice. Her basic premise is that people have the potential to take care of themselves in health as well as in illness and that the self-care capacities of the clients can be strengthened through education and guidance. The core of Orem's philosophy is the belief that people have an innate ability to care for themselves. According to that philosophy, the concept of self-care becomes the focal point of the nurse's thinking and behavior. Self-care contributes in specific ways to human structural integrity, human functioning, and human development.[14]

Self-care is defined by Orem as activities a person initiates and performs on his own behalf to maintain life, health, and well-being. Self-care agency is the individual's own ability to perform self-care. Agency includes decisions about self-care and the actions required to accomplish self-care.[22] Nursing, therefore, is required when a deficit exists between individual's self-care needs and self-care abilities.

Nursing interventions vary according to the client's deficits identified. The methods used to help clients are:

- Acting or doing for another
- Supporting physically or psychologically
- Guiding and teaching
- Providing a physical or psychological environment that promotes personal development

The nursing plan is implemented by the nurse who will assess and evaluate the client's progress. As needs and abilities change, the plan is modified. The client should progress until self-care deficits no longer exist and nursing actions are no longer needed.[3,13]

In the self-care process, five components can be identified:

1. Health promotion: The health promotion activities are geared toward maximizing well-being; for example, exercising regularly.
2. Health maintenance: The health maintenance activities are geared towards maintaining the health status, such as getting enough sleep.

3. Prevention of health problems: Disease prevention activities seek to eliminate risk factors of specific health problems, such as eating a low-cholesterol diet to reduce heart disease risk.
4. Detection of health problems: The disease detection activities seek to increase the consciousness of the individual in regard to signs and symptoms. It includes learning of certain self-examination techniques, such as breast self-examination to detect breast lumps.
5. Disease management: This pertains to learning to follow instructions of the health team and early detection of complications or side effects of treatments.

QUALITY IN HEALTH CARE: A CONCEPTUAL APPROACH

Quality in health care has been defined as the *provision of high-level professional services* that are accessible to the population and that, through the use of the existing resources, attain compliance and satisfaction of the clients.[15] This definition of quality implies that the services delivered are the measure rather than increased capacity of the individual to participate in the care process.

Donabedian defines quality of health care services as the type of care expected to maximize the well-being of patients, once the balance between gains and costs has been considered in all parts of the process.[5]

The concept of quality in health care originated in the world of clinical medicine. Most of the existing studies have been done in hospitals, especially in industrialized countries, and the collection of data is centered around diagnoses, treatments, or results of patient care.

In developing countries, great importance is given to primary health care, and the main concern of the governments is to increase accessibility to health services and improve the problem-solving capacity of the first level of care. In these countries, there is a need to evaluate quality of care from a population or group perspective as well as from the perspective of an individual client of the health system. The standards to evaluate quality in health care in developing countries are very modest because information systems are scarce, unsophisticated, and not dependable, thus increasing the difficulties in obtaining reliable quality measurements.

According to the literature, different dimensions or elements can be considered to measure quality in health care. We will define eight dimensions and comment on how a self-care nursing model can affect these elements, improving quality in health care. These dimensions are: scientific and technical expertise, accessibility, satisfaction or acceptability of health care services, effectiveness, efficiency, continuity of care, timeliness of care, and job satisfaction of health care providers.

Scientific and technical expertise. This dimension considers the competency of professional and nonprofessional health personnel in applying advances in knowledge and technology within the existing resource base to produce health and satisfaction in the attended population. Expertise is measured not only in the strict technical sense but also incorporates into the concept the quality of interpersonal relationships established between the clients, families, or community and the health care providers.

Accessibility. The facility by which health care services are obtained by the population are critical. Accessibility measures consider geographical, organizational, economic, cultural, and emotional barriers. The question to be answered is: Is health care available for whoever needs it, when it is needed?

Satisfaction or acceptability of health care services. This measures the degree which health care services satisfy the expectations of the clients (individuals, families or communities). These expectations do not necessarily coincide with those of the health care providers; this means that care based on scientific and technical expertise is not always acceptable and does not necessarily produce high satisfaction in the client.

The concept of acceptability deals with at least three basic components:

- The effect of health care actions on the specific health problem of the client, family, or community.
- How organizational factors (physical atmosphere, waiting time, schedules, visiting hours, continuity of care by the same professional, etc.) affect acceptability of care.
- How the interpersonal relationship established between the client and the health care providers affects acceptability of care. Studies show that the establishment of a good interpersonal relationship between the health care provider and client is associated with higher satisfaction. If this positive relationship is established, the gap between the client's and the health care provider's perceptions and expectations with regard to health care delivery can be minimized.

There is evidence that satisfaction with health care is influenced by client-related variables such as demographic characteristics, attitudes, previous experiences with health services, and the perception of his or her health status. For example, an obese person with hypertension who expected to obtain medications to reduce his weight may be unsatisfied with the health care provided if the physician recommends to reduce the caloric intake and to exercise and tells him that medication is unnecessary or even harmful for his health. A person who has sleeping difficulties due to a problem at work might be very unsatisfied with the health care if he did not receive the medication and the sick leave he expected to get.

Within the concept of acceptability, the factor of compliance—the degree in which the patient or client accepts and does what the health care team has recommended—is also present. Self-care education tends to improve compliance by increasing the level of knowledge, motivation, and skills of the client and his family to make health-related decisions.

Effectiveness. This measures the degree to which a certain health care activity, which is practiced in a specific health care setting, produces an improvement in the health status of the patient, family, or community.

Efficiency. This measures the degree to which the highest level of quality can be obtained, with the existing resources.

Continuity of care. This dimension of quality can be defined as the degree to which needed care is provided in an uninterrupted and coordinated manner.[18] In this definition, it becomes evident that quality of care depends upon the health care providers as well as the consumers of care. In order to have uninterrupted care, self-care is essential.

Timeliness of care. The JCAHO has incorporated into the definition of quality care the dimension of timeliness of care, defined as the degree by which care is provided when it is needed, at the right moment.[8]

Job satisfaction. Some authors[1] consider job satisfaction of health care providers as another measure of quality in health care because it influences the quality of interpersonal relationships between providers and clients and, consequently, their satisfaction with the health care provided.

WHY IS A SHIFT NEEDED FROM A TRADITIONAL HEALTH CARE DELIVERY SYSTEM TOWARD ONE BASED ON SELF-CARE?

Research done in Santiago, Chile, shows that approximately half of the health events in the community are solved by the people themselves without the support of the health services.[12] About 14% of the population suffers from chronic diseases that require professional assistance; nevertheless, the reduced resources within the health institutions, high medical costs, and other access problems to obtain health services limit the population from attaining timely professional health care. These data are not too different from studies done in industrialized countries, where it has been found that only 25% to 50% of the people who are sick have contact with professional health care providers.[4] For this reason, health self-care practices of individuals and families have to be recognized as the first level of care and as part of the primary health care system.[12,21] If we believe that self-care is part of the base of the health care pyramid, then we can say that to improve health and life expectancy of the people, it is not only necessary to modify the organization and structure of health services but also essential to increase the motivation, knowledge, and skills of individuals, families, and communities to take better care of themselves and to obtain professional help when needed. Hospitals and other health services need to share responsibilities as an integrated system that offers health care and self-care education to the population in search for improvement of the health of the population.

In Latin America, the main reasons for incorporating the self-care concept into the health care system are:

- Life expectancy has increased, as well as the incidence of chronic diseases in the adult population.[20] To manage these health problems, compliance to treatment and healthy self-care behaviors is essential.
- The dissatisfaction of the population to be exposed to highly specialized medical care, with a somatic and pathophysiologic approach, by which the patient is not considered a holistic human being with psychological, social, and spiritual needs, has increased the population's interest in participating in health care decisions.
- The recognition that the majority of health problems are solved in the community without the participation of the health care institutions confirms that there is a need to help the population to improve its knowledge, attitudes, and self-care skills and to learn when and how to better use the health services.
- The awareness of the existing relationship between unhealthy life styles and the morbidity and mortality patterns in the country, the main causes of death being cardiovascular diseases, cancer, accidents, and liver cirrhosis, all of which are related to health risk behaviors that can be reduced by healthy self-care practices.

Concern has arisen lately among health professionals, the public, and administrators in the developing world about how to improve quality in health care. Professionals are concerned about how to improve their scientific and technical expertise and how to correct certain deficiencies in the health system. The public is worried about the lack of accessibility to health care services and is not satisfied with the interpersonal relationship established with the health personnel. Administrators are preoccupied with how health care resources are allocated and distributed, how the health system can be made more accessible and equitable for the population, and how health costs can be reduced.[17]

In institutions where self-care is considered a permanent component of health care delivery, all activities performed by the health care providers, mainly by nursing personnel, are geared towards obtaining and maintaining clients' autonomy, respecting their needs and preferences, and strengthening knowledge, motivation, and skills that they need to be able to make adequate health-related decisions. In this health delivery model, the clients and their families are considered part of the health care team, and every interaction between nursing personnel and clients is used to strengthen their self-care capacities and to increase their health promotion and disease prevention behaviors (Fig. 49-2).

In this model, the clients are taught and encouraged to define their own health status, identify health problems when they arise, and make health-related decisions, either through self-care actions or getting professional help.

The health care providers consider the clients' self-care practices, their lifestyles, beliefs, myths, and values that will undoubtedly affect the way they participate in health care decisions, comply to medical treatment, or change behaviors. The client's participation in health care and the horizontal provider/client relationship in which both parties share and learn from

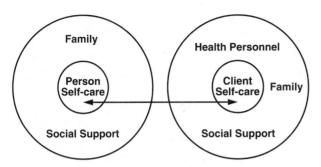

Person in the community · Client in the health service

Fig. 49-2 Health care delivery model with emphasis on self-care.

each other, with clear communications and mutual trust, helps to overcome cultural, emotional, and organizational barriers, facilitating accessibility to health care.

The described model was developed by the Nursing Service of the Outpatient Clinic of the Catholic University Hospital in Santiago, Chile (CEDIUC), in partnership with the School of Nursing with the financial support of the Kellogg Foundation (1983-89). In regard to job satisfaction of the health personnel (another dimension of quality in health care), this experience has shown that this working philosophy improves the morale of the nursing personnel and decreases their turnover. In this institution, emphasis not only is given to self-care of "external clients" (patients) but also to self-care practices of the health care workers, the "internal clients" of the institution. These practices are fostered during working hours, providing time for regular exercise during lunch breaks, organizing stress management activities, and self-care continuing education programs.[9] The nursing personnel feels proud of this model, has clarity of mission, and helps to lead the effort of improving the eight dimensions of quality in health care. In this system, everyone has two jobs: their own job and the job to help improve the patient's job of taking care of himself.[2]

At CEDIUC, the assumption that quality only fails when health personnel do the right thing wrong has been questioned. Experience has shown us that frequently quality fails when nursing personnel do the wrong thing right. For example, in the traditional nursing model, the nurse or nurse's aid of a clinic or hospital controls the child's temperature correctly. In the self-care model, this is done by the mother, because it

is expected that she will control the temperature correctly at home. In this case, the wrong thing to do is to control the temperature; the right thing is to let the mother do it and have the nurses or nurse's aide supervise the procedure and teach or reinforce her as necessary.

CONCLUSIONS

Self-care nursing improves quality of health care as it works towards a holistic approach of health care and emphasizes human values. It changes the passive role of the clients to a more participative attitude, increasing compliance towards the recommendations of the health team and empowering the population to demand their rights, to recognize their responsibilities, and to identify their needs and priorities in regard to their personal and community health.

The self-care approach fosters the continuity and timeliness of care (dimensions of quality health care) by promoting self-responsibility and self-efficacy of clients, families, and communities. It tends to the democratization of professional knowledge. As the model is centered around the clients' opinions and practices, it increases their satisfaction and acceptability of health services.

Action research is needed in Latin America to measure and improve quality of care: the client/provider relationship has to be explored as a quality measurement and more clarification is needed on the roles of providers and clients as a means of improving health care. Also, much work still has to be done to educate the clients and the health care providers toward a more participatory style of health care delivery in which they work together as a real team.

REFERENCES

1. Batalden P., Goldfield, N., & Buchanan, E. (1989). Industrial models of quality improvement. In D. B. Nash (Ed.), *Providing quality care: The challenge to physicians.* Philadelphia: American College of Physicians.
2. Berwick, D., Godfrey, A., & Roessner J. (1991). *Curing health care.* San Francisco-Oxford: Jossey-Bass.
3. David, J. A., Christensen, D., Hohon, S., Ord, L., & Wells, S. (1978). Implementing Orem's conceptual framework. *The Journal of Nursing Administration, 8*(11), 8-11.
4. De Friese, G., Sehnert, K., & Barry, P. (1982). Medical self-care instruction for lay persons: A new agenda for health. *Möbius, 2*(1).
5. Donabedian, A. (1980). *The definition of quality and approaches to its assessment.* Ann Arbor, Mich: Health Administration Press.
6. Hill, I., & Smith, N. (1985). *Self-care nursing: Promotion of health.* Norwalk, Conn: Appleton-Century-Crofts.

7. Huw, R. (1988). *A Population geography*. London: Paul Chapman.

8. Joint Commission on Accreditation of Healthcare Organizations. (1990). *Quality assurance in ambulatory care* (2nd ed.). Chicago: Author.

9. Lange, I., & Campos, C. (1989). Atención de salud con énfasis en autocuidado [Health assistance with emphasis on self-care]. *Educación para el Autocuidado en Salud, 6*(4), 10-15

10. Levin, L. (1983, February). Self-help: One way to health. *World Health,* 24-29.

11. Maglacas, A. (1988). Health for all: Nursing's role. *Nursing Outlook, 36*(2) 66-71.

12. Medina, E. (1984). Importancia de la educación para el autocuidado del paciente [The importance of education for the patient's self-care]. *Educación para el Autocuidado en Salud, 1*(12) 11-15.

13. Morse, W., & Werner, J. (1988). Individualization of patient care using Orem's theory. *Cancer Nursing, 11*(3), 195-202.

14. Orem, D. (1991). *Nursing: Concepts in practice* (4th ed.). St Louis: Mosby.

15. Palmer, R. H. (1990). *Evaluación de la asistencia ambulatoria: Principios y prácticas* [Ambulatory assistance evaluation: Principles and practices]. Madrid: Ministerio de Sanidad y Consumo.

16. Rey, C. J. (1989). *Método epidemiológico y salud de la comunidad* [Epidemiological method and community health]. Madrid: Ed. Interamericana, McGraw-Hill.

17. Saturno, P., Imperatori, E., & Corbella, A. (1990). *Evaluación de la calidad asistencial en atención primaria* [Evaluation of the quality of assistance in primary health care]. Madrid: Ministerio de Sanidad y Consumo.

18. Shortell, S. M. (1976). Continuity of medical care: Conceptualization and measurement. *Medical Care, 14,* 377-391

19. Steiger, N., & Lipson, J. (1985). *Self-care nursing: Theory and practice*. Bowle, Md: Brady Communications Company.

20. Valdivieso, V. (1992). Medicina interna en Chile *[Internal medicine in Chile]. Revista Médica de Chile,* 120(5), 503.

21. Williamson, J. D., & Danaher K. (1978). *Self-care in health*. London: Croom Helm.

22. Woods, N. (1989). Conceptualization of self-care: Towards health-oriented models. *Advanced Nursing Science, 12*(1), 1-13.

PART SIX

GOVERNANCE

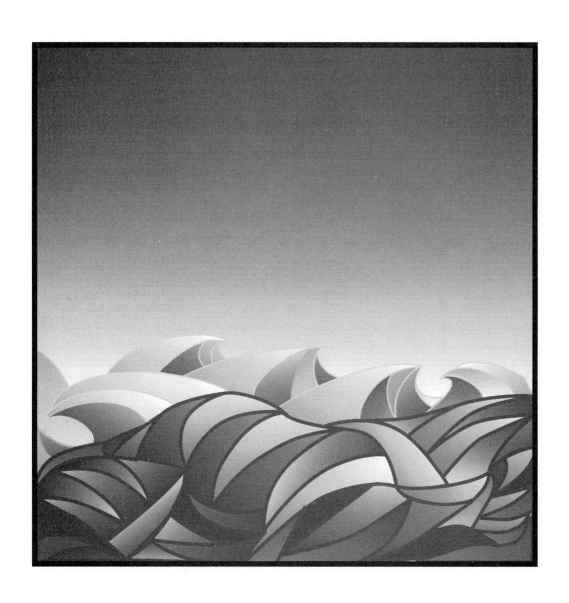

Shedding dependency

JOANNE COMI McCLOSKEY, HELEN KENNEDY GRACE

Throughout the history of nursing, the dependency position of the profession has remained a consistent topic of debate and concern. In the previous sections, the concerted efforts to establish the knowledge base for the field and concerns for assuring quality and the advances that have been made in the practice realm speak to the internal strengthening of the profession. Yet, in some respects, the influence of nursing in the broader realm of the health care system as a whole remains limited. In this section, the debate chapter poses the question of whether nursing has the power to change the health care system. Subsequent chapters look at practice, education, and the profession itself to explore the question of nursing's increased power in governance at various levels.

In the debate chapter, Sweeney and Witt suggest that since this question needs to be raised once more in this edition, the answer to it obviously must be "no." From this beginning point, however, they note that the current focus on the health care crisis in this country potentially is an opportunity for nursing to increase its influence. Joining a traditional definition of power with a human action model, the authors provide a new framework for analyzing this question. Factors that limit nursing's power to change the health care system are identified as (1) the lack of a brief, concise, and comprehensive *mission* statement that communicates to the public, (2) the inability to energize *commitment* of the members of the profession, (3) *structures* as represented in nursing organizations that, instead of having unique functions, compete with each other for the same constituencies, and (4) the inability to mobilize *resources* of the profession as a whole as represented in the numbers of nurses in the field. Turning to the pro side of the argument, the authors argue that the sheer numbers of nurses, numerically the largest group in the health field, constitute the collective power to create

change. With a clear sense of mission, a positive self-image, empowered with positive self-confident attitudes, and with respect for the abilities of other nurses, the potential power base of nursing can be developed. Actualization of this power base requires reexamining past relationships between nurses and physicians and working together in a new alignment to meet the needs of the patients they collectively serve. By joining together with a shared mission, self-confident in the contributions that nurses make to patient care, nurses collectively do have the power to change the health care system.

Gaining power through collective bargaining has been one approach used by nursing, but this has not been without controversy. The controversy over collective bargaining revolves around the professional status of nursing—trade union approaches are viewed by many to be in conflict with the basic values of a profession. O'Connor argues that the increase in nurses involved in collective bargaining units is a reflection of the contribution that unionization is making to the evolution of nursing as a profession. Changes in the environment, such as prospective payment systems that have increased the demands for nurses both in acute and home and long-term care settings, have resulted in a tendency for employers to make unilateral decisions about the deployment of nurses in a way that is counter to values within the profession. One response to this trend is an increased involvement of nurses in unionization. Bargaining is increasingly viewed as a way of equalizing power between administration, with its goals of operating at a profitable or at least at a break-even level, and nurses, who are the backbone of the system.

More evidence of the increased power of nursing is seen in the development of nursing organized practice settings. Lundeen sees community nursing centers as a significant force influencing health care reform. A tracing of the history of community nursing centers from the pioneering work of Wald in 1915 to the present, with some 250 nursing centers in existence, shows them to be a significant force for change. Given the current health care crisis with the concerns about cost, quality, and accessibility of care, community nursing centers provide significant opportunities for nurses to have an impact on health care reform. Nursing's strength lies in the ability of its practitioners to provide consumer-oriented preventive and early intervention services at reasonable cost and to appropriately refer patients in need of medical care. While nursing has the power to provide models of care that provide alternatives to our current medical care system, making this transition will require significant shift in public policy. The challenge facing nursing is to use the current health care crisis as an opportunity for change.

Forming organizations is one way of promoting survival and protecting groups from external threats, as Hegyvary notes. Nursing organizations are one way of mobilizing the inherent power of the profession. There are two multipurpose organizations: the American Nurses Association, with membership consisting of registered nurses only, sets standards for the profession and represents the economic interests of nurses; and the National League for Nursing, with membership outside of the profession, which has eight designated functions. With membership declining in the multipurpose nursing organizations, clinical specialty organizations, in contrast, are experiencing a rise in membership. A third type of organization represents functional specialty interests of nursing administration and nursing educational administration. A fourth type of emerging organization is found in liaison groups that bring together the interests of the multiple nursing organizations. By building links between and among the multiple organizations, the inherent power of the profession may be realized; without these links the existence of multiple organizations can lead to fragmentation and can lessen the potential influence of a united profession.

The next two chapters turn from the general issue of the profession as a whole to more specific issues related to governance of nursing faculty and then of nursing practice. As nursing education becomes more fully integrated into higher education, governance of nursing educational programs necessarily is changing. Ostmoe addresses the question of whether increased involvement of nursing faculty in decision making necessarily

implies reduced power of deans. Noting nursing education's historically strong autocratic and bureaucratic roots, she writes that the evolving models of shared governance and political models, with multiple committees vying for decision-making power, are more typical. Declining resources place increased pressure on governance processes, in turn placing increased pressure on both faculty and deans. Leadership, as distinguished from control, involves a "purposive exchange of influence in decision making." With this as a perspective, Ostmoe concludes by describing the dean of the future as a "transforming leader" who engages with faculty in a shared governance process.

Within organizations in which nursing is practiced, the governance of nurses becomes an even more complex issue. Maas and Specht argue that shared governance systems are necessary to accommodate two systems of authority, that of the profession with responsibility for the conduct of its members and that of the employing organization. Shared governance systems require shared decision making by professional nursing staff and nursing management. Such a system requires that concepts be operationalized in a structure that clearly delineates responsibility for professional nursing practice on the one hand, responsibility for management of a system of nursing services within an institution on the other, and a structure for bringing the two together to achieve shared governance. Effective functioning of a shared governance system requires nurses skilled in negotiative, consensus building, and decision-making skills. The role of management within such a system becomes one of consulting, teaching, collaborating, and creating a positive work environment in which the skills of professional nurses are maximized.

In this section's final chapter, by Styles and Ohlson, the focus turns once more to an international perspective and to the responsibility of nurses to see themselves as part of a broader international community. The structure of the International Council of Nurses (ICN) as a federation of national nurses associations is described, and the functions of the ICN to strengthen nursing internationally and to unify the profession are detailed. The World Health Organization (WHO), as a specialized intergovernmental agency of the United Nations, has as its primary mission the coordination of international health work. The chief scientist for nursing is the primary voice of the profession within WHO. Working through ministry of health structures in countries throughout the world and working through committees established to address specific issues relevant to nursing, the voice of the nursing profession is being heard in broader discussions and approaches to improvement of health around the world. While the functions of these two international organizations are different, with the ICN linked to the profession of nursing around the world and WHO linked to delivery of health care services, interactions between the two serve to unify nursing around the world.

Do nurses have the power to change the health care system? The advances reported within this section hold promise for the future. The most promising developments are those that show the increased understanding of governance processes that entail negotiation, compromise, consensus building, and capacity building, in contrast to our long history of autocratic, bureaucratic organizational structures and the accompanying dependency themes that have, for so long, dominated our systems.

CHAPTER 50

Debate

Does nursing have the power to change the health care system?

SANDRA S. SWEENEY, KAREN E. WITT

This is the third time this book has addressed and debated the question: Does nursing have the power to change the health care system? As such, revisiting the question for this edition presented us with an ubiquitous challenge: Is the question answerable or even feasible given a decade's passage of time without precise evidence toward resolution? One could argue, for example, merely posing the question once again serves as de facto proof that nurses do, indeed, lack the power to change the health care system. However, one could also argue that preceding debates have served a useful purpose by identifying and providing a philosophical foundation from which new frameworks and opportunities can now be used to convert crisis-ridden realities into tangible expressions of effective and efficient action.

Each of the chapters that appeared in earlier editions also debated the question, Does nursing have the power to change the health care system? Those debates occurred at critical periods throughout the past decade and attempted to relate both the prevailing posture of power and the context of its meaning to nursing in an evolutionary fashion. This chapter builds upon our previous efforts to frame the debate, not only by examining its positive and negative perspectives, but also by accommodating the philosophical structures previously identified to explicate a contemporary model designed to link action with authenticity. Thus, this chapter extends our previous work by offering an agenda for substantive action from which nurses can authentically embrace the elusive concept of power and marshal the resources necessary to transform illusive idealism into pragmatic realism.

One needs only to glance at the headlines of newspapers or news journals or hear the top stories featured on television and radio to become acutely aware of the existing health care crisis in this country. It seems more difficult, however, for most of our citizens (including nurses) to truly comprehend the extent to which this crisis will affect all levels of American society—not just the "known" populations at risk. The crises are happening *now,* and nurses must capitalize on their power base *now,* if they are to prevent their roles from becoming further blurred. Nurses must seize present opportunities, forge their contributions, and make their distinctness known if they are to be included as part of the emerging revolutionary paradigm of health care.

Nurses and their profession are embarking on a new era in which traditional concepts such as change and power are taking on new definitions, dimensions, conceptualizations, and meaning. Indeed, Toffler[16] suggests that the entire structure of power as previously known is disintegrating and yielding to new forms, new relationships, strange alliances, and catastrophic collisions. This transformation of power is recognized and used in reorganizing, reconceptualizing, and extending this debate to better reflect the emerging changes in the nature of power and how nurses can

We wish to acknowledge and thank Dr. Robert Terry for allowing us to utilize two of his prepublished chapters from his forthcoming book titled *Leadership: The Courage to Be Authentic,* scheduled for publication in 1993. His collegial cooperation enabled us to structure this debate in a new framework, and we are most appreciative of his assistance and trust.

make it work for them. If nurses are to achieve status as valued members of the health care system, they must be open to and endorse new missions and visions as they confront new realities.

The framework used to organize and structure previous debates was one Berle published in 1969. This chapter views Berle's[4] seminal work as having provided the philosophical base from which power can be framed, while incorporating a new, more reality-based, conceptual framework that is easily operationalized.

Berle argued that power is a universal experience and attribute of human beings with "five discernible natural laws":

1. Power invariably fills any vacuum in human organization.
2. Power is invariably personal.
3. Power is invariably based on a system of ideals or a philosophy.
4. Power is exercised through, and depends on, institutions.
5. Power is invariably confronted with, and acts in the presence of, a field of responsibility.

Laws, by definition, allow for generalizations while providing a structure for logical reasoning. Berle's laws provide an appropriate philosophical structure for debate, and previous chapters have briefly stated each law followed by: (1) an amplification of the law itself and (2) an argument in which power and its relationship to the profession of nursing is made relative to nursing's role in the contemporary health care delivery system. Berle's laws have been fully explicated in previously published editions and are not duplicated here, even though they continue to constitute the philosophical premises from which this debate is structured.

This chapter accepts Berle's five laws as givens but differs from previous debate arguments by revisiting and augmenting them using a model proposed by Terry[14] to incorporate operational dimensions of power for structuring the debate in this chapter. Terry's human action model provides an attractive, reality-based, viable, and easily integrated framework upon which to structure this debate, since its key concepts address "action" and "authenticity"—criteria that will not only be expected but demanded by both providers and consumers of future health care delivery in this country. Any unit of action, Terry suggests, such as just showing up and being willing to engage others, makes it possible to construct new perspectives and practical actions for the involved parties. Authenticity is further assured when one shows up and engages others with the logic and courage necessary to face important issues and resolve difficult problems. Indeed, Terry's work employs an "experiential realism" approach in that major components of action not only emerge from one's lived experience but also serves to further inform it. This perspective is closely aligned with other initiatives and changing directions in generating and refining the structure and syntax of nursing's knowledge through humanistic, phenomenological, and hermeneutic methodologies.

Terry's human action model fuses action and authenticity into a consummate relationship in which logic and courage form the connections between action and authenticity. He also identifies seven generic features that exist in his model, each of which are briefly defined as follows:

1. *Fulfillment* is an embodiment term denoting that *into which* human action moves.
2. *Meaning* is a significance term justifying the *for which* human action moves.
3. *Mission* is a direction term identifying that *toward which* human action moves.
4. *Power* is an energy term signifying that *by which* human action moves.
5. *Structure* is an organizing term denoting the *through which* human action moves.
6. *Resources* is a material term connoting that *with which* human action moves.
7. *Existence* is a limiting and possibility term outlining that *from which* human action moves.

Thus, while Berle's[4] work focuses exclusively on five invariant laws of power, Terry's[14] model provides a personal and organizational context in which to organize this revised debate. Finally, the conceptual definition of power synthesized for use in earlier chapters has also been revised to better reflect how our perspective of power has changed and is now used in this chapter. Power is conceptually defined as:

The ability to employ energized and committed efforts toward the attainment of "being fulfilled." It is situation specific and exists as either a stimulus or state of being in which conscious authentic action is experienced internally and purposefully directed toward meaningful and fulfilled existence. It takes on specific form(s), emerges, can be used or diffused, has sustenance requirements, is subject to challenge and spiritual questioning. Power can be gained or lost by election, expiration, resignation, or expulsion; it is a universal attribute of human beings and is governed by five invariant laws.

Power, as conceptually defined in previous chapters, tended to portray power as *Power,* that is, a concept whose meaning reflected a capital *P*—a concept capable of and deserving a forceful and freestanding status. Certainly, there has been a tendency to interpret power as being closely aligned to using force or control to influence or make others conform. Terry's[14] model, however, addresses power from the perspective of a small *p*—a significant concept that, when combined within a context, synthesizes the energy and commitment needed to accomplish a mission while simultaneously allowing one to realize a meaningful and fulfilling existence.

Perhaps *Power* as previously perceived is unable to function as a freestanding phenomenon, whereas *power* as partner within the context of mission, structure, and resources can provide an avenue on which meaning, existence, and fulfillment become the final destination and when achieved culminate in an all-at-once experience.

Terry's model[14] has been adapted by the authors and is schematically represented in Fig. 50-1.

Fulfillment, as defined in Terry's[14] human action model, refers to the completed act—the simultaneous culmination of meaning, mission, power, structure, resources, and existence at any given moment and place. Fulfillment signifies the coming together of three distinct processes: (1) thinking, (2) doing, and (3) being. Thus, completed acts may be integral or separate and actual, implied, or virtual.

Meaning, another of the model's seven generic features, addresses the *whys* that underlie actions—the reasons, rationalizations, justifications, and value orientations—that serve to explain particular actions. Meaning makes sense out of daily life and provides the context within which it exists. Meaning is confirmed publicly and is the vehicle for dialog between two or more people. Meaning is the innate part of our past that we bring with us to every situation that, when confronted with new contexts, either forces us to cope using our familiar contexts of meaning or requires us to create new contexts. When the process works, one has invention and creativity; when the process fails, one is left with stereotyping and prejudice.[14]

Spiritual questioning is a subset of the larger question of meaning and intercepts the model at the juncture of meaning and existence. Spiritual questioning addresses the challenges of faith-based actions that encourage us to live our lives fully without knowing the ultimate answers to all of life's questions. Spiritual questioning transcends both meaning and existence enabling one's sense of fulfillment to be fully exploited (in a positive sense) and perceived.[14]

Mission refers to the *toward which* of action—any action that implies direction. Mission statements provide the necessary guidance needed to galvanize resources toward the achievement of common goals. Mission statements are: (1) future oriented; (2) societal, organizational, and/or personal in nature; and (3) either mega or mini in scope. They become the visions from which the direction and goals for either individual or collective entities emerge.[14]

Power, according to Terry,[14] is used to connote energy—the actual not potential expenditure of energy, the *by which* of human action. Power is the dimension, decision, or commitment that energizes one's ability to accomplish any given mission. If an individual, organizational, or societal entity lacks power (energy and commitment), then nothing happens and inertia ensues, leaving behind only unfulfilled expectations. Terry[14] also argues power is closely tied to mission and resources, and chooses to focus on power as the expenditure of energy rather than the value-laden attitudes and confused, if not polemic, definitions of

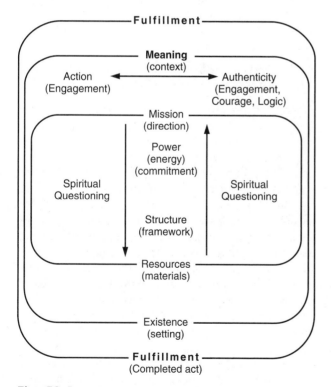

Fig. 50-1 Fulfillment model. (Adapted from Terry's Human Action Diagnostic Tool. Used with permission.)

power one finds in much of nursing's contemporary literature. Viewing power as an energy source (a vital life force) provides synergy (positive flow) and enhances decision-making efforts.

Structure refers to the *through which* of action—the organizing framework, the plan, form, process, the map upon which activities, once energized, are propelled toward accomplishment of the mission. Structure is essential for the accomplishment of tasks, whether simple or complicated, habits or rituals, and comprises the basic unit of both formal planning and predictability equations. While structures may lack perfection, function differently than originally intended, or need revision, they are necessary for action to occur.[14]

Resources comprise the *materials and products* of action, that is, those items, services, actions, and so forth essential to the accomplishment of the mission. Resources are not only essential, but they must also be appropriate for the mission. Unusable, inappropriate, or otherwise unwanted resources have to be discounted when attempting to complete a mission. Resources, as defined by Terry,[14] must meet six criteria. Resources must be: (1) recognized as potentially *usable*; (2) selected for the mission at hand; (3) able to be put to use; (4) manageable; (5) quantifiable; and (6) available.

Existence addresses the foundation, the setting for action. Terry[14,15] defines existence as constituting the parameters of an entire range of possible action(s). It is the ecological and historical context within which actions occur. It includes language and inherited artifacts, rituals, and routines. It is particular, unique, and the base upon which an organization exists, grows, and accomplishes its purpose. What meaning is to the context of action, so existence is to the setting for action. Thus, when the known becomes unknown and the certain uncertain, existence and all that it means become threatened and frantically searches for stability.

As stated earlier, fulfillment refers to the product(s), the act(s) or action(s) itself; thus, fulfillment represents the finished product, the point at which meaning, mission, power, structure, resources, and existence converge at a given time and place. If the mission is to prepare a class, the class itself is the completed act. If a mission is to heal the sick, then when sickness is healed, the healed being constitutes the completed act. Likewise, if a mission is to prevent illness, then the absence of illness—as a state of being—becomes the fulfilled act. Completed acts can exist separate from the being, exist within a being, or can exist actually or virtually. Fulfillment, then, refers to the explicit combination the previously identified seven elements of human action adopt as peculiar unto themselves. The model therefore seems particularly appropriate to nursing because of the integral involvement of nurses who often seek fulfillment of their own beings while performing specialized acts with or for other human beings.

One of the major premises of Terry's[15] theory suggests the identification and diagnosis of problems, issues, or concerns usually occurs one or two levels below the area at which resolution to the problem rests. Thus, if one diagnoses resources as the major issue, attending to it at that level will not resolve the issue. Rather, if the problem is located at the resource level, the solution is generally found at higher levels of the hierarchy, such as reexamining the notions of structure, power, or mission. Terry asserts individuals, organizations, and societies often seek to identify and solve problems at or below the level of concern, whereas the satisfactory solution(s) are generally found to exist one or two levels above the identified level of concern. This premise is, we think, particularly applicable to nurses and provides great promise as a way with which to meet the profession's contemporary concerns.[14]

NURSING DOES NOT HAVE THE POWER TO CHANGE THE HEALTH CARE SYSTEM

Nursing cannot change the health care system because it does not have a brief, concise, and comprehensive mission statement clearly specifying the parameters governing its meaning, existence, and realm of practice. The profession of nursing lacks a mission statement that completely and concisely communicates its reason(s) for being to clients, the general public, other health care professionals, or even nurse themselves. Without a clear mission statement, nursing remains without direction. It is unable to articulate its purpose, goals, and objectives, let alone the direction toward which it can or should move. Without a clear mission statement, nurses and nursing remain aimless, lack clearly defined prescribed boundaries and are subject to manipulation from outside forces. Justification for nursing's existence, in the absence of a visionary mission statement, remains difficult to articulate and defend. Given the present chaotic status of health care in this country, if nursing continues to remain missionless, there can ultimately only be one consequence for the profession as we know it now—death by self-inflicted ambiguity.

The health care industry in this country is in deep and profound trouble. The era of public-supported expansion and freedom of self-governance for health care institutions is no longer a reality. Instead, the health care industry now finds itself facing increasing demands for change—radical change, in some areas—from all sectors and levels of American society. The question as to whether health care is a right, a privilege, or a commodity to be owned and sold remains a core issue, as are the closely associated questions regarding access, finance, ownership, payment, and length of hospital stay. The existing system is being perceived as no longer adequate or capable of providing necessary illness care, let alone administer to essential health care needs of most American citizens and our guests. A current election year campaign theme—questioning the priorities surrounding health care in the United States asks why we, as communities, guarantee the provision of attorneys for the legal defense of those accused of committing crimes but are unable or unwilling to provide health care professionals to care for the members of our society who are in need.

Increasingly complex technologies continue to be designed to preserve and prolong the human life span. This prolongation of life has significant effects on a society due to the need to protect the lives of those whose conditions at birth are fragile and vulnerable, to the quite different but equally important needs of a chronically ill and aging population. Augment these concerns with the needs of the homeless, individuals with AIDS, the uninsured, the underinsured, pregnant mothers, young children, and victims of war and disasters, and the collage becomes depressing, hopeless, and overwhelming. Previous conceptualizations of a nurse healing the sick, injured, and dying are no longer appropriate for this new order of health care. Previously dominant places of employment such as hospitals and acute care settings are rapidly yielding to new opportunities for nurses, in such areas as nurse-operated clinics and centers, community health programs, occupational health programs, schools, outpatient care, churches, and homes.

Certainly, given the context of the challenges just identified, is it feasible for nursing to articulate a mission, a direction, or a prescribed line of movement? Recently, a group of graduate students was asked to participate in an exercise—to write brief mission statements for the profession of nursing. Collectively

their suggestions provided the following list of mission statements:

1. Promotion of individual and environmental well-being
2. Promotion of healthy lifestyles over the lifespan
3. Shape the future of health care
4. Use knowledge for quality patient care
5. Health care's future
6. Provide professional, humanistic, holistic, knowledgeable nursing care
7. Provide expert knowledge to individuals, groups, and communities
8. Health care for all
9. Holistic care of patients and families
10. Promotion of health now and for the future
11. Help human beings live life more fully
12. United effort to exert a positive influence
13. Professional interaction toward human responses
14. Work smarter, not harder
15. Light the way to health (use F. Nightingale's lamp or a candle for symbolism)
16. Health care benefits for all, emphasizing health promotion
17. Humanize the process toward global quality

The assignment was rated as difficult, and the results, while believable and applicable to nursing generally, could also apply to a variety of other health care professionals. Obviously, the statements were unable to clearly capture a "unique" mission for nursing. Unless this ambiguity is resolved at mega- and mini-levels, the profession will continue to suffer a lack of direction regarding its personal, organizational, and societal dimensions. A mission statement must be forthcoming from the leadership of the profession, that is, capable of providing direction for all of its practitioners, as well as the membership of the 49 distinct organizational segments purporting to represent nurses throughout the United States and its territories. There needs to be a clear statement describing what nurses (and nursing) are doing if we are to: (1) promote a collective image, (2) become a recognizable force in the rapidly changing and emerging health care arena, and (3) consolidate our energies under the direction of leaders dedicated to accomplishing mission statements within the scope of their organizational contexts.

Clearly, until nursing establishes precise mission statements, it cannot generate or utilize its power and energized commitment toward purposeful goals and objectives. Left purposeless, nursing's only alternative will be to remain dormant, underutilized, and marginalized as a segment of existing health care professions. Thus, when new opportunities emerge and require a commitment of power and energy, nursing may fail to respond to such initiatives.

The litany of lament regarding nursing's history of oppression continues to reinforce and inhibit nurses and the profession from articulating new missions and pursuing new opportunities. Nurses remain at risk and are easy prey—often succumbing to perceptions held by others that their work is low in value and that they can be easily replaced by family members or less-educated, minimally trained health care workers. As long as the energy and power invested by the total aggregate of nurses continues to exist amidst such self-destructive behaviors and conflicts, nurses and nursing will remain preoccupied with reactionary thinking and its consequent behavior. These patterns of reaction prevent nurses achieving any sense of self-fulfillment. Subsequently, these patterns remain circular and their focus introspective, leaving nurses even more vulnerable to the forces of external threats that inhibit or confiscate the power nurses need to propel themselves and their profession forward in a growth-producing manner.

The third component of Terry's model relates to structure—the organizational processes through which human actions move. The profession of nursing has well-defined structures and processes; however, the extent to which many are related to a clear mission statement is often not clear. The profession has, for example, a legal structure embodied in the state board examination and various legislative acts governing the parameters of practice. Each state also has a state board of nursing charged with granting licenses and monitoring the activities of nurses to assure standards of safe practice for the publics nurses serve. Each state, however, establishes its own rules and regulations governing the practice of nurses which diffuses, if not diminishes, the power held by these organizational structures.

The American Nurses Association originally perceived itself as the primary professional organization representing the profession and its members. It was so structured that additional representation was managed through statewide and district level branches as the means through which nurse members were represented throughout all levels of the organization. Another organization, the National League for Nursing, originally viewed its tasks as performing the monitoring and surveillance functions accompanying the governance and maintenance of quality educational programs for the preparation of safe practitioners of nursing. This organization also incorporated state offices; however, its real effect upon nurses and nursing remains vested at the national level because it relates to its accreditation role in postsecondary nursing education and community health programs.

Sigma Theta Tau represents a third organization whose task is to support and promote the scholarship and leadership arm of the profession. It was to be a forum for scholarship in which nurses could validate and test research-based assessment and intervention strategies as part of conducting research-based nursing practice.

The *Social Policy Statement,*[2] adopted by the American Nurses Association in 1980, specifies the following structural components: (1) the social context of nursing, (2) the nature and scope of nursing practice and (3) specialization in nursing practice. Other structures guiding the profession include codes of ethics relative to research, practice, and education, roles such as care provider, teacher, manager, investigator, and member of the discipline,[5] and the organizations reputed to represent specialties with the profession. While most of these structures were originally designed to assist nurses in unique and specific ways, such particularity seems to have been foresaken in recent years. Now, instead of representing nursing's unique and purposely diverse needs by means of specific organizations, these structures seem to have kept their organizational titles while relinquishing their unique functions.

All of nursing's structures now compete with each other for the same constituencies and financial sources. All concern themselves with legislative and licensing issues, political influence, research and scholarship, education and practice and compete for the right to represent all nurses. Thus, rather than having distinct avenues of representation serving singular purposes and goals, nurses find themselves confronting divided loyalties unable to stretch either themselves or their finances across all of the structures currently in place. The continued dilution of resources and permeability of organizational boundaries readily fosters an environment of underrealized and underutilized power and energy and as such negates the potential power, energy, and strength that is usually vested in structural components such as organizations.

Resources comprise the next dimension of Terry's[14] model and refer to the materials and products essential to the accomplishment of any mission. Given the large number of nurses prepared for the practice of nursing, one can easily argue nursing has more than enough human resources with which to accomplish any mission regardless of scope. Nurses, as resources, certainly meet the six criteria specified by Terry.[14] Nurses are usable resources. They are educated and selected for their ability to provide safe quality care. They are used in a wide variety of occupational and professional contexts. They are, in general, managed resources quantifiable in number and readily available.

Nurses are, however, more often than not viewed as being interchangeable; that is, an associate degree-prepared nurse is a nurse, a baccalaureate degree-prepared nurse is a nurse, a master's degree-prepared nurse is a nurse, and/or a doctorally prepared nurse is a nurse. Thus, when considered as being the same or similar rather than unique and distinct, nurses can be erroneously perceived as being equal in their knowledge base and capability for providing care. Unfortunately, position descriptions detailing salary and expectations relating to job performance often confirm this phenomena. Nursing continues, therefore, to suffer the effects of functional redundancy currently imposed and maintained by many health care institutions. Aaronson[1] states, "Since the 1950s the functions of different types of nursing workers have been defined and redefined . . . while hospital administrators have been successful in keeping the boundaries of occupational responsibility purposely ambiguous to permit flexibility in allocation of tasks." This self-fulfilling prophecy is bound to persist; therefore, until nurses can be and are used appropriately by being given roles, responsibilities, and performance guidelines commensurate with their credentials.

Nurses are not generally active in developing new occupations or professional contexts despite the entrepreneurial atmosphere surrounding professions in evolution. Rather, some nurses continue to seek employment in traditional institutional settings upon graduation from school, continue working in nursing for a year or two to "gain experience," and then often return to school. Others continue changing the focus of their practice or leave the profession without realizing what other directions their special knowledge, expertise, and talent could have taken them.

Nurses, as managed resources, also seem content to support the status quo. Rarely are nurses perceived as risk takers or leaders within hospitals or other medically dominated organizations. Instead, institutional policies seem insistent on keeping nurses as managed resources even when institutional policies may jeopardize safe quality care. Nursing assistants, for example, are now giving intravenous medications to patients in acute and chronic institutional settings at the direction of institutional administration. Nurses employed in such institutions supervise and assume full responsibility for the actions and judgments of those nursing assistants, who are neither prepared for nor licensed to practice nursing. Why? Why do nurses risk losing their licenses and the right to practice their profession? Nurses to whom we have spoken argue they did not have any input into the decision-making process and are now afraid to oppose administrative dictates for fear of risking their job. How ironic! Nurses are willing to accept responsibilities to keep a job which, if and when a client would be harmed, could result in their losing the right to practice that job. Nurses, it seems, prefer compliance to confrontation—regardless of the consequences.

While the preceding argument has focused primarily on four specific areas—mission, power (energy, commitment), structure, and resources—these components articulate within the broader context of meaning, existence, and fulfillment.[14] Mission, power (energy, commitment), structure, and resources might be analogous to the management dimension of nursing; that is, the action(s) and processes through which action(s) occur while the concepts of meaning, existence, and fulfillment may serve to represent the soul of nursing. Thus, when both dimensions exist simultaneously, nurses remain attracted to and actively participate in their profession. When either dimension is absent, nurses leave and refocus their talents into other areas or professions or remain captive in a profession no longer capable of providing them with a meaningful and fulfilling existence.

Meaning, as defined by Terry,[14] addresses the reasons, rationalizations, justifications, and value orientations that nurses use to explain their actions toward or on behalf of clients. Nurses are too often unable or unwilling to explain why a particular action or intervention has been used with a patient. The legacy of explanation and justification for explaining the reasons of nursing is often strongly steeped in traditional rhetoric with statements like: "because the doctor ordered it done/given this way," "because this is the institutional policy," or "because this is the way I learned how to do it." Nursing's historical tradition of being subservient to physicians, educated on the job, and working primarily in and for bureaucratic, rule-bound institutions has often sabotaged the true "meaning and context" of nursing.

Wiens[18] notes that in hospitals, performance levels expected of nurses are often reflected by the weakest link in the chain, the blue-collar nurse. She concludes hospital bureaucracies thereby impede accountability and autonomy in practice by those professional nurses who seek it. Therefore, rather than being appreciated and respected as logical and courageous members of a profession, nurses often continue to be perceived in stereotyped and prejudicial images communicated through the media. Another difficulty nurses have regarding the aspect of "meaning" rests with their inability or unwillingness to share meaningful moments with other colleagues. Thus, the meaning of nurses' work often remains a private, personal moment rather than a shared experience. This tendency toward private moments of "meaning" may be personally satisfying; however, they lessen the professional pride that comes from experiencing uniqueness as a unit of health care providers.

Elliott[8] notes that nursing has routinely been excluded from official levels of discourse regarding health care and, therefore, is often barred from influencing health policy. Nursing's problems with discourse are rendered even more complex by the many value conflicts it encounters with the society within which it practices. Mason et al.[11] describe nursing as existing in two different worlds, where the values of one world (cure) are acknowledged as being superior to those of the other (care). She indicates that nursing embodies the values of caring while the systems in which most nurses work value economic efficiency and high-tech cure. The outcome is defined as the marginalization of nursing.

The conclusion of World War II offered the profession of nursing new opportunities and contexts for meaning. The introduction of the scientific method and the development of nursing research as a means by which nursing actions could be explained and/or outcomes predicted opened up new avenues on which nursing could begin to relate action(s). However, nursing practice continues to reflect a lack of applied research-based findings being routinely incorporated into the daily care of clients. Only since the profession has begun to teach research methods to baccalaureate students and expect research studies as an outcome of master's and doctoral programs have significant gains in identifying and utilizing research-based practice modalities become more of a reality.

Nursing as an "action" has existed since the beginning of time, although the meanings ascribed to its existence have varied over time. Existence, according to Terry[14] defines the parameters of practice within which an organization operates. Throughout nursing's history, clear parameters defining the practice of nursing as being distinct from the practice of medicine have remained illusive and poorly defined. Additionally, nursing's attempts to define the parameters of its knowledge and practice base have been ravaged by the realities imposed by phrases such as "under the direction and supervision of a physician" or under the guise of "operating within preexisting policy statements." Aaronson[1] described this situation as nested differentiation, a structural arrangement in which one party (i.e., physicians) arranges for the other party (i.e., nurses) to provide services to the third party (i.e., patients). She notes this practice allows physicians to control access of nurses to patients and of patients to nurses. Patients then view nursing's services as a subset of physician's services.

Certainly, the introduction of concepts unique to nursing and methodological strategies, such as conceptual analysis, grounded theory, reformulation, and qualitative research, can infuse new meaning into the knowledge, practice, attitudes, and settings being used by nurses. Until fully incorporated into nursing, however, existence as an independent and autonomous profession will remain unattainable. Nursing as it exists today remains under siege more than ever before during its history and does not have the power to change the health care delivery system.

NURSING DOES HAVE THE POWER TO CHANGE THE HEALTH CARE SYSTEM

Nursing—in its collective self—does have the power to change the health care system. Indeed, there is no question as to the critical importance nurses and nursing have relative to their roles in the health care delivery systems of this country. Since nurses comprise the largest group, numerically, among all categories of health care workers, they have the numerical advantage. Given their visibility and presence in more areas of responsibility than other health care professionals, so too do they have a visibility advantage. Given their numbers, their visibility, and their increasingly advanced educational preparation, nurses have tremendous opportunities to utilize their power and energy toward changing the health care system.

All nurses must begin to believe in themselves, their profession, and the importance of their work if they expect to mobilize their collective power, create new structures, and capitalize on their resources. The first step toward establishing a belief system rests upon the ability to clearly define and adopt a mission statement that promotes creative and lasting change(s) while simultaneously organizing and galvanizing the collective whole (of nurses) toward well-articulated purposes and endorsed goals.

Mission statements attempt to answer three basic questions: (1) Who are you? (2) Whom do you serve? and (3) What do those you serve get? The determination of an appropriate mission statement to fit these turbulent times is not an unfamiliar experience since nursing as a profession has had mission statements formulated in the past. Nightingale,[6] for example, stated nursing's mission was "to serve humanity through the prevention of needless illness and death." Another early mission statement was to alleviate human suffering. These missions statements, reflective of nursing's concern for humans and humanity within an illness-oriented frame of reference, have served nursing well. However, given nursing's rapidly changing and expanding fields of responsibility, it is perhaps time to revisit and revitalize our mission(s). Currently, there is a need to devise a mission statement that provides direction for nurses now involved in the dual domains of illness care and health promotion.

A decade ago the profession proposed the following definition of nursing: "Nursing is the diagnosis and treatment of human responses to actual or potential health problems."[2] This definition has been very helpful in providing directions for nursing education, research, and practice. Nurses have begun to focus on clients as individuals, families, or communities, and have adopted "caring" as the basis of their unique modalities accompanying ministrations and interventions. However, Wesorick[17] states, "Saying we care and not delineating what that means is not sufficient." New mission statements, clearly articulated, will provide the guidance needed by nurses as they explore and expand their arenas for practice. Now is the time for a creative overhaul of the American health care delivery system. Nursing as a profession—in concert with its leadership core—is capable of acting on this exigency now by marshaling its power and reawakening, fully engaging, and evoking a new sense of energized commitment from its members. Such actions are necessary and essential if nursing is to seek and own its place in the new order of health care.

Power, within a context whereby nurses possess the ability to employ energized and committed efforts toward fulfillment, presents nurse(s) with awesome realities. Imagine for a moment, the power realized when one or more completed acts provide a nurse with a meaningful existence because of being fully engaged in logical, courageous, and authentic actions. Nurses already possess this power, and if they would permit themselves to recognize, rejoice, and enjoy these moments, they would slowly but surely begin to build images that foster renewed pride in being a professional. Rather than discounting their importance and their power to affect and effect people during critical periods, nurses need to internalize and appreciate those precious times when they can and have utilized their power to influence another human being.

Recently, the nursing literature has seen a significant increase in the number of publications addressing the need to empower nurses and foster a sense of pride and accountability. Indeed, 1992 witnessed the introduction of a new journal titled *Revolution: The Journal of Nurse Empowerment.*[13] The use of the word *revolution* in the title stimulated our curiosity. *Empowerment,* in our view, refers to a complete cycle of events as differentiated from the more limited phases of revolution and rebellion. If nurses choose to pursue the utilization of empowerment, it is critical that they perceive empowerment as a process whereby nurses adopt the attitudes and characteristics of an empowered group capable of managing its own profession while simultaneously providing for the needs of society. Gibson[10] used a conceptual analytical methodology to study the attributes, characteristics, and uses of empowerment. Results suggested empowerment was a process whereby people were assisted to assert control over factors that affected their lives generally, but more specifically, empowerment also exists within individuals or with members of institutional, organizational, or societal groups. Copp[7] has identified the characteristics of those who empower as including people who are "open and receptive; excitedly alive; reasonably free from undue bias, prejudice, and stereotyping; believe in justice and equity; and have resources, connections, networks, and contact loops."

If empowerment is to be useful in mobilizing and actualizing nurses, then the following facets must be addressed and insured: characteristics identified by Copp[7] must be representative of and shared among all professional nurses in this country. Nurses and nursing must develop mission statements. Nurses must energize and harness their collective power and commit themselves to convergent missions and activities. They must empower colleagues who possess the insight and articulate the visions by identifying what needs to be done and must empower nurses who possess positive professional self-images and self-confidence. And, finally, nurses must be empowered so they can share and rejoice in the success of their colleagues. Nurses must be willing to let go of control and trust shared decision making. Only nurses who endorse and live these behaviors, continually reaffirming them through personal example, remain free and capable of empowering not just themselves but others. Gibson[10] argues that if nurses are to adopt an empowerment model with their profession, such a move will require a paradigm shift in existing patterns of thought and behavior. Such a possibility exists now and should be evoking vigorous responses throughout the profession. Reformulating attitudes will occur within clearly articulated mission statements because nurses will endorse new concepts of their importance to each other and the profession. Once nurses accept their mission(s), they will engage and accomplish them in energetic, powerful, and committed ways. Elliott[8] maintains that nurses caring for patients must be considered by nurses and others as doing the most prestigious work possible. Only then can the importance of nursing's "care" work add to the integrity of health care and be reinforced and valued by all members of society. Currently, new initiatives are being made to promote this change in attitude by encouraging closer collegial ties among nurses in practice, education, and research.

Nurses can empower themselves and their colleagues by developing bonds with each other as professionals whose shared interests and meanings hold more value than individual personal interests. An empowered community of nurses will, in time, prove to society the value associated with the provision of quality nursing care. The nursing profession has a long history of dedicated pioneers whose leadership has served the needs of all nurses, not just specialized segments. Aston and Leland's[3] study of women leaders concluded that there are three distinct groups of leaders: 1) instigators—women who are visible change agents and who have been recognized for their significant accomplishments; 2) predecessors—women who had served in leadership roles during the 1940s and 1950s; and 3) inheritors—women who assumed leadership roles during the modern phase of the women's

movement. Certainly, nurses have had and continue to have numerous role models with which they can identify from all three classes of leaders. Our legacy of leadership is rich. Appreciation of the work of those who have preceded or who travel with us is essential if we are to sustain or capitalize on it. We must learn to appreciate the work of others if we are to maintain and promote positive attitudes towards the work of today. Finally, those who accept the mantle of leadership among nurses today must be dedicated toward achieving accomplishments that are collective in nature and focused on advancing the profession along a trajectory toward autonomous but interdependent collegially shared practices. Likewise, nurses who chose to be followers must be willing to empower those who lead in order to form a unified coalition among all nurses. Once united, nurses can consolidate their energies and demonstrate their commitment toward securing a unique and significant place in the emerging revolutionized health care system of this country.

Thus, the power invested in small but focused efforts and the dedicated but collective action that enhances the capacity of nurses to improve their self-image by developing a positive attitude relative to themselves and their profession will, given the contexts of practice, education, or administration, allow the profession to reenergize itself and renew its commitment to the individuals, groups, and communities they serve. The collective power of many can enhance and validate the power of one whereas the power of one often fails to excite the power of a collective whole.

Nursing, as a discipline, has witnessed significant changes in its knowledge base during the past 40 years. Tremendous strides, based upon research validated in practice, has provided the profession with a reliable knowledge base through the concepts, theories, and models derived from borrowed or unique domains of science. Nurses need to build upon this existing knowledge by continuing to research the boundaries of their profession while simultaneously incorporating valid and reliable interventions into their realm of practice. Once the power of implementing one's own knowledge base is fully realized, nursing's power to change the health care system will become self-evident.

Nursing may wish to consider establishing new relationships and alliances with physician colleagues to better assure the provision of safe patient care—particularly in those instances when business-oriented administrators look for areas within the system to initiate budget reductions by substituting minimally educated and trained workers to provide "nursing care." Nurses and physicians must begin to view each other as professional colleagues who value and trust each other's mutual concerns for clients entrusted to their care.

This means, then, that nurses and physicians must be prepared and willing to reexamine the nature of their past and present relationships on behalf of their clients. Addressing this challenge, Fagin[9] states that continuing to hold "a single-discipline, self-centered view of the future will be destructive to both professions, to the newly emerging health care system and most of all, to those who must be healed." Current economic and political pressures have created a health care environment that has been described as hostile by many who work within it. Productivity, defined in economic terms, is concerned solely with the diagnosis and treatment of health problems, activities for which nurses interact interdependently with medicine. Changes in the health care system will demand collaborative, rather than competitive, behavior among professional colleagues and between professional disciplines. Therefore, nurses need to endorse and support their collective interests more so than ever before in their history.

Structure, the third component of Terry's model,[14] addresses the organizational processes through which human actions move. The organizational structures now present throughout the profession of nursing have made important contributions in assuring safe practice and in representing nursing to its many publics. However, to ensure that they remain effective and efficient, existing organizations must reexamine their mission statements and (1) develop statements that convey their unique purpose and function, (2) offer nurses organizational structures that are diverse but supportive of nursing's collective agendas, and 3) eliminate organizations that duplicate missions and serve to diffuse nursing's energy, power, and commitment among its membership on artificial rather than real points of difference.

State boards of nursing must distinguish between the licensing examinations given to two-year and four-year graduates of nursing programs. The prevailing posture of providing one examination for both levels is an injustice to the applicants, the profession, and the society nurses serve.

Finally, some observations and comments relating to the resource component needed to accomplish missions. Nurses outnumber all other health care groups of professionals; therefore, it is a profession that is re-source rich and capable of accomplishing any mission presented it. Nurses can expect differential treatment when seeking employment opportunities in the discipline. Nurses can voice their polite disapproval of hiring practices that do not discriminate on the basis of educational preparation or accumulated experience. If renegotiation of salary or benefits is not permitted at hiring, then nurses who possess higher degrees and more experience should perhaps negotiate for earlier performance reviews and/or evaluations. Resources must be usable, wanted, and appropriate for the mission at hand. For example, given a particular staffing plan for a nursing unit, one might need a ratio of three professional nurses to each LPN in order to provide quality and safe nursing care. However, if the staffing request is filled with one professional nurse to three LPNs, while a resource allocation has, indeed, been made, it is clearly not the desired ratio, and it becomes an unwanted or inappropriate resource. This distinction between wanted and unwanted resources is often applicable to the professional dilemmas nurses confront on a regular basis throughout their practice and warrants receiving fastidious attention whenever, wherever, and however nurses attempt to provide safe care.

Nurses need to acknowledge the strength provided to the profession and each other when each level of practitioner shares his or her particular talents with each other in an interdependent fashion. Nurses must learn to value each other and their level of contribution and refer clients to each other when appropriate. Nurses need to enlarge their scope of practice by including a health orientation in addition to the more familiar illness-driven protocols.

Nurses who respond to their mission(s) will recognize the incredible power they have regarding the provision of care from either a health or illness paradigm. They will relate to organizational structures that represent both their common and distinct needs as professionals. They will realize the critical role they have relative to the entire health care delivery system and develop a deep appreciation for the meaning of their work, the importance of their existence, and a realization of the full measure of fulfillment.

Nurses and the profession of nursing no longer have to justify or rationalize the importance of their work. The meaning of their work is present in every interaction and intervention used in diagnosing and treating human responses. Being able to assist others cope with the realities of human condition is a unique gift that epitomizes nursing and is a major aspect of realizing and experiencing a sense of fulfillment.

As nurses, we must begin to celebrate the gifts of our profession and their effect on humanity. We must begin to appreciate ourselves, particularly knowledge and skill in practice, as being worthwhile and capable of working miracles when directed toward caring for clients. We must proclaim the value of our work and cultivate an atmosphere in which we work collectively toward common missions with unbounded power, energy, and commitment. Let us adapt our structures, especially those of an organizational nature, to better reflect and enhance the utilization of our vast array of resources. Finally, let us herald the influence individual contributions have to the collective whole, as paraphrased in the following anecdote:

Long, long ago, the Greek gods lived on Mt. Olympus. According to their history and tradition, these gods created the world. They brought not only the world into being, but also created nurses. And they decided it would be good to make nurses in their own image—to be as powerful as they were. But the problem was where to place this power. If the gods made it too easy for nurses to find, would not the nurses rise up one day and overthrow them?

For many months they pondered over where to hide nurses power so that they wouldn't find it easily. Each god had his own ideas. One said, "Let's place it in a cave and put a big boulder outside so they can't get in." Another suggested they hide it at the top of the highest mountain in the world. "They'll never get up there." Some said the power should be buried under the ocean. Others thought it should be hidden deep in the forest where no one had ever been. "But," it was argued, "if we're going to give them the same power as we have, surely they'll find it in all those places."

Finally one god came up with the most brilliant idea of all. He said, "I have the answer. I've thought of the one place nurses would never think of looking!" "Where's that?" the gods all asked eagerly. "Well," he replied, "It's very simple. Let's hide the power of nurses right inside themselves. They'll never ever think of looking there."[12]

Nurses do have the power to change the health care system. All we have to do is look within ourselves and to those we serve to actualize our potential into authentic action.

REFERENCES

1. Aaronson, L. (1989). A challenge for nursing: Reviewing a historic competition. *Nursing Outlook, 37*(6), 274-279.
2. American Nurses Association. (1980). *Nursing: A social policy statement.* Kansas City, Mo: Author.
3. Aston, H. S., & Leland C. (1991). *Women of influence, women of vision.* San Francisco: Jossey-Bass.
4. Berle, A. A. (1969). *Power.* New York: Harcourt, Bruce, and World.
5. Briggs, N. (1982, September). Report of statewide task force on nursing competencies. University of Wisconsin-Eau Claire.
6. Cohen, I. B. (1984, March). Florence Nightingale. *Scientific American,* 128-137.
7. Copp, L. A. (1989). That which empowers. *Journal of Professional Nursing, 5*(4), 169.
8. Elliott, E. (1989). The discourse of nursing: A case of silencing nursing. *Nursing & Health Care, 10*(10), 539-43.
9. Fagin, C. (1992). Collaboration between nurses and physicians: No longer a choice. *Nursing & Health Care, 13*(7), 354-363.
10. Gibson, C. H. (1991). A concept analysis of empowerment. *Journal of Advanced Nursing, 16,* 354-361.
11. Mason, D., Backer, B., & Georges, A. (1991) Toward a feminist model for political empowerment of nurses. *Image: The Journal of Nursing Scholarship, 23*(2), 72-77.
12. Nightengale/Conant. (1991). Advertisement.
13. Revolution. (1992). *Journal of Nurse Empowerment, 2*(2).
14. Terry, R. W. (1993). *Leadership—the courage to be authentic.* San Francisco: Jossey-Bass.
15. Terry, R. W. (1991). *Class notes.* Minneapolis: University of Minnesota.
16. Toffler, A. (1990). *Powershift.* New York: Bantam.
17. Wesorick, B. (1991). Creating an environment in the hospital setting that supports caring via a clinical practice model. In D. Gout & M. Leininger (Eds.), *Caring: The compassionate healer,* (pp. 135-49). New York: National League for Nursing.
18. Weins, A. (1990) Expanded nurse autonomy: Models for small rural hospitals. *Journal of Nursing Administration, 20*(12), 15-22.

CHAPTER 51

Viewpoints

Why are we seeing more unionization?

KAREN S. O'CONNOR

Nurses have been effectively addressing professional and economic issues through collective bargaining for more than 40 years. Recent legal advances make this a time of dynamic expansion in unions' ability to negotiate for health care workers. The majority of nurses, however, have only general knowledge about the process or its achievements. In spite of this relative lack of information, unionization in health care is increasing at a time when union strength in other sectors is generally declining. Nurses are contributing significantly to the growth of collective bargaining.

This trend in health care is the opposite of trends in other industries, where unions lose most of the representation elections. In health care, unions currently win approximately 50%. Unionized health care workers (including nurses) totaled only 14% of the total in 1980, 20% to 25% of the 3.3 million acute care hospital workers now belong to unions, although in 1990 the proportion of unionized workers in U.S. private industry dropped to 12.1%. The number of registered nurses (RNs) covered by collective bargaining agreements had grown to approximately 239,000 by 1987; the 1991 Supreme Court decision upholding maximally efficient separate bargaining units for RNs, physicians, and other specialized employee groups makes it likely that the percentage of organized health care workers will soon rise sharply. There are an estimated 500,000 RNs still eligible to be organized.

Nurses' growing awareness of and participation in collective bargaining is indisputable. Thus, the question to be analyzed is not "whether" but "why" and "how." This analysis must consider the impact of the current economic and political environment—on health care, on consumers, on individual practitioners, and on the nursing profession. An understanding of these factors clearly suggests that nurses will continue to seek out collective bargaining in ever-increasing numbers.

This conclusion has far-reaching implications for the profession. For much of the period following its formal inception, nursing has been reluctant to question the system in which it practices. Such reticence is rapidly crumbling as the profession strives to meet the increased demand for nursing services and as nursing moves into a leadership role in the health care industry.

The 1991 Supreme Court decision upholding specialized all-RN bargaining units greatly facilitates union activity on behalf of nurses. The actual processes of collective negotiation need revision, however, to accommodate new developments in society and in the work environment. The approach chosen by nursing and its representatives to meet the challenges of rapid change driven by technological capacity and demographics will strongly determine the profession's continuing success. This success or failure will have direct, immediate consequences for patients and clients.

Nursing's commitment to quality patient care is indisputable. Indeed, it is this commitment that leads nurses to choose collective bargaining. Nurses have always known that working conditions and their ability to provide quality care are inextricably intertwined. In the past, collective bargaining has proven to be an effective tool for shaping a workplace that supports practice. To continue such success, the process needs to be reexamined in the context of an evolving milieu.

ENVIRONMENT

Health care in the United States has changed profoundly since the introduction in 1983 of Medicare's prospective payment system (PPS). Cost containment was a growing concern throughout the 1970s, but despite various initiatives, costs continued to spiral. The theory of PPS was radical: prospective fixed pricing rather than unlimited retroactive billing. Competition was to be introduced into the system with resultant savings to the consumer. Health care providers began focusing on marketing a product to a customer rather than delivering needed care to a patient. Hospitals shifted their efforts toward pleasing the payers. Many believe this resulted in a major power shift from physicians to hospital administrators, insurers, and other reimbursing entities.

Although health care has always been a business, the ramifications of being a competitive business are becoming increasingly clear. The for-profit sector in health care has become prominent. Shareholders who expect dividends of necessity affect the mission of such entities. Although the not-for-profit institution technically does not make money, many factors are driving even that sector to maximize revenue over expenses. Corporate restructuring is common as facilities seek to expand their market and limit financial losses and tax consequences. Health care managers and workers alike are now accustomed to discussing competition, productivity, and marketing.

Corporate restructuring has simultaneously produced trends toward centralization and decentralization. Centralization of institutional control has emerged most prominently in multifacility chains, whether profit or not-for-profit. Centralized control moves the locus of decision making farther away from the bedside. The result is decision makers with little direct contact with the patients or the nurses responsible for providing care. Decentralization has been seen as a cure, yet it carries complications of its own. Moving the locus of decision making nearer to the bedside, decentralization enables flexible and rapid adaptation to individual circumstances. It also creates opportunities for inconsistent policies, however, and for inconsistent execution of policies within a single institution. Optimization of the benefits of decentralization increases the need for collective organization and clearly articulated aims and principles within the nursing profession.

Concurrent with these developments, theories of human resource (HR) management have become increasingly important over the last decade. The goal of human resource management is to create a positive and productive labor relations or personnel environment through the establishment of extensive communication channels facilitating creative exchange between management and employees, greater on-site decision making by employees, pay structures with fewer job classifications and wage grades, and extensive internal dispute-resolution systems.

Some observers have described human resource management as seeking to coopt unionization by providing unorganized workers with many of the benefits of a union. It is correct to say that these management techniques have become prominent in health care at a time when health care employees have increasingly sought out unionization. It is difficult to draw cause-and-effect conclusions—in either direction—from such relationships, however, in a complex and dynamic climate of global influence. For example, Japan—where management techniques giving rise to the human resources approach were developed—is far more heavily unionized than the United States; Japanese-style management was initially known here for its impact on quality and productivity.

U.S. companies are increasingly aware that in the absence of forums stimulating communication of employees' perspectives, interests, and input, competitiveness is hobbled and processes of adaptive change are arrested. Regardless of motivation, the human resources phenomena reflects a growing desire on the part of management and workers to engage in dialogue for mutual benefit. A contributing influence may be seen in the dissolution of old, traditionally divisive class boundaries; equal access to education and the resultant acceleration of vertical mobility now places former employees in management roles.

The approach does bring significant benefits to the workplace, particularly where the HR staff conceives itself to be neutral representatives of the employees. A major breakdown occurs in situations of profound conflict, however. No corporation is able to stay neutral in such circumstances, and no corporation will sacrifice the perceived interest of shareholders for those of employees. Human resource networks give employees some influence within a company. Unlike unions, however, they are not a source of power.

CONSUMER CHARACTERISTICS AND SOCIETAL DEMAND

Large-scale demographic and societal changes are placing more demands on nursing. During the course of this century, life expectancy has shown a dramatic increase. Americans lived an average of 47.3 years in

1900. By 1988, the average person could expect to live almost 28 years longer, with a life expectancy of 74.9 years. The boom-bust birth trend of the second half of the twentieth century greatly multiply the impact of increased life expectancy on health care. Nearly one third of the current population—approximately 75 million Americans—were born between 1946 and 1964. The baby boomers themselves have had relatively few children; the birth rate from the mid 1960s through the late 1970s was exceptionally low. The United States is "graying," with the proportion of older people increasing yearly. There are relatively fewer young adults to provide care.

More than 9000 Americans per day are now turning 40. In 1996, the first baby boomer will reach 50. By the year 2050, one in three Americans will be over 55.[8] As this large postwar generation ages, health conditions will typically require increased intervention. This need is compounded by the shortened length of stay mandated by Medicare's PPS. Patients are hospitalized for the most acute stages of illness and then discharged to recover at home, perhaps with temporary nursing care.

Demand for nursing personnel is high in today's acute care settings. Concurrent advances in health care technology have supported two separate but related trends: more complex, technically advanced care and simpler, more mobile, less tertiary-centered care. Both trends result in a broader spectrum of care being delivered across the lifespan. The technical advances supporting more complex care are turning hospitals into a conglomerate of special care units. Registered nurses are also playing larger roles in care management and care-quality assessment. In 1972, hospitals employed an average of 50 nurses for every 100 patients; by 1985, that average had risen to 91 nurses for every 100 patients. Approximately two thirds of all nurses practice in acute care settings, despite expansions of demand in other arenas.

The refinements in management of both chronic and recovery phases of acute illness have increased the demand for nursing care at home. Long-term care facilities are also providing a broader spectrum of care delivered across the lifespan, with resultant needs for more trained personnel. Because the availability of technically adept individuals to provide high-quality nursing care is critical, particularly for a society whose population will include an increasing and proportionally dominant sector of older individuals, the nursing profession is experiencing both increased bargaining power and a weighted investment in progressive change.

THE CHANGING NATURE OF THE PRACTITIONER

Aggregate characteristics of the nursing profession are changing. The demographic profile of individual nurses also reflects societal change.

Nursing remains predominantly female. Approximately 97% of employed RNs are women. Historically, many nurses have chosen to continue working after the birth of children. However, that trend is even more pronounced as the proportion of nurses who continue to work after having children parallels the increasing proportion of working mothers in the general population. More practitioners than ever before are likely to be single heads of household or to have income coequal in importance to their spouses. The average age of practicing nurses is now approximately 39 years. Although no clear data are yet available, the average number of years worked is probably increasing.

The trends for individual practitioners, like the large-scale societal ones, increase the investment of nurses in their profession. Older, more experienced personnel with long-term work commitments have a strong incentive to positively influence their employment setting through such means as collective bargaining.

Demographic factors also mean that individual nurses have a broad range of economic factors to consider. Child care and health insurance have emerged as high-priority issues. Salary competitiveness for nurses with 15 to 20 years of experience is a critical concern. The ability to provide elder or respite care is becoming an issue for nurses with aging parents. Pension portability and retirement issues are gaining increased attention. Today's practitioner is obviously, and necessarily, concerned about the economic return from work.

THE GROWING AUTONOMY OF THE PROFESSION

To provide high-quality, consistent care with the ability to evolve with changing social needs, the nursing profession must autonomously control not only (1) the designation and performance of professional services and (2) the physical and psychological environment in which the services are delivered, but also (3) the philosophical premises determining these service and environment factors. To the degree that any of these three highly interrelated elements are controlled by external agencies, the ability for sensitive response to needs is slowed, and care is subject to inconsistency.

Nursing employs a variety of sophisticated strategies to regulate and promote autonomous professional practice. Nurses are increasingly successful in managing institutional politics (within organizations) and traditional politics (external to organizations). Coalitions unifying the profession with a wide variety of health care and consumer groups are being used to move legislative and regulatory initiatives vitally important to nursing. These mechanisms all exert oblique impact on the workplace. Collective bargaining is being increasingly seen as a medium in which to directly shape the workplace and control practice.

WHY UNIONIZATION?
Historical perspective of employment

Nurses' decision to seek collective bargaining is complex. To fully understand the choice, one must recall the traditions of nursing and nurses' experience as employees in health care.

Nursing's traditions are firmly rooted in religious and military antecedents, as well as its ethos of service. Loyalty and obedience were historically emphasized. The role has been characterized in the past as that of mother surrogate. Nurses believed that the client's or patient's needs were superior to their own and precluded concern about economic and working conditions.

Since the late 1930s, the vast majority of nurses have been employees in health care institutions. Employers have emphasized loyalty and obedience. The implicit quid pro quo was that the employer would then attend to the needs of the nurse. However, this quid pro quo went largely unfulfilled. Congress enacted the Social Security Act in 1935, yet it took another 30 years for unemployment insurance to be mandated in all sectors of health care. The Fair Labor Standards Act was adopted in 1938 to set a ceiling on hours of work and a minimum wage level, among other things. Amendments to cover health care workers were not adopted until 1966.

In addition to institutionalized assumptions of self-sacrifice, most nurses face special challenges in the workplace. They must function simultaneously as independently licensed professionals and as employees subject to the direction of an employer. Individual practitioners have an obligation to those in their care. Failure to fulfill that obligation may result in administrative action affecting a nurse's license or a civil lawsuit alleging negligence. Conflicts arise regularly between nurses and employers over business decisions that adversely affect the delivery of care.

The collective bargaining process

Collective bargaining as a process must also be considered when analyzing nurses' choices regarding unionization. The Labor-Management Relations Act defines collective bargaining as "the performance of the mutual obligation of the employer and the representatives of the employees to meet at reasonable times and confer in good faith with respect to wages, hours, and terms and conditions of employment, or the negotiation of an agreement or any question arising thereunder, and the execution of a written contract incorporating any agreement reached. . . ." The fundamental or mandatory subjects of employment about which labor and management may bargain are (1) the price of labor; (2) rules that define how labor is to be utilized, including hours, job practices, and job classifications; (3) individual job rights; (4) union and management rights in bargaining relationships; and (5) methods of enforcement, interpretation, and administration of the agreement, including resolution of grievances.

Within this legal framework, nurses, through their elected representatives, are empowered to meet with employers and bargain for a legally enforceable agreement or contract on the above subjects. Issues such as orientation for new nurses, floating, and nursing practice committees may also be subjects of bargaining. Additionally, the parties can mutually decide to bargain on items beyond the scope of mandatory subjects and include any agreed-upon provisions in the contract.

In the recent past, conflicts between employer and nurses have usually been settled through a contractual grievance procedure that could end in arbitration by a neutral third party. Principles of equity and due process are at the heart of this method. The human resources approach is opening the way to an alternative approach for settlement, however, through well-defined channels of cooperative internal dispute resolution, generating direct or indirect mutual benefits for management and employees that extend beyond those derived from external adversarial arbitration.

Collective bargaining delivers

Bargaining on a collective basis was originally developed in the industrial settings of the 1930s as a way to equalize the differences in power between employees and employers. The collective bargaining process has proved to be equally applicable to professionals, and many groups of white collar professionals, including physicians, have engaged in it.

Collective bargaining has been the defined means that ensured nurses' participation in the delineation of employment policies. As stated, it has been used for more than 40 years to address practice and economic issues. The leaders of state nurses' associations (SNAs) initially focused on the salaries, benefits, and working conditions they knew influenced recruitment, retention, and delivery of care. Over time they begin to address increasingly complex work and practice issues.

Today SNA contracts are driving the source creating improvements in the workplace that support nursing practice and benefit patient care. SNAs have used collective bargaining to improve orientation for new nurses and nurses required to float. Some contracts have eliminated floating entirely. Other improvements include input into patient classification systems that determine staffing levels; in-house per diem pools providing flexible scheduling and compensation while maintaining a nursing staff knowledgeable about the facility; diversion of ambulances and admissions if staffing falls below agreed-upon levels; and elimination of or limitations on nonnursing activities that keep nurses away from the bedside.

Contractually mandated nursing practice committees are now almost universal in SNA contracts. Similar to the internal dispute or problem resolution teams of human resources settings, these committees provide for ongoing communication and problem solving related to employment and professional issues between nurses and management. Backing cooperative interaction with union power, they may be seen as a progressive step towards what Porter-O'Grady[15] refers to as a newer model of collective relationship.

A new model of collective relationship

Historically, the union-management relationship has been a polarized one, conceptually rooted in an assembly-line paradigm that assumes identical, interchangeable workers performing identically mechanistic and interchangeable tasks. Such adversarial, mechanical models of collective bargaining are no longer appropriate, however, particularly in human services, and may be profoundly limiting in a context where information, flexibility, and speed are primary determinants of effective function.

The profile of the nursing profession has changed since initial utilization of collective bargaining, reflecting societal shifts. Members of the profession are increasingly educated. Registered nurses are increasingly involved in management or supervisory positions rather than providing direct patient care. As nursing has turned from a task focus to a service orientation, job descriptions and expectations have become much more fluid. Individual creativity, adaptability, and decision-making capacities are increasingly necessary job skills in a workplace where mind is progressively replacing muscle.[17]

The old dichotomy that shuts a door between the thinkers and the doers in an organization no longer holds. New approaches to management now invest the worker as a partner in the operational process, delivering such incentives as joint management-labor work teams, self-managing work teams, shared governance, and profit-sharing.

Traditional unionism has had one source of power: the negative, reactive ability to thwart management decision, to slow and obstruct work by saying "no." There has not been a widely institutionalized forum within which unions were able to influence work through the positive generation of innovative advance.[10]

To continue as effective mediators of change, organizations representing health care workers must acknowledge the altered relationship between employees and management. Management, in turn, must accept union negotiations into the cooperative partnership they have formed with employees, rather than regarding unions as an unwelcome and threatening third party. By taking the unprecedented step of integrating management into the collective, health care unions will enable an expansion beyond the traditional limits into applications now made possible by cooperative interaction and the computerized manipulation of data.

Industrial unionism modeled itself—with great success—on the rigid categorizations of the assembly line and early twentieth century "scientific management." Such models are not merely metaphors, but guidelines or maps of systems that pervade and dominate a time. The late twentieth century is not defined by the machine, but by electronic transfer; its functions shape the workplace and the worker.

Unions' ability to impact work has expanded beyond the organization of workers to include the organization and dissemination of information. While continuing to drive progressive change, unions can function as the agency that links employee-management problem-solving teams from individual organizations to a network, facilitating rapid information exchange and the wide-scale testing and locally tailored establishment of successful solutions.

As cooperative participants in the operational process, employee representatives on hospital boards will facilitate integration of union philosophy and policies into management decision processes. Early and continuous access to information will enable union think tanks to anticipate change and take the lead in important issues, developing and effecting productive contributions as well as alternative strategies.[2]

By seeking to be an innovative force working directly on the behalf of hospitals and health care employees, unions will benefit nursing practice, quality of worklife, and care quality to an even greater degree than previously possible.

To remain functionally useful, union contracts must reflect the paradigm shift that has already begun to transform the worker. A major conceptual and practical revision is necessary for contracts to accommodate the flattening hierarchies, increased flexibility, and situation-specificity of contemporary work roles and conditions.

Rather than fragmenting work in myriad catalogues of detail, enumerating multiple job categories with rigidly associated particulars of staffing, scheduling, role description, and hours, contracts must establish the parameters of responsibility within the employee-management relationship. The defining conditions that must be considered include policy making, goal setting, work design, change management, and an articulated human resource philosophy whose principles serve as guidelines in decision making. Flexible process should be established within work groups to accommodate conflict resolution, problem solving, and innovation. Union contracts should clearly define the structural guidelines within which work roles, activities, and relationships occur or evolve, allowing the concrete details of operation to be designed within the specific and unique context of each individual work unit.[15]

FUTURE DEMANDS
The nursing shortage

Nurses today continue to work under conditions of a personnel shortage that is increasing demands on the profession. The U.S. Bureau of Labor Statistics has identified nursing as one of the fastest-growing fields of employment and projects that by the year 2005, the number of available positions for registered nurses will have increased 40% over 1990 to 2.5 million.

The rapidly expanding demand for nursing services is attributed to at least two factors: advances in technology requiring delivery of increasingly complex care, which necessitates specialized training and denser staffing patterns; and the aging population producing growing health care needs.

In 1991, 35% of hospitals reported a moderate shortage of registered nurses, with 8% of hospitals indicating severe shortage and an associated vacancy rate of 20%. In 1990, RN vacancy rates were 11% overall; the 1991 figure of 8.7% shows a drop in average vacancy rates reflecting both the general economic recession of that period and salary increases delivered as part of hospitals' struggle to keep staff positions filled.

Because there are invariably year-to-year fluctuations in any quantified phenomena, including levels of nurse employment, it is difficult to determine trends from such short-term data as a change between one year and the one immediately following. The overall 8.7% of total available RN positions in hospitals that went unfilled in 1991 remains above the 5% level considered average for the majority of occupations. Technologically demanding medical-surgical and intensive care areas showed the greatest RN shortages in 1991, with vacancy rates of 11.6% and 11.1%, and this is consistent with conclusions that technological advance is a factor in shortage conditions.

It should also be noted that current hospital vacancy rates, while important, do not reflect the entirety of RN work settings. The tremendous growth in outpatient and home care means that many more registered nurses will be needed in these areas. Nursing homes have shown the highest vacancy rates, by far, of any employment context. Even though hospital stays have shortened in response to Medicare cost-containment mandates, the ratio of nursing personnel to patients continues to rise, and the number of full-time equivalent registered nurse positions in hospitals increased 9.6% in 1990 and an additional 6% in 1991.

Evidence of the strain that the shortage places on the existing work force has filled the nursing and non-nursing literature for the last several years. Nurses reported a lack of adequate orientation for new graduates, floating of experienced nurses to unfamiliar clinical areas, and many hours of mandatory overtime. Patient caseloads or assignments allowed nurses to respond only to the most basic or urgent needs of patients and families.

Competitive salaries are a major influence in the recruitment and retention of nursing professionals. State nursing associations began to bargain for better salaries in the mid-1960s, when staff nurses were averaging less than $4,500 per year. Although SNAs made significant early gains, salary growth was unable to keep pace with the demand for nursing services during the time. NLRB rulings handicapped union activities.

Survey figures show an increase in average starting pay from $8,172 in 1972, to $23,488 in 1989. The highest pay rates rose from $10,152 to $35,300 during the same time period. When inflation is factored into those salary figures, however, the increases are seen to be illusory. By 1989, starting salaries had actually dropped 9% in functional terms. Highest-level salaries increased only 10% over the 17-year period between 1972 and 1989.[6]

By 1992, the relationship of salaries to inflation had changed markedly. According to data from the Consumer Price Index for urban settings, the increase to $32,000 average base salary for Level 1 RNs placed them 20% ahead of inflation-driven increase; average base salaries for Level 4 RNs, at $39,000, placed somewhat lower, at 15.7% ahead of inflation. While these figures are an improvement over earlier ones, salary potentials over the course of a career in the traditionally female fields of both nursing and teaching are in no way comparable to those associated with seniority in other professions.

The seeds of tomorrow

The values of college-age students have shifted markedly in a direction which is the reverse of that several years ago, when studies demonstrated that college freshmen were primarily motivated by the economic return from a particular career rather than its social value. Students concerned about long-term career prospects are also aware of the aging-population bell curves transforming health care into a growth industry. Nursing programs now have waiting lists in many areas of the country, and recent graduates and hospital incentive strategies have helped to soften the shortage from its recent alarming proportions. But the number of entering RNs is still not adequate to meet greatly increased needs.

The youngest baby boomers are now entering their thirties. The baby bust extending from the mid 1960s to the late 1970s makes probable a scarcity of young workers in comparison to the expanding number of available positions. The most recent Report to Congress projects decreases in the supply of registered nurses within the next 15 years and forecasts severe upcoming shortages.[13]

Not only are there fewer individuals in the 18 to 24 age bracket now, but nursing is no longer one of the few career options available for young women. While nursing continues to be dominated by women, a recent study documented that for the first time, more female college freshmen planned a career in medicine than in nursing. Current trends suggest that by the middle of the twenty-first century the majority of physicians will be women, and this is only one of the numerous professions in which gender barriers are dissolving. Hospitals are increasingly aware that they will be competing for women workers with many other sectors.

For health care employers, this means that being an attractive workplace for women will be critically important. This does not mean simply adequate income; other sectors will pay as well as or better. Creating an environment that is secure, safe, supportive of women—rewarding to women who choose to stay in health care and receptive to women's ambitions—will serve hospitals best.[8]

Hospitals are fighting the RN shortage with incentives that include wage and benefit structures designed to address the salary compression of staff nurses, permanent shift choice rather than rotating shifts, collaborative practice committees, and tuition assistance to workers enrolled in RN programs.

In spite of these attempts to recruit and retain RNs, stepped-up efforts to reduce health care costs through the legislation of factors that will increase provider competition carry with them the likelihood that hospitals may feel pressured to economize in ways that have direct economic impacts on registered nurses. If this occurs, recent gains might be frozen or reduced and the shortage will be further exacerbated. Nurses' unions will be the central players in an effort to deflect such pressures into an opportunity for health care organizations to maximize efficiency through increased utilization of highly educated, skilled, and cost-effective advanced practice nurses in place of expensive physician-centered health care.

All indicators suggest that the current shortage will continue for some time, fueled by ever-increasing demands for complex care, a demographically shrinking pool of qualified applicants and recruits, poor working conditions, and developments within the health care industry.

FUTURE POTENTIALS: THE NEW LEGAL ENVIRONMENT

In April 1991, the Supreme Court voted unanimously to uphold a 1989 National Labor Relations Board regulation providing for eight separate and distinct collective bargaining units in private acute care hospitals:

- RNs
- Physicians
- Other professionals
- Technical employees
- Business office clericals
- Skilled maintenance
- Non professionals
- Guards

American Hospital Association attorneys argued that the regulation would raise labor costs and increase strikes and organizing with resultant disruption of patient care. The Court's ruling ended 17 years of conflict, dating from a 1974 labor law that allowed the NLRB to determine the composition of bargaining units.

The American Nurses Association supported all-RN bargaining units on the basis that the profession's interests are subject to factors that are unique and specific to nursing. These factors include direct, frequent, and repeated patient contact; licensure requirements; 24-hour scheduling; and compressed wage structures. Although RNs have historically formed their own units, between 1984 and 1988 the NLRB and federal courts approved only units that lumped RNs with other health care professionals. When the NLRB approved small, homogeneous employee units in April 1989, the American Hospital Association (AHA) immediately sued, contending that the law required the board to determine a unit's composition on a case-by-case basis. By July, the AHA had won a federal injunction barring use of the new rule.

Union efforts were critically impeded during this time by the difficulties of organizing large groups of diverse professionals with divergent workplace and practice concerns. The Supreme Court affirmation that homogenous units are appropriate accelerates unions' ability to recruit members, determine bargaining issues, and develop negotiating tactics.

Hospitals have most often sought to hamper union activity by raising obstacles and demanding hearings that may go on for months or years. Policy shifts that the Supreme Court upheld dramatically expedite the unionization process, reducing the allowable delay period between petition filings and elections from 30 to 45 days.

Before the AHA-driven injunction, the 1989 ruling resulted in a rapid increase of organizing drives leading to union victories. Leaders from both the American Nurses Association and the American Hospital Association agree that the 1991 Supreme Court decision makes it probable that state nurses' associations and unions will increasingly negotiate on behalf of nurses.

CHALLENGES FOR THE PROFESSION

Periods of social, political, and economic transition are invariably difficult, and the nursing profession is facing major challenges and opportunities. The benefits derived from collective bargaining provide an unequivocal answer to the question, "Why more unionization among nurses?" Collective relationship has contributed substantially to nursing's evolution as a profession, and there is more to accomplish.

An effective response to pressures in the economic and political environment hinges on the ability of nurses' representatives to document and demonstrate the effect of nursing care in improving patient outcomes. To further nurses' control of practice in the workplace, a clear and accurate definition of contemporary nursing practice must be conveyed to public and private policy makers and to purchasers of health care services.

Retaining experienced nurses in the work force is an issue of pressing concern. Recruiting new applicants will be crucial. New approaches to compensating nurses must be devised, and salaries must become competitive with those of other professions. The U.S. Health and Human Services Commission on Nursing has called for a improvement of the attractiveness of nursing as a career.

The reduction of health care costs must be accomplished not by reducing the salaries of valuable, highly-trained personnel but through the initiation of new forms of work organization that utilize registered nurses more effectively. Appropriate nursing skill mixes must be developed for health care delivery.

The establishment of self-managing work teams in health care facilities is central to progressive work restructuring. Self-managing teams have been shown to generate the most profound innovations in approach and to produce the highest levels of quality and productivity.[2] In spite of this superior function, they are rare in the United States, where authoritarian assumptions pervade the work environment, dominating management and remaining for the most part unquestioned by employees. California Nurses Association President Mary Foley has declared the 1991 Supreme Court decision an "historic juncture for nurse empowerment."[18] The new legal guidelines for bargaining units dramatically impact negotiation's effectiveness. With assumptions rethought and methods expanded, health care unions are in a strong position to meet present and future challenges. The aims of unionization continue to serve a useful and necessary function in the dynamic political and economic environment surrounding professional nursing practice. Increasingly turning to the strength of collective relationship to improve the environment for nursing, nurses are demonstrating their commitment to improving practice where they work. And patient care will benefit as a result.

REFERENCES

1. AHA threatens fight to finish over bargaining. (1990, September). *American Journal of Nursing,* 11.
2. Altman, S. (1990, April 5) Health care in the '90s: Not more of the same. *Hospitals,* 64.
3. American Hospital Association. (1992). *Executive summary: Report of the [April] 1991 hospital nursing personnel survey. Talking points: The 1991 hospital nursing personnel survey.* December, 1992.
4. Buerhaus, P. (1992, December 18). *Managed competition and nursing.* Cambridge, Mass: Harvard School of Public Health.
5. Burda, D. (1992, April 20). Nursing shortage! Nursing shortage? It seems to depend on who's talking. *Modern Health Care.*
6. Flanagan, L. (1986). *ANA's economic and general welfare program, 1946-1986.* Kansas City, Mo: American Nurses Association.
7. Freeman, R. B., & Medoff, J. L. (1984). *What do unions do?* New York: Basic Books.
8. Friedan, E. (1991, April 5). Health care's changing face: The demographics of the 21st century. *Hospitals,* 36-40.
9. *Health care organizing: The NLRB rule in practice—A BNA special report.* (1991). Washington D.C.: The Bureau of National Affairs.
10. Hoerr, J. (1991, May/June). What should unions do? *Harvard Business Review,* 30-45.
11. Industrial Union Department (AFL-CIO). (1986). *The inside game: Winning with workplace strategies.* Washington D.C.: Author.
12. Lehr, R. I., & Middlebrooks, D. J. (1987). *The new unionism—A blueprint for the future.* New York: Executive Enterprizes.
13. Moses, E. (1992). Nursing shortage. *Nursing: Health personnel in the United States; 1991. The 8th report to Congress.* Washington, D.C.: U.S. Department of Health and Human Services, Bureau of Health Professions.
14. NLRB approves rule for unit composition in health care facilities; RN unit presumed to be appropriate. (1989, March 31). *SNA Legal Developments,* 1-3.
15. Porter-O'Grady, T. (1992, May/June). Of rabbits and turtles: A time of change for unions. *Nursing Economic$,* 177-182.
16. Supreme court hears debate on all-RN units. (1991, May). *American Journal of Nursing,* 11.
17. Toffler, A. (1990). *Powershift.* New York: Bantam.
18. Unanimous Supreme Court vote for all-RN units ignites a major campaign to organize nurses. (1991, June). *American Journal of Nursing, 95,* 103-104.
19. Unions focus on statistics in support of NLRB's proposed health care unit rules. (1987, October 26). *Daily Labor Report,* A11-A14.
20. Unions place priority on organizing, target nurses. (1989, May 12). *E&GW Update,* 1.
21. *Unions today: New tactics to tackle tough times—A BNA special report.* (1985). Washington D.C.: The Bureau of National Affairs.
22. Unions seek ways to address nursing shortage in bargaining. (1988, April 27). *Labor Relations Week,* 401-402.
23. Wilson, N., Hamilton, C. L., & Murphy, E. (1990, February). Union dynamics in nursing. *Journal of Nursing Administration,* 35-39.
24. *Work and family: A changing dynamic—A BNA special report.* (1986). Washington D.C.: The Bureau of National Affairs.

CHAPTER 52

Community nursing centers

Implications for health care reform

SALLY PECK LUNDEEN

The health care delivery system in the United States is broken. We pay too much for too little compared to other industrialized nations. Fundamental changes in the conceptualization of the delivery of care will be required if we are to address adequately the issues of cost, quality, and access. Real and lasting change in health care delivery in this country will require a fundamental shift in the paradigm upon which the current delivery system is based.

Nursing's Agenda for Health Care Reform[19] has outlined just such a paradigm shift. This proposal calls for "a restructured health care system that will focus on the consumers and their health with services to be delivered in familiar, convenient sites, such as schools, workplaces, and homes . . . a shift from the predominant focus on illness and cure to an orientation toward wellness and care." One of the cornerstones of *Nursing's Agenda* is the enhancement of consumer access to services by delivering primary health care in community-based settings.

Community nursing centers (CNCs) are key examples of the community-based settings identified in *Nursing's Agenda for Health Care Reform*. This chapter will briefly review the history of CNC development and discuss the contributions that CNCs can make to health care reform in the critical areas of increased access, improved quality, and reduced cost.

HISTORY OF NURSING CENTERS MOVEMENT

As noted by Glass,[8] CNCs have their historical roots firmly planted in the traditions of Lillian Wald at the Henry Street Settlement in New York,[24] Myra Breckenridge at the Frontier Nursing Service in Appalachia,[4]

and other nursing leaders. The recent community nursing centers movement began with renewed pioneering efforts in the mid to late 1970s in widely disparate locations, including Freeport, New York,[11] Lehman College,[17] Chicago, Illinois,[13] University of Wisconsin–Milwaukee,[23] Montana State University,[9] and Arizona State University.[3]

Henry's[10] landmark address at the 1978 Annual Meeting of the American Public Health Association offered both affirmation to these early centers and a blue print for action. In this presentation, she outlined the potential for nursing centers to promote change in the areas of nursing practice, education, and research. Additional reflections on these issues were published in an earlier edition of *Current Issues in Nursing*.[15]

Development of additional nursing centers continued into the 1980s and nearly 200 nurses attended both the First and Second Biennial Conferences for Nurse Managed Centers held in Milwaukee in 1982 and 1984. Early enthusiasm for the potential for these centers to contribute to a gap in the health care delivery system was reported by Selby.[21] Work at these first two national conferences included attempts to clarify the nature of "nurse-managed centers." The results of a Dephi survey conducted at the second conference in 1984[7] were further modified by a 1986 ANA task force and resulted in the following definition:

Nursing centers—sometimes referred to as nursing organizations, nurse-managed centers, nursing clinics, and community nursing centers—are organizations that give the client direct access to professional nursing services. Using nursing models of health, professional nurses in these centers diagnose and treat human responses to actual and potential health problems, and promote health and optimal functioning among target populations and communities. The services provided in these centers are holistic and client centered, and are reimbursable at a reasonable fee level. Accountability and responsibility for client care and professional practice remain with the professional nurse. Overall accountability and responsibility remain with the nurse executive.

Nursing centers are not limited to any particular organizational configuration. Nursing centers may be freestanding businesses or may be affiliated with universities or other service institutions, such as home health agencies and hospitals. The primary characteristic of the organization is responsiveness to the health needs of the population.[1]

The need for a more concrete organizational structure was discussed by participants at both the Third and Fourth Biennial Conferences (Scottsdale, Arizona, in 1986 and Milwaukee, Wisconsin, in 1988). As a result, the Council for Nursing Centers was formed within the National League for Nursing (NLN) in 1989. This more formalized structure has facilitated increased involvement of nurses affiliated with the development and operation of CNCs in the national debate on health care policy reform.

It has always been difficult to determine the actual number of nursing centers. In a survey of all NLN–accredited baccalaureate nursing programs, Barger[2] reported that 51 schools of nursing were operating a center at the time of the survey. It has always been difficult to identify centers not directly affiliated with academic settings. A survey conducted by the National League for Nursing, with support from the Metropolitan Life Insurance company, identified nearly 200 nursing centers nationally (academically and non-academically affiliated) in 1991.[18] In addition, the Parish Nurse Resource Center[6] indicates that at least 40 parish nurses (a special CNC model) were practicing in Midwest parishes in 1991. Although current counts are not accurate, it is clear that development of and interest in CNCs continues to grow.

COMMUNITY NURSING CENTERS AND PRIMARY HEALTH CARE

The definition of primary health care developed at the World Health Organization Alma Alta Conference in 1978 states:

[Primary care is] essential health care based on practical, scientifically sound and socially acceptable methods and technology made universally accessible to individuals and families in the community through their full participation and at a cost that the community and country can afford to maintain at every stage of their development in the spirit of self-reliance and self-determination. . . . It is the first level of contact of individuals, the family and community with the [national] health system bringing health care as close as possible to where people live and work, and constitutes the first element of a continuing health care process.[26]

Collado[5] notes the continuing challenges inherent in altering policy to incorporate an emphasis on primary health care. This is not the paradigm that guides the reform proposals being debated by policy makers, consumers, and practitioners across this country. Most of the current U.S. health care reform proposals extant continue to take for granted an emphasis on a basic system of delivering fragmented, highly bureacratized, institutionally based services to individuals. These reform proposals struggle to develop payment or rationing strategies that address "high-tech," cure-focused solutions in spite of the fact that the overwhelming body of evidence supports the needs for "high-touch," care-focused solutions.

The goals outlined in *Healthy People 2000* acknowledge the ineffectiveness of the current system in the United States and speak to the need to develop alternative delivery models. These goals identify the need to:

- Increase the span of healthy life by preventing premature death, disability, and disease and enhancing quality of life.
- Reduce health disparities among Americans; that is, improving the health of population groups that are now at highest risk of premature death, disease, disability—the economically and politically disadvantaged.
- Achieve access to preventive health services for all Americans. Approximately 18% of all Americans and 31% of those without either private or public health insurance have no source of primary health care. These inequities must be addressed and the disparities eliminated to decrease our health care costs.[22]

The primary health care paradigm is being explored and implemented in many countries throughout the world as the most rational solution to health care equity. For the past 15 years, the community nursing centers movement has paralleled and reflected efforts to develop strategies to more effectively deliver primary health care. Several key phrases in this definition of primary health care are essential principles of CNC practice models:

- Essential health care
- Socially acceptable methods

- Universally accessible
- At a cost the community can afford
- As close as possible to where people live and work

Community nursing centers provide delivery models that are suited to the WHO definition of primary care, and they can play a key role in achieving the goals in *Healthy People 2000* in the United States. Nurses involved with the implementation of CNCs have much to contribute to the health care reform debate on issues related to access, quality, and cost.

COMMUNITY NURSING CENTERS AND ISSUES OF ACCESS

Much is made about improving access to health care by providing health insurance to the 38 to 40 million Americans who are uninsured. National health insurance proposals and initiatives to modify and/or expand current entitlement programs and reimbursement mechanisms frequently focus on the extension of "coverage" to this population. While the challenge to include the uninsured in the mainstream of health care delivery system in this country is an important one, it falls far short of addressing the real issue. Many Americans with insurance coverage do not find health care, particularly primary health care, accessible. Data indicate that families covered by Medicaid are significantly more at risk for health problems than other families.[20] For example, women receiving Medicaid (a form of public health insurance) initiate prenatal care later and receive fewer visits than other women.[25] *It is clear that increased insurance coverage alone will not solve the issues of access.*

Improving access to health care for all will require more than simply making insurance coverage, private or public, available to every resident. CNCs can significantly improve access to primary health care for insured and uninsured alike in a number of specific ways. These include:

- Providing services in *community-based settings* which are already identified by consumers as accessible (i.e., worksites, neighborhood centers, schools, churches, day care centers, recreation centers, and homes).
- Increasing the *flexibility* of provider organizations by extending or changing hours of service delivery, providing additional support services that are responsive to consumer needs, and reducing bureaucratic red tape that may impede a productive client/provider interaction.

- Increasing the *acceptability* of the services provided by (a) developing culturally appropriate intervention strategies, (b) providing services in the primary language of the client population served, and (c) involving consumers in the development and evaluation of services.
- Providing *outreach, support,* and *follow-up services* designed to meet the needs of the populations being served including transportation, outreach, follow-up calls or visits, on-site child care, crisis or information telephone services, and so forth.

The establishment of a viable network of CNCs as the first link in the delivery system could dramatically increase access to primary health care in this country. The integration of CNCs with existing human service agencies, worksites, churches, day care centers, and schools would address the issue of equal access for even the most vulnerable members of society.

COMMUNITY NURSING CENTERS AND ISSUES OF QUALITY

Quality primary health care is much more than medical care. The major health-related problems in most communities will never be solved by simply implementing medical interventions. The major health-related problems of this nation have little to do with specific illnesses and cures. They have much more to do with people learning how more effectively to (a) prevent or cope with common problems, (b) provide care for themselves or a loved one, and (c) cope with existing chronic conditions.

Quality primary health care demands that teaching, counseling, guidance, care coordination, and surveillance to assure continuity be improved for all. For the most part, these are nursing interventions. Professional nurses have always assumed the role of teacher and care coordinator in health care practice settings. The provision of continuity, care coordination, and surveillance have been basic principles of community health nursing practice since the turn of the century. CNCs build upon these traditions and improve the quality of health care delivery by providing consumers with providers that are a continuous, community-based presence for all families' members across the lifespan.

Although specific delivery models may differ, professional nurses practicing in CNCs involve consumers as active partners in the health care process. The increased self-sufficiency of clients is viewed as a primary goal in CNC settings. Nurses are approachable and accessible providers of primary health care and as care coordinators and advocates, they can assist individuals and families to more effectively utilize a wide array of existing health and human services. CNCs thus provide consumers support to reach higher levels of self-care autonomy and wellness.

COMMUNITY NURSING CENTERS AND ISSUES OF COST

Significant cost reduction in the overall health care budget in this country will require nonmedical solutions. The astronomical rise in health care costs in this country are related directly to the extensive emphasis on high-technology medical interventions and the burgeoning administrative costs of a bureaucratic system out of control. As a result, specialized, procedure focused, diagnostic, and "fix-it" interventions claim a high percentage of the health care dollar. While current managed care solutions may provide short-term relief in some segments of the system, no long-term cost savings will be realized until we implement more comprehensive health care delivery models. CNCs are an important element of a redesigned system that will effectively reduce costs.

Most of the expenditures for medical care that are bankrupting this nation can be prevented if people are supported to modify their lifestyles in favor of more healthy life options. CNCs emphasize health promotion and disease prevention activities. The goal of CNCs is to improve the overall health status of individuals, families, and communities while reducing the need for expensive medical interventions.

The impact of prevention and early intervention strategies on the overall cost of providing medical care has been well documented. One simple example will be offered here. Each time the birth of an early-term, low-birth-weight infant is prevented through either pregnancy prevention or early and effective prenatal education provided at a CNC, the overall national health care budget is saved approximately $200,000 in high-technology medical interventions during the neonatal period alone. Since that is over half the annual budget of the average CNC, it is not difficult to establish the cost effectiveness of the CNC model.

Another important goal of community nursing centers is to assist clients who need medical services to obtain those services as efficiently and effectively as possible. CNCs provide an unparalleled primary health care

mechanism for the early identification of health care problems and the provision of the support necessary to assure that clients seek early medical intervention when appropriate. This also has important implications for overall health care expenditures in this country.

Comprehensive, collaborative, coordinated, community-based models of health care delivery such as CNCs offer humanistic, consumer-focused alternatives to the current fragmented, inhumane, costly "nonsystems" in place in communities across the country.[16] It is possible to control health care spending, but not without a dramatic restructuring of the health care deliver paradigm. Community nursing centers are well positioned to provide leadership in addressing these important issues of cost.

OPPORTUNITIES AND CHALLENGES

Community nursing centers provide several important opportunities for professional nurses to have an impact on health care reform. First, CNCs demonstrate the commitment of professional nurses (specifically nurse educators in the case of the academic nursing centers) to actually struggle in a concrete way with the complex and frustrating policy issues facing providers and policy makers. This increases both the knowledge base and the professional credibility that nurses carry with them into the health policy debate.

Second, CNCs provide the appropriate environment to integrate education and research agendas into a futuristic practice environment. They provide a very effective base for the development of innovative educational strategies that will better prepare the primary health care practitioners necessary to accomplish a restructuring of the system. CNCs also offer the opportunity to generate new knowledge about the nature of vulnerable populations, their perception of their health-related needs, and more effective strategies for best addressing those needs.

Third, CNCs serve to strengthen the natural partnership between consumers and nurses. Direct access to professional nurses services through CNCs will allow consumers to experience and evaluate the relative importance of these services within the total health care environment. In the long term, consumer groups will be our greatest allies in the policy struggle to reallocate an appropriate share of available resources into *health,* rather than medical care, and the concomitant issues of autonomous nursing practice roles and direct nursing reimbursement.

Finally, CNCs can serve as concrete examples of the models that we seek to define and explain to policy makers. There is nothing more effective following presentation of legislative testimony than to offer a blanket invitation to all those present to visit an existing CNC to "see for themselves." Seeing professional nursing practice in place in a CNC model, legislators can experience the significant impact that the center has on specific individuals and populations of interest. Such experiences can serve to bring important issues and potential solutions into focus for many policy makers.

A major challenge to community nursing centers currently is survival in an environment where the fiscal incentives favor more medical model treatment-oriented organizations. CNC survival in the coming decade will be directly linked to the ability of these centers to develop and test more appropriate health care delivery and cost-containment strategies. Issues of funding for this alternative delivery model were apparent early in the recent movement[12] and continue to plague the viability of CNCs.[14] Recent legislative efforts focused on direct reimbursement strategies for nurses in advanced practice are important initiatives that will contribute to stabilization of these organizations, but continued efforts are needed. Ultimately, the impact of CNCs will be determined, in large part, by the ability to develop creative funding strategies and to link current or newly defined reimbursement mechanisms directly to these change-oriented organizations.

SUMMARY

There has never been a better time to move forward with a thoughtful health care reform agenda that addresses the health concerns that threaten a generation. The current chaos of the health care delivery system and the frustration of policy makers had created an environment ripe for policy change. If professional nursing is to make a significant and lasting impact on the development of policies that alter the current allocation of health care resources, we must be prepared to offer innovative and effective models that do restructure health care delivery in this nation. Community nursing centers are leading the way.

REFERENCES

1. American Nurses Association. (1987). *The nursing center: Concept and design.* Kansas City, Mo: Author.
2. Barger, S. E. (1986). Academic nursing centers: A demographic profile. *Journal of Professional Nursing, 2,* 246-251.
3. Branstetter, E., & Holman, E. (1989). A nursing model of health care: A 10-year trend analysis. In A. Arvonio (Ed.), *Nursing centers: Meeting the demand for quality health care* (NLN Pub. No. 21-2311). New York: National League for Nursing.
4. Breckenridge, M. (1952). *Wide neighborhoods: A story of the frontier nursing service.* New York: Harper.
5. Collado, C. B. (1992). Primary health care: A continuing challenge. *Nursing & Health Care, 13*(2), 408-413.
6. Djupe, A. M., & Lloyd, R. C. (1992). *Looking back: The parish nurse experience.* Park Ridge, Ill: The National Parish Nurse Resource Center.
7. Fehring, R. J., Schulte J., & Riesch S. K. (1986). Toward a definition of nurse-managed centers. *Journal of Community Health Nursing, 3*(2), 59.
8. Glass, L. K. (1989). The historic origins of nursing centers. In A. Arvonio (Ed.), *Nursing centers: Meeting the demand for quality health care* (NLN Pub. No. 21-2311). New York: National League for Nursing.
9. Hauf, B. (1977). An evaluation study of a nursing center for community nursing student experiences. *Journal of Nursing Education, 16*(8), 7-11.
10. Henry, O. M. (1978). *Demonstration centers for nursing practice, education, and research.* Paper presented at the Annual Meeting of the American Public Health Association, Los Angeles, California. October 15, 1978.
11. Jones, A. (1976). Nursing center for family services. Overview of a nursing center for family services in Freeport. *Nurse Practitioner, 1*(6), 26-31.
12. Lang, N. (1983). Nursing centers: Will they survive? *American Journal of Nursing, 83*(9), 1290-94.
13. Lundeen, S. P. (1986). An interdisciplinary nurse managed center: The Erie Family Health Center. In M. D. Mezey & D. O. McGivern (Eds.), *Nurse, nurse practitioners: The evolution of primary care* (pp. 278-288). Boston: Little, Brown.
14. Lundeen, S. P. (1989). Strategies for community nursing center survival. In A. Arvonio (Ed.), *Nursing centers: Meeting the demand for quality health care* (NLN Pub. No. 21-2311). New York: National League for Nursing.
15. Lundeen, S. P. (1990). Nursing centers: Models for autonomous nursing practice. In J. C. McCloskey & H. K. Grace (Eds.), *Current issues in nursing* (3rd ed., pp. 304-309). St Louis: Mosby.
16. Lundeen, S. P. (1992). Comprehensive, collaborative, coordinated, community-based care: A community nursing center model. *Journal of Family and Community Health.*
17. McEvoy, M. D. (1986). A college nursing center: Idea to implementation. In M. D. Mezey & D. O. McGivern (Eds.), *Nurse, nurse practitioners: The evolution of primary care.* Boston: Little, Brown.
18. National League for Nursing. (1992). *MetLife survey of community nursing centers.* Unpublished study.
19. National League for Nursing & American Nurses Association. (1991). *Nursing's agenda for health care reform.* New York: Author.
20. Nelson, M. (1992). Socioeconomic status and childhood mortality in North Carolina. *American Journal of Public Health, 82*(8), 1131-1133.
21. Selby, T. (1984). Nurse-managed centers show their potential. *American Nurse, 16*(5), 19-21.
22. Sullivan, L. (1991). Partners in prevention: A mobilization plan for implementing Healthy People 2000. *American Journal of Public Health, 5*(4), 293.

23. Riesch, S., Felder, E., & Stauder, C. (1980). Nursing centers can promote health for individuals, families and communities. *Nursing Administration Quarterly, 4*(3), 3-4.

24. Wald, L. D. (1915). *The house on Henry Street.* New York: Holt.

25. Wisconsin Department of Health and Social Services. (1989). *Obstetrical care in Wisconsin, 1989.* Madison, Wis: Author.

26. World Health Organization/UNICEF. (1978). *Primary health care.* Geneva: Author.

CHAPTER 53

A guide to nursing organizations

What they are and how to choose them

SUE THOMAS HEGYVARY

Humans and most other forms of life exhibit a consistent tendency to organize themselves. Types of organizations vary with regard to their purpose. The most basic type of organization exists to promote survival and protect the group from external threats.

As human societies developed over time, population subgroups began to perform specialized functions. Practitioners of a particular trade found it desirable and sometimes necessary to organize itself for various reasons—a sense of identity and social support, the delineation of standards, and control of the trade. This focus of human organization continued to develop in sophistication in industrialized societies.

The development of occupations and professions has been accompanied by the continued evolution of trade associations. This chapter explores the formation of professional organizations in nursing and the continuing development of four types of nursing organizations: multipurpose, clinical specialty, functional specialty organizations, and the recently formed interorganizational alliances. This discussion contrasts existing organizations and projects aspects of the future of nursing organizations. The overall picture is of a diversity of personal and professional choices. A more extensive review of these topics may be found in a publication of the American Academy of Nursing.[6]

THE FORMATION OF PROFESSIONAL ORGANIZATIONS

In previous decades, the literature on professional organizations has centered on the development of standards of practice and alliance, control, and promotion of practitioners in a particular trade or profession. A predominant focus was the delineation of characteristics of occupations and professions and of the appropriate activities of the professional organization. That focus has shifted in recent years. Hall[5] notes the shift toward emphasizing linkages among occupational groups and between the organization and other parts of the social structure. He concludes that "obtaining and maintaining power in the broader social context . . . would be the major activity or goal for a professional organization." Hall states further:

The professional organization would appear to be the only source of power for establishing nurses as a profession and supporting its members as paid professionals. It would appear that the empowerment of nursing as a profession and of nurses as individuals can only come about through the actions of the professional organizations.[5]

Although it is clear that professional organizations need to serve the purposes of self-regulation, representation, and organizational development,[10] the current trend is to focus less on structure and definitive static purposes. Increasingly, professional organizations are concerned about interorganizational linkages and changing activities in response to changing environments. This discussion of the past, present, and future of nursing organizations reflects that changing focus.

Studies of the development of formal organizations cite three major themes, the first of which is differentiation. Lawrence and Lorsch[7] note that as groups become larger, they tend to differentiate into specified parts. The result is increasing differences within the organization, both in the orientation toward goals and in the formal status of subunits within the structure.[7]

The development of specialized subunits gives rise to the second theme in organizations, the need for integration. Integration refers to the processes and methods used to increase collaboration among functional departments in working toward common goals. The nature and extent of integration presents the third theme of interdependence among units. The integration of differentiated units requires linkages based on the type and extent of interdependence.

The issue of interdependence is of more than academic concern in nursing. Because of the very large number of nursing organizations, their overlapping memberships, and their parallel attention to issues of common concern, their activities certainly influence each other. When the views and goals of nursing organizations are shared and jointly promoted, the result can be the increased strength of the profession. An example is the response of organized nursing to the American Medical Association's intent to create three new categories of care givers. When the interests and activities of nursing organizations are in conflict, however, the perception both within and outside nursing may be of trouble within the profession. An example of an issue generating considerable conflict is entry into practice.

The following description of nursing organizations portrays differentiated units within nursing, not necessarily by rational design. Each of the organizations described below has evolved from other organizations as a response to changes in the organizational environment. Some of those pressures for change, coming both from within and outside organizations, are evident in nursing today. An individual nurse's choice of membership in professional organizations very likely will be based on the historical image, perceived goals and functions, and trends and probable future directions of each organization.

Multipurpose organizations

Two national nursing organizations are categorized as multipurpose organizations. This section describes the American Nurses Association (ANA) and the National League for Nursing (NLN) as umbrella organizations that serve a variety of functions and constituents.

American Nurses Association (ANA). For many nurses, the American Nurses Association is *the* professional organization. It is the only multipurpose organization solely for registered nurses. Its origins can be traced to 1893, through several other organizations. Its most recent merger was with the National Association of Colored Graduate Nurses in 1950.

ANA activities range from those considered typical of a professional association, such as setting standards for practice, to those considered typical of a labor union, for example, ensuring a collective bargaining program for nurses. The ANA also includes two semi-autonomous organizations: the American Academy of Nursing and the American Nurses Foundation.

The purposes of the ANA as stated in its bylaws are (1) to work for the improvement of health standards and the availability of health care services for all people, (2) to foster high standards of nursing, and (3) to stimulate and promote the professional development of nurses and advance their economic and general welfare. The bylaws of the ANA designate 15 functions related to standards of nursing practice, education and nursing services, code of ethics, credentialing, legislation, health policy, evaluation, research, economic and general welfare, professional leadership, professional development of nurses, affirmative action, collective bargaining, communicating with the membership, consumer advocacy, and representation of the profession.[4]

The ANA's achievements over the decades are remarkable, particularly in view of its internal diversity, combined with increasing professional, social, and political turbulence. In 1985, 12.1% of the registered nurses in the country were ANA members, down from a peak of 24.1% in 1970. The ANA has successfully represented the profession in many ways, despite the small percentage of nurses who are members.[2]

The ANA is the only U.S. nursing association with official representation in the International Council of Nurses. Although its approximately 200,000 members do not comprise a majority of the profession, it is still the most visible, active, and comprehensive of all American nursing organizations.

National League for Nursing (NLN). The National League for Nursing was incorporated in 1952 by a merger of the National League of Nursing Education, the National Organization of Public Health Nurses, and the Association of Collegiate Schools of Nursing. The creation of a second multipurpose organization, in addition to the ANA, was based on a decision made at the 1950 ANA convention. Because of the perceived need to restructure national organizations, the members voted for the ANA to continue as the membership association for registered nurses. The NLN, as a new multipurpose organization, would include nurses, interested nonnurses, and relevant institutions to strengthen nursing education and service.

Unlike the ANA then, membership in the NLN is open to both individuals and agencies. The inclusion of nonnurses as members adds a new perspective, as well as some controversy about control of the profession. Agency membership includes organizations providing nursing services or nursing educational programs.

The eight designated missions and functions of the NLN include strengthening and supporting nursing services, promoting research for the knowledge base of nursing education and practice, maintaining responsiveness to its membership, promoting public understanding and support of nursing, and exploring new avenues for promoting nursing such as alternative health care settings.[9]

Like the ANA and multipurpose organizations in other professions, the NLN has suffered a decline in membership in recent years. Currently it has approximately 1700 institutional members and 1500 individual members.

Clinical specialty organizations

As specialization in health care has become more pronounced, specialty organizations have gained strength and membership. This trend is evident in both nursing and medicine. Undoubtedly the growth of clinical specialty organizations has contributed to the declining membership of multipurpose organizations such as the ANA and the NLN. Membership in these organizations, however, is overlapping. Many nurses retain membership in the large multipurpose organizations and also express their clinical identity through a specialty organization.

Clinical areas around which specialty organizations have formed include critical care, nephrology, nurse anesthesia, neuroscience, occupational health, nurse-midwifery, ophthalmology, plastic and reconstructive surgery, postanesthesia, urology, infection control, operating room, pediatric oncology, rehabilitation, emergency, enterostomal therapy, orthopedics, pediatric associates and nurse-practitioners, school nurses, intravenous therapy, addictions, oncology, obstetrics and gynecology, and public health.

Nursing specialty organizations serve a variety of purposes, differ in organizational structure, and vary greatly in membership size. Some specialty organizations, such as the American Association of Critical Care Nurses, have a large number of members. Others, such as the National Nurses' Society on Addictions, have few members and offer much more limited services to their memberships.

The concern shared by these organizations—that is, promoting the identity and professional interests of nurses in specialty areas—led to the formation in 1981 of the National Federation of Specialty Nursing Organizations (NFSNO). By 1984, the NFSNO reported that it represented 400,000 nurses through its 27 constituent organizations. The nature of representation through this national federation has been very limited, however, as the NFSNO has maintained the role of a voluntary alliance of organizations and does not have the intent of formalizing any control of constituent organizations. Individual nurses are members of the constituent organizations, just as the national federation is comprised of members' organizations.[8]

The NFSNO represents a significant chapter in the history of nursing organizations in the United States. Not only does it present a challenge to the two large multipurpose organizations, it also illustrates changing trends in the profession and in society at large. Nurses have indicated through their membership in specialty organizations that they want to be identified with a clinical specialty area. At the same time, they recognize the necessity of a national alliance of nurses with common interests. Since the mission and goals of the NFSNO parallel some of the functions and activities of the ANA and the NLN, they compete to enlist members as well as to represent the profession. In a later section, this chapter further discusses the trend toward national alliances.

Functional specialty organizations

This section differentiates organizations that center on a "functional role" as opposed to a specialty area of practice. The two major examples of this type of national organization are the American Association of Colleges of Nursing (AACN) and the American Organization of Nurse Executives (AONE).

American Association of Colleges of Nursing (AACN). The American Association of Colleges of Nursing exists to improve the practice of professional nursing through (1) advancing the quality of baccalaureate and graduate programs in nursing, (2) promoting research in nursing, and (3) providing for the development of academic leaders. AACN was established in 1969 in response to the need for a national organization devoted specifically to baccalaureate and graduate education in nursing. Schools of nursing in all 50 states and Puerto Rico are represented by the AACN. In 1986, there were 383 member schools of nursing in senior colleges and universities, and the membership has since continued to grow.

The AACN has an institutional membership and does not provide for individual membership. Its activities focus on all aspects of academic concern and development, including governmental affairs.[1]

American Organization of Nurse Executives (AONE). Formerly known as the American Society of Nursing Service Administrators, the AONE has grown rapidly to a membership of over 3700 members. Initially one of 156 personal membership groups in the American Hospital Association (AHA), the AONE has continued to distance itself from the umbrella of the AHA. In doing so, it has maintained an alliance with hospital administration but also has positioned itself for more autonomy as a professional nursing organization.

The central purpose of the AONE is to promote safe and effective patient care. Its designated functions center on influencing health care delivery in nursing practice, participating in the formulation of public policy related to health and nursing, promoting nurse-executive practice, supporting nursing research and education, providing information and data for members regarding analysis, and contributing to policy formation and strategic planning at local, state, and national levels.[6]

The AONE is an individual membership organization that continues to grow in size and national influence. Its increasing identity as a professional nursing organization, combined with continued ties to hospital administration, position the AONE as a relatively small but focused and powerful national organization.

Developing alliances among nursing organizations

Several of the nursing organizations mentioned above illustrate the formation of coalitions and alliances that produce new organizations. These coalitions and alliances occur for varying reasons. One reason is the proliferation of organizations with common purposes, so that reason suggests combining forces. Another driving force can be perceived threats, either from other nursing organizations or from forces external to the nursing profession.

In addition to the existing formal alliances (the NFSNO and the alliance of state organizations that now constitute the ANA), there are two existing alliances of nursing organizations: the Tri-Organizational Nursing Council and the Nursing Organization Liaison Forum (NOLF), which are growing in strength.

Tri-Council. The Tri-Council now formally includes four nursing organizations: the ANA, the NLN, the AACN, and the AONE. Organizations such as the American Association of Critical Care Nurses, the American Academy of Nursing, and the National Council of State Boards of Nursing, among others, also may meet with the Tri-Council. Most recently, under the pressure of the national nursing shortage and the proposal of the American Medical Association for three new categories of care givers, the Tri-Council invited all national nursing organizations to participate in a summit meeting. Both the precipitating factors and the success of that meeting illustrate the recognition of the need for national coalitions in response to a changing environment.

The Tri-Council, formed in 1972, emerged as a response of nursing organizations to their multiple interdependencies and the need for a unified nursing approach to issues of mutual and national concern. It is composed of the presidents, presidents-elect or vice presidents, and executive directors of the member organizations. The Tri-Council lacks a formal organization and legitimacy as a single umbrella organization. Its success is based on shared interests and goals and on the mutual consent and benefit of the participants. Given the current pressures and directions in nursing organizations, it appears possible and even likely that the Tri-Council as an interorganizational alliance will continue to grow in strength and perhaps to evolve further as a formal alliance of nursing organizations.[6]

Nursing Organization Liaison Forum (NOLF)

Another example of an organizational alliance has occurred under the auspices of the ANA. The NOLF was formed in 1982 to provide a forum for discussion among nursing organizations and the ANA and to promote concerted action among national nursing organizations. The NOLF currently claims 41 participating organizations.

It is clear that the agenda of the NOLF has many similarities to those of the NFSNO and the Tri-Council. These common agendas and overlapping interests illustrate both the need and the probability of increasing organizational alliances in the future.[3]

THE FUTURE OF NURSING ORGANIZATIONS: PERSONAL AND PROFESSIONAL CHOICES

This brief overview has presented some of the major nursing organizations; it certainly is not a complete list. Among those not included in the discussion are Sigma Theta Tau, the international honor society of nursing that selects individuals for membership; a number of regional nursing associations, such as the Western Institute on Nursing; and the National Council of State Boards of Nursing.

Individual nurses and institutions have a variety of choices for organizational membership, depending on their interests and desires for affiliation. Nurses tend to join professional organizations for two major reasons: to gain a stronger sense of professional identity and to support an organization that represents nurses' personal and professional goals.

It is likely that nursing organizations of the future will represent greater alliances than exist at present. Such alliances, analogous to formalized networks or systems in other sectors of society, may result in greater national control of the nursing profession and in less autonomy for the many individual organizations. At the same time, however, such alliances may be essential for the future of the profession. Individual nurses influence these developments by their membership and participation in national nursing organizations.

REFERENCES

1. American Association of Colleges of Nursing. (1981). *Bylaws.* Washington, D.C.: Author.
2. American Nurses Association. (1985) *Facts about nursing, 1984-1985.* Kansas City, Mo: Author.
3. American Nurses Association. (1984). *Operating guidelines: The Nursing Organization Liaison Forum.* Unpublished document. Kansas City, Mo: Author.
4. American Nurses Association. (1983). *Staff organization, philosophy, and functions.* Kansas City, Mo: Author.
5. Hall, R. H. (1982). *Organizations: Structure and process,* (3rd ed). Englewood Cliffs, N.J.: Prentice-Hall.
6. Hegyvary, S. T., Duxbury, M. L., Hall, R. H., Krueger, J. C., Lindeman, C. A., Scott, J. M., & Scott, W. R. (1986). *The evolution of nursing professional organizations: Alternative models for the future.* Kansas City, Mo: American Academy of Nursing.
7. Lawrence, P. R., & Lorsch, J. W. (1967). *Organization and environment: Managing differentiation and integration.* Cambridge, Mass: Harvard University Press.
8. National Federation of Specialty Nursing Organizations. (1984). *The first ten years.* Washington, D.C.: Author.
9. National League for Nursing. (1983). *NLN mission and goals, 1983-1985.* New York: Author.
10. Ryan, J. A. (1983). *Force of professional control: Determinants of member orientation to internal and external program strategies of the American Nurses Association.* Ann Arbor, Mich: University Microfilms International.

CHAPTER 54

Faculty governance and strong deans

Are they compatible?

PATRICIA M. OSTMOE

Informed faculty governance processes and strong deans are not merely compatible. The survival of nursing education programs within institutions of higher education in the twenty-first century will depend to a large extent on the existence of both a strong visionary dean and a strong participative faculty.

GOVERNANCE

Governance is essentially the process of decision making in institutions of higher education. The governance of colleges and universities and, therefore, any unit or subunit of a college or university historically has been a delicate and often fragile pattern of authority, power, and influence.[12] Governance within schools and colleges of nursing has tended to reflect the typical models of university governance that have been evident throughout the history of higher education. These models appear to be evolutionary, and since nursing education entered the system of higher education relatively late, governance structures in nursing programs did not, and even today may not, reflect the structures of the university or college as a whole. Dressel[6] described four typical governance models: (1) benevolent anarchy, (2) autocratic, (3) collegial, and (4) political. In the benevolent anarchy model, individuals and units go their diverse ways with only a few common policies and rules. Few, if any nursing programs reflect this model. The roots of nursing education in the autocratic and bureaucratic organization of hospitals, in addition to the offering of prescriptive undergraduate curricula, make the benevolent anarchy model almost an impossible option for nurse faculty and administrators.

The second model of university governance, the autocratic model, is very familiar to most nurse faculty.

While this model was popular in higher education in the late 1800s, it was still a prevalent model in nursing schools in the 1960s. Many deans of nursing schools modified the model, and nursing schools were, therefore, often administered by *benevolent* autocrats. (One might speculate that the nurturing and feministic attitudes and characteristics of the deans made the benevolent autocrat model more palatable for them and their faculties.) While faculties in schools and colleges of nursing were operating under the autocratic model, the rest of the university community was adopting the now familiar collegial model of shared governance. During the late 1960s and early 1970s, faculty governance was a burning issue for many American colleges and universities, and the collegial model flourished.[3] However, it should be noted that it was not until the mid 1980s that Kritek[10] advocated for and explained the benefits of the shared governance model of governance in academic nursing. Ideally, governance under the collegial model results in joint decision making and frequent consultation among all interested parties within the university community: faculty, students, administrators, and boards of trustees. However, as Dressel[6] noted:

Unfortunately, as institutions become larger and more complex, the interests and needs of various faculty units differ. Consensus seldom exists or is achieved only after conflict or compromise. Fatigue, disgust, and the pressure of other matters often play a major role in acquiring the votes needed for majority acceptance of some policy. In large institutions, attempts to maintain collegiality have led to innumerable committees at various levels, with excessive involvement of time by administrators and faculty sitting with the various committee.

The scenario described by Dressel is one very familiar to faculties associated with schools and colleges of nursing, even those that are composed of just a relatively few faculty and staff. Faculties in nursing programs are renowned for their committee structures. Perhaps this is why Baldridge[2] postulated the existence of the political model. In this view of university governance, conflict situations result in a series of political maneuvers aimed at negotiating compromise.

In reality, no one model adequately explains governance processes within universities or schools and colleges of nursing. In fact, several models probably operate simultaneously. Unfortunately, little research on nursing faculty governance has been reported in the literature. O'Kane[15] conducted a study of the extent of faculty participation in decision making in associate and baccalaureate schools of nursing. Among O'Kane's primary study results were: (1) "Faculty reported that their participation in decision making was primarily in the area of making recommendations, not final determinations" and (2) "Faculty stated that they were usually involved in classroom-oriented, decision-making areas but desired increased faculty involvement in administration and facilities utilization."[15].

Bahrawy[1] surveyed 294 faculty employed full-time in baccalaureate nursing programs in Connecticut, New Jersey, and New York to determine actual and ideal levels of nursing faculty participation in five areas of governance: academic, student, personnel, public, and financial affairs. Bahrawy's findings were somewhat consistent with those of O'Kane. She found that the faculty believed they had substantial decision-making participation in academic affairs, somewhat lower participation in the areas of public and personnel affairs, quite low in the area of student affairs, and virtually nonexistent in the area of financial affairs. These findings are of particular interest because governance issues are again becoming more of a focus of attention in higher education. Birnbaum[3] speculates that the resurgence of interest in governance may be due in part to concerns related to declining resources. Gilmour[8] also found that budget was among the top issues of presidents and governance chairs in universities to be addressed in the next three years. It seems imperative then that nursing faculty governance structures be modified so that faculty perceive their involvement more positively in all areas but especially in fiscal decision making.

Characteristics of effective governance systems

What are the prerequisites to an effective governance system in schools and colleges of nursing? Before speculating on this point, an important disclaimer seems relevant. Birnbaum[3] reminds us that the governance system of every institution is—and should be—different from that of every other because their histories, cultures, and relationships are different. The following discussion then is more about process and goals than about specific structures and procedures.

In the ideal organization, in an ideal world, one might expect to find decisions made that maximized the goals of the organization, were supported by all constituents, contributed to the job satisfaction of employees (faculty, staff, and administrators), and met all the needs of those served by the organization (students, parents, and the public). It is my opinion that any attempt to reach for this ideal must reflect a valuing of shared governance and shared authority and, at the same time, an acceptance of the normalcy of conflict. Conflicts over role and authority occur because faculty, administrators, and students perceive the educational enterprise from different vantage points and because they have unique responsibilities.[12] The challenge then for effective governance is to design a process that helps one group or individual to clearly understand the perspective of the other group or individual. McConnell and Mortimer[12] argue effectively that it is important to accept and institutionalize conflict through open debate and democratic processes. They believe doing so will serve six important purposes:

1. Encourage not only orderly, but also reasonably rapid change
2. Promote more responsive organs of government representative of a broader range of constituencies
3. Stimulate more diverse inputs leading to the substantive consideration of a wider range of alternatives and more persuasive proposals for change
4. Reduce pressure on committees to reach artificial consensus, ignore or suppress dissenting views, and resist debate over opposing views and alternative courses of action
5. Strengthen the legitimacy of structures and processes of governance and make them responsible to a wider range of constituencies
6. Direct debate to substantive educational issues instead of toward relatively inconsequential administrative details[12]

One of the most important aspects of institutionalizing conflict is to clarify lines of responsibility and authority. The kinds of decisions to be made by the dean, other administrators, departments or divisions, committees, and campus-wide bodies should be specified. "A central element in the clarification of responsibility and authority is the recognition that both the product and the process of governance are important. This means that decisions will be evaluated not only on their substance, but also on how they were reached."[12]

Lee conducted a qualitative study of eight institutions of higher education to assess the "interplay between leadership and governance and, more specifically, on how leadership both affected governance and was affected by it." She identified several variables that affected the perceived effectiveness of university senates. Although her study looked at governance from the perspective of university senates, the variables she identified seem relevant for any governance structure. Lee's major findings are summarized as follows:

1. Senates that included large numbers of nonfaculty (this category included academic administrators) were viewed by both faculty and administrators as less effective than faculty-dominated or all-faculty bodies.
2. Senates that included a large number of committees were perceived to be less efficient and therefore less effective than those with a few committees.
3. Unilateral framing of issues, either by administrators or faculty, was often counterproductive; interaction between the two groups was perceived to produce better quality decisions.
4. Old disputes between administration and faculty shaped the governance system in ways that even two or more decades could not change.
5. The quality of the faculty who chose to participate in governance was critical to governance effectiveness.
6. The development of governance leadership continuity was a significant factor to a governance systems success.
7. On campuses where governance was viewed as relatively effective, there was a routinized formal relationship between faculty governance leaders and the administration. Regular interaction appeared to result in greater trust and more inclination on the part of both sides to resolve problems informally.
8. In effective systems, the administration's accountability to the senate was perceived to be

genuine. Acceptance of the senate's recommendations was not as important as the administration's practice of explaining why, on occasion, it could not accept the senate's recommendation or why it felt that some modification was necessary.[11]

These findings offer both faculty and administrators in colleges of nursing, who are sincerely interested in effective governance, concrete guidance toward improving their governance processes. Honest reflection and assessment of governance as it currently exists and operates must occur before the system can be improved. It will take both strong deans and strong governance leadership to subject themselves to this self-examination. Deans and faculties must consider tailoring the reward system to encourage higher-quality faculty participation in governance. This is no small undertaking especially in institutions where the reward systems have traditionally favored primarily researchers or outstanding teachers only. The problems facing health care and nursing education require the best and the brightest of the faculty be involved in addressing their solution. Governance leaders must be encouraged, developed, and rewarded for their efforts and contributions.

STRONG DEANS

What characterizes a strong dean? The title assigned to this chapter *could* imply an underlying assumption that somehow a strong dean uses *power* to attempt to control the faculty with or without a functioning faculty governance system. Certainly, those of us that have been either students or faculty in schools of nursing understand authoritarian administrators or teachers. Many nurse administrators, students, and faculty have never experienced any organization that was anything but benevolently autocratic. The curriculum revolution in nursing education reflects our authoritarian roots and is really all about learning to teach and interact in ways that are more collegial and less controlled and controlling. The difficulty that many nurse educators have had in understanding and adapting to the basic tenets of the curriculum revolution give evidence that many, if not most, of us do not understand the fundamental distinction between leadership and control. The organizational literature abounds with discussions and definitions of leadership and control. But, simply stated, leading is about guiding; and controlling is about dominating. The dictionary defines the verb *lead*, as "to show the way."[14] *Control,* on the other hand, is defined as "to exercise authority or dominating influence over."[14]

McConnell and Mortimer[12] believe that leadership "inheres in reciprocal relationships between administrators and faculty," and that "the act of leadership requires the purposive exchange of influence in decision making." What needs to be understood and accepted, perhaps more by deans than by faculty, is that leaders come from among both the faculty and the administration. The 1990s have brought a changed environment for leadership. The atmosphere of growing external controls, decreased institutional and school autonomy, and generally scarce resources require that academic leaders be able to clarify missions, articulate an academic vision, and be accountable for the quality of their programs and graduates.[9] This challenge requires not only strong administrative leadership but recognition and utilization of strong faculty leadership.

The strong dean of the twenty-first century will share common values and goals of the faculty. This dean will be a futurist, an opportunist, and a pathfinder. The dean will need to be a transforming leader who engages with others in such a way that the dean and the faculty raise one another to higher levels of "motivation and morality."[4] Green[9] argues that leaders in the late twentieth century and beyond will be required to perform five tasks: serve as a symbolic leader, achieve workable unity, serve as a team leader, function as an information executive, and operate as a future agent. If these tasks characterize a strong dean, then such a dean will be very effective in working with the faculty governance system in schools and colleges of nursing.

STRONG FACULTY

The compatibility of a strong dean and the faculty governance system rest not only on the abilities, interaction style, and vision of the dean but also on the expertise, interaction style, broad perspective, and leadership talents of a strong faculty. Ostmoe and Sparks[16] described the need for faculty who are scholars and demonstrate their scholarship not only in research but also in their teaching, practice, and service. Other researchers have found that faculty with highest rates of published research show a statistically greater preference for institutional service than faculty who are less productive.[13] Almost 20 years ago, Fulton and Trow[7] also found that in leading universities more than

half of the highly active researchers spent more than 10% of their time on administration compared with one third of the "inactives." These findings are encouraging because they lead one to conclude that those faculty who are the most up-to-date in their area of expertise are also those most likely to be concerned about and involved in faculty governance and faculty leadership. It is becoming increasingly clear, however, that the rewards to faculty who spend their time in governance affairs and faculty leadership must be direct rather than indirect. Faculty who are visionary, who have an institutional perspective, who take risks, who inform themselves and others, who listen, who speak, and who care must be rewarded by the dean, by department and division chairs, and by their colleagues in personnel committees. Not only should such faculty be rewarded, but a dean who sincerely wants to promote faculty leadership development will keep faculty well informed, seek faculty's advice on all significant issues, especially those involving personnel and fiscal matters, and use their faculty's initiatives as part of the college's strategic planning.[17] Conversely, faculty leaders will likewise keep the dean informed, seek the dean's perspective on significant issues, and contribute to the strategic plan of the college.

A well-informed organization is able to respond intelligently and wisely to the changing economic, political, and social influences that constitute a school/college's future challenges.[17] Openness, honesty, sharing of information, and collaborative leadership among all significant players in the school or college will benefit everyone. Even the most complex colleges will be responsive to change and embrace innovation. Students will flourish, the work environment will be exciting and satisfying, and the health care of the clients will be improved.

Pollock's[18] research appears to confirm the value of the approach suggested in this chapter. Her top-ranked schools of nursing study was designed to delineate a composite of elements that constituted a top ranked school. She found a "clear separation between administrative decisions and faculty decisions;" "an atmosphere of freedom and challenge;" "good working relations between faculty and their administrators; they worked together toward common goals, and there was mutual trust;" "there was mutually consistent planning for organizational and individual growth which benefited both the faculty and nursing program;" and "faculty had opportunities for input without excessive meetings."

SUMMARY

In summary, faculty governance and strong deans are compatible if the organizational culture ascribes to and implements DePree's[5] beliefs about leadership. He writes,

A future leader has consistent and dependable integrity, cherishes heterogeneity and diversity, searches out competence, is open to contrary opinion, communicates easily at all levels, understands the concept of equity and consistently advocates it, leads through serving, is vulnerable to the skills and talents of others, is intimate with the organization and its work, is able to see the broad picture, is a spokesperson and diplomat, tells why rather than how.

Our education and attributes as nurses have prepared all of us for this form of leadership. If we can overcome our traditions and past acculturation, we can have dynamic and productive leadership and governance in all our colleges and schools of nursing. Deans and faculties can and must work together if our schools are going to flourish into the twenty-first century.

REFERENCES

1. Bahrawy, A. A. (1992). Participation of nursing faculty in university governance. *Journal of Nursing Education, 31*(3), 107-112.
2. Baldridge, J. V. (1971). Introduction: Models of university governance—bureaucratic, collegial, and political. In J. V. Baldridge (Ed.), *Academic governance.* Berkeley, Calif: McCutchan.
3. Birnbaum, R. (Ed.). (1991). *Faculty in governance: The role of senates and joint committees in academic decision making.* San Francisco: Jossey-Bass.
4. Burns, J. M. (1978). *Leadership.* New York: Harper & Row.
5. DePree, M. (1989). *Leadership is an art.* New York: Doubleday.
6. Dressel, P. L. (1981). *Administrative leadership.* San Francisco: Jossey-Bass.
7. Fulton, D., & Trow, M. (1974). Research activity in American higher education. *Sociology of Education, 47,* 29-73.
8. Gilmour, J. E. (1991). Participative governance bodies in higher education: Report of a national study. In R. Birnbaum (Ed.), *Faculty in governance: The role of senates and joint committees in academic decision making.* San Francisco: Jossey-Bass.
9. Green, M. F. (1988). Toward a new leadership model. In M. F. Green (Ed.), *Leaders for a new era.* New York: Macmillan.
10. Kritek, P. B. (1985). Faculty governance: A key to professional autonomy. *Journal of Nursing Education, 24*(9), 356-359.
11. Lee, B. A. (1991). Campus leaders and campus senates. In R. Birnbaum (Ed.), *Faculty in governance: The role of senates and joint committees in academic decision making.* San Francisco: Jossey-Bass.
12. McConnell, T. R., & Mortimer, K. P. (1971). *The faculty in university governance.* Berkeley, Calif: University of California Center for Research and Development in Higher Education.
13. Megel, M. E., Langston, N. F., & Creswell, J. W. (1988). Scholarly productivity: A survey of nursing faculty researchers. *Journal of Professional Nursing, 4*(1), 45-50.
14. Morris, W. (Ed.). (1976). *The American heritage dictionary of the English language.* Boston: Houghton Mifflin.
15. O'Kane, P. K. (1984). Faculty and administrator perceptions of decision making. *Journal of Nursing Education, 23*(8), 329-331.
16. Ostmoe, P. M., & Sparks, R. K. (1990). Issues related to promotion and tenure, revisited. In J. C. McCloskey & H. K. Grace (Eds.), *Current issues in nursing* (3rd ed.). St Louis: Mosby.
17. Plante, P. R. (1988). In support of faculty leadership: An administrator's perspective. In M. F. Green (Ed.), *Leaders for a new era.* New York: Macmillan.
18. Pollock, S. E. (1986). Top-ranked school of nursing: The role of the dean. *Journal of Nursing Education, 25*(8), 315-318.

CHAPTER 55

Shared governance in nursing

What is shared, who governs, and who benefits?

MERIDEAN L. MAAS, JANET P. SPECHT

Governance or self-regulation has long been recognized as a privilege given to professions that earn the public trust by demonstrating accountability for their specialized practice.[26] To assure that professionals will not misuse autonomy for their own rather than their clients' interests, society requires professionals to demonstrate accountability for their actions.[19] Nursing has developed many self-regulating mechanisms (codes of ethics, standards, credentialing and accreditation criteria, and guidelines for peer review) demonstrating the ability to govern its members in the public interest;[23] however, gaining the privilege of governance has been slow. Professional nursing governance in practice settings, where medicine and administrators who benefit from the subordinate employee status of nurses have dominated, has been especially constrained.

Although there have been isolated examples of the implementation of models of professional nursing governance in organizations over several decades,[10,11,14,19,24,33] recognition of the need for nursing governance in hospitals has been most focused since the 1980s. The value of nursing to the delivery of health care in hospitals has risen and become more visible because of relentless technological and medical advances and costs. After a period of widespread use of registered nurses to provide a variety of services to allow the downsizing of other departments and workers that assist nurses, hospitals began to reconsider the best use of nursing knowledge and skills. The folly of using nurses to perform the functions of a number of other workers and to do work for which they are highly overqualified became clearer as the undersupply of nurses compared to demand reached critical proportions. While the demand for nurses grew, increasing numbers of nurses demonstrated dissatisfaction with their jobs and careers by moving to part-time work, leaving nursing for other careers, or moving to other practice settings after a brief period of employment.[32] A decreasing number of persons entered the nursing field due to low pay, limited career advancement opportunities, and a greater number of career options for women.[3]

Finally, demands for more accountability for the outcomes of care have accompanied the pressures to control costs. As a result, nurse and hospital administrators are recognizing that the staff nurse, at the point of contact with the patient, is in a critical role to assure the delivery of quality care.[35]

These and other factors have encouraged nurse executives in hospitals to move to models of nursing practice that increase nurse autonomy for clinical decision making and participation in decision making throughout the organization. Shared governance models have been a popular strategy in the 1980s and early 1990s to increase nurse job satisfaction and retention and to achieve cost effective quality outcomes.[36] Empowering nurses within the hospital decision-making system, particularly with regard to increasing nurses' authority and control over nursing practice, has been the stated aim of shared governance models. There are a number of issues, however, that are apparent as increasing numbers of hospitals initiate changes to implement shared governance. These issues include: (1) lack of clearly defining criteria for shared governance, (2) mixed motives for the implementation of nursing shared governance, (3) disagreement about how shared governance can and should be implemented, and (4) concerns about the effects of shared governance on different roles within nursing and hospital systems.

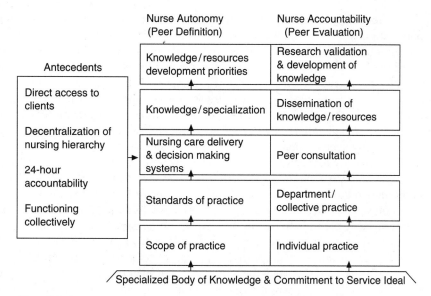

Fig. 55-1 Iowa Veterans Home model of professional nursing practice. *(From Maas, M. L. [1989]. Professional practice for the extended care environment: Learning from one model and its implication.* Journal of Professional Nursing 5(22), 66-76.) © W. B. Saunders Company. Used with permission.

SHARED GOVERNANCE – WHAT IS IT?

There is need to clarify the concept of shared governance and the structures and processes that must be in place for implementation in employing organizations if the nursing profession is to honor its contract with society as described in the American Nurses Association's *Social Policy Statement.*[1] The concept of shared governance comes from recognition of the need to accommodate two systems of authority when professionals are employed in organizations. In organizations, authority is ordinarily vested in positions arranged in a hierarchy, with positions higher in the hierarchy assigned a greater scope of authority than positions below them. Although professionals employed by organizations occupy positions with corresponding organizational authority, they also have authority as a function of membership in their profession.[25] For a profession, authority is based on specialized knowledge. To get important jobs done effectively by experts who are also competent judges of the needed expertise, society gives professionals autonomy. When professionals are employed by organizations, there is always the danger that the societal needs that are entrusted to the profession will become subordinated to the organization's needs. This is the critical reason why governance shared by the organization and its employed professionals has evolved.

Nursing-shared governance in organizations is synonymous with professional nursing practice in organizations that employ nurses.[21] In nursing, shared governance means that nurse employees and the organization are partners in meeting the goals of the organization and the mandates of the nursing profession.[29,30] However, descriptions of the requisite structures and processes for claimed shared governance models are often incomplete or unclear. Unless the individual and collective authority and accountability of professional nursing staff for decisions that define and regulate nursing practice and for decisions shared with management, including the management of resources, are codified with decision-making structures and processes in place in the organization, nursing shared governance does not exist.

As illustrated in Fig. 55-1, specialized knowledge and commitment to a service ideal are the foundation for professional nurse autonomy and accountability.[21] Professional nursing autonomy means that professional nurses have the authority to define and decide what services they will provide and what constitutes safe and effective practice. Professional accountability means responsibility and answerability to authority for the services rendered. That is, the profession takes action to assure that the practice of its members is safe and effective. Thus, organizational structures of decision making, coordination, and control, set forth in a constitution and by-laws, are needed to: (1) enable nurse peer definition of the scope of nursing practice, standards of practice, nursing delivery system, qualifications for selection of staff, and knowledge and resources required; and (2) enable peer evaluation of the practice, promotion, and retention of individual nurses; evaluation of the department (collective) practice; peer consultation; dissemination of knowledge and development of knowledge through research. Contrary to some definitions that describe shared governance as a structure for staff nurse autonomy,[27] the structure must enable professional autonomy and accountability of all professional nurses, as individuals and as a collective, if governance is shared by the organization and employed professional nurses.[20] All registered professional nurses, regardless of position in the organization (e.g., staff nurse, clinical specialist, nurse researcher, nurse educator, nurse manager, or nurse administrator), must have professional autonomy and accountability as individuals and as a collective of peers.[19]

There is much variation in the organizational models implemented under the label of shared governance. A number of different terms, such as participation in decision making, participative management, self-governance, empowerment, and professional practice, are used that are, at times, intended to be synonyms for shared governance and, at other times, to indicate different organizational models with varying degrees of nurse participation in decision making. There appears to be consensus that shared governance means some amount or type of shared decision making by nursing staff and nursing management. There is less clarity and agreement regarding what specific decisions are made or shared by nurses and management, what nursing staff are included in the shared governance, and whether nurses as individuals and/or as a collective have authority and accountability for certain decisions. Thus, models of practice implemented under the label of shared governance include those with minimal, ad hoc, or informal participation of some or all nursing staff in a very limited number of decisions with little or no expectation for nursing staff accountability for decisions and range to models where the profession and the organization truly share authority and accountability for the profession's mandates and organization's mission.

Because all nursing staff do not have the specialized knowledge and socialization to the service ideal that professional nurses do, it should be obvious that de-

mocracy in the workplace is not nursing shared governance. Nursing staff who assist registered professional nurses in the delivery of care are clearly not qualified to govern the profession, although they can participate in decisions. It is less obvious and more controversial to assert that all registered nurses (RNs) are qualified to assume professional autonomy and accountability. All RNs share the profession's mandate; however, there is a great variation in their knowledge, education, and experience. Implementation of shared governance requires that RNs who are expected to assume professional autonomy and accountability are prepared to do so. This means that initial shared decisions of organization and nursing leadership who are implementing shared governance must be the definition of criteria for admitting RNs to professional decision-making privileges and agreement on the programming and resources needed to assist RNs who desire to meet the criteria.

The controversy over what decisions professional nurses and organization management should make mostly focuses on a debate about whether nurses who are not managers can decide matters of resource distribution. This is simply a concern about loss of control on the part of managers and reflects a lack of commitment to professional nursing governance. Professional shared governance requires that all nurses in the organization develop a consensus about goals and priorities and the expectations that available resources will be allocated accordingly. All nurses are kept aware of the available resources and share the planning of their allocation and the responsibility to develop alternatives when there is shortfall. Specific areas of authority and responsibility for different roles (e.g., managers, educators, and clinicians) are defined in writing in a constitution, and by-laws and control for decisions is placed with those who carry them out.[13] Disagreements about decisions are resolved through negotiation. Although the development of the consensus, structures, and expectations for shared governance is not easy, resistance to doing it because of concern about who will make what decisions is most often a lack of commitment to professional nursing practice and an unwillingness to relinquish control.

Professional nurse participation in decision making, empowerment of nurse professionals, participative management, and work redesign each are coincident and necessary for professional shared governance, but none are synonymous with it. Often, but not always, the goals of work redesign are to enhance the authority of nurses and rectify organizational problems that con-

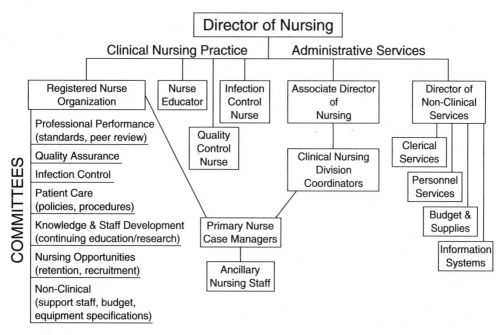

Fig. 55-2 Iowa Veterans Home department of nursing. *(From Maas, M. L. [1989]. Professional practice for the extended care environment: Learning from one model and its implications.* Journal of Professional Nursing 5(22), *66-76.)* © W. B. Saunders Company. Used with permission.

tribute to suboptimal use and turnover of professional nurses.[37] Thus, the goal of work redesign efforts may be directed towards implementation of shared governance models. However, the goals of many work redesign efforts are also to increase the participation of nurses in decision making without providing the structures whereby nurses have professional authority and accountability for all decisions affecting nursing practice. It is nurses who must be astute about the distinctions among these concepts, so that they are not misled into believing they are sharing governance with management as professionals, when in fact they are not equal partners in meeting the mandates of the profession or the goals of the organization. If the structures enabling professional autonomy and accountability outlined in Fig. 55-1 are not implemented, nursing shared governance is not operational. Fig. 55-2 provides one example of decision making, coordination, and control structures defined in a constitution and by-laws that enable nursing shared governance in an organization.[21]

Clarity about nursing shared governance is essential if it is to be more than one more "bandwagon" that is jumped on without being anchored to a clear theoretical base and commitment to enabling professional nursing practice. Some argue that nursing's knowledge base is insufficient to support control of practice as

professionals and that the majority of nurses do not want more professional authority and accountability. Others complain that shared governance is little more than a philosophy, just a fad, or a nursing self-aggrandizement and that there is no empirical evidence that benefits accrue when nurses have more professional autonomy.[34] A few even assert that shared governance tends to sound like a religion when the convicted argue its merits. Admittedly, the recent description of change to shared governance in hospitals as "transformation" may sound a bit like "being born again," connoting a spiritual experience rather than a functional model of social organization that has been derived from sound theory and empirically validated.[31]

The claim by some that nurses are unwilling to exercise self-discipline and act in the public's interest is unfounded. As a profession, nursing has demonstrated over and over again that it is worthy of the public's trust and that it is able to govern its members in accord with that trust.[26] Nurse administrators who observe that staff nurses appear to be unwilling to assume professional authority and accountability are too often noting the behaviors of nurses who have been used and abused to benefit others. These nurses have typically experienced capricious changes, a lack of power and control over a heavy workload, and a lack of socialization in the knowledge and skills needed for organizational and interdisciplinary politics. There is evidence that professional nurses welcome shared governance if it is implemented with their participation, with ample opportunity to gain the needed knowledge and skills for consensus decision making, and with the appropriate organizational structures for professional authority and control of practice in place.[18] Further, there is evidence that nursing's knowledge base is sufficient to support control of practice and that nurses participate more actively in the development and dissemination of knowledge in a professional model of practice.[18,24]

If nursing is to achieve professional practice in employing organizations, nurses in all roles must be clear about what it is. Equally important is the need to examine the motives of those who say they have implemented or seek to implement shared governance models.

MOTIVES FOR SHARED GOVERNANCE: IS IT THE "OPIATE FOR THE NURSES?"

While it is assumed that the motives for implementing all shared governance models are to enhance the delivery of care, these motives are mixed in regard to commitment to enabling the work of the professional nurse. Because shared governance is currently a popular concept among nurses, many hospitals boast shared governance as a desirable feature of their organization with minimal structures of shared governance in place. In some cases, the motive seems to be to increase nurses' perceptions of empowerment for practice without actually divesting power from the organization hierarchy to nurses as professionals.[29,30] Clearly, organization and nurse managers have been reluctant to relinquish power and control over decisions that influence nursing and the organization. Recently, because of nurse dissatisfaction with the practice environment, collective bargaining and collective action have become more of a perceived threat to nurse and hospital administrators.[15] Thus, administrators' decisions to implement shared governance may be based on selection of the better of two less than desirable choices: shared governance rather than collective bargaining. When collective bargaining or some other collective threat is perceived, wise nurse administrators seek models that integrate the "threat" with structures of shared governance.[5]

Too often, nurses have had their hopes raised that they are gaining authority and control over the circumstances of their work and their ability to effect patient care priorities, only to have these hopes dashed by the whims of those who hold the real power in the organization. Implementation of shared governance may simply be a strategy to gain what management wants without actual gains in decision making authority for nurses. Nurses may not initially recognize that what is portrayed as shared governance does not provide them with authority and control over their practice or enable nursing and the organization to meet the professional mandate and organizational goals as partners. However, they soon recognize their lack of power and become frustrated and disillusioned. This is when nurses are apt to leave employment or withdraw to the safety of the traditional hierarchy, where they seek minimal accountability and investment of time, energy, and risk in their jobs. These circumstances underscore the importance of nurses' understanding of what shared governance is, what it entails in terms of nurses' authority and accountability for decision making, and how shared governance is best implemented in organizations.

IMPLEMENTATION OF SHARED GOVERNANCE: IS THERE A BEST WAY?

It has been noted that shared governance models are not the same in all settings and that this variation is appropriate because of cultural and system operational differences.[28,38] However, there is a current debate about whether implementation is best orchestrated from the top down or from the bottom up and whether shared governance can be operational as separate unit-based models as opposed to whole system models. Certainly, there is agreement that the nursing and hospital administrations must be supportive of the changes in any case.[12,18,29,30] There is less agreement, however, about how to involve the whole staff in the change process and about which is better, unit by unit implementation or simultaneous, phased-in implementation of change to shared governance throughout an entire nursing department.[4,6,29,30] Although unique issues must be addressed with each approach, it is the view here that either approach is appropriate, depending on the situation and assuming that principles of participative change and socialization of nurses are not violated.

Leadership from nursing administration and from clinical nurses who have a vision regarding nursing shared governance is essential. These persons must begin to define the objectives and expectations of nurses and create the organizational circumstances whereby all nurses can participate to conceptualize and implement shared governance. Planned change, rather than directive change, is necessary.[8] Paradoxically, bureaucratic methods are used at the outset to reinforce expectations about professional practice, participation, and change. However, participation of all nurses to gain an understanding of shared governance and new organizational goals, develop new meanings about the nurse's role and work, and acquire new skills and behaviors needed to enact shared governance soon shifts the predominate decision making methods to collaboration, negotiation, and consensus. Whether implementation of shared governance is top down throughout the whole organization or bottom up, unit by unit, nursing administrators and managers become consultants, teachers, coaches, and facilitators.

In either approach, nurses must be assisted to learn the skills of confrontation, negotiation, collaboration, and consensus decision-making.[18] They must also understand the requirements of professional practice and what it means to be accountable as a professional.[38] Through consensus decision making, combined with the expectation of accountability, nurses must develop shared beliefs and values about standards of practice and the structures and processes that will best assure their enactment.[18] Consensus decision making promotes collegiality and the responsible use of collective action by all nurses, regardless of position.

If the unit-based approach to the implementation of shared governance is chosen, one advantage is that more nurses involved in the change will likely be committed to it from the outset. Implementation is more focused and involves fewer nurses. Following success on one or more units, other units are apt to become interested, choose to implement shared governance, and profit from the experience of the pioneering units. However, nursing administration and the nurses on the pioneering units will need to be cognizant of the effects of shared governance in one or a few units on the rest of the nursing department and organization. Different patterns and modes of communication and decision making will necessarily exist between the nurses on units with shared governance and nurses on other units, nurse administrators and managers, persons in other departments, and members of other disciplines. Finally, the scope of shared governance implemented on single units will be constrained at the outset because collective authority and accountability cannot include all nurses in the organization. With unit-based shared governance, the collective, central power and influence

of nursing is diluted. Nursing administration will need to retain the prerogative for any decisions that affect the nursing department or organization as a whole until all units implement shared governance and the partnership for decisions between all nursing professionals and the organization is defined. For this reason, unit-based implementation may be more appealing to some nurse administrators who wish to dilute the collective power of nurses. Because of the limited scope of unit-based shared governance, progress to a full partnership of shared governance between nursing and the organization may be very slow or may never evolve. Shared governance is not fully implemented until there are structures for all professional nurses to collectively make department wide decisions and negotiate these decisions with administration.[7]

With the whole-system approach, the issues focus on how to involve large numbers of nurses in the change process so that they learn the skills of consensus decision making, participate in decision making, develop shared meanings, and actualize the behaviors of professional autonomy and accountability. If shared governance is implemented throughout an entire system, individual nurses should be deprived the choice to not participate and to not be accountable professionals. This can present difficult problems because nurses will have different amounts of understanding and commitment to professional practice. Nursing administration must expect all nurses, regardless of position, to plan and implement the changes needed for nursing to share governance with the organization. In this regard, nursing administrators must depend on middle and first line managers to support the change to shared governance and to alter their roles to become facilitators, teachers, and consultants for each other and for staff nurses. If middle managers are not committed to shared governance and resist the needed changes, many problems will ensue. The effects of shared governance on middle- and first-line managers, as well as on nursing and organization line and staff roles, staff nurse roles, and the roles of members of other disciplines have to be anticipated with plans carefully made to prepare position occupants for the needed changes and skills.[38]

ROLE AND SYSTEM EFFECTS OF SHARED GOVERNANCE

Little empirical data has been reported about the effects of implementation of shared governance models on individual staff nurses' roles, the roles of managers and administrators, or on organizational systems, their structures, and processes.[38] Most literature focuses on the effects of shared governance on the role of the nurse manager and on the authority and accountability of the staff nurse.[17,19,29,30]

There is agreement that management styles have to change along with organizational structures that enable professional nursing shared governance.[19,29,30] As stated above, the role of management becomes one of consulting, teaching, collaborating, and creating an environment with the structures and resources needed for the practice of nursing and shared decision making between nurses and the organization.[36] This new role is foreign to many managers. Although managers will retain responsibility for specified functions, they will share accountability with all nurses and act in accord with the consensus among nurses about goals and priorities. Because rules about sharing decisions between management and the profession are ambiguous, managers experience stress and anxiety especially in the early stages of implementing shared governance.[38]

Managers also experience role stress because of the added time and costs required to enable consensus decision making among nurses.[12] If not supported by organization and nursing administration, middle- and first-line managers, even though committed to shared governance, may not choose to expend the effort or take the risks needed to enable nurses to develop the needed consensus. Nurses need to be able to meet together for consensus decision making, and it is managers who must facilitate their doing so. Administrators who are serious about implementing shared governance will prepare managers for the new role and support them throughout the lengthy change process. Administrators who are serious about implementing shared governance will also relinquish control of the decisions for which professional nurses are accountable.

For staff nurses, the critical role changes with shared governance are increased accountability and risk. All problems can no longer be blamed on others because all nurses share decisions and accountability for their outcomes. As noted earlier, new understandings and skills are needed. Perhaps most stressful to nurses is the accountability for knowledge to support the decision-making authority of professionals. However, role conflict and ambiguity are also stressors. An important example of role conflict with management is when resources are not considered appropriate for quality care.[29,30] Rather than being avoided or ignored as sources of dissatisfaction, shared governance pro-vides the structures and processes for conflict resolution and role clarification through confrontation, negotiation, and consensus decision making.

Staff nurses should be salaried rather than paid an hourly wage, with salaries set commensurate with the added accountability and investment required of a participant in shared governance.[16] Further, salaried staff nurses should have more flexible hours and greater control over their time with accountability shared among nurses for patient care coverage. Staff nurses often fear being salaried because they believe administration may take advantage of them and make inordinate demands for their time. Administrators also often resist changing from hourly wages to salaries for staff nurses. Administrators fear that they will lose control and will not be able to hold nurses accountable for an equitable exchange of investment and productivity for salary. Shared governance, with staff nurses salaried, provides the means for the most benefits to accrue to all parties—nurses, the organization, and patients—if nurses are also afforded the rights and privileges ordinarily enjoyed by salaried professionals and are held accountable for cost effective practice.

CONCLUSION

Because almost all practicing nurses are employed, nursing shared governance in employing organizations is imperative if the profession is to fulfill its social contract.[1] Implementation of shared governance models that enable professional nursing practice is jeopardized, however, when there is lack of clarity about what shared governance is and when shared governance is confused with other organizational innovations that are similar but not the same. Likewise, it is important that the motives of those who implement nursing shared governance be consistent with a commitment to professional nursing authority and control over nursing practice so that the profession can meet its commitments to clients in all practice settings. Shared governance requires that nurses are accountable to define and control nursing practice. Nurses must also be accountable to understand what shared governance is, expect that the necessary structures and processes are present if implementation of shared governance is claimed, be discerning about the motives for implementation, and take the risks and develop the knowledge to support the privilege of professional practice. If the aim of all nurses in an organization is to implement structures that enable the profession to define and control practice, the approach to implementation, unit-based versus whole system, does not matter as long as mechanisms for collective nursing authority and accountability are developed for the nursing department as a whole. Nurses committed to professional nursing practice will also be committed to the role adaptations and corresponding stresses that accompany implementation of shared governance, recognizing the benefits of supportive collegial relationships and consensus decision making among nurses in all roles.

Finally, nurses must also be accountable for demonstrating the benefits of shared governance to patients, nurses, and the employing organizations. While there is some research linking shared governance to improved job satisfaction and social integration of nurses,[9,19,22] improved patient outcomes,[18,19] and cost to the organization,[12] more systematic investigation of these effects is needed. As with all organizational innovations, strategies and tools must be developed so that nurse administrators and clinicians can conveniently initiate the collection of data to systematically evaluate the outcomes of shared governance.[23] Accountability for systematic evaluation of innovations would prevent the adoption of every "new idea" presented as a panacea for nursing and provide the data to refine innovations and their implementation.

REFERENCES

1. American Nurses Association. (1980). *Nursing: A social policy statement.* Kansas City, Mo: Author.
2. American Nurses Association. (1983). *Peer review in nursing practice.* Kansas City, Mo: Author.
3. American Nurses Association. (1992). Standards of nursing practice. Code for nurses with interpretive statements. The nursing shortage in the 1990's: Realities and remedies. In *Best sellers.* Kansas City, Mo: American Nurses Publishing.
4. Carmanica, L., & Rosenbecker, S. (1991). A pilot unit approach to shared governance. *Nursing Management, 22*(1), 46-48.
5. Crocker, D. G., Kirkpatrick, R. M., & Lentenbrink, L. (1992). Shared governance and collective bargaining: Integration, not confrontation. In T. Porter-O'Grady (Ed.), *Implementing shared governance: Creating a professional organization.* St Louis: Mosby.
6. Fagan, M. J. (1991). Can unit-based shared governance thrive on its own? *Nursing Management, 22*(7), 104L-104P.
7. Foster, B. E. (1992). Models of shared governance: Design and implementation. In T. Porter-O'Grady (Ed.), *Implementing shared governance: Creating a professional organization.* St Louis: Mosby.
8. Hersey, P., & Blanchard, K. (1986). *Management of organizational behavior; Utilizing human resources.* Englewood Cliffs, N.J.: Prentice-Hall.
9. Hinshaw, A. S., Smeltzer, C. H., & Atwood, J. (1987). Innovative retention strategies for nursing staff. *Journal of Nursing Administration, 17*(6), 8-16.
10. Horvath, K. J. (1990). Professional nursing practice model. In G. G. Mayer, M. J. Madden, & E. Lawrenz (Eds.), *Patient care delivery models.* Rockville, Md: Aspen.
11. Jacoby, J., & Terpste, M. (1990). Collaborative governance: Model for professional autonomy. *Nursing Management, 21*(2), 42-44.
12. Jenkins, J. E. (1988). A nursing governance and practice model: What are the costs? *Nursing Economic$, 6*(6), 302-311.
13. Jenkins, J. E. (1991). Professional governance: The missing link. *Nursing Management, 22*(8), 26-30.
14. Johnson, L. M. (1987). Self-governance: Treatment for an unhealthy nursing culture. *Health Progress, 5,* 41-43.
15. Kerfoot, K. (1992, March). *Unit-based shared governance: The federation model.* Paper presented at conference. Shared Governance: Sailing toward success. San Diego, California.
16. Lawrenz, E., & Mayer, G. G. (1990). In G. G. Mayer, M. J. Madden, & E. Lawrenz (Eds.), *Patient care delivery models,* Rockville, Md: Aspen.
17. Ludemann, R. S., & Brown, C. (1989). Staff perceptions of shared governance. *Nursing Administration Quarterly, 13*(4), 49-56.
18. Maas, M. (1989). Professional practice for the extended care environment: Learning from one model and its implementation. *Journal of Professional Nursing, 5*(2), 66-76.
19. Maas, M., & Jacox, A. (1977). *Guidelines for nurse autonomy/patient welfare.* New York: Appleton-Century-Crofts.
20. Maas, M., Jacox, A., & Specht, J. (1975). Nurse autonomy: Not rhetoric but for real. *American Journal of Nursing, 20,* 2201-2208.
21. Maas, M. L., & Specht, J. P. (1990). Nursing professionalization and self-governance: A model from long-term care. In G. G. Mayer, M. J. Madden, & E. Lawrenz (Eds.), *Patient care delivery models.* Rockville, Md: Aspen.
22. McCloskey, J. C. (1990). Two requirements for job contentment: Autonomy and social integration. *Image: The Journal of Nursing Scholarship, 22*(3), 140-143.
23. McCloskey, J. C., Gardner, D., & Maas, M. (1992, May). *Assisting managers to assess effectiveness of innovations in patient care services.* Proposal submitted to Robert Wood Johnson Foundation.
24. McDonagh, K. J., Rhodes, B., Sharkey, K., & Goodroe, J. H. (1989). Shared governance at St. Joseph's hospital of Atlanta: A mature professional practice model. *Nursing Administration Quarterly, 13*(4), 17-28.
25. Mintzberg, H. (1979). *The structuring of organizations.* Englewood Cliffs, N.J.: Prentice-Hall.
26. Peplau, H. (1985, February). Is nursing self-regulatory power being eroded? *American Journal of Nursing,* 141-143.
27. Pinkerton, S. E. (1988). An overview of shared governance. In S. E. Pinkerton & P. Schroeder (Eds.), *Commitment to excellence: Developing a professional nursing staff.* Rockville, Md: Aspen.
28. Porter-O'Grady, T. (1987). Shared governance and new organizational models. *Nursing Economic$, 5*(6), 281-286.
29. Porter-O'Grady, T. (1991). Shared governance for nursing. Part I: Creating the new organization. *AORN Journal, 53*(2), 458-466.
30. Porter-O'Grady, T. (1991). Shared governance for nursing. Part II: Putting the organization into action. *AORN Journal, 53*(3), 694-703.
31. Porter-O'Grady, T. (1992). Shared governance: Looking toward the future. In T. Porter-O'Grady (Ed.), *Implementing shared governance: Creating a professional organization.* St Louis: Mosby.

32. Prescott, P. A. (1987). Another round of nurse shortage. *Image: The Journal of Nursing Scholarship, 19*(4), 204-209.

33. Rose, M., & DiPasquale, B. (1990). The Johns Hopkins professional practice model. In G. G. Mayer, M. J. Madden, & E. Lawrenz (Eds.), *Patient care delivery models.* Rockville, Md: Aspen.

34. Schwartz, R. H. (1990). Nurse decision-making influence: A discrepancy between the nursing and hospital literatures. *Journal of Nursing Administration, 20*(6), 35-39.

35. Spitzer-Lehmann, R. (1989). Middle management consolidation. *Nursing Management, 20*(4), 59-62.

36. Stichler, J. F. (1992). A conceptual basis for shared governance. In T. Porter-O'Grady (Ed.), *Implementing shared governance: Creating a professional organization.* St Louis: Mosby.

37. Strasen, L. (1989). Redesigning patient care to empower nurses and increase productivity. *Nursing Economic$, 7*(1), 32-35.

38. Wilson, C. K. (1989). Shared governance: The challenge of change in the early phase of implementation. *Nursing Administration Quarterly, 13*(4), 29-33.

CHAPTER 56

International nursing

The role of the International Council of Nurses and the World Health Organization

VIRGINIA M. OHLSON, MARGRETTA MADDEN STYLES

Does nursing have the power to change the health care system? There are two major organizations—one governmental and one nongovernmental—whereby nursing's influence can be mobilized at the international level and throughout the world.

The International Council of Nurses (ICN) and the World Health Organization (WHO) play significant roles in nursing and health care worldwide and in promoting the global goal of health for all by the year 2000. Yet in view of questions frequently raised by nursing students and practicing nurses, it seems that some nurses know relatively little about either of these international organizations. Common remarks include: "I would like to attend an ICN congress. How can I become a member of the ICN?" and, "I am interested in working with the WHO some day. How do I apply for membership?"

Usually the inquirer is surprised to learn that direct membership in either of these organizations is not open to them as individuals. Members of the ICN are national nursing associations (NNAs); when an individual nurse holds membership in a NNA belonging to the ICN, that individual is qualified to participate in many of its activities and programs. Similarly, members of the WHO are affiliated by country. Although certain WHO activities are at the government level, opportunities exist for individual health professionals to participate in working assignments in various parts of the world and to utilize many programs and resources of the organization.

This chapter provides a brief description of the ICN and the WHO and their respective roles in international health and nursing. Selected examples from the current agendas of the two organizations will be used as a case study of the healthy interaction between the professional and governmental sectors in bringing about needed change. In combination, we draw from a wealth of experience in international nursing through ICN, WHO, and other agencies.

It is not difficult to discuss the role of the ICN in international health from a nursing perspective because it is a federation of nursing associations managed by nurses and financed primarily by nurses. The WHO, in contrast, is an organization of many health disciplines; nevertheless, nursing always has had an active role within the WHO and its influence has been felt in numerous ways worldwide.

INTERNATIONAL COUNCIL OF NURSES

The ICN was founded in 1899 as an independent, nongovernmental federation of national nurses' associations. It is the oldest international professional organization in the health care field and the only body representative of the total nursing profession worldwide.

Organization and administration

The NNAs of 111 countries comprise the 1993 membership of the ICN. In addition, the organization is in contact with nursing bodies or groups of nurses in many countries, including those of the former USSR. Only one NNA per country can belong to the ICN. For example, the American Nurses Association is the sole U.S. member of the ICN. However, as nursing and the conditions under which nurses practice have continued to change, consideration is being given to possible adjustments in the organizational structure that might more appropriately accommodate the ICN's growing relationships with other organizations. In 1991, the first international specialty organization was qualified as a resource group to the ICN, an official designation recently approved by the ICN.

The governing body of the ICN is its Council of National Representatives (CNR), composed of two delegates from each of the member associations. Each member association has one vote in the conduct of the ICN business, regardless of the membership size. Currently the largest NNA belonging to the ICN is the United Kingdom's Royal College of Nursing, followed by the nurses' associations of Japan and the United States. The CNR meets every two years. In the interim periods, program decisions are made by an elected board of directors that meets annually or as frequently as necessary. Membership on the board includes a president, three vice presidents, seven area representatives, and four members at large. Area representatives are elected from the seven ICN areas—Africa, Europe, North America, South and Central America, Southeast Asia, the eastern Mediterranean, and the western Pacific. The ICN has only one standing committee, the Professional Services Committee, a very active group vested with responsibility to consider problems and trends in nursing education and practice and to make recommendations to the board for further exploration by the CNR. Ad hoc committees or task forces are appointed as needed to deal with matters pertinent to the concerns of the ICN.

Headquartered in Geneva, Switzerland, the ICN employs an international corps of five nurse consultants and other professional and support staff. Constance Holleran of the United States has served as the organization's executive director since appointment by the board of directors in 1981.

Purpose and objectives

The purpose of the ICN is the same today as it was at the time of founding: "to provide a medium through which the interests, needs, and concerns of member national nurses' associations can be addressed to the advantage of the public and nurses." The ICN's program is based on four objectives:[16]

1. To promote the development of strong nursing associations

2. To assist national nursing associations to improve the standards of nursing and the competence of nurses
3. To assist national nurses associations to improve the status of nurses
4. To serve as the authoritative voice for nurses and nursing internationally

Objective one: the national associations. Promotion of the development of strong national nurses' associations is a prime objective of the ICN. All the ICN programs and activities are planned by the member associations, their elected representatives (the CNR), and the highly qualified staff persons at headquarters. Collectively, the member associations and their representatives set goals for nursing education, practice, and research and authorize the staff to use resources to assist member associations, singly and collectively, in ways that will enhance or strengthen their development. Staff consultation is provided on request to member associations by telephone, correspondence, or in person, as well as through assistance with the implementation of projects pertinent to the ICN goals. Manuals, guidelines, and other resource materials are made available to member associations. All aspects of the ICN's programs and activities are directly or indirectly related to the attainment of the organization's prime objective—the development of strong NNAs.

Objective two: education and practice. Since 1978, a main program emphasis of the ICN has reflected the organization's commitment to primary health care and the global goal of health for all by the year 2000 (HFA/2000)—the goal adopted by 134 nations at the WHO/UNICEF conference convened in 1978 at Alma-Ata in the then-Soviet republic of Kazakstan. In collaboration with its member associations, the ICN has endeavored to influence and prepare nurses and nursing services to participate more effectively in a primary health care system. Recognizing that nursing has the potential to influence decision making for health at all levels of government and in the society at large, the ICN committed staff and resources to the sponsoring of numerous workshops in primary health care in all of the seven ICN regions. Workshops were directed to the NNAs' potential for leadership in their countries, with the purpose of strengthening nursing's role in achieving the goal of health for all. Great emphasis is placed in ICN workshops on the continuing education needs of nurses working in rural primary health care settings.

Throughout its existence, ICN has maintained an interest in the regulation of nursing education and practice worldwide. High priority has been given to encouraging and assisting NNAs in their efforts to establish and update nursing standards. Periodically, the ICN has conducted studies and seminars related to nursing regulations and standards and published reports on these efforts.[5,8,9,12,13,14] In recognition of the need for an official statement of position regarding regulatory mechanisms affecting standards for nursing education and practice, an ICN study was conducted by Styles in 1983 and 1984. The study was made at the request of the Professional Services Committee (PSC) and accepted as policy by the CNR in 1985.

The purpose of the study was twofold: (1) to collect, organize and report data on how nursing currently is regulated worldwide, and (2) to derive guidelines that might be helpful to ICN in the development of an official position for assisting member associations in the evaluation and development of a regulatory system for nursing. Overall findings of the study revealed that:

the structure of the profession is ill-defined and diverse; educational requirements and legal definitions of nursing are generally inadequate for the complexity and expansion of the nursing role as it is emerging in response to health care needs; and the goals and standards of the profession worldwide are less apparent than one-half century ago, although they may be well crystalized in some countries, the conclusion is inescapable that the welfare of the public, the profession, and the practitioner will be better served if greater relevance, rationality, consistency, and clarity are brought to bear on the regulatory system.[8]

In response to these findings, the CNR in 1987 adopted an official statement of position on regulation of nursing, guided by 12 principles of professional regulation and associated policy objectives for nursing.[8] An opportunity to test and implement these guidelines has been provided through a series of workshops held in all of the ICN's regions from 1986 to 1992, with funding from a variety of governmental and philanthropic organizations. As a result of these efforts over a period of a decade, nursing laws, regulations, and standards have been enacted or revised in many countries, providing greater uniformity and authority for nursing to reach its potential impact upon health care.

Objective three: social and economic welfare of nurses. The ICN gives high priority to assisting national nurses' associations in matters relating to the socioeconomic welfare (SEW) of nurses. Major stress is placed on the importance of providing assistance and resources to those associations that are able to initiate and implement SEW programs in their countries through collective bargaining and other approaches, as appropriate.

The SEW program of the ICN has four major objectives: (1) to identify information and data about socioeconomic welfare; (2) to provide information, educational programs, and consultation on SEW to national nurses' associations; (3) to work and communicate with other international organizations in regard to the social and economic welfare of nurses—particularly the International Labor Organization (ILO) and WHO; and (4) to examine and determine how the present socioeconomic situation affects health services and the lives and working conditions of nurses.[6] Pertinent information about SEW is shared with member associations through a regularly published newsletter, the *Socio-Economic News*. The association's dedication to the socioeconomic status of nurses has had a tremendous influence on the improvement of working conditions of nurses worldwide.

Objective four: a unified voice for nursing. The ICN, composed of 111 member associations, has the unique potential, opportunity, and responsibility to serve as the authoritative voice for nursing and nurses internationally. The extent to which it honors and accepts this responsibility has been demonstrated and documented on many occasions and in various ways. Frequently at the WHO's World Health Assembly, which convenes annually in Geneva, Switzerland, ICN has presented position statements on issues relevant to health care and nursing. Examples are: the ICN's statements on infant feeding, nursing in primary health care, the role of nursing in WHO, and the state of the health of women in today's world. Although the ICN is a nursing organization and the WHO is an interdisciplinary health organization, the high degree of camaraderie and collaboration that exists between these two organizations and their nursing staffs has contributed immeasurably to a unified voice for nursing in the international arena.

The ICN has maintained an active publishing program, issuing books, manuals, monographs, reports, and guidelines relative to nursing education, practice, and research. Its official organ is the *International Nursing Review,* a bimonthly journal published in Switzerland.

The ICN has published (in English, French, and Spanish) numerous statements reflecting the organization's stance on issues related to nursing, health care, and societal matters of concern to the profession. Periodic listings of these position statements in the *International Nursing Review* reflect the ICN's broad range of concerns.

Primary emphasis has been placed on the ways in which the ICN carries out its work in relation to its four primary objectives. It is important to recognize the extent to which its staff must interact with numerous other international organizations and agencies—including such organizations as the WHO, UNICEF, ILO, and other governmental and nongovernmental philanthropic agencies—to achieve these objectives.

Recognition also should be given to the ICN's work with the International Committee of the Red Cross (ICRC), the International Commission of Health Professionals for Health and Human Rights, Amnesty International, and other organizations, in efforts to trace nurses who have disappeared or have been imprisoned because of their work.

Blueprint for future action

In view of the ICN's many programs and nursing's pressing needs, in 1989 the CNR approved a five-year plan of action. Nine priority areas were identified.[7]

- Continue efforts to strengthen the effectiveness of national nurses' associations (NNAs)
- Support the work of NNAs to improve employment conditions for nurses in all settings and to promote the social and economic welfare of all nursing personnel
- Strengthen the ICN and NNAs in ways oriented to promote participation in effective relationships with interdisciplinary, interprofessional, and international government agencies, for the purposes of improving the health of the public
- Review changes and adjustments in the organizational components and relationships of the ICN
- Encourage NNAs to be more active in setting and enforcing standards for nursing education and nursing practice, leadership, and management in their countries
- Assist NNAs and others in bringing about more appropriate regulatory mechanisms for nursing practice, thus making it possible for the knowledge and skills of nurses to be more effectively utilized and recognized within the health system
- Orient NNAs to promote and assist as feasible with health personnel planning and development for nursing in all its areas of practice

- Ensure that the ICN Code for Nurses continues to provide the ethical guidance required by nurses in a rapidly changing world with constant social, technological, genetic, and pharmacological advances
- Work with NNAs to encourage and facilitate the development of research in nursing and by nurses and the dissemination of research findings

Although this blueprint was set down as a five-year plan of action in 1989, activities related to the plan will not cease at the close of the five-year period, since they are basically related to the four objectives which the ICN regards as central to its primary purpose. However, at the 1993 quadrennial congress convened in Madrid, Spain, the CNR adopted a new five-point strategic plan to guide its activities for the next five years.

In 1991, the ICN board approved a projected long-term project referred to as the International Classification of Nursing Practice (ICNP)—a project designed to make nursing practice more understood and visable in health care settings and reimbursement systems. The intent of the project "is to describe what nurses do relative to certain human needs, to produce certain outcomes or to explain what nurses do in response to particular human situations which enable people—as individuals, families, and communities—to achieve and maintain good health."[18]

Another new promising ICN initiative has established the International Council of Nurses Foundation (ICNF), which aims to raise the necessary funding base for educational programs to prepare nurses to assume new leadership roles. Information and advice for individuals and national nursing associations interested in assisting with this endeavor are available from the ICN headquarters office in Geneva, Switzerland.

THE WORLD HEALTH ORGANIZATION

The World Health Organization was established in 1948 as a specialized agency of the United Nations in Geneva, Switzerland, where it is still headquartered. It came into existence as the world was attempting to recover from World War II and as millions were falling victim to poverty and disease.

It was in these troubled times that the constitution of the WHO was formulated. The preamble of that historic document gives evidence of the concern for social justice on which the organization was founded and has firmly stood for more than 40 years. Its succinct statement of beliefs is widely known: "The enjoyment of the highest attainable standard of health is one of the fundamental rights of every human being without distinction of race, religion, political belief, economic, or social condition."

Organization and administration

The WHO is an intergovernmental agency. In 1948, there were 56 member countries; by 1993, membership had increased to 185. The highest policy-making body of WHO is the World Health Assembly (WHA), which is responsible for the execution of WHO policies in collaboration with its employed staff, referred to as the WHO secretariat. The highest officer in the WHO is the director general, elected for a five-year term by the WHA on nomination by the executive board. Currently, this position is held by Dr. Hiroshi Nakajima of Japan. Numerous administrative and technical personnel and diversified knowledge and skills are employed at WHO headquarters in Geneva.

WHO's program is decentralized into six regional offices: AFRO, the African regional office, in Brazzaville, Congo; PAHO/AMRO, the Pan American Health Organization, which serves as the regional office for the Americas, in Washington, D.C.; EMRO, the eastern Mediterranean regional office, in Alexandria, Egypt; EURO, the European regional office, in Copenhagen, Denmark; SEARO, the Southeast Asian regional office, in New Delhi, India; and WPRO, the western Pacific regional office, in Manila, Philippines.

WHO's activities are financed by annual mandatory contributions from its member countries and by voluntary contributions from government and private agencies.

Functions of WHO

The WHO constitution specifies 22 functions, summarized as follows:

1. Coordinating international health work undertaken by national and international groups, both governmental and voluntary, or by scientific and professional groups
2. Assisting governments in strengthening health services through technical assistance, through direct aid as requested, or through providing counseling or personnel support in the development of programs
3. Fostering action in specific fields of particular need such as maternal and child health and welfare, mental health, disease eradication, nutrition, and improvement of water supplies

4. Developing or promoting international agreements and standards including policies and regulations; standards of teaching and training in health, medical, and related fields; standardization of the international nomenclature of diseases and of diagnostic procedures and standards
5. Conducting, encouraging, and supporting studies and research in the field of health, including studies of administration and social techniques for health care[3,27]

Although the constitution of WHO was written more than 40 years ago, its 22 statements of functions have not changed. However, the programs necessary for their implementation have been modified considerably with increased understanding of the world's health problems. Similarly, the administrative structure of WHO and the size and nature of the secretariat also have changed as new policies have been formulated by the WHA and new priorities established.

Health for all by the year 2000

Fulop and Roemer[4] describe the ways in which WHO's policies and programs have been influenced over time by the variety of social forces operating within the organization and its member countries. Certainly, the changing nature of WHO membership has influenced program directions. In 1948, 57% of WHO member states were developed countries, and 43% were developing countries. By 1978, many new countries had become sovereign states and joined WHO, considerably changing the nature of its membership. Currently, over 75% of the members represent the developing countries. Interestingly, it was not until 1977 that growing concern over the health conditions in many countries resulted in establishing the year 2000 as the target date for reaching WHO's long standing objective, "the attainment of the highest possible level of health for all people."[4]

In the following year, an international conference on primary health care was convened by WHO and UNICEF in Alma-Ata, bringing representatives of 134 governments and 67 United Nations' organizations and other specialty agencies and nongovernmental organizations. It was at this conference that the now-renowned Declaration of Alma-Ata was formulated, recognizing primary health care (PHC) as the key to attaining health for all by 2000. The conference declared that the health status of hundreds of millions of people was unacceptable and could only be rectified by a new, equitable approach to health and health care that would close the gap between the world's haves and have-nots. In 1979, the Thirty-Second World Health Assembly endorsed the Declaration of Alma-Ata.[26] In 1981, the WHA established the Global Strategy for Health of All by the year 2000 (HFA/2000),[25] and countries were encouraged to formulate their own national policies, strategies, and plans of action for attaining this goal. Since that time, the pursuit of health for all, and the PHC approach, has continued to be a central focus for WHO policies and program strategies. However, it is increasingly being recognized that social, economic, and political changes in the world, as well as changing patterns, have had implication for the countries' development. Therefore, WHO's program of work for 1995-2001 will need to place emphasis on providing universal access to care, including promotive, preventive, and curative services, with priority given to countries and people in greatest need.[18]

Nursing in WHO

Where does nursing fit in this complex intergovernmental, interdisciplinary health organization? What is nursing's role in the WHO in this decade, and what will it be by the year 2000? Some understanding of the structure of nursing within WHO could assist in answering these questions.

Structure for nursing in WHO. The highest administrative post for nursing in the headquarters of the WHO is the position designated as "chief scientist for nursing." Dr. Miriam Hirschfeld from Israel currently holds this position. As the chief administrator for nursing in WHO, the nursing chief reports to the director general through the assistant director general, as do other administrative position chiefs. Simultaneously, the nursing chief also holds a position in the Division of Development of Human Resources for Health and in this role reports to the director of that division. A few other nurses are employed at WHO headquarters assigned, not to nursing, but in positions dealing with program areas concerned with specific diseases such as AIDS, immunizations, maternal and child health, and employee health services.

The chief scientist for nursing is the primary voice for nursing in the organization and, in this capacity, must interpret the potential, contributions, and needs of nursing within an interdisciplinary context. In carrying out the responsibilities of the office, the chief scientist for nursing maintains contact with numerous international agencies and organizations concerned directly or indirectly with nursing, and with nursing personnel in the six WHO regional offices. The administrator reviews program plans and projects of the regions, provides technical assistance as feasible, and participates in conferences and workshops at the request of the regional offices. Possibly the greatest responsibility of the nursing administrator in this interdisciplinary organization is that of communicating, interpreting, stimulating, and planning nursing's contributions to various WHO programs.

Each WHO regional office has its own nursing and other health-related personnel whose responsibilities and programs of work are designed and implemented within the regional areas. The relationship between the WHO headquarters and the regional offices is advisory rather than administrative, since WHO operates on a decentralized basis that permits autonomy within broad policy guidelines. As a result, nursing may be organized quite differently in each region. The WHO's primary commitment at all levels is to its member countries and to the strengthening of those countries' institutions. Although problems in nursing in various countries are to some extent quite similar, they differ significantly in degree in various areas of the world. WHO nurses in the regions deal with a wide range of programs and problems related to nursing practice, education, training, organization, administration, and research. Duties have encompassed such activities as the analyses of nursing needs in a country or area, the design of projects to meet a particular need, the recruitment or assistance with recruitment of personnel for various projects of the organization or a member country, and evaluation of project outcomes.

Nature of nursing in WHO. Nursing has had an important role in WHO from the time of the organization's founding. The programs of nursing have been carried out through (1) long- and short-term projects in many parts of the world with goals and objectives that have varied according to place and time; (2) workshops, conferences, and committees that have enabled the development and dissemination of reports, recommendations, and guidelines; and (3) a wide variety of administrative functions and activities.

Projects have been developed for implementation at the local, regional, and interregional levels. Although some projects have related specifically to nursing, many have been interdisciplinary. In the early years of WHO, nurses were involved in projects as members of specialized teams concerned with treatment and control of diseases such as malaria, venereal diseases, and tuberculosis, and also with maternal and child health programs. In later years, a higher priority was placed on programs of nursing and midwifery education. Although consideration is still given to such projects, a prime emphasis in recent years has been on projects particularly relevant to the achievement of the goal of HFA/2000 through primary health care (PHC).

WHO maintains a system of expert panels, representative of the various disciplines, that function as advisory bodies to the organization. The expert panel in nursing includes representatives of various specialty areas in nursing and of the geographic regions. The panel does not meet as a group, but from time to time representatives from the panel meet to deliberate and make recommendations on a matter of concern to nursing and WHO. An example of their action is reflected in the report of the expert committee of 1984, *The Education and Training of Nurse Teachers and Managers with Special Regard to Primary Health Care.*[23,24] Each time an expert committee on nursing is convened, a report summarizing its deliberations and recommendations is published and made available to governments, professional organizations, educational institutions, and other interested agencies and individuals. A "Study Group on Nursing Beyond 2000" was scheduled to convene in 1993, and papers were proposed by various experts on pertinent issues.

Throughout the years, a wide variety of guides, reports, and materials relevant to nursing practice, education, administration, and research have been prepared and disseminated by WHO headquarters and the regional offices. Numerous statements have been developed and published as summaries and recommendations of conferences or workshops convened to deliberate on some specific aspects of nursing.[17,20,23] Frequently, these publications represent the work of an individual or group commissioned by WHO to conduct a specific study. Many of these publications are available through the headquarters and regional offices; in some of the regional areas, bibliographies of studies are available.

As a discipline within WHO, nursing supports and affirms the programs of the organization and the attainment of its goals. Health care planning and implementation uses the team approach, and within this context nursing must carve out its directions, its functions, and its role.

WHO collaborating centers for nursing development

For many years, WHO has designated a number of health professional colleges or departments in universities and other health-related agencies and institutions as WHO Collaborating Centers. This designation has been given in recognition of the institution's or agency's potential to participate in the furtherance of WHO goals and objectives. The first nursing centers to be so designated were in Europe. Two of these centers were named in 1980: the Collaborating Center for Nursing Research and Education, located at the Danish Institute for Health and Nursing Research in Copenhagen, Denmark; and the Collaborating Center for Nursing associated with Hospices Civils de Leon, in Lyon, France. Now more than 26 such centers have been designated as WHO nursing centers or are under consideration in various parts of the world, including Australia, Bahrain, Botswana, Brazil, Canada, Colombia, Denmark, Finland, France, India, Japan, Kazakhstan, Korea, Philippines, Solvenia, Thailand, the United Kingdom, the United States, and Zaire. Six WHO Collaborating Centers for Nursing Development in the United States are as follows: the College of Nursing of the University of Illinois at Chicago (1986); the School of Nursing of the University of Pennsylvania, Philadelphia (1988); the School of Nursing of the University of Texas Medical Branch at Galveston (1988); the School of Nursing at the University of California, San Francisco (1991); the School of Nursing at George Mason University, Fairfax, Virginia (1991); and the School of Nursing at Case Western Reserve University, Cleveland, Ohio (1993).

In April 1988, the first general annual meeting of the Global Network of the WHO Collaborating Centers for Nursing Development was convened in Maribor, Yugoslavia. Representatives of the designated and potential collaborating centers were in attendance. It was a historic meeting. The work of the network is facilitated by WHO, although the network itself is not a component part of the WHO. When the Global Network was first established, the College of Nursing of the University of Illinois at Chicago (UIC) was voted as the first secretariat of the Network, and will continue to function in this role until 1994, when another elected center of the Network will assume this responsibility. From the time of its beginnings, the Network has served as a conduit for information sharing and the exchange of materials and expertise between members and their individual centers. Two new publications, available through the Office of the Secretariat describe the work of the individual centers which has been initiated since their designation as a WHO Collaborating Center and their membership in the Global Network. It is anticipated that member centers representing all areas of the world eventually will be able to set down common goals of high priority and plan collaborative action toward their realization. Achievement of these goals would strengthen the capacity of each center, as well as the Network, to move forward with the particular primary health care mission for which they were established.[2]

INTERACTING ICN AND WHO AGENDAS

Throughout their history, ICN and WHO have pursued mutual goals and engaged in collaborative projects. Only two contemporary examples, among many, will be mentioned here.

In 1982, ICN and WHO—recognizing that regulatory reform was essential to maximize nursing's role in primary health care—undertook parallel and cooperative initiatives in nursing regulation. ICN commissioned the study outlined previously,[8] and WHO convened an expert group on nursing regulation to which the ICN consultant was appointed. Complementary sets of guidelines ensued. The regional workshops on nursing regulation conducted by ICN from 1986 to 1992 included teams of representatives from the two sectors, the NNAs and the ministries of health. Only through such cooperation could the profession demonstrate its accountability for standards of nursing practice and governments evidence their commitment to nursing's contribution toward health for all.

In 1989, the 42nd World Health Assembly (WHA) adopted a very significant resolution on "Strengthening Nursing and Midwifery in Support of the Strategy of Health for All." The resolution called upon WHO and member nations to engage in strategic planning of their nurseforce; to develop sound policy, management, and supervision at all levels; and to improve standards of nursing education along the lines of primary health care. The resolution further mandated a progress report in 1992. ICN mobilized its NNAs to bring this resolution to the attention of their governments, to press for action on the specific recommendations, and to pursue every avenue to achieve more representation on the member delegations to the 1992 WHA. Nurses showed up in force in close to 20 delegations at the 45th Assembly and were very active and effective throughout the discussions. With respect to the report on strengthening nursing, they were successful in getting facts on the table regarding nursing's involvement in health care policy and planning throughout WHO and its member nations. As a consequence, a global advisory group on nursing and midwifery, reporting to the highest level of the WHO secretariat, was established.[19]

SUMMARY

This chapter has described the role of ICN and WHO in relation to nursing internationally. Much more could be said of the many ways in which the nurse leaders of these two organizations work collaboratively in their office headquarters in Geneva and in the many regions and countries of the world. Nurses in these two organizations are few in number, yet their accomplishments on behalf of nurses and for nursing and health care are far-reaching and impressive.

Does nursing have the power to change the health system? In their crucial positions, WHO and ICN are influencing directions for nursing and patterns of health care delivery all over the world. Individually and collectively, we too, as nurses of the world, have a role in this global endeavor. Health for all by the year 2000: the year for attainment of this goal is not far away! If not in the year 2000—when?

REFERENCES

1. Bridges, D. (1965). *A history of the International Council of Nurses, 1899-1964*. Philadelphia: J. B. Lippincott.
2. Duxbury, M. (1988). *The global network of World Health Organization collaborating centers for nursing development*. Unpublished manuscript.
3. Freeman, R. (1965). *Nursing in the World Health Organization*. Geneva: World Health Organization.
4. Fulop, T., & Roemer, M. (1982). *International development of health manpower policy*. Geneva: World Health Organization.
5. International Council of Nurses. (1992). *Nursing regulation guidebook: From principle to power*. Geneva: Author.
6. International Council of Nurses. (1987). *Report of the Social Economic Welfare Committee, Council of Nurse Representatives*. Geneva: Author.
7. International Council of Nurses. (1987). Nursing's priorities set at New Zealand. *International Nursing Review, 34*(6),276.
8. Styles, M. (1986). *Report on the regulation of nursing: A report on the present, a position for the future*. Geneva: International Council of Nurses.
9. International Council of Nurses. (1975). *Nursing legislation in Latin America the last half of the 20th century*. Geneva: Author.
10. International Council of Nurses. (1975). ICN adopts definition of nursing. *International Nursing Review, 22*(6),184.
11. International Council of Nurses. (1973). *Report of the professional services committee*. Geneva: Author.
12. International Council of Nurses. (1970, 1971). *Report on an international seminar on nursing legislation, Warsaw*. Geneva: Author.
13. International Council of Nurses. (1969). *Principles of legislation for nursing education and practice: A guide to assist national nursing associations*. New York: S. Karger.
14. International Council on Nurses. (1960). *Nursing legislation: Report on survey of nursing legislation*. London: Author.
15. Mussalem, H. (1983). *Succeeding together: Group action by nurses*. Geneva: International Council of Nurses.
16. Quinn, S. (1981). *What about me? Caring for the careers*. Geneva: International Council of Nurses.

17. Storey, M., Romer, R., Mangay MagLacas, A., & Paloscia Riccard, E. A. (1988). *Guidelines for regulatory changes in nursing education and practice to promote primary health care.* Geneva: World Health Organization.

18. Voltaire, F. (1992). *Report of proceedings of the fifth general meeting of the global network of WHO collaborating centres for nursing development.* Unpublished report.

19. World Health Organization. (1992). *Strengthening nursing and midwifery in support of strategies for health for all.* Geneva: Author.

20. World Health Organization and Pan American Health Organization. (1987). *Meeting on planning for change in nursing development.* Washington, D.C.: Pan American Health Organization.

21. World Health Organization and University of North Carolina. (1987). *Health manpower for primary health care: The experience of the nurse practitioner.* Chapel Hill, N.C.: University of North Carolina.

22. World Health Organization. Regional Office for Europe. (1988). *Postbasic and graduate education for nurses.* Copenhagen: Author.

23. World Health Organization. (1982). *Division of health manpower development: Nursing in support of the goal of health for all by the year 2000.* Geneva: Author.

24. World Health Organization. (1984). *Education and training of nurse teachers and managers with special regard to primary health care* (Tech. Rep. No. 708). Geneva: Author.

25. World Health Organization. (1981). *Global strategies for health for all by the year 2000.* Geneva: Author.

26. World Health Organization. (1978). *Alma-Ata, 1978: Primary health care.* Geneva: Author.

27. World Health Organization. (1948). *Constitution of the World Health Organization.* Geneva: Author.

PART SEVEN

HEALTH CARE REFORM

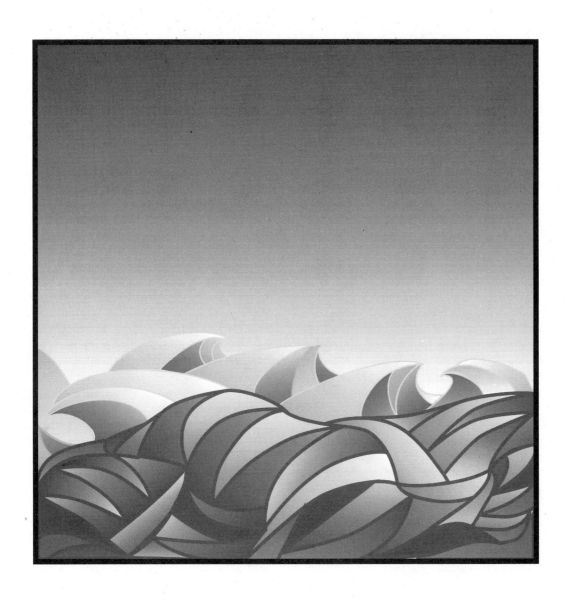

The role of nursing in achieving health care reform

JOANNE COMI McCLOSKEY, HELEN KENNEDY GRACE

Turning to yet a broader context, this section addresses the role of nursing in contributing to health care reform. In the debate chapter, Grace and Brock summarize some of the facets of the health care crisis that has emerged as a major concern in the past several years.

The fact that the cost of health care is increasing—at the same time that access is decreasing and the quality of health care services, particularly primary preventive services, is declining—is of major concern to individuals, employers, and public policymakers. Multiple proposals for health care reform have been put forward. Most address reform in terms of paying for access to the system as it is now constituted. In the debate chapter, Grace and Brock argue that these approaches are not likely to result in significant reform, particularly in light of their cost, at a time in which expenditures for health care services are growing more rapidly than the economy as a whole. Alternative approaches of working from state and local levels to achieve more fundamental change in the system itself are described. The authors propose an approach that would involve restructuring the system around primary preventive and primary health care services linked to secondary and tertiary levels of care, reducing administrative costs, redirecting financing streams for support of the restructured system, and engaging the community in an active process of ethical decision making regarding distribution of health care dollars. Nurses, in such a system, would constitute the core of the delivery system, and they are central in achieving these fundamental reforms.

In the first viewpoint chapter, Maraldo asserts that the time is right for health care reform and that nurses have a major role to play. This assertion is built upon the observation of increased consumer interest in health care reform coupled with the galvanizing effect of the nursing shortage of the late 1980s upon nursing. For the first time, nurses were asked what they wanted to see changed within the health care system. Out of this, the National League for Nursing (NLN), through an extensive process involving nurses and nursing organizations, developed Nursing's Agenda for Health Care Reform. Four elements for change are part of this agenda: (1) payment for services of nonphysician providers; (2) medical effectiveness testing; (3) encouragement of managed care options, and requirement for the uninsured; and (4) public disclosure of vital health information. Noting that most of the major proposals for health care reform at the national level do not address reforms in the system, Maraldo argues that the time is right for the nursing profession to join with consumers in achieving more fundamental reform.

Turning to the financing of health care, Davis first provides an overview of Medicare and Medicaid. With the growth of the elderly population, and the government funding programs that provide coverage, the federal share of health care expenditures is progressively increasing. Through a variety of cost-cutting measures such as encouragement of managed care, incentive-based prospective payment systems, and medical effectiveness testing for various procedures, progress is being made in reducing the costs of care. But this cost cutting is outpaced by the growth of the population in need of federal funding for its care. In such a climate, important opportunities are open for nurses to demonstrate the contributions that they can make to reducing length of hospital stay and to maintaining people in community care settings, thereby improving quality of care while reducing overall costs.

Nurses have had difficulty achieving recognition for the role that they can and do play in the delivery of health services. This is reflected in the way in which nurses have been paid. Traditionally nursing services have been paid for in the form of salaries provided by the institutions in which the nurses work. As nurses have become increasingly visible in their own right as providers of needed health care services, direct reimbursement for their services has become a prominent issue. Streff provides a comprehensive overview of the current status of direct reimbursement for nursing services. Tracing the history of efforts to gain third-party reimbursement, the author shows that significant progress has been made, with a large number of states now providing direct reimbursement for nurse practitioners. The current status of reimbursement from a variety of sources is provided, and strategies are suggested for influencing legislative changes. Negotiation with managed care systems is described as a current challenge. The chapter ends on an optimistic note and provides useful suggestions to nurses for costing out their services to maintain financially viable practices.

Another suggested route to reform is advocated by Fagin and Binder, who recommend a closer alliance between nurses and consumers in assuring that health promotion and disease prevention are prominent features of a restructured health care system. Collaboration between nurses and consumers is part of a longstanding tradition in the field, as evidenced in the early structure of the National Organization for Public Health Nursing. Alliances between consumers and nurses have been a powerful influence in the past, and these should be built upon in the present efforts directed toward health care reform. The challenge is to move from a system in which patients are passive recipients of care that is disease focused and prescribed by the physician to one in which consumers are active participants in maintaining their health and are knowledgeable regarding treatment; and nurses are central to this transition.

Changing the focus to the acute care hospital, Curran discusses work redesign as a key to health care reform. Increasingly, hospital organizational restructuring centered around the needs of patients is occurring. Patient-focused care, case management approaches, and total quality management are all approaches to such restructuring. While such restructuring is designed to improve patient care, it is also essential in assuring the financial viability of hospitals that are faced with the need to control ever-escalating costs. Restructuring the health care process around the client allows the nurse to focus attention on clinical care rather than on the many other functions that nurses have traditionally performed. The restructuring process requires a high degree of leadership from nursing and requires full use of the professional expertise of nurses, expertise that has too often been squandered in our prior patterns of organization.

In the international chapter in this section, Kerr provides an overview of the Canadian health care system. Tracing the development of health care within the Canadian context from the 1800s, we see that the Canada Health Act of 1984 put in place the medicare program that remains intact today. Provisions of the Canadian plan include universality of coverage to all people, comprehensiveness of medically necessary services, accessibility of the services to all segments of the population, portability of coverage from one province to another, and public administration of the program at the provincial level. Introduction of the Canadian plan has produced stability in health care costs in relation to the gross national product, in contrast to the situation in the United States, where health care costs are escalating at a far more rapid pace. Noting that the Canadian system has been built primarily around medical services, Kerr points out that nursing has been most affected in relation to hospital services, where nursing is viewed as one of the high costs of hospitals. Nurses are currently vulnerable within the system. However, there is a growing emphasis on maintaining patients in community-based settings, stressing prevention and health promotion. It is expected that, as this change in emphasis develops, the impact upon nursing will be great and that opportunities for nurses will be opened up.

While the need for health care reform is obvious, the shape of that reform is not yet clear. Although there are numerous proposals, most address only approaches to providing coverage for the uninsured and the underinsured. Fundamental reform, involving a shift from emphasis upon the medical care system to a broader focus upon health, is necessary. If this shift is to occur, nursing must be an active and vocal participant in the process. Building coalitions with patients, whether at the community level or in acute care settings, will be an essential part of the process. Reform is possible if nurses become an active part of the solution.

CHAPTER 57

Debate

Solving the health care dilemma

What will work?

HELEN KENNEDY GRACE, ROSLYN McCALLISTER BROCK

Concern over ability to pay for health care costs in case of illness is a major concern of U.S. citizens. In a recent survey, workers indicated that fear of losing health care coverage was one of their major concerns, even greater than that of losing their jobs.[3] The concerns of citizens are joined by those of employers who are putting out an increasingly high percentage of their profits to pay for insurance for their employees. In the economic summit convened by then President-elect Clinton, the chief executive officer (CEO) of Ford Motor Company reported that the costs for health care coverage of workers exceeded the cost of steel for building automobiles.

While concerns over adequate health care coverage for those who are employed and insured are one matter, increasingly large numbers of Americans find themselves with limited coverage through federal programs such as Medicare or Medicaid or having to provide their own coverage for themselves and their families. For this ever-increasing pool, finding access to health care services is becoming more and more difficult. Their illnesses are allowed to progress to an acute stage before medical care is sought, and at that time, care is most frequently obtained through emergency rooms, thus continuing the cost escalation of health services. While these individuals may be unable to pay for the services they receive, they cause hospitals, struggling to survive, to increase charges for all who use emergency room and acute care services. These increased charges get passed on to others who use the emergency room and hospital services, and thus the cost to employers continues to escalate to accommodate this cost shifting.

In the meantime, lacking primary preventive and health care services readily accessible at the community level, increasing numbers of people do not receive assistance in maintaining their health and that of their families. Expectant mothers do not receive adequate prenatal care and deliver low–birth weight, impaired infants requiring days, weeks, and sometimes years of expensive neonatal intensive care; children do not receive care for typical infectious diseases such as ear infections and later develop hearing loss, which then requires special remedial programs in the schools and permanently impairs the individuals in a competitive work environment; adults receiving little assistance in health promotion maintain unhealthy lifestyles contributing to development of costly chronic diseases; and the elderly with an accumulation of problems that could have been prevented end up in nursing homes to live out their last years in settings that are costly both materially and in quality of life. Lack of availability of and access to low-cost health services at the community level results in the need for expensive, acute care services to treat problems after they develop, and the costs are likely to continue to escalate.

While there is widespread recognition of the problems as evidenced by the almost daily news stories about some aspect of the "health care crisis," the viable solutions being put forward to address the problems are limited. The last presidential campaign elicited a number of proposals for health care reform. This chapter will first analyze these proposals and assess the likelihood that these top-down approaches could achieve health care reform. Alternative approaches of working from state and local levels to achieve more fundamental reform are then described. Most recently, the American Hospital Association (AHA) and the American Medical Association (AMA) have joined in the reform movement by placing on the table their own proposals for reform. Much earlier, the National League for Nursing, joined by other nursing organizations, placed its proposal for health care reform in the public domain. Concluding this chapter, a more radical approach for health care reform pushed from the community level is described. Participation of nurses in achieving affordable, acceptable, accessible health care services is key in resolving this health care crisis.

TOP-DOWN APPROACHES TO HEALTH CARE REFORM

National health care reform proposals fall into four categories: employer-mandated insurance, single-payer proposal, market-based reform, and managed competition.

Employer-mandated insurance, commonly known as "play or pay," is a reform proposal tied to the workplace. Employers are given two options in the provision of health coverage: either provide coverage to all full-time employees or pay a tax. Those who work for employers that "play" are covered under this proposal, while those who work for employers that "pay" are often left to find coverage under government-sponsored programs, further contributing to the development of a two-tier health care system.[4] Taxes from employers who pay are used to subsidize health coverage for other workers whose employers did not provide a health plan.[6] The major advantage of this proposal is that it increases the number of persons insured. However, it does not address the needs of the unemployed, or of self-employed or seasonal workers. Small businesses with fewer than five employees would be adversely affected under this plan because of the high costs of premiums.

The single-payer proposal suggests a government-administered plan modeled after the Canadian health care system. The government would be the administrative insurance agent and would set rates and issue payments to health providers and facilities. A federal tax would be levied on all residents to pay for this form of universal coverage. One of the major disadvantages of the proposal is that it may require large tax increases and put private insurers out of business, replacing them with government bureaucracies.[5] Also, some have argued that rationing of care and long waiting lines for

desired services would be logical outgrowths of a government-sponsored health plan because of its limited funding capacity to provide comprehensive coverage and sustained funding for needed high-technology equipment.[9]

Market-based reform is an approach that would relieve employers of the responsibility of providing health insurance coverage. Individuals would have the flexibility to purchase their own health coverage and then receive tax credits or vouchers in relation to the amount of coverage they received. This approach is similar to the British system that requires physicians to become government employees.[5] An advantage of this plan is that it may promote price competition among providers for delivery of care. A significant disadvantage is that it does not consider the unemployed, seasonal workers, or domestics who do not have a steady workplace for acquiring resources to purchase needed health coverage.

Managed competition is a reform plan developed by Alain Enthoven of Stanford University. The Clinton administration is currently reviewing some facets of its design for restructuring the health care system. It proposes that individuals be grouped into health maintenance organizations (HMOs) that are managed by a single entity—either the government or employers. The administrator of the HMO would become a consumer advocate on behalf of its membership for low-cost, high-quality health services, thus entering into a free-market "managed" competition for health services delivery. One major disadvantage of managed competition is that it does not work well in rural areas where competition among physicians and provider organizations is limited or virtually nonexistent.

The major deficit in all of these top-down approaches for health care reform is that all are addressing the financing of the system, without proposing fundamental reform within the system itself. There is a dire need to redirect health care reform discussions to concentrate on health promotion and disease prevention as the cornerstones of an affordable, accessible health care delivery system, rather than on the current medical system that overtreats illness.

STATEWIDE INITIATIVES

According to the American Public Health Association's national publication, *The Nation's Health,* 1992 was "a watershed year for state health care reform."[8] The state legislatures of Alaska, Colorado, Florida, Minnesota,

Vermont, and Oregon all tossed their health care reform hats into the political arena in an attempt to tackle the problems of access and escalating costs of health care services.

Alaska

Health care reform reports issued by the Alaska state legislature[1] outlined the following as components of a comprehensive health care reform package:

- Establish a single entity to oversee the cost containment, access, and pooling initiatives
- Control health care costs by establishing a global spending limit for all health care expenditures in Alaska and a reimbursement system for all health care payers
- Increase access by reforming the small group insurance market, creating pools, and providing subsidies to certain uninsured individuals
- Reduce medical malpractice costs
- Reduce the "excess capacity" in Alaska's health care facilities by strengthening the certificate of need process

Colorado

ColoradoCare is the health reform plan advocated by the governor of Colorado. The plan calls for a statewide insurance program that would be managed by a state health authority.[7] The health authority would determine the health benefits to be provided to all citizens and would negotiate with insurance companies and health providers to deliver services to all participants in the program. Each year, citizens would be able to select their health plan from the list of insurers provided by the state health authority. Insurers would have to enroll all applicants, provide full coverage without waiting periods or preexisting condition exclusions, and use uniform billing, payment, and reporting forms.[7] All insurers would be paid the same amount for enrollees in their programs. The plan would be financed by taxes, and the state legislature would set the budget and have the authority to place limits or caps on health care expenditures.

In keeping with the National Governors' Association's declaration that "health care must be available and affordable for all Americans," the Colorado legislature[4] further promulgates the following as the principles necessary for health care reform:

- Cost containment—the system must control costs for the system as a whole and for individual families

- Universality—the system must cover all Americans
- Prevention—the system must give access to preventive care, including prenatal care, immunizations, early detection, and guidelines for healthy living
- Portability—the system should not limit access to care according to job or income; coverage should travel with individuals as they change jobs, and no one should have to stay in a particular job to keep insurance
- Low administrative costs—the system must spend less on administration and more on health
- Quality and choice—the system must build on the best features of the current system, including high-quality care and freedom of choice among providers

Florida

In the state of Florida, the governor has taken a very proactive stance and proposed legislation that mandates that all Floridians have universal access to health care by 1994. The plan is innovative in that it brings state and local governments, employers, and citizens to the table to try to solve the access problem in the state by promoting wellness. If the discussions prove fruitless, a state health agency would be established and would take the leadership in developing a health care reform plan. The plan would focus on providing coverage to typically overlooked populations such as low-income and unemployed individuals and small business owners. A health care data system is also being proposed that would allow for tracking and analysis of statewide health access and insurance information.

Minnesota

The Minnesota plan is keenly oriented toward cost containment. The plan proposes to provide extended coverage and access to low-income children and their families and then phase in all other categories of the uninsured and the general population. Small businesses would participate in insurance pools that would allow them to provide health benefits to their employees. Regional boards would be established to monitor how the program was working and to set limits on health expenditures.

Oregon

All residents in the state of Oregon would be covered under its health care reform plan. In brief, under this plan, medical conditions would be ranked according to severity and outcomes of treatment. The state legislature would determine how much would be paid for health care expenditures and would in effect set limits on health service delivery. Conditions ranked above a determined line would be covered; those below the line would receive no coverage. Implementation of this plan has serious ethical implications in that it promotes "rationing" of health services.

Vermont

There are three major principles in the Vermont health care reform plan: universal access to care, global budgeting for all health expenditures, and an overall statewide plan for allocation of health care resources.[7] Like Florida, the state has issued legislation for the creation of a health authority whose mission would be to design a comprehensive health care reform package. The state's plan would provide extended Medicaid coverage for low-income children. Global budgets would facilitate cost containment measures by linking health resources to hospital budgets and certificate of need requests. Insurance pools would be created to provide greater incentives to enhance the purchasing power of participating groups.[7] Another added feature of the plan requires that uniform medical claim forms be instituted to control rising administrative costs.

Deficiency of statewide initiatives

These statewide approaches to addressing the health care crisis are all directed toward various aspects of the problem, including access for all residents, dealing with multiple insurers, approaches to managed care, and capping of costs. None directly address the need for fundamental reform of the substance of health care, the delivery system itself.

REFORM PROPOSALS OF PROFESSIONAL ORGANIZATIONS

The American Hospital Association[2] has come forth with its own health care reform strategy. The AHA's proposal is based on eight principles:

1. There should be guaranteed universal access to a package of basic health care benefits.
2. The health care system should be financed by both government and private sources.
3. The health care delivery and health care financing systems should be restructured so that incentives are consistent for all parties to achieve cost controls.
4. Health care delivery should be established using community care networks.

5. Payments by purchasers should be based on capitated fees to community care networks in concert with incentives given to providers.
6. Cost shifting should be avoided.
7. Maximum flexibility should be maintained to ensure success.
8. Formation of networks should be promoted in the public sector by encouraging the Medicare and Medicaid programs to use and advocate the use of networks for their beneficiaries.

The most recent professional group to enter the dialogue related to health care reform has been the American Medical Association. Sensing the tides of change, after the election of President Clinton, the AMA came forth with its proposal, which advocates that employers be required to pay medical bills of uninsured workers, plus a penalty. Other components include tax incentives for health individual retirement accounts; extension of medical benefits to part-time workers using vouchers equal to a set percentage of gross pay; support for managed care as an option in a pluralistic delivery system; incentives to switch to uniform electronic billing; and tax credits for small employers spending more than a set percentage of wages and pretax income on health benefits.

The National League for Nursing, joined by other nursing organizations, placed its agenda for health care reform on the public agenda in 1991. This plan calls for four actions: (1) payment for nonphysician providers; (2) medical effectiveness testing; (3) encouragement of managed-care options, and requirement for the uninsured; and (4) public disclosure of vital health information. This agenda for health care reform involves joining with consumers as a force for health care change.

Not surprisingly, the proposals emanating from professional associations have embedded within them some elements that serve to advance the goals of the professional associations and their responsibilities to member organizations.

MORE FUNDAMENTAL HEALTH SYSTEM REFORM

While clearly the issue of reform in health care is the topic of the day, the component most noticeably lacking in the approaches related is fundamental restructuring of the system itself. Our current system is structured around a medical model designed to treat disease. All of the incentives in the system are built to reinforce this orientation. Until the system is restructured to emphasize health promotion and primary prevention to reduce disease, and the incentives redirected to support this emphasis, it is unlikely that any significant change will occur. But such a redirection is likely to have major repercussions, particularly to vested interests who potentially have much to lose in a restructured system, such as hospitals, physicians, and insurers. These are extremely powerful lobbying groups, and it is easy to understand why the multiple proposals for health care reform tiptoe around these special interest groups with their potential for financing political action committees. Health care reform is a highly charged political matter, and it is highly unlikely that solutions to the current crisis will come through governmental action or through the public policy process. The public policy arena responds to the pressures of political constituencies, and the process militates against comprehensive change. Changes that occur through natural public policy processes are incremental and in many instances serve to compound the problems rather than resolve more fundamental problems. And the solutions offered by professionals and professional interest groups address the problems through the eyes of the providers, and not through those of the community. How are more fundamental approaches to addressing the health care crisis to be achieved?

Through experience with a broad cross section of demonstration projects across the country directed toward underserved populations and vulnerable population groups (infant-child, adolescent, elderly, and family), the Kellogg Foundation has had the opportunity to gain a somewhat different perspective on the health care crisis within this country. From this experience, we have learned to appreciate the rich reservoir of resources represented by people living in communities across the country as being part of the solution, rather than the problem, in addressing high-priority health concerns.

Grandmothers who make it their business to teach adolescent girls about sexual matters and thus reduce adolescent pregnancy, community health advocates who serve as bridges between formal health care providers and the health needs of communities, and young people who are volunteering time and talent to help elderly people in rural areas of the South are but a few examples of what can be achieved through local initiatives. The solution to the current health care crisis cannot be achieved by the politicians or the providers, but requires the participation of a broad cross section of constituencies across this country in initiating true change.

To accelerate this process, the Kellogg Foundation is now attempting to collaborate with selected communities within Michigan that wish to work toward fundamental reform of their health care systems. The primary goal of the comprehensive community health model (CCHM) is to assist these Michigan communities in making their health care systems more accessible, affordable, and acceptable to local residents, employers, and providers. Using community-based demonstration sites, the CCHM will test its assumption that health care is a local matter and that communities need to play preeminent roles in design, implementation, and management of fundamental health care reform. The CCHM will work with communities to develop local solutions and to achieve the following objectives:

- Extend universal coverage communitywide
- Eliminate adverse selection in the insurance market
- Increase local control of health decision making
- Enhance the accountability, quality, and effectiveness of the health care delivery system
- Reduce the inefficiency of the system and reduce overhead costs through streamlining administration
- Develop an integrated delivery system emphasizing primary prevention, primary care, and health outcomes

Through establishment of a community board that is responsible and has authority for decision making regarding how all health- and human service–related dollars are spent, the CCHM offers communities an opportunity to achieve fundamental reform of their health care delivery systems by greatly increasing control at the local level. Creation of health enterprise zones to allow for demonstration of a restructured system of health care under management of a community board holds promise that communities can greatly increase the efficiency of the system through a single administrative structure that reduces cost shifting and other wasteful gaming that is currently prevalent. As a community's health system becomes more integrated and organized around primary prevention and primary care, the care provided will be more cost effective. Ultimately, use of high-cost tertiary care will be reduced. In the process, the health of the community will be improved.

If these demonstration models prove to be successful, it is hoped that they may serve as a model for more extensive and fundamental health system reform at the state and national levels.

SUMMARY

Can the health care crisis be resolved so that all Americans have access to health care at costs that are affordable to those who pay the bills? The issues cannot be resolved through approaches to ensuring the system that is currently in place. Given the economic climate, approaches that do not address more fundamental issues are likely to fail. Similarly, issues that do not address the fundamental problem of a medically driven, disease-oriented approach are unlikely to yield appreciable gains. The health care crisis confronting us can only be resolved by engaging the people who pay the bills (the employers) and the people who use the services (the consumers) to be major participants in solving the problems. The entire system must be reshaped and the focus changed, along with the incentives, to maintain the health of people and engage them as active participants in the process. At the center of this reform are nurses. It is nursing that has the knowledge base and the skills necessary for engaging with people in the community in effective approaches to health promotion and disease prevention. And nurses can be the monitors of health and the frontline identifiers of problems in need of treatment.

But without these frontline workers, and the active involvement of people in being the keepers of health in the community, the system will continue to focus upon disease and its treatment. If our system can change its focus to become a true health care system, the strengths of our medical care system and our high-technology hospitals can be used more effectively; in the end, a restructured system has the potential for gain benefiting everyone involved.

REFERENCES

1. Alaska State Legislature Health Resources and Access Task Force. (1992, March). *Health care reform final recommendations to the governor and the seventeenth Alaska legislature.* (Report). Adopted March 14, 1992.
2. American Hospital Association. (1992, January 25). *Key concepts underlying AHA's national health care reform strategy* (Approved by the AHA Board of Trustees).
3. Eckholm, E. (1991, September 26). Health benefits found to deter switches in jobs. *New York Times,* p. 1.
4. *Governor Romer's Colorado health care reform.* (1993, January). *Health Care Reform Initiative, 1,* 1–4.
5. McNeil, D. G., Jr. (1991, November 17). Washington tries to sort out health insurance proposals. *New York Times,* p. 3.
6. *New School Commentator, 3*(6), 3. (1992, March).
7. *State initiatives in health care reform.* (1992, October). Newsletter for the Robert Wood Johnson Foundation's State Initiatives in Health Care Financing Reform Program. Published by Alpha Center in Washington, D.C.
8. Three additional states pass health care reform plans. (1992, July). *Nation's Health,* p. 17.
9. The three routes to health care reform. (1992, February 15). *National Journal,* p. 381.

CHAPTER 58

Viewpoints

Nursing's agenda for health care reform

PAMELA J. MARALDO

LAUNCHING A NATIONAL MOVEMENT FOR REFORM

In 1961 John Kennedy told Americans that it was time to reach for the moon; it took just eight years. In the 1990s it seems we have a new challenge tantamount to reaching the moon: can the nation adopt a workable national health plan?

In fact the barriers to advancing a national health proposal appeared until recently even more substantial than those faced by early astronauts seeking to penetrate beyond the Earth's atmosphere. What the space program had that health care has traditionally lacked is committed leadership capable of advancing the nation forward, undaunted by the inevitable naysayers. Most policymakers and pundits observing health care scoffed openly at the idea that meaningful national health reform was possible or plausible. The American people want it, but aren't willing to pay the costs, they said. Too many complex political scores to settle in order to hold the thing together, too many competing interests, not enough real desire, they shrugged.

By 1990 the shrugs ended. Daily accounts in the media exhorted policymakers to rectify the ills of a health care system that was failing. Public criticism of American hospitals became more and more prominently featured in the popular press. Polls were released indicating strong public sentiment in favor of major reform—and a willingness to pay for it. A *New York Times*/CBS News poll[5] indicated that voters were willing to embrace a broad range of possible solutions to the health care problem, including compelling employers to extend health benefits, imposing a tax increase if it would address the problem of skyrocketing medical costs, and even adopting a Canadian-style

government-paid health system. In 1991 pollsters Daniel Yankelovich and John Immerwahr identified an "expert/public gap"—deep divisions between the way experts analyzed health care and the way the public saw the issue. "In essence," said Yankelovich, "the public defines the health care crises as an old problem: An age-old human failing—greed—has taken over."[7] Numerous other polls and surveys conveyed public outrage at the health system and demands for change.[2]

Despite a growing avalanche of opinion surveys and media attention, policymakers still resisted serious action toward reform. Conventional wisdom in Washington now held that although Americans were concerned about health care and willing to accept change, they were nonetheless preoccupied with a wide range of issues and would not necessarily hold legislators accountable on this one complaint. The process of reforming health care appeared laden with land mines, and without a decisive public mandate, action seemed too dangerous for the individual policymaker.

Conventional wisdom was turned on its head in 1991. In that year Pennsylvania held a special election to fill the seat vacated by the untimely death of U.S. senator John Heinz. Running against two-time Pennsylvania governor and odds-on favorite Richard Thornburgh was candidate Harris Wofford, a relative unknown with no elective political experience. After polls put Wofford 40 points below Thornburgh in September before the election, Wofford's handlers decided to conduct a somewhat unorthodox poll of their own. Instead of preparing a complex questionnaire and instructing paid pollsters to read it to statewide respondents, Wofford's staff personally called a few hundred Pennsylvanians and asked only one question: "What issue matters the most to you and why?"

The answer surprised them. Over 70% of the respondents volunteered that they were most worried about health care. Health care outranked the economy, unemployment, the environment, drugs, and every other major issue facing the state and the nation. This despite the relative inattention to the subject in the media and by other politicians. For although diseases and new treatments make the news, structural issues of high costs, inadequate quality, and lack of access rarely appear as page-one stories. They were page-one issues to Pennsylvanians.

As a result of the survey, Wofford centered his campaign on a promise to reform health care. Nearly all of his advertisements, announcements, and speeches were dominated by the pledge to fight for change in the health care system. Despite the fact that he had no background in health care and no details of what kind of change he intended, the promise to do *something,* anything, about health care as a top policy priority resonated with Pennsylvanians. Thornburgh was put on the defensive, forced to explain what he had accomplished for health reform, which caused him to underestimate the power of the issue and refuse to commit to a policy of reform. This proved his downfall. Despite endorsements and visits to the state by President Bush and other prominent Republicans, Wofford defeated Thornburgh and sent a powerful message to Washington that health reform was an idea whose time had come. In the wake of the surprise election results, President Bush immediately canceled a trip to Japan to work with advisers fashioning his long-awaited national health plan.

With the Wofford victory, the nation moved into "Phase 2" of the reform process. No longer debating whether or not reform is necessary, possible, probable, or appropriate, now Americans are arguing what kind of reform they will implement. Not even the most conservative or change-aversive pundits dare to suggest that reform might not be necessary. No politician interested in reelection will sit on the fence on the issue of health reform, as Thornburgh attempted so unsuccessfully.

THE NURSING SOLUTION

While public opinion brewed and politicians hesitated, nurses were rolling up their sleeves to try and solve the problem. Two events converged in the late 1980s that galvanized nurses to join together as never before in hopes of leading the way toward national reform. First, the structural problems of health care became the subject of scrutiny and debate by a newly powerful stakeholder in the health care dynamic: the consumer of health care. Groups such as the American Association of Retired Persons, the People's Medical Society, and the National Consumers' League suddenly became major players in the health policy game—players with as much power as traditionally omniscient provider groups like the American Medical Association. This occurred for several reasons, including the implementation of diagnostic-related groups (DRGs), which released patients from hospitals sooner and sent consumers grappling for hospital alternatives like home health care; the unseemly conditions in many nursing homes; the growing demographic presence of the elderly in society; and the growing number of chronically ill Americans who needed expensive and too-often unavailable care.

The message to consumers was this: doctor doesn't know best any more and maybe never did. Consumers had to become involved as participants in health care, not passive recipients, or else desperately needed care might become unaffordable, of poor quality, or simply nonexistent. For nurses, this growing consumer activism was more than welcome. The battle to recognize the health needs that expand beyond the incidentals of cure—the majority of health needs, and the needs most appropriately addressed by nurses—was a battle nurses could not fight alone anymore. For indeed nurses have battled since the turn of the century to assign priority to preventive care, ongoing care for the elderly and chronically ill, prenatal care, and health promotional education. The drama and true accomplishments of the biomedical enterprise notwithstanding, nurses knew from professional experience and consumers knew from personal experience that basic care needs have been too often overlooked in the delivery of health care in the nation.

The second major event galvanizing nurses in the late 1980s was the onset of the worst nursing shortage in the twentieth century.[6] By 1988, enrollments in nursing were 184,924, down 23% from a decade earlier.[3] Numerous press reports revealed the human drama behind the numbers: dangerously understaffed hospitals, where registered nurses (RNs) worked without a break for 12 or more hours, serving twice their normal load of patients with occasional dire consequences.[6] Consumers feared hospitals more than ever; hospitals and long-term care facilities turned to temporary nurses, underqualified nursing staff, and other stopgap measures to alleviate the effects of the shortage.[6]

Commissions and studies examined the problem of the nursing shortage and came up with a few reasons for it and recommendations for amelioration. Salaries were a problem, said the U.S. Health and Human Services' secretary's Commission on Nursing, which released a definitive report on the nursing shortage and recommended a point-by-point strategy for alleviating it. But the salary issue arose not at the entry level, as many thought, but at more advanced levels of experience. A nurse on the job 20 years earned little more than an entry-level nurse, a very different scenario from that found in other professions such as law and medicine. Media image was another challenge. Americans grew up with distorted and even meanspirited images of what nurses and nursing involved, from "Hot Lips" Hoolihan to Nurse Ratchet.

But everyone agreed that the number one cause of the nursing shortage was poor utilization of nurses. Health care facilities required as part of nursing responsibilities nonnursing tasks that took nurses away from patients and caused stress and dissatisfaction. Even in many facilities complaining bitterly of the nursing shortage, nurses reported spending 50% or more of their time on nonnursing tasks such as clerical work, serving food, cleaning, and other important work not efficiently completed by scarce RNs. Not only did the ill-defined scope of nurses' job descriptions discourage people from aspiring to a nursing career and cause practicing nurses to give up in despair, but it also had a severe impact on the quality of care delivered in the nation.[6]

Although there had been shortages in the past, none had ever sustained such ongoing public scrutiny and vigilance, in part because none had had so much attention from organized consumers. So in the late 1980s, health policymakers, prodded by increasingly powerful consumers troubled by the quality of care in America's health system, asked nurses for the first time, "What do you want?"

The adage "be careful what you ask for, you might get it" haunted nurses. Yes, nurses wanted career ladder salaries, more media role models, better utilization—but this wouldn't be enough to solve the shortage in the long run nor enough to satisfy nurses in the short run. Nurses wanted fundamental change in the health care delivery system—change that would value those priorities that nurses and consumers shared but that had been placed on the back burner by the mammoth biomedical machine. Nurses wanted to provide prenatal care in communities, to promote home care, to see the health care system centered on the vibrant needs of communities.

Nurses sought to actualize the nursing model of health care, the model that defines health needs first and foremost based on the experience of the individual, and only then at the event of a disease.[1] Nurses wanted to integrate within the scope of the health care system issues like drug abuse, alcoholism, poverty, and homelessness—in hopes of contributing the enormous expertise and resources of the nation's health system to be a partner with the American people instead of a technician interested only when physiological failures occur. Yet how would we explain to policymakers, colleagues, and the American public what this nursing vision entailed?

AN AGENDA IS BORN

The challenge and opportunities sparked by events in health care in the late 1980s represented a turning point in the nursing community. We held in our hands exciting potential to make lasting change in health care. It made no sense to continue haggling over issues of past dissension that found nurses battling each other instead of standing up for what we had in common. The nursing heritage was too precious to waste on contending among ourselves. So at the 1987 National League for Nursing (NLN) convention in Washington, D.C., the membership passed the first resolution of its kind in the nation, calling for nurses to develop a national health proposal.

In the ensuing months, NLN board members and staff met with consultants, economists, nurse leaders, nurses from all segments of the delivery setting, and policymakers to develop a foundation for the plan. How should health care be financed? Who would be eligible for what benefits? In discussions, what appeared to matter most to nurses was not what nurses preferred, but what consumers wanted. Asked about health reform, nurses would invariably explain how consumers seem to prefer home care, but can't get it, or how consumers would like to have preventive care available, but have difficulty finding the services in their communities.

So a coalition of nursing organizations hired nationally known polling firm Peter Hart Associates to conduct a public opinion poll to tell us how the public felt about health care. What the Hart survey found was serious concern among Americans about the quality of health care in the nation and fear about escalating costs, which consumers by a vast majority blamed on physician fees. Respondents recommended expanded utilization of nurses for primary care, home care, and other needed services. Most of all, more than any other provider, the public identified nurses as the solution to the problems in health care.

The results of the poll were more than enlightening; they proved a clarion call for America's nurses. Not only were the people seriously disenchanted with business as usual in health care, but they were anxious for solutions and saw nurses providing them. Given the strong message from the Hart survey, advancement of a national health plan emerged as a number one policy priority among nursing organizations.

The National League for Nursing developed a draft and then sought endorsement from the American Nurses Association (ANA) and other nursing organizations. After considerable discussion and fact-finding, a final draft was prepared and endorsed by the NLN, the ANA, and, eventually, over 45 nursing organizations representing a membership of 1 million.[4]

NURSING'S AGENDA FOR HEALTH CARE REFORM

Nursing's Agenda for Health Care Reform includes four vital elements of change proposed by nursing.

Payment for services of nonphysician providers

Nurses are, of course, the primary cost-saving mechanism to provide basic health services. All the major studies looking at nursing effectiveness confirm that nurses provide high-quality, cost-effective care equal, and often superior in calibre, to physician services.

Nurses should not apologize anymore or hide their light under a bushel. There is no system of primary care in America. Nurses could provide affordable basic health care to those who need it—and are in fact doing so, despite restrictions, in communities throughout the nation. In Nursing's Agenda for Health Care Reform, nurses would be positioned as mainstream providers of care—in primary care, preventive health services, home care, and long-term care—with payment from all customary sources for nursing services in those settings. As the Peter Hart poll confirmed, the public is clamoring for primary care systems and supports nurses in those roles.

Medical effectiveness testing

Instead of leaving it to the prerogative of individual physicians to order the appropriate tests, procedures, surgeries, and the like, interventions could only be ordered after they had been demonstrated to be medically effective. Physicians call this "cookbook medicine;" it is really just the application of basic research principles—such as how many times on average a given procedure was performed effectively.

Managed care options encouraged, and mandated for the uninsured

Managed care—the best package of services for a given population at the lowest price—should be encouraged for employees as well as the uninsured. Some community nursing centers (CNCs) are examples of managed care, providing a point of entry into the delivery setting where overall care can be monitored and planned.

In a system serious about prevention, CNCs could be located in postsecondary schools or workplaces. Nurses could identify health problems and, with the diagnostic and prescriptive authority to treat them on the spot, offer preventive care to intervene against the development of a more acute phase of the disease or the need for hospitalization. Nursing's agenda recommends establishment of a national network of CNCs and other kinds of community primary care centers to offer needed services throughout the nation.

Public disclosure of vital health information

If health care institutions and providers, as well as accrediting bodies, are required to release data about quality to the public, individuals will be able to make intelligent choices between competing alternatives. Information subject to disclosure in nursing's agenda would include evidence of outcome, alternatives to prescribed procedures, and differences among possible interventions, as well as experience and track record of health providers.

It is important to recognize that the roots of many of the inefficiencies in health care are in the curtailment of the free market in health care. Consumers choose providers and accept treatment regimens with less information than they would select a new automobile or even a brand of cereal. This means that competition among providers is not based on quality or cost considerations, and inefficiency ultimately results. Currently, the main force consumers exercise to redress problems of quality is not the power of the purse, but the power of the courts. Malpractice is an expensive, unsatisfactory solution to the problem of quality, but it is the only solution available when information with which to choose providers is so scarce. Until the health system is reformed, malpractice must remain as the last resort for dissatisfied consumers.

THE NATIONAL DEBATE

Nursing is not alone among those proposing plans to reform the delivery system. A number of reform proposals circulating in Washington and elsewhere also provide ideas for reforming health care. Most of them center on expanding access to cover all Americans or at least more of our citizens than currently are included. With a single-minded determination to expand health insurance coverage, many health proposals lack interest in determining what kind of health care system should be purchased with the recommended infusion of funds.

One of the issues strongly emphasized by nursing's agenda is that the nation's health care system must be restructured to meet the current and evolving demand for health care. This element is missing from other plans. For instance, the problem of uneven geographical distribution of health facilities and services in the nation is one that has long perplexed policymakers and has not been easily amenable to solution. This has been particularly true in rural areas, where physicians are scarce and patient volume is often not high enough to justify the cost of establishing adequate acute care health facilities by restructuring the delivery setting to appropriately meet the demand for services.

As mentioned earlier, nursing's agenda would address the problem of uneven access with incentives for creation of community health facilities providing preventive and ongoing basic services to discourage to the extent possible the need for crisis intervention. It is not enough to mandate health benefits for the uninsured, because the health system is simply not prepared to provide care to them all. Nursing's agenda is designed to address the problem of access on a more fundamental level.

CONCLUSION

Given the tenor of public opinion in the nation favoring health care reform, nurses have an extraordinary opportunity to bring real change to the health care system. While the American public demands change to lower costs, enhance access, and improve the quality of care, only nursing's agenda includes all the interlocking elements of change necessary to meet this surge of public sentiment. Indications are that if the American public will be expected to pay added taxes or the indirect added costs of employer coverage, they will also expect fundamental change of the magnitude nursing proposes.

The health care system must be restructured to meet the demands of the consumer of care, not the needs of providers. Health care reform will not satisfy the public otherwise. Furthermore, the problems of cost and quality that plague health care derive from waste and inefficiency of a system not driven by customer service considerations or real competition. By expanding both coverage and access at the community level, addressing the overuse and regulation of technology, mandating public disclosure, and proposing proved cost-cutting innovations that the public supports, nursing's agenda gets at the roots of the challenges ahead and offers real solutions.

Like those who would conquer space in the 1960s, in the 1990s it is nurses and their supporters poised to conquer the newest frontier in American life: the re-creation of the health care system. If we remain true to our mission, not rankled by the pessimists, and courageous in our commitment to the American people, we have the opportunity to create a new health care system that truly serves the health of the public.

REFERENCES

1. Aiken, L., & Fagin, C. (1992). *Charting the future of health care.* Philadelphia: J. B. Lippincott.
2. Health care costs top "worry list" again. (1991, October 1). *The Wall Street Journal,* p. C-22.
3. National League for Nursing. (1992). *Nursing data source, vol. I.* New York: Author.
4. National League for Nursing & American Nurses Association. (1991). *Nursing's agenda for health care reform.* New York: Author. Endorsed by:
   Advocates for Child Psychiatric Nursing, Inc.
   American Academy of Ambulatory Nursing Administration
   American Academy of Nursing
   American Association of Colleges of Nursing
   American Association of Critical Care Nurses
   American Association of Neuroscience Nurses
   American Association of Nurse Anesthetists
   American Association of Occupational Health Nurses
   American Association of Spinal Cord Injury Nurses
   American Holistic Nurses Association
   American Nephrology Nurses Association

American Psychiatric Nurses Association
American Radiological Nurses Association
American Society of Ophthalmic Registered Nurses, Inc.
American Society of Plastic and Reconstructive Surgical Nurses
American Society of Post Anesthesia Nurses
American Urological Association Allied
Association of Black Nursing Faculty in Higher Education, Inc.
Association of Community Health Nursing Educators
Association of Operating Room Nurses, Inc.
Association of Pediatric Oncology Nurses
Association of Rehabilitation Nurses
Association of State and Territorial Directors of Nursing
Chi Eta Phi Sorority, Inc.
Coalition for Psychiatric Nursing Organizations
Dermatology Nurses Association
Emergency Nurses Association
Florida Organization of Nurse Executives
Intravenous Nurses Society, Inc
Leukemia Society of America
Midwest Alliance in Nursing
NAACOG, The Organization for Obstetric, Gynecologic, &
   Neonatal Nurses
National Association for Health Care Recruitment
National Association of Hispanic Nurses
National Association of Neonatal Nurses
National Association of Nurse Practitioners in Reproductive
   Health
National Association of Orthopaedic Nurses
National Association of School Nurses, Inc.

National Black Nurses' Association, Inc.
National Conference of Gerontological Nurse-Practitioners
National Federation for Specialty Nursing Organizations
National Flight Nurses Association
National Nurses Society on Addictions
National Nursing Staff Development Organization
National Organization of Nurse Practitioner Faculties
New Jersey Association of Directors of Nursing
   Administrators/Long Term Care Facilities, Inc.
New Jersey College Health Association
North American Nursing Diagnosis Association
Nurse Consultants Association
Nurses House Incorporated
Oncology Nursing Society
Philippine Nurses Association of America, Inc.
Society for Education and Research in Psychiatric-Mental Health
   Nursing
Society for Peripheral Vascular Nursing
Society of Gastroenterology Nurses and Associates
Society of Otorhinolaryngology and Head-Neck Nurses, Inc.
Southern Council on Collegiate Education for Nursing
Western Institute of Nursing

5. *New York Times/CBS News health care poll.* (1991, August 18-22).
   Storrs, Conn: Roper Center.

6. U.S. Department of Health and Human Services, Secretary's Commission on Nursing. (1988, December). *Support studies & background information, volume II.* Washington, D.C.: Author.

7. Yankelovich, J. I. (1991, Third Quarter). A perception gap. *Health Management Quarterly.*

CHAPTER 59

Financing of health care and its impact on nursing

CAROLYNE KAHLE DAVIS

HEALTH CARE FINANCING

With the advent of Medicare and Medicaid in 1965, the federal government embarked on a significant subsidy of health care. Today 35 million Americans are enrolled in Medicare, a program for the elderly, the disabled, and those with end-stage renal disease, and 25 million indigent qualify for Medicaid. It is easy to see why a significant proportion of health care services are now paid for by these programs. The initial thrust of the program during the 1970s was concern for access to care, but this focus has changed to one of concern for escalating costs. By the 1980s it was apparent that structural changes in both payment and delivery of services needed to occur. To understand the impact of fiscal policy on the delivery system and on nursing, we must first have a basic understanding of Medicare and Medicaid.

Medicare, as envisioned in its original legislation in 1965, was to assist people over the age of 65 to pay for their acute care illnesses. Additional coverage was provided later that recognized the unique needs of disabled individuals as well as people with end-stage renal disease. For more than two decades the decisions about which services would be covered reflected almost totally payment for care received in hospitals as well as payments to physicians. During the early 1980s it was recognized that many ambulatory-type services not previously provided by Medicare should be covered so that there would be attractive alternatives to expensive inpatient hospitalization. For example, ambulatory surgery was approved in 1981, and now over 50% of a hospital's surgical interventions are done in same-day surgery facilities that cater to ambulatory care procedures. As more elderly citizens receive care for their acute health needs, their lifespans have been length-ened so that now the average life expectancy is 75 years. Indeed, we now have 3.3 million Americans over the age of 85 and 45,000 over the age of 100.[1] Projections are for these two groups to grow considerably over the next two decades.

As our elderly live longer, they suffer from more chronic diseases that require different therapeutic care. Many more people now need skilled nursing home care or continued therapeutic support in the home with or without community support services. Medicare has been under constant pressure to expand its coverage of these services. Congress introduced legislation annually to expand home care programs and nursing home care, but until the Medicare Catastrophic Illness Protection Act of 1988, little legislation was ever successful. With the passage of this landmark legislation, Congress did indeed expand both home care and skilled nursing home services to further protect the elderly from devastating financial problems brought on by their chronic care needs. This legislation was short lived, however, as Congress responded to the elderly group's unhappiness with a "means test" for increased premiums to pay for expanded services by repealing the entire act the following year.

At the same time, the enormous growth in Medicare outlays has put the Health Insurance Trust Fund in danger of bankruptcy by 2005 unless the payroll contribution to Medicare is increased by 47% or outlays reduced by 32%. Increasing payroll taxes is not viewed as a popular move by either the administration or Congress. The Medicare program's budget is in danger of further reductions to protect the basic solvency of the program. Clearly, neither alternative of payroll tax increases or decreased outlays alone will ensure the long-range solvency of Medicare. A reform of the entire

Medicare program will undoubtedly occur in the late 1990s that will probably require increased contributions by wealthier beneficiaries (means test).

Despite the previously mentioned concern, the public-sector share of our national health care expenditures is expected to grow from its current 40.6% to 42.5% by 2000, with the federal share increasing from 28.7% to 32.6%.[4] Most of these projected increases in both Medicare and Medicaid are due to the increased number of elderly who need care, coupled with the very heavy costs of highly sophisticated technology developed to treat many of the acute care problems. Because of the projected dramatic increases in outlays to these two programs over the next decade, health care providers must anticipate changes in payment for health care services that embody the concepts of cost constraints to protect the integrity of these programs. For example, Medicare payments nearly doubled between 1981 and 1985 and are projected to increase from $131 billion in 1992 to $320.8 billion by 2000.[9] Medicaid too will increase more than 50% every 5 years from its fiscal year 1992 base of $65 billion to $138 billion by 2000.

Medicaid is a jointly sponsored state-federal program that provides both acute and long-term services for about 20 million poor. Each state may set its own criteria for eligibility based on income standards that have been broadly determined by federal guidelines. Federal guidelines also define a mandatory scope of covered services, such as hospital, physician, and skilled nursing facility care. Although services such as eyeglasses are optional, coverages are determined individually by each state legislature. In 1981 Congress passed legislation that approved Medicaid payment for nurse-midwife services directly. Recent years have seen an expansion in recognition of coverage of payment to nonphysician providers such as nurse practitioners, certified nurse-midwives, and certified registered nurse anesthetists for Medicare and Medicaid.

Primarily, single-parent children and unwed mothers eligible for Aid to Families with Dependent Children (AFDC) are the ones who benefit mostly from acute care and preventive services. Although the elderly are less than 20% of the enrollees, the outlays for long-term care for them average about 45% of all payments. Since 1981 there has been continued emphasis on cost containment within the Medicaid program. This has given rise to intergenerational debates about the appropriateness of services available between acute and long-term care.

Looking only at health care, statistics show that the poor and elderly accounted for 44% of all admissions to hospitals in 1986, up from 40% in 1981. As the trend continues, the government's influence on health care delivery systems will continue to escalate, and shortfalls in payments to hospitals by Medicare and Medicaid will compound the current payment problems. The government's search for further efficiencies will cause even further restructuring in the delivery of services. More attempts to rationalize the delivery of adequate care will lead more providers to negotiate with preferred provider organizations (PPOs) and health maintenance organizations (HMOs). One of the major attractions of managed care is the reduction in utilization of selective services without an appreciable denial of access to quality service.

According to the National Center for Health Statistics, inpatient hospital days per 1000 population have already declined since 1980 by 27%, from 1134 days per 1000 to under 700.[6] Many HMOs report usage rates of around 400 inpatient days per 1000 population. As we move into an era of even more managed care, one can anticipate a continued movement to less care in our high-cost hospitals and more services provided in other patient care settings. Expansion of services in home care is reflected in the enormous growth in the number of home care agencies between 1981 (3169) and 1987 (5887), an 85% increase; skilled nursing facilities expanded 39%; and ambulatory surgical centers, virtually unknown before 1981, grew at a 516% rate.[3] These increases have had an enormous impact on nursing, because each agency needs registered nurses to supervise and give care. The rapid increases in these alternatives in health care have helped to increase the demand for nurses.

In the acute care hospital sector, payments have been controlled since 1983 by the initiation of an incentive-based prospective payment system utilizing diagnostic-related groups (DRGs). This system has enabled the government to reduce its payment outlays to hospitals by many billions of dollars. For example, the hospital market-basket inflation increased 18% between 1984 and 1987, yet Medicare, whose beneficiaries account for 39% of hospital revenues, raised prices paid to hospitals only 9%. This has caused hospital net profit margins to decline precipitously since 1984, with small rural hospitals experiencing the most problems. The American Hospital Association (AHA) recently reported that more than half of all community hospitals actually lost money on Medicare inpatient care in recent years, a fact that the AHA cites as a reason some hospitals have closed or merged.

Meanwhile, employers have grown increasingly concerned about payments for health insurance to cover their employees and retirees. Within 7 years, employer payment for health insurance doubled,[2] spurring interest by businesses in cost containment measures such as those initiated by the federal sector. Utilization review has emerged as a major enterprise among businesses, along with coverage options that encourage the use of PPOs and HMOs.

The blending of both private-sector and public-sector concern for financing escalating health care services has led to a new emphasis on productivity and the need for more information to better manage the delivery system. Although hospitals have initiated major marketing strategies and developed contractual relationships with multiple PPOs and HMOs to assure an adequate group of patients, they are only now beginning to measure productivity and quality of care through the use of new hospital information systems. The Department of Health and Human Services' new initiative to determine medical effectiveness of specific procedures should, over the next decade, produce some startling savings—as much as $20 billion to $50 billion—and change the way health care is delivered in our country.

The strategy to study the medical effectiveness of physician practice decisions grew out of the work of Wennberg, a physician who found major variations in practice patterns between different communities, even those within the same state. Robert Brooks, MD, of the Rand Corporation, has also investigated selected procedures, such as coronary artery bypass grafts, cataract surgery and carotid, and endarterectomy, and concluded that as much as 20% to 30% of these procedures may not be necessary and may not improve the quality of a person's life.

The Department of Health and Human Services is now planning to invest between $75 and $200 million over the next several years in research to analyze the outcomes of selected procedures to determine the best practice patterns by comparing large volumes of claims data with actual outcomes for patients. Although the focus thus far has been on medical decision making related to patient outcome, new interdisciplinary research studies are beginning to indicate a significant relationship with nursing. Nursing practice should initiate further interdisciplinary studies related to outcome of care.

The Cleveland business community, together with hospitals and physicians, has formed a privately sponsored organization to collect and analyze data from all regional hospitals related to quantifying outcomes of care. This data has been released publicly and is expected to be utilized to influence business leaders' selection of health care providers in the Cleveland region. Other business groups around the country are watching this activity very closely and may try to replicate it in other communities.

HEALTH CARE REFORM

The economic slump of 1990 to 1992 caused serious unemployment, which catapulted the concerns for cost of health care services and access to appropriate low-cost health services into the public consciousness. With the elections of 1992, health care reform became a major concern for politicians everywhere; both major political parties identified strategies for health care reform. Expansion of coverage to those currently not insured could be by vouchers or tax credits coupled with small group health insurance reform or by mandating that employers provide coverage to all their workers. Both parties also talked about the need for health insurance networks or purchasing co-ops to strengthen the small businesses' ability to purchase group health insurance through managed care given by community providers. Since the general public has very little understanding of the advantages and disadvantages of all these proposals, there is as yet no approach that has emerged as having support from a majority of Americans. It is likely that much discussion and study of other countries' models of delivery of care and cost containment will occur in the near future.

One clear lesson that is likely to emerge from these studies is that other countries such as Canada and the Netherlands utilize public health nurses to provide most primary care services. The combination of access to primary care and emergency care appears to be the trade-off that other populations have accepted to guarantee access, with queuing for elective service viewed as a necessary part of cost controls.

Whether Americans can change their values to endorse waiting remains to be seen since we are a country that values immediate gratification of our needs (fast foods, automated teller machines, and drive-in banking). We also place a high value on technology and appreciate advanced high technology in selecting our care providers. Controlling costs could cause significant restrictions in capital, which could decrease our available investments in high technology.

IMPACT ON NURSING

From the beginning of the Medicare prospective payment system, immediate changes were noted. Length of hospital stay dropped precipitously, and review for appropriateness of admission caused a concomitant decrease in admissions, thus causing occupancy to plummet in many hospitals. As hospital budgets became tighter, new responsibilities were defined for the nursing staff. Registered nurses (RNs) were utilized to deliver total patient care, and nurse's aides and licensed practical nurses (LPNs) were laid off because of declining occupancies.

Cost of nursing services began to be examined more closely, because these services represented a large share of the hospital budget. Discharge planning assumed a major new role in importance as patients were discharged to aftercare facilities, such as home care and skilled nursing facilities. Within several years, the hospitals diversified into major new ambulatory services, and all these settings demanded registered nurses, causing an increase in demand for RNs just as enrollments into schools of nursing were experiencing sharp declines. As the impact of these increased demands were being felt, hospitals began to request that nursing leadership take a new look at the appropriate utilization of nursing personnel. Nursing has recognized the enormous impact of "substitutions" for other care givers and is beginning to restructure the nursing environment to better utilize the skills of both clinical and nonclinical care givers, while retaining the primary role of case manager for the registered nurse.

As quality-of-care issues became a central concern to hospital trustees and management, the role of nursing was highlighted. The enormous role that nurses play in assisting patients to recuperate is finally being recognized. Concern has escalated over patient complications that cause increased lengths of stay that affect a hospital's fiscal stability, especially when the extended stay results in an "outlier" (an extended stay costing the hospital more than the amount Medicare pays); registered nurses are a valuable asset that can prevent these occurrences. Nurses are using their clinical skills at the bedside to monitor and spot complications and intervene appropriately to prevent complications serious enough to alter a patient's treatment pattern or length of stay. Ever so slowly the contem-

porary image of nursing is changing to recognize this vital role that nurses have in the provision of care.

The central value in the health care system seems to be the maintenance of a proper balance between quality of care, access to care, and cost. Ideally, quality of care should be increased, access should be increased, and cost should be decreased. Some people do not believe this is possible, and others believe that by restructuring the system and demanding more productivity, along with more appropriateness of therapeutic interventions, quality can be increased while reducing cost and enhancing access.

Hornback[5] wrote that the value of nursing and hence its economic rewards ought to be derived from its contributions to access, quality, efficiency, equity, and health status.[3] During hearings on the nursing shortage, the Commission on Nursing heard many nurses testifying to the need to pay more for experienced clinical nurses. One of the 16 recommendations of the commission suggests that attention be given to fixing the "wage compression" problem to retain nurses at the bedside. Indeed, some hospitals have recognized the problem and are designing clinical career ladder programs with salaries approaching $50,000 to $60,000 for selected nurses with significant clinical experience. This is an important breakthrough for nursing because it recognizes the enormous contribution nurses are making to the patients' care regimens. However, hospital administrators are becoming uneasy thinking about the fiscal problems they already have, even without these salary increases. Thus it is up to the nursing leadership to demonstrate that the nursing department is willing to restructure itself to become as efficient and productive as possible and that not all nurses will be paid the $50,000 figure.

Some hospitals will continue to use all registered nurses because of the type of patients and the care that is needed, but many other hospitals will redistribute the care-giving functions among many levels of nursing personnel. Demonstration projects are already being designed to encourage hospitals to evaluate these restructured delivery systems focusing on the quality of care being delivered by these nursing units.

To assist nursing in its management of patient care services, hospitals may need to introduce computerized patient care management information systems. Nurses must recognize the need to utilize modern management tools such as information systems in order to better track patient care and account for errors of omission in care. By enhancing productivity through restructuring the patient care environment and using new technology, nurses may have more time to focus on case management of their patients. Unless nursing is willing to embrace these recommendations, the shortage of nurses will probably continue, causing some hospitals to reduce services, close beds, or incur higher operating costs in overtime and agency fees. Concern for bottom-line budgets could cause some organizations to lower their standards of care unknowingly and thus jeopardize their fiscal situation even further, because the government can deny payments to hospitals for substandard care.

As hospitals track patient care, it will become more apparent that nurses have a major role in preventing poor care. Nurses may be able to win a larger role in decision making about therapeutic care plans once they quantify the cost benefits of their activities.

Managed care has long recognized the talents of nurse practitioners as cost-effective care givers, especially for maintenance of chronic care, and will continue to seek qualified individuals to deliver these services. Because business and industry are now encouraging the use of managed care, it follows that nurses will be increasingly recognized as cost-effective providers of services. The decade of the 1990s will be an important era for nurses, as we will see continued awareness of the importance of nursing in the delivery of health care services. Nurses' increased political awareness and activism should enable nursing to help to shape future health care reforms.

A rational allocation of resources means changing expectations. Expectations need to be changed about the length of stay in an inpatient care setting as well as whether inpatient care is the most appropriate choice. Consumers, providers, and payers must adjust their expectations. Technological change has forced physicians and nurses to examine their practice patterns and adjust to sweeping psychological changes demanded by the new delivery system. Nurses must be willing to change their expectations about how and where health care services are to be provided, insisting only on cost-effective quality services that promote optimum outcomes in the quality of life for patients.

REFERENCES

1. Dychrwald, K. (1989). *Age wave.* Los Angeles: Jeremy Tarcher.
2. Employee Benefit Research Institute. (1987). *The changing health care market.*
3. Health Care Financing Administration. (1987). *Health Care Financing Review, 9*(2).
4. Health Care Financing Administration. (1987). National health care expenditures 1986-2000. *Health Care Financing Review, 8*(4).
5. Hornback, M. (1988). Economic models of nursing practice. In *Alternate conceptions of work and society: Implications for professional nursing.* Washington, D.C.: American Association of College of Nursing.
6. U.S. Department of Health and Human Services. (1987). *Health in the United States* (Pub. No. 88-1232). Rockville, Md: National Center for Health Statistics.

CHAPTER 60

Third-party reimbursement issues for advanced practice nurses in the '90s

MAUREEN BEIRNE STREFF

This chapter describes third-party reimbursement issues identified and confronted during 9 years of extensive on-the-job experience in designing, lobbying for, and implementing third-party reimbursement for certified psychiatric clinical specialists in Massachusetts. In this chapter we will review the history of third-party reimbursement, both public and private; examine both the nonlegislative and legislative strategy processes; and explore more fully the managed-care vehicle for providing health care specifically for nurse clinicians in the institutions or private sector from an optimal patient care focus as well as professional and financial stability for the nurse clinician.

HISTORY OF THE THIRD-PARTY REIMBURSEMENT IMPACT ON THE NURSING PROFESSION

In 1948 the American Nurses Association (ANA) identified third-party reimbursement for nursing services as a priority and included it in the association platform. However, the issue of reimbursement did not fully bloom until the nurse practitioner (NP) movement toward role autonomy pointed to the identification of potentially reimbursable services. The ANA House of Delegates (in 1972, 1974, and 1976) adopted resolutions urging vigorous support of direct reimbursement for the services of nurses by both public and private third-party payers. The state nurses' associations also began to explore possible avenues to accomplish that goal. The process, on the national level of the ANA and on the level of the state associations, evolved through the formation of groups to research current reimburse-

ment policies and potential effects of third-party reimbursement of nurses on the health care system. The ANA in a report in June 1983, "Third-Party Reimbursement Legislation for Services of Nurses. . . A Report of Changes in State Health Insurance Laws," addressed the reimbursement status of nursing services in particular states. In 1984 the ANA[1] published the work of the Council of Primary Health Care Nurse Practitioners and the Joint Task Force on Third-Party Reimbursement for the Services of Nurses. This publication has been a useful tool for designing a route to reimbursement. At the time of that publication, 14 states had legislation affecting specific or all-inclusive nurse groups. By 1986 a review of the national precedents set by the federal and state governments and private commercial insurance carriers added 18 states. The nursing specialty affected by the legislation is spelled out specifically by each state. Even in 1988 the concept of reimbursement for nursing services was revolutionary in a number of states. Some states continue to choose the incremental approach of one group per piece of reimbursement legislation because legislators in some states (e.g., Massachusetts) continue to be concerned about the projected cost of services by the numerous types of nurse practitioners and are still reluctant to pass reimbursement legislation. These nurse practitioners are currently working on approaches to illustrate cost savings that can be achieved for their particular specialty. Since 1948 the ANA has continued to pursue third-party reimbursement and provide educative experiences as in the January 1992 conference in Washington, D.C., entitled "Nursing Reimbursement: How to Get Paid for Your Services."

Table 60-1   States mandating third-party coverage for nurses, by year enacted

State	All registered nurses	Nurse practitioners	Psychiatric nurses
Alabama			
Alaska		88	
Arizona		85	
Arkansas			
California			82
Colorado	87/90		88/90
Connecticut		84	84
Delaware		90	
Florida			
Georgia			
Hawaii			
Idaho			
Illinois			
Indiana			
Iowa	89		
Kansas			
Kentucky			
Louisiana		84	
Maine			83
Maryland		79	83
Massachusetts			86
Michigan			
Minnesota		88	
Mississippi		80	
Missouri			
Montana		87	
Nebraska			
Nevada	85		
New Hampshire		85	
New Jersey	84		
New Mexico			
New York	84		
North Carolina			
North Dakota	85	85	89
Ohio			
Oklahoma			
Oregon		80	
Pennsylvania	86	86	
Rhode Island			
South Carolina			
South Dakota		80	
Tennessee			
Texas			
Utah		79	
Vermont			
Virginia			89
Washington	81	81	
West Virginia			77
Wisconsin			
Wyoming			

Adapted from: *Blue Cross and Blue Shield issue brief: State mandated health insurance laws.* (1990, September). Washington, D.C.: American Nurses Association.

Table 60-2 Nurse-midwife practice legislation, by state

Jurisdiction	Year effective
Alaska	1981
California	1991
Colorado	1987
Connecticut	1984
Florida	1982
Maryland	1979
Massachusetts	1985
Minnesota	1983
Mississippi	1979
Montana	1983
New Hampshire	1985
New Jersey	1982
New Mexico	1979
New York	1983
Nevada	1985
North Dakota	1986
Ohio	1985
Oregon	1979
Pennsylvania	1981
Rhode Island	1990
South Dakota	1980
Utah	1979
Washington	1973
West Virginia	1983

Compiled by American Nurses Association, Washington, D.C., 1991.

Table 60-3 States requiring direct private insurance reimbursement to CRNAs by statute

Alabama	New Jersey
Alaska	New Mexico
Arizona	North Dakota
Colorado	Pennsylvania
Delaware	South Dakota
Kansas	Washington
Maryland	West Virginia
Minnesota	
Mississippi	
Montana	

Compiled by American Nurses Association, Washington, D.C., 1991.

PUBLIC AND PRIVATE COMPONENTS OF THIRD-PARTY REIMBURSEMENT
Public component

The public component of the third-party reimbursement system includes Medicaid, Medicare, the Civilian Health and Medical Program of the Uniformed Services (CHAMPUS), and the Federal Employees Health Ben-

efits Program (FEHBP). Medicaid and Medicare are administrated at the federal level by the U.S. Department of Health and Human Services, Health Care Financing Administration (HCFA). CHAMPUS is administered by the Department of Defense.

Medicaid. Medicaid is a federally assisted and state-administered program providing medical assistance to members of families with dependents who are aged, blind, disabled, or under the age of consent (minors). Each state designs and administers its own program and can designate health care providers as long as the state design complies with federal guidelines; by state legislation the general law can be amended, as it was in Massachusetts in 1987 to include podiatrists' services. In 1988 a bill was filed to include the private practice services of certified clinical specialists in psychiatric and mental health nursing. This legislation died in committee each year.

Nurse-midwifery services to Medicaid subscribers have been reimbursable since 1982 when the Medicaid law changed and required all states to meet the needs of pregnant women. In 1977 the Rural Health Clinic Services Act was passed, which provides Medicaid and Medicare reimbursement for services provided by nurse practitioners and physician assistants in health centers located in medically underserved rural areas with or without a supervisory physician on-site. Twenty-eight states reimburse nurses in advanced practice under Medicaid; 31 states reimburse certified nurse anesthetists under Medicaid.

Medicare. Medicare is a nationwide health insurance program authorized under Title 18 of the Social Security Act, which provides benefits to persons 65 years of age or older. Medicare Part A is the hospital insurance program; Part B is the supplementary medical insurance program. As a result of the Omnibus Budget Reconciliation Act (OBRA) of 1989, the employer of a nurse practitioner may bill a Medicare carrier for the NP services delivered to a resident in a skilled nursing facility. This coverage became effective in April 1990.

The Omnibus Budget Reconciliation Act of 1990 covers services of NPs and clinical nurse specialists (CNSs) performed in collaboration with an MD in the rural setting. Specific guidelines and instructions for filing claims are listed in Medicare carrier manuals (MCMs) available in regional offices across the country. Nurse practitioners and clinical nurse specialists were able to bill directly for services rendered on or after January 1, 1991. A listing of rural areas may be obtained from the Health Care Financing Administration.

Table 60-4 States with health insurance laws providing for reimbursement by category

	Registered nurse	Certified registered nurse anesthetist	Certified nurse-midwife	Nurse practitioner*	Psychiatric mental health specialist
Alabama		x			
Alaska		x‡	x	x	
Arizona	x†	x	x	x	x
Arkansas		x	x		
California		x	x	x	x
Colorado	x	x‡	x‡		
Connecticut			x	x	x
Delaware		x	x	x	x
Dist. of Columbia					x
Florida			x		
Georgia					
Guam					
Hawaii					
Idaho				x	
Illinois					
Indiana					
Iowa	x	x	x	x	x
Kansas		x	x	x	x
Kentucky				x	
Louisiana			x		
Maine					x
Maryland	x	x‡	x‡		
Massachusetts			x		x
Michigan			x	x	
Minnesota		x	x	x	x
Mississippi		x	x	x	
Missouri			x	x	
Montana		x	x	x	x
Nebraska					
Nevada			x‡	x	
New Hampshire		x	x‡	x	
New Jersey	x†	x	x	x	x
New Mexico	x†	x	x	x	x
New York	x		x		
North Carolina					
North Dakota		x‡	x‡		x
Ohio		x	x		
Oklahoma					
Oregon			x	x	
Pennsylvania	x†	x	x	x	x
Rhode Island			x‡		x
South Carolina					
South Dakota		x	x	x	
Tennessee		x	x		
Texas					
Utah	x	x	x	x	x
Vermont			x		x
Virginia					x
Virgin Islands					
Washington	x	x	x	x	x

Table 60-4 States with health insurance laws providing for reimbursement by category—cont'd

	Registered nurse	Certified registered nurse anesthetist	Certified nurse-midwife	Nurse practitioner*	Psychiatric mental health specialist
West Virginia	x	x	x	x	
Wisconsin					
Wyoming	x				

*Includes variations of advanced, certified, etc.
†Certified.
‡Added by ANA data compiled in 1991.
Information obtained October 1990 from ANA constituent members.

Table 60-5 Legal titles and state requirements for advanced nursing practice

State/jurisdiction	Titles not specified	Titles specified		
		Title	Requirement	Regulatory agency
Alabama		CRNA;NP;CNM	1	BON
Alaska		NP	1	BON
Arizona		CRNA;CNM;NP	1	BON
Arkansas		CRNA;CNM;NP		BON
California		CRNA;CNM;NP	2	BON
Colorado	x		2	BON
Connecticut		ARNP	1	DOHS
Delaware		ARNP	1,2,3	BON
Dist. of Columbia		NP;CNM		BON
Florida		ARNP;CNM;CRNA	1,2,3	BON, BOM
Georgia				
Guam		NP;CRNA;CNM;CRNP	1,2,3	BON
Hawaii	x			BON
Idaho		NP	2	BON, BOM
Illinois	x			BON
Indiana		NP;CNM	2	BON, BOM
Iowa		ARNP	1,2	BON
Kansas		CRNA;NM;CNS;NP	1,2	BON
Kentucky		ARNP;CRNA;CNM;NP	1,2,3	BON
Louisiana		NP;CNM	1 or 2	BON
Maine		NP	1	BON
Maryland		NP	1,3	BON
Massachusetts		CRNA;CNM;PMH;NP	3	BON, BOM
Michigan		CRNA;CNM;CNP	1,2	BON
Minnesota	x			BON
Mississippi		NP;CNM;CRNA	3	BON
Missouri	x			BON
Montana		CRNA;CNM;NP	1	BON
Nebraska		NP	1,3	BON, BOM
Nevada		APN	1,2,3	BON
New Hampshire		ARNP	1,2	BON, BOM
New Jersey		NP;CRNA;CNM	1	BON
New Mexico		NP;CNS;CRNA	2,3	BON
New York		NP	1,3	BON
North Carolina		NP;CNM	1,2,3	BON, BOM
North Dakota	x	CRNA;CNM;NP;CNS	1,2	BON
Ohio	x		1,2	BON
Oklahoma		NP;CRNA;CNM	2	BON
Oregon		NP	2	BON

Continued

Table 60-5 Legal titles and state requirements for advanced nursing practice—cont'd

State/jurisdiction	Titles not specified	Titles specified		
		Title	Requirement	Regulatory agency
Pennsylvania		CRNP	1,2,3	BON, BOM
		CNM	1,2	BON, BOM
		CRNA	1,2	BON
Rhode Island		CNP	2	BON
South Carolina	x			BON
South Dakota		CNP;CNM	1,3	BON, BOM
Tennessee	x	CNP	1,2,3	BON, BOM
Texas		ARNP;CRNA;CNM;NP	1,2	BON
Utah		NP;CRNA;CNM;NS	1,2,3	BON
Vermont		NP	1,2,3	BON
Virginia		CNM;NP;CNS	1,2,3	BON, BOM
Virgin Islands				BON, BOM
Washington		ARNP	1,2	BON
West Virginia		CRNA;CNM		BON
Wisconsin	x	CRNA;CNM	1,2,3	BON
Wyoming	x	ANP	1,2,3	BON

Abbreviation Key
NP = Nurse Practitioner
ANP = Advanced Nurse Practitioner
ARNP = Advanced Registered Nurse Practitioner
APN = Advanced Practitioner of Nursing
CNP = Certified Nurse Practitioner
CRNA = Certified Registered Nurse Anesthetist
CNM = Certified Nurse-Midwife
CNS = Clinical Nurse Specialist

PMH = Psychiatric Mental Health Specialist
1 = Certification
2 = Advanced Education
3 = Protocols or MD Collaboration
BON = Board of Nursing
BOM = Board of Medicine
DOHS = Department of Health Services
Information obtained October 1990 from ANA constituent members.

Medicare fee schedule changes in relation to physicians began in January of 1992 as a result of the Omnibus Budget Reconciliation Act of 1989 that established a resource-based fee schedule for payments to physicians under Medicare Part B. Nonphysician practitioners payments are currently being studied. Nurses need to be aware of current procedural terminology (CPT) codes used in filing claims so that correct payment is received for each procedure or service rendered. It is highly recommended that nurses review documents available from the HCFA regarding Medicaid and Medicare rules and regulations and confer with the American Nurses Association for updates on the status of these reimbursement policies, as they are in active revision. The ANA filed, for the 1992 legislative year, a bill to provide direct Medicaid reimbursement to nurse practitioners and clinical nurse specialists for services they are legally authorized to perform under state law. This measure expands the provision enacted as part of the Omnibus Budget Reconciliation Act of 1989 as previously mentioned. The ANA also filed, for the 1992 legislative year, a bill entitled the Primary Care Health Practitioner Incentive Act, to provide direct Medicare reimbursement to NPs, CNSs, and certified nurse-midwives. This bill would issue payment to these nurses at 97% of the physician's fee schedule for services that they are legally authorized to perform under state law, regardless of location or practice setting and regardless of whether or not they are under the supervision of or associated with a physician (according to information provided by Marjorie Vanderbilt at the ANA Washington, D.C., office). Passage of this Medicare legislation would provide a necessary vehicle for the certified psychiatric clinical specialists who were not included in the Omnibus Budget Reconciliation bill signed by President Bush in December 1989 that gave clinical psychologists and licensed clinical social workers access to providing outpatient mental health services to the elderly.

CHAMPUS. CHAMPUS recognizes and provides payments to certified nurse-midwives, nurse practitioners, and psychiatric nurse specialists and certified nurse anesthetists for services rendered to spouses and children of active-duty or retired program uniformed-services personnel, and to family members of deceased active-duty or retired personnel.

Table 60-6   Medicaid reimbursement of nurses in advanced practice by state*

States	Nurses in advanced practice		States	Nurses in advanced practice	
	Nurse practitioner*	Clinical nurse specialist		Nurse practitioner*	Clinical nurse specialist
Alabama			Missouri		
Alaska			Montana	x	x
Arizona			Nebraska	x	
Arkansas	x		Nevada	x	
California	x		New Hampshire	x	
Colorado	x	x	New Jersey	x	
Connecticut			New Mexico	x	
Delaware	x		New York	x	
District of Columbia	x		North Carolina	x	
Florida	x	x	North Dakota		
Georgia			Ohio		
Hawaii	x		Oklahoma		
Idaho	x		Oregon	x	
Illinois			Pennsylvania	x	
Indiana			Rhode Island		
Iowa			South Carolina	x	
Kansas	x		South Dakota		
Kentucky	x		Tennessee		
Louisiana	x		Texas		
Maine			Utah		
Maryland	x		Vermont		
Massachusetts			Washington	x	
Michigan			West Virginia	x	
Minnesota	x	x	Wisconsin	x	
Mississippi	x		Wyoming		

*All states by federal mandate must cover the services of certified pediatric and family nurse practitioners.
Adapted from the American Nurses Association's *1990 study of state nurse associations;* and Pearson, L. (1991, January). 1990–91 update: How each state stands on legislative issues affecting advanced nursing practice, *Nurse Practitioner.*

FEHBP. The Federal Employees Health Benefits Program (amended effective November 5, 1990) allows federal employees enrolled in FEHBP health plans direct access to nurse- midwives, nurse practitioners, and nurse clinical specialists. The U.S. Office of Personnel Management (OPM) in Washington, D.C., monitors the upholding of this law.

Private component

Private insurance companies were initially established to sell life insurance and expanded into including health insurance. The purpose of a private insurance company is to make money for owners and investors. Many of them are willing to abide by state-mandated mental health coverage rules and therefore reimburse nonphysician providers. Another third-party payer group, known as health care services contractors,

Table 60-7   31 states that reimburse CRNAs under Medicaid

Alaska	Nebraska
Arizona	Nevada
Arkansas	New Mexico
California	Ohio
Colorado	Oklahoma
Florida	Oregon
Illinois	South Carolina
Iowa	South Dakota
Kansas	Tennessee
Kentucky	Texas
Louisiana	Utah
Maryland	Washington
Minnesota	West Virginia
Mississippi	Wisconsin
Missouri	Wyoming
Montana	

Compiled by American Nurses Association, Washington, D.C., 1991.

Table 60-8   Current direct federal reimbursement for nursing services

Federal programs	Nurse practitioner	Certified nurse-midwife	Certified registered nurse anesthetist	Clinical nurse specialist
Medicare				
Part A	No	No	No	No
Part B	Yes[1]	Yes	Yes	Yes[2]
Medicaid	Yes[3]	Yes	State discretion	State discretion
CHAMPUS*	Yes	Yes	Yes	Yes[4]
FEHB†	Yes	Yes	Yes	Yes

[1]Limited to nursing facilities and rural areas.
[2]Limited to rural areas.
[3]Limited to Pediatric NPs and Family NPs.
[4]Limited to certified psychiatric nurse specialists.

*Civilian Health and Medical Program of Uniformed Services.
†Federal Employee Health Benefit Program.
Compiled by the American Nurses Association, Washington, D.C., 1991.

Table 60-9   CRNA reimbursement under four federal payers

Medicare

1. The Omnibus Budget Reconciliation Act of 1986 gave CRNAs the authority to bill directly for their services under Medicare Part B, effective January 1, 1989.
2. The Omnibus Budget Reconciliation Act of 1990 created a fee schedule with new conversion factors for medically directed CRNAs and nonmedically directed CRNAs, effective January 1, 1991.
3. The HCFA final rule, published in the August 7, 1990, *Federal Register,* addressed the uniform relative value guide for anesthesia services, base units, time units, and modifiers.
4. The HCFA final rule, published in the November 25, 1991, *Federal Register,* regarding payment for physicians' services has a great impact on payment for CRNAs and anesthesiologists.

Medicaid

There is no federal Medicaid mandate that states must reimburse for CRNA services. However, 31 states reimburse CRNAs at varying rates under Medicaid.

Champus

CRNAs are directly reimbursed under CHAMPUS, like anesthesiologists. CHAMPUS mandates that separate prevailing profiles be developed for different classes of providers, such as anesthesiologists and CRNAs. The Department of Defense final rule, published in the September 6, 1991, *Federal Register,* noted that the prevailing charges for all anesthesiology services are being frozen in 1991, because of data limitations that prevent comparison of CHAMPUS prevailings to the new Medicare fee schedule.

FEHBP

CRNAs are directly reimbursed for their services under FEHB, like anesthesiologists.

Compiled by American Nurses Association, Washington, D.C., 1991.

includes such companies as Blue Cross/Blue Shield. These groups are not insurance companies in the same sense as private insurers; rather they were established by medical societies or hospitals, which are connected with a group of providers to deliver health care to clients who have prepaid on an insurance plan for services they may need. The traditional insurance programs have become more costly in the past few years, and there has been an enormous shift to health main- tenance organizations (HMOs), which were created in the 1970s as an alternative to traditional health care plans. Even Blue Cross/Blue Shield has created some HMOs within its organization while maintaining its traditional indemnity plans. Other companies such as Travelers, Aetna, and John Hancock also created new systems.

The HMOs are currently being identified with *managed health care* (MHC), a term used to describe a variety of health care plans designed to contain the cost of health care services delivered to members while maintaining the quality of care. Current trends across the country indicate that probably only 19% of mental health services will be delivered through the traditional fee-for-service model. The remainder will be divided among HMOs, MHCs, and other organizations. After the January 1992 enrollment a company in Massachusetts reported 80% of its employees enrolled in managed care programs and 15% in indemnity plans. Prior to January 1991, 30% of the employees were enrolled in managed care, with 60% enrolled in indemnity plans.

The managed care system has created a new language for nurses in advanced practice to add to their glossaries. A few of the new terms follow, with brief explanations.

Health maintenance organization. An HMO is an entity that is neither a private insurance nor health care contractor but that can be operated by some for-profit or not-for-profit organization that provides health care in an organized system to subscribing members in a geographical area with an agreed-upon set of basic and preventive supplemental health maintenance and treatment services for a fixed, prepaid charge.

Preferred provider organization. A preferred provider organization (PPO) is a health care financing and delivery program with a group of providers such as physicians and hospitals who contract to give services on a fee-for-service basis that provides financial incentives to consumers to utilize a select group of preferred providers and pay less for the services. Insurance companies usually promise the PPO a certain volume of patients and prompt payment in exchange for fee discounts.

Independent practice association. The Independent Practice Association (IPA) has a contract with a managed care plan to deliver services in return for a single capitation rate (fixed fee). The IPA then contracts with individual providers either on a capitated basis or on a fee-for-service basis.

Self-funded plan. Another form of private reimbursement is the self-funded plan, which emerged as a result of rapidly increasing health care costs and high insurance premiums that were paid by employers. In a self-funded health plan the risk for medical cost is assumed by the employing company rather than an insurance company or managed care plan. Under the Employment Retirement Income Security Act (ERISA),

self-funded plans are exempt from certain requirements such as premium taxes and mandated benefits. These self-funded plans often contract with insurance companies or third-party administrators (TPAs) to administer the benefits. In Massachusetts many businesses, particularly those with fewer employees, have become self-funded. Since such companies are not obliged to follow mandated mental health benefits, many certified psychiatric medical specialists are not currently being reimbursed. The companies have set policies covering the services of psychiatrists and psychologists either because these were the only known providers at the time the policies were written and the policies have not been updated, or because the companies are not aware of the scope of practice of the certified psychiatric clinical specialists.

Mental health care providers in Massachusetts are concerned because the legislators have asked the division of insurance to study the cost of mandated benefits to companies that currently provide a basic $500 mental health benefit. If this mandated mental health benefit law is repealed, it will greatly affect the mental health delivery service in the private sector.

DESIGN OF STRATEGIES FOR REIMBURSEMENT POLICY

The enactment of a reimbursement policy requires a design that addresses the credentials and the scope of practice of the nurse, the responsibility and accountability of the nurse to the patient and the third-party payer, the relationship of the nurse to other providers with whom he or she might need to collaborate, and a projected cost analysis of the policy. There is general agreement among health care providers that graduate-level (i.e., master's degree) preparation is mandatory for nursing specialists, as it is for other health care specialists. In addition, it is presumed that each profession establishes its standards and policies for practice and methods for licensure and the granting of credentials within the states. The legislators are concerned about the needs of the consumer as well as the wishes of their constituents. Consumers have the right to select from many providers, individuals, or groups that might best meet their health care needs and from which they can be assured of receiving competent services. The consumer's right to choose health care services is enhanced by a reimbursement policy that includes services within the scope of practice of professional nursing.

In establishing eligibility to be a provider and receive reimbursement, the nurse has created an atmosphere in which certain services can be rendered to patients that will be documented and evaluated as designed by the standards for practice, and for which the nurse is responsible and accountable to the patient and third-party payer, as agreed upon in a contract. Nurses practicing independently do establish collaborative relationships with other health care providers as may be required to maximize treatment benefits. Institutions readily provide that opportunity for nurses as members of interdisciplinary teams, as well as occasions for networking within the institution.

Nurses interested in reimbursement are attempting to make available to the consumer nursing services that are unique and different from those of physicians, psychologists, social workers, or any other health care providers. The nursing specialist, regardless of particular practice, has training and experience in physical health and medical sciences. The practical skills in all of the nursing specialties and the knowledge of psychopharmacology assure the consumer as well as the third-party payer that the nurse is prepared to assess, diagnose, treat, teach disease prevention, and promote self-help. The latter two services will require more documentation to convince insurers that those services should be reimbursable. The assignment of fees for nursing services should be based on the kind of service offered, the level of expertise of the provider, and the responsibility incorporated in the delivery of the services; the assignment of fees should also take into account a just and equitable income for the provider as a professional who wishes to continue to offer such services.

Nonlegislative strategies for third-party reimbursement

The nonlegislative strategies for third-party reimbursement require a major commitment on the part of the leadership and membership of the ANA and the state nursing associations to interact effectively with elected officials in government, as well as with administrators of major corporations who have or should have an investment in advocating cost-effective health care for all.

In addition, networking with the national insurance organizations such as the National Association of Insurance Commissioners (NAIC) and the Health Insurance Association of America (HIAA) is of major importance. A state insurance commissioner promulgates regulations that are meant to protect the consumer as

well as the provider. In 1987 the commissioner of insurance sent directives to HMO directors that outlined mandated benefits available and also listed the four mandated mental health professionals (i.e., psychiatrists, psychologists, licensed independent clinical social workers, and certified clinical specialists in psychiatric and mental health nursing). Members of the nursing profession should attend meetings of these associations, serve on task forces and boards, and present written or oral testimony at hearings. These particular approaches will educate the public about the scope of practice of a credentialed professional nurse and illustrate the services that warrant reimbursement.

Many community action groups want the support of nurses and want to join with nurses to lobby for consumer services. Such groups are very important to the nursing profession because they represent the consumer's viewpoint on nursing services to the legislators.*

Nonlegislative strategies are encouraged whenever possible, as long as it is understood that companies can alter reimbursement plans when leadership changes occur; in legislative reimbursement, changes can only be made by repealing an old law. Thus with legislation the risk of losing what has previously been enacted is less.

Legislative strategies for third-party reimbursement

Developing a legislative strategy for third-party reimbursement is a major task. This is the most effective path to reimbursement because it is a more permanent solution. Receiving reimbursement based on a waiver or petition could be subject to change when the leadership of a particular agency or organization changes.

The ANA has recommended guidelines for the development of legislative strategies. One of these guidelines deals with seeking reimbursement for services of all registered nurses, not merely those of a specific group. Nurses in each state must assess the political climate when preparing to submit a reimbursement bill and must know who the proponents and opponents of

---

*In Massachusetts, for example, this community support was especially effective in gaining passage of the reimbursement bill for psychiatric clinical specialists, because patients did not give testimony for ethical reasons. Another group that helped was the Friends of the Nurse-Practitioners who wrote letters to legislators in support of the prescription writing bill. A uniformed police officer who had received health care services from this group came to the State House to testify at a health care hearing, and his testimony carried weight with the committee.

such legislation will be. In Massachusetts an all-inclusive bill proved to be a mistake and was defeated at the first hearing because of concern about the broad financial implications, educational preparation of nurses, and quality care issues. The greatest opposition came from the medical associations and the insurance associations. In mental health and other specialties, turf issues surfaced, and rivalry among specialties has been acute in relation to fees assigned for nursing services. Any nursing practice act has to be interpreted clearly to the legislators so that the role of nursing can be properly defended. The federal and state insurance laws and codes need to be reviewed so that decisions can be made about amending existing laws. It is advisable to have legal counsel from within the association or hired by the group filing the legislation to review the current statutes.

Decisions about which insurers will be affected and whether the reimbursement will be mandatory or optional are crucial in getting the legislation passed and must be kept in mind when filing. The more insurance companies that are included, the more options the consumer has to choose specific plans and still be assured of access to the provider of choice. However, the group filing the legislation should be willing to omit a specific payer if it appears that the bill would be defeated with that inclusion. For example, in Massachusetts a decision was made to delete Medicaid because the reimbursement law in the state did not address Medicaid's exclusion of nonmedical mental health providers.

In considering mandatory reimbursement versus optional reimbursement, mandatory reimbursement was selected because it assured payment for services and, just as important, because it assured recognition by colleagues and consumers as being qualified to provide such services. For the most part, insurance companies and business organizations were opposed to the mandatory reimbursement concept, claiming that an increase in the number of providers increased the demand for the services. It was necessary and helpful to meet with representatives of these groups to present data, to educate them regarding our role and scope of practice, and to better understand their position. These meetings set the tone for potential negotiation.

Selecting bill sponsors from among the senators and representatives was a key element in designing effective strategy. Sponsors were selected on the basis of their support of the role of the professional nurse who is qualified to practice at an advanced level. The particular political affiliation of the legislators and their positions on relevant committees through which the bill would have to pass received prime consideration.

The legislative process

Vigilance best describes the position that the bill's sponsors and supporters must assume throughout the legislative process. Passage of a reimbursement bill requires a clearly stated fact sheet, a definition of the scope of practice, a cost analysis, and a projection of the impact of the bill. Each legislator must have this information because the bill's opponents will be developing their own fact sheets and information to present.

A grass roots organization called Nurses United for Reimbursement of Services (NURS), made up primarily of psychiatric clinical specialists, was begun in Massachusetts in 1975; this group took the initial steps toward proposing reimbursement legislation for mental health services by nurses. The leaders and members were a major force in lobbying for this piece of legislation, offering support to one another and networking extensively with the state nurses' association, legislators, other health care providers, and community groups. They did not give up, even after the bill had been left in committee for several years in a row despite valiant efforts to move it along. Victory came when Blue Shield of Massachusetts, one of the strongest opponents, finally acknowledged that nurses could provide cost-effective, quality health care.

IMPLEMENTATION OF REIMBURSEMENT LEGISLATION AND NEGOTIATION WITH MANAGED-CARE SYSTEMS

NURS now stands for Nurses United for Responsible Services in Massachusetts, and the role of the group has been expanded to include not only the previous intent to implement the reimbursement bill but also to continue to work with other nursing groups to achieve reimbursement and to file additional legislation that gives consumers access to cost-effective health care rendered by credentialed providers. The implementation of the reimbursement bill, as well as the other pieces of legislation, is an ongoing process. Insurance companies continue to deny claims outright or stall payment with excuses such as "We do not acknowledge certified psychiatric clinical specialists among our providers." We have had to send copies of the statute to insurance companies and in some cases invoke the assistance of the insurance commissioner to convince companies to accept nurses as eligible providers.

Becoming part of the managed-care systems has required persistence. It also requires understanding of words such as *closed panel,* which may either mean that a managed-care company is no longer accepting applications from new providers (a reason frequently given to nurses) or that a managed-care plan, usually an HMO, obtains services only from health professionals contracted with the managed-care plan. It is also important to understand terminology such as *at risk* when the provider agrees to accept a fixed amount of money in a capitated agreement. If the cost of providing services exceeds the agreed-upon amount, the provider is at risk for, and must cover, the overage. The positive side is that if the cost of providing services is less than the amount of money received, the provider has additional profit.

When considering membership as providers in managed-care systems (whether by invitation or by pursuit), nurses should consider several important factors: Since managed care is a fast-growing reality and some companies have had financial difficulties and had to merge with others or go out of business, it is essential for nurses to be vigilant in pursuing a clear definition of the managed-care system. Particulars to be considered before joining might include the philosophy of the organization, standards of care, credentials of leadership, fees for joining, process for submitting claims, and rate and frequency of payments. And there are other questions to be asked. How is patient confidentiality handled in the utilization review process? How is the decision made on number of sessions allowed, and by whom? Is there an appeals process? How comfortable are you with the policies? And is the orientation focused on brief, short-term psychotherapy, as most of managed care is oriented to that type of treatment?

FINANCIAL SURVIVAL FOR NURSES IN THE WORLD OF THIRD-PARTY REIMBURSEMENT AND MANAGED CARE

Nurses working in salaried positions in institutions—whether hospitals, clinics, or HMOs—need to negotiate salaries that provide them with a lifestyle that enhances physical and mental health and facilitates their reaching their optimal potential as a person and as a professional. Nurses choosing to work in private practice and be self-employed have these same needs. The myth that self-employment or being in private practice ensures making a lot of money needs to be viewed in the context of third-party reimbursement and managed-care contract rates, because many patients are not paying out of pocket exclusively for services in times of financial recession. It is essential for nurses to ask themselves the basic question, How much net and gross income do you want to earn from your private practice? This question is followed by, How many hours are actually billable? The nonbillable hours usually include those spent on preparation of client reports for insurance companies, case records, marketing and networking, and attendance at professional meetings for continuing education, as well as sick days, holidays, vacation days, and natural emergencies that might prevent clients from getting to an office. The addition of actual patient hours and nonbillable hours gives a total of an actual workweek. In addition to the number of hours it is necessary to work, the costs of maintaining a practice must be given a thoughtful, accurate assessment. These costs include rent, utilities, phones, answering services, insurance (malpractice and liability, as well as life, health, and disability), office supplies, equipment, consultation, journals, bookkeeping, secretarial services, and memberships in professional organizations. The reality is different for each of us. The considerations are universal to all of us. Are the fees paid for our services adequate to meet personal and professional needs while providing cost-effective care?

CONCLUSION

Third-party reimbursement for nursing services either by insurance companies directly or by managed-care systems will benefit consumers in their search for cost-effective, quality health care by a competent, credentialed provider group. Nurses need to continue working together with their professional associations, with special interest groups, and with federal and state agencies to design health care policy that ensures delivery of services to all people needing health care, in addition to designing, lobbying for, and implementing legislative activity that ensures this goal. Nurses, because of both their training and their ability to improvise, have been known for their design of treatment plans that go beyond the walls of a hospital or office. Innovative, cost-effective treatment plans for meeting the health care needs of the '90s and beyond will be of great interest to third-party reimbursers and managed-care corporations.

RECOMMENDED READING

American Nurses Association. (1984). *Obtaining third-party reimbursement: A nurse's guide to methods and strategies.* Kansas City, Mo: Author.

American Nurses Association. (1988). *1988 legislative and regulatory fact sheets*. Kansas City, Mo: Author.

American Nurses Association. (1989, May). *Report in the 1988 state nurses association survey on nursing practice*.

Aydelotte, M. K., et al. (1988). *Nurses in private practice: Characteristics, organizational arrangements and reimbursement policy*. Kansas City, Mo: American Nurses' Foundation.

Cooper, R. G., & LeJa, J. A. (1990). An investigation of managed health care case managers. *Journal of Allied Health, 19*(3), 210-225.

Hogue, E. E. (1989, May/June). Opportunities for nurses seeking third-party reimbursement using existing mechanisms. *Pediatric Nursing, 15*(3), 279-280.

LaBar, C. (1990). The issue of third-party reimbursement: Advice for nurse practitioners from a nation expert. *Nurse Practitioner, 15*(3), 46-47.

LaBar, C. (1985, November/December). Third-party reimbursement status of legislation. *Oncology Nursing Forum, 12*(6), 53-58.

Oss, M. E. (1991, September/October). Managed health benefits—trends in buying, packaging, and delivery. *Employee Assistance Digest,* 36-40.

Scott, C. L., & Harrison, D. A. (1990). Direct reimbursement for nurse practitioners in health insurance plans of research universities. *Journal of Professional Nursing, 6*(1), 21-32.

CHAPTER 61

Nursing and consumerism

How can we get decision making closer to the consumer?

CLAIRE M. FAGIN, LEAH F. BINDER

Today there is widespread consensus among health providers and consumer interests that health promotion and disease prevention are vital elements in a high-quality, cost-effective health care delivery system. Numerous campaigns dealing with one or another health problem are ongoing or episodic. But consensus splits on the question of how to most effectively convince consumers to respond to these campaigns by altering behaviors.

The delivery system as it is currently structured contains few incentives for providers to contribute to preventive and/or promotional efforts. On the contrary, the health care system frequently offers incentives for implementation of high-technology, high-skill operations, procedures, and interventions without addressing the preventive mechanisms that would eliminate some of the demand for such services.[12] As a result, millions of Americans have little contact with the health care system until they land in the emergency room, and millions more partake in dangerous behaviors—such as failing to obtain appropriate vaccinations or continuing sexual encounters when suffering from a sexually transmitted disease—that could be discouraged with appropriate noncoercive professional help.[31] This chapter will examine effective efforts to provide for the public health—both within the context of the health care delivery system and outside—and recommend strategies for change that involve integrating consumers more fully into the decision-making fabric of the health care system.

It is important to recognize that despite its flaws, health care in the United States is not without successes in the arena of preventive and promotional health. Efforts to discourage smoking have resulted in the decline in smoking among Americans, and attempts to encourage behaviors that defend against heart disease, such as healthier diets and exercise, have similarly shown promise. Nonetheless, on key international indicators of health quality, notably longevity and infant mortality, the United States competes poorly with other industrialized nations despite health expenditures second to none.[15] There is much more work ahead, and for a variety of reasons, nurses are in a unique position to forge the way forward.

BACKGROUND

In 1984 I was fortunate enough to have been granted one of the first two Distinguished Scholar Awards from the American Nurses' Foundation for a project to investigate the links between nursing and consumerism. I set out to develop a model of effective collaboration between organized consumers and nursing. What emerged from this project were two welcome surprises. First, although it seemed at the start that consumers and nurses might have distinct goals in health care that might not be congruent—nurses seeking to advance the profession, consumers aiming for self-help within or without the health system—it soon became clear that the two groups shared very powerful common interests with explosive potential. Indeed, the origins of the nursing profession in the United States were influenced to a large extent by consumer involvement. The influence of volunteers in hospital schools of nursing was extremely important, and the quality of schools was often a direct result of the priorities these women placed on service, training, and student life.[23]

An intraorganizational collaboration that could be said to be a direct historical antecedent of the current project was the National Organization for Public Health Nursing (NOPHN).

Consumer involvement was an integral part of the philosophy on which NOPHN was founded. Lay membership—at first non-voting, but very soon fully participatory—was considered a radical idea, but the insistence of the NOPHN on inclusion of lay members was based on the belief that nursing is a problem of the community as well as of the profession. [Though] early activities of lay members were heavily slanted toward fund-raising, their responsibilities were constantly broadened as time went on and soon included policy-setting and directional areas.[5]

In 1952 seven organizations decided that they could best be served by a single organization "in which nurses and others interested in health services could work together." The National League for Nursing was composed of nurses, allied professionals, and interested citizens as individual members, and of nursing schools and public health nursing agencies as agency members. Of the nurse members, only those who had belonged to NOPHN had previous collaborative experience as equals with nonnurses.[25] NOPHN's 40-year history provided convincing evidence of the strength of collaboration between nurses and nonnurses both in the development of nursing as a community service and in improving the welfare of society.

The volunteer tradition, and the organizational experience of the NOPHN laid the groundwork for collaborative activities that were to come in the fields of mental health, maternal health and midwifery, child health, hospice care, and other significant movements in service and education—which became the second surprise finding in my study. The extent to which nurses and consumers were collaborating in a variety of effective initiatives was remarkable, and it provided a framework of past success that I believe offers insight as we move forward with new collaborative efforts.

Today, perhaps no group of nurses has stronger organized ties with consumers than nurse-midwives. There is no question that one of the reasons for the success of midwives in achieving reimbursement earlier than other nurses is the consumer desire for midwives' care. Consumers faced with the threat of having midwife services curtailed collaborate with each other and with midwives to pressure for their choice of services. Because midwife services are reimbursed, more people are able to experience this care and hence strengthen their preference for these kinds of services.

One of the initiatives I examined that exemplified this support for midwifery was Consumers for Choices in Childbirth, a citizens' action group that arose from the need to support midwives' practice at Yale in the late fall of 1976. The Yale nurse-midwifery practice began in 1975 with an agreement with Yale's department of obstetrics and gynecology. Not anticipating that the practice would be extremely successful, there was considerable surprise about the number of clients interested in the practice and subsequently a lack of interest on the part of physicians in serving as consultants or backups to the practice. When complaints came from clients about the discontinuity of medical consultation, the department of obstetrics and gynecology decided to close the practice. Much to the surprise of physicians, the decision to close the practice created havoc in the community. There was an outpouring of consumer sentiment regarding midwives and expressions of great enthusiasm about their care. The clients involved in the consumer coalition made it clear that their concerns had to do with consistent obstetrical consultation that was supportive of midwifery care.

Citizen outrage at physicians' derogatory remarks about clients of midwifery services and about the midwives was channeled into constructive, assertive behaviors to enable others to receive the high-quality care they had received from the midwives in the past. The committee sent letters, circulated petitions, and elicited support from others by publishing a newsletter to report their activities. They discussed issues of importance to pregnant women and parents, and sent representatives to the health systems agency. The midwifery practice was reinstated with adequate physician backup.[4]

In other areas of nursing care, people have not been as likely to establish a preference for health care provided by nurses because information and reimbursement are not as readily available. This is changing, however, for two reasons. First, the growth of managed care and preferred provider arrangements has frequently entailed increased employment of nurse practitioners and clinical nurse specialists to provide ongoing, primary health care and other services.[22] Second, state and federal reimbursement laws are changing, and nurses may now practice autonomously in many rural areas and selected additional sites. In response to the expansion of consumer access to direct nursing services, the linkages between consumers and nurses on the political and individual levels have become more sophisticated and more identifiable in the seven years since I first examined collaborative opportunities between nurses and consumers.

The best example of the growth in consumer-nurse relations is embodied by one nurse, Terry Chalich, RN.

In the early 1980s, on her own time and funds, Chalich developed a program to help unemployed workers find health care.[24] Her belief that nurses have a great responsibility in dealing with the present health care crisis was translated into action: not only did she volunteer but she stimulated volunteerism within her community and among her colleague providers. She set up offices where providers offer free or low-cost care, established a resource list of other health care services for the unemployed, disseminated literature outlining help available to the unemployed, and even negotiated with hospital billing offices to reduce fees. Chalich's network proved very successful in meeting critical needs in her community, and it earned her a strong reputation in the community. In 1990 Chalich was an unsuccessful candidate for Congress, but she was successful in raising issues in nursing and health care reform. In a 1992 article describing her campaign, Chalich[2] identified other nurse activists involved in community change, among them Sharon Malhotra, who has taken national leadership in exposing risks associated with lawn care pesticides.

THE CHALLENGE BEFORE US

My study and subsequent developments indicate that bringing nurses together with consumers on the political and community level works best when consumers are already organized and informed, and when nurses are both active participants and knowledgeable resources moving forward with consumers in the same direction. This train is on the tracks and rolling.

Currently, one of the problems of involving consumers actively in decision making is that public health campaigns—efforts to encourage healthy lifestyles—are often considered in isolation from the experience of consumers within the entire health care delivery system. Part of the reason for separating the two issues has been that different people dominate in the two aspects of health efforts: coalitions of professionals and lay people from a variety of backgrounds—from social workers to public health specialists to community leaders—tend to advance public health campaigns, while the delivery setting is more hierarchical and dependent on perceived professional status. Nurses tend to be present as leaders and/or experts in both contexts.

In fact, from the nursing perspective, public health campaigns and the delivery setting are not separate spheres of action but interrelated agendas, and the problems of the delivery setting plague public health movements. At the heart of the problem is the medical model and consequent public mythology about the role of the delivery system. According to the myth, which has been portrayed in numerous media outlets, the health care system consists of an assembly of physicians who take charge of people's lives when an unfortunate incident occasions the need for a cure. Occasionally the cure is not forthcoming, but often enough physicians are able to stem the tide of tragic consequence. Either way, the physician, and the health care system he or she represents, is an episodic occurrence that retreats into oblivion once the cure issue is settled.[30] What people discover when they encounter the real health care system is that the majority of providers are not physicians, the majority of health care needs are not amenable to cure, and the majority of consumers should be availing themselves of some form of regular, as opposed to episodic, contact with providers.

The contrast between the myth and the reality has in the past proved difficult for Americans to accept, or even acknowledge. Perri Klass[9] received angry letters and even a death threat when she noted in her memoirs of medical residency that most people admitted to a hospital cannot be cured. The concept that, for all its impressive accomplishments, medical science is severely limited in scope troubled many of her readers. The image of the kindly physician dispensing problem-solving drugs and cures is so powerful that it is the image most parents encourage their children to view as reality and take for granted as the building block relationship at the foundation of the health care system.

It is not quite like believing in Santa Claus to believe in physicians like Marcus Welby and the medical model he exemplifies, because some physicians and medical interventions clearly save lives and make people feel better. Even health problems that do respond to medical interventions, however, are not treated with provider intervention alone. On the contrary, no broken leg will become whole, no disease will enter remission, no wound will heal without the preeminent authority and power of the human body. Diseases like acquired immunodeficiency syndrome (AIDS), which attack the body's immune system, demonstrate in tragic ways the limits of medical science—not only medicine's inability to cure the particular virus, but also medicine's inability to fend off disease in the absence of bodily mechanisms that enable interventions to work.

But the fact that providers merely assist the body in healing itself has been obscured by the romanticized concept that providers are in charge of the curative function. The power dynamic implicit in the idealized doctor-patient relationship is a dominant-subordinate one, and as a result the idealized role of health care consumers negotiating the health care system has been a subordinate, passive role. For the consumer, interaction with the health care system becomes an exercise in vulnerability and even humility, rather than a consultation with professionals on achieving one's optimal health. The results are often unhealthy: some consumers avoid health services until the last possible moment; others do the opposite, compulsively clinging to health providers expecting cures for myriad often-undefinable ailments.

The habits of passivity, of regarding one's health as something to be addressed episodically by omniscient others, create a climate where public health education and promotion is difficult. Furthermore, within the delivery setting, consumer passivity enables some of the most pressing problems in the health care system—cost overruns, inadequate quality, and inefficiencies—to propagate without check.

Thus the challenge for improving the public health goes beyond imparting information about healthy lifestyles, preventive care, or even quality of care. At its roots, the challenge of public health calls for consumer participation as full partners in the health care system, actively responsible for their own ongoing health maintenance and vigilant in demanding quality and cost effectiveness. This is the nursing model of care.

PROMOTING CHANGE

Recently, significant changes have occurred that indicate progress will be rapid in the coming decade toward a more powerful role for consumers. Our health care system is in the midst of revolutionary change. Contributing to this are an increasingly older population; necessary changes in primary focus away from cure to care because of lowered mortality rates and higher morbidity and chronicity; changing values regarding who gets how much care, permitting major reallocations of economic risk; alternative health care systems and providers; and extraordinary growth in for-profit health care in segments of the enterprise. The consumer as represented by the large employer or corporation can and has exercised considerable clout in these enormous changes.

But the process has only begun. Numerous factors, such as the unusually high rate of unnecessary surgeries and procedures,[32] suggest that consumer vigilance

and other regulatory checks and balances are not what they should be. Most important for the public health will be a philosophical change on the part of the consumer with regard to the locus of control in health matters: away from the physician to the consumer, with the simultaneous development of personal accountability for one's health and medical choices. This will require change in fundamental aspects of human behavior. Such a challenge cannot be underestimated. Changing behaviors and mind-sets, even when they are clearly in the self-interest of targeted populations, is an agenda that has perplexed governments and philosophers since Stone Age policymakers tried to induce people to use the wheel.

As the decade proceeds, however, signs are evident that a positive shift in public attitudes is occurring that may mean a change in the way people perceive health care in their lives. Numerous public opinion polls demonstrate increased distrust of the health care system and vigilance on the part of consumers in evaluating the health care they are receiving,[18] which may mean fewer passive, "doctor knows best" patients in the future. Consumers are also acting on the political level to enforce change in the delivery system. Groups such as the American Association of Retired Persons (AARP) and the National Consumers' League emerged from relative obscurity to become by the mid-1980s major forces in national health policy making.[28] Some congressional campaigns have in recent times turned on the candidate's position on health reform.[7]

EMPOWERING COMMUNITIES

As we examine strategies for achieving transition in the public posture with regard to health care, it is instructive to bear in mind the social and political context in which significant change must occur. Policymakers are approaching questions of social welfare differently than in the past, which will likely have an impact on the outcome and velocity of health care reform. They are important strategies for nurses to consider.

The 1992 riot in Los Angeles, sparked by what was widely perceived as a racist verdict in a police excessive-force case, killed more than 50 people, injured hundreds more, and resulted in millions of dollars worth of damage to inner-city communities. In the wake of the riot, partisan accusatory fingers began assigning blame. From Republicans came an attack on the Great Society programs begun in the Johnson administration, which pundits on the right accused of creating and sustaining a "culture of dependency" among inner-city residents;[10] from Democrats arose denouncement of the Reagan and Bush administrations' cuts to federal entitlement and urban development programs that, claimed the left, exacerbated poverty and hopelessness in the community.[21]

In some sense, both sides were correct: lack of federal attention in the 1980s to urban poverty contributed to community decay, and at the same time the approach of the Great Society programs has tended to disempower those it was intending to serve. But partly in the process of rebuilding Los Angeles, new ideas arose about the role of the public and private sectors in stimulating growth, opportunity, and hopefulness in poor areas. In a best-selling book published around the time of the Los Angeles riot, David Osborne and Ted Gaebler exemplified the new thinking by identifying models of what they called "entrepreneurial governments," which

promote competition between service providers. They empower citizens by pushing control out of the bureaucracy, into the community. They measure the performance of their agencies, focusing not on inputs but on outcomes. They are driven by their goals—their missions—not by their rules and regulations. They redefine their clients as customers and offer them choices. . . . They prevent problems before they emerge, rather than simply offering services afterward. . . . And they focus not simply on providing public services, but on catalyzing all sectors—public, private, and voluntary—into action to solve their community's problems.[14]

According to this model, governments steer rather than row,[19] lending direction and support to local communities, citizens, businesses, and nonprofit organizations, which are then responsible for providing the substantive essence of community needs. Instead of direct services, governments will move toward more participatory government models.

The Osborne and Gaebler model was applied, though not deliberately, by columnist and politician Alan Keyes, who suggested that inner-city development must begin by empowering neighborhoods and communities to create their own governing bodies that would administer social welfare programs, operate a sheriff's department, and authorize a community justice of the peace. The most important weakness of many poor communities, said Keyes, "may be the fact the community itself has no authority over the many government programs that affect its individual inhabitants. Because of this deficiency there is no connection between the help the individual receives and the decent

mores the community needs to encourage."[8] When responsible citizens in a community have some authority to regulate conditions and rules in the neighborhood, adds Keyes, youngsters are provided with constructive, instead of destructive, role models. Communities set their own standards and enforce them through peer pressure as well as laws.[8]

PUBLIC HEALTH IN THE COMMUNITY

The approach of the reinvented government model mirrors in many respects the recommendations of Nursing's Agenda for Health Care Reform (see Chapter 58). Nurses, too, recommend shifting activity away from large acute care settings and toward smaller community settings for the delivery of health services, and encouraging a free-market competitive environment by revealing to consumers information and data about quality of care not previously available.[17] In the end, the philosophical approach of nursing's agenda and the reinvented government model are identical: empower citizens by creating avenues of participation, and promote higher accountability between providers and recipients of services.

The dual issues of citizen empowerment and community-level approaches to policy making offer important possibilities for meeting public health needs and ought to guide us as we formulate a model for bringing consumers into the fold. The community-based perspective appears to be a major determinant in the success of public health efforts. For example, a wide-ranging analysis of three studies that investigated community-based cardiovascular disease prevention programs found that when practitioners gained collaboration from residents and community leaders, the campaigns could be effective.[14] Numerous other examinations of the trend toward health promotion in the community have revealed similar positive results. An analysis of the trend by communications specialist John L. McKnight concludes by recommending continued efforts on the community level, pointing out that "to enhance community health, we need a new breed of modest health professional. They are people with a deep respect for the integrity and wisdom of citizens and their associations."[13]

Luckily, the members of this "new breed" of unassuming, respectful health professionals qualified to provide care at the community level are graduating from nursing school—and practicing for years in a variety of settings in communities across America. Indeed, nurses are active participants in many of the most successful community health campaigns.

The definition of community need not be limited to precise neighborhood parameters. In a study conducted by Motivational Educational Entertainment, investigators found that teenagers in inner-city neighborhoods in Philadelphia; Camden, New Jersey; New York; Washington, D.C.; and Oakland, California, had been raised in a milieu so removed from American mainstream culture that no medium except rap music was credible enough to convey effective messages on improving or escaping life in the ghetto.[34] Researchers explained that the youth "have leaders, a social structure" and derided national public service campaigns aimed at curbing drug use or advocating safer sex practices as "mainstream assumptions that these are rudderless, leaderless young people yearning for a catch phrase upon which to focus their lives."[34] Researchers believed that rap music represented a way to reach inner-city teens on their own terms, within the reputation of the community they identified with—a larger national community of black, alienated teens. The public health message could only reach them through the avenues defined as most reputable within that community.

Another community without walls is the gay community, which has responded in exemplary ways to the scourge of the AIDS epidemic. According to the Centers for Disease Control, community demonstration projects revealing the most positive changes in sex practices were in "cities with strong gay communities and positive images of gay men."[20] Unfortunately, this is one bright spot within a discouraging context. Studies on the national level indicate a large proportion of individuals with AIDS remain sexually active,[26] and studies by the National Institutes of Health and the Centers for Disease Control suggest that knowledge of human immunodeficiency virus (HIV) status does not in itself produce appropriate behavioral change.[20] Thus the community structure and its propensity to accept a new message are vital links in efforts to promote healthful behaviors.

TARGETED CAMPAIGNS FOR HEALTH PROMOTION

Why does the community presence appear to correlate with the impact of public health ventures? In part the reason is rooted in classical understanding of effectiveness in public health campaigns, which was described most efficaciously by investigators in a Stanford study

on the role of communications in health. Researchers concluded that possession of favorable attitudes about the message of a public health campaign does not in itself ensure the adoption of the practice recommended: people need in addition the skills and resources to undertake a behavioral modification. "It is essential in planning any health intervention to consider kinds of changes expected," the researchers warned. "Be skeptical of any health program that assumes that informing people will be enough to win their cooperation."[27] The study cited the example of smoking cessation campaigns: programs that point out the gravity of the health risk have limited success; programs that advise and assist smokers on the process of living without cigarettes may see better results.[27]

The problem of providing an effective solution-based approach to health promotion may explain the difficulty of national or broad-based mass media campaigns. Campaigns that simply offer information about a health problem are likely to have minimal impact, but the state of the art in public health is advanced enough that these are now relatively rare. Most campaigns are instead designed to advise people on taking steps to solve the identified problem. But broad-based campaign recommendations have to straddle a fine line between on the one hand offering broad advice applicable to a wide variety of targeted audiences and on the other hand offering some form of step-by-step approach that appears to be most effective in altering behaviors. The specified, step-by-step approach runs the risk of being too narrow in focus to apply to a diverse audience; the broad approach might not be helpful to anyone.

This problem of recommending practicable behaviors for a diverse audience has plagued many mass media campaigns. A study of mass media antismoking campaigns in Australia aimed at informing smokers of risks and suggesting they avoid smoking concluded that while the campaigns managed to educate people of the health risks, they did not appear successful in convincing people to quit.[11] Another study with similarly discouraging results was conducted by psychologists in South Carolina who examined the effects of an alcohol education presentation aimed at adolescents. Though the tenth and eleventh grade students in the study exhibited enhanced knowledge of the topic, there was no observable change in attitudes or alcohol involvement.[13]

Mass media campaigns that include detailed recommendations for consumer response have shown success.

A campaign in Connecticut offered low-cost screening mammograms to women over the age of 34 who had not been previously examined, and it resulted in 2500 inquiries over a 7-day period.[6] In Australia investigators examined the outcome of a television show that gave instructions on recognizing signs of melanoma and recommended visiting a physician if signs were present. An increase of 167% was observed in the number of melanomas diagnosed in the 3 months after the show was aired, including a significant shift in the proportion of tumors removed in the thin, easily treated stage.[29]

Another mass media campaign that appears to have demonstrated remarkable success is the "designate a driver" campaign of the Harvard School of Public Health.[1] Utilizing a variety of mass media outlets, including public service announcements and entertainment media, the campaign has been effective because it offers a solution to the problem of drunk driving that is specific, memorable, and applicable to most populations. A broader approach to the problem of drunk driving might be "don't drink and drive," or the even broader "don't drink," which are clearly difficult for consumers to undertake when alcohol consumption is a problem. The Harvard campaign thus narrowed its focus to suggest a simple, relatively easy way to address the problem that would likely be workable for virtually every audience reached by the mass media. The slogan also made its way into the cultural language and thus achieved some community reinforcement.[1]

It seems obvious there is a need for practical public health campaigns targeted with recommendations for action that specific populations will be able to access. The community-based model would likely be able to target particular identified populations more efficiently and directly than the mass media strategy, which is an important component of effective public health efforts. While health problems in and of themselves do not usually vary from a purely scientific point of view, the behavioral changes and personal initiatives required of populations facing the challenges are often vastly different. For instance, family planning in a poor inner-city neighborhood requires different kinds of services and counseling than in a suburban middle-class community.

Thus many public health initiatives may prove most effective when targeted to meet the specific needs and skill levels of particular populations and aimed at introducing practical solutions to health problems.

People may also be less resistant or distrustful of the message when conveyed within the community, using reputable community outlets (such as rap music to reach inner-city teens). Furthermore, participation within the community in reinforcing behavioral change can, as previously discussed, be a powerful catalyst for behavioral change. Researchers at the University of New Mexico School of Medicine conducted an analysis of the literature on community-based public health and examined case studies to propose a model of "empowerment education," which suggests participation of people in group action and dialogue efforts directed at community targets and shows considerable promise.[33]

INFORMATION AND EMPOWERMENT

Information about health promotion is not the only kind of information consumers need to become powerful participants in their own health maintenance. Consumers also need knowledge of the health system, its constraints, its options, varieties of insurance benefits available, and cost-effective providers, as well as information about the most common health problems affecting them in their age group and appropriate self-care. Consumers should be informed about known evidence of outcome of procedures and operations they consider, and have access to information they need to select providers and settings on the basis of qualitative criteria. We cannot make intelligent choices in a competitive health care system without such information being widely available through an array of media and spokespersons. Ultimately, without a range of information, consumers cannot effectively pressure for change, because it is difficult to know which changes are beneficial to them and which are not.

But just like information provided for health promotion purposes, the availability of information about the range of options in the delivery setting depends on the willingness of consumers to do something with the new knowledge. Will consumers exercise the power of the purse to create the changes necessary in the delivery system? Will they use information about quality to choose appropriate providers and settings? Will they demand changes in the delivery setting and outside it that will refocus health care toward the real needs of consumers? Will they move from the prescribed mythological role of passive recipient of cure to the powerful role of participant and guardian of their own health?

NURSES: STEERING TOWARD CONSUMER EMPOWERMENT

The role suggested for "reinvented government" of (1) steering but not rowing, (2) emphasizing prevention of crisis, and (3) being mission-driven in our approach to public business applies to nurses interested in reinventing health care. As consumers achieve new confidence and competence in negotiating health care, evaluating options, and maintaining their own health, nurses have an unusual opportunity to move consumers toward empowerment—not by achieving it for them, but by steering consumers forward. We can do this in a variety of ways. First, in advancing Nursing's Agenda for Health Care Reform, we advocate positioning nurses as "gatekeepers" within the delivery setting, monitoring prescribed care regimens across providers and settings and aiding consumers in choosing among recommended procedures, prescriptions, and care.[17] In this position, nurses can function as patient advocates, translating complex information into concrete options and formulas for consumer decision making. The consumer makes the decision, but nurses are in the position of (1) spearheading consumer usage of valuable information, which if implemented on a widespread basis would likely lead to innovations in the delivery setting aimed at enhancing efficiency, quality, and cost effectiveness and (2) discouraging on a mass scale the habits of patient subordination that are ingrained in consumers and perpetuated in part by the current health system structure.

Nurses are also challenged on the community level to continue the innovations in health promotion and create new models for health service delivery that will reach the public more effectively. This is especially true in poor communities, where access to health services is often extremely limited, but it is equally valuable for middle-class communities, where cost-effective health services and enhanced consumer vigilance are also needed.

Consumer-nurse alliances at the community level are feasible, desirable, and, as we have seen from the efficacy of community-level action in general, strategically effective. When starting such a coalition, it is best to begin with one or two specific goals, instead of a broad agenda. Goals might include any of the following:

- *Releasing information about quality of care.* A community group could dedicate itself to publicly revealing information about the quality of care delivered by local hospitals, nursing homes, community health care agencies, and private practice providers. Some information, such as hospital mortality data, is readily available.* Most critical information is not released to the public, however, and a community-based coalition to press for announcement of key quality indicators might succeed not only in unveiling hidden information of import, but also in implementing a campaign to politically involve consumers in the policies and procedures of health care delivery.

- *Promoting the public health–healthy lifestyles.* A number of initiatives, such as smoking cessation, fitness, and disease prevention, are excellent targets of community campaigns. The key, as discussed earlier, is to suggest alternative behaviors to targeted populations and then help them access these alternatives to the extent possible.

- *Setting up community nursing centers.* A National League for Nursing study revealed a fast-growing trend of community nursing centers opening in hundreds of communities from California to New York.[16] These centers are trying innovative approaches to encouraging citizen participation in the process of delivering health care within the community with promising results.[16] Some are private practice arrangements with nurses providing direct care; others are affiliated with nursing schools, hospitals, or other agencies to provide care in the community. Some target particular populations, such as the elderly or adolescents, while others provide a variety of services to a broad population. There are a variety of funding options available to help nurses start community nursing centers, including foundation support, federal and state grants, and university subsidies. Nurses seeking to start a center should start at the level of the community they intend to serve, connecting with citizen groups that might be interested in helping get a center off the ground. The community nursing center is the essence of Nursing's Agenda for Health Care Reform and is almost exclusively advanced at the community level.

- *Advancing nursing's agenda for health care reform.* Nursing's agenda does not exist in a vacuum. It is wholly dependent upon citizen support and initiative

---

*For information on hospital mortality rates contact: Health Care Financing Administration, Office of Public Affairs, 435H Hubert H. Humphrey Bldg., 200 Independence Avenue, S.W., Washington, DC 20201.

on its behalf—and the community will again be critical in that effort. A coalition of groups and/or individuals interested in promoting the agenda could hold functions and speaking engagements to discuss the agenda's approach to various issues of concern to the community's health needs. A community with a large elderly population might be interested in how increased access to home care services might affect citizens in the community; a younger population might explore options in the agenda for prenatal care provided by nurses.

All community consumer-nurse collaborative efforts should aim to generate not only increased general knowledge about possibilities in health care, but actual changes in the way health care is experienced in communities. Build a center. Start a home care agency. Create a new insurance plan for local employers to buy into. While in many cases state and federal laws will restrict creation of new models, it is important that communities try to bang down the legal doors slammed shut on communities suffering from health hazards that are preventable, treatable, and/or affordably dealt with.

Ultimately, by maintaining a presence in schools, community centers, and communities throughout the nation, and upholding the nursing model of care that specifies patient empowerment and respect for individuality, nurses can break the model of dominant-subordinate provider-patient relations that has discouraged so many Americans from utilizing the system appropriately.

The time is ripe for transformation in the health care system that will bring consumers into the fold as equals in the delivery of health care and leaders in the promotion of their own care. It will be up to nurses and others to couple health promotion efforts and traditional public health messages with a campaign to empower consumers within the delivery system and expose the mythology of enforced passivity that many Americans believe is endemic to receiving health services. So far only nurses have stepped forward to promote such changes in the delivery of health care.

Nurses have traditionally viewed clients as equals—partners in the delivery of health care, not subordinates to be given orders. We must continue to take that philosophy into American communities and into Congress. Given the emerging role of consumers individually, within communities, and nationally, the potential for change is enormous, and nurses will be instrumental in its effectiveness.

REFERENCES

1. Carter, B. (1989, September 11). Television: A message on drinking is seen and heard. *New York Times.*
2. Chalich, T., & Smith, L. (1992). Nursing at the grassroots. *Nursing and Health Care, 13,* 242-244.
3. Collins, D., & Cellucci, T. (1991, August). Effects of a school-based alcohol education program with a media prevention component. *Psychology Reports, 69,* 191-197.
4. Fagin, C. (1984). *A model for the effective collaboration between organized consumers and nursing—Report of an American Nurses' Foundation sponsored project.* Unpublished report.
5. Fitzpatrick, L. (1975). *The National Organization for Public Health Nursing (NOPHN) 1912-1952: Development of a practice field* (pp. 163-164). New York: National League for Nursing.
6. Gregario, D. I., Ikegeles, S., Parker, C., & Benn, S. (1990, July). Encouraging screening mammograms: Results of the 1988 Connecticut breast cancer detection awareness campaign. *Connecticut Medicine, 54,* 370-373.
7. Its eye on election, White House to propose health care changes. (1991, November 12). *New York Times.*
8. Keyes, A. (1992, June 8). Restoring community. *National Review, 44*(11), 38-41.
9. Klass, P. (1987). *A not entirely benign procedure: Four years as a medical student.* New York: Putnam.
10. Kramer, M. (1992, May 18). Two ways to play the politics of race. *Time, 139,* 35-36.
11. Macaskill, P., Pierce, J. P., Simpson, J. M., & Lyle, D. M. (1992, January). Mass media-led anti-smoking campaign can remove the education gap in quitting behavior. *American Journal of Public Health, 82,* 96-98.
12. Maraldo, P. (1989, Fourth Quarter). The nursing solution. *Health Management Quarterly,* pp. 18-19.
13. McKnight, J. L. (1992, February 6). Remarks made at the Medicine for the 21st Century Forum conference, sponsored by the American Medical Association and the Corporation for Public Broadcasting, Rancho Mirage, Calif.
14. Murray, D. (1992, February 6). *Lessons learned from the NLHBI sponsored community based cardiovascular disease prevention studies.* Paper presented at the Medicine for the 21st Century Forum conference, Rancho Mirage, Calif.
15. National Center for Health Statistics. (1988). *Vital statistics 1988.* Rockville, Md: U.S. Department of Health and Human Services, Public Health Services.
16. National League for Nursing. (1992, May 13). *Community nursing centers: A promising new trend in American health.* Paper presented at the National League for Nursing conference, Washington, D.C.
17. National League for Nursing & American Nurses Association. (1991). *Nursing's agenda for health care reform.* New York: Author.
18. *New York Times/CBS News health care poll.* (1991, August 18-22). Storrs, Conn: Roper Center.
19. Osborne, D., & Gaebler, T. (1992). *Reinventing government: How the entrepreneurial spirit is transforming the public sector.* New York: Addison-Wesley.
20. Patton, C. (1990). *Inventing AIDS* (p. 29). New York: Routledge.
21. Race against time. (1992, May 25). *New Republic, 206,* 7-9.
22. Schull, D., Tosch, P., & Wood, M. (1992). Clinical nurse specialists as collaborative care managers. *Nursing Management, 23,* 30-34.

23. Sheahan, D. (1981, May 22-23). *Influence of occupational sponsorship on the professional development of nursing.* Paper presented at the conference on the history of nursing to Rockefeller Research Center, Pocanizo-Hills, N.Y.

24. Sleby, T. L. (1984). RN helps unemployed find health services that are affordable. *American Nurse, 16,* 1-24.

25. Sleeper, R. (1972). *Changing years of National League for Nursing, 1952-1972.* New York: National League for Nursing.

26. Smith, H. L., Peragallo, N., Ferrer, X., Lake, E. T., & Aiken, L. H. (1987). *AIDS prevention research: Population-based and epidemiological perspectives, as applied to the AIDS epidemic in Chile.* Interim report.

27. Solomon, P., McAnany, E., Goldschmidt, D., Parker, E., & Foote, D. (1979, January). *The role of communication in health. Stanford University Institute for Communications Research.* Washington, D.C.: U.S. Agency for International Development.

28. Starr, P. (1982). *Social transformation of American medicine.* New York: Basic Books.

29. Theobald, T., Marks, R., Hill, D., & Dorevitch, A. (1991, October). Goodbye sunshine: Effects of a television program about melanoma on beliefs, behavior, and melanoma thickness. *Journal of the American Academy of Dermatology, 25,* 717-723.

30. Turow, J. (1989). *Playing doctor: Television, storytelling, and medical power.* New York: Oxford University Press.

31. U.S. Congress, Joint Economic Committee, Subcommittee on Education and Health. (1989). *Medical alert, A staff report summarizing the hearings on health care in America.* Washington, D.C.: Institute of Medicine, National Academy Press.

32. U.S. Congress, Joint Economic Committee, Subcommittee on Education and Health. (1989). *A staff report summarizing the hearings on the future of health care in America.* Washington, D.C.: Institute of Medicine.

33. Wallerstein, N., & Bernstein, E. (1988, Winter). Empowerment education: Freire's ideas adapted to health education. *Health Education Quarterly, 15,* 379-394.

34. Young, S. T. (1992, May 25). Urban blacks: A study in alienation. *Philadelphia Inquirer,* p. A14.

CHAPTER 62

Work redesign

The key to true health care reform

CONNIE R. CURRAN

Since the late 1980s a silent revolution has occurred in American health care. Work redesign, or the restructuring of care delivery around the patient, has become the newest form of organizational restructuring being undertaken by American hospitals. The goal of work redesign is to improve continuity and reduce fragmentation of care delivery. Pulling from the tenets of management science, production management, statistics, and economics,[2] the desired outcomes of hospital work redesign are improved patient outcomes and improved hospital outcomes, including reduced cost of care delivery.

NATIONAL TRENDS AFFECTING HOSPITALS

There is a need to reform the delivery of health care in hospitals, a need driven by the continuing federal budget deficit coupled with the escalation in health care costs. Currently, health care's share of the gross national product (GNP) has risen beyond predictions of national experts. The GNP is the dollar value of all final goods and services produced in an economy in a year.[1] Predicted by a group of health care executives to be 14% of the GNP by the year 2000, the Commerce Department reported that health care's share of the GNP was already 14% in April 1992.[3,12,29] The growth in the GNP in 1992 makes it the fifth straight year of double-digit increases. Further, the Commerce Department expects average annual increases of 12% to 13% over the next 5 years, with the potential for health care's share to reach 25% to 26% of the GNP by the year 1997. The growth in costs has been attributed to expensive high-technology equipment and treatments, an aging population, and malpractice-related costs.

But the need for restructuring hospital care is driven by more than simply growth in costs. Various alternative delivery systems and health care reforms practically mandate restructuring to ensure the financial viability of hospitals.

Expectations of universal health insurance are increasing, and futurists predict that it won't happen by 1996 but will by the year 2000.[3,12,30] Institution of universal health insurance would essentially mean a fixed fee paid to hospitals for all potential care. Regardless of the prospective payment mechanism, universal health insurance will be spurred by increasing national expenditures on health care. National health care expenditures in 1990 were $670.9 billion and are expected to almost triple to $1615.9 billion by the year 2000.[12] Universal health insurance coupled with the predicted growth in managed care will necessitate cost-efficient care delivery to ensure financial viability.

Managed care has grown and will continue to grow. The percentage of Medicare and Medicaid beneficiaries will continue to grow; pilot managed-care projects for Medicare are currently being funded by the Health Care Financing Administration,[17] and some states are funding Medicaid trials.[11] There is a high probability that both Medicare and Medicaid will be capitated in the next 5 years. And where Medicare leads other payers will follow.[15] Under a capitated reimbursement system hospitals remain viable by reducing costs of care related to delivery as well as by determining when and where the least costly setting for care delivery exists. Hospitals and payers are increasingly turning to case managers and CareMaps or critical pathways as a means to encourage review and reduction in unnecessary care and costs. Alexander[2] cautions that true savings in health care cannot be limited to only one profession. Rather, the whole process of patient care delivery must be restructured to deemphasize the "professional" as opposed to "patient" mentality.

There is a growing reorientation of the health care system from a focus on individual patient needs to an emphasis on societal needs and preventive measures. This is evidenced by the more than 45 national health care bills introduced for legislation. Virtually all include a significant role for managed care.[30] Again, for hospitals to remain financially viable under an increasingly prospective health care system, costs must be cut.

The shift from inpatient to outpatient care delivery will continue and is fired by the shift toward minimally invasive surgical procedures and the growth in prospective payers. "Current experts forecast that 'Nintendo' surgery could shift 5% to 15% of inpatient surgeries to ambulatory care within the next 5 years."[30] The shift from inpatient to outpatient care will mean a decrease in inpatient hospital admissions per 1000 population, a decrease in average length of stay, and decreasing revenues from inpatient care. Hospitals will need to determine how to deliver inpatient care in the most cost-efficient manner possible.

Payers will attempt to limit access to technology as a cost control strategy for those institutions with high utilization and/or costs. This will be demonstrated by a substitution of home care services for inpatient care, shorter lengths of stay, encouragement of professional extenders (i.e., nurses' assistants, nurse practitioners, and physician assistants), refusal to pay for advanced technology, travel to centers of excellence, decreased reimbursement of indirect costs of care, and less time with physicians.

More hospitals are predicted to close. As a matter of fact, 80 hospitals per year were predicted to close between 1991 and 1993, with 66 hospitals per year expected to close between 1994 and 1996.[3] The remaining hospitals will become more collaborative and less competitive in order to make the best use of scarce resources.[30] Increasing attention will be paid to restructuring the fragmented, inefficient delivery system, as the only way to contain costs and ensure access.

In the future, hospitals will be asked to disclose increasing amounts of information to accrediting agencies such as the Joint Commission on Accreditation of Healthcare Organizations, payers, and the public. Disclosure requirements will relate to a variety of information including patient care quality indicators, patient care outcomes, medical and other professional qualifications, overall hospital utilization, hospital mal-

practice claims settled, amount of charity care provided, and amount of community services provided. Cost data are already reported by hospitals in many states. Patients and payers will be able to choose hospitals and, eventually, health care providers based on cost and clinical data.

Hospitals are being challenged to demonstrate their community service mission because of escalation of costs, the need for increased sources of new revenue, and declining fiscal position of many city and state governments. Hospitals must take specific action to demonstrate this commitment to retain physicians and patients as well as to maintain not-for-profit status according to new legislation before Congress. To provide community service, hospitals must provide some inpatient and outpatient services even if they take losses on these services. In order to take losses on some services, hospitals must be as efficient as possible on nonloss services because cost shifting is becoming less and less tolerated by payers.

Losses arise from a variety of community services including community health areas that emphasize society over the individual patient. These services include radon screening, child health and immunization programs, eldercare programs, sick child care programs, and environmental health issues such as hazardous waste and air-water quality programs.[16] Again, hospitals must finance these programs out of their own funds and cannot cost shift these expenses to other inpatient or outpatient programs. To do this, hospitals must be cost efficient in their increasingly prospective payment environment.

Population demographics are also changing. Hospitals will have to take care of increasingly older patients. The median age of the U.S. population was 33 in 1990 and is expected to be 36.3 in the year 2000.[12] The number of people more than 100 years old will grow from 54,000 in 1990 to 108,000 in the year 2000.[12] These changing demographics indicate the direct increase in the Medicare health care burden in the years to come and point to the need to determine how care will be provided to the aging population in the most cost-efficient manner. The long-term care issue will become increasingly important to health care providers and consumers and still needs to be addressed. Executives who start to address these issues before the issues attack them will really capture the market in health care.

Physicians and chief executive officers (CEOs) agree that the quality of nursing staff is a major factor for physicians seeking affiliation with a hospital. Because nursing is critical to attracting and retaining physicians and hence patients, hospitals must remain competitive in their recruitment and retention of nurses. Hospitals that have instituted work redesign have documented improvement in patient and nurse satisfaction levels.[21] Restructuring allows the nurse to spend more time at the bedside and less time on nonnursing activities. Cross-trained personnel pick up activities such as housekeeping, clerical, and nursing aide functions in order to free the nurse for patient care.

A predicted short supply of nurses in the future necessitates redesign of hospital services in order to attract and retain nurses. Besides nursing, shortages exist in medical technology, pharmacy, physical therapy, occupational therapy, radiology technology, and respiratory therapy.[3,6,22] For hospitals to attract and retain these professionals, they must redesign care around the patient to facilitate their work.

IMPLICATIONS OF NATIONAL TRENDS

In the next 5 years government, employers, consumers, providers, and payers will experience significant pressure as a result of the rising cost of health care. The federal government will continue to shift more of the health care burden to the states and the private sector. In turn, providers and consumers will resist these attempts and exert pressure on government to increase their payment and services. State and local governments will attempt to deal with the federal government's share of the burden by instituting rationing programs for scarce state dollars. Oregon currently has submitted such a proposal for consideration.[23]

Payers will attempt to decrease their portion of the health care dollar by increasing deductibles and copayments or by eliminating some services such as vision or dental services. Consumers, the weakest lobbying voice, will pay an increasing portion of the health care cost out of their own pockets. Many will forgo coverage rather than pay out of pocket for private coverage. Others will seek managed-care plans to limit their personal losses and decrease their risk of exposure to catastrophic loss or financial devastation.

Providers will need to act strategically and attempt to decrease their costs of inpatient care through operational improvements or restructuring of care. An increasing proportion of inpatient care will be prospectively reimbursed. Therefore the only way for hospitals to maintain their margin is to reduce costs. Cost control becomes particularly critical in light of declining resources, increasing patient acuity, the aging population, the rapid deployment of expensive medical technologies, and the continued burden of medical and professional malpractice and liability costs.

By the year 1996 the marketplace will become more controlled. Managed-care principles will have been adopted by all payers, and payers will seek to work with only the most efficient hospitals and with those with dominant market shares.[3]

Hospitals will have to learn to make more intelligent use of their increasingly scarce and expensive human resources.[3,14] The future availability of nurses is even less optimistic because of the decrease in population growth between 1965 and 1975. This puts hospitals on a collision course with the "age wave," which alone may capsize the system.[14]

For hospitals to be appealing to patients, nurses, other health professionals, and physicians, they must restructure the health care process around the client and reduce the work of providing patient care. In one hospital, a simple chest X-ray for a patient required 64 steps, only 7 of them related to the X-ray itself.[21] In the same hospital, nurses found themselves devoting only 20 minutes of each hour to actual patient care. Nothing could be more frustrating to care providers than to have to fight constantly to schedule simple tests or lab work for their clients. The mounting dissatisfaction of nurses saluted as professionals yet reduced to stocking supplies has accelerated their exodus from hospitals.[14] Peter Drucker stated that there are many different motivations to become a nurse but he doesn't think anyone ever goes into nursing to become a clerk.[9]

INTRODUCING WORK REDESIGN

Work redesign is simply the redesign of care delivery and provider roles around the needs of patients, rather than around the needs of providers. The process of work redesign is usually very individualized; there is no boilerplate that fits each and every institution. Work redesign encourages the elimination of the departmental model or professional focus and instead focuses on the patient. It encourages cross-training and new or modified care delivery roles. It challenges the very basis of some professional licensure laws.

Various terminology for work redesign is found in the literature and includes the following: patient-centered care; patient-focused care (PFC); work redesign; operational restructuring or simply restructuring;

work flow; integrated care; operations improvement; new practice models; differentiated nursing practice; total quality management–continuous quality improvement; and the patient-focused hospital.* There is even a Patient-Focused Care Association.†

The various forms of work redesign cluster into three broad categories: (1) patient-focused care, (2) case management–differentiated nursing practice, and (3) total quality management.

Patient-focused care

Patient-focused care encompasses all forms of patient-centered work redesign and essentially restructures the delivery system at the unit level. PFC almost always includes a cross-trained care provider–clerical person and restructures patient units so that a variety of centralized services such as registration, medical coding, respiratory therapy, electrocardiogram (ECG), physical therapy, dietary, laboratory, X-ray, and pharmacy are relocated to the patient care unit.

Responsibility for all the decentralized services may lie in the hands of the new unit manager, who may be a nurse, or may be restructured in a matrix format. Staff nurses have an expanded role as the leaders of care teams composed of themselves and the cross-trained personnel, who have typically been licensed practical nurses, former nurses' aids, ECG technicians, or phlebotomists.

Education of the cross-trained personnel is usually conducted collaboratively by the various licensed professionals delegating tasks to that role. For instance, nursing teaches basic patient care, laboratory teaches phlebotomy and the performance of simple laboratory procedures, and so on. Units do not have to undergo reconstruction to accomplish PFC, but many have. Physical reconstruction allows units to eliminate the typical nurses' station and restructure the floor so that substations, cubicles outside the patient room, or movable carts hold patient supplies, charts, and medications. Health care providers no longer have to walk 10 miles a day to the nurses' station to communicate; rather they wear message-sending beepers or even headphones with a belt pack that enable them to communicate and free their hands.

---

*References 5,7,8,10,13,18,19,24,27,28.
†The Patient-Focused Care Association (1-800-877-PFCA; 4239 Farnum, Suite 28, Omaha, NE 68131) published the *PFCA Review.*

Case management

Case management or differentiated nursing practice is the second form of work redesign. Case management can be very different from PFC. Not only can it encompass all the changes included in PFC, but it also usually entails the use of CareMaps, created collaboratively by various health care professionals, which detail the care to be delivered for an entire hospital stay. The CareMaps identify the multidisciplinary standard of care and form a standard against which all health care professionals can document. The CareMaps enhance the potential for exception-based charting by all professionals, a problem not tackled in PFC. Once CareMaps are created, the variances from the standard can be tracked and reduced, thereby standardizing care delivery and reducing costly quality and cost outliers. The CareMaps can be used along with continuous quality improvement in order to achieve drastic reduction in variances.

In addition to the cost and quality standards achieved under case management, the nurse's role at the clinical level can be enhanced. The typical role of the nurse continues in the form of a care associate, but an enhanced case manager role emerges that provides more depth to current clinical ladders. This new role may help reduce the salary compression typical in the clinical hierarchy of nursing. Further, it provides a role that coordinates the functions of the many health care providers.

Total quality management

Total quality management–continuous quality improvement (TQM-CQI) is the third form of work redesign that is being attempted by U.S. hospitals. Hospitals not taking to the new philosophy of TQM of their own accord will eventually do so because of the 1993 Joint Commission on Accreditation of Healthcare Organizations standard that mandates that hospitals incorporate an improvement philosophy.

TQM builds on the tenets of Edward Deming's 14 basic principles. These 14 principles are broad and encourage a focus on quality, statistical process control, communication, breaking down barriers between staff areas, education and self-improvement, and a customer focus.[20] The difference between TQM and PFC is that the PFC literature is more prescriptive than the TQM literature. TQM fosters incremental change or continuous improvement as a philosophy, rather than the drastic changes that appear to be going on with PFC. But TQM is not limited to incremental change, and PFC or case management could be a TQM project.

Phases of work redesign

Whether hospitals choose to pursue operational improvements on their own or bring in outside consultants, they must go through four phases: preparation, analysis, generation of ideas, and implementation.[5,7] During the first phase, it is essential that hospital and nursing administration commit to keeping all parts of the organization involved and apprised of progress. Critical tasks to address in this first phase are deciding on the project's organization, developing an approach to human resources, preparing a communication plan, and making operational improvement the top management priority.

During the second phase of implementation, analysis, hospitals review and set targets for change based on an extensive internal and external comparison of cost and quality data. During the third phase, generation of ideas, hospitals assign personnel from various levels of the organization to work in multidisciplinary task forces to generate ideas for achieving the targets. During this stage of the operational improvement process, it is vital that radical ideas not be squashed or rejected. For each idea generated as a solution, the cost, risk, and obstacles to implementation of the idea are documented as criteria for senior management to use in the selection of the final solution.

The final phase of operational improvement, implementation, consists of the development and institution of a plan based on the ideas selected by senior management. The plan should include specific steps, responsibilities, timetables, and layoff schedules, if necessary. After approving the plan for implementation, top management asks all those departments affected to meet and review it. Human resources ensures that the plan addresses personnel changes, and the finance department ensures that the plan meets budgetary requirements. Only then does implementation occur. Many hospitals implement operational improvement slowly in pilot units to ensure that future full-scale implementation is debugged. Quantitative measures or targets should be evaluated at prespecified intervals to ensure that the change process is progressing as planned. If targets are not being met, administration needs to determine the cause.

Outcomes of work redesign

Patients in hospitals that have completed work redesign report higher patient satisfaction, reduced lengths of stay, and decreased adverse occurrences.[21] Further, these same patients request to be readmitted to the redesigned units with the same care teams they had on previous admissions.

Hospitals that have redesigned the care delivery process have experienced several changes, including the following: process simplification or improved work flow; dramatically reduced turnaround times on tests or procedures; fewer job classifications; flattened organizational structures; elimination of some schedulers, coordinators, documenters, and transporters; decentralization of ancillary and support services to point-of-service delivery on patient care units; exception-based charting; redefinition of everyone's job (e.g., administration and care givers); and, ultimately, lower cost of care delivery.[19,24] Lower costs result from reducing transaction volume, structuring idle time, and avoiding the costs of poor communication related to centralization and specialization.[19]

STRATEGIES FOR THE FUTURE

Whether work redesign is accomplished using case management, patient-focused care, shared governance, decentralization of ancillary services, total quality management, continuous quality improvement, critical pathways for selected diagnoses, or redefinition of care episodes, the scope of implementation throughout the United States is small but growing at an exponential rate. Nineteen pioneering models of operational restructuring were featured in the July/August 1992 issue of *Healthcare Forum Journal;*[2] at least 12 cases of operational restructuring have been documented in *Strategies for Healthcare Excellence* in 1991 and 1992;[25,26] seven major consulting firms are offering patient-focused care products; the Healthcare Forum had sold-out attendance at the first two national conferences on patient-focused health care delivery in 1991 and 1992;[4] and many hospitals are attempting to restructure on their own.

The heightened interest in work redesign is more than the latest passing craze. To become part of the organizational culture, redesign will require substantial time and leadership from the CEO and nursing administration. Work restructuring requires a commitment to stable and effective change, not just change for the sake of change. The implementation process for even one pilot unit may take up to a year. Full-scale implementation throughout a hospital may take up to 5 years.[21]

Hospital and nursing administrators must establish their vision of the future, based on the present and probable environment, to determine if work redesign is an appropriate strategy for them. Given the national trends affecting hospitals, a key tactic for maintaining a hospital's margin is to improve overall operational efficiency and effectiveness. In other words, restructure care, thereby improving quality and reducing costs.

There is a growing gap between the organization's need for nursing to assume an enlarged role in the redefined care delivery system and the traditional task-oriented role decreed by influential elements of the medical profession.[14] Because nursing and ancillary services are a key factor in attracting physicians and patients, nursing must implement recruitment and retention programs that emphasize a new broader role to retain the highest-quality professional in nursing.

Differentiated nursing practice and case management both have had good success with improving satisfaction and retention.[13] Through a case management system, nursing's role evolves to be the coordinator of care delivery. In essence, nurses become the engineers of care, coordinating the tasks of the various professions in the development of CareMaps, and then fine-tuning and adjusting the standard process rather than starting from scratch with every patient. Case management moves nursing away from its traditional role to one of educator, advocate, and coach. This new role is also compatible with the transagency role that nurses will have to fill in order to smooth and facilitate patients' progress in and out of the hospital.

Hospitals will have to ensure that nurse executives and managers are integrated into all aspects of the hospitals' operations. Every effort must be made to strengthen the collaboration between nurses and other professionals so that effective management of all aspects of patient care and utilization are achieved. With work redesign, vice presidents of nursing typically assume a greater role within hospital executive management than in the past and, in doing so, must expand their vision beyond nursing to one that encompasses the full range of patient care services and operations. Hospitals will place a greater value on the nurse executives' clinical and business orientation and their ability to coordinate the two functions in order to achieve new levels of efficiency and service.

Nurse executives should prepare to accept a broader role in the hospital by becoming better acquainted with issues in health care reform, financing, and care delivery. To do this, nurses must extend and maintain their professional relationships outside of their profession, read widely, and extend their professional memberships to national nonnursing organizations. They should extend their influence beyond nursing to total patient care.

Other roles and relationships also vary in a redesigned workplace. Decentralizing services such as dietary, laboratory, pharmacy, physical therapy, and ECG to the patient care level decreases the amount of steps, personnel, and time needed to collaborate on patient care. Cross-training of hospital personnel will improve staffing flexibility and productivity and eliminate downtime and the amount of communication needed to complete simple tests for patients. Licensure laws may need to be challenged and altered in order for hospitals to implement cross-trained personnel.

Hospital and nursing administrators that anticipate the need for operational restructuring will have to convince physicians, nurses, and payers of the need for this change and be prepared for resistance. A survey of health care executives indicates that the simple notion of cross-training is more readily accepted by hospital administrators than physician respondents.[3] While the challenges are large, the motivation and possible outcomes require the effort.

CONCLUSION

Radical methods must be developed to abate the growth in health care costs and to ensure quality outcomes. One suggested method is the operational restructuring of health care delivery around the patient as opposed to organization of health care around increasingly fragmented providers of health care. Redesigning care delivery around the patient, rather than around professions, is a major strategy for ensuring quality and service while reducing cost. The work redesign process is an essential element in bringing about the much-needed reform in health care delivery.

REFERENCES

1. Albrecht, W. (1986). *Economics* (4th ed.). Englewood Cliffs, N.J.: Prentice-Hall.
2. Alexander, J. (1992). Operational restructuring: 19 pioneering models. *Healthcare Forum Journal, 35*(4), 43-63.
3. Andersen, A., & American College of Healthcare Executives. (1991). *The future of healthcare: Physician and hospital relationships.* Chicago: American College of Healthcare Executives.
4. Back by popular demand. (1992). *Healthcare Forum Journal, 35*(4), 94.
5. Baronas, A. (1991). Dollars and sense: Achieving lasting organizational improvements through employee involvement. *Nursing Economic$, 9*(4), 277-280.
6. Burda, D. (1992). Nursing shortage! Nursing shortage? It seems to depend on who's talking. *Modern Healthcare, 22*(16), 34-35.

7. Curran, C., & Smeltzer, C. (1991). Operation improvement: Efficiencies and quality. *Journal of Nursing Quality Assurance, 5*(4), 1-6.

8. Dienemann, J., & Gessner, T. (1992). Restructuring nursing care delivery systems. *Nursing Economic$, 10*(4), 253-310.

9. Flower, J. (1991). It's late in the day. *Healthcare Forum Journal, 34*(4), 58-62.

10. Fralic, M. (1992). Creating new practice models and designing new roles: Reflections and recommendations. *Journal of Nursing Administration, 22*(5), 7-8.

11. Freund, D., Rossiter, L., Fox, P., Meyer, J., Hurley, R., Carey, T., & Paul, J. (1989). Evaluation of the Medicaid competition demonstrations. *Health Care Financing Review, 11*(2), 81.

12. Gardner, E. (1992). Hospital of the future. *Modern Healthcare, 22*(30), 34-65.

13. Goertzen, I. (1991). *Differentiating nursing practice into the twenty-first century.* Kansas City, Mo: American Academy of Nursing.

14. Hanrahan, T. (1991). New approaches to caregiving. *Healthcare Forum Journal, 34*(4), 33-38.

15. Herr, W. (1991). Taking a deep breath over capital payments. *Healthcare Financial Management, 45*(3), 19-32.

16. Hudson, T. (1992). Hospitals strive to provide communities with benefits. *Hospitals, 66*(13), 102-110.

17. Langwell, K., & Hadley, J. (1989). Evaluation of the Medicare competition demonstrations. *Health Care Financing Review, 11*(2), 65-81.

18. Lathrop, J. (1991). The patient-focused hospital. *Healthcare Forum Journal, 34*(4), 17-20.

19. Lathrop, J. (1992). The patient-focused hospital. *Healthcare Forum Journal, 35*(3), 76-78.

20. Neuhauser, D. (1988). The quality of medical care and the 14 points of Edward Deming. *Health Matrix, 6*(2), 7-14.

21. Ollier, C. (1992). Ambitious "Care 2000" initiative decentralizes work processes at San Diego Mercy Hospital and Medical Center. *Strategies for Healthcare Excellence, 5*(8), 1-7.

22. Rodgers, J. (1992). Nursing shortage continues despite what data may say. *Modern Healthcare, 22*(25), 56.

23. Ryan, M. (1992). Oregon's Medicaid waiver denied. *Medical Group Management Update, 31*(9), 3.

24. Strasen, L. (1991). Redesigning hospitals around patients and technology. *Nursing Economic$, 9*(4), 233-238.

25. *Strategies for Healthcare Excellence.* (1991). *4*, pp. 1-12.

26. *Strategies for Healthcare Excellence.* (1992). *5*, pp. 1-8.

27. Tarte, J., & Bogiages, C. (1992, February). Patient-centered care delivery and the role of information systems. *Computers in Healthcare,* pp. 44-46.

28. Tonges, M. (1992). Work designs: Sociotechnical systems for patient care delivery. *Nursing Management, 23*(1), 27-32.

29. Updata. (1992). Healthcare spending to reach 14 percent of GNP in 1992. *Healthcare Financial Management, 46*(2), 7.

30. Wachel, W. (1992). As they see it: Experts forecast trends and challenges. *Healthcare Executive, 7*(4), 16-20.

CHAPTER 63

The Canadian health care system

Overview and issues

JANET C. ROSS KERR

In a society in which life is deeply valued, the health of people becomes an issue of fundamental importance. Responsibility for health was granted to the provinces in the British North America Act that established the Canadian Confederation in 1867. Health was reserved as a federal prerogative for marine hospitals and quarantine and for aboriginal peoples. The Constitution Act of 1982, which superseded the original legislation, confirmed and continued this division of powers. Social democratic traditions along with Canada's growth and development as a colonial empire perhaps contributed more than other factors to the perception of the need to ensure the availability of health care for the population. In the aftermath of social upheavals created by the Depression and two world wars, many factors converged to create a receptive climate for consideration of public financing of individual health care expenditures. Federal-provincial agreements emerged from public debate and discussion and culminated in the implementation of a system of national health insurance to cover health care costs for all Canadians.

THE ESTABLISHMENT OF THE CANADIAN HEALTH INSURANCE SYSTEM

Although the Canadian program of insurance for hospital services at the federal level was not enacted until 1957, the stage was set for the federal legislation in previous supportive developments in the provinces. Saskatchewan was clearly in the forefront of provincial developments and, after World War I, passed legislation enabling municipalities to raise taxes to support the employment of physicians (the municipal doctor plans), the establishment of hospitals, and the development of hospitalization plans. The window of op-

portunity created by firm support from the Canadian Medical Association (CMA) for publicly financed health insurance in 1934 was lost through government inaction, as the CMA later withdrew its support in favor of private plans initiated by physicians in several provinces. Saskatchewan decided to "go it alone" when it became the first jurisdiction in North America to enact legislation establishing a prepaid plan of hospital insurance in 1947. The federal government passed its first legislation dealing with health in 1948, although it fell short of the objective of establishing a prepaid hospital insurance plan; the National Health Grants Act included funds for hospital construction, professional training, public health, and other provincial services, areas seen as providing the basis for the later establishment of national health insurance.

When the Hospital Insurance and Diagnostic Services Act was passed in 1957, it provided for comprehensive inhospital patient care services with universal coverage for residents of participating provinces. Because health fell within provincial jurisdiction, the government of each province had the right to decide whether or not to develop a plan to insure hospital services conforming to the federal guidelines outlined in the legislation. However, because the plan involved 50/50 cost sharing with the provinces, any province deciding to opt out of the arrangement would forgo tax dollars the federal government would otherwise contribute to health care in that province and would, in opting out, effectively subsidize the plans of other provinces. Initially five provinces agreed to participate when the act came into force in 1958, and by 1961 all provinces were full participants in the program. Excepted from the national hospital insurance program were tuberculosis and mental hospitals and certain other institutions.

In adding prepayment for medical services to the hospitalization plan in 1962, the province of Saskatchewan again became the first jurisdiction to implement such legislation. It did so over the loud protestations of Saskatchewan physicians who went on strike for 23 days beginning July 1, 1962, the date the legislation was implemented. In the face of vehement opposition from physicians, the Saskatchewan government was forced to make concessions to the medical profession in the form of allowing opting out of the plan and extrabilling. Implementation of the federal agenda to add medical services to its program of prepaid health insurance was undoubtedly hastened and facilitated by the lessons learned from the Saskatchewan experience. The federal Medical Care Act was thus passed in 1966, and the controversial nature of the legislation may explain the participation of only two provinces at the time the legislation came into force on July 1, 1968, as well as the 5-year length of time it required for all provinces to enter into an arrangement with the federal government for the prepayment of medical services. The plan allowed for coverage of physicians' services in and out of hospital, but did not prevent the provinces from allowing physicians to opt out of the plan, bill patients directly, or impose surcharges on the established fee for a particular service.

In the early part of the 1970s the escalation of expenditures and the growing size of the federal deficit caused concern over the open-ended nature of some health expenditures, in particular those for physicians' services. In 1977 the arrangements for federal-provincial cost sharing were amended with the passage of the Fiscal Arrangements and Established Programs Financing Act. This ended the open-ended 50/50 cost sharing and introduced block funding that involved transfer of some tax points to the provinces and reduced the federal contribution to health care to 25% with additional federal contributions based on increases in the gross national product (GNP). In the years following the passage of this legislation, concern mounted over the increased use of copayments termed user fees for institutional services and extrabilling practices among physicians in provinces where this was allowed. The federal government's response to these perceived erosions of Medicare was the Canada Health Act of 1984, through the provisions of which extrabilling and user fees were disallowed. Although physicians mounted a strong and vocal campaign to prevent the prohibition of extrabilling, it was to no avail, and the act was implemented by the liberal government of the day. A measure of the popularity of Medicare in Canada may be seen in the fact that the progressive conservative government elected later in 1984 did not make any attempt either to amend the legislation or to develop new proposals, either immediately or in the 8 years to follow. As of 1992 the provisions of the Canada Health Act remained intact.

THE PHILOSOPHICAL BASIS OF HEALTH CARE LEGISLATION

Canadians have come to believe in health insurance coverage as a right of citizens, and this translates into support for Medicare; support is reported to be as high as 85%.[4] The rationale for the evolution of the federal health legislation program can be found in five basic principles of health care from which the standards for the legislation are derived. The first principle, universality, means that coverage is offered to the population as a whole rather than to selected population groups. The principle of comprehensiveness ensures that all medically necessary services included in the plan are covered. Although extrabilling and user fees were allowed in the initial stages, differential charges may no longer be applied on a private basis for services covered by the plan. The principle of accessibility is perhaps the most difficult to satisfy, particularly with a sparse population scattered over a vast amount of territory. However, reasonable access to services is seen as essential even in view of the need to constrain costs. Portability, or coverage for residents of one province when they require services just after a move or during a visit to another province, is the fourth principle that must be assured in plans. And finally, public administration, nonprofit operation by an organization fiscally responsible to the provincial government, is required. In the various acts passed by the federal government relative to health insurance since 1957, progressive refinement of the standards applicable to provincial health plans based on the basic principles has been evident.

The incorporation of a system of health care in legislation ensures that certain defining characteristics will emerge from the philosophy and principles upon which it is based. Because the system itself is entrenched within the law, if change is desired, full legislative review will be needed. This might be either an advantage or a disadvantage depending upon the issue of concern and the nature of any change deemed necessary. At the outset, the Canadian health care system evolved in a manner not unlike systems in other Western countries. The fact that the provincial plans insure hospital care and physicians' services means that the hospital and the physician are paramount in the system. It is not surprising to find that the number of hospital beds increased at a rate much higher than the rate of population increase until legislation appeared to end the 50/50 federal-provincial cost sharing. Outpatient care, home care, and community health services were areas not eligible for federal cost sharing at the outset. The exclusion of these forms of care from federal financing encouraged physician-centered, in-hospital care during the first 35 years of health care legislation in Canada.[5] The high cost of these methods of providing care has led to a search for more effective and efficient lower-cost alternatives. The consumer movement has also heightened awareness of the need for consumers to be active participants in matters pertaining to their health. The "Alma Ata" agreement by countries who are members of the World Health Organization of health for all by the year 2000 has carried with it an implicit challenge to encourage genuine community involvement in planning for health in ways that have not been either recognized or explored previously in health care delivery systems. The challenge for health care in Canada is to tailor the legislative arrangements for health care to encourage community-based measures facilitating health maintenance, health promotion, and prevention of disease and to balance these with measures to restore health. Thus, "many believe that it will not be possible to sustain the current system without major modifications. Task forces and commissions in most provinces are looking at ways to shift the heavy focus on physician and institutional care to 'community based' alternatives and non-physician providers."[2]

ISSUES IN COST CONTAINMENT
Costs of medical care

Analyses of the Canadian experience with Medicare have concluded that introduction of a system of universal health insurance has led to relative stability in health care costs in reference to the gross domestic product.[1,7] Whereas Canadian health care costs were equivalent to those in the United States before the full implementation of Medicare in 1971, "by 1985 the United States was spending over two percentage points of GNP more (and growing) on health care." Despite the Canadian record, it is widely concluded that fine-tuning is required to control escalation of costs in the system. The area that is the focus of the most attention is that of physicians' fees: "Payments for physician services, which in most countries run a significant second to institutional care in their share of total health costs, tend to be the most difficult and controversial to control."[1] Since physicians are remunerated primarily on a fee-for-service basis in Canada, "the rate of increase of those fees is a natural target."[1]

Although physicians are reimbursed for their services on a fee-for-service basis, they bill the health insurance plan in each province for their fees rather than the individual patient. Since it is the health insurance plan that is billed, physicians' fee schedules have been the subject of negotiation between provincial governments and the medical profession in each province since the full implementation of Medicare in 1971. In the interest of containing costs, there is considerable pressure in most provinces to keep the rates of increase in physicians' fee schedules to a reasonable level. Expenditures for physicians' services constitute approximately 16% of health expenditures, a figure that is considerably higher at 20% in the United States.[1] Analyses of fee increases have noted that "since 1971 physicians' fees in all the provinces of Canada have risen no more rapidly than general inflation rates, and in some provinces and/or time periods have lagged well behind."[1]

The negotiation of fee schedules between governments and physicians has often produced considerable conflict and from time to time is carried out in the public eye with intense media attention. Although strikes are rare, physicians have not hesitated to employ threats of service withdrawal in negotiations in order to support their fee demands. A strike lasting 25 days occurred in Ontario in 1986; however, as in the 1962 Saskatchewan physicians' strike, it "failed in its fundamental political objective—the obstruction of government's resolve to extend its control over health insurance."[6] However, the notion of solidarity within physician ranks to maintain "autonomy and dominance in the health care system"[6] has been challenged. It has been suggested that "the degree of organization and commitment of the medical profession is less than is commonly assumed, and that the political weight of the profession is greater than it need be because governments and other political actors hold exaggerated assumptions about its organization and commitment."[6] The national survey of Canadian physicians conducted in 1986 to 1987 found that 61% agreed that "Medicare 'has positively influenced the health status of Canadians' by improving access to medical services."[6] It also found that just over "60% of physicians are satisfied 'in the practice of medicine' under Medicare and only 24% are dissatisfied."[6] Finally, a finding that "60% of physicians disapprove and only one quarter approve of 'the withdrawal of nonemergency services' in support of income demands" lends credence to the premise that solidarity and commitment among physicians to "an unregulated medical marketplace"[6] is not as firm as is commonly believed.

Other concerns in relation to costs of physicians' services are physicians' billing activity, the supply of physicians, and specialization. Controls on fees produced increased billing activity, as physicians sought to respond to fee controls by increasing their activity. However, a number of studies have shown that physicians have not been able to offset the impact of fee controls on their incomes, and "the extent to which they are able to do so depends critically on the fee negotiation context."[1] Also, since fees are negotiated between physicians and provincial governments on an annual basis, there is an ongoing opportunity for removing " 'loopholes' in the fee schedule that provide the opportunities for procedural multiplication."[1] The supply of physicians is another factor that interacts with other variables relative to containment of medical costs. Thus while "billing activity per physician has increased more rapidly in Canada [than in the United States], utilization per capita has not, at least since 1975. In that year Canada cut back sharply on physician immigration, with the result that while prior to 1975 physician supply was growing more rapidly in Canada, since then it has grown more slowly."[1] Access to specialization has been strictly limited in Canada, and as a result of this one half of all physicians in Canada are general practitioners, as compared with 10% in the United States.[8] Since specialists perform more procedures and carry out more tests, allowing the ratio of general practitioners to specialists to change will cause increases in costs and may not serve the public good. Indeed, the optimal size of medical school enrollments is an issue that is currently being debated in Canada, because if the physician-population ratio increases, it is likely that medical services and costs will also increase. However, it must be recognized that all of the variables of concern in containing physician costs become more difficult to deal with because of the open-ended nature of expenditures for medical care.

Cost of hospitalization

The problems relative to the escalation of the cost of medical services are not of the same magnitude in ex-

penditures for hospitalization and other areas of health spending, as budgets are established and strictly followed. There are important issues of cost control here, but provincial governments hold responsibility for establishing and maintaining a health system that will not only serve consumer needs, but also be affordable. Hospitals are provided with a global budget to cover operating costs on an annual basis by provincial governments. Capital expenditures are considered separately, but the process is again one of negotiation with the government. This does not allow for expansion of hospitals or the purchase of expensive equipment without a process of rationalization. Although hospitals operate under the direction of boards of directors, in this matter of annual budget determination and approval, the government clearly has the upper hand. This centralized process by which the annual total expenditures of hospitals are established is clearly a political one, and the debate is often highly public. Hospital administrators are increasingly going public with their case for maintenance of or increase in funding. This can sometimes paint a false picture of the situation, as what appears in the media may be simply posturing in a public debate over the advisability of expenditures in one area or another. Thus, "the difficulty for health policy and funding is that, since the boy always cries wolf (and must do so, given the political system of funding), one does not know if the wolf is really there. The political dramatics should not mislead external observers into believing that the wolf is always at hand."[3]

Costs for nursing form a significant portion of the costs of hospitalization, although they are hidden within the global budget of the hospital. Although the public debate over hospital costs is intense and prolonged, the nursing work force forms the element of hospital expenditures that can perhaps be most easily manipulated. The all too familiar scenario of closing beds and laying off employees, principally nurses, in response to government cost-cutting measures is played out frequently in tough economic times. However, in view of changing emphases in the health system, with the focus moving from acute, inhospital care to community-based care and treatment emphasizing prevention, promotion of health, and consumer initiative, nurses must face the prospect of radical changes in the nature and structure of care that will have a profound impact upon the profession. All too often nurses are not at the table when cost containment decisions are made, or, if there, they may find themselves in vulnerable and compromised positions in relation to the hard decisions that are being made. In contrast to the process of determining remuneration for physicians where the fee schedule is directly negotiated between physician organizations and the government, the situation is very different for nurses. Since nurses are largely employees of hospitals, they answer to their superiors, nursing administrators, and ultimately the chief executive officer of the employing institution. While nursing unions exist in all provinces with a mandate from nursing members in local hospitals to bargain collectively for salary levels for various categories of nursing employees, individual hospital administrators acting on direction from boards have the right to determine the number of nursing positions needed in an institution. Under enlightened administrations, representatives of nursing unions may sit on advisory councils that consider nursing issues and recommend solutions to the chief nursing administrator; however, it is unlikely that this is the case in the majority of hospitals. Therefore the nursing work force in hospitals can be made to contract or expand rather quickly by changing the number of positions. Issues relative to the supply of nurses are important, as it is essential to prepare an appropriate number of nurses with the educational background necessary to allow them to contribute to the health system in an important and meaningful way.

Nurses are likely to find themselves in the forefront of the increasing emphasis upon community-based care. While community health agencies have employed a small part of the nursing work force, nurses working in the community form a highly educated group and have historically worked relatively autonomously in collaboration with other health professionals. Although initial health legislation only allowed for remuneration in provincial plans for physicians and dental surgeons, the Canada Health Act of 1984 contained a provision to allow for payments to "health practitioners." The Canadian Nurses' Association lobbied intensively and successfully for the inclusion of this clause, which, to date, no provincial government has implemented as part of its plan. However, the opportunity is there for the development of community health centers that could be reimbursed for the services of a variety of health professionals including nurses. A small group of nurses is engaged in independent practice in most provinces; however, a nurse in independent practice must bill the client directly for services, as no provincial plan will currently allow this. In any move to an increased focus upon community-based health care

services, nurses will undoubtedly be called upon to play an important and continuing role.

FUTURE DIRECTIONS

The tax-supported system of health care that has evolved in Canada over a period of some 35 years, while not flawless, is nevertheless highly regarded by consumers who react negatively to any suggestion that the system is imperiled. Such suggestions are the order of the day and simply part of business as usual in a not-for-profit system operated in the public sphere where interest groups and institutions alike have the opportunity to argue for funds and/or programs that they see as beneficial. It is recognized today that there are limits to the nature and amount of care that can be provided and limits to growth. To ensure the continuation of the system, measures must be taken to ensure that universal availability and access to needed services are balanced by the provision of reasonably comprehensive services in a publicly funded, nonprofit, and affordable system.

The system must respond to perceptions of a need for change in the nature and context of health care. It has been pointed out that Canada "provides a test case in the limits of medical care *per se,* and the health problems which still confront Canadians cannot, in general, be improved merely by improving access to medical care."[2] Canada has had a hospital- and physician-centered system of health care entrenched in its universal health care legislation for some 35 years. The social determinants of health such as income, education, employment, and others are important elements in the health of a nation. Universal health insurance has provided some assistance to vulnerable population groups, but other measures to address some of these problems are needed. Health is increasingly seen more broadly than simply the absence of illness, and in the presence of new approaches to the meaning of health, the nature and context of health care must change as well.

The needs of professional groups must be balanced by the needs of society. In the evolving health care system in Canada, there is a need for the health professions to work collaboratively in the best interest of the consumer. The system that has developed in Canada has provided high-quality medical and hospital care and has contributed significantly to improvements in the health of people. However, despite new and impressive technological adjuncts to care, rational judgments must be made concerning the nature and context of health and health care. Social and cultural determinants of health require much study and attention in order to produce improved health outcomes. The political framework within which the issues relative to health care insurance plans are debated and determined will be conditioned by the economic and social realities of effecting fundamental change in the system. Decisions to move to a community-based model emphasizing prevention of disease, promotion of health, and partnerships between professionals and consumers will be difficult ones, but they are those that will ultimately hold the greatest potential for impacting health positively. Issues surrounding hospital governance, education of health professionals, the integration of boards of health agencies on a regional basis, and restructuring the systems for providing care and for remunerating health professionals in a reasonable and rational way must be considered in a collaborative manner to allow the health care system in Canada to meet the challenges that are ahead in this century and beyond.

REFERENCES

1. Barer, M. L., Evans, R. G., & Labelle, R. J. (1988). Fee controls as cost control: Tales from the frozen north. *Milbank Quarterly, 66*(1), 1-64.
2. Deber, R. B., Hastings, J. E. F., & Thompson, G. G. (1991). Health care in Canada: Current trends and issues. *Journal of Public Health Policy, 12*(1), 72-82.
3. Evans, R. G., Lomas, J., Barer, M. L., Labelle, R. J., Fooks, C., Stoddart, G. L., Anderson, G. M., Feeny, D., Gafni, A., Torrance, G. W., & Tholl, W. G. (1989). *New England Journal of Medicine, 320*(9), 571-577.
4. Inglehart, J. K. (1990). Health policy report: Canada's health care system. *New England Journal of Medicine, 315*(12), 778-784.
5. Kerr, J. R. (1991). In J. R. Kerr & J. MacPhail (Eds.), *Canadian nursing: Issues and perspectives* (2nd ed.). Toronto: Mosby.
6. Stevenson, H. M., Williams, H. P., & Vayda, E. (1988). Medical politics and Canadian Medicare: Professional response to the Canada Health Act. *Milbank Quarterly, 66*(1), 65-104.
7. Van Loon, R. J. (1980). From shared cost to block funding and beyond: The politics of health insurance in Canada. In C. Meilicke & J. L. Storch (Eds.), *Perspectives on Canadian health and society services policy: History and emerging trends.* Ann Arbor, Mich: Health Administration Press.
8. Terris, M. (1991). Global budgeting and the control of hospital costs. *Journal of Public Health Policy, 12*(1), 61-71.

PART EIGHT

HEALTH CARE COSTS

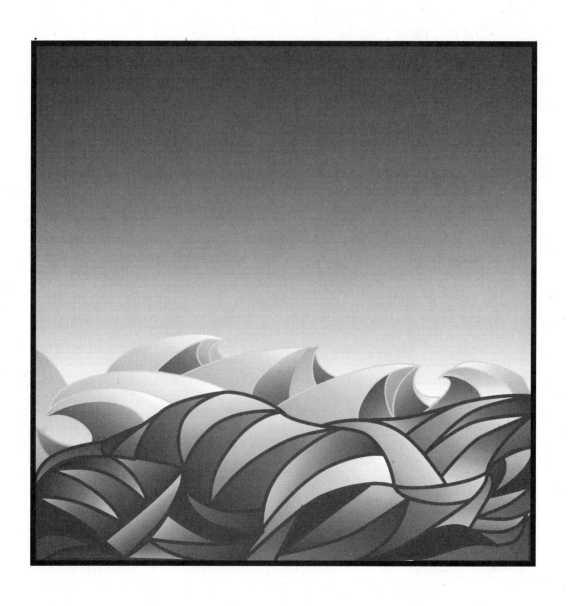

Nursing's part in health care costs

JOANNE COMI McCLOSKEY, HELEN KENNEDY GRACE

The cost of health care is a concern for all health care providers in these times. While nursing care is a major part of health care, the impact of this care on the costs of health care is virtually ignored in discussions of this matter. What impact does nursing have on the cost of health care? Do we help to lower costs? Or are we part of the reason for runaway costs? This section addresses some of the issues around the costs of nursing care.

In the debate chapter, Grace addresses the pressing problem of rising health care costs. While health care costs are expected to rise to 15% of the gross national product (GNP) by the end of the century, one in four Americans is uninsured or underinsured and many people are in poor health. Grace first analyzes four factors contributing to the high costs of health care: an excess of hospital beds, a surplus of highly specialized physicians who have too much say in treatment plans, insurance plans that benefit hospitals and physicians rather than patients, and lack of consumer involvement in health care decisions. Grace distinguishes between medical care, which "focuses on the diagnosis and treatment of disease," and health care, which has as its aim "the well-being of the individual and family at an optimal level of health." We currently have a system of medical care. Her proposal for change to a system of health care includes returning the responsibility for health care to the individual and family, using health care providers to support the family, demystifying health and illness through education, and using the acute care system appropriately. She outlines some of the steps toward change to a comprehensive health care system, including the need to dispel the myth that anything less than care provided by a physician is second-best. Nurses, she says, are central in making the difference, and this can happen if we can become "one strong voice."

The importance of identifying nursing costs is evident in efforts since diagnostic-related group (DRG) implementation to cost out nursing service. Scherubel briefly reviews the history of nursing in this area and then reviews several methods used to identify the costs of direct (hands-on) nursing care. These include relative intensity measures (RIMs), nursing care categories, the GRASP classification system, patient management categories, nursing diagnoses, and the nursing intensity index. Scherubel also points out that there are many methods for measuring indirect costs such as nursing support services and institutional overhead costs. She discusses the value of knowing nursing costs and spells out dilemmas and future needs. Her chapter includes an impressive reference list that those interested in studying or determining nursing costs will find helpful.

When one looks at cost, one also needs to look at quality. In the next chapter, McCormac Bueno and Fralic describe a cost-quality measurement index called QualDex that was developed and is used at Robert Wood Johnson University Hospital. The system quantifies the performance of quality and cost on each nursing unit. It consists of an analysis of five quality elements and five cost elements. The authors review each element and define its measures. While others may prefer a less quantitative approach, they will find the authors' choice of variables and structure very helpful. As the authors point out, "Although the contribution of nurses to the maintenance of quality is widely recognized, the additional association of nursing with cost containment is essential and warrants acknowledgment." This report of one effort to measure both quality and cost outcomes of nursing care is impressive.

In the next chapter, Alfano discusses costs of health services in long-term care. She points out that the need for long-term care is not confined to the aged; it is also needed by a growing number of others, including those with acquired immunodeficiency syndrome (AIDS) and children who survive acute illnesses. She says that one of the stumbling blocks to reduced costs is the current requirement for physician determination that services are necessary. Nursing, she says, ought to have assumed the leading role in the improvement of long-term care but, other than a few notable efforts, has dragged its feet. She points out that the most frequent services needed in the home for the chronically ill and frail elderly are support services such as assistance with shopping and housecleaning. These social services (not health services) ought to be dependent, not upon the recommendation of a physician, but upon that of a responsible "primary care giver." The author recommends a case management approach with professional nurses as case managers. She questions the move to develop home health nursing programs and challenges public health nurses to refocus and "get back on target." Alfano also raises many other challenging and controversial points. At the end of the chapter she proposes that nurses grapple with the difficult questions related to rationing of care. This is an insightful and provocative chapter. Alfano raises our consciousness of these difficult issues. Not that we know, what will we do about them?

The many issues surrounding health care reimbursement in the United States are addressed next by Collard. Several factors accounting for a rise in health care expenses are discussed, including financing, relative price of health care, aging population, malpractice litigation, technology, lack of primary care, excess capacity, and administrative costs. Collard's chapter contains many interesting facts, such as the fact that 24% of today's health care dollars are spent on administrative costs and the fact that there are over 1500 different insurance forms. She also discusses current financing mechanisms, the rising numbers of uninsured, outcomes of health care spending, and the state of the U.S. health care system. She concludes with policy recommendations for the future that include identifying a basic package of health services for all citizens, outcomes research to identify what works, identifying centers of excellence, restructuring reimbursement for physicians, and setting limits on lawyers' fees in malpractice settlements. Finally, she proposes greater reliance on nurses who are cost effective and underutilized. The topic of reimbursement is filled with terms often unfamiliar to nurses. A glossary of common financing and reimbursement terminology is included in this informative chapter.

The costs of a specific regulation are addressed in the next chapter. McPherson and Jackson address the costs of safety precautions to protect health care workers from bloodborne pathogens. This is a confusing situation, as the guidelines from the U.S. Centers for Disease Control (CDC) and the Department of Labor's Occupational Safety and Health Administration (OSHA) address different aspects of infection control and have changed over time. Health care agencies are faced with the dilemma of implementing CDC universal precautions for everyone while also implementing another isolation system. One system expects health care workers to act the same for all patients, while the other expects caution only when caring for patients with suspected or known infections. Costs of complying with the OSHA regulations are estimated at $146 per employee per year or around $813 million per year. The chief cost is the necessary protective equipment, especially gloves. The annual cost for implementing CDC universal precautions is estimated at about $336 million. Universal precautions use chiefly barrier techniques (gloves, gowns, masks, eyeglasses) based on traditional isolation techniques. While these may minimize nosocomial infections, there is little evidence to support the effectiveness of universal precautions in preventing bloodborne infections in health care workers. These authors say that the best risk reduction strategies to prevent human immunodeficiency virus (HIV) or hepatitis B infection are engineering controls to reduce risks from needles and other sharp equipment, and work practice modifications in the use of sharp devices. They give an example of using injury data to change products and practice associated with intravenous access devices. The costs of administering a dose of hepatitis B vaccine and the costs of a follow-up program for an employee exposed to hepatitis B are addressed in detail.

A cost population is defined a bit differently in the next chapter. Meadows examines the issues and costs surrounding mothers and their infants exposed to cocaine. Her general thesis is given in the chapter's subtitle: "a broader perspective." We need, she says, a broader perspective on what has been dehumanizingly and narrowly addressed as "crack babies." The exact scope of the problem is difficult to know, but there is agreement that drug addiction among pregnant women is a serious problem, both for the mother and the unborn fetus. The National Institute on Drug Abuse reports that as many as 350,000 infants annually have been born to mothers using cocaine, but data reflecting the number of infants with cocaine effects are not available. Meadows reports and examines the research, which, she notes, has concentrated on describing the problem and has several limitations. She points out that "the more we focus on gathering information, the further we seem to move away from prevention-oriented interventions." After an examination of the complex issues, she turns to addressing the costs in four areas: direct, indirect, intangible, and comparative. The exact costs associated with cocaine exposure, she concludes, are not known and may be incalculable. Efforts need to be directed toward preventing drug use and toward treatment before pregnancy. Readers will find this chapter interesting in its relation of the specifics of cocaine exposure and of the approach used to begin to address costs for a particular diagnostic population.

One of the chief costs of health care is the salaries of providers. Havens and Mills address the wage and remuneration practices in nursing. They address the question, Are nurses paid what they are worth? They present data and examine issues so that readers will debate the question and search for answers. The authors present many interesting facts including the following: most staff nurses are paid according to an hourly wage, with only 6% of hospital nurses salaried in 1990; nurses working in the Northeast earn 39% more than those employed in the west central states; and differences among specialties amount to less than $1 per hour. Nurses, they say, are paid for the time they work, rather than for their skills, expertise, or accomplishments. Employers value *when* a registered nurse (RN) works (shift) more than knowledge, skills, and job requirements. The authors compare the salary gains of nurses to those of other occupations. While nurse salaries have improved dramatically in the past 5 years, nursing still lags behind in overall gain. Nursing salary increases are slowing. The authors also discuss the labor market for nurses and its imperfections, and the issues involved in economic equity.

Turning to the costs of nursing education, Forni and Burns present multiple strategies for increasing revenues and reducing expenditures in nursing education programs. They point out that in 1993, 42 states cut budgets for higher education. As governments can be relied on less for sources of money, nursing programs are developing other options, both external and inter-

nal. External sources include private foundations, individual donors, Medicare pass-through funds, special arrangements with health care agencies, and grants and contracts. Internal sources include student tuition, faculty practice, continuing education offerings, royalties, inventions, and nurse-managed clinics and centers. The authors discuss each of the sources. They also discuss sources of cost savings and some of the advantages and disadvantages associated with each. Finally, they point out that the cliche "it takes money to make money" is true for nursing programs. In these tough economic times, this chapter provides many ideas on ways to generate and save money in higher education.

Lastly, the issue of government involvement in paying for health care costs is addressed by Biscoe in the concluding chapter. She says that the degree to which an individual agrees with the national approach to health care depends on that individual's perspectives. No country can please all its citizens. There may be an infinite demand for health care, but what direction should governments take in fulfilling this demand? Biscoe takes a world view, reviewing the health care and financing patterns of several countries: Singapore, Belgium, Japan, Canada, France, Switzerland, Sweden, and Australia. Readers will find it interesting to compare the health care practices of these countries with those of their own. Few nations, says Biscoe, know what they are trying to buy for their health care money. In all countries there is debate over the amount of money allocated to health promotion and prevention versus illness and curative care. Biscoe points out that politics is a major variable in any plan and no one model is right for all countries.

Taken together, the chapters in this section raise many interesting issues and challenges for nursing. A partial list might include rationed care, government involvement in health care, types of practitioners for the chronically ill and aging, reliable measures of quality and cost, relationships with physicians, benefits and burdens of regulations, and costs of nursing education. Nursing's ability to identify and deal with economic issues has come a long way in the past decade. The current concerns about the costs of health care open up many opportunities for nursing. Are we ready?

CHAPTER 64

Debate

Can medical care costs be contained?

HELEN KENNEDY GRACE

Medical care costs continue to rise at a rate of 10% per year—far exceeding the inflation rate. Medical care costs consume 12.7% of the gross national product (GNP) and are expected to rise to 15% by the end of the century. The increasing consumption of the GNP for medical care services means that resources are being shifted from other areas of need, such as housing and social services. While the costs of medical care have escalated for some time, it is only recently that the general public has become visibly concerned. As Reinhardt[6] summarized the situation, "The notion continues to spread that health care is one of those commodities to which every citizen in a civilized society is entitled regardless of ability to pay. This sentiment now threatens to engulf all technically available health care regardless of its costs."

Despite the continued rise in the costs of medical care, it is estimated that 65 million Americans, or one in four, are either uninsured or underinsured. Thirty-five million Americans have neither private nor public insurance, and another 30 million have minimal coverage.

Ironically, despite this high rate of expenditure for medical care in the United States, the health of the people as measured by a number of standards is not good. Infant mortality rates, particularly among blacks, are alarmingly high.

Assessment of progress in meeting health goals for the nation points to similar problems in the health of adolescents, minorities of all age groups, and the elderly.

This chapter will first analyze the factors contributing to the high cost of medical care. It will then offer what this author is convinced are the only viable, long-term solutions if medical care costs are to be contained.

THE HIGH COST OF MEDICAL CARE

There are four major contributors to the escalation of medical care costs:

1. The overcapacity of hospitals
2. A surplus of highly specialized providers
3. The inequitable financing of health care services
4. The passive role of the health care consumer

Hospitals

The first hospitals were designed to care for those who had no families. They were directed toward care of patients and not cure. After World War II, with advances in technology and anesthesia and the inflow of public dollars, the focus of hospitals quickly shifted to cure.

The Hill-Burton program, begun in 1946, provided a massive infusion of federal and state governmental monies, and helped construct over 400,000 hospital beds between then and the early 1970s. The most current data indicate that there are now just under 5800 community hospitals containing nearly 1 million beds. Community hospitals admitted slightly less than 36 million patients in 1985 . . . with an average length of stay of 7.4 days. The average hospital's occupancy rate, a measure of the industry's capacity being utilized, was 64 percent. Hospitals now employ 3.6 million people, or about one out of every 30 U.S. workers.[8]

Until 1977, there was a continuing increase in demand for hospital beds; the demand plateaued in 1982, and since that time there has been a steady decline in both number of admissions and length of stay. Renn[8] attributes this decline to four factors:

1. The change in incentives to a prospective payment system that provides payment based upon average costs of treatment for patients within a particular diagnostic category

2. Growth in capitated financing arrangements that provide disincentives for admitting patients to hospitals
3. A proliferation of treatment settings that can substitute for hospitalization
4. The increased burden of cost sharing, which shifts part of the cost of care directly to the patient

Despite decreased use of hospitals, profit in the overall hospital industry has increased. Schramm and Gabel[9] report, "Although hospital occupancy declined by 12% in the first year of prospective payment, profits doubled and reached record levels. In 1984, hospital profits were 6.2% of total revenues—three times higher than a decade earlier."

How can the increase in profitability of hospitals be explained? First, the estimated costs of treatment for diagnostic-related groups overestimated the actual costs, and certain hospitals profited on the treatment of particular categories of patients. Fast turnover of patients increase the profitability of hospitals. And even though the number of hospital beds being occupied was lower, most hospitals remained open. Costs of patient care cover the overhead for keeping these facilities open and were included in the rate-setting formulas. Renn[8] estimates that in 1984 there was an excess of 140,000 beds, or roughly 800 average-sized community hospitals.

The decline in numbers of patients in private hospitals has been achieved, in some instances, by keeping out patients likely to be most costly; shifting costs for the care of patients from private nonprofit hospitals to public hospitals; and discharging patients earlier, shifting costs from the hospital to the family and community.

Providers

Factors contributing to the escalating cost of medical care are the high incomes that physicians make, the increase in numbers of physicians, overspecialization of practice, and the phenomenal power physicians have over patients in the decision-making process. In noting that medical care costs in the United States are 3 times those in Britain and 5 times those of Japan, Menzel[4] raises the question of whether or not we are getting our money's worth. He notes that physicians make twice and sometimes up to 5 times that of other professionals with equal training. Menzel concludes, "It is utterly hypocritical for doctors, health care administrators, academic analysts, and policymakers to close their eyes to the level of doctors' income amidst an otherwise vigorous concern for making health care worth the increasing money we pay for it."

Under normal marketplace conditions, an increase in the supply of physicians would serve to drive the income of physicians downward and also address another problem, that of maldistribution of physicians. For example, Massachusetts has 308 physicians per 100,000 residents, while Mississippi has less than half that number per resident, 122 per 100,000. A Michigan study of the health professions indicates that increases in the total number of physicians result in a concentration of physicians in urban areas. The costs of medical care rise proportionately to the number of physicians practicing in an area. While the number of physicians has increased dramatically in Michigan since 1960, there were more counties in Michigan without physicians in 1985 than there were in 1960.

One of the reasons for the escalation of costs is the increased specialization of physicians. The more highly specialized the physicians, the higher the consumption rate of medical care services to support specialty practice. Renn[8] cautions:

If physicians continue to make most of the allocative decisions in the delivery system, if the emphasis on treatment in acute care inpatient settings persists, and if payment mechanisms continue to insulate physicians from the financial risks associated with their decisions—then growth in the supply of physicians will probably translate into corresponding growth in health care spending.

While the fees charged by physicians for services account for only 20% of medical costs, decisions made by physicians represent 80% of expenditures. Physicians decide when, how, and for how long patients are to be hospitalized and medically treated. One of the problems related to the physician's decision-making and health care costs is that the physician holds that the physician-client relationship is "sacred" and that no one should interfere with the physician's rights to care for each individual patient, including ordering the tests and treatments defined as necessary for "good" patient care regardless of their costs. The problem with this is that the physician is looking at care from the perspective of only the individual patients that come through the door to his or her practice and does not have to weigh the values of individual patient treatment against the broader question of the need of all people within the United States, including the privileged and the poor.

Financing

A further complication in controlling medical care costs surrounds the way in which medical care services are financed. Payment usually comes from a third party rather than from the individual. Public payers—federal, state, or local governments—paid slightly more than 40% of medical care expenditures in 1985, while private insurance supplied an additional 31%. Direct out-of-pocket payments by patients accounted for 27%.

One of the unique features of U.S. medical care financing has been the role of private insurance. Starting in 1929, Blue Cross plans became a major force in the financing of medical care. One of the unique features of these plans was that they were originally provider based and involved service agreements with all of the providers in an area. Rashi Fein[2] clarifies, "Blue Cross and similar plans were brought into being by hospital representatives with active support of the AHA [American Hospital Association] acting in response to serious problems they and their patients faced: how should hospital bills be paid and how should stable hospital revenues be assured?" The insurance plans were largely for the benefit of hospitals and physicians, and only secondarily for the welfare of patients.

The interlocking relationships between physicians, hospitals, and insurers have dominated decision making regarding the financing of medical care rather than the interests of the patient, Renn[8] notes. "Physicians and hospital representatives often dominate the plans' boards of directors and see the plans, like most participants, as a means of ensuring the financial solvency of the community's providers." Blue Cross established the approach of reimbursing hospitals on a retrospective, cost-plus basis, thus building in disincentives for economy. Payment of bills related to hospitalization also built in incentives for physicians to hospitalize patients and thus contributed to the overbuilding of hospital facilities.

Another complicating facet of this scene was the ability of insurance companies to link with businesses so that the provision of medical insurance became a major part of the benefits paid to workers. Thus the worker began to see the provision of medical care insurance and, thereby, the assurance of the economic viability of hospitals and of physicians, as part of the benefits to be expected. Until recent years, the employer has accepted this obligation, until the costs have escalated to a point beyond the ability of the employer to pay. Currently, 10% of the cost of a U.S. automobile goes to pay the health care costs of workers. Employers

are saying that they can no longer pay the cost and are requiring the employees to pay a portion of their medical care costs. This is a factor considered partially responsible for reduced utilization of medical care services. Initiated in 1966, the Medicare program provides a number of benefits to the elderly covered by the Social Security system. Medicare currently provides 28% of the income of hospitals. Medicare extended to the elderly the concepts established by Blue Cross/Blue Shield for working people and brought the financing for these services into the federal government. Thus public funding was used to support the private offering of services of physicians and hospitals. Fein[2] writes:

Medicare paid hospitals retrospectively on the basis of the costs incurred by covered beneficiaries at participating providers and paid physicians their reasonable, customary, and prevailing fees. While originally resisted by organized medicine as an instance of the federal government becoming an intervening force between the physician and his or her patient, Medicare payments have become a major source of income for both physicians and hospitals. In addition to paying physicians and hospitals, Medicare became a major stimulant for capital growth without reference to community needs and priorities or regional planning efforts.

While insurers of public sources pay for over 70% of health care costs, Renn[8] points out, "Ultimately individuals pay for all health care expenditures . . . consumers, workers, and taxpayers, with the dollars taking merely different routes to the providers." If this is so, why are consumers not more involved in the debates about reducing medical care costs?

Consumer participation

Since much of the cost of care for those without adequate insurance coverage under the prospective payment system was paid for by overcharging for the actual costs of care, much of this cost was subsidized by insurers and indirectly by consumers. This was a hidden problem until the change to a prospective payment system. Now the costs of care for the uninsured and underinsured cannot be paid for this way. As a result, some worry that a two-, three-, and four-tier system of medical care is emerging. Thurow[10] has labeled three levels as follows: one for people on government assistance, a second for workers having employer-paid plans, and another for the wealthy who can afford the private health care market. To this Reinhardt[7] has added a fourth tier at the bottom for indigent patients who have no insurance. The result of this separation into tiers, according to Morreim,[5] is that each tier is increasingly forced to care for its own patients using only the resources available to that tier. And as each lower tier is less well-funded than that above, a serious question arises: Should physicians still be expected to deliver the (roughly) same standard of care to all patients regardless of their resources?

As this debate regarding differential treatment dependent upon ability to pay emerges, medical care costs continue to escalate far beyond other costs in our economy.

Since physicians and hospitals primarily control the goods of medical care, the consumer has little choice over the types of treatment he or she receives. Although there are a number of options, the consumer is purposefully kept ignorant, and, therefore, the decision-making control is in the hands of the provider. As a result, the most costly form of treatment is usually that provided. Too often even with basic medical care knowledge, the consumer assumes that the "doctor knows best" and rarely challenges the prescriptions that are made. Reinhardt[6] further observes that while physicians are always resisting intrusion of government into their relationships with patients, they are not averse to using regulations to restrict the practice of other less costly practitioners. Restriction of licensure and controlling payment for other service providers constrains less costly care.

Increasingly, the public is becoming more knowledgeable about the issues related to costs of medical care. We are confronted by hard choices. Do we continue to address problems of medical care costs by withholding services from those who cannot pay? What are the long-range consequences of this approach? What is the legacy that we will leave our children if we opt to deny services that could prevent illness and instead pay the costs associated with chronic illness and disability? Fein[2] summarizes the challenges for us:

Health care and the way we pay for it is a matter of efficiency, and today's system is inefficient. Health care and the way we pay for it is a matter of equity, and today's system is inequitable. We can do better; and, since we can, we should. Will we? It depends upon whether enough of us are concerned about costs, recognize that a less costly system will free resources for other private and public purposes, and support the notion of health care budgets. It also depends upon whether enough of us care enough to work at translating concepts of decentness, humaneness, cooperation, universality, and justice into actions that would protect all members of the American family. At stake is not only your health care

system, but the very nature of our society. While it may appear that in this scenario the consumer is a passive participant, the health care dilemma has indeed been consumer driven and is a reflection of (1) the American inclination to prefer being "fixed" as opposed to "avoiding getting broken," and (2) the American inclination to deify doctors and to assume that the most expensive advice/care is the best. This fascination with high technology continues to fuel the system and technology creates its own demand.

FROM MEDICAL CARE TO HEALTH CARE

Enthoven and Kronick[1] have characterized the situation of rising health care costs and decreased access as a "paradox of excess and deprivation." While it is possible to describe the current situation in great detail, what are the avenues for addressing the problem? Two recent proposals have been set forth and have received widespread attention, particularly in the medical community.

Enthoven and Kronick[1] have proposed universal health insurance coupled with managed competition in which the insurers (private and public) contract with competing plans to "manage a process of informed cost-conscious consumer choice that rewards providers who deliver high quality care economically." The costs of implementation of their plan would be $15 billion in additional costs in the first year (3% of GNP) as a one-time increase. Long range, this approach is projected to decrease the rate of escalation of health care costs, but does not hold forth the promise of decreased cost.[1]

An alternative approach, a national health program for the United States, has been proposed by Himmelstein and Woolhandler[3] on behalf of a working group of physicians. To summarize the central elements of this proposal:

We propose a national health program that would (1) fully cover everyone under a single, comprehensive public insurance program; (2) pay hospitals and nursing homes a total (global) annual amount to cover all operating expenses; (3) fund capital costs through separate appropriations; (4) pay for physicians' services and ambulatory services in any of three ways: through fee-for-service payments with a simplified fee schedule and mandatory acceptance of the national health program as the total payment for a service or procedure (assignment), through global budgets for hospitals or clinics, or on a per capita basis (capitation); (5) be funded, at least initially, for the same sources as at present with all payments disbursed from a single pool; and (6) contain costs through saving on billing and bureaucracy, improved health planning, and the ability of the national program, as the single payer for services, to establish overall funding limits.

It is important to note that this proposal does not address any changes in practices of either hospitals or physicians, but merely proposes a way of paying for them. Neither does this proposal address anything other than the payment for physicians, hospitals, and nursing homes.

While both proposals contain very important potential strategies for paying for the high cost of medical care, it is important to bear in mind that both continue to emphasize the interests of the providers, the hospitals, and physicians in how the bills will be paid as business as usual; the interests of the consumer regarding more appropriate care are secondary. Second, these proposals continue to focus upon medical care. Although the term *health care* is used, these proposals do not address broader issues of health care. While some might argue that truly expanding the definition from medical to health care would further escalate the problem, an alternative argument is that if health care were provided, the medical care system would be utilized more appropriately, thereby reducing costs.

Medical care focuses on the diagnosis and treatment of disease, while health care has as its aim the well-being of the individual and family at an optimal level of health. Within this broader framework, the individual and the family have primary responsibility for maintaining health with support from health care specialists. While individuals still will experience illness that will require expert care and treatment, a broader orientation to health care would result in earlier identification of problems at a less acute stage, and, therefore, the treatment would be less costly. Furthermore, a reduction in chronic diseases, most of which are preventable, and maintenance of mobility as people age would do much to reduce costs of care in the long run. For example, in the area of maternal child care, there is growing evidence that early prenatal care that is comprehensive in nature, including provision for adequate nutrition, social services support, and health education, reduces infant mortality, increases infant birth weight, and reduces numbers of damaged (mentally and physically) infants. Rough data drawn from one midsize community indicate that providing such comprehensive services to about 500 uninsured and underinsured mothers by a nurse-managed clinic using nurse-midwives will cost about

$250,000 over the available compensation for such care from both public and private sources. However, the local community hospital has experienced a total decline in demand for a neonatal intensive care unit, a "savings" to the hospital of $650,000. While simple mathematical calculations would lead to a conclusion that $400,000 has been saved, if one looks at this from a provider perspective (hospital and physician), the conclusion is somewhat different. The hospital looks at this scenario as a loss of revenue, in that the $650,000 previously spent on neonatal intensive care was collectible revenue. From the physicians' point of view, these "savings" were largely a result of services provided by nutritionists, social workers, nurses, and midwives. Physicians' revenues, both for obstetrical and pediatric care, were reduced.

Similar examples could be drawn from well-child care, women's health, and care of the elderly. Returning responsibility for health care to the individual and family, engaging a wide range of specialists in supportive roles to the individual and family, demystifying health and illness through education of the public, and using the medical care system appropriately to treat only acute diseases are the long-range solutions to the problem of escalating medical care costs.

If this be so, what are the steps toward change in this direction? First, there need to be some carefully controlled demonstration projects, such as that described earlier, that illustrate the benefits to be achieved by comprehensive health care. Some examples of such studies are beginning to appear in the literature. Producing data, however, is merely the first step. These data then must be made known to those who pay the bills—ultimately, everyone in this country. In the scenario related to prenatal care, nothing will change in the community if the financing for expanded prenatal care to create this degree of long-range improvement is left to the decision making of the providers. These data need to be translated and publicized so that citizens of the community know the choices that are open to them, so that ultimately they can make informed decisions as to how health care is to be provided. In this community, the $400,000 that could be saved through adequate prenatal care could result in reduction of dollars going for insurance, either directly or indirectly, and it could be redirected toward other pressing societal issues.

Nurses have a crucial role to play in creating change. First, movement from a medical care system to health care requires nursing intervention and leadership.

Nurses can set up the demonstrations that lead to necessary data and publicize these findings to individuals and policymakers. Ultimately, a revolution of the citizenry is the only force to create change in a democracy. Nursing has the capacity to educate the consumer to create such changes.

A second essential step is to articulate clearly the components of health care, enlist individual responsibility for maintenance of health, and clearly describe the supportive roles of health specialists in promoting individual health, including that of nurses. The myth that anything less than medical care provided by physicians is second-best must be dispelled. In fact, there is mounting evidence that for health care, the physician is perhaps the least qualified. At the heart of change is the need for the consumer to be educated, and nurses have the expertise to provide this education.

What hinders this type of change? First, nurses have been socialized to be co-conspirators with hospitals and doctors in maintaining the current medical care system. They have been reticent to let the public know of the unnecessary and damaging high-technology invasive procedures that are being done every day in the interests of the medical care system. Nurses are intimidated and fearful of loss of jobs when the hospital is their main employer, and all avenues for practice independent of physicians or hospitals are constrained. With nurses comprising the largest number of health care workers in the United States (1.8 million, estimated), collectively the profession has the capacity to speak with one loud voice. Second, energies of the profession have become focused on the profession itself rather than on the issues of health care for people. Fragmentation of the profession results in a feeling of abandonment on the part of nurses engaged in practice, who feel that leadership is preoccupied with the self-interests of the profession. If nurses can unite, with a common concern for health care for people at affordable costs, they have the capacity to join with consumers to create such change and thereby "heal" themselves.

In summary, change is possible. Such change depends on (1) a fundamental change from a focus on a medical care delivery system to participatory health care for people; (2) breaking the monopoly of hospitals, physicians, and insurers in the decision-making process that preserves the current system; (3) engaging the consumer in assuming greater responsibility for personal health and decision making regarding broader health policy issues; and (4) greater involvement of nurses and other health-related specialists in joining with the consumer in supportive roles and relationships with an emphasis upon health promotion–disease prevention. Nurses are central in making the difference. The ability to become one strong voice on behalf of the U.S. public is essential if nursing is going to be a force for positive change.

REFERENCES

1. Enthoven, A., & Kronick, R. (1989). A consumer-choice health plan for the 1990's. *New England Journal of Medicine, 320*(1), 30.
2. Fein, R. (1986). *Medical care medical costs: Search for a health insurance policy.* Cambridge, Mass: Harvard University Press.
3. Himmelstein, D. U., & Woolhandler, S. (1989). A national health program for the United States: A physician's proposal. *New England Journal of Medicine, 320*(2), 102-108.
4. Menzel, P. T. (1986). *Medical costs, moral choices.* New Haven, Conn: Yale University Press.
5. Morreim, E. H. (1988). Cost containment: Challenging fidelity & justice. *Hastings Center Report, 18*(6), 22.
6. Reinhardt, U. W. (1981). Health insurance and cost containment policies: The experience abroad. In M. Olson (Ed.), *A new approach to the economics of health care* (p. 151). Washington, D.C.: American Enterprise Institute for Public Policy Research.
7. Reinhardt, U. W. (1987). Health insurance for the nation's poor. *Health Affairs, 6*(1), 101-112.
8. Renn, S. (1987). Health care delivery in the 1980s. In C. Schramm (Ed.), *Health care and its costs: Can the U.S. afford adequate health.* New York: W. W. Norton.
9. Schramm, C. J., & Gabel, J. C. (1988). Prospective payment: Some retrospective observations. *New England Journal of Medicine, 318*(25), 1682.
10. Thurow, L. C. (1985). Medicine vs. economics. *New England Journal of Medicine, 313*(10), 611-614.

CHAPTER 65

Viewpoints

Costing out nursing services

Is it happening?

JANET C. SCHERUBEL

The advent of diagnostic-related groups (DRGs) signaled a new phase in health care reimbursement; yet health care costs continue to rise and now represent a major economic issue in the United States. Across the country, providers grappling with rising costs and decreasing revenues are reexamining patient care delivery systems and their costs. Nurses and nursing organizations have placed renewed emphasis on identifying nursing care costs and demonstrating fiscal accountability for nursing practice.[43,58,60,65,95]

In this chapter, efforts to define and measure the costs of nursing care are described. Examples illustrate nurses' use of the knowledge of these costs to demonstrate the cost effectiveness of nursing practice, improve service delivery, and decrease health care costs.[16,19,31,77,91,104] As such strategies are applied on a broad scale, nursing can contribute to a better, more effective and efficient health care delivery system.

HISTORICAL DEVELOPMENT OF COSTING

Historically, hospitals used the patient day as the unit of measure to quantify services. Under this system it was difficult to allocate expenses to specific departments, particularly those associated with nursing services. Despite these difficulties, nurses, primarily independent nursing practitioners, have sought reimbursement from third-party payers for services since the late 1940s.[48,70,72,78,109,110] In addition, nurses have successfully utilized a fee-for-service approach for hospital-based nurse specialists and nursing education departments.* Concurrently, future-oriented nursing administrators identified and separated nursing costs from other hospital services and in some cases billed patients for these services.[8,23,30,97,102,111]

Today, with improved cost accounting practices, providers have a better understanding of resource consumption in health care delivery. Methods have been developed to determine the profitability of patient services, highlight wasteful practices, and streamline service delivery. Nurses now have access to more accurate information and are able to identify nursing costs and isolate them from costs of other health care services. This information makes possible monitoring and managing of nursing budgets, as well as strategic planning.†

METHODS OF COSTING NURSING SERVICES
Direct nursing care costs

A number of methods have been developed to quantify the costs of nursing services. An early system was based on the New Jersey relative intensity measure (RIM).[12,38,49,50,65] Designed to work within the DRG structure of patient classification, RIMs assigned relative values based upon minutes of time to homogeneous clusters of nursing care activities. This approach allowed appropriate cost allocations for nursing care within the nursing resource clusters.

---

*References 24, 31, 55, 57, 73, 74, 78, 80.
†References 4, 14, 29, 44, 64, 83, 90, 96, 105.

Nonetheless, there were critics of the RIM system. One criticism regarded the linkage to patient length of stay rather than to patient acuity.[17,106] Grimaldi and Micheletti[38] cited other deficiencies in the RIM studies, particularly limitations in the methodology. They noted that small numbers of patients from limited geographical areas were used in generating costing equations. In addition, one quarter of the equations generated were estimates derived from others due to small sample sizes. Thompson[103] and Trofino[106] concurred, adding that little was done to test the reliability and validity of the RIM methodology. These methodology problems created difficulties in data analysis. For in initial reports, hypothesized relationships between nursing intensity and length of stay were not supported by the actual data.

A somewhat different method, also based on DRGs, was proposed by Curtin.[15] Curtin suggested development of 23 major nursing care categories (NCCs) divided into 356 general nursing care strategies (NCSs) to parallel major diagnostic categories and DRGs. Nursing care strategies would in effect be the detailed nursing care plans that included both direct and indirect patient care activities. The NCSs were graduated in terms of increasing nursing time required by patients. The system was attractive in that the NCC and the NCS complemented the DRG model. However, as Curtain noted, it was necessary to integrate DRG coding and nursing classification systems.

Several systems have been developed that do not rely on either the DRG classification system or traditional patient classification systems.[67] One well-known system is the GRASP classification system. The GRASP classification system has several advantages. First, patients are classified on an individual basis, rather than being aggregated into composite levels. Second, the system allows for recording of substantially more nursing activities per patient. Although this approach has advantages, record keeping may become complex and cumbersome. To address this problem, some classification systems employ selected key indicators to represent many nursing activities.

Yet another approach involves patient management categories.[117] Developed by physician panels to represent clinically discrete patient types, the system incorporates severity of illness throughout the model. Patient management paths identify a variety of treatment modalities. Nursing services are allocated to the categories either by the use of a patient classification system or through identification of nursing "intensity" as determined by the physician management strategies.

Two systems have been developed based totally on nursing frameworks. Halloran advocated documentation of nursing care based on nursing diagnoses.[40] In his work, he demonstrated that nursing diagnoses were twice as effective as DRGs in explaining nursing work loads. Reitz based her nursing intensity index on a prototype nursing classification system.[84] Using the nursing process, the index includes 11 functional categories encompassing both biophysical and behavioral health parameters.

There is widespread agreement that to accurately cost nursing services it is necessary to use a reliable and valid system for the identification of nursing services provided to patients.[16,27,45] Perhaps the most frequently used is the patient classification system. Originally developed for the allocation of nursing staff to patient care units, these systems are now being employed to identify the costs of services.[30,46,99,106] Use of an acuity-based system to allocate costs has many proponents.[33,34,47,83,106,112] Acuity systems allow the nurse to retrospectively tally nursing care needs for each patient daily. Costs, determined from work-sampling studies, are generated for the services delivered to patients and assigned on an individual basis.

Another method of apportioning costs is initiated using aggregate patient data. Ratings obtained from patient classification systems are compiled to determine the total direct nursing care costs for all patients in an institution during a given period of time. Costs may then be allocated to future patients based on their classification scores for the total length of stay.

Indirect care costs

A variety of classification systems have been developed to identify the costs of direct care needs of patients. However, there is a second component of nursing care costs that must be identified: the indirect costs of patient care, including nursing support services and institutional overhead costs allocated to the nursing department. Several methods have been developed for this purpose.[27,30] Indirect costs may be determined for the total patient population or for the total patient days in a given time period. Then these costs are equally divided among all patients on a per capita basis. Using this approach, indirect costs may be divided based on the length of stay of individual patients. In other systems, indirect costs are allocated based on the level of the patient's need for nursing care as determined through a patient classification system. In some instances, combinations of these approaches may prove more useful to the institution, depending on the sources of indirect costs and the characteristics of the cost accounting system.[100]

Regardless of the method selected for cost allocation, it should accurately measure the costs incurred in the delivery of care. Further, the method chosen must be employed consistently across all departments within the institution to ensure equitable allocation of expenses. Each institution must carefully examine the alternatives available and select the most appropriate method for its needs.

USES OF COSTING NURSING SERVICES
Identifying costs of specific populations

A major outcome of costing nursing services has been the quantification of services nursing provides.[68,98] Nursing care costs may be determined for specific patient groups (e.g., DRGs) within institutions. Lagona and Stritzel[53] used a patient classification system to determine the differences in the costs of nursing care for patients with myocardial infarction classified in two DRGs. Data derived from the classification system were utilized to calculate the hours of nursing care and associated salary costs required for each DRG. Lagona and Stritzel demonstrated that nursing costs were in fact different for the two DRGs, with complicated myocardial infarctions (DRG 121) costing $1000 per case, while the average cost of caring for patients with uncomplicated infarctions (DRG 122) was less than $800. This information proved valuable to nursing management for planning and decision making.

Using a slightly different methodology, McClain and Selhat[63] determined average direct nursing costs for three different DRGs (DRG 88, DRG 195, DRG 197). In their study, nursing costs were calculated not only for registered nurses, but for each level of personnel: costs for registered nurses, those for licensed practical nurses, and an aggregate cost determined by staff mix.

Other nurse researchers have successfully extended this methodology to compare nursing resource consumption between different health care institutions.[3,87,107] In Sampson's study[87] of nursing costs for care of newborns in 70 institutions, she was able to explain over 95% of the variability in costs. Perhaps more important, she demonstrated that large preexisting data sets may be used to determine nursing costs. This finding has ramifications for nurse administrators. Too often nurses overlook the extensive data sources available within their health care

system. By using existing data, administrators may analyze previous costs of service before implementing new systems.

Recognizing variability in patient needs

A second outcome of quantifying nursing services is that the quantity and quality of these services may be compared for different patients.[6,62,81,107] Identification of the costs of nursing care has led to a better understanding of the variability of nursing needs and their costs for different patients with similar problems, or for individual patients over time.*

For example, Giovannetti and her associates[35] found wide variability in nursing hours for patients within DRGs. Giovannetti noted that chronic obstructive pulmonary disease (COPD) patients required fewer hours of care when hospitalized for 2 weeks, while those hospitalized for only 1 week required more nursing care. This pattern was reversed in patients hospitalized for hysterectomies. For these patients, nursing care hours increased with length of stay. Similarly, many nurse researchers have described changes in patient care needs over time.[3,53,63,66]

The results of fiscal studies undertaken to determine the costs of nursing care are important for management decisions ranging from establishment of daily staffing patterns to long-range program-planning and budgeting activities. For example, the development of product line, or service line, management has been enhanced by the identification of needed resources and the appropriate allocation of these resources.[2,10,23]

Demonstrating cost effectiveness of nursing services

A third benefit of identifying nursing costs is the ability to recognize nursing as a source of revenue rather than expenditure within the hospital.[3,37,39,85,86,97] Some nurses have extended this position and proposed the organization of independent nursing staff corporations to make nursing a for-profit entity.[101,106] Others feel a need to define the nursing product and demonstrate that it may be offered at a competitive price.[101]

Through the identification of nursing costs, it has been possible to evaluate current practices in nursing care delivery. For example, nurses have compared the costs of team and primary nursing care delivery systems.[6,18,77,116] With increasing frequency the costs of nursing care are included as an important variable for

---

*References 3, 11, 39, 66, 69, 71, 79, 92, 93.

analysis as new methods of patient care delivery are tested.[1,32,59,75]

Costing activities have been extended beyond the acute inpatient environment. Ambulatory nursing services, emergency departments, nursing centers, and home health agencies have all recognized the need to quantify the costs of their services to maintain a sound financial basis.[42,51,61,81,113] Cost identification is essential in nursing homes to respond to regulatory definitions of skilled and intermediate nursing care classifications. Systems have been developed to identify these nursing costs and outcomes of care.[42,51]

Improving patient care delivery

A further advantage of costing nursing services has been the development of more cost-effective techniques in nursing care delivery. Nursing practices have become more efficient and streamlined.* More productive methods of care delivery have been instituted. The development of nursing case management has improved the continuity of patient care without undue expenses.[26] The institution of unit assistant programs and family care giving has led to better utilization of professional nursing staffs and a decrease in nursing performance of nonnursing duties.[28,88,114] Through these and other innovations, nursing has made valuable contributions to improved health care delivery and has participated in controlling the rising costs of health care.[36,93]

There is a growth in the entrepreneurial efforts of nurses.[13] Nursing students are encouraged to pursue expanded nursing opportunities.[76] As nurses establish freestanding businesses, the costing of services provided is an essential component of their business plans.[5,115] Efforts to quantify the costs of nursing services are not limited to direct patient care delivery costs. In a period of increasing fiscal constraints, nurse executives are reexamining the costs of all nursing activities, especially those not involved in direct patient care. Nurses have measured the costs of continuing education, management, and nursing research.[7,22,25,56,108] Studies report the cost effectiveness of continuing education programs, particularly when these programs contribute to improvements in nursing practice.[22,56] These activities will continue and expand to include other nursing support services.

---

*References 21, 41, 42, 44, 71, 77, 82, 89.

DILEMMAS OF COSTING NURSING CARE

Costing nursing care services is not without it problems. Identifying the actual costs of care may create difficulties for the nurse executive. Costing services carries the potential for decreased allocations of resources to nursing departments.[85] If nurses are able to provide services with decreased costs, nursing budget requests may be reduced.

There are limitations to the use of patient classification systems for deriving costing formulas.[27,46] Many systems base their classifications on nursing care delivered, not nursing care required. Thus if nurses are unable to provide necessary care, for whatever reason, be it staffing, available support services, or time, this care—or lack thereof—is not documented. If budgeting decisions are based on care delivered, rather than on nursing care normally required by patients, the decisions may not accurately reflect the true costs of nursing care.[27]

Nurse executives must acquire new skills to successfully manage the nursing department budget. A sound working knowledge of cost accounting and budget management is essential in today's health care environment. Nurse executives need productive working relationships with colleagues in finance and hospital administration, and the ability to clearly articulate the goals of and resources needed for cost-effective, quality nursing care.

Furthermore, the process of costing nursing services may be resisted by some, due to the potential for power inherent in the establishment of nursing as a revenue-producing health care service.[60,64] Other disciplines may view the establishment of independence as an encroachment on their territory.

Finally, as Sherman[94] points out and as is evident from the studies described in this chapter, it is difficult to compare the results obtained from different settings.[64] Small sample sizes, variability in data collection tools, and the question of reliability of the data collected all present problems to researchers and administrators alike. Nevertheless, it is possible to use existing data sets. Another approach is to establish national norms for data collection. Nurses need to agree on the definitions of nursing care and appropriate means to collect these data. Nursing costs should be included in a nursing minimum data set.[44,52,95]

Despite the potential problems inherent in costing of nursing services, the benefits are considerable. In the current health care environment, cost-effective and efficient care has become essential. Identifying the costs generated in providing nursing care is the first step in the costing process.

SUMMARY

The process of identifying nursing costs began as a response to cost containment efforts. Activity accelerated as reimbursement programs shifted from a retrospective to a prospective basis. Great strides have been made in quantifying nursing services and the costs of these services. At the same time, nurses have gained new knowledge of the patterns and variations in care required by patients. Patient care delivery has been streamlined, and the cost effectiveness of nursing has been demonstrated repeatedly. Nurses may well be proud of these accomplishments.

However, the work is not done. Changes in funding and the increased focus on alternative health care delivery systems will dictate additional studies of the costs and outcomes of nursing care in all settings.[20,52,54,72] Costing out nursing service: is it happening? The answer is a resounding yes, and it will continue to happen as nurses describe the unique and special services they provide to consumers.

REFERENCES

1. Aiken, L. H. (1990). Charting the future of hospital nursing. *Image: The Journal of Nursing Scholarship, 22*(2), 72-78.
2. Anderson, R. (1985). Products and product-line management in nursing. *Nursing Administration Quarterly, 10*(1), 65-72.
3. Arndt, M., Skydell, B. (1985). Inpatient nursing services: Productivity and cost. In F. A. Shaffer (Ed.), *Costing out nursing: Pricing our product*. New York: National League for Nursing.
4. Bargagliotti, L., & Smith, H. (1985). Patterns of nursing costs with capital reimbursement. *Nursing Economic$, 3*(5), 270-275.
5. Bennett, S. J. (1990). Blending the entrepreneurial and faculty roles. *Nurse Educator, 15*(4), 34-37.
6. Betz, M., Dickerson, T., & Wyatt, D. (1980). Cost and quality: Primary and team nursing compared. *Nursing and Health Care, 1*(3), 150-157.
7. Boston, C. M. (1986). Justifying costs for continuing nursing education departments. *Nursing Economic$, 4*(2), 83-85.
8. Brewer, C. (1984). Variable billing: Is it viable? *Nursing Outlook, 32*(1), 38-41.
9. Bruekner, S. J., & Blair, E. (1977). Cost of education in a department of nursing service at a university medical center. *Journal of Nursing Administration, 8*(3), 21-27.
10. Bruhn, P., & Howes, D. (1986). Service line management: New opportunities for nursing executives. *Journal of Nursing Administration, 16*(6), 13-18.
11. Caterinicchio, P. P. (1983). A defense of the RIMs study. *Nursing Management, 14*(5), 36–39.
12. Caterinicchio, P. P., & Davies, R. H. (1982). Developing a client-focused allocation statistic of inpatient nursing resource use: An alternative to the patient day. *Social Science and Medicine, 17*(5), 259-272.
13. Crowley, M. A. (1989). The entrepreneurial nurse consultant: A Marxist analysis. *Journal of Advanced Nursing, 14*(7), 582-586.
14. Curran, C. R. (1992). An interview with Sharon Lynn Hollander. *Nursing Economic$, 10*(1), 9-14.
15. Curtin, L. (1983). Determining costs of nursing service per DRG. *Nursing Management, 14*(4), 16-20.
16. Curtin, L. (1986). Who says "lean" must be "mean"? *Nursing Management, 17*(1), 7-8.
17. Curtin, L. L. (1984). DRG creep, DRG weights and patient acuity: Determining costs of nursing services. *Nursing Management, 15*(10), 7-9.
18. Dahlin, A., & Gregor, J. (1985). Nursing costs by DRG with an all RN staff. In F. A. Shaffer (Ed.), *Costing out nursing: Pricing our product*. New York: National League for Nursing.
19. Davis, C. (1983). The federal role in changing health care financing. *Nursing Economic$, 1*(2), 98-104, 146.
20. Davis, C. (1986). Health care reform: What can we expect? *Nursing Economic$, 4*(1), 10-11.
21. del Bueno, D., & Bridges, P. (1985). Providing incentives while reducing costs: An employee suggestion plan. *Nursing Economic$, 3*(4), 212-215.
22. del Bueno, D., & Kelly, K. (1980). How cost effective is your staff development program? *Nurse Educator, 5*(5), 12-17.
23. de Mars, M. P., & Boyer, F. (1985). Developing a consistent method for costing hospital services. *Healthcare Financial Management, 39*(2), 30-37.
24. Derby, V. L. (1980). Financing nursing education. *Nurse Educator, 5*(2), 21-25.
25. Deremo, D. Z. (1989). Integrating professional values, quality practice, productivity and reimbursement for nursing. *Nursing Administration Quarterly, 14*(1), 9-23.
26. DeZell, A. D., Comeau, E., & Zander, K. (1988). Managed care via the nursing case management model. In J. Scherubel (Ed.), *Patients and purse strings II*. New York: National League for Nursing.
27. Dijkers, M., & Paradise, T. (1986). PCS: One system for both staffing and costing. *Nursing Management, 17*(1), 25-34.
28. Donovan, M. I., Slack, J., Robertson, S., & Andreoli, K. G. (1988). The unit assistant: A nurse extender. *Nursing Management, 19*(10), 70-71.
29. Edwardson, S. (1985). Measuring nursing productivity. *Nursing Economic$, 3*(1), 9-14.
30. Ethridge, P. (1985). The case for billing by patient acuity. *Nursing Management, 16*(8), 38-41.
31. Fagin, C. (1986). Opening the door on nursing's cost advantage. *Nursing and Health Care, 7*(7), 353-357.
32. Farren, E. A. (1991). Effects of early discharge planning on length of hospital stay. *Nursing Economic$, 9*(1), 25-31.
33. Flarey, D. C. (1990). A method for costing nursing service. *Nursing Administration Quarterly, 14*(3), 41-45.
34. Giovannetti, P. (1979). Understanding patient classification systems. *Journal of Nursing Administration, 9*(2), 6+.
35. Giovannetti, P. (1985). DRGs and nursing workload measures. *Computers in Nursing, 3, 2+*.
36. Grace, H. K. (1985). Can health care costs be contained? Nursing's responsibility. In J. C. McCloskey & H. K. Grace (Eds.), *Current issues in nursing* (2nd ed.). Boston: Blackwell Scientific Publications.

37. Griffith, H. M., Thomas, N., & Griffith, L. (1991). MDs bill for these routine nursing tasks. *American Journal of Nursing, 91*(1), 22-6.

38. Grimaldi, P., & Micheletti, J. (1982). DRG reimbursement: RIMs and the cost of nursing care. *Nursing Management, 13*(2), 12-22.

39. Grohar, M., Myers, J., & McSweeney, M. (1986). A comparison of patient acuity and nursing resource use. *Journal of Nursing Administration, 16*(6), 19-23.

40. Halloran, E. J. (1985). Nursing workload, medical diagnostic related groups, and nursing diagnoses. *Research in Nursing and Health, 8,* 421-433.

41. Harrell, J., & Frauman, A. (1985). Prospective payment calls for boosting productivity. *Nursing and Health Care, 6*(10), 535-537.

42. Harris, M., Santoferraro, C., & Silva, S. (1985). A patient classification system in home health care. *Nursing Economic$, 3*(5), 276-282.

43. Hartley, S. (1986). Effects of prospective pricing on nursing. *Nursing Economic$, 4*(1), 16-17.

44. Hayes, S. H., & Carroll, S. R. (1986). Early intervention care in the acute stroke patient. *Archives of Physical Medicine and Rehabilitation, 67*(5), 319-321.

45. Herzog, T. (1985). Productivity: Fighting the battle of the budget. *Nursing Management, 16*(1), 30-34.

46. Higgerson, N. J., & VanSlyck, A. (1982). Variable billing for services: New fiscal direction for nursing. *Journal of Nursing Administration, 12*(6), 20-27.

47. Hoffman, F. (1988). Costing out nursing services. In *Nursing productivity assessment and costing out nursing services* (pp. 227-245). New York: J. B. Lippincott.

48. IRS challenges the "independent contracting" option for nurses. (1990). *American Journal of Nursing, 90*(11), 78, 89-90.

49. Joel, L. (1983). DRGs: The state of the art of reimbursement for nursing services. *Nursing and Health Care, 4*(10), 560-563.

50. Joel, L. (1984). DRGs and RIMs: Implications for nursing. *Nursing Outlook, 32*(1), 42-49.

51. Joel, L. (1985). Costing out nursing in nursing homes. In F. A. Shaffer (Ed.), *Costing out nursing: Pricing our product.* New York: National League for Nursing.

52. Johnson, M. (1989). Perspectives on costing nursing. *Nursing Administration Quarterly, 14*(1), 65-71.

53. Lagona, T., & Stritzel, M. (1984). Nursing care requirements as measured by DRGs. *Journal of Nursing Administration, 14*(5), 15-18.

54. Lauver, E. (1985). Where will the money go? *Nursing and Health Care, 6*(3), 132-135.

55. Lazinski, H. (1979). The effects of clinical teaching on the budgets of schools of nursing. *Journal of Nursing Education, 18*(1), 21-24.

56. Lesser, J. E. (1985). Cost effectiveness of continuing education. In J. C. McCloskey & H. K. Grace (Eds.), *Current issues in nursing* (2nd ed.). Boston: Blackwell Scientific Publications.

57. Lubic, R. (1985). Reimbursement for nursing practice: Lessons learned, experiences shared. *Nursing and Health Care, 6*(1), 23-25.

58. Lynaugh, J. E., & Fagin, C. M. (1988). Nursing comes of age. *Image: The Journal of Nursing Scholarship, 20*(4), 184-190.

59. Mallock, K. M., Milton, D. A., & Jacobs, M. O. (1990). A model for differentiated nursing practice. *Journal of Nursing Administration, 20*(2), 20-26.

60. Maraldo, P. J. (1985). DRGs: Implications for nursing practice. In J. C. McCloskey & H. K. Grace (Eds.), *Current issues in nursing* (2nd ed.). Boston: Blackwell Scientific Publications.

61. Martin, K., & Schut, N. (1985). The Omaha system: Implications for costing community health nursing. In F. A. Shaffer (Ed.), *Costing out nursing: Pricing our product.* New York: National League for Nursing.

62. Mason, E., & Daugherty, J. (1984). Nursing standards should determine nursing's price. *Nursing Management, 15*(9), 34-38.

63. McClain, J. R., & Selhat, M. S. (1984). Twenty cases: What nursing costs per DRG. *Nursing Management, 15*(10), 27-34.

64. McCloskey, J. C. (1989). Implications of costing out nursing services for reimbursement. *Nursing Management, 20*(1), 44-49.

65. McCloskey, J. C., Gardner, D. L., & Johnson, M. R. (1987). Costing out nursing services: An annotated bibliography. *Nursing Economic$, 5*(5), 245-253.

66. McKibbin, R. C., Brimmer, P. F., Clinton, J. F., & Galliher, J. M. (1985). *DRGs and nursing care.* Kansas City, Mo: American Nurses Association.

67. Meyer, D. (1985). Costing nursing care with the GRASP system. In F. A. Shaffer (Ed.), *Costing out nursing: Pricing our product.* New York: National League for Nursing.

68. Mezey, M. (1983). Securing a financial base. *American Journal of Nursing, 83*(10), 1297-1298.

69. Mitchell, M., Miller, J., Welches, L., & Walker, D. (1977). Determining cost of direct nursing care by DRG. *Nursing Management, 15*(4), 29-32.

70. Mittlestadt, P. (1992). Bill would increase reimbursement for advanced practice nurses. *American Nurse, 24*(1), 3.

71. Mowry, M., & Korpman, R. (1985). Do DRG reimbursement rates reflect nursing costs? *Journal of Nursing Administration, 15*(7, 8), 29-35.

72. Mundinger, M. (1985). DRGs: A glass half full for nursing. *Nursing Outlook, 33*(6), 265.

73. National League for Nursing. (1982). *Analyzing the cost of baccalaureate nursing education.* New York: Author.

74. National League for Nursing. (1982). *Cost effective management in schools of nursing.* New York: Author.

75. Naylor, M. D., Brooten, D., Brown, L., & Borucki, L. C. (1991). Institutional yield on research: A case study. *Nursing Outlook, 39*(4), 166-169.

76. Norris, D. A. (1989). Nurse entrepreneurs: The quiet revolution. *Imprint, 36*(5), 56-59.

77. Olsen, S. (1984). The challenge of prospective pricing: Work smarter. *Journal of Nursing Administration, 14*(4), 22-26.

78. Palcini, J. (1984). Perspectives on level of reimbursement for nursing services. *Nursing Economic$, 2*(2), 118-123.

79. Piper, L. (1983). Accounting for nursing functions in DRGs. *Nursing Management, 14*(11), 26-27.

80. Powell, P. (1983). Fee for service. *Nursing Management, 14*(3), 13-15.

81. Ransien, T. (1982). Recognizing emergency department price components. *Healthcare Financial Management, 38*(12), 12-29.

82. Redford, J. B., & Harris, J. D. (1980). Rehabilitation of elderly stroke patients. *American Family Physician, 22*(9), 153-160.

83. Reitz, J. (1985). The development of a cost allocation statistic for nursing. In F. A. Shaffer (Ed.), *Costing out nursing: Pricing our product.* New York: National League for Nursing.

84. Reitz, J. A. (1985). Toward a comprehensive nursing intensity index: Part I. Development. *Nursing Management, 16*(8), 21-30.

85. Reschak, G., Biordi, D., Holm, K., & Santucci, N. (1985). Accounting for nursing costs by DRG. *Journal of Nursing Administration, 15*(9), 15-20.

86. Riley, W., & Schaefers, V. (1983). Costing nursing services. *Nursing Management, 14*(12), 40-43.

87. Sampson, L. F. (1991). Predicting the marginal cost of direct nursing care for newborns. *Journal of Nursing Administration, 21*(3), 42-47.

88. Selby, T. L. (1988). Nurses find ways to ease shortage; recruit, retain. *American Nurse, 20*(10), 1, 9-10.

89. Servellen, G. M., & Mowry, M. M. (1985). DRGs and primary nursing: Are they compatible? *Journal of Nursing Administration, 15*(4), 32-37.

90. Shaefers, V. (1985). A cost allocation method for nursing. In F. A. Shaffer (Ed.), *Costing out nursing: Pricing our product.* New York: National League for Nursing.

91. Shaffer, F. (1983). Nursing power in the DRG world. *Nursing Management, 15*(6), 28-30.

92. Shaffer, F. (1984). A nursing perspective of the DRG world: Part I. *Nursing and Health Care, 5*(1), 48-51.

93. Shaffer, F. (1984). Nursing: Gearing up for DRGs: Part II. Management strategies. *Nursing and Health Care, 5*(2), 93-99.

94. Sherman, J. J. (1990). Costing nursing care: A review. *Nursing Administration Quarterly, 14*(3), 11-17.

95. Simpson, R. L., & Waite, R. (1989). NCNIP's system of the future: A call for accountability, revenue control, and national data sets: National Commission on Nursing Implementation Project. *Nursing Administration Quarterly, 14*(1), 72-77.

96. Sovie, M. (1985). Managing nursing resources in a constrained economic environment. *Nursing Economic$, 3*(2), 85-94.

97. Sovie, M., & Smith, T. (1986). Pricing the nursing product: Changing for nursing care. *Nursing Economic$, 4*(5), 216-226.

98. Stanley, M., & Luciano, K. (1984). Eight steps to costing nursing services. *Nursing Management, 15*(10), 27-34.

99. Stevens, B. (1981). What is the executive's role in budgeting for her department? *Journal of Nursing Administration, 11*(7), 22-24.

100. Strasen, L. (1990). Implementing salary cost per unit of service productivity standards. *Journal of Nursing Administration, 20*(3), 6-10.

101. Strong, B. (1985). Nursing products: Primary components of health care. *Nursing Economic$, 3*(1), 60-61.

102. Thomas, S., & Vaughan, R. G. (1986). Costing nursing services using RVUs. *Journal of Nursing Administration, 16*(12), 10-16.

103. Thompson, J. D. (1984). The measurement of nursing intensity. *Health Care Financing Review, 11* (Annual Suppl.), 47-55.

104. Thompson, J. D., & Diers, D. (1985). DRGs and nursing intensity. *Nursing and Health Care, 6*(8), 435-439.

105. Toth, R. (1984). DRGs: Imperative strategies for nursing service administration. *Nursing and Health Care, 5*(4), 196-203.

106. Trofino, J. (1985). RIMs: Skirting the edge of diaster. *Nursing Management, 16*(7), 48-51.

107. Trofino, J. (1986). A reality based system for pricing nursing service. *Nursing Management, 17*(1), 19-24.

108. Urquhart, A. L., Wooding, G. M., Budinger, K. M., & Henry, B. M. (1986). Perspectives on nursing issues and health care trends. *Journal of Nursing Administration, 16*(1), 17-24.

109. Vanderbilt, M. (1992). Bills would benefit advanced practice RNs. *American Nurse, 24*(1), 7.

110. Vanderbilt, M. W. (1990). Budget provisions are victory: Advanced practice nurses to benefit. *American Nurse, 22*(1), 1, 17.

111. Vanderzee, H., & Glusko, G. (1984). DRGs variable pricing and budgeting for nursing service. *Journal of Nursing Administration, 14*(5), 11-14.

112. Vanputte, A., Sovie, M., Tarcinale, M., & Studen, A. (1985). Accounting for patient acuity: The nursing time dimension. *Nursing Management, 16*(10), 27-36.

113. Verran, J. (1986). Patient classification in ambulatory care. *Nursing Economic$, 4*(5), 247-251.

114. Weis, A. (1988). Cooperative care: Innovative care in a time of change. In J. Scherubel (Ed.), *Patients and purse strings II.* New York: National League for Nursing.

115. Welton, J. M. (1989). Going into business as a nurse. *American Journal of Nursing, 89*(12), 1639-1641.

116. Wolf, G. A., Lesic, L. K., & Leak, A. G. (1986). Primary nursing: The impact on nursing costs within DRG's. *Journal of Nursing Administration, 16*(3), 9-11.

117. Young, W., Patterson, M., & Groetzinger, S. (1985). Patient management categories and the costs of nursing services. In F. A. Shaffer (Ed.), *Costing out nursing: Pricing our product.* New York: National League for Nursing.

CHAPTER 66

Balancing cost and quality

A model for action

MAUREEN McCORMAC BUENO, MARYANN F. FRALIC

Today's nurse executives and managers are faced with the challenge of balancing the quality and cost of care in health care organizations. While the systematic evaluation of quality and analysis of the cost of providing care have occurred as separate entities in the past, "it is a relatively new process to analyze the cost of providing care and determine if the cost of providing care can be reduced without negatively affecting the quality of care."[6] In fact, the possibility of improving quality while reducing costs has recently been considered.[6,16]

A variety of systems and agencies have impacted the quality and cost of health care. The prospective payment system, for example, has influenced an increase in efficiency and a reduction in the cost of hospital operations. In addition to private payers, regulatory agencies, such as Medicare's Peer Review Organization (PRO) and the Joint Commission on Accreditation of Healthcare Organizations (JCAHO), have focused on the definition, measurement, and evaluation of operations in terms of quality and cost factors. The Peer Review Organization screens Medicare hospital admissions to determine if patients receive quality health care in a cost-effective manner. The JCAHO has recently supported a total quality management (TQM) approach to patient care that is centered around customer satisfaction, increased productivity, and lower costs.[2,25] Organizations of this magnitude are expeditiously mandating and defining quality and cost for health care organizations. It is unrealistic to expect a perfect measure of either in the immediate future. The time is right for organizations to build on the foundations already established and in operation, despite the limitations of present systems.

Nursing management systems must be quickly established to define, monitor, analyze, and display the components of the cost-quality equation. Nurses are critically important in influencing the quality of health care and the nature of patient outcomes.[1] According to a national survey of hospital chief executives, nurses were identified as one of the most important factors in maintaining the quality of care.[27] Research studies have documented the valuable role of nurses in the attainment of quality patient care.[5,19] Although the contribution of nurses to the maintenance of quality is widely recognized, the additional association of nursing with cost containment is essential and warrants acknowledgment. Quality and cost are "two implacable imperatives" that require skillful management.[9]

The quantification of both quality and cost elements provides a foundation for effective decisions by nurse executives and managers. "It is both expedient and necessary to have the right information, in the right format, in the right time frame, and in the right amount."[13] In the words of Peter F. Drucker,[10] an appropriate measurement is the "hinge" of an effective decision.

THE COST-QUALITY MODEL

The purpose of this chapter is to describe a cost-quality measurement index called QualDex, which was developed at Robert Wood Johnson University Hospital (RWJUH), a 416-bed academic teaching institution in New Brunswick, New Jersey. The QualDex system provides a numerical indicator of both quality and cost performance of each nursing unit. This chapter includes (1) a review of the quality and cost elements included in the model; (2) the process of data collection, analysis, and report generation; (3) significance of the model; and (4) implications for practice. The qual-

---

**QUALITY AND COST ELEMENTS
FUNDAMENTAL TO THE
COMPREHENSIVE NURSING
MANAGEMENT MODEL QUALDEX**

Quality elements

Compliance with standards of nursing practice (nursing process)
Compliance with standards of nursing care (patient outcomes)
Occurrence of untoward patient incidents*
Occurrence of hospital-acquired infections*
Patient satisfaction

Cost elements

Compliance with budget (salary)
Compliance with staffing format
Nursing hours per patient day
Compliance with budget (nonsalary)
Work load (patient days, occupancy, acuity)

---

*Attributable to nursing care.

ity and cost elements fundamental to this comprehensive nursing management model are presented in the box above. The original research study that guided the development of QualDex was described by Fralic and Brett[14] in an earlier publication.

QUALITY ELEMENTS

Donabedian[8] outlined a model for optimal quality assessment that includes three components: structure, process, and outcome. Examples of structure assessments include the evaluation of administrative organization, determination of staff qualifications, and inspection of the physical facility.[31] The other two components, process and outcome, are well known to the nursing profession. Standards for nursing practice (nursing process) guide the provision of care, and standards of care (patient outcomes) foretell expected outcomes. In addition to the measurement of compliance with these standards, the measurement of patient incidents, hospital-acquired infections, and patient satisfaction are also necessary for the evaluation of quality health care.

Compliance with standards of nursing practice (nursing process)

The providers of patient care are the focus of standards of nursing practice. That is, process standards describe

the expectations of nurses in the delivery of safe, quality patient care.[29] They "specify the expected level of performance that nurses need to demonstrate to ensure that the standards of care will be achieved and represent the institutions' definition of what the nurse can do."[7]

Nursing standards at RWJUH are derived from expert opinion, research findings, other scientific literature, consultation, policies, procedures, regulatory agencies, and published standards from professional organizations. They are developed for each of the nine nursing diagnostic and management categories of the nursing division's conceptual model (Fig. 66-1). These are (1) activity, (2) comfort, (3) elimination, (4) nutrition, (5) oxygenation, (6) protection, (7) coping, (8) growth and development, and (9) management of health. The nursing standards committee includes clinical nurse specialists, nurse managers, and staff nurses who develop, approve, and revise standards for all areas where nursing care is delivered. Nursing standards provide the basis for the development of quality indicators that examine compliance with standards. The activity standard (see the box on page 493), for example, provided the basis for the development of a quality indicator that measures compliance with standards for immobilized patients (see the box on page 494).

Quality data, based on nursing standards, are collected by staff nurse quality analysts as part of the Professional Practice Analyst Program in nursing at RWJUH.[15] Quality data are analyzed and reported through the quality program and are also integrated into the QualDex system on a monthly basis. The QualDex system utilizes existing data from established systems whenever possible to prevent duplication of work.

Compliance with standards of nursing care (patient outcomes)

Standards of care focus on what the patient can expect from individuals who deliver nursing care.[26] Health care consumers are increasingly involved in the care they receive, and they expect optimal outcomes. "Outcomes are the products of action"[4] and include mortality, complications, adverse effects, other indicators of morbidity, and patient satisfaction.[3,24,29] The emphasis of outcome research is placed on strengthening the relationship between nursing interventions and specific patient outcomes.

Standards of care at RWJUH are developed, approved, monitored, and reported in the same manner as standards of practice.

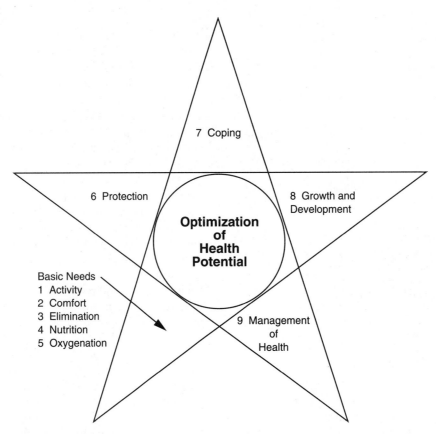

Fig. 66-1 The conceptual model for nursing (developed by the standards committee at Robert Wood Johnson University Hospital in collaboration with Margaret Lunney).

Occurrence of untoward patient incidents

An adverse occurrence is considered "an event, involving the patient directly or indirectly, that is either a mistake in judgment or performance or is an accident."[20] Medication errors and patient falls are examples of incidents that may result in negative patient outcomes. The systematic collection, analysis, and evaluation of incidents is needed to promote the identification and resolution of problems.

Members of the risk management department and safety committees (hospitalwide and nursing division) at RWJUH screen incident reports completed by hospital employees and managers. Nursing representatives assist in determining if the incident is attributable to nursing and make decisions concerning the type of corrective action needed. Incident data are integral to examining the cost-quality relationship and are included in the monthly QualDex reports.

Occurrence of hospital-acquired infections

Surgical wound infections, urinary tract infections, bacteremias, and pneumonias are typical examples of hospital-acquired or nosocomial infections.[22] Nosocomial infections "affect at least 6% of individuals admitted to U.S. hospitals, adding an average of 4 days to each patient's length of stay at an average of $1800 per infection."[22] To address the alarming rate of nosocomial infections, the Joint Commission on Accreditation of Healthcare Organizations[17] identified nosocomial infection rates as an outcome indicator of quality care that requires attention.

A major national study was initiated by the Centers for Disease Control (CDC) from 1974 to 1985 to evaluate the effects of infection control programs on nosocomial infection rates.[22] The study identified interventions performed by health care practitioners that reduce the patient's risk for acquiring infection. Proper

Nursing Diagnosis & Management Category
(Aspect of Care)

ACTIVITY: A motion of action that is produced dependently or independently.

STANDARD OF CARE (OUTCOME)

STANDARD OF PRACTICE (PROCESS)

1. The patient maintains or improves functional body
   alignment, joint motion, muscle strength and/or body
   tone.

- Assess activity limitations considering present physical
  status and pertinent history.
- Assess requirement for restricted activity or rest due to
  disease process or condition.
- Formulate an individualized exercise/toning plan, as
  needed, in collaboration with patient/significant
  others/physician/physical and/or occupational therapist.
- Set up realistic, progressive goals which include:
  —timing, frequency and duration of exercises.
  —timing of analgesics with exercise.
  —rest periods interspersed with activity.
  —teaching family members program specifics.
  —consideration of progress impediments (i.e., physical
    deficits, environmental constraints).
- Utilize support devices to maintain/support limits in
  functional position.
- Implement planned exercise/toning program with pa-
  tient and/or significant others:
  —Develop, schedule and initiate program according to
    the nature of limitations.
  —Ensure family/significant others are capable of carry-
    ing out the plan of care via return demonstrations.
  —Provide family/significant others with information re-
    garding available community resources to assist with
    home program.
  —Evaluate patient for proper body alignment, joint mo-
    tion and body tone after the program is implemented.
  —Adjust therapy/regimen according to patient's re-
    sponse.

2. The patient performs ADL(s) dependently or independently.

- Assess the patient's ability to perform ADL considering
  his/her present physical/psychological status and pertinent history.
- Assess the patient for S/S of fatigue and/or tiring upon
  performing ADL.
- Assess for ADL intolerance due to inadequate sleep, energy consuming treatments, medications or pain.
- Assess impact of patient's nutritional status on ADL.
- Formulate a plan of ADL activity in collaboration with
  the patient, physician, physical therapist, dietician
  and/or psychiatric nurse clinical specialist.
- Implement an ADL program which attempts to increase
  energy expenditure and considers the patient's tolerance.
- Encourage family/significant others to participate with
  the patient in an ADL program which promotes independence.
- Evaluate the therapy program and adjust the regimen
  according to the patient's response.

From: American Nurses Association and National Association of Orthopaedic Nurses. (1987, March-April). Orthopaedic nursing practice: Process
and outcome for criteria for selected diagnoses. *Orthopaedic Nursing,* 6(2), 11-16. Revised by Clinical Nurse Specialist, Surgery; Approved by
Standards Committee, June 1991.

QUALITY INDICATOR: COMPLIANCE WITH STANDARDS FOR IMMOBILIZED PATIENTS

ROBERT WOOD JOHNSON UNIVERSITY HOSPITAL NURSING DIVISION

QUALITY INDICATOR—Compliance with Standards for Immobilized Patients

NURSING DIAGNOSIS & MANAGEMENT CATEGORY—Activity

DATA SOURCES—(N)Nsg Hx, (FS)Flowsheet, (OB)Observe, (C)Care Plan, (P)Progress Notes, (I)Interview, (K)Kardex

FREQUENCY & AMOUNT—Each unit assesses ten patients per assigned month.

THRESHOLD FOR EVALUATION—85% YES

NURSING PRACTICE STANDARD—(PROCESS)

- The nurse assesses the patient for immobility according to assessment guidelines and "Activity" Standard.
- The nurse identifies immobility problems and documents plan of care.
- The nurse implements measures to promote activity that is realistic and progressive.
- The nurse considers the use of analgesics, rest periods, support devices, exercise/toning program, etc., to improve patient activity.
- The nurse evaluates patient response to interventions and adjusts care accordingly.
- The nurse involves patient/family in care to fullest extent possible.

NURSING CARE STANDARD—(OUTCOMES)

- The patient maintains or improves funtional body alignment, joint motion, muscle strength and/or body tone.
- The patient performs ADL(s) dependently or independently.

DEVELOPED BY/DATE:

APPROVED BY/DATE:

PPAC—3/88, 2/91

REVISED BY/DATE:

Indicator Committee—2/88

Clinical Nurse Specialist, Surgery and Chair, PPAC Committee—1/91

SOURCES:

—Adapted in 2/88 from indicators "Appropriateness of Care for the Immobilized Patient"
(Medical/Surgical)—2/88 & "Appropriateness of Care for Decubitus Prevention with Immobilized Patient" (Critical Care)—2/89

—Nursing Division Standards, "Activity"—rev. 6/91

—ANA & NAON, 1986, *Core Curriculum for Orthopaedic Nursing,* Anthony J. Janetti, Inc., Pitman, N.J. From Nursing Concepts: Immobility section.

PROCESS

—Is the patient assessed & reassessed as needed for:

(FS,P)1. ability to turn, transfer or walk prn?

(FS,P)2. functional ROM prn?

(FS,P)3. muscle strength/tone prn?

(FS,P)4. coordination prn?

(FS)5. Was turning done as needed during current shift?

(OB)6. With turning, is the skin assessed and interventions done as necessary (i.e., clean, massage, check bony prominences/pressure points)?

(OB)7. Is active or passive ROM encouraged and done prn?

(OB)8. Are isometric/isotonic exercises encouraged and done prn?

(OB)9. Are extremities/body kept as much as possible in proper alignment (i.e., proper positioning, use of pillows, splints, braces)?

(OB)10. Are heels and elbows monitored and protected from skin breakdown prn?

(OB)11. Are measures taken to prevent sheering (i.e., trapeze, draw sheet, encourage pt. to help as much as possible)?

(OB)12. Is the patient kept clean and dry as much as possible?

(OB)13. Is the patient provided with sensory stimulation (i.e., pictures, magazines, mobiles, imagery, radio)?

(C)14. Is there an "Activity" or "Protection" plan of care (i.e., problem identified, interventions & pt. response noted) for patients w/a significant/persistent immobility problem?

(K,P)15. Is the patient premedicated as needed for pain prior to activity?

(OB)16. Patient OOB as ordered & as able?

(OB)17. Nurses use proper body mechanics when moving or assisting patient?

(OB)18. Nurse encourages proper use of assistive equipment (i.e., walker, crutches, trapeze)?

(OB)19. Does the nurse have equipment necessary to get patient OOB (i.e., Geri-Chair, Hoyer Lift, wheelchair)?

QUALITY INDICATOR – Cont'd

(OB)20. Is the nurse able to get a team of people together within a reasonable period of time to get the patient OOB and/or back into bed?

(P,FS)21. Have other health professionals (i.e., PT, OT) been consulted as needed?

OUTCOMES

(I)22. Has the nurse discussed with you, your expected activity (progression of, limitations, restrictions, interventions/response) during your hospitalization?

(P)23. As available, has the family been informed of patient's activity (progression of, limitations, restrictions, interventions/response) during this hospitalization?

(OB)24. Is the patient's ROM, muscle strength/tone, body alignment at an acceptable level (concurrent w/patient's medical condition and optimal nursing care)?

*(OB)25. Does the patient verbalize and/or demonstrate compliance with mobility interventions, limitations, restrictions?

Sources: (FS)Flowsheet, (P)Progress Notes, (OB)Observe, (C)Care Plan, (K)Kardex, (I)Interview

hand washing, skin preparation, and wound dressing using aseptic and antiseptic techniques;[21] proper handling of diagnostic and therapeutic devices such as catheters;[23,30] and proper use of sterile barriers are interventions under the control of nursing personnel.

At RWJUH, nosocomial infection rates are monitored for 2 of 4 quarters during the calendar year. Infections associated with cardiac surgery, for example, are monitored by focus survey during the other 2 quarters. Data are provided by the infection control nurse and practitioner on a quarterly basis for inclusion in the QualDex analyses and reports.

Patient satisfaction

Patient satisfaction is commonly considered an outcome indicator of quality.[4,16,18] Customer satisfaction is inherent in the total quality management philosophy put forward by Deming and others.[2] While satisfaction is considered a measure of quality by many, Eriksen[11] cautions nurse administrators against considering patient or customer satisfaction as the sole evaluation mechanism for determining quality.

Patient satisfaction is one of the five quality indicators in use at RWJUH. A 20-item satisfaction questionnaire, developed by representatives from the nursing division and guest relations department, is administered on a monthly basis to patients and visitors by staff nurse quality analysts. Data are collected, analyzed, summarized, and integrated into the QualDex system.

COST ELEMENTS

Cost management is increasingly critical to the financial well-being of health care organizations. The role of nurse executives and managers in meeting the hospital's financial objectives has expanded over time. Timely information on salary and nonsalary budgets, nursing care hours, and work load contributes to the effective and efficient allocation and utilization of hospital resources.

Compliance with budget (salary)

The salary budget represents the greatest expenditure within a nursing cost center.[12] It includes base salaries, shift differentials, premiums, fringe benefits, and sick, holiday, seminar, vacation, and overtime pay.

Salary data at RWJUH are collected, analyzed, and reported each pay period by payroll personnel and finance managers from the finance department and nursing division. Labor distribution reports are reviewed by nurse managers and data abstracted for inclusion in the QualDex system.

Compliance with staffing format

A full-time equivalent (FTE) is widely considered the standard for comparing hours worked that allows for comparison across employees and units, and over time.[12] The calculation of FTEs includes all levels of health care providers, such as registered nurses, licensed practical nurses, nursing assistants, unit clerks, technicians, and others. Monitoring compliance with budgeted FTEs is a high priority for nurse managers. Full-time equivalents are analyzed and reported using the same mechanisms as described for the salary budget.

Nursing hours per patient day

Nursing hours per patient day (NHPPD) are determined by dividing paid nursing hours by actual patient days for a particular time period. While it is an established standard for comparing nursing units and institutions to each other, nurse managers should exercise caution due to common variations in staff mix and patient populations.

At RWJUH, labor distribution reports provide data for determining nursing hours. Patient days are provided by the hospital's admitting department. The two components are integrated as NHPPD on a monthly basis into QualDex.

Compliance with budget (nonsalary)

Nonsalary expenses are an essential component of the cost of providing care. Adequate patient care supplies of acceptable quality and quantity are necessary for the delivery of patient care. Nurse managers in today's cost-conscious environment cannot afford to tolerate waste or inefficiency.

Monthly nonsalary usage reports are distributed to nurse managers for evaluation and are then integrated as an important cost element into QualDex.

Work load (patient days, occupancy, acuity)

Work load is typically expressed in terms of acuity and census measures such as average daily census, patient days, or occupancy rates.[12] These quantitative indicators of work load guide the identification of personnel requirements for a particular patient care unit. Nurse managers frequently utilize this information when making staffing and budget decisions.

Patient days and occupancy rates are typically generated by hospital admitting departments. The Navy Workload Management System for Nursing, developed by the Navy,[28] is a reliable and valid factor-evaluative patient classification system in use at RWJUH. While acuity and census data are collected and reported on a daily and monthly basis as part of routine patient classification procedures, monthly summaries are included in QualDex reports.

UNITS OF MEASUREMENT: QUALITY AND COST

Compliance with standards of nursing practice (process): the number of nursing process criteria achieved divided by the number applicable

Compliance with standards of nursing care (patient outcomes): the number of patient outcome criteria achieved divided by the number applicable

Occurrence of untoward patient incidents: the number of incidents attributable to nursing (e.g., medication errors and patient falls)

Occurrence of hospital-acquired infections: the number of infections attributable to nursing

Patient satisfaction: patients' scores on the patient satisfaction instrument developed by the hospital; higher scores represent higher levels of satisfaction

Compliance with budget (salary): all salary dollars paid, including sick, holiday, seminar, vacation, and overtime pay

Compliance with staffing format: full-time equivalents for all nursing personnel, including nurses reassigned from other units

Nursing hours per patient day: calculation of paid nursing hours and actual patient days

Compliance with budget (nonsalary): costs of unit supplies and patient care supplies that are not charged to a particular nursing unit

Work load (patient days, occupancy, acuity): the patient days, occupancy, and average acuity points for all patients

---

THE QUALDEX PROCESS

Systems exist in most health care organizations for capturing many if not all of the quality and cost elements described. The box above summarizes the units of measurement for each of the elements at RWJUH. While the collection of data is becoming a routine component of nursing operations, systems that integrate quality and cost, such as the QualDex system, are not yet commonplace.

The process of integration developed at RWJUH involves the following steps:

1. Quality and cost data are generated by individuals in several hospital departments (e.g., infection control, guest relations, risk management, payroll, and finance).
2. Data are sent to the nursing systems coordinator and finance manager for nursing, who input it into LOTUS 1-2-3 for analysis each month.

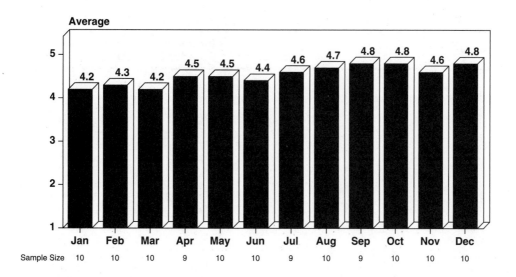

Fig. 66-2 Example of patient satisfaction over time for a particular nursing unit.

3. Actual values are compared to established standards for quality elements or budgeted numbers for cost elements to determine variances that are reported in numerical and percentage formats. Historical hospital data are commonly utilized to determine standards and budgets.

4. An overall quality and cost score is computed for each nursing unit each month and is used for comparison across units.

5. A monthly unit report is distributed to head nurses. A sample report is presented in Table 66-1.

6. A monthly report is distributed to the directors of each nursing service; it includes the director's areas of responsibility.

7. Monthly quality and cost summaries are distributed to nursing directors and senior nursing management. Table 66-2 depicts a sample quality summary that is used to compare the performance of nursing units.

8. The development of trended data in graphic format is in process as a means of improving readability and interpretability. Fig. 66-2 provides a graph of patient satisfaction data over time for a particular nursing unit. Graphs that include multiple quality and cost elements are also being introduced.

SIGNIFICANCE OF THE MODEL AND IMPLICATIONS FOR PRACTICE

The QualDex model enables nurse managers to "see how their own units have performed against each individual measure during the month, with respect to previous months, and as compared to other nursing units."[14] Each element can be evaluated and discussed, and corrective action targeted if necessary. The relations among elements can also be evaluated and altered to improve nursing practice, and thus, patient care delivery. A variety of questions can be answered. Is compliance with standards of nursing practice and care related to the number of professional nurses involved in direct patient care? What happens to the rate of hospital-acquired infections as acuity increases on a nursing unit? What is the relationship between compliance with staffing formats and patient satisfaction?

A comprehensive report is useful for nurse managers and executives who manage multiple priorities. Systems need to be designed and implemented to provide nurse managers and executives with performance data. According to Drucker,[10] "a manager analyzes performance, appraises it, and interprets it." In addition, managers act on information to improve performance. The QualDex model at RWJUH provides the basis for such action. It quantifies the contribution, value, and worth of professional nursing practice in today's challenging health care environment.

Table 66-1   Sample monthly QualDex report for a particular nursing unit*

	Actual	Budget or standard	Variance from standard	Percentage variance
Cost				
Compliance with budget				
Salary	$82,760	$ 89,521	$6,761	7.6
Nonsalary	$15,081	$ 11,489	($3,592)	−31.3
TOTALS	$97,841	$101,010	$3,169	3.1
Workload				
Patient days	946	862	84.0	9.7
Occupancy	95.6%	87.1%	8.5%	9.7
Acuity level—points/patient	33.0	30.1	2.9	9.6
Compliance with staffing format				
Paid full-time equivalents including overtime	30.08	31.2	1.12	3.6
Total full-time equivalents	30.08	31.2	1.12	3.6
Nursing hours/patient day				
Actual versus budget	3.92	4.42	0.50	11.3
Corrected for acuity	3.92	4.85	0.93	19.2
Quality				
Process (weighted average)	98%	92%	0.06	7
Outcome (weighted average)	96%	88%	0.08	9
Incidents/patient day	0.01	0.69	0.68	99
Infections	0.0	0.2	(0.20)	−100
Patient satisfaction	4.8	4.3	0.50	12
Cost score	3.1%			
Quality score	6.9%			

*Fictitious data.

Table 66-2   Sample monthly QualDex report summarizing unit-based indicators*

	Quality analysis†					
	Process			Outcome		
Unit	Standard percentage	Actual percentage	Percentage variance from standard	Standard percentage	Actual percentage	Percentage variance from standard
1	79	74	−6	77	87	13
2	77	—	—	75	—	—
3	74	92	24	85	79	−7
4	79	74	−7	76	89	17
5	90	86	−5	86	95	11
6	87	88	1	86	74	−14
7	87	89	3	87	89	3
Medical/Surgical	81	85	5	82	82	−0
Total division	84.0	88.2	5.0	83.0	87.0	4.9

*Fictitious data.
—, Data not available.
†July: new standard 1988 and 1989 cumulative.

Table 66-2 Sample monthly QualDex report summarizing unit-based indicators*—Cont'd

Incidents per patient day‡

Unit	Standard ratio	Actual	Actual ratio	Percentage variance from standard
1	0.77	10	1.01	−31
2	0.73	6	0.60	17
3	0.56	2	0.24	56
4	0.55	2	0.21	61
5	0.44	6	0.72	−65
6	0.38	1	0.11	71
7	0.67	1	0.13	80
Medical/Surgical	0.59	4	0.06	89
Total division	0.56	56	0.55	2

Infections§

Unit	Standard	Actual	Percentage variance from standard
1	12.0	18.0	−50
2	17.0	42.0	−147
3	7.0	15.0	−114
4	8.0	14.0	−75
5	9.0	6.0	33
6	4.0	7.0	−75
7	4.0	1.0	75
Medical/Surgical	8.7	14.7	−69
Total division	5.4	8.3	−55

Patient satisfaction scores‖

Unit	Standard	Actual	Percentage variance from standard
1	4.6	4.4	−4
2	4.5	—	NA
3	4.4	—	NA
4	4.4	4.3	−2
5	4.5	4.5	0
6	4.3	4.6	7
7	4.4	4.4	0
Medical/Surgical	4.4	3.2	−29
Total division	4.5	4.5	0

*Fictitious data.

‡July: actual not applicable; new standard 1988 and 1989 cumulative.

§July: actual not applicable; new standard.

‖Guest relations; July: new standard not applicable.

REFERENCES

1. Aiken, L. H. (1990). Charting the future of hospital nursing. *Image: The Journal of Nursing Scholarship, 22*(2), 72-78.
2. Arikian, V. L. (1991). Total quality management: Applications to nursing service. *Journal of Nursing Administration, 21*(6), 46-50.
3. Balit, H., Lewis, J., Hochheiser, L., & Bush, N. (1975). Assessing the quality of care. *Nursing Outlook, 23*(3), 153-159.
4. Brett, J. L. (1989). Measure and validation of the practice of nursing and nursing administration: Outcome indicators of quality care. In B. Henry, C. Arndt, M. DiVincenti, & A. Marriner Tomey (Eds.), *Dimensions and issues in nursing administration* (pp. 353-369). Boston: Blackwell Scientific Publications.
5. Chassin, M. R., Park, R. E., Lohr, K. N., Kelsey, J., & Brook, R. H. (1989). Differences among hospitals in Medicare patient mortality. *Health Sciences Research, 24*(1), 1-31.
6. Curran, C., & Smeltzer, C. H. (1991). Operation improvement: Efficiencies and quality. *Journal of Nursing Quality Assurance, 5*(4), 1-6.
7. Dang, D., & Callahan, B. (1991). Standards of practice and standards of care: Developing a successful model in a large division of nursing. In P. Schroeder (Ed.), *The encyclopedia of nursing care quality: Vol. 2. Approaches to nursing standards* (pp. 121-132). Gaithersburg, Md: Aspen.
8. Donabedian, A. (1966). Evaluating the quality of medical care. *Milbank Memorial Fund Quarterly, 44,* 166-203.
9. Donabedian, A. (1984). Quality, cost, and cost containment. *Nursing Outlook, 32*(3), 142-145.
10. Drucker, P. F. (1966, 1967). *The effective executive.* New York: Harper and Row.
11. Ericksen, L. R. (1987). Patient satisfaction: An indicator of nursing care quality? *Nursing Management, 18*(7), 31-35.
12. Finkler, S. A. (1984). *Budgeting concepts for nurse managers.* Orlando, Fla: Grune and Stratton.
13. Fralic, M. F. (1989). Decision support systems: Essential for quality administrative decisions. *Nursing Administrative Quarterly, 14*(1), 1-8.
14. Fralic, M. F., & Brett, J. L. (1990). Nursing's newest mandate: The cost-quality imperative. In J. C. McCloskey & H. K. Grace (Eds.), *Current issues in nursing* (3rd ed, pp. 399-404). St Louis: Mosby.
15. Fralic, M. F., Kowalski, P. M., & Llewellyn, F. A. (1991). The development of an evaluation tool for unit-based quality assurance. *Journal of Nursing Quality Assurance, 4*(2), 63-70.
16. Helt, E. H., & Jelinek, R. C. (1988). In the wake of cost cutting, nursing productivity and quality improve. *Nursing Management, 19*(6), 36-48.
17. Joint Commission on Accreditation of Healthcare Organizations. (1992). *Strategies for quality improvement in nursing.* Oak Brook Terrace, Ill: Author.
18. Jones, K. R. (1991). Managing quality in a changing environment. *Nursing Economic$, 9*(3), 159-164.
19. Knaus, W. A., Draper, E. A., Wagner, D. P., & Zimmerman, J. E. (1986). An evaluation of outcomes from intensive care in major medical centers. *Annals of Internal Medicine, 104*(3), 410-418.
20. Larrabee, J. H., Ruckstuhl, M., Salmons, J., & Smith, L. (1991). Interdisciplinary monitoring of medication errors in a nursing quality assurance program. *Journal of Nursing Quality Assurance, 5*(4), 69-78.
21. Larson, E. (1985). Handwashing and skin: Physiologic and bacteriologic aspects. *Infection Control, 6,* 14.

22. Larson, E., Oram, L. F., & Hedrick, E. (1988). Nosocomial infection rates as an indicator of quality. *Medical Care, 26*(7), 676-684.

23. Maki, D. G. (1981). Nosocomial bacteremia. *American Journal of Medicine, 70,* 719.

24. Marek, K. (1989). Outcome measurement in nursing. *Journal of Nursing Quality Assurance, 4*(1), 1-7.

25. Masters, F., & Schmele, J. A. (1991). Total quality management: An idea whose time has come. *Journal of Nursing Quality Assurance, 5*(4), 7-16.

26. Patterson, C. H. (1988). Standards of patient care: The Joint Commission focus on nursing quality assurance. *Nursing Clinics of North America, 23*(3), 625-638.

27. Quality—thy name is nursing care, CEOs say. (1989, February 5). *Hospitals, 5,* 32.

28. Rieder, K. A., & Jackson, S. S. (1985). *An evaluation study of the Navy medical department's patient classification and staffing allocation system: The Workload Management System for Nursing* (Report No. 5-85). Annapolis, Md: Navy School of Health Sciences Research Department.

29. Smith, T. C. (1991). Nursing standards: The basis of professional practice. In P. Schroeder (Ed.), *The encyclopedia of nursing care quality, Vol. 2. Approaches to nursing standards* (pp. 7-18). Gaithersburg, Md: Aspen.

30. Stamm, W. E. (1978). Infections related to medical devices. *Annals of Internal Medicine, 89* (Pt. 2), 764.

31. Ullmann, S. G. (1985). The impact of quality on cost in the provision of long-term care. *Inquiry, 22,* 293-302.

CHAPTER 67

Long-term care

Overpriced and underrated

GENROSE J. ALFANO

HEALTH CARE: QUESTIONS OF COST AND NEED

Is long-term care costing us too much? And how much is too much? Too much is whatever amount we are unwilling to pay, and oddly enough quality usually doesn't enter into it. Our reaction to health care costs stems from a belief that we can't afford health care. But affordability is usually based on where we are willing to spend whatever money we have.

All signs indicate that we are not willing to spend our money, or for that matter any of our other resources, on long-term illness care. That is why third-party payers, such as the federal, state, and local governments along with private insurance investors, are comfortable in keeping benefits and reimbursement levels for the long-term care population at the lowest possible levels. Despite all the rhetoric, enriched health care budgets are not seen as critical to the nation's welfare.

The all-inclusive generic term *health care* has in fact increased not only the cost of illness care but of health and maintenance care as well.

Health care is an all-encompassing term. There is the broad spectrum of prevention of disease; the maintenance of well-being and striving to improve physiological function, physical competencies, and psychological stability; the incidents of illness and the breakdown of physiological and/or psychological function resulting in dysfunction, threat to life, and threat to future function; and the recovery or restorative period during which functions return to the preillness phase. The restorative period may also involve rehabilitative efforts to help the body and the person to regain full capacity to function, or to function at optimum capacity in the face of competency losses.

The rehabilitative phase usually moves out of the medical sphere and becomes more focused on retraining for development of specific skills necessary to daily living or to career involvement.

It is during the rehabilitative phase as well as in the initial phase of prevention that we find the most blurring of health versus social services. Should the cost of providing a homemaker to prepare food and clean a home, as well as to provide some personal assistance with carrying out activities for daily living, be considered a health care cost or a social welfare cost? Should the monies for care of the acutely ill and the monies for maintaining individuals safely in their own homes come out of the same pocket?

The need for long-term care

The tendency to assume that only the aged require long-term care and services is being rapidly refuted by the number of persons with illnesses or disabilities related to acquired immunodeficiency syndrome (AIDS), and the number of children and young and middle-aged adults who are surviving acute illnesses with residual functional and health problems. Long-term care needs are present in every age group and stratum of our society.

Criteria for determining costs

Caps for home care costs have been determined by prorating them against the costs of hospital illness care and institutional nursing home care. Yet the nature of the care and the system of delivery are totally dissimilar. Home care is not a substitute for either of these services but an appropriate choice of service for the needs of the individual involved.

Increasing complexity and deteriorating service

Long-term care services can be broken down into those that involve extensive medical procedures with continuing medical interventions and close supervision, those that involve periodic technical procedures and medical evaluation, those that require physical assistance and supervision throughout each 24-hour period, and those that require supportive help on an as-needed basis.

When we examine how these services are being provided, we find high costs, inadequate personnel both in numbers and in competency, deficiencies in the services being offered, and unnecessary time delays due to a snarl of red tape.

One of the most common stumbling blocks is the need for physician determination that the services are necessary. In fact, because a good number of physicians tend to base their evaluation of patient capacity upon the seriousness of the illness and because as a group they are among the least informed of the health professionals about availability of support services and community resources, necessary and appropriate help is often not recommended.

Consequently, not only has the cost continued to escalate but also the nature of the care and services has not improved greatly over the past 5 to 6 years, either in the home or in institutions.

Fluctuation of individual care needs

Chronic illness poses an interesting challenge to the health care system because the care required by individuals is not constant and often runs a cycle of acute medical and acute intensive nursing to maintenance medical and intensive rehabilitative and supportive nursing. The individual's ability to carry out activities of daily living may fluctuate. Thus the need for services and assistance may also vary. Eligibility requirements for care and services that are subject to acts of the legislature may impede timely intervention at a lesser cost and result in a need for more extensive care and services at a later date.

Despite the fact that we have been aware of these factors for more than 20 years, there is still considerable confusion about how to deal with them. Debate has centered around what services are necessary, rather than focusing on developing criteria for where and by whom services could most appropriately be delivered.

Nursing, which ought to have assumed the leading role in the improvement of long-term care in all settings, has dragged its feet. Despite efforts such as the teaching nursing home project cosponsored by The Robert Wood Johnson Foundation and the Academy of Nursing, and the community college–nursing home partnership sponsored by the Kellogg Foundation, long-term care is still a low priority on the nursing association's agenda.

By and large the best-prepared individuals among nurses and physicians have not seen care and involvement with the chronically ill, particularly the aged, as a rewarding or exciting specialty. Consequently this population has had to rely on well-intentioned minimally prepared health workers. Those nurses who have chosen geriatrics as a specialty have been more involved with working with the healthy aged than with the ill, and geriatric nurse clinicians have become so disenchanted with their inability to change institutional long-term care systems that they have often left to go into private practice or home care.

Providing services appropriate to needs

Ideally, the best place for people to live is in their own homes, close to those for whom they care and who care for them. They may maintain the lifestyle most comfortable and familiar to them and have near to them those things that are part of who they are. It is assumed that necessary care given in the home will be less costly than if it were given in the institution. However, depending upon the amount of care needed, the frequency and the nature of the care, and the number of persons being served within a given area, the cost may in fact be greater.

Surveys continue to show that the most consistent need of the chronically ill and the infirm, frail elderly is assistance with activities of daily living.[1] Most of these services do not require a full-time homemaker or personal attendant. Nor do they usually require a nurse, a social worker, or a physical therapist, and (in most instances) certainly not all three. For the most part, these chronically ill and frail elderly require only periodic services of a physician, some of them not needing to see a physician for months at a time.

The most frequent services needed are support services brought into the home, such as shopping, housecleaning, meals on wheels, and friendly visits, especially when there are no immediate family members or friends. In many instances, chauffeur service to do the shopping and various personal errands may be all that is necessary to provide a good quality of life and maintain the health status.

These are not "health services" although they support health. They are social services. The ability to attain such services through public programs ought not to be dependent upon the recommendation of a physician, but rather upon that of a responsible primary care provider—a health care professional qualified to assess competencies and mobilize available resources.

Case management and cost effectiveness

The primary care provider would in effect be a case manager responsible for ensuring individuals' access to and attainment of necessary services in a timely fashion. I personally opt for professional nurses as case managers and primary care providers in long-term care. Nurses are prepared in health teaching and illness prevention, as well as in the performance of various "technico-medical" skills and assessments. They are also prepared in helping people to identify and work through psychosocial problems. A nurse who is performing at maximum capacity ought to be able to help people to work through the services they need and help them gain access to those services and then coordinate the services so the person doesn't get lost in the shuffle. Public health nurses have traditionally played this role, and it is time for them to get back on target.

The functional capability of each individual may be initially assessed by a nurse, a physician, a physical or occupational therapist, and/or a social worker. Joint assessment or team consultation may be indicated. Potential for improvement or change can be evaluated, and periodic reassessment can occur based upon intervals determined by the clinical history, the existing illness, or any new crisis or exacerbation of the original illness.

Technical procedures related to illness care or illness prevention would be carried out by the health professional qualified to deliver that care.

It could be possible to allocate cost of these services to a social welfare rather than a health care budget, thereby allowing social need to determine rendering of services, rather than health status.

REFOCUSING PUBLIC HEALTH AND COMMUNITY NURSING

Public health and visiting nurses have long been the bulwark of care of the chronically ill in the community in relation to health teaching, family counseling, and morbidity care. Now the home health nurse has been added to those who provide care in the home. Unlike their public health colleagues, these nurses visit to carry out specific care techniques or treatments and do not concentrate on overall health or family care issues. Consequently a whole spectrum of community health care and disease prevention is going unattended. This is a wasteful use of nursing personnel and a loss of opportunity to carry out timely health teaching.

Proliferation of health workers

The growth of job titles in the field of long-term care is phenomenal. The result has been fractionalization of care with increasing numbers of people to carry out similar and closely related responsibilities. Such systems have always resulted in duplication of effort, poor communication, and increased costs, with no appreciable improvement in care and services received by patients/clients. We keep trying to solve personnel shortages by adding personnel. We are facing shortages because of the ever-increasing role specificity for health professionals. What we need are larger numbers of broadly prepared generalists in nursing and in medicine—people who know how to care for people instead of parts.

Quality versus quantity in nursing homes

Understanding of motivation for living, individual differences among people even in the same age group, and value systems of others; knowledge of the interrelational effect of psyche and soma, and the complexities of physiological response and reaction to external and internal stimuli, real or perceived, are important competencies in the day-to-day care of the long-term chronically ill person.

There is a prevailing myth that hiring professional registered nurses (RNs) would be more costly than hiring licensed practical nurses (LPNs). However, if the RNs were expected and permitted to function with a scope and span of responsibility commensurate with a professional level of practice rather than that of a technical apprentice and gatekeeper, then the preponderance of care delivered would be nurturing and rehabilitative in nature rather than caretaking or custodial. While such care might not result in a larger number of discharges from institutions, it could mean more functional residents, resulting in less of a drain on resources. If RNs were the care coordinators, there would be less need for so many health workers.

It is ridiculous to argue that RNs are more expensive. Once the LPN becomes the preferred worker by virtue of availability and then experience, it is foolish to assume that this group will be content to receive less money. They will expect to be paid a salary equal to their responsibility.

And what about the nurses' aides? As of April 1992, they are required to have at least 70 hours of training before employment and must be certified as aides for nursing home care.[2] In some states licensure is being required, under boards of either education or nursing, although this is not a federal stipulation. The original reason for hiring aides for long-term care was that they were inexpensive, unskilled labor, easy to procure and plentiful; so it will be interesting to see what happens to salaries when this group of personnel becomes certified, and how quickly hospitals facing a shortage of qualified, suitably prepared nurses will rationalize that aides certified in long-term care with just a little extra in-service and supervision by RNs or LPNs will be good substitutes for professionally licensed nurses. Thus the nursing home and home health industry will be under added pressure to pay higher salaries for this group of workers.

There is a common saying that points out that "the more things change, the more they stay the same." The issue is still whether or not adequate or even safe nursing care can be given by minimally prepared people, particularly when there is little or poor supervision. My conviction is that it cannot be and that the care and cost for long-term care will never be different until we are able to recruit and retain broadly prepared persons to deliver day-to-day nursing care and services. Whatever their title, they must have the knowledge, skills, and competencies to do the job that needs doing.

There is only one certainty about cost for the long-term care of patients in institutions: it will go up. The critical issue is whether it will go up accompanied by dramatic qualitative improvements in the method of delivering care and the competencies and characteristics of the personnel most immediately involved, or go up without any appreciable improvement in care.

Cost reduction through flexibility

The trend toward multiservice centers, regardless of type, must be examined very closely. Costs of affiliated outreach programs often run higher than those of freestanding or unipurpose facilities. Often those programs that cost less to operate have costs allocated from the more expensive services or must pay a proportion of the cost of services for the entire corporation, many of which the smaller unit does not use.

The rationale is always that the affiliation or relationship permits the patient or client to have access to total services and the care given is of higher quality. While in some instances this may be true, there is also the danger that this out-reach unit can in effect become the step child receiving less than it contributes, or receiving more sophisticated services than it needs. And the third party or individual payer is paying for hidden services rarely received.

Well-run and organized freestanding unipurpose units with good working relationships with medical centers may constitute the most cost-effective and qualitatively good situations.

As the long-term care facility becomes essentially a residence that provides necessary clinical and personal care, unit structures and allocation of staff will vary, and patients or residents can be assigned to units based upon their most immediate clinical or physical need. Some residents might be able to go out to work after receiving the needed assistance to get ready. When residents required treatment, they could attend the nursing clinic within the facility, or, if necessary, be transferred to the infirmary for a course of treatment and care.

Such an arrangement would make possible a base rate relevant to room and board charges, with specific charges for nursing or medical care and treatment added when required. With such a system, daily rates for room and board would be constant, while other charges would vary. This could preclude the need to transfer individuals to skilled nursing units when temporarily in need of more intensive nursing services, provide a more efficient use of beds by introducing the element of flexibility, and lead to a more explicit and accurate cost accounting approach to care.

Respite care

The day-care hospitals that can supply needed daily assistance and facilities with beds allocated for respite services to provide relief to the primary care provider or family are other alternatives. These can either defer or avoid nursing home or hospital admission.

Vacation camps for the cognitively or physically impaired who have no active illness not only serve to enhance quality of life but also serve to maintain individuals in the home setting and provide needed relief for the family or care givers.

Allocating costs: How do we pay?

The inability of hospitals and nursing homes (which represent the bulk of long-term care facilities) to identify their specific costs has led to the predetermined payment based on diagnostic-related groups and, in nursing homes, based upon the resource utilization groups. While the prospective payment system presumably discourages abuse, it also encourages overpayment and waste when only minimal services are required.

It is time for us to examine alternative methods for assisting people with the cost of their illness and health care. In my opinion, the practice of reimbursing the institution for services rendered to patients inflates costs and is disadvantageous to the patient, who is seen only as the user and recipient of services rather than the chooser and payer of services. It is the third-party payer the institution is interested in pleasing, not the patient. I think organized nursing must concentrate more of its energies on using its political clout to work for a system in which government pays the health insurance premiums on behalf of the aged and the medically indigent to cover a variety of programs for both health and illness care. Such a system would be similar in principle to a health maintenance organization (HMO), except the insured would be free to choose their own providers. The policies could be underwritten by a number of solid and well-established insurance companies. Companies such as Aetna and Travelers have long-term care policies, but the premium is prohibitive for many. Unlike Medicare, Medicaid, or present hospitalization policies, the payment would go to the insured and the insured would pay the provider.

The American Association of Retired Persons' Health Care America proposal recommends a health insurance access card—"Medicard"—to present to the provider.[3] I am pleased to note that this idea is beginning to gain some attention. I believe that organized nursing would do well to join forces with groups such as this in formulating health care proposals. Self-interest by the profession is important, but attention to the interests of the needy is ultimately in our own best interests. I think we need to concentrate our efforts not on who will be paid for services but how services will be paid.

Rationing care

Unpleasant questions we must still grapple with are the following: Can we afford to offer care indiscriminately to all who seek it? Isn't it time we begin to ration health services? Perhaps we should stop paying for extraordinary care for those whose lives are limited to bed or chair, or to pain and confusion. Perhaps we must refuse to pay for extraordinary measures or any care for those whose illnesses are a direct result of unhealthful behaviors and who refuse to alter that behavior even after they have been warned or advised to change.

If such a course were adopted, then the government or other health insurers would have a moral responsibility to provide for payments for health teaching and health maintenance or behavior modification counseling.

Rationing care could mean that those who could afford to pay for their own health care could receive services despite the rationing. And, if so, would the wealthy then drain the existing services to the extent that those who are eligible for services would not receive them?

We must seek ways to safeguard the quality of care by strengthening moral and ethical codes within the professions, and to police and maintain the integrity of the individuals who practice within each discipline. Peer pressure must be the watchdog for good quality care, not regulations.

Ultimately it all comes down to where and how we want to spend our money and concentrate our resources. We can waste it or spend it wisely.

The cost of long-term care for the aged infirm or permanently impaired will still represent a major chunk of health care expenditures for this society. And, as long as we continue to hire minimally competent personnel, it will cost more than it should. It takes knowledgeable, committed nursing care to bring about quality, cost-effective long-term care.

REFERENCES

1. Highlights of AARP health care American proposal. (1992, March). *AARP Bulletin, 33*(3).
2. Proposed rules. (1992, February 5). *Federal Register, 57*(24).
3. U.S. General Accounting Office. (1983). *Medicaid and nursing home care: Cost increases and the need for services are creating problems for the states and the elderly.* Report to the chairman of the subcommittee on health and the environment, Committee on Energy and Commerce House of Representatives.

CHAPTER 68

Paying for health care

Trends, issues, and future directions

ANN F. COLLARD

Today our health care system is under siege. Three main problems plague the system, forming a trilogy of troubling issues: inadequate access to services, rising costs, and unknown quality. While some may debate the causes of these problems, none will debate their severity nor the resulting widespread concern. As responsible providers of health care, and as interested stakeholders in the system, it is incumbent upon nurses to acquaint themselves with current issues under debate in the health care arena. The purpose of this chapter is to provide a brief overview of health care financing and reimbursement issues. In it I describe health care expenditures and trends, factors associated with rising health care costs, and current financing mechanisms; I also include a description of the uninsured population and who pays for specific health care services. I conclude with several recommendations for the future. Since specific terms and definitions may be unfamiliar to the reader, a glossary of common financing and reimbursement terminology is included, in the appendix to the chapter.

TRENDS IN HEALTH CARE EXPENSES

Health care spending is out of control in the United States. By all measures, the current system is unsustainable and requires radical change in order to prevent eventual system collapse.

Since the 1960s we have witnessed a steady increase in health care spending. According to government figures[13,21] in 1970, the United States spent $74 million dollars on health care—7.3% of the gross national product (GNP). This figure was expected to reach a staggering $809 billion (13.4% of the GNP) during 1992. If the present trend continues, by the year 2000 the United States will spend $1616 billion on health care—16.4% of the GNP.[7] Such unchecked growth cannot continue.

FACTORS ACCOUNTING FOR RISE IN EXPENDITURES

A number of factors have contributed to this unparalleled growth in health care expenditures. Briefly described here, these factors include the financing of health care through the extension of third-party payment through private insurance and public programs; an increase in the relative price of medical services; an aging population; malpractice litigation; burgeoning growth in technologies and an emphasis on high-technology tertiary care; an increase in the supply of trained specialists and hospital beds; a lack of emphasis on prevention and primary care; and rising administrative costs.

Financing

The rise in private insurance for hospital and physician care, which began in the 1950s, effectively reduced the price of care to patients at the time of the illness episode, thus reducing the level of out-of-pocket expenditures. This resulted in an increase in the demand for health care, and research has demonstrated an inverse relationship between demand and price.[12] The Medicare and Medicaid programs were implemented in 1965 under the Johnson administration. These public programs reduced the price of health care to the elderly, the disabled, and the poor and are discussed in more detail later in this chapter.

Relative price increase

The relative price of health care services, compared to other goods, has increased dramatically. Rising wage rates for health care workers partly account for this price increase. For example, between 1963 and 1989 salaries of head nurses rose 76% and those of nursing supervisors rose 63%,[24] far outstripping increases in earnings in other areas such as manufacturing. While price increases may reflect improved quality, the value of that improvement is not accounted for in the price index, and thus the additional expenditure is attributed solely to inflation.[15]

Aging population

Not surprisingly, per capita spending on health care for the elderly is higher than spending for the young, and health care expenditures increase sharply with age.[25] The U.S. population is growing older, and this trend will continue well into the next century,[23] thus further increasing health care spending. Simultaneously, the birth rate has dropped, resulting in the elderly's representing a larger proportion of the entire population than ever before. Increasing life expectancy of the elderly also contributes to increased health expenditures. Today technological advances and improved medical care are extending the lives of people who previously would have died from illnesses. However, large expenditures during the last several years of life are common and account for significant health care spending associated with age.

Medical malpractice litigation

Increasing medical malpractice claims result in rising insurance premiums, which in turn are passed along by health care providers to the consuming public. Some allege that fear of litigation distorts the behavior of physicians, causing them to practice "defensive medicine" by ordering more tests and procedures than are necessary, while others argue that the effect is marginal and that some benefit is derived from the practice of defensive medicine.[20]

Technology

The proliferation of medical technology is another major factor in rising health care costs. The range of diagnostic and therapeutic advances has expanded greatly during the last 20 years. Costs increase as more interventions become available, often replacing previously existing, more invasive therapies. Once these new technologies become available, they are increasingly utilized because they reduce risk to the patient; as this occurs, health care costs are driven higher.

Lack of emphasis on primary care and prevention

Technological advances encourage a greater reliance on expensive tertiary care to the detriment of prevention and primary care. Perverse reimbursement incentives within the system also reinforce such behavior. Since providers are paid according to what they do, it is in their economic best interest as income maximizers to do more. Thus in a traditional fee-for-service model, the more care that is provided, the higher the level of reimbursement. Not surprisingly, this encourages providers to do more. Specialists are typically the providers who prescribe and perform the newest tests, procedures, and surgeries; and the greater the volume, the higher their salary. Thus inequities in income distribution encourage physicians to select the more lucrative specialties; this is a particularly compelling consideration when newly trained physicians are often faced with educational debts exceeding $100,000. As a result, there is a current glut of specialists who typically earn considerably higher salaries than their primary care colleagues.

Finally, a preoccupation with improved technologies and the pursuit of "magic bullets" to fight disease has always been a driving force in the U.S. health care system. Developing and mastering such new technological advances pose new challenges that peak physicians' interest and may provide more intellectual stimulation than primary care areas such as immunization and cholesterol reduction.

Excess capacity of the system

System capacity also affects costs. It is a common axiom of health planning that if a hospital bed exists, providers will strive to fill that bed. The same holds true for technologies. If a hospital purchases a magnetic resonance imaging (MRI) machine, it will utilize that equipment both as a revenue-generating center and as a drawing card to capture market share of patients and providers, even if the need for that technology is not apparent.

Administrative costs

Because our current health care system is comprised of multiple insurers, considerable administrative costs are incurred. Today 24% of health care dollars are spent on administrative costs.[2] Each insurance plan generates its own special form—today there are over 1500 different insurance forms—thus creating a maze of requisite paper work. Since providers must cope with multiple payers, each with their own set of rules and reporting guidelines, the providers are forced to hire more administrative staff so that they can comply with these multiple reporting requirements. Overhead expenses are increased and subsequently passed on to the consumer in the form of higher charges and, ultimately, higher insurance premiums. The potential savings that could be generated (some estimates exceed $100 billion)[2] by streamlining administration are enormous.

FINANCING HEALTH CARE

Today roughly six out of seven Americans have some type of health insurance.[1] Some receive insurance through employer-sponsored plans, while others pay for it themselves or receive it through government-sponsored programs such as Medicare or Medicaid. Payment structures differ enormously, as does the range of benefits that is covered under each policy. Almost all plans cover hospitalization and associated physicians' charges, although the extent of coverage varies. Plans differ in the services covered, payment for a given service, and whether or not the physician can bill the patient for the potential shortfall. A brief overview of the major insurers follows.

Medicare provides health insurance coverage to the elderly and disabled. Because the program is federally sponsored, Medicare benefits do not vary among states. The Medicare program has two parts. Part A, which pays for hospital care and limited nursing home benefits for the elderly and disabled and patients with end-stage renal disease, is financed through a payroll tax. Part B covers the physicians' charges and is primarily financed through federal budget support, with partial financing provided through an annually adjusted premium. Because Medicare covers only a portion of personal health care costs of the elderly—85% of hospital costs and 64% of physicians' services[25]—most beneficiaries purchase supplemental coverage called "medigap" insurance.

Medicaid is a state-administered program that operates under loose federal guidelines. Under Medicaid, states pay for acute care services and long-term care for low-income individuals. Eligibility criteria and benefits vary enormously among states. The federal government provides matching grants—from 50% to 80% of program costs—to states that provide specified benefits to particular populations. Participating states must provide certain benefits to "categorically needy" individuals, including those receiving benefits through the Aid to Families with Dependent Children (AFDC) and supplemental security income (SSI) programs, and the poor blind, aged, and disabled individuals receiving cash assistance. As of July 1, 1990, states also cover pregnant women and young children in families with income and assets low enough to qualify for AFDC, or limited benefits to all pregnant women and mandatory benefits to children under 1 year of age living in families with incomes below the poverty level threshold.[18] Additionally, states have the option to cover "medically needy" individuals. These include anyone covered by AFDC or SSI whose income or assets exceed the eligibility limits for cash assistance but whose income is less than 133.33% of the maximum AFDC payment for families of the same size.

Two thirds of Americans under age 65 and nearly three fourths of employees are covered by employer-sponsored programs.[5] Each private insurance plan has its own limits, and many employers offer more than one plan. Approximately 32.5 million people receive care from health maintenance organizations (HMOs)[11] that provide a stated range of services to an enrolled population on a prepaid, capitation basis. Choice of providers is also restricted in an HMO. Another popular provider option is the preferred provider organization (PPO), which combines limits on cost sharing with restricted choice of providers.[10]

DISTRIBUTION OF PAYMENT FOR HEALTH CARE SERVICES

How is the health care expenditure pie divided? In 1989, hospital spending accounted for nearly half of health care expenditures, and hospitals and physicians taken together accounted for two thirds.[9] While dollars flowing to hospitals rose gradually from 1960 until 1980 and have declined slightly since then, payment to physicians has remained consistent at about 20%.[9] Spending for nursing home care, as a percentage of overall health care spending, more than doubled between 1960 and 1980[9] (4.2% to 9.2%) due to a rise in the population more than 80 years old and the introduction of the Medicaid program, which pays for nursing home care for the aged and disabled poor, in 1965.

The distribution of payment sources also varies according to health care service.[9,17] For example, in 1989, 54% of hospital revenues came from government sources, while private insurance accounted for 41% of hospital revenues and out-of-pocket expenses accounted for only 5% of hospital revenues. In that same year, government sources paid 33% of physician bills, while private insurers accounted for 48% and patients' out-of-pocket expenses accounted for 19%. The government programs also paid for 56% of all payments to nursing homes, while out-of-pocket expenses covered 45%. Private insurance financed only 3% of nursing home care. Finally, the majority of payments for pharmaceuticals were out of pocket (72%), while government programs accounted for 12% of pharmaceutical payments and private insurance accounted for 16%.

THE RISING NUMBER OF UNINSURED

According to the Employee Benefit Research Institute, in 1990 16.6% of the nonelderly population—35.7 million people—did not have private or public health insurance. This figure represents an increase from 34.4 million in 1989 and 33.6 million in 1988.[6] Although some of this increase can be attributed to population growth, the percentage of all Americans who are uninsured increased as well, indicating a real change in insurance status. Among the 35.7 million uninsured, most were working adults (55.7%), while the remainder were nonworking adults and children. Of the uninsured, 85% lived in families headed by workers, and nearly 50% were either self-employed or working in firms with fewer than 25 employees. Nearly 29% of workers in firms with fewer than 25 employees were uninsured in 1990. The number of children who were uninsured in 1990 was 9.8 million, or 15% of all children.

What are the implications of so many Americans having no health insurance? The interaction between health insurance and health status is difficult to interpret. On one hand, individuals who are sick may be unable to work and therefore be ineligible to receive employer-based health care benefits. On the other hand, lack of health insurance may contribute to illness. However, recent research in this area offers disturbing results.[8] Uninsured patients admitted to hospitals were more likely than insured patients to be admitted on weekends, which indicates that the admissions were not discretionary and the patients were seriously ill. Uninsured patients were also less likely to receive specific therapies such as coronary bypass surgery and joint replacement and more likely to have abnormal test results and die in the hospital. While

these results cannot be unequivocally explained on the basis of insurance status alone, the evidence strongly suggests that lack of insurance makes a significant difference not only in therapies provided but also in outcomes of treatment for the uninsured.

THE STATE OF AMERICAN HEALTH CARE

Although the United States spends more per capita on health care than any other country, among developed countries we have only an average life expectancy rate and a much higher than average infant mortality rate.[19] Admittedly, these measures represent crude indicators of health status. However, they do provide a method for comparing selected outcomes across countries. Our disappointing outcomes coupled with high costs lead many observers to conclude that U.S. health care spending is misdirected. According to the Centers for Disease Control, while the United States recorded its lowest infant mortality rate ever in 1989 (the most recent year for which we have statistics), black babies still die at more than twice the rate of whites, and the nation trails much of the developed world in this regard. The leading cause of death for white infants has been birth defects; for black infants it has been prematurity or low birth weight. While the white infant mortality rate dropped 4% from 1988 to 1989, the black rate increased slightly, indicating an even greater disparity between blacks and whites.[26]

Overall consumer satisfaction with the U.S. health care system could also be improved. In a recent survey[16] of randomly selected adults, despite high levels of satisfaction with their own medical care and their own insurance programs, Americans tended to rate the overall health care system unfavorably. While 54% of Americans rated the U.S. health care system as either fair or poor, only 7.9% rated it as excellent. Also, three quarters of all Americans supported adoption of some form of national health care system, and over half of all Americans said they would support a national health care system even if it meant increasing taxes.

Many consider health care reform to be the major social issue of the 1990s. For many reasons, the major stakeholders in the system—hospitals, physicians, businesses, and consumers—are becoming increasingly dissatisfied with the current system. For nearly a century federal lawmakers have debated the pros and cons of national health insurance. The debate focuses on four main issues: whether health insurance should be voluntary or compulsory; how costs would be distributed between the public and private sectors; how the program would be financed; and finally, whether spending should be controlled through market forces or government regulation or a combination of both.[22]

While interest and activity in this area have heated up during the last years, consensus concerning a course of action still does not exist. Currently there are several models of health care reform that are being proposed. These include a universal health care plan modeled on the Canadian system; a "play or pay" program that would require employers to provide minimum health care coverage to all employees or pay new taxes to finance a government-run plan; a tax credit of up to $3750 a year for low-income families and deductions for the middle class with the goal of helping many of the uninsured purchase basic health insurance; a consumer choice model that would provide a tax credit allowing individuals to purchase health insurance on their own or through employers; and finally, a managed competition model in which employers would have to offer, and workers would be required to join, one of several comprehensive health plans.

WHERE DO WE GO FROM HERE?

There is a broad consensus that we spend too much on health care, but what is less clear is how much we *should* spend and *for what* services. It is imperative that the strong voice of nursing be represented at the health care discussion table. There may not be one definitive answer for solving the health care crisis. Rather, it is likely that health care reform will require a hybrid approach that will be implemented incrementally. However, we can identify important questions to be answered: What benefits should be covered and for whom? What services should comprise a basic health care package? And how will access to technology be controlled?

Some states have already started to grapple with these questions. For example, while many may disagree with its approach to rationing health care, Oregon did take on the difficult challenge of attempting to define what the state would and would not pay for. Nursing was present in this decision-making process. While Oregon and others propose rationing health care, I believe that *rationing basic health care services is not necessary.* However, I also believe that more rational allocation of existing resources is urgently required. In the remaining paragraphs of this chapter, I offer suggestions for incrementally improving the U.S. health care system.

In any discussion of reforming the U.S. health care system, the example of Canada inevitably arises. Some suggest that the United States should emulate the Canadian health care system. I believe that this system has several important strengths—it provides primary health care to all its citizens and it uses only one universal administrative form. However, it has serious shortcomings in other important areas that I believe limit its broad appeal in the United States.

For example, the average American does not want to wait 6 to 12 months for a surgical procedure, even if the problem is not life threatening in nature. Nor would the average American be comfortable with requiring a child needing open-heart surgery to wait for extended periods of time to have this life-saving surgery. The existence of queues for such special procedures is an apparent reality in Canada today. Because supply may not always match demand, Canadians, who can afford to do so, travel across the U.S. border to obtain these services more expeditiously.

Americans are unaccustomed to waiting for extended periods of time to obtain services that they want and need. We believe that the American way dictates that if your child requires heart surgery, you should not be denied access to that procedure for any reason—even if you are poor. For these reasons, I believe that Americans are not likely to embrace a health care system that is philosophically different from our own. Also, Americans fundamentally see themselves as "innovators"—not "imitators" of other countries' programs.

However, this does not mean that there are not valuable lessons that can be learned from the experience of other countries. One such lesson is how to reduce our administrative costs. The potential for savings in this area alone is enormous, and the savings generated through streamlining and improving efficiency could pay for important health care services such as prenatal care for all women.

As is the case in Canada, I also believe that the U.S. health care system should provide a *basic package* of health care services to which all citizens are entitled. This package should include services that we *know* make a difference in the quality of individuals' health status such as immunizations, prenatal care, and other primary health services including programs for smoking cessation and weight control, and vigilant monitoring of chronic illnesses such as hypertension, diabetes, and glaucoma. While it is not realistic to believe that our system can provide *all* services to *all* people, it is shameful that in a country such as ours more than 35 million people have been allowed to fall through the cracks of our health care system and are denied access to basic health care services. It is time for our nation to make the provision of basic health care services to all citizens a priority of the highest order.

However, providing basic services is not the entire solution to our health care crisis. We must also redirect our resources to pay for what really works. Until recently we did not have a reliable handle on what works in health care and what doesn't work because little research focused on outcomes of treatment. However, there is a visible shift in priorities in Washington toward conducting outcomes and effectiveness research that indicates this is no longer the case. The Agency for Health Care Policy and Research (AHCPR) is the government's arm for general health services research, including outcomes and effectiveness research. The shift in priorities for the government emerged from a growing body of research that indicated that as much as one fourth of all medical care provided today may be unnecessary and that a substantial number of procedures are unnecessary or of little value.[4,27] Creation of the AHCPR provides a home base for determining what really works and also for answering the growing concern about the quality of care provided under Medicare and Medicaid. Although the process for conducting such research is rigorous and some critics believe it takes too long, it offers the most promising approach to appropriate allocation of our resources.

Outcomes research will also enable us not only to identify the centers of excellence (and those centers whose outcomes are unacceptable), but also to develop standards against which to compare outcomes of treatment at various institutions. For virtually every other product that consumers purchase (the majority of which cost far less than health care), consumers have access to information that will assist them in assessing the quality of that product. Remarkably, to date, this has not been the case in health care—but it should be. For example, as educated consumers of health care, we deserve to know the "batting average" of a specific surgeon performing a specific procedure at a given hospital before we go to that hospital. And the system should reward, by authorizing payment, only those centers that perform adequately against an accepted standard of practice. If a hospital operates at a consistently low capacity and its staff members do not perform specific procedures in sufficient quantity to remain proficient, then that institution should not receive reimbursement

for performing those procedures until its batting average improves.

I also believe we can make other changes in the health care system that will improve care and ration the use of precious resources. For example, there needs to be a more equitable distribution of income among physicians. Physicians should be reimbursed so that they are rewarded for thinking and not just doing. We need to pay primary care physicians more and specialists less, thus reducing the tremendous income disparity between these providers. Medicare has moved in this direction through the development of the resource-based relative value scale (RBRVS). This system pays physicians based on the resources required to provide the service, and it is likely that private insurers will follow this trend.

Physicians should also be reimbursed fairly for providing services to poor patients. While the topic of physician salaries stirs up considerable emotion, physicians actually lose money providing health care to some patients. Such is frequently the case with Medicaid patients. The tremendous paperwork requirement, coupled with grossly inadequate reimbursement levels, makes many physicians think twice about serving this population. In practices where there are sufficient caseloads of other patients with private insurance, some of these shortfalls can be cross-subsidized. However, in practices comprised primarily of Medicaid patients, this ability to cross-subsidize does not exist. Thus the reimbursement system itself becomes a barrier to access to health care for the Medicaid population, who may have no other option except to seek care at a significantly more expensive tertiary care center emergency room.

We can reduce health care spending by protecting physicians who adhere to acceptable standards of practice (and have the equivalent of "safe driving records") from unfair malpractice charges. Medicine is an art as well as a science. Human errors are made and a positive outcome cannot be guaranteed in all instances. For those cases with negative outcomes, a risk pool should be established to appropriately compensate patients for their pain and suffering. In cases of negligent practice, appropriate awards to patients should be set depending on the extent of the loss, and the percentage of the award accruing to the attorney should be capped. The threat of being sued has forced physicians to practice "defensive medicine," which encourages them to order unnecessary tests and procedures that drive up health care costs.

Finally, we should utilize nurses more effectively within the health care system. Despite their considerable expertise in many areas, nurses are underutilized in the health care arena. Although making up the largest group of providers of health care, nurses have long suffered under the monopolistic practice of physicians despite compelling evidence that they offer cost-effective alternatives to traditional medical care. In study after study, nurses working in expended practice roles as midwives, nurse anesthetists, clinical specialists, and nurse practitioners have demonstrated that they provide safe and effective care to patients, often at lower cost than their physician counterparts. In fact, during the 1980s, it was the preoccupation with reducing costs that fueled the support for non-physician health care providers. However, the pricing factor will be less important in the future because the new RBRVS physician payment system will pay "equal value for equal service." This means that nurses and physicians performing the same task will be paid the same rate, thus removing the distinction based on credentials.[3]

Today nurses must maximize their visibility to consumers, who are frequently their greatest allies. In a national study conducted in 1990,[14] nurses far outshone any other medical personnel in the minds of patients. Of the respondents, 77% felt that nurses played a valued and constructive role in health care, compared with only 42% who felt the same about physicians. It is time to acknowledge that if nurses were utilized to their fullest potential and were reimbursed according to the services they provide, patients would surely benefit. If nurses could practice all the skills they have learned both inside and outside hospitals, it could profoundly change the shape of health care in this country.

APPENDIX: GLOSSARY OF REIMBURSEMENT TERMS

Aid to Families with Dependent Children (AFDC)

A program of income support for low-income families that was established by Title 4 of the Social Security Act.

access The ability to obtain needed medical care.

ambulatory visit groups (AVGs) Analogous to DRGs for acute hospital care, a system for classifying ambulatory visits for the purpose of reimbursement.

assignment The process in which an enrollee agrees to assign benefit rights to the provider, who agrees to accept as the total charge for the covered service the amount that is approved by the carrier as the reasonable charge. The provider may then charge the enrollee only for the coinsurance and unmet deductible.

balance bill The portion of the physician's charge that exceeds the allowable charge.

beneficiary A person eligible for benefits under an insurance plan.

benefit period The period used to limit benefits in the Medicare hospital insurance program.

bundling The use of a single payment for a group of related services.

capitation A health insurance payment mechanism in which a fixed amount is paid per person to cover services over a period of time; a fixed per capita payment.

case mix The illness severity among a group of patients.

categorically needy Under Medicaid, those aged, blind, or disabled individuals or families and children who meet financial eligibility requirements for AFDC, supplemental security income, or an optional state supplement.

charge The bill that is generated for a given service and submitted for payment to an insurer or individual (e.g., the charge for a computerized tomography [CT] scan). A charge may be different from a cost.

coinsurance The percentage of the balance of covered medical expenses that a beneficiary must pay after payment of the deductible.

copayment The sum of coinsurance and deductibles; alternatively, a fixed dollar amount per service that is the responsibility of the beneficiary.

cost The real expense that is incurred in providing a given service (e.g., the true cost to the institution of providing a CT scan).

cost sharing The portion of payment for health expenses that the beneficiary must pay, including copayments (deductibles and coinsurance) and balance bills.

cost shifting A situation in which a health care provider compensates for the effect of decreased revenue from one payer by increasing charges to another payer.

covered services Services and supplies for which the insurer will reimburse.

customary, prevailing, and reasonable (CPR) The method of paying physicians under Medicare from 1965 until January 1992. Payment for a service was lim-

---

Modified from: Physician Payment Review Commission. (1992). *Annual report to Congress* (pp. 363-374); and (1990). *Medicaid and Medicare Data Book: Health care financing program statistics* (pp. 129-133).

ited to the lowest of (1) the physician's billed charge for the service, (2) the physician's customary charge for the service, or (3) the prevailing charge for that service in the community. This is similar to the usual, customary, and reasonable system used by private insurers.

deductible A specified amount of covered medical expenses that a beneficiary must pay before receiving benefits.

diagnostic-related groups (DRGs) A system of classifying patients on the basis of diagnoses for purposes of payment to hospitals.

direct cost The labor, supply, and equipment costs directly attributable to the provision of a specific service.

fee for service A system of paying physicians for individual medical services rendered, as opposed to paying them salaries or capitation payments.

fee schedule A list of predetermined payments for units of medical service.

gaming Gaining advantage by using improper means to evade the letter or intent of a rule or system.

global service A package of clinically related services treated as a unit for purposes of billing, coding, or payment.

Group HMO An HMO that pays a medical group a negotiated per capita rate, which the group distributes among its physicians, usually on a salaried arrangement.

health maintenance organization (HMO) A prepaid organized health care plan. Individuals are enrolled in the plan, and services are provided through a system of affiliated providers. Comprehensive benefits are financed by prepaid premiums with limited copayments.

independent practice association (IPA) An HMO that contracts with individual physicians to provide services to HMO members at a negotiated per capita or fee-for-service rate. In this model, physicians maintain their own offices and can contract with other HMOs and see other fee-for-service patients.

indirect cost Those costs that cannot be easily traced to particular services, but that must be assigned using explicit accounting methods; sometimes referred to as common or overhead costs.

Medicaid A joint federal-state program of federal matching grants to the states to provide health insurance for categories of the poor and medically indigent. Individual states determine eligibility, payments, and benefits consistent with federal standards.

medically needy Under Medicaid, those aged, blind, or disabled individuals or families and children whose income resources are above the limits for eligibility as categorically needy but who, after deduction of incurred

medical expenses, fall within limits set under the Medicaid state plan and therefore become eligible for Medicaid benefits.

Medicare fee schedule The resource-based fee schedule used by Medicare to pay for physicians' services.

medigap insurance Private health insurance policies designed to supplement Medicare coverage. Benefits may include payment of Medicare deductibles, coinsurance, and balance bills, and payment for services not covered by Medicare.

outcome The consequence of a medical intervention on a patient.

outcomes and effectiveness research Medical or health services research that attempts to identify the clinical outcomes (including mortality, morbidity, and functional status) of the delivery of health care.

paid amount The portion of a submitted charge that is actually paid, by either third-party payers or the insured, including copayments and balance bills.

pass-through amounts The costs such as capital, direct medical education, and organ procurement that are reimbursed by Medicare on a reasonable cost basis and are "passed through" directly to the hospitals on a periodic (e.g., quarterly) basis apart from the payments for actual medical care for Medicare beneficiaries.

preferred provider organization (PPO) A financing arrangement in which networks of panels of providers agree to furnish services and be paid on a negotiated fee schedule. Enrollees are offered a financial incentive to use doctors on the preferred list.

premium An amount paid periodically to purchase medical insurance benefits.

prevailing charge One of the screens that determined a physician's payment for a service under the Medicare CPR payment system; it was the 75th percentile of customary charges, with annual updates limited by the Medicare Economic Index (MEI).

professional component The part of a relative value or fee that represents the cost of a physician's interpretation of a diagnostic test or treatment planning for a therapeutic procedure.

prospective payment system (PPS) The Medicare system used to pay hospitals for inpatient hospital services based on the DRG classification system.

reasonable charge The lowest of the actual charge billed by the physician, the charge the physician or supplier customarily bills for the same service, or the prevailing charge.

reasonable cost Prior to the institution of the Medicare prospective payment system, the payment mechanism for hospital care that was constructed retrospectively and was based on criteria applied to direct and indirect costs.

relative value A value that reflects a comparison to an arbitrary standard.

relative value scale (RVS) An index that assigns weights to each medical service; the weights represent the relative amount to be paid for each service. (The RVS used in the development of the Medicare fee schedule consists of three cost components: physician work, practice expense, and malpractice expense.)

resource-based relative value scale (RBRVS) A relative value scale that is based on resources involved in providing a service.

spend-down A method by which an individual establishes Medicaid eligibility by reducing gross income through incurring medical expenses until net income (after medical expenses) meets Medicaid financial requirements.

submitted charge The actual charge submitted to the patient or insurer.

supplemental security income (SSI) A program of income support for low-income aged, blind, and disabled persons that was established by Title 16 of the Social Security Act.

tort reforms Efforts to change the procedural or substantive rules for malpractice claims in the court system (e.g., reductions in statutes of limitations, limits on attorneys' contingency fees, and caps on settlements).

upcode To bill for a service that is paid at a higher rate than the actual service provided.

REFERENCES

1. Aaron, H. (1991). *Serious and unstable condition: Financing America's health care.* Washington, D.C.: Brookings Institution.
2. A conversation with C. Everett Koop, MD (1992). *Business and Health, 10*(3), 55–56.
3. Bradley, P. (1991, September). Physician payment: Why it matters to nurses. *American Nurse, 8.*
4. Brook, J., & Vaiana, M. (1989, June). *Appropriateness of care: A chart book.* Report prepared for the national health policy forum, George Washington University, Washington, D.C.
5. Employee Benefit Research Institute. (1990, July). *Issue Brief Number 104.*
6. Employee Benefit Research Institute. (1992, February). *Issue Brief Number 123.*
7. Faltermayer, E. (1992, March 23). Let's really cure the health care system. *Fortune Magazine,* p. 47.
8. Hadley, J., Steinberg, E., & Feder, J. (1991, January 16). Comparison of uninsured and privately insured hospital patients: Condition on admission, resource use, and outcome. *Journal of the American Medical Association, 265*(3), 374-379.
9. *Health and Human Services News.* (1990, December 20).
10. Health Insurance Association of America. (1990). *Providing employee health benefits: How firms differ: Results of a 1989 national survey of employers* (p. 49). Washington, D.C.: Author.
11. Health Insurance Association of America. (1990). *Source book of health insurance data* (p. 31). Washington, D.C.: Author.
12. Keller, E., & Rolph, J. (1988). The demand for episodes of treatment in the health insurance experiment. *Journal of Health Economics, 7,* 263-277.
13. Levit, K., Lazenby, H., Cowan, C., & Letsch, S. (1991). National health expenditures, 1990. *Health Care Financing Review, 13*(1), 16.
14. *National survey commissioned by Nurses of America.* (1990).
15. Newhouse, J. (1989). Measuring medical prices and understanding their effects: The Baxter Foundation prize address. *Journal of Health Administration Education, 7,* 24.
16. Novalis Corporation. (1992, January). *The state of American healthcare.* Unpublished survey.
17. Office of National Cost Estimates. (1990). National health expenditures, 1988. *Health Care Financing Review, 11,*(4), 26–28.
18. Rovner, J. (1990, November 3). Families gain help from Hill on child care and Medicaid. *Congressional Quarterly Weekly Report,* p. 3721.
19. Schieber, G., & Poullier, J. P. (1989). Overview of international expenditures. *Health Care Financing Review* [Annual Supplement], pp. 1–9.
20. Sloan, F., Bovberg, R., & Githens, P. (1992). *Insuring medical malpractice.* New York: Oxford University Press.
21. Sonnefield, S., Waldo, D., Lemieux, J., & McKusick, D. (1991). Projections of national health expenditures through the year 2000. *Health Care Financing Review, 13*(1), 46.
22. Thorpe, K. (1991). The national health insurance conundrum: Shifting paradigms and potential solutions. *Journal of American Health Policy, 1,* 17.
23. U.S. Department of Health and Human Services. (1989, June). *Social security area population projections: 1989* (Actuarial Study 105), p. 14.
24. U.S. Department of Labor, Bureau of Labor Statistics. (1989, March). *Industry wage survey: Hospitals, United States and selected metropolitan areas.* Unpublished survey.
25. Waldo, D., Sonnefeld, S., McKusick, D., & Arnett, R. (1989). Health expenditures by age group, 1977 and 1987. *Health Care Financing Review, 10,* 111-120.
26. *The Wall Street Journal.* (1992, February 7).
27. Wennberg, J. (1990, October 25). Outcomes research, cost containment, and the fear of health care rationing. *New England Journal of Medicine,* pp. 1202-1204.

CHAPTER 69

The costs of safety precautions to reduce risk of exposure to bloodborne pathogens

DIANA C. McPHERSON, MARGUERITE M. JACKSON

It has long been recognized that health care workers (HCWs) are at risk for a variety of bloodborne infections, but the epidemic of human immunodeficiency virus–acquired immunodeficiency syndrome (HIV-AIDS) has brought this issue to the forefront.

In late 1986 several labor unions petitioned the Occupational Safety and Health Administration (OSHA) to establish emergency regulations to mandate health care employers to provide a variety of safety measures for health care workers. OSHA did not agree to the emergency regulations, but it did initiate a rule-making process that culminated in the publication of the OSHA bloodborne pathogens standard on December 6, 1991.[26] The standard marked the completion of more than 4 years of work by OSHA and verbal and written testimony by thousands of health care professionals, labor union representatives, and members of a concerned public. In 1987 when the standard was first proposed, there was a great deal of emphasis on barriers, such as gloves, gowns, masks, and protective eyewear as safety measures; however, as the standard evolved, it became apparent that other strategies were much more likely to reduce bloodborne pathogen risks to HCWs.[18]

WHAT ARE SAFETY PRECAUTIONS?

Safety precautions for bloodborne pathogens include a variety of strategies that are intended to reduce or eliminate the risk of exposure of health care workers or patients to potentially infectious biological agents.

Using the traditional industrial hygiene approach, the risk reduction hierarchy of controls is as follows: (1) engineering controls (design out the problem), (2) work practice controls (modify the behavior), and (3) personal protective equipment (barriers).

Engineering controls are controls that isolate or remove the bloodborne pathogen hazard from the workplace. Examples include sharps disposal containers, self-sheathing needles, and needle-free intravenous access devices.

Work practice controls are modifications in procedures that reduce the likelihood of exposure by altering the manner in which a task is performed. Examples include using a one-handed recapping technique for used needles; requiring any person (whether nurse, physician, or technician) who uses a sharp to discard it into a sharps disposal container immediately after use; providing adequate lighting for tasks involving sharps; and lifting all bags of trash and linen so that they are always away from the body in case a sharp has been incorrectly discarded into the bag.

Personal protective equipment is specialized clothing or equipment worn by an employee for protection against a hazard. Examples include gloves, gowns, masks, eye protection, and devices that permit resuscitation without mouth-to-mouth contact.

Universal precautions are an approach to infection prevention and control that was developed by the Centers for Disease Control[9,10] in 1987 to 1988. Universal precautions treat all human blood and certain body fluids as if they are infectious for hepatitis B virus (HBV), human immunodeficiency virus, or other bloodborne pathogens. Universal precautions do not apply to feces, nasal secretions, saliva, sputum, sweat, tears, urine, or vomitus (unless they contain visible blood) because these body substances have not been associated epidemiologically with transmission of bloodborne pathogens. The OSHA standard applies only to blood and body fluids to which universal precautions apply. That is, other body substances are not *regulated* under the standard.

There is little evidence to support the effectiveness of universal precautions in preventing bloodborne infections in health care workers.[13] Universal precautions have their origins in traditional isolation techniques intended to reduce risks of cross-transmission of organisms between and among patients and personnel.[5,7] The primary strategy for traditional isolation techniques is the wearing of personal protective equipment, especially gloves, gowns, and masks. In 1987 the Centers for Disease Control responded to increasing concern of health care workers about bloodborne diseases by recommending that the precautions outlined in the 1983 isolation category "blood and body fluid precautions" be used consistently for all patients rather than only for those patients in whom a bloodborne infection had been diagnosed or was suspected. They titled these new recommendations "universal precautions" or "universal blood and body fluid precautions."[9] Originally these precautions also applied to all blood and body fluids (feces, urine, saliva, etc.) but in 1988 were modified to *exclude* those body substances that had not been associated epidemiologically with transmission of bloodborne pathogens.[10] Universal precautions recommend specific precautions to be taken with soiled linen, trash, and used sharps, as well as a comprehensive postexposure management strategy for persons experiencing mucous membrane, parenteral, or nonintact skin exposures to blood or body fluids. Universal precautions also emphasize the importance of hepatitis B immunization, employee education and training, and monitoring for compliance. *Engineering controls and work practice modifications are not strongly emphasized in isolation precautions because the intent is to use a barrier to interrupt transmission of organisms from one person to another.*

An important aspect of universal precautions, as defined by the Centers for Disease Control, is that they must be combined with another strategy of precautions intended to reduce risks of infection of patients and HCWs with other types of biological agents. Thus health care agencies are faced with the dilemma of implementing universal precautions for everyone, based on taking specific precautions with certain body fluids of all patients, while also implementing another isolation system. The traditional isolation systems commonly in use involve assigning a patient to a category of isolation (category-specific isolation precautions) or using specific barriers based on the diagnosis or suspected diagnosis of a particular disease in the patient (disease-specific isolation precautions). Thus

one system expects HCWs to act the same for all patients when handling blood or certain body fluids, while the other system expects HCWs to act with caution only when caring for patients with diagnosed or suspected diagnosed infections caused by other infectious agents. This leads to considerable confusion!

Many health care agencies have elected to consider *all* blood and body substances as potentially infectious because infectious agents other than HIV, HBV, and bloodborne pathogens may be transmitted by feces, urine, saliva, sputum, vomitus, wound, and other drainage. This broader strategy of generic infection precautions has been named body substance isolation (BSI)[14,15,17,21,22] and is also called body substance precautions, universal body substance precautions, or a variety of other names. When evaluated, body substance isolation has proved to be much easier to teach and implement than a combination of other strategies. In addition, its primary purpose is to reduce risks of cross-transmission of organisms among and between patients, with the secondary benefit of reducing risks to health care workers.[4,16,19,20,25]

COSTS OF SAFETY PRECAUTIONS

There are a variety of ways to calculate costs for safety precautions. Costs are incurred when vaccines are administered, tests are performed, supplies are purchased, and treatment and follow-up for exposures are prescribed. These costs are usually referred to as direct costs. Direct costs attributable to safety programs also include the salaries and benefits for personnel who provide training, monitor for compliance, and provide the services of postexposure follow-up. In addition, the costs of space to provide the services and equipment needed to maintain the office (e.g., computers and telephones) are also measurable costs.

Indirect costs include the cost of illness incurred primarily due to lack of implementation of risk reduction strategies. Indirect costs include decreased earnings resulting from lost time from work and lost wages due to premature death or disability from occupational illness or injury.

Cost savings from prevention of avoidable injuries, exposures, infections, and illnesses are difficult to measure. Although it is possible to measure the costs of providing prevention services (e.g., the personnel, space, and equipment for an employee health service and a hospital epidemiology unit), it is not possible to directly assess savings from an infection prevented in either a patient or an employee. McPherson, Jackson, and Rogers[23] stated it well:

What is it worth to a worker *not* to get an infection? We can measure the cost of hepatitis B vaccine and the compliance rate. We cannot measure the value of life lost due to hepatitis B because the worker failed to get hepatitis B vaccine. What does it cost to provide other prevention strategies to reduce worker risk? How well do they work? Again, because the outcomes (infections in workers) are so rare, it is nearly impossible to measure a before-and-after change in worker infection rates.

It is also difficult to measure the positive effects of educational programs about safety. Common strategies include pre- and post-test measurement of knowledge of the information presented, but observation of behavior change is rarely done because of the costs of the labor required for such observational evaluations. Nonetheless, when observational studies have been done,[20] it has been clearly shown that education and monitoring for compliance can have a positive effect on employee behavior.

The Occupational Safety and Health Administration[26] included costs of compliance in their rule-making process. Annualized costs of compliance were estimated in association with the following components of the standard:

$ 97,523,109	Engineering and work practice controls
106,710,705	Vaccination and postexposure follow-up
32,587,446	Exposure control plan
101,937,270	Housekeeping
326,877,357	Personal protective equipment
134,405,018	Training
17,253,151	Record keeping
$812,703,560	Total

OSHA also estimates that there are 5,576,026 health care workers in the United States to whom the OSHA standard will apply. This means that the annualized cost per health care worker for compliance with the standard is $145.75. Of the affected health care worker population, 68% is employed in hospitals, physicians' offices, dentists' offices, and nursing facilities (nursing homes). These settings also represent about half of all affected establishments. Other settings where the standard applies include medical and dental labs, residential and hospice facilities, home health agencies, drug rehabilitation centers, hemodialysis centers, government and industry clinics, blood-plasma-tissue centers, and sites performing personnel services for temporary

help, funeral services, medical equipment repair services, and linen services. Also affected are public service workers in law enforcement, fire and rescue, correctional facilities, lifesaving, schools, and waste removal.

The cost of providing personal protective equipment is clearly one of the major expenses of implementing the OSHA standard. Several years before implementation of the standard, McPherson, Jackson, and Rogers[23] evaluated the cost of supplies associated with implementation of the body substance isolation system at a large teaching hospital. The system was fully in place by May of 1987. In this study of changes in supply costs before, during, and after implementation of the BSI system, we found that about 80% of the costs were for nonsterile gloves. Glove use, estimated on a per patient per day basis, increased from 7.8 pairs per patient per day before implementation to 15.7 pairs per patient per day when the system was fully implemented. The use of gloves in the BSI system is primarily intended to reduce risks of cross-transmission of organisms between and among patients, and secondarily to reduce risks to health care workers. The positive effect of appropriate use of gloves in reducing risks of cross-transmission between and among patients as evaluated by Lynch and co-workers[20] was evidenced by a measurable decline in the frequency of certain marker organisms during and after implementation of the BSI system at their large teaching hospital.

Several investigators have evaluated the costs of supplies associated with implementation of the Centers for Disease Control's universal precautions.[9,10] Doebbeling and Wenzel[12] studied the direct costs of universal precautions in a large teaching hospital by calculating costs per patient admission. Costs increased from $13.70 to $22.89 per admission after implementation of universal precautions. Two thirds of the increase was due to the cost of nonsterile gloves. Extrapolating the data to all U.S. hospitals for fiscal year 1989, they estimated total costs to be at least $336 million. This is very close to the $322 million estimated for hospitals by OSHA.[26]

Stock, Gafni, and Bloch[24] conducted an economic analysis of universal precautions in a large hospital in Canada. They estimated the incremental cost of implementing universal precautions to be about $315,000 for their hospital for 1 year. Using these data combined with estimates of the low frequency of occupationally acquired HIV infection among health care workers, they estimated that more than $8 million

Table 69-1 Estimated cost per dose for hepatitis B vaccine*

Element of cost	Time involved per dose (min)	Cost per dose ($)
Vaccine	—	$37.00
Supplies, forms, immunization record, etc.	—	1.00
Nurse practitioner: salary = $24/hour; benefits (25%) = $6/hour[†]	10	5.00
Practical nurse: salary = $12/hour; benefits (25%) = $3/hour[‡]	10	2.50
Clerk: salary = $9/hour; benefits (25%) = $2.25/hour[§]	12	2.25
TOTALS	32	47.75

*Estimated costs of administering a single dose of hepatitis B vaccine to a health care worker in an employee health service of a health care facility in a metropolitan area on the West Coast of the United States. This estimate does not include overhead costs such as space, computers for scheduling and data management, refrigerator space for storage of vaccine, and physician backup for the nurse practitioner. These additional overhead costs for administration of hepatitis B vaccine by a private physician's office can add an additional 40% to 60% to the overall cost per dose, making it $75/dose or more.

[†]Nurse practitioner functions: Medical evaluation, interview for contraindications, record completion (including consent) consistent with requirements of OSHA. Note: Nurse practitioner may not need to see employee for second and third doses; initial intake may take longer than 10 minutes; employees may call nurse practitioner for questions before or during vaccine series.

[‡]Practical nurse functions: Preparation and administration of vaccine, completion of immunization record for medical record and for employee, blood drawing for postvaccine screening (if requested by employee or nurse practitioner).

[§]Clerk functions: Scheduling of initial and subsequent appointments, data entry into employee health data base, pulling and refiling medical records, completion of other forms as required by agency, reordering vaccine from supplier.

would be spent to prevent one case of HIV seroconversion. *These costs are well above the usual amount our society spends on prevention of death from any other disease.* Most importantly, Stock, Gafni, and Bloch concluded that the universal precautions implemented in their hospital were neither efficacious nor cost effective if their purpose was to prevent bloodborne infections in health care workers. However, they noted that the impact of universal precautions on nosocomial infections in patients may be the most appropriate and effective measure of their usefulness. Proponents of the BSI system have made this point consistently since 1987.[16,17,21]

McPherson, Jackson, and Rogers[23] and Stock, Gafni, and Bloch[24] suggested that rather than placing emphasis on barriers that have little proved efficacy in reducing risks of HIV infection or HBV infection, prevention strategies should focus on those circumstances where risk is greatest: puncture injuries. *Strategies to reduce these risks primarily include engineering controls to reduce risks from needles and other sharp equipment, and work practice modifications in the use of sharp devices.*

HEPATITIS B AND HEPATITIS B VACCINATION

Thousands of HCWs have been infected with hepatitis B over the years, and HCWs are a primary target for the hepatitis B vaccine, first licensed in the United States in 1982. A number of studies have quantified the risk of hepatitis B infection from a single needle puncture to be between 6% and 30%;[8] yet as recently as 1990, researchers at the Centers for Disease Control estimated that fewer than half of all at-risk HCWs had been immunized against hepatitis B.[1] The Occupational Safety and Health Administration bloodborne pathogens standard[26] mandates that employers provide the vaccine at no expense to the employee, beginning in 1992. It is anticipated that this action will increase the proportion of HCWs protected against hepatitis B. The costs for this safety measure are variable, ranging from $40 to $75 per dose or more. To be fully protected, each employee should receive the three-dose series; some will need a fourth dose. Table 69-1 presents an estimate of cost per dose for hepatitis B vaccine that can be applied generally to this issue.

HUMAN IMMUNODEFICIENCY VIRUS AND POSTEXPOSURE MANAGEMENT

The first case of occupational transmission of HIV to a HCW was reported in England in 1984.[2] Since that time 14 studies have enrolled about 2000 HCWs at the time of an HIV exposure and followed them for at least 90 days up to more than 1 year after the exposure.[3] In these studies through 1990, six HCWs were reported to have seroconverted, for a seroconversion rate of 0.32% or about 1 chance in 300. All of these exposures were percutaneous; none of the subjects in the studies have seroconverted from mucous membrane or nonintact skin exposures. There are also case reports of HIV-infected HCWs identified in prevalence surveys or as incidental findings when blood was tested for other reasons (e.g., for blood donation). By April 1990, 27 documented seroconversions had been reported in the medical literature or to the Centers for Disease Control, including the 6 seroconversions in the 14 studies.[3] When the routes of exposure were evaluated, 22 of 27 were found to have resulted from percutaneous exposures (punctures or cuts). Mucous membrane or cutaneous exposures were implicated in the 5 remaining cases. Almost all of the cases (25 of 27) were associated with blood or a body fluid containing visible blood; the other cases were in laboratory workers exposed to concentrated virus. In many of these cases, it is difficult to be certain that the only exposure is an occupational one. In addition, because there are many workers' compensation issues, including financial compensation, that are associated with attribution of an illness or injury to the workplace, case reports must be evaluated with caution.

Postexposure management for HIV exposures is variable, largely because of the controversy about whether or not azidothymidine (AZT), zidovudine or retrovir, should be offered as a prophylaxis. Although it is not yet clear whether or not AZT administration will prevent HIV infection in health care workers, it is clear that if it is to be of any value, it must be initiated as soon as possible after the exposure event. Guidelines for administration of AZT have been published by the Centers for Disease Control.[11] Table 69-2 presents estimated costs for postexposure management of exposures to HIV with and without the costs of AZT. Because AZT administration requires laboratory testing at several intervals, as well as purchase of the drug itself, the overall postexposure costs with AZT are considerably higher than those without AZT.

It is also important to realize that even if engineering and work practice controls result in a reduction in the number of needle puncture injuries, it is unlikely that the personnel required to run programs for employee health, hospital epidemiology, and postexposure follow-up can be eliminated from the payroll. The major costs for these programs are personnel costs (salaries and benefits). Accordingly, the principal direct cost savings from reducing the numbers of puncture injuries will be costs of laboratory tests and drugs (e.g., AZT). A benefit of fewer injuries to employee health programs is that if fewer HCWs need to be seen for postexposure management, the time saved can be used by program personnel to provide health promotion and disease prevention services and perform other activities usually relegated to less important time slots than acute and follow-up management of injuries. In other words, if there are fewer injuries to care for, the program manager might be able to get "caught up" on his or her other responsibilities!

USING DATA TO REDUCE INJURY-EXPOSURE RISKS

What kind of a price tag does an agency put on disease prevention when measured against the bottom line? One consideration is regulatory requirements. That is, the agency has no choice but to comply with the OSHA bloodborne pathogens standard.[26] Other federal agencies, such as the Food and Drug Administration and the Centers for Disease Control, can also have considerable influence on decisions made by health care agencies. Requirements for accreditation by the Joint Commission on Accreditation of Healthcare Organizations (JCAHO), as well as state licensing and certification requirements, are also influential factors.

OSHA has given some latitude in choices of engineering controls, work practice controls, and personal protective equipment. Clearly, if the best risk reduction strategies are provided by engineering controls, then emphasis should be placed on selection and evaluation of newly designed products intended to reduce percutaneous injury risks. We and others have used our own data to direct selection of risk reduction products. By analyzing our puncture injury-exposure data for 1989 to 1990, we determined that many of our injuries were associated with intravenous access devices. In 1990 to 1991, we obtained information on the devices available and conducted product trial evaluations that led to selection of several risk reduction devices. During late 1991 to early 1992, these devices were purchased, training was provided, and supplies were made available throughout the facility. In addition, a major training program in the OSHA bloodborne pathogens standard was initiated in early 1992 that will be repeated annually. The effects of these risk reduction strategies were seen in 1992 in a reduction of reported puncture injuries-exposures.

Table 69-2 Estimated costs for postexposure management of HIV exposures (with and without AZT)*

Visit	Postexposure follow-up costs($)	Postexposure follow-up and AZT prophylaxis costs ($)
Initial visit	Visit[†] = 125 Lab[‡] = 50	Visit = 125 Lab[§] = 80 AZT[‖] = 450
Week 2		Visit = 50 Lab = 30
Week 4		Visit = 50 Lab = 30
Week 6	Visit = 50 Lab = 50	Visit = 50 Lab = 80
Week 8		Visit = 50 Lab = 30
Week 12 (3 months)	Visit = 50 Lab = 50	Visit = 50 Lab = 50
Month 6	Visit = 50 Lab = 50	Visit = 50 Lab = 50
Month 12 (1 year)	Visit = 50 Lab = 50	Visit = 50 Lab = 50
TOTALS	TOTALS Visits = 325 Lab = 250 575	TOTALS Visits = 475 Lab = 400 AZT = 450 1325

*Estimated costs of a postexposure follow-up program for an employee exposed to blood or body fluids who is known to be immune to hepatitis B, either due to completion of the hepatitis B vaccine series or with evidence of natural hepatitis B disease. This program for postexposure follow-up is consistent with requirements of OSHA[26] and CDC.[9] These estimates are for an occupational health specialist's office located in a metropolitan area of the West Coast and include overhead, salaries, benefits, computer support, and confidential storage and maintenance of medical records for the exposed employee.
†Costs of office visit; primary care provider is nurse practitioner working under physician-approved protocol.
‡Cost for an HIV antibody test.
§Cost for an HIV antibody test ($50) plus laboratory costs for monitoring AZT use according to CDC protocol.[11]
‖Estimated costs for the drug administered for 4 to 6 weeks, depending upon protocol followed.

These injury-exposure data are collected continuously and will be analyzed carefully to direct our risk reduction interventions in the future. This is an important example of continuous quality improvement (CQI) to make the health care workplace a safer one for health care workers.

REFERENCES

1. Alter, M. J., Hadler, S. C., Margolis, H. S., Alexander, W. J. Hu, P. Y., Judson, F. N., Mares, A., Miller, J. K., & Moyer, L. A. (1990). *Journal of the American Medical Association, 263*(9), 1218-1222.
2. Anonymous. (1984, December). Needlestick transmission of HTLV-III from a patient infected in Africa. *Lancet,* 1376-1377.
3. Beekmann, S. E., Fahey, B. J., Gerberding, J. L., & Henderson, D. K. (1990). Risky business: Using necessarily imprecise casualty counts to estimate occupational risks for HIV-1 infection. *Infection Control and Hospital Epidemiology, 11,* 371-379.
4. Birnbaum, D., Schulzer, M., Mathias, R. G., Kelley, M., & Chow, A. W. (1990). Adoption of guidelines for universal precautions and body substance isolation in Canadian acute-care hospitals. *Infection Control and Hospital Epidemiology, 11,* 465-472.
5. Centers for Disease Control. (1970). *Isolation techniques for use in hospitals.* Atlanta: Author.
6. Centers for Disease Control. (1975). *Isolation techniques for use in hospitals* (2nd ed.). Atlanta: Author.
7. Centers for Disease Control. (1983). Guideline for isolation precautions in hospitals. *Infection Control, 4,* 245-325.
8. Centers for Disease Control. (1985). Recommendations for protection against viral hepatitis. *Morbidity and Mortality Weekly Report, 34,* 313-335.

9. Centers for Disease Control. (1987). Recommendations for prevention of HIV transmission in health-care settings. *Morbidity and Mortality Weekly Report, 36*(Suppl. 2S), 3S-18S.

10. Centers for Disease Control. (1988). Update: Universal precautions for prevention of transmission of human immunodeficiency virus, hepatitis B virus, and other bloodborne pathogens in health-care settings. *Morbidity and Mortality Weekly Report, 37,* 378-388.

11. Centers for Disease Control. (1990). Public Health Service statement on management of occupational exposure to human immunodeficiency virus, including considerations regarding zidovudine postexposure use. *Morbidity and Mortality Weekly Report, 39*(Suppl. RR-1), 1-14.

12. Doebbeling, B. N., & Wenzel, R. P. (1990). The direct costs of universal precautions in a teaching hospital. *Journal of the American Medical Association, 264,* 2083-2087.

13. Gerberding, J. L., & Henderson, D. K. (1987). Design of rational infection control policies for human immunodeficiency virus infection. *Journal of Infectious Diseases, 156,* 861-864.

14. Jackson, M. M. (1989). Implementing universal body substance precautions. *Occupational Medicine: State of the Art Reviews, 4*(Special issue), 39-44.

15. Jackson, M. M., & Lynch, P. (1984). Infection control: Too much or too little? *American Journal of Nursing, 84,* 208-210.

16. Jackson, M. M., & Lynch, P. (1991). An attempt to make an issue less murky: A comparison of four systems for infection precautions. *Infection Control and Hospital Epidemiology, 12,* 448-450.

17. Jackson, M. M., Lynch, P., McPherson, D.C., Cummings, M. J., & Greenawalt, N. C. (1987). Why not treat all body substances as infectious? *American Journal of Nursing, 87,* 1137-1139.

18. Jackson, M. M., & Pugliese, G. (1992). Regulations: The OSHA bloodborne pathogens standard. *Today's O.R. Nurse, 14*(7), 11-16.

19. Lee, J. J., Marvin, J. A., Heimbach, D. M., Grube, B. J., & Engrav, L. H. (1990). Infection control in a burn center. *Journal of Burn Care and Rehabilitation, 11,* 575-580.

20. Lynch, P., Cummings, M. J., Roberts, P. L., Herriott, M. J., Yates, B., & Stamm, W. E. (1990). Implementing and evaluating a system of generic infection precautions: Body substance isolation. *American Journal of Infection Control, 18,* 1-12.

21. Lynch, P., Jackson, M. M., Cummings, M. J., & Stamm, W. E. (1987). Rethinking the role of isolation practices in the prevention of nosocomial infections. *Annals of Internal Medicine, 107,* 243-246.

22. McPherson, D. C., & Jackson, M. M. (1987). Isolation precautions for a changing environment . . . a new approach. *Journal of Healthcare Material Management, 5*(6), 28-32.

23. McPherson, D. C., Jackson, M. M., & Rogers, J. C. (1988). Evaluating the cost of the body substance isolation system. *Journal of Healthcare Material Management, 6*(6), 20-28.

24. Stock, S. R., Gafni, A., & Bloch, R. F. (1990). Universal precautions to prevent HIV transmission to health care workers: An economic analysis. *Canadian Medical Association Journal, 142,* 937-946.

25. Troya, S. H., Jackson, M. M., Lovrich-Kerr, M., & McPherson, D. C. (1991). A survey of nurses' knowledge, opinions, and reported uses of the body substance isolation system. *American Journal of Infection Control, 19,* 268-276.

26. U.S. Department of Labor, Occupational Safety and Health Administration. (1991). Occupational exposure to bloodborne pathogens: Final rule, 29 CFR Part 1910:1030. *Federal Register, 56,* 64003-64182.

CHAPTER 70

The costs of cocaine (crack) exposure

A broader perspective

PHYLLIS D. MEADOWS

What are the costs of "crack babies?" The question in itself poses a number of concerns for today's practitioners in health and human services. The term *crack babies* and the poorly defined issues that form the narrow categorical focus it implies have created the basis for much-needed discussion. First and foremost is a need to dismiss the dehumanizing label of "crack babies." In keeping with the value placed on individualized care, these babies will hereinafter be referred to as "infants exposed to cocaine."

To more fully understand the dynamics of infants exposed to cocaine, an emphasis must be placed on summarizing the most current information on the problem. To study the problem, a framework must be developed that views the mother and infant as an interconnected and inseparable dyad. The effects upon one unit within the dyad will compound those upon the other. Females who are of childbearing age, preconceptual, pregnant, or parenting are included within this framework because of their relationships to probable, potential, or actual live births.

The current perspective regarding infants exposed to cocaine is extremely limited in scope. The most common viewpoints suggest severe outcomes and long-term expenditures for exposed infants. These views have been oversensationalized yet effective in alarming an array of professionals into arming themselves with state-of-the-art interventions and techniques. While we should be concerned about the growing incidence of infants exposed to crack cocaine, we should be more concerned about the public overreacting to the problem without data and research to substantiate the level of concern. If we want to determine the true costs associated with infant exposure to crack, we must begin to examine the problem from a very broad context.

A valid understanding of the costs associated with infant exposure to crack cocaine demands an accurate awareness of the problem viewed within a broader context. An examination of costs should extend beyond basic financial issues and incorporate the complex series of escalating or influencing factors involved.

The level of the expense for infants exposed to cocaine is best determined by a review of the scope of the problem, its prevalence and growth, and the degree of severity of short- and long-term effects. The outlay for health care is of great significance, but professional and social expenditures also require close examination.

The deliberate concentration on cost containment has driven health professionals to value economic descriptions of physical conditions. It is unrealistic to assume that the costs associated with drug exposure can ever be finitely measured. The problem is too complex and the related issues are too immense. Therefore, the goal within this context is to decipher the problem, frame the issues and research, and determine reasonable focal points for potentially reducing associated costs.

SCOPE OF THE PROBLEM

Cocaine use among childbearing-aged females (between 15 and 44 years of age) is considered to be highly prevalent. The National Institute on Drug Abuse (NIDA)[7] estimated in 1989 that there were approximately 60 million females of childbearing age in the country, and roughly 15% were substance users. Some reports estimate usage rates among females to be as high as 20%.[10] More than 6 millon women use illicit drugs and 14% have tried cocaine.[5] While the evidence suggests that an alarming number of females use illicit drugs, it is generally believed that these numbers underestimate the prevalence and the degree of drug use. Most will agree, however, that cocaine use among women and pregnant women has risen dramatically over the last decade.

Studies have a limited ability to reflect drug usage accurately. Many studies have relied heavily upon the methodology of self-reporting from substance-using pregnant women. "Estimates that rely on self-reporting of drug use by pregnant women probably reflect underestimates of actual usage when compared with chemical drug testing."[5] Pregnant women who fear legal punishment may deny their drug use or simply avoid the mainstream health care system. Chavkin[3] reported that there had been at least 50 efforts to prosecute pregnant women for using drugs. Some women have actually been convicted, and many states are seeking penalties for pregnant women using illegal substances. These barriers make it extremely difficult to determine the extent of the problem and limit the capacity to determine the number of infants who could potentially be exposed.

The data on infants exposed to cocaine are equally confounding. NIDA[7] reports that as many as 350,000 are affected annually. These numbers are echoed by many of the experts in the field and appear to be astounding when compared with the limited resources and treatment available. The current data have failed to reflect the actual number of infants with cocaine-specific effects. The numbers are difficult to ascertain because of the use of multiple drugs that is typical among pregnant women using cocaine.[2,4,5,10] However, these figures would be significant in computing the costs associated with cocaine-exposed infants.

Comparative data are essential for understanding the costs associated with drug exposures. The severity of the estimated number of infants exposed to cocaine when compared to the actual number of infants born with fetal alcohol syndrome (FAS) presents an interesting perspective. While we are still attempting to determine the number of infants affected by cocaine exposure, we know that annually 10,000 infants are born with FAS. This becomes a critical point, as the focus of attention shifts from the more widely used legal drugs of known deleterious effects (e.g., alcohol and cigarettes) to illicit drugs such as cocaine.

Cocaine use among women has not reached the proportions of alcohol and tobacco use, but it is becoming far more popular and newsworthy. The effects of alcohol and tobacco on infants in utero are defined and conclusive and therefore raise a series of interesting questions. Comparatively, to what extent is it necessary to expend our efforts on infants exposed to cocaine at this juncture? Do we know enough about the specific effects of exposure to cocaine on infants to refocus scarce resources? Are the effects of cocaine exposure conclusive enough that we can prescribe categorical care? Is it more practical to focus on the substance-using female before she becomes pregnant? Answers to these questions are best derived from a clearer understanding of the effects of cocaine on the mother-and-infant dyad.

EFFECTS ON MOTHER AND INFANT

A focal point for measuring the effects of cocaine is the mother-and-infant dyad. The physical, psychological, and environmental effects of cocaine usage and exposure are significant in determining overall costs. The physical effects of cocaine on pregnant women largely relate to the vasoconstrictive properties of the drug. The effects of cocaine use during pregnancy include increased risk of premature separation of the placenta and associated hemorrhaging, miscarriage, and severe hypertension. Premature rupture of membranes, early onset of labor, and preterm delivery have also been reported with usage during the prenatal period.[5] Cocaine alters neurotransmitters, resulting in cardiovascular changes that may lead to myocardial infarction and cardiac arrhythmias. The impact of cocaine is extremely hazardous for women of childbearing age, particularly those who are pregnant. Again, the effects of cocaine use are further compounded in women who use multiple drugs. Pregnant women with poor prenatal nutrition and complicating medical histories, and those failing to obtain adequate prenatal care are at significant risk for poor pregnancy results. "The exact dosage necessary to produce these results is unclear, and may vary from individual to individual, and within the same individual across time."[10] While it is clear that there are physical implications associated with the use of cocaine, the depth to which these factors influence costs is not clear.

The psychological effects of cocaine on pregnant women are equally disturbing because the drug is highly addictive. The compulsive behaviors associated with addiction complicate the environment for both user and infant. Cocaine use becomes the priority, and all other social and personal issues are secondary. Drug use may precipitate a crisis or occur as a result of a crisis within the user's home or immediate environment. Individuals who return to a drug-intensive environment, whether in a home or a community, are particularly at risk.

The research describing the physiological and psychological effects on infants has grown and changed tremendously over the past 10 years. Exposed infants have been described as hypersensitive, irritable, inconsolable, and unable to focus. Cocaine exposure has been linked to sudden infant death syndrome and an array of congenital anomalies. Neonates were reported to have lower birth weights, sleep and feeding disorders, and cognitive and developmental delays caused by intrauterine drug exposure. However, the recent research does not support these findings for all infants. In studies conducted by Chasnoff,[1] it was found that fewer than half of the cocaine-exposed infants tested experienced low birth weight, prematurity, intrauterine growth retardation, and small head circumference.

Each year researchers are identifying potentially new effects on infants exposed to cocaine. One study suggests that infants may experience effects from passive inhalation of crack cocaine.[6] Although these new findings contribute to the growing body of knowledge, they also create new tangents that lead us off on the pathway of more information seeking. The more we focus on gathering information, the further we seem to move away from prevention-oriented interventions.

Few studies have examined the long-term effects of cocaine exposure on infants. Many experts in the field have predicted that there will be serious long-term implications for care, treatment, and education of children with a history of exposure. There is currently no information or research, however, to support this hypothesis.

The limitations within the existing research have made it difficult to specify the effects of cocaine exposure on infants. The issues surrounding cocaine use and exposure are complex and dynamic. The validity of research findings are lessened by (1) methodological issues, (2) the number of confounding variables, (3) conflicting and biased reports, and (4) the prevalence and patterns of cocaine use.[4] Most significant among these factors is the reporting of conflicting and biased information. These issues will be explored in more detail in the discussion on direct and indirect costs.

An accurate awareness in areas involving the physical, psychological, and environmental effects of co-

caine use and exposure is important. In order to determine the extent of investment needed for pregnant women and infants, each of these areas warrants equal consideration when reviewing costs. However, the physical effects of cocaine on women (addiction) and infants (low birth weight) require special attention because of the demand they place on the health care system.

Drug addiction resulting from cocaine use and low birth weight (LBW) among exposed infants are two of the unchallenged areas appearing consistently in the literature describing the drug's effects. Jointly these areas provide the most reasonable focal points for discussion. They significantly contribute to a comprehensive view of the problem, and they provide the basis for determining fiscal and/or cost-related issues.

The long-term impact of drug addiction and LBW among infants, regardless of the cause, has significant implications for determining overall costs. Both conditions require at some point an assessment, diagnosis, treatment, and special care. The expenses for these interventions are reflected in direct and indirect costs, and they are inflated or minimized by a number of influencing factors. The costs of one condition should also be compared to the costs of similar conditions. Though some of the costs are not measurable, all are important when calculating expenditures incurred when addressing the focal points of the mother-and-infant dyad and its conditions of addiction and low birth weight.

UNDERSTANDING COST LEVELS

Costs that affect the mother-and-infant dyad occur on four basic levels that heavily impact health, social, and human service systems. These levels are defined as follows. The first level involves direct costs. Direct costs are incurred through the expenditure of time, effort, and/or resources applied to or directly affecting a focal point. These include investments from individuals, communities, agencies, institutions, and systems.

The second-level expenses are referred to as indirect costs. Indirect costs are those expenditures that are not directly applied to a focal point but that help to shape the framework for addressing a problem. Indirect costs are closely related to direct costs. The application of resources can be augmented or diminished depending on the functional capacity of indirect cost mechanisms.

Intangible costs are represented in the third level. These are primarily reflected in costs to society and are determined by the resulting status of communities impacted by a problem. Intangible costs increase direct and indirect expenditures. They are often immeasurable but can serve as a basis for determining future costs for society.

Finally, the fourth level refers to comparative costs. This aspect of cost is useful in determining the relative degree of impact of expenses within a broad area of focus. Long-term financial costs are compared to determine whether it is feasible to direct efforts toward one focal point versus another.

Each of these aspects of cost helps to broaden the perspective on the problem and determine the extent of its overall impact on society. The following sections briefly describe various aspects within each level. The information is not intended to be all-inclusive but should serve as a basis for further discussion.

Direct costs

The cost of treatment represents the greatest expense for the cocaine-exposed mother-and-infant dyad. The focal points of LBW and addiction greatly elaborate upon this view.

LBW refers to infants who are small for their gestational age or premature. A representative proportion of these infants are born to women addicted to cocaine. LBW is the leading cause of infant mortality and morbidity. The expense of advance technology and its capability to maintain life contribute significantly to the dollars spent on neonatal health care. "Given the strong relationship between birth weight and the cost of care, it is probable that reductions in birth weight due to cocaine use increase the costs of newborn care."[8] Recent studies found hospitalizations for cocaine-exposed infants to be more lengthy and costly than those for infants who were not exposed.[11]

It is very difficult to determine the specific effects of cocaine as opposed to those of other variables; therefore, it is virtually impossible to determine to what degree exposure to cocaine influences costs. However, the relationship of cocaine use and exposure is relatively significant. Bearing this in mind, it is only reasonable to surmise that cocaine-exposed infants increase the risk of higher health care expenditures.

Childbearing-aged women and pregnant women who are addicted to cocaine could potentially influence health care costs in a number of ways. First and foremost are the needs for additional treatment and services during the prenatal period. Many addicted pregnant women will require considerable expenditures of time and expertise. Case management may be necessary, and drug treatment and intense monitoring will be required to support improved birth outcomes. "Lack of prenatal care among drug-using women was a major and significant factor in neonatal costs."[1] Women who seek little or no prenatal care are considered to be at extremely high risk. Those who avoid the health care system until delivery impose additional costs on the health care system, especially in the area of emergency room care.

Treatment and care for the mother-and-infant dyad are the most notable expenses, but there are other direct costs not widely publicized. There are personal expenses that we all contribute as people, family members, and professionals. Time and effort are invaluable gifts, whether they are directed toward individuals who need our support or toward taking the time to learn and build expertise in an area of focus. It is also important to mention that among the personal expenses are contributions of tax dollars.

The dyad of mother and infant exposed to cocaine has garnered considerable attention from agencies focusing on high-risk groups. A multiplicity of agencies are likely to become involved if the dyad returns to its home environment. Protective services, social services, developmental specialists, and crisis interventionists provided from both the public and private sectors will add to the costs. The more comprehensive the needs, the more expensive will be the care.

Indirect costs

Training for professionals and practitioners represents a significant indirect cost, particularly when viewed within a framework of constantly changing information about cocaine exposure and treatment. Information and interventions that are current one year are outdated and dismissed as irrelevant the next year.

The tangential nature of the research contributes to this problem and adds to the costs. Investments in research are often too open and flexible, allowing investigators to pursue their own interests rather than clarifying information in a focused area. This "scatterbrain" approach to financing and conducting research is expensive. The professionals that rely on this information must bear the costs along with the recipients of their care. It takes time to learn and unlearn techniques that have not been adequately studied or presented in the literature. Conversely, the potential effects of carrying out inappropriate interventions on the consumer could result in costly professional and legal errors. This may be considered the extreme, but it is consistent with the research results to date.

Crack cocaine has been oversensationalized in the media and professional literature. As a result, addicted pregnant women and later, their newborn infants are stigmatized. From many perspectives, the pregnant drug user is seen as a criminal. Society's denial that the majority of women used drugs before becoming pregnant has brought a number of pregnant drug users to trial. Indirect contributions of tax dollars have financed several convictions to date.[3] Indirectly these social factors have a grave impact on the costs associated with the dyad.

The overwhelmingly negative view of pregnant drug users will precipitate a sum of costly reactions. First, a number of pregnant drugs users will avoid treatment and prenatal care for fear of punishment. Second, those who seek treatment will place additional stress on an already-overtaxed system. Finally, while this framework assumes that the mother and infant will return home as a unit, in many instances this does not occur. Adding to the indirect costs are infants left in hospitals as "boarder babies," or placed within the foster care system. Both situations are fiscally demanding and contribute to the scope of indirect costs.

Intangible costs

Intangible costs are often immeasurable, but they are reflected in the emotional outlay of those directly and indirectly affected by drug use. These are the internal expenditures of physical energy, mental activity, decision making, and response to events. Drug use adds continuous and ongoing stress to the environment. All systems are disrupted by this stress and must constantly pay a price to regain or maintain stability.

Comparative costs

Briefly, cocaine use and exposure within the mother-and-infant dyad represents one of many illegal drugs that influence costs in our society. When compared to the effects of legal drugs such as alcohol and tobacco, the costs to society are minimal. A focus on drugs such as cocaine and the acceptance of alcohol and smoking have diverted a number of resources from fighting the devastating effects of FAS. Comparatively, NIDA reports that an estimated 10,000 infants *will* be born with FAS each year, whereas conflicting reports are not certain how many infants *may* be affected by cocaine use. "The cost to society is enormous, estimated at $596,000 per FAS child throughout his or her life-

time."[9] The costs for cocaine-exposed infants are not known, although figures about LBW are available. FAS is known to cause mental retardation resulting in expensive long-term care and treatment. The long-term effects of cocaine exposure are not known at this time.

INFLUENCING FACTORS

Overall costs are influenced by factors such as poverty, racism, access barriers, and a focus on treatment versus prevention. Costs escalate among disenfranchised groups. Individuals within these groups (primarily people of color) must not only deal with the problem in question, but must also address their problems with limited resources, facing barriers to access and decreasing availability of services.

A focus on the pregnant substance abuser creates a different set of barriers. These barriers typically present themselves in the form of stereotypes and displays of offensive attitudes among professionals and practitioners.

Although drug treatment is more costly, it is often chosen over prevention strategies. A focus on the pregnant drug user is also a costly decision because of the comprehensiveness of required care. A preventive focus on childbearing-aged females not only costs less to deliver but also has the potential for reducing costs in the long run through early intervention.

CONCLUSIONS

To formulate an appropriate view of the costs associated with cocaine-exposed infants, the focus must include the mother-and-infant dyad. The issues surrounding this dyad are constantly changing and present a challenge in determining costs. The exact costs associated with cocaine exposure are not clearly known and may be virtually incalculable.

Efforts need to be directed toward preventing drug use among females of all ages and ensuring that adequate resources are available to treat them before they become pregnant. Labels and categories will need to be removed, with a renewed focus on individualized care. Research is important for describing conditions and forming strategies for treatment; however, it should be linked to practice and serve a directed purpose of clarifying information through replication.

An awareness of the costs is important, but the goal should be to minimize unnecessary expenditures. We can begin to accomplish this by focusing on each cost level and determining specific areas that demand immediate attention.

REFERENCES

1. Chasnoff, I. J. (1991). Drugs, alcohol, pregnancy and the neonate: Pay now or pay later. *Journal of the American Medical Association, 266*(11), 1567-1568.
2. Chasnoff, I. J., Griffith, D. R., Freier, C., & Murray, J. (1992). Cocaine/polydrug use in pregnancy: Two-year follow-up. *Pediatrics, 89*(2), 284-289.
3. Chavkin, W. (1991). Mandatory treatment for drug use during pregnancy. *Journal of the American Medical Association, 266*(11), 1556-1560.
4. Frank, D. A., Zuckerman, B. S., Amaro, H., Aboagye, K., Bauchner, H., Cabral, H., Fried, L., Hingson, R., Kayne, H., Levenson, S. M., Parker, S., Reece, H., & Vinci, R. (1988). Cocaine use during pregnancy: Prevalence and correlates. *Pediatrics, 82*(6), 888-894.
5. Horgan, C., Rosenbach, M., Ostby, E., & Butrica, B. (1991). *Targeting special populations with drug abuse problems: pregnant women* (National Institute on Drug Abuse Research Series, No. 1). Rockville, Md: U.S. Department of Health and Human Services.
6. Mirchandani, H. G., Mirchandani, I. H., Hellman, F., English-Rider, R., Rosen, S., & Laposata, E. A. (1991). Passive inhalation of free-base cocaine ("crack") smoke by infants. *Archives of Pathology and Laboratory Medicine, 115,* 494-498.
7. National Institute on Drug Abuse. (1989). *Drug abuse and pregnancy* (DHHS Pub. No. C-89-04). Washington, D.C.: U.S. Government Printing Office.
8. Phibbs, C. S., Bateman, D. A., & Schwartz, R. M. (1991). The neonatal costs of maternal cocaine use. *Journal of the American Medical Association, 266*(11), 1521-1526.
9. Streissguth, A. P., & Kinney, J. (Eds.). (1991). *Clinical manual of substance abuse.* St Louis: Mosby.
10. Thurman, S. K., & Berry, B. E. (1992). Cocaine use: Implications for intervention with childbearing women and their infants. *Children's Health Care/Journal of the Association for the Care of Children's Health, 21*(1).
11. U.S. General Accounting Office. (1990). *Drug exposed infants: A generation at risk* (Pub. No. HRD-90-138). Washington, D.C.: U.S. Government Printing Office.

CHAPTER 71

Are nurses getting paid what they are worth?

DONNA SULLIVAN HAVENS, MARY ETTA MILLS

The purpose of this chapter is to provide recent data describing wage and remuneration practices in nursing and to present key issues in determination of the worth of nursing work. The question is not, Are nurses paid enough? but, Are nurses paid what they are worth? From this perspective, the goal is to present relevant data and examine issues that can assist readers to knowledgeably participate in the debate and search for answers to the question.

COMPENSATION FOR NURSING WORK

Salaries are frequently viewed as a reflection of everything from social values to business and market economics. The value that a society places on a particular job is most often demonstrated by the salary and benefits assigned to it. Salary is measured through a combination of elements including tangible remuneration (salary and benefits), professional rewards, and personal satisfaction. Traditional registered nurse (RN) compensation has included hourly wage, benefits, overtime, differentials, and holiday pay. More recent additions to this list are bonuses, incentive pay, and pay for performance programs.[1,10,11,21,25]

Benefits such as time available to meet personal needs (i.e., annual leave, sickness leave, personal, education, and retirement needs); reimbursement for work-related efforts such as education, research, and clinical development; and incentives such as paid transportation, housing, and child care options also have monetary value. The discussion in this chapter, however, will focus primarily on base wages (excluding benefits) for registered nurses working in acute care hospitals—two thirds of all employed RNs.[12] Since data pertaining to this group are uniformly collected across national samples by professional organizations, corporate analysts, and the U.S. government, the chapter will focus on this population.

Salary determination

There are several means to determine salaries. Some of these include job worth evaluation using a criterion-based rating system developed around knowledge, skills, responsibilities, effort, and working conditions; pay according to productivity; pay according to supply and demand; and same pay for all, in which employees receive the same wages without regard to the nature of the job or level of productivity.[2,25] Negotiation through collective bargaining and methods that employ a combination of these strategies may also be used.

While a variety or combination of methods may be used to determine rate of pay, most staff nurses today are paid according to an hourly wage.[10] The findings of a 1990 randomized national study with 221 responding acute care hospitals suggested that only 5.9% of staff RNs were salaried, with that number projected to increase to 19.0% by 1995.[10] This implies that generally, as of this writing, nurses are paid for the time they spend at work, not necessarily for their skills, expertise, or accomplishments.

Salary levels

Available salary data for RNs generally represent only the 68% of staff RNs working in hospitals and usually do not include the other 32% of RNs working in other settings that have traditionally been paid lower salaries.[12] With this caveat in mind, the 1992 annual *American Journal of Nursing* salary survey[4] of hospitals in 17 major urban areas reported staff RN salary data based on a 40-hour workweek and excluding differentials. Starting hourly rates were reported from a high range of $18.94 to $22.02 per hour ($39,395 to

$45,802 annually) in San Francisco to a low range of $10.25 to $12.60 per hour ($21,320 to $26,208 annually) in St. Louis. Top rates were reported from a high range of $23.51 to $31.25 per hour ($48,000 to $65,000 annually) in New York to a low range of $16.97 to $19.76 per hour ($35,299 to $41,100 annually) in Cleveland.[4]

The Bureau of Labor Statistics also reported 1991 hourly ranges for staff RNs. Data were collected via a national survey of private hospitals. Reported hourly wages did not include premium pay for overtime or for work on weekends, holidays, and late shifts. Also excluded were bonuses such as performance bonuses and profit-sharing payments. Pay increases under cost-of-living allowances and incentive payments were included. Hourly rate ranges were broad, from $8 an hour ($16,640 annually) to $40 an hour ($83,200 annually). Average rates also varied by area of the country, from a low in Dallas of $15.17 per hour ($31,553 annually) to $21.82 per hour ($45,386 annually) in San Francisco.[20]

The geographical variability in RN salaries, apparent in both the *American Journal of Nursing* and the Bureau of Labor Statistics data, suggests a "territorial market" in terms of salaries and salary gains.[4,12] According to Brider,[4] RNs working in the Northeast earned nearly 39% more than those employed in the west south central states in 1991. Therefore, when interpreting regional variations, geographical cost-of-living differences need to be considered.

Due to the need to limit the growth of health care costs, there is now an increased focus on ways in which health care delivery might be restructured. This restructuring has generally involved using a smaller core of professional staff with redesigned roles supported by a larger cadre of nonprofessional assistive care personnel.[9,13] Adjunctively, some institutions have implemented pay for performance and incentive-based professional practice programs.[11] These latter arrangements are not included in base wage rates and, as a result, are not reported as part of salary statistics normally collected by salary surveys such as those conducted by Monitrend II and the Bureau of Labor Statistics.

Because salary advances are viewed as economy driven,[4] most forecasters are now suggesting that they will continue to slow. While gains made through contract negotiations that extend several years into the future will continue to increase salaries, there are indications that the trend toward raising nursing salaries may be leveling off. Increases were being projected in the area of 5.2% for medical-surgical nurses in 1992, with a 6.4% raise being budgeted for all nursing personnel, compared with the previous year's 6.9% rise.[4]

Differentials

The survey data indicated that hourly earnings also varied according to five different specialty areas (medical-surgical, intensive care unit [ICU]–coronary care unit [CCU], maternal-child, outpatient, and psychiatric), with staff RNs working in ICUs and CCUs earning the highest mean average hourly wage— $14.98.[4] However, hourly wage differences between the five specialty areas amounted to less than $1 per hour within the lowest, average, and highest hourly wage categories. The specialty area in which an RN worked did not influence hourly pay as much as number of years of experience. Interestingly, while there were hourly differences according to different lengths of service within a specialty area, on average, over a career, an RN could expect to earn only a maximum of $4 to $5 more than the starting hourly rate.[4]

While many nurses have the opportunity to work more lucrative (often undesirable) shifts and overtime hours, this is not an option for all, due to age, health status, or family responsibilities. For instance, the nurse who works the night shift for 1 year might add $4000 to $5000 to his or her annual salary.[12] What this might imply is that in general those able to enhance their base wages by adding the differentials and bonuses are those who do not have additional responsibilities, such as family, outside of the work arena. It has been suggested that those most apt to take advantage of these salary enhancements might be the younger, less experienced nurses. The implication is that, on an annual basis, younger, less experienced RNs may earn as much or more than their more experienced colleagues.[4]

Differentials may also be offered for education and/ or specialty certification. In 1990 only 20% to 27% of hospitals offered salary differentials for the baccalaureate or master's degree.[10] The reported increase to the base hourly wage for baccalaureate education ranged from 10 cents to $1 per hour, with $1 reported most often.[4,10] Of note is the fact that attainment of educational credentials may be built into clinical ladder advancement criteria, and often ladder advancement is associated with higher hourly earnings. Nevertheless, while some institutions report a variety of means to recognize the RN for this educational achievement, the

Table 71-1   Salary progression in selected occupations (salary in dollars)

	1986			1991			Percentage rate of gain or loss
Occupation	Average starting salary	Average maximum salary	Percentage of salary progression	Average starting salary	Average maximum salary	Percentage of salary progression	
Attorney	31,014	101,189	226.2	40,302	125,855	212.3	(6.1)
Chemist	22,539	74,607	231.0	27,162	88,749	226.7	(1.9)
Accountant	21,024	61,546	192.7	24,809	75,347	203.7	5.7
Engineer	27,866	79,021	183.6	32,459	95,058	192.9	5.0
Purchasing clerk	13,994	29,834	110.0	16,395	34,515	110.5	0.5
Computer programmer	20,832	42,934	106.1	26,103	42,533	62.9	(40.7)
Buyer	21,242	41,304	94.4	24,766	47,997	93.8	(0.6)
Personnel director	39,817	75,170	88.8	45,618	101,922	123.9	39.5
General clerk	10,478	19,332	84.5	11,791	23,113	96.0	13.6
Accounting clerk	12,517	21,872	74.7	14,639	24,787	69.3	(7.2)
Secretary	16,326	28,051	71.8	19,844	34,085	71.8	0.0
Personnel clerk	14,193	23,702	67.0	15,659	27,599	76.3	13.9
Registered nurse	20,340	27,744	36.4	27,225	48,924	79.7	119.0

Modified from: U.S. Department of Labor, Bureau of Labor Statistics. (1986, October). *National survey of professional, administrative, technical & clerical pay* (Bulletin 2271), Washington, D.C.: Author; and U.S. Department of Labor, Bureau of Labor Statistics. (1992, January). *Occupational wage survey: Hospitals* (Bulletin 2392), Washington, D.C.: Author.

attainment of a baccalaureate degree is at best considered to add $1 per hour to the worth of the work of nursing. In general, educational differentials are less than shift differentials, implying that *when* an RN works may be more valued by employing institutions than the knowledge, skill, and credentials possessed by the practitioner.

Specialty certification may also be rewarded in a variety of ways including financial support for preparatory courses and bonuses and awards for passing. Upon certification, bonuses were reported to range from $150 to $1000 annually.[10]

COMPARISON OF NURSING SALARIES WITH THOSE OF OTHER PROFESSIONS

The U.S. Department of Labor, Bureau of Labor Statistics surveys wages for selected professional, administrative, technical, and clerical occupations in private hospitals and private industry. A comparison of average starting salaries and average maximum salaries for selected occupations is reported in Table 71-1 for the years 1986 and 1991.

It is interesting to note that over the 5-year period between 1986 and 1991 nursing as a profession showed the most significant rate of salary gain (119.0%) when compared to other selected occupa-

tions listed in the table. The percentage of salary progression for nurses, while lowest of the rates reported in 1986 (36.4%), had risen to the second highest quartile by 1991 with a rate of 79.7%. Further examination, however, reveals that the mean rate of salary progression for the selected occupations equaled 124.6%. Applying this figure to the starting average nursing salary would create a maximum average salary of $61,147, suggesting that while nursing has made advances in salary levels, it still lags behind the average occupational progression level. In addition, the notable salary gains are seen only in certain geographical areas, suggesting a territorial market.[4,12]

Other interesting comparisons can be made between the educational requirements and salaries of RNs and other health care professionals as depicted in Table 71-2. Examination of this table suggests that RNs have the lowest minimum educational requirements to practice and the lowest average 1991 salary.

Combining this with salary data that demonstrate the relatively minor influence of education on current nursing salary levels, there does not appear to be a direct meaningful relationship between the two. Educational level seems to be a greater factor in obtaining promotional positions such as middle manager or clinical specialist for which salary levels have not been reported here.

Table 71-2   Educational requirements and salaries in selected health care occupations

Occupation	Educational requirements	1991 average salary ($)	2000 average salary ($)
Registered nurse	Associate degree, diploma, baccalaureate, or master's degree	27,000	50,000
Physician assistant	2 years of college and 2 years of physician assistant study (baccalaureate and graduate study available)	35,000-60,000	47,250
Physical therapist	Baccalaureate—master's degree preferred	31,421-66,150	45,000-96,000
Pharmacist	Graduation from a 5-year college of pharmacy	44,000	60,605
Occupational therapist	Baccalaureate or master's degree	29,796	51,000
Speech pathologist	Master's degree	31,421	46,000
Dietitian	Baccalaureate	27,562-71,662	40,000-80,000

Compiled from information in: Kleiman, C. (1992). *The 100 best job for the 1990s and beyond.* Dearborn, Mich: Dearborn Financial Publishing.

FACTORS AFFECTING THE WORTH OF NURSING WORK

Worth is defined as "monetary value . . . the value of something measured by its qualities or by the esteem in which it is held."[22] Calculation of worth here may be dependent on the perspective of the individual or entity making the determination of monetary value, usefulness, etc., of nursing. Factors that may influence determination of the value of the services of the nursing profession include the nursing labor market and the concept of economic equity.

The nursing labor market

In an ideal situation, the value or worth of a good or service (here, the professional nursing practice) is determined by the demand for that good or service. Before 1988, the shortage of nurses was a key factor in driving salary considerations relative to the recruitment and retention of staff. Since that time, several factors have combined to impact the way in which salaries are viewed. Salaries have, in fact, increased in response to a growing hospital demand for staff who can care for an ever-increasing population requiring acute care of patients.[19] However, the labor market in health care, and in particular in nursing, is not perfect. Potential nursing labor market imperfections affecting the worth of nursing work include (1) an undervaluation of the work of nursing,[7] (2) the existence of a monopsony, and (3) the mobility factor.

The general public does not clearly understand the education needed, the skills required, and the hazards associated with professional nursing practice.[7] Confusion may also exist among the public and employers when not all nurses can clearly describe the nature and value of the services provided. The existence of mul-

tiple educational pathways leading to practice of a single role compounds the confusion both internally and externally to the profession. As a result, when performing a wage evaluation of nursing work, it is difficult to build a case for enhanced job worth due to the need for a rigorous educational background when those with and without baccalaureate degrees perform the same role. Strasen[18] noted that "nursing compensation is equitable with other professions that require two years of college education." This multiplicity in educational requirements, with the minimum educational requirement factored into the job worth equation, is not in the best interest of nursing when worth of the work is analyzed.

A second imperfection in the nursing labor market is the existence of a monopsony. A monopsony exists when there is one buyer or supplier of goods or services. In today's health care arena, hospitals are the prime employer for over 68% of professional nurses.[12] This fact carries great importance, especially considering evidence that wages paid to nurses in hospitals often determine noninstitutional nursing wages.[8] In some geographical areas, there is only one hospital that employs nurses. Even in cases where there are several hospitals in a geographical region, the literature suggests that agreements have been made between institutions to set nursing wages at a particular level.[19] When formal agreements are not made, it is not unusual for nursing wages to be set based upon the market value of the wages paid by others[2,25] in a particular region. This has the effect of determining nursing wages according to what is currently paid (whether or not the level is appropriate) rather than assessing critical factors to determine the actual worth of the service.

A third imperfection in the nursing labor market is the fact that the majority of professional nurses are women (98%). Some argue that as women, many nurses are geographically limited in terms of employment. Dawes[7] pointed to the fact that many nurses grow up, attend school, and eventually work in the same geographical area. This "immobility factor" may serve to further promote monopsony in the nursing labor market.

Economic equity

According to Brider,[3] women and nurses have been struggling for equitable compensation for many years. The National Committee on Pay Equity reported that in 1990 women earned 66 cents for every $1 earned by men, and in general, according to Dawes,[7] "women with a college education earned the same as a male high school dropout." Sex-based wage discrimination may occur when less than 30% of either sex is employed in a certain job.[23] In the nursing profession, 98% of all workers are female.

Pay equity is "a broad concept [and] refers to the movement to assure that all disadvantaged groups . . . are compensated on the basis of the inherent value or worth of the work they perform, rather than on the basis of historically depressed pay levels or other discriminatory factors."[3] Pay equity is often used to encompass the concepts of comparable worth, sex-based wage discrimination, and equal pay for equal work.[16]

The Equal Employment Act of 1972 focused on "comparable pay for comparable work," and this is the crux of the problem—how and by whom is comparability of work determined? Comparable worth "refers to equal pay for work done by females and males that is of comparable value to the employer. Value to the employer is defined by skill, effort, and responsibility required to do the job."[16]

Nursing salaries have been affected by pay equity issues. Examples include the following: Minnesota, 1982—RN work was rated equivalent to that of vocational instructors, but RNs were paid $537 less per month; California, 1980—electrical foremen were paid $2268 per month for work rated equal to that of nurses, who were paid $839 per month; Washington, 1982—RNs received $1368 per month for work rated higher than that of highway engineers, who were paid $1980 per month (from testimony of American Nurses Association president Eunice Cole to the U.S. House of Representatives Subcommittees on Human Resources, Civil Service, and Compensation and Civil Service, September 21, 1982) cited by Brett.[2]

The comparability of nursing wages to those of other professions has also served as the focus for litigation.[5,6,16] In a landmark comparable worth case (*Lemmons v. City and County of Denver*, 1980)[15] in which the ruling went against nurses, the judge claimed that the comparable worth issue had the potential to "disrupt the entire economic system of the United States." This is symbolic of the environment in which nursing is addressing issues of compensation relative to worth.

CONCLUSIONS

The measure of job worth has often been described in terms of salary. There is evidence that health care organizations have addressed salary levels through an examination of the effect of wage compression within and between professions, use of job evaluation methods, and implementation of programs such as pay for performance.

These factors have been instrumental in changing the dynamics of nursing compensation. The situation is still very fluid, but there are indications that nursing salary ranges have dramatically widened over the past 3 years. For example, in 1986 an average starting salary for RNs of $20,340 with a maximum of $27,744 was reported. In 1991, starting salaries were averaging $27,225 and averaging a maximum of $48,924. This represents a 34% increase in starting salaries and a 76% increase in average maximum salaries over a 5-year period.

Still, there appears to be little relationship between salary and educational level or work experience. Furthermore, a comparison of the average rate of salary progression for selected occupations suggests that, while advances have been made, the rate of nursing salary level increases still lags behind the progression rate averaged across occupations.

The real question is how to establish an appropriate means to measure job worth other than "current market rates." Wage levels are currently the best standard measure of comparability. However, they do not account for the variable trends impacting compensation. These might include business-specific demands or downturns, auxiliary roles subsumed by specific careers that impact perceived worth, and changes in professional autonomy. Furthermore, additional means of calculating comprehensive benefit packages inclusive of available bonuses, gain sharing, and other options having a monetary benefit should be developed.

REFERENCES

1. Bell, E., & Bart, B. (1991). Pay for performance: Motivating the chief nurse executive. *Nursing Economic$, 9*(2), 113.
2. Brett, J. (1983, June). How much is a nurse's job really worth? *American Journal of Nursing,* pp. 877-881.
3. Brider, P. (1980, October). The struggle for just compensation. *American Journal of Nursing,* pp. 77-88.
4. Brider, P. (1992, March). Salary gains slow as more RNs seek full-time benefits. *American Journal of Nursing,* pp. 34-42.
5. Cook, A. (1990). Comparable worth: An economic issue. *Nursing Management, 21*(2), 28-30.
6. Creighton, H. (1984). Comparable worth cases. *Nursing Management, 15*(11), 20-22.
7. Dawes, R. (1989). The economics of comparable worth. *Nursing Management, 20*(1), 80B, 80F-80H.
8. Dean, R., & Yetter, T. (1979). Nurse market policy simulations using an econometric model. In R. Scheffler (Ed.), *Research in health economics,* (pp. 255-300). Greenwich, Conn: JAI Press.
9. Eastaugh, S. (1990). Hospital nursing technical efficiency: Nurse extenders and enhanced productivity. *Hospital and Health Services Administration, 35*(4), 561-573.
10. Havens, D. (1990). *Analysis of the nature and extent of implementation and projected implementation of a model proposed to support professional nursing practice in acute care hospitals.* Unpublished doctoral dissertation, University of Maryland, Baltimore. (University Microfilms No. 91-100096).
11. Havens, D., & Mills, M. (1992). Professional recognition and compensation for staff RNs: 1990 and 1995. *Nursing Economic$, 10*(1), 15-20.
12. Joel, L. (1992). Nursing salaries: Recurring themes and new insights. *Journal of Nursing Administration, 22*(3), 13, 15, 17.
13. Kirby, K., & Garfink, C. (1991). The university hospital nurse extender model. *Journal of Nursing Administration, 21*(1), 25-30.
14. Kleiman, C. (1992). *The 100 best jobs for the 1990s & beyond.* Dearborn, Mich: Dearborn Financial Publishing.
15. Lemmon v. City and County of Denver, 620 F.2d 288 (U.S. 10th Cir. Ct., 1980). Cert. denied 499 U.S. 880 (1980).
16. Mahrenholz, D. (1987). Comparable worth: Litigation and legislation. *Nursing Administration Quarterly, 12*(1), 25-31.
17. Prescott, P., Phillips, C., Ryan, J., & Thompson, K. (1991). How nurses spend their time. *Image: The Journal of Nursing Scholarship, 23*(1), 23-28.
18. Strasen, L. (1992). Nurses' salaries are adequate! *Journal of Nursing Administration, 22*(3), 12, 14, 16, 18.
19. Styles, M. (1985). The uphill battle for comparable worth. *Nursing Outlook, 33*(3), 128-132.
20. U.S. Department of Labor, Bureau of Labor Statistics. (1992, January). *Occupational wage survey: Hospitals* (Bulletin 2392) Washington, D.C.: Author.
21. Wasylak, T. (1991, April). Pay for performance. *Canadian Nurse,* pp. 30-31.
22. *Webster's Ninth New Collegiate Dictionary.* (1988). Springfield, Mass: Merriam-Webster.
23. Weingard, M. (1984). Establishing comparable worth through job evaluation. *Nursing Outlook, 32*(2), 113.
24. York, C., & Fecteau, D. (1987). Innovative models for professional nursing practice. *Nursing Economic$, 5*(4), 162-166.
25. Youngkin, E. (1985, January-February). Comparable worth: Alternatives to litigation and legislation. *Nursing Economic$, 3,* 38-43.

CHAPTER 72

How can nursing decrease the costs of nursing education?

PATRICIA R. FORNI, PAULETTE BURNS

Higher education is not experiencing the levels of funding achieved in past decades, nor will it in the foreseeable future. This forecast includes nursing education, which will continue to be faced with fluctuating enrollments and decreasing sources of revenue. Budgetary adjustments will have to be made if nursing is to meet its goals. The fact is that 33 states experienced budget cuts in higher education in fiscal year 1992 and 42 states are cutting budgets in fiscal year 1993.[11] With the federal budget deficit increasing annually, little help from the government can be expected. Pressures from state legislators and higher education coordinating agencies for cost effectiveness and accountability are mounting.

Faculty productivity is being scrutinized in many states as a natural consequence of tightening resources. Patrick M. Cullan, former vice president of the education commission of the states, speaking on this issue, said, "Higher education is not going to be exempt from the economic, technological, and demographic pressures that are causing every type of institution we have to reconsider how to organize itself to get the job done."[12] Nor is it any wonder that policymakers and taxpayers expect a reasonable return on their investment dollar when one considers that a sizable portion of state budgets go to higher education. Over $38 billion was spent in fiscal year 1991 for public colleges and universities, according to Research Associates of Washington.[14]

Faculty work load and productivity is only one facet of accountability that is being examined. Educational institutions across the nation are being asked to demonstrate "outcomes" as a requirement for academic accreditation as well as for funding allocations from legislatures and governments. Departments, schools, and colleges, by discipline, are being judged on numbers of students, numbers of graduates, student credit hour production, faculty-student ratios, funded research dollars per square foot of space, and the like. These challenges are being brought to bear while attempting to maintain quality of programs without regard to resources needed and justified by tradition.

Academic programs are being called upon increasingly to demonstrate innovative ways to achieve their goals within budget limitations. As a first step, the educational program must decide how a budget reduction will be absorbed in relation to the three university missions of teaching, research, and service. The goals for productivity among the three missions must be determined as well. For example, faculty teaching work load could be increased to allow fewer faculty members to teach the same number of students. In this example, however, faculty research and service activities would of necessity be reduced to accommodate higher teaching loads. This issue is especially important to nursing, as many nursing schools are at a critical point in building research programs.

There are at least two strategies for addressing the challenge of shrinking budgets: (1) increase revenue streams from other sources and/or (2) decrease expenditures. These strategies must be considered in tandem with assumptions and goals regarding productivity and outcomes of the educational unit. For example, does a budget reduction mean decreased enrollment, or could the status quo be maintained by doing the same with less?

For discussion purposes, we have made the following assumptions about the higher education funding picture:

1. For the foreseeable future, allocations of state and/or federal funds for higher education will not see great increases and, in fact, may be reduced.
2. Accountability for use of public funds for education will take on paramount importance in the public view.
3. The trend toward privatization of public-supported institutions of higher education will continue.
4. Higher education institutions will be forced to adopt new ways of acquiring budgetary resources.
5. Part of the costs for higher education will be passed on to students through higher tuition and fees.
6. Demographic changes in society will have significant consequences for higher education.
7. Issues of program quality will have to be addressed in the face of shrinking budgetary resources.
8. Educational institutions and/or programs that fail to respond to the herein-identified changes will be forced to close or to significantly reduce operations.
9. The present focus on outcomes as a measure of productivity and quality will continue to be of importance for program funding.

Insofar as the strategies and assumptions discussed in this chapter apply to private institutions of higher education, they may be considered for their use as well.

Nursing educators must begin to address how they will meet these challenges if program viability is to be maintained. There is a general perception among some university administrators that nursing programs are expensive compared with other academic disciplines. However, Melvin[15] found in a study of three baccalaureate nursing programs that program costs were lower than the average instructional expenditures for full-time equivalent students in the respective universities. Roberts,[18] in a Canadian study, found that the cost of a bachelor of nursing (BN) degree was not significantly different from the mean cost of an honors arts degree and was below the cost of an honors science degree. In 1986 the American Association of Colleges of Nursing (AACN) undertook a study of the costs of generic baccalaureate nursing education. According to Kummer, Bednash, and Redman,[13] the study found that the three most important groups of variables in constructing costs were as follows:

(1) faculty size and instructional costs including teaching load, salaries, and benefits; (2) student enrollment and curriculum patterns including student attrition; and (3) other institutional costs including support staff costs, direct instructional costs for non-nursing courses taken by nursing students, and indirect costs.

A question is on the minds of educators and administrators: Can nursing decrease the costs of nursing education and, if so, how? This question will be explored under the two strategies of increasing revenues and decreasing expenditures.

INCREASING REVENUES

Given the first assumption stated previously, any increase in revenues is not likely to come from tax-supported sources. What, then, are the possible sources of revenue streams for nursing education? Sources of revenue are those external to the nursing unit and those that can be generated within the nursing unit. External sources include private foundations; individual donors, including alumni and friends; Medicare pass-through funds; special arrangements with hospitals and health care agencies; and extramural grants and contracts. Internal sources of revenue include student tuition, faculty practice, continuing education offerings, royalties, inventions, and nurse-managed clinics and community nursing centers. See Fig. 72-1 for suggested sources of revenue streams.

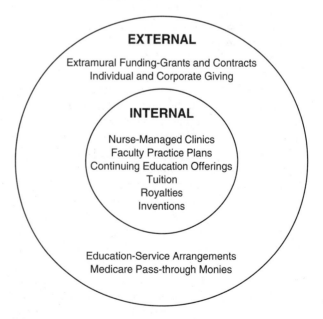

Fig. 72-1 Sources of revenue streams.

External sources of revenue

A number of large private foundations, such as W. K. Kellogg, Robert Wood Johnson, and Helene Fuld, typically fund programs of interest to nursing. Additionally, there are numerous small foundations that have funds for nursing education. Library resources containing data on funding priorities, amounts, application deadlines, and proposal formats can be consulted for more information. One such source is *The Foundation Directory,* edited by Stan Olson,[17] which provides authoritative sources of information on private philanthropic giving in each state.

Another revenue stream consists of monies and gifts from donors such as alumni, friends of nursing, and corporations. Most nursing education programs probably have not promoted such activity to the fullest potential. As part of their education, nursing students should be socialized to believe that annual giving is a professional responsibility of alumni. Special fundraising events such as banquets, galas, and athletic events serve as revenue streams that can tap into donors other than alumni and gross considerable returns. Gifts such as bequests of property should not be overlooked as sources of revenue.

The phenomenon of privatization of public institutions is being discussed in many circles. This term refers to the fact that public-supported institutions are increasingly turning to private donors, money-making enterprises, and tuition for support, as state allocations continue to shrink.[4]

Medicare pass-through monies are available to some nursing programs through their affiliated hospitals. This money is derived from Medicare funds "for those portions of direct education costs that reflect the average Medicare patient population of hospital services."[7] Funds are allocated to hospitals and are used to help defray the costs of educating health professionals. There are five demonstration projects nationwide in which graduate nursing education programs are receiving these pass-through monies.[2]

Education-service arrangements provide linkages between nursing programs and hospitals or other service agencies for purposes of funding faculty-staff positions, for example, to provide clinical supervision of students, for academic advisement, or for other academic needs. The University of Oklahoma College of Nursing has such an arrangement with its university-affiliated hospital to fund an academic counselor's position and for clinical supervision of two groups of undergraduate students.

Endowments are sources of money from generous benefactors that are set up in perpetuity. Income from endowments is derived from the interest earnings on the principal. Endowed monies usually are earmarked for purposes specified by the donors. Some states have matching fund programs whereby private donations are matched with state funds. Endowed chairs in nursing are on the increase. According to data on institutional resources and budgets, 57 schools of nursing reported endowed chairs, ranging from one to six, with a range of monies from $10,000 to $2,137,225.[1] Endowments, while providing additional support, do not provide predictable funding in that interest income fluctuates with the economy.

Extramural funding through research and training grants and contracts is another source of revenue. This funding can provide both direct cost recovery funds and indirect cost recovery (ICR) funds. Direct costs are those associated with the conduct of the grant or contract, such as salaries, equipment, travel, and supplies. Indirect costs are administrative costs and are figured as a percentage of the direct costs. These monies are intended for use to support grant activities. For example, ICR monies may be allocated throughout the institution to extend support of other research efforts in order to generate more funds. These monies may be used for secretarial assistance, research assistants, purchase of equipment, and other support of further research efforts.

Internal sources of revenue

The sources of revenue streams discussed so far have been external to the institution and the nursing unit. What revenue streams can the nursing unit generate?

Tuition is the major source of revenue for educational institutions, and more students mean more tuition. Nationwide there is a growing dependence on tuition as a major source of income. Yet in most state institutions, tuition covers only a small percentage of total costs for "instate" students. In 1960 tuition accounted for 17.7% of the total costs of instruction and support, rising to 24.8% in 1990.[4] In general, tax-supported institutions are formula funded, which means that they are tied to student enrollments in terms of full-time equivalents (FTEs) and student credit hours produced. Unlike most other academic disciplines, but not unlike many health profession disciplines, nursing is limited in the number of students it can enroll, primarily because of the required student-faculty ratios for clinical experiences and the availability of clinical sites for practicums. Over time, enrollments in nursing programs have vacillated from extreme declines experienced in the mid 1980s to record highs experienced in the early 1990s. Billingsley[3] reports that some colleges have assessed students in the health professions for additional costs and concludes that this may be a future trend for nursing.

Traditionally, medical schools have relied on income from faculty practice plans to support large portions of medical school budgets, whereas nursing has relied solely on allocations from the parent institution for budget support. In the future, nursing faculty practice plans may be looked upon as a major source of income for the nursing unit. In the Houston linkage model at the University of Texas School of Nursing, Houston, faculty practice occurs on a contractual basis and amounted to $601,408 in 1990 to 1991.[21] Dean Patricia Starck in a personal communication in June 1992 reported, "Faculty practice coupled with revenues from the newly opened University of Texas Nursing Services in Houston is projected to be $1,000,000 in fiscal year '93." The American Association of Colleges of Nursing[1] reports that 53 schools have had written practice plans.

Continuing education offerings, if carefully managed, may provide another source of income to nursing programs. Many continuing education programs are self-supporting and realize profits. Contracting with large organizations, for example, to provide learning packages for employees is a revenue source. These contracts can serve as a major source of income for nursing education as service agencies decrease their in-house staff development programs. In states where continuing education in nursing is mandatory, universities have a potential earning opportunity.

Royalties from publications, and production of computer software programs, videos, and packaged learning materials developed by faculties also could serve as a revenue source for the nursing unit. Patents for inventions are another source of revenue. However, they are subject to the rules and regulations of the governing institution, and revenues derived from this source may have to be shared.

Nurse-managed clinics operated on a fee-for-service basis are growing in numbers. The potential for income generation from nurse-managed clinics is on the increase. This is in part due to the reimbursement for nursing services that is available from third-party payers, including Medicare and Medicaid. According to the AACN,[1] nurse clinics and centers were operant in 76 schools of nursing with sources of support from

---

SOURCES OF COST SAVINGS

Organizational structure
Curriculum organization
Student body size and characteristics
Faculty-staff size and characteristics
Work load policy
Material resources
Instructional costs
Staffing practices
Teaching methodologies

---

internal school of nursing funds, fees for service, grants, free space, and other. Increasing revenue streams is in consonance with Hegevary's ideas[10] for diversifying schools' funding to survive economic slumps. An additional resource on nursing centers is a National League for Nursing (NLN) publication[16] of the 1989 proceedings of the National Conference on Nursing Centers.

REDUCING EXPENDITURES

Expenditures are a function of many factors including mission and goals, type and size of parent institution, nursing organizational structure and curriculum organization, and number and level of programs offered by the academic unit. See the box above for suggested sources of cost savings.

Nursing units that exist in large research institutions have different expectations for scholarship than do those that are located in small liberal arts colleges. Accordingly, the costs for meeting their respective missions and goals are different. In institutions where the major focus is on teaching, the costs of operating the nursing program are generally less.

Organizational structure

The organizational structure of the academic unit determines how many administrative and support staff members are required to carry out the functions of the program. As a general rule, the more complex the structure, the more costly. Reductions can be achieved by simplifying the structure and reducing administrative and staff positions. How much administrative time is allocated to carry out the mission of the academic unit? Can responsibilities be consolidated? Does the nurse administrator have instructional responsibilities as well as administrative responsibilities?

Consortial arrangements whereby several institutions get together to offer a degree program have been developed in some states. These arrangements are cost effective in that they avoid duplication of programs and conserve state resources. The University Center at Tulsa (UCT) is such an arrangement. UCT is a consortium of four state universities offering unduplicated undergraduate and graduate programs at a single site. Each institution is designated to offer specific programs. The University of Oklahoma College of Nursing is designated to offer the master's degree in nursing at this site.

If the nursing unit has a continuing education program or nurse-managed center, are they self-supporting or do they require funding from the nursing budget? How are the faculty members organized? How many committees are there, what are their membership requirements, and what is the frequency of meetings? Faculty time (as spent in committee meetings) is a valuable resource. A school should calculate the number of hours spent in meetings, place a dollar figure on this use of time, and then ask the question, Does the outcome justify the cost? All of these questions have a bearing on costs associated with organizational structure.

Curriculum organization

Curriculum organization, including length of the nursing major, number and type of specialties, and levels of programs, affects costs in many ways. The lengthier the program, the more costly it is in terms of personnel requirements. The more career tracks that are offered within a program level, the more costly. For example, the master's curriculum at the University of Oklahoma College of Nursing requires 45 semester credit hours, but a total of 77 credit hours are required for 6 specialty areas and 3 role preparation areas. Master's programs in the United States offer from 1 to 24 specialty areas and from 1 to 19 functional role areas.[5] The more specialty tracks that are offered, the smaller the class size per course. Small classes are expensive. Costs also are related to levels of programs offered. Master's and doctoral programs, requiring low student-faculty ratios with doctorally prepared faculty, are more costly than undergraduate programs. Thesis and dissertation guidance is labor intensive for faculty and thus incurs costs. It would be interesting to compare thesis versus nonthesis costs in master's curriculums.

Frequency of course offerings is another cost consideration. Traditionally low-enrollment master's courses could be scheduled less frequently, such as every other year, to provide for a larger enrollment and to free faculty for other activities. Multiple teaching sites and multiple clinical sites also require additional resources.

Teaching methodologies can have a great impact on the budget. A plethora of nursing electives, with low enrollments, is a luxury most programs can no longer afford. Offering electives for nonnursing majors is a way to increase student credit hours generated.[19] Team teaching, whereby a number of faculty members sit in on all classes of one course, is expensive and outdated. The least expensive, most credit hour–producing method is that whereby one professor lectures to a large class. Expensive methodologies are those that require special equipment and low enrollments and thus increase faculty requirements.

Class size and mix are important cost factors. Class size may be increased by offering courses open to non-majors. Some nursing programs have developed nursing courses that are required of nonnursing majors. This strategy would be a consideration for increasing student credit hours that are in turn tied to formula-funded budgets. On the other hand, costs can be reduced by limiting class size and downsizing programs.

Another cost consideration in undergraduate education is student mix in relation to generic versus RN students. In general, it is less costly to educate RNs because they do not require laboratory instruction skills as extensive as those required by generic students. Moreover, clinical supervision of RNs is not as labor intensive in most clinical areas.

Student-faculty ratios are cited as the most costly component of nursing education. According to the 1974 Institute of Medicine study on health professions education costs, student-faculty ratios were found to be the major source of variation in baccalaureate nursing program costs. Higher costs were associated with lower student-faculty ratios.[15] Because of the nature of the nursing discipline, requiring close supervision of students in the clinical setting, the ratio cannot be increased significantly without jeopardizing safety and quality. Furthermore, boards of nursing in each state generally specify a maximum number of students per faculty member.

The ratio of laboratory to credit hours is another cost factor. The more contact hours faculty members spend in clinical laboratory, the more costly. A related factor is the number and ratio of clinical credits required in the curriculum. Using a 1:3 ratio, a course with 4 credit hours of clinical credit would require 12 contact hours of supervision per week per academic term, whereas using a 1:4 ratio, a course with 4 credit hours of clinical credit would require 16 contact hours per week per academic term. In the future, a more efficient method of achieving clinical learning objectives may be through clinical simulations using advanced technology. The concept of "virtual reality" as discussed by Sigma Theta Tau librarian Debra Schneider[20] is another strategy that may help to reduce faculty work load strain in regard to helping students meet clinical objectives. "Virtual reality . . . is a three-dimensional, computer-generated or computer-managed interactive environment" in which the participant is included within the simulation.[23]

Insofar as students require remediation, cost factors increase as more faculty time is devoted to helping students. However, student retention and graduation rates are extremely important in an era in which outcome measures are being used to evaluate program effectiveness and to determine funding.

Personnel costs

The largest cost category in any educational budget is personnel. Dienemann[6] suggested at least five options for reducing faculty work load including the following: changing class size, supplementing full-time faculty with other types of personnel, and changing classes from one location to another. Cost variables include number of faculty members, faculty rank mix, faculty tenure mix, faculty turnover and longevity, and length of contracts. Faculty salaries are related to all of these variables. One can assume that tenured faculty members at the higher ranks who have the longest time in service will usually be paid most. Mix refers to the proportion of individuals in each category, so that a large proportion of professors would cost more, as would a large proportion of tenured faculty. High faculty turnover is expensive because replacement is costly. Faculty contracts may vary in length from 9 to 12 months, and costs vary proportionately. The same considerations apply to the mix of full-time versus part-time employees, in relation not only to salaries but also to fringe benefits covered.

Cost also is related to the number and type of staff members required to meet program goals. The use of graduate teaching assistants as assistive to teaching is cost effective because it frees more highly paid faculty members for other activities. How much of the academic support services does nursing provide for its programs? If the nursing unit has responsibility for recruitment, advisement, and financial aid, for example, then the costs will be greater than for programs in which this is handled centrally.

Faculty requirements (numbers) are closely tied to work load. When faculty members carry heavy teaching loads, fewer faculty members are required for instruction. Work load policies should permit attainment of the mission and goals of the nursing unit, as well as the requirements for faculty promotion and tenure. To illustrate, in a 36–credit hour master's curriculum with one specialty track using a teaching work load of 6 credit hours per semester for graduate faculty, six faculty members would be required. Using a work load of 9 credit hours, four faculty members would be required. Assuming faculty members were at the associate professor rank at salaries of $45,000, the cost savings in the latter example would be $90,000.

The use of part-time faculty to provide clinical supervision of students is cost effective. In many situations, staff nurses serve as mentors and preceptors at no cost to the academic unit. The benefits to service agencies when staff nurses serve as mentors and preceptors need to be taken into account when negotiating these arrangements. Studies reported by Hawken and Hillestad[9] and Starck and Williams[22] conclude that service agencies gain tangible resources through these collaborations.

Other cost factors

A number of expense categories can be manipulated to reduce costs. These include instructional materials, computer hardware and software, library and laboratory expenses, research, equipment, supplies, communications, travel, printing, renovation, and repair.

Factors external to the institution that affect costs are NLN accreditation and requirements imposed by state boards of nursing under rules and regulations of the nursing practice acts. Accreditation is an expensive but necessary condition and state board requirements are not negotiable.

OTHER CONSIDERATIONS

"It takes money to make money" may be a cliché, but it is true. To generate revenue, it is sometimes necessary to spend money up front. For example, student recruitment is a necessary first step in attracting students to an institution for purposes of increasing enrollment. Costs associated with recruitment include travel, development of brochures or other promotional materials, personnel time, and communication costs. Fund-raising can be profitable but requires similar resources in terms of personnel, communications, and public relations activities. Grantsmanship is a labor-intensive endeavor with associated costs. The payoff in terms of funded grants and contracts is well worth the effort.

Demographic changes will have important effects on higher education in the following ways. The number of people 18 to 22 years old is decreasing, so that universities and colleges are having to recruit other population age groups. The average age of students in nursing is on the increase. Registered nurses and licensed practical nurses are returning to school in increasing numbers to attain higher degrees. These factors are forcing nursing programs to develop innovative means for nontraditional students to meet their educational goals, such as weekend and evening classes, accelerated tracks, and tracks for second-career students.

Moreover, funding is affected in another way, in that older taxpayers are exhibiting reluctance to support a system of education that competes with dollars for health care, an area of more immediate concern to them.[24] Nursing educators should not lose sight of the fact that investors in higher education (taxpayers) want an accounting of the returns on their investments and want to know that their tax dollars are being used in the most efficient manner. In the future, accountability for faculty time and effort will be scrutinized more closely. Productivity will be measured in outcomes, such as graduation rates, student credit hours produced, and funded research dollars. Geitgey[8] urged nursing educators to become more involved in politics and public policy formation in order to influence state and federal funding decisions.

Any discussion of cost cutting should take into consideration quality issues. It is incumbent upon the individual institution to determine which cost-effective measures can be undertaken without compromising the educational outcomes of the program. In this chapter, we have demonstrated that there are sources of revenue streams for nursing educational programs to pursue and that there are cost-saving measures to be employed. Nursing can respond creatively to the budgetary challenges of the future through implementation of innovative strategies and ideas.

REFERENCES

1. American Association of Colleges of Nursing. (1991). *Institutional resources and budgets.* Washington, D.C.: Author.

2. American Association of Colleges of Nursing. (1992). Dean's summer seminar set for Big Sky. *Syllabus, 18*(2), 2.

3. Billingsley, M. (1991, Winter). Hard times all around [From the editor]. *Nursing Connections, 4*(4), 13-14.

4. Blumenstyk, G. (1992, May 13). College officials and policy experts ponder implications of "privatizing" state colleges. *Chronicle of Higher Education,* pp. A25-A27.

5. Burns, P. G., Nishikawa, H. A., Weatherby, F., Forni, P. R., Moran, M., Baker, C. M., Booton, D. A., & Allen, M. E. (in press). Master's degree nursing education: State-of-the-art. *Journal of Professional Nursing.*

6. Dienemann, J. (1983). Reducing nursing faculty workloads without increasing costs. *Image: The Journal of Nursing Scholarship, 15*(4), 111-114.

7. Frank, K. M. (1990). Funding for nursing education: Passthrough or pass over? *Nursing Economic$, 8*(3), 132.

8. Geitgey, D. (1982). Financing nursing education—a public perspective. In *Economics of higher education in nursing* (pp. 13-14). Washington, D.C.: American Association of Colleges of Nursing.

9. Hawken, P. L., & Hillestad, E. A. (1987). Weighing the costs and benefits of student education to service agencies. *Nursing and Health Care, 8*(4), 223-227.

10. Hegevary, S. T. (1992). Funding of schools of nursing. *Journal of Professional Nursing, 8*(3), 142.

11. Hines, R. (1992). State higher education appropriations: A retrospective of fiscal year 1993. *Grapevine, 34*(384), 3137.

12. Jacobson, R. L. (1992, April 15). Colleges face new pressure to increase faculty productivity. *Chronicle of Higher Education,* pp. A16-A18.

13. Kummer, K., Bednash, G., & Redman, B. K. (1987). Cost model for baccalaureate nursing education. *Journal of Professional Nursing, 3*(3), 176-189.

14. Layzell, D. T. (1992, February 19). Tight budgets demand studies of faculty productivity. *Chronicle of Higher Education,* pp. B2-B3.

15. Melvin, N. (1988). A method for the comparative analysis of the instructional costs of three baccalaureate nursing programs. *Journal of Professional Nursing, 4*(4), 249-261.

16. National League for Nursing. (1989). *Nursing centers: Meeting the demand for quality health care.* New York: Author.

17. Olson, S. (Ed.). (1992). *The foundation directory* (14th ed.). New York: Foundation Center.

18. Roberts, P. M. (1989). An estimate of the cost of educating a BN graduate and graduates of other disciplines at a Canadian university: A case study. *Journal of Nursing Education, 28*(3), 140-143.

19. Santo-Novak, D. A. (1990). P.R.I.C.E.—a funding model for educational viability. *Journal of Nursing Education, 29*(3), 142-144.

20. Schneider, D. (1992). Virginia Henderson Library leads nursing to new age. *Reflections, 18*(1), 9-10.

21. Starck, P. L., Walker, G. C., & Bohannan, P. A. (1991). Nursing faculty practice in the Houston linkage model: Administrative and faculty perspectives. *Nurse Educator, 16*(5), 23-28.

22. Starck, P. L., & Williams, W. E. (1988). What does nursing education cost? Turning the question around. *Journal of Professional Nursing, 4*(1), 38-44.

23. Virtual reality: A technology in nursing education's future? (1991). *Nursing Educators MicroWorld, 5*(3), 17, 19.

24. Yudof, M. G. (1992, May 13). The burgeoning privatization of state universities. *Chronicle of Higher Education,* p. A48.

CHAPTER 73

Who pays for the costs of care in other countries?

GILLIAN BISCOE

At one end of the continuum of health care financing is the marketplace approach; at the other end, government monopoly. Each country's position on this continuum arises from a complex interaction of culture, politics, economics, and management ability. No model in the world is agreed upon as the best for health care delivery and financing. The models used by various countries have their own particular advantages and disadvantages and are developed for a particular socioeconomic, cultural, and political environment.

There are also marked differences between developed and developing countries in terms of financing health care systems. Mortality is much higher in developing countries, as is morbidity. However, both developed and developing countries face an increasing gap between the costs of health care and the money available to meet those costs. There is increasing critical analysis of how health care might best be financed to reduce this gap. In some countries this has resulted in the rationing of services. Around the world there is concern for problems that may arise in the future because of the increasing elderly population and a declining number of taxpayers contributing to health care costs.

The World Bank[4] has defined three main problems in the health care sector: allocation issues, such as insufficient spending on cost-effective health programs; internal inefficiency issues, such as wasteful public programs of poor quality; and inequity issues, such as inequitable distribution of the benefits of health services. The World Bank's view is that the fundamental cause of these problems is inappropriate approaches to health care financing.

In low-income developing countries (for example, Ethiopia, Uganda, and Pakistan) the average spending on health is about $9 per capita per year. In middle-income countries (Poland, Thailand, and Greece) the figure is $31. In developed countries (Singapore, France, and Japan) the average figure is $670.[4]

The percentage of gross national product (GNP) spent on health in 1984 ranged from 2% by Ethiopia to 9.3% by the United States. In terms of total government spending, this figure becomes 3.4% for Ethiopia (the most recent figures available are from 1980) and 11% for the United States. In addition to government financing sources, more than half of the health care costs in developing countries are borne directly by individuals. In developed countries this fraction is less than one fourth.

The problem with using macroindicators such as GNP and GDP (gross domestic product) is that they give no indication of how well the money is spent nor on what it is spent. A large amount of effort in most countries is going into the development of outcome measures. The only other measures we have are aggregate measures of things like infant mortality and life expectancy. While these give good intercountry comparisons, they do not tell us what we should spend our money on and what really works in improving health.

Most would expect that the more money spent, the better the health of people. This is not the case. Americans spend most on health care and have the worst rates in the developed nations of infant mortality and life expectancy. Japan spends the equivalent of $978 per person on health and 6.7% of its GDP and has the highest life expectancy and the lowest infant mortality rate when compared to Canada, the United States, Great Britain, and Sweden.

Vietnam's major health issues have to do with the macrodeterminants of health: clean air, clean water, clean food, nutrition in general, and socioeconomic, employment, and education issues. The hospitals in Vietnam are poorly staffed and very poorly equipped. Modern textbooks are hardly available. The figures on health care spending there are focused more on hospitals and community health centers and mask the beginnings of international support to rebuild Vietnam's infrastructure.

In the People's Republic of China much has been done to improve the health of citizens through improvement in living conditions, education, and employment since the end of the cultural revolution. Again, their costs of health care mask large amounts of money spent on other determinants of health.

In all countries there is increasing tension between spending money to promote health and prevent illness and satisfying the voracious appetites of hospitals for money to spend on curative care and research.

Health care can therefore be said to cover an indefinable range of needs and services. The general view is that there is also an infinite range of demands made by consumers on any health care system. This issue can be put in a philosophical perspective: Is equity and access to health care a right, or should it be contingent on the ability of the consumer to pay?

An analogy might be found in the demand for luxury automobiles. A survey in the United States might result in 100% of the respondents replying yes to the question, If you could afford a Mercedes-Benz, would you want one? Not everyone drives a Mercedes-Benz because not everyone can afford one. The desire for a Mercedes-Benz does not entail satisfaction of that desire. Similarly, there may be an infinite demand for health care, but does that mean that countries have to fill that demand? The issue of need versus demand, and the associated ethical debates, is receiving increased attention from both health care providers and consumers.

This argument cannot be fully developed in this chapter, but such issues are already influencing decisions on how health care is financed. Philosophical and ethical issues of needs versus rights, together with economic factors, will shape the future of health care financing.

The World Health Organization's 1981 goal of health for all by the year 2000 has resulted in increased attention to raising health status as distinct from providing curative services. Curative services are in many cases necessary precisely because both society and the individual do little to maintain health. At the crux of the issue of achieving health for all is the question of how to finance primary health programs while maintaining curative services in the transition period between an illness-oriented health system and a health-oriented system. In its simplest form the issue can be viewed as how to redirect the financing of expensive, hospital-based curative care to health promotion and health prevention strategies, in order to reduce the need for curative care.

INTERNATIONAL OVERVIEW
Singapore

Singapore's system of health care financing is based on aspects of its cultural philosophy. In Singapore the family is the basic social and economic unit. Although there is a collective responsibility on the part of society to care for the family, Singaporeans believe that personal responsibility also exists. Singapore is particularly concerned with the imbalance between an aging population and its younger members, and it hopes to promote financial independence among the future elderly so that they may shoulder their own health costs.

Since 1984 employees and employers in Singapore have been required to make equal payments to employees' personal saving accounts. Interest is paid on the money deposited, the balance is the property of the account holder, and it can only be used to pay for the medical expenses of employees or their families. At retirement age (55 years), the holder can access the account, but a minimum balance must be maintained. On the death of the account holder, any balance remaining in the account is paid to the estate's beneficiaries, free of estate or death taxes.

In 1983 health expenditures in Singapore were 6.4% of total government expenditures. The ratios of physicians and nurses to the general population were 1:1100 and 1:340, respectively, and the corresponding ratio for hospital beds was 1:340.

Belgium

Belgium is a hereditary, representative, and constitutional monarchy. Belgian law largely reflects the national philosophy of liberalism and individualism. Paradoxically, Belgium's legislation on health financial matters, including physician reimbursement, is highly detailed and regulatory, to the extent that it covers issues that in other Western European countries might be regarded as infringing on ethical matters.

As in most industrial countries, health care costs in Belgium have been difficult to contain. Health insurance is compulsory, with individuals paying little if anything from their own pockets for treatment or consultation. This has resulted in a situation in which it is the norm to press for second opinions, which tends to overburden diagnostic facilities and increase costs.

Japan

Japan has a nationwide social health care system, but the delivery of health care services relies heavily on the private sector. The social health care system is based on the West German model.

The Japanese Medical Association is particularly strong and has considerable influence on national medical policy. Physician income is very high compared to that of other professional groups. Japan's health care system is extremely complex, reflecting the complex nature of its society.

As with other nations, Japan faces steep increases in health care costs. Quality and availability of health facilities are assured in Japan. The combination of accessibility, availability, and health insurance programs results in an expensive system.

Japan's citizens all have public health insurance coverage, 52% through Health Insurance for Employees (HIE) and 48% through National Health Insurance (NHI). Both insurance schemes, however, leave the individual paying out-of-pocket expenses for his or her health care. For example, HIE covers 90% of employees' hospital expenses and 80% of the expenses of their dependents, with an out-of-pocket maximum equivalent to $392 per month.

In general, good quality care is received and there are minimal waiting times for personal appointments. The view of the Japanese, however, is that too much money is spent on hospital care, advanced technology, and treatment of the terminally ill. Physician costs are also considered to be high.

Canada

Canada's system of health care financing is based on equity and access, with means testing considered anathema and anything less than 100% participation inequitable.

The Canadian constitution limits the federal parliament to implementing national programs through provincial governments. Private insurance is allowed only for services not covered under the provincial health services plan. Persons may not be excluded on the basis of preexisting conditions.

Canada spends 8.5% of its GDP on health and the equivalent of $1554 per capita. Inflation in Canada

from 1977 to 1987 was 6.4%. Health care costs have increased by 8.5% in the same period.

The 100% public health insurance coverage is automatic for all residents and is financed through national taxation (38%) and provincial taxation (62%). In addition, 90% of Canada's residents have private insurance coverage. The main source of payment is through employers. Private insurance cannot cover anything that is already covered by public insurance. Typically it covers things like some prescription drugs, ambulance service, nursing home care, and private hospital rooms.

Canada's infant mortality rate is 7.3% and its life expectancy is 79.2.

France

Since the French socialist party came to power in 1981, there have been many changes to the laws and regulations affecting health. The socialist government has attempted to tackle health expenditures and to permanently modify the health care system through structural reforms such as decentralization and departmentalization. Again, as in most developed countries, health costs have in general risen faster than the nation's ability to pay. The government has sought to halt the rising costs of health care by limiting supply.[3]

France's social insurance system strongly reflects various occupational and class interests. Thus conflict arises along class lines more frequently than in other welfare states where social insurance systems tend to blur class conflict.

France spends 8.7% of its GDP on health and the equivalent of $1178 per capita. Its infant mortality rate is 8.2 per 1000 live births, and the life expectancy is 77.6.

Switzerland

Since 1848 Switzerland has been a federation with cantons forming its federal structure. Responsibility for health care falls first on the cantons. Unlike Germany or Canada, Switzerland has no political ideology dictating equal access to health care.[2] Cantons therefore draw up plans to suit their own needs. There is frequent duplication of services, giving rise to additional and unnecessary expense. Some cantons are richer than others, resulting in further inequities. On the other hand, the Swiss view is that decentralization of decision making means that health care services can be adapted with considerable flexibility to the differing cultures and philosophies of the various cantons.

Health care spending in Switzerland is 8.7% of GDP and the equivalent of $1301 per capita. The infant mortality rate is 4.9% and the life expectancy is 78.9.

Sweden

Sweden's population has 100% automatic public health insurance coverage. There are small copayments (for example, for hospital care, the copayment is equivalent to $10 per day up to $150 per year). The insurance is financed 65% by local tax, 10% by employer payroll tax, and 6.5% by federal tax and some government subsidies. About 7% of the population have supplementary private insurance. The majority of those with private insurance are highly paid executives and their families. The insurance covers such things as private hospital accommodations and private elective surgery, which can be done more quickly than surgery in the public system.

Sweden's infant mortality rate is 5.9% and the life expectancy in 1990 was 79.3 years of age.

Australia

Australia has universal public health insurance paid for by a levy (the Medicare levy) on gross taxable income. In addition, 42% of the population have supplementary private insurance. There is currently debate over the relative roles of the public and private sectors based on ideological issues. Doctors' fees are paid through Medicare, but many doctors charge above the scheduled fee, with individuals having to make up the difference.

No charges are raised for public patients in public hospitals: a 5-year Medicare agreement is the funding mechanism between the commonwealth government and the state and territory governments. There are complex interrelationships between the commonwealth government, state and territory governments, and local governments in the funding and provision of health care.

Australia's health care spending as a percentage of GDP is 7.0% and the per capita expenditure is equivalent to $990. The infant mortality rate is 8.2% and life expectancy is 76.6.

SUMMARY

The structure and financing of national health care systems are the result of complex interactions of culture, politics, and economics. For all countries, the growth in national resources allocated to health care outweighs the growth in available resources.

The World Health Organization's philosophy of health for all strongly emphasizes equity.[1] There is, however, a basic economic principle having to do with choice. Choice means that not everything is available, that resources are limited, and that trade-offs must be made. Few countries have a strategic plan for health care. Few countries know what it is they are trying to buy with the large amounts of money expended on health care. Few countries measure what it is they have bought for those large amounts of money.

There are many who say that health care is first and foremost about care, that its social benefits outweigh any costs. There are others who respond that that may be so, but that decisions have already been made that result in the fact that some people have access to treatment and others do not (examples are age restrictions for admission to coronary care units and labor restrictions in delivering community-based health care).

There is no one model of health care that is right for all countries. Each different culture requires that health care delivery be tailored to those cultural needs. Each country's economy will determine to a large extent how much money is available to purchase health care. Politics is a key variable. The purchase of health care is expensive, and the effective management of that purchasing process is critical.

Notwithstanding these complexities, the key to health cost containment is the national definition of milestones to be achieved and health goals to be attained. Strategic plans can then be developed that address allocation, efficiency, and equity issues in achieving those goals. A clear road map will then emerge, enabling each country to restructure health care to best suit its own unique situation.

REFERENCES

1. Andreano, R. (1988). *The challenges to health for all and primary health care: An economist's perspective.* Unpublished background paper to joint WHO/ICN consultation on nursing for primary health care: 10 years after Alma-Ata and perspectives for the future.
2. Veska. *Health services in Switzerland, AARAU and the Swiss Hospital Association.*
3. Walliman, I. (1986). Social insurance and the delivery of social services in France. *Social Science and Medicine, 23*(12), 1305.
4. World Bank. (1987). *Policy study: Financing health services in developing countries.* Washington, D.C.: Author.

PART NINE

PERSONAL AND PROFESSIONAL ASSERTIVENESS

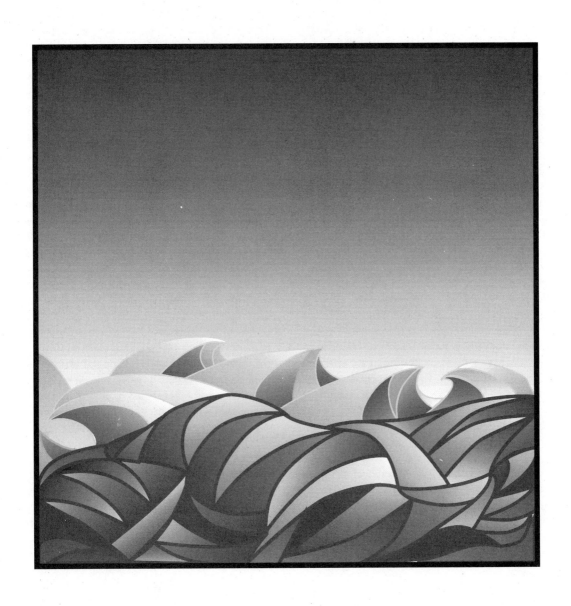

The winds of change

JOANNE COMI McCLOSKEY, HELEN KENNEDY GRACE

While nursing has always been predominantly a women's profession, the impact of changing roles of women in the broader society has not, until recent years, been reflected in nursing. In fact, in the early years of the women's movement, nurses were perceived to be part of the problem, in that nursing was viewed as a profession that reinforced traditional women's roles in society. Caring for the sick was equated with the mothering role of women in the family. Women's rights activists have never truly joined with the profession to secure greater independence and recognition of the significant contributions made by nurses. As opportunities for women opened up in a wide range of professions, women were encouraged to enter the "real" professions—that is, medicine, law, business, and computer science—rather than pursue careers in the more traditional fields for women such as teaching and nursing. Nursing schools saw a dramatic decrease in applicants as women moved into other fields. Nurses moved out of the profession to other fields of endeavor where they could achieve greater recognition and independence. However, in recent years these trends appear to be reversing. A large number of students are now entering nursing after they have "sampled" careers in other fields. An increasing number of men are entering the field. And the profession itself is increasingly incorporating values that support career development within the field. This section looks at issues related to the evolving profession and the impact of internal and external forces in the process of change.

In the debate chapter, Swanson focuses upon the internal structure of the profession as reflected in approaches to career development. After an extensive review of theories related to career development, Swanson first argues that career development is not possible within nursing, primarily because of the emphasis upon entry-level employment, limited opportunity for

career advancement in the field, work conditions within the field, and lack of support and recognition from hospital administration and medical staff. Disenchanted with the field, many nurses have moved to part-time employment or to employment outside of nursing. On the pro side of the debate, new opportunities for assisting graduates to secure appropriate positions, assessment processes that allow nurses to formulate career paths within the field, a changing work environment with greater emphasis upon clinical career paths, and developing counseling and mentoring programs are all presented as evidence of support of career development within the field.

A historical perspective on nursing's quest for professionalism is provided next by Brodie. Nursing has gone through a series of steps in the process of becoming a profession: (1) domestic art, (2) religious calling, (3) skilled discipline, (4) pool of expert managers, and (5) pool of expert clinicians. Interlacing the development of nursing organizations and refinements in nursing education through the years with these phases, Brodie concludes that "much of nursing's current claim to professionalism is based on mastery of medical knowledge and skills." The challenge of the future is to continue to build upon the strong traditions within the field to move toward greater self-direction.

Donley and Flaherty assert that the nursing shortage of the 1980s highlighted the imagery problems of nursing. The imagery problems of nursing are reflected in the mixed symbols that are presented in the media. Nurses are depicted as caring, compassionate persons, which implies weakness and powerlessness; and yet they take on medical (masculine) symbols such as the white coat and stethoscope. Rather than relying upon the imagery of nursing that is being communicated through the media, Donley and Flaherty speak to the potential power of nurses as individuals to convey accurate information to the public. Ironically, the nursing shortage of the 1980s demonstrated that, unlike other fields, nursing was experiencing poor employment conditions and growing employee dissatisfaction at that time. The lack of differentiation in nursing and substitution of nurses for other health workers remain problems within the field and, coupled with lack of autonomy for nurses, continue to blur the public's perceptions of the vital role of nurses in providing quality health care. Nurses are pawns of the broader health care system and its financing. The authors conclude: "The story of the image of nursing is very much like the story of Cinderella. When the real image of nurses is acknowledged, the reflecting mirror of power and greed that has distorted nursing's image will be broken."

Part of the imagery problem of nursing is the overlap with traditional roles of women. Shea makes the linkage between feminism and nursing and describes the historical trends that have now made it possible to join feminist ideology with the nursing profession. The current emphasis on caring as a central focus of the profession dovetails nicely with changes in the feminist perspective, which has become "kinder and gentler." The author traces the history of feminism, through the early emphasis on gaining equal rights and suffrage (nineteenth century), through the '60s, with the emphasis on the equality of women to men, to today's feminism, which draws upon a theoretical perspective that stresses differences between genders rather than similarities. These differences are being reframed as positive attributes. This change in feminist ideology coincides with the current emphasis in nursing on the caring process. Women's health is presented as an example of an area where feminist ideology and nursing practice logically come together in a complementary way. Suggesting that the third wave of the women's movement is just around the corner, Shea challenges nurses to become part of a positive force for change.

The next two chapters in this section focus upon collaboration between physicians and nurses. The first, by Baggs, is focused upon collaboration within acute care practice settings, while the second, by Lenz, is directed toward community-based multidisciplinary educational settings. Baggs begins by noting that the terminology of collaborative practice has different meanings in medicine and nursing. Most of the writing related to collaborative practice has been done by nurses. Loss of power by physicians and gaining of power by nurses is a threat to traditional medical prac-

tice. Collaborative practice was advanced through the National Joint Practice Commission some 20 years ago. Yet the guidelines developed then are not implemented to any marked degree in practice settings today. Despite evidence that collaborative practice results in improved patient outcomes, an astoundingly low percentage of physicians (14%) and an even lower percentage of nurses (7%) report using collaborative problem solving in clinical settings. Obstacles to collaborative practice include traditional communication patterns, decision-making prerogatives of physicians, and a reluctance on the part of nurses to accept greater responsibility for decision making. Changes in educational programs to promote collaborative learning and changes within practice settings to facilitate collaborative problem solving are beginning to emerge.

Turning to the community practice side, Lenz focuses her views on collaboration on multidisciplinary community-based education and practice. Basing multidisciplinary health professions education within the community, in settings where the community is more than a passive recipient of the byproducts of the educational-service process, creates a powerful new dynamic to foster collaboration between medicine and nursing. Development of such an educational-practice model is not without a set of challenges. The nurse educator within the community setting must be both a provider and an educator. Although less than 20% of all health care occurs in hospitals, most clinical nursing education is based in tertiary care settings. Lenz argues that nursing has a pivotal role to play in the community and can potentially be a significant force in health system reform. Barriers to moving toward these expanded horizons arise from within the profession— from our lack of skills in the political domain and from the behavior of nurses as oppressed persons. External barriers come from the financing of health care, male dominance of medical practice, and a conflict of perspectives between nursing and medical education. Nursing education, with its emphasis on an educational model that values research and teaching over practice, is in basic conflict with the medical apprenticeship model. To bring nursing and medical education together requires a new degree of involvement of nursing educators in clinical practice, working side by side with medical educators. The community, working with health professions educators in programs focused on real-life needs of people, can do much to forge new relationships and build upon the contributions of nursing to improving the health of people.

In the international chapter in this section, the focus shifts to nursing in Russia, which is a reality jolt, given the real advances that are being made in nursing in the United States. Smith, as founder of the U.S.-Russian Nurse Exchange Consortium, provides current insights into the challenges facing nursing in the context of economic and political realities. Faced with desperately inadequate facilities and resources, nurses in Russia are the backbone of the health services system. Yet they face the same prejudices and constraints as their fellow nurses around the world. Low salaries, poor working conditions, and expectations that they will perform menial work such as cleaning and washing walls in addition to caring for 30 patients per day—all of these make the lives of nurses difficult. Despite these conditions nurses are beginning to organize, and links between the East and West are being forged. Nurse-to-nurse international exchanges are proposed as a means of supporting efforts by nurses to improve their lot and thus to improve patient care in the changing context of Russia today.

This section provides an interesting overview of the processes of change within nursing and the potential for joining with forces outside of nursing. Are we on the threshold of major breakthroughs that will allow nurses to demonstrate fully their contributions to health care both within and without hospital settings? The potential of joining forces with the changing feminist movement and of achieving peer relationships and true collaboration with physicians is clearly on the horizon. Whether or not nursing moves forward to achieve this new degree of professionalism depends to a great extent upon the acceptance of the responsibility that accompanies increased authority. Clearly the winds of change are blowing. Will nursing ride the currents and move toward changes that are inevitable, to become part of the solution of our current health care crises, or will we continue to wallow in a past of grievances and wrongs and miss this golden opportunity?

CHAPTER 74

Debate

Career development

Its status in nursing

ELIZABETH A. SWANSON

In the United States, almost every individual has an opportunity to select an occupation. Adolescents are trying to figure out who they are and what they want, as well as to get an idea of what is available in the surrounding environment. Parents wonder how involved they should be, while friends and teachers willingly give advice about making career choices.

It is very important to remember that many individuals making these occupational choices *are* adolescents—individuals who are still developing, both intellectually and emotionally.[46] The ability to make a sound occupational choice is thus very closely related to the general maturation of the individual.[14]

For the purpose of this writing, the theoretical focus will be on developmental theories that deal with the way in which career decisions of maturing individuals evolve. By definition, a career implies a developmental sequence of activities, not just a one-time decision. The developmental notion is also supported by a career characteristic, namely that it is an organized effort or array of jobs within a plan. But women appear to approach career development differently.[41] As Henning and Jardin[17] point out, women in management positions view a career from a psychological perspective relating to personal growth, making a contribution to others, and doing what one wants to do. Men are advancement oriented, with a series of events in mind that will result in recognition and reward.

Nursing is a predominantly female profession and, as such, reflects the female approach to career development.[17] Generally, nurses seek to change jobs only after dissatisfaction has set in. But the job change may not always result in advancement of professional development. Nurses appear to have relatively low career aspirations, and frequently when vacancies occur, there are very few qualified individuals to fill them.[22] Thus a question needs to be raised as to whether career development exists or is even possible within nursing. Kleinknecht and Hefferin[23] contend that the career development models within nursing can assist individuals to identify interests, values, and aspirations as well as help them define the manner in which goals can be achieved. Furthermore, they say, these models can serve to enhance a nurse's job satisfaction by making the work more challenging, interesting, and rewarding, and by incorporating opportunities for policy making. With this background information in mind, I will briefly summarize the classic maturation theories of career development and use aspects of that presentation to debate the status of career development within nursing. The interested reader can refer to the original works or the previous edition of McCloskey and Grace for a more extensive discussion of the classic theories of career development.

REVIEW OF LITERATURE
E. Ginzberg and associates

Ginzberg and associates[14] have a three-period process of career development, which they contend is based on a series of irreversible compromises. The first period is one of fantasy, focusing on the desire for and pleasure of work. An outcome of this period is that children recognize that they will be working someday.

The second period, the tentative period, is a four-part period of development occurring between the ages of 11 and 18. During the part called "interest," students identify occupational choices based on activities, interests, and work of parents. "Capacity"—the second part of this period—is when the individuals display an intensification of trends established earlier. The third part of the tentative period is "value," in which the individual realizes that much consideration goes into making a vocational choice and that goals and values have a significant impact on that choice. "Transition" closes out the tentative period. The individual is beginning to move from a focus on predominantly subjective factors to trying out skills, studying various careers, recognizing financial rewards, and evaluating life circumstances of these careers as a means of making an occupational choice.

The third, realistic, period, takes place between the ages of 18 and 22 and is divided into the three parts of exploration, crystallization, and specification. Throughout the realistic period, individuals assess their past and future and examine the many factors that influence occupational choice. This period concludes with the selecting of a specific job or graduate education.

Since the origination of the general theory, Ginzberg[13] has suggested three conceptual changes. First, occupational decisions are a life-spanning phenomenon, not a short-term event restricted to adolescence and early adulthood. Second, irreversibility has been modified to encompass the idea that it exists for some people at selected times in their life. Finally, the element of compromise has become one of optimization, in which the individual searches for the most appropriate fit between the preferred career avenues and the accessible opportunities.

Empirical evidence regarding the theory is mixed. Some evidence exists that students emphasize different kinds of experiences in their vocational development at various age levels.[5] There is also empirical support for the idea that students realign their career preferences in response to the reality of the outside world.[18] But the data are inconclusive as to what the stages are, when they occur, and in what order they occur.[21]

In summary, Ginzberg and his colleagues[14] have developed an approach to career development that defines the vocational choice process as a specific behavior. They propose a systematic and predictable series of tasks that young people face during adolescence, which ends with the selection of a specific vocational choice.

D. Tiedeman

The second developmental theory to be reviewed was created by Tiedeman.[49] Stimulated by the writings of Ginzberg and Super, Tiedeman views career development as a function of the emerging self, becoming increasingly differentiated and comprehensive.

Tiedeman views decision making as crucial to the individual's career development. The decisions made daily are as significant as those made to dissociate oneself from the past. Focusing on the decision framework, each decision includes two periods with several substages.

The first period is anticipatory. Anticipatory behavior is broken down into the stages of exploration, crystallization, choice, and specification. During the exploration stage, the individual reviews aspirations, present and future opportunities, interests, capabilities, disagreeable elements of a career choice that could be tolerated, and the manner in which the choice is viewed by persons near the individual. As the choices become clearer, the person enters the stage of crystallization. With the choice made and goals defined, the person's behavioral system becomes oriented to vocational development. Not only does the image of self in the occupational position become perfected during the choice stage, but doubt about the occupational choice diminishes, leading to the stage of specification. If this dissipation of doubt does not occur, the individual will return to a more basic stage of this decision-making process.

The second period involves implementation and adjustment. With the closure of the anticipatory period, the period of implementation and adjustment emerges. The vocational concerns come face to face with reality and induction begins. This is the first of three stages within Tiedeman's period of implementation and adjustment. During this stage, the individual is involved in fitting goals and the field into the broader context of society.

In summary, Tiedeman[49] views career development as a function of the developing self, which becomes more differentiated and complete. Osipow[30] contends that the theory is very complicated and hard to understand, has few practical applications, and is more philosophical than career development oriented, but he does state that the work appears to bridge the gap between the developmental formulations of Ginzberg and Super.

D.E. Super

The third and final developmental theory to be reviewed was constructed by Super.[48] A brief presentation of the 10 postulates developed by Super and the stages of the theory will be the basis for discussion.

To begin, one basic postulate recognizes that people differ in their abilities, interests, and personalities and that, as one experiences life, these factors come to identify the individual's uniqueness. Thus individuals are qualified by virtue of these characteristics for a number of occupations. Thus individuals' inabilities to perform a particular skill would only disqualify them from their selected occupation *if* that skill were of extreme importance to successful performance.

Another postulate is that all occupations require a set of abilities, interests, and personality traits—with tolerances wide enough to allow some variety of occupations for each individual and some variety of individuals in each occupation. Thus workers could have differing levels of a trait or skill appropriate for a selected occupation and still be able to perform the work.

Vocational preferences and competencies—the situations in which people live and work, and hence their self-concepts—change with time and experience, making choice and adjustment a continuous process. Super believes that these changes impact the skill level of workers, the work environment, and the self-concept of workers. With any of these changes, workers who were once satisfied with their work may become dissatisfied later and seek new employment.

Self-concept is a significant element and is defined generally as the individual's perception of the circumstances or conditions of existence. Super states that it is imperative to define self-concept in this way because the situation surrounding an individual always affects one's behavior and understanding.

The entire process of career development is a series of life stages characterized by growth, exploration, establishment, maintenance, and decline. These stages are subdivided into (1) the fantasy, tentative, and realistic phases of the exploratory stage and (2) the trial and stable phases of the establishment stage. The growth stage refers to the physical and psychological dimensions of development. Self-concepts are forming during this stage, and individuals are involved in numerous experiences that assist them in making their tentative and final occupational determinations.

In the exploration stage, individuals understand that work is part of life. But their verbalized choices may be unrealistic, especially if they are expressed during the fantasy phase. After the fantasy phase, individuals advance into the tentative phase, in which occupational choices are limited to a few alternatives. During the final phase or the realistic phase, the list of occupational choices consists of those that individuals perceive as being realistic for them to attain.

The establishment stage involves early efforts in actual work situations. Using these work experiences as a testing ground, individuals evaluate whether the choices made in the previous exploratory stage have any merit. Generally, gains are made in confidence, experience, and proficiency, and the individuals become stabilized.

On advancing through the stabilizing phase of the exploration stage, individuals enter the maintenance stage. As a part of this stage, individuals continue in or improve their occupational situation. Because the work situation is always changing, individuals try to alter those components of their work that are less than satisfying, but in general they do not continually try to change the work situation.

During the decline stage, individuals work to keep their jobs and are not concerned about enhancing their positions. This period ends at retirement, the last stage of career development proposed by Super.

Murphy and Burck[28] propose an addition to Super's developmental theory. They suggest that the stage of renewal be added between the stages of establishment and maintenance. They contend that this is natural, because individuals reevaluate earlier goals and plans and either recommit to those goals or decide to refocus and make a midlife career change.

The nature of the career pattern is determined by individuals' parental socioeconomic level, mental activity, personality characteristics, and opportunities.[48] Some factors may be more significant than others, and parental socioeconomic level may be one of the most important. This particular factor exposes individuals in the earliest stages of development to their parents' work, associates, and family, all of which can greatly influence later work patterns. Additional factors that may be important are an individual's mental abilities and subsequent academic successes, the ability to work with others, and the gift of being in the right place at the right time.

Development through the life stages can be guided, partly by facilitating the maturation of abilities and interests and partly by aiding in reality testing and the development of the self-concept.[48] Thus the secondary education system and its guidance system are important in helping individuals to develop abilities and interests and to obtain a perspective of their own strengths and weaknesses so they can make appropriate occupational choices.

The process of compromise between individual and social factors and between self-concept and reality is one of role-playing, whether the role is played in fantasy, in the counseling interview, or in real-life activities such as school classes, clubs, part-time work, and entry-level jobs.[48] Individuals may seek out related experiences to evaluate the match between the occupations of choice and their self-images. Perhaps individuals interested in a health care occupation would volunteer at day-care centers, senior citizens' centers, or hospitals.

Work and life satisfaction depend on the extent to which individuals find adequate outlets for their abilities, interests, and values; individuals depend on their establishment in a type of work, a work situation, and a way of life in which they can play the kind of role that is appropriate.[47,48] Super states that when experiences encountered at work correspond to the individuals' images, there is ample opportunity for individuals to be as they wish to be. In contrast, if work does not afford opportunities for individuals to act in accordance with their mental images of themselves, they are discontented. This dissatisfaction could easily provoke them to look for work situations in which their work experiences would be more in line with their mental images.

Many studies have been conducted to evaluate Super's developmental theory and supporting concepts. In general, the research findings confirm the idea that occupational choice represents the implementation of a self-concept. The results also provide an impressive volume of empirical support for the general aspects of Super's theory.

Career theories and women

Although the three theories just covered are of primary importance in understanding the process of career development, some researchers contend that they do not adequately explain the vocational behavior of women.[30,32] For instance, these stages may be delayed or interrupted due to marriage and child rearing responsibilities. Fitzgerald and Crites[9] contend that the development of a vocational self-concept for women may be very complex due to the divided role expectations of wife, mother, and worker.

With the paucity of theories directly applicable to women, other efforts have generated constructs relevant to a woman's career development. Psathas[35] delineated some of the factors affecting women's entry into occupational roles and stated that gender is the most noticeable of all factors.

A second attempt at constructing a career development framework for females can be attributed to Zytowski.[52] His nine postulates attempt to take into account the distinctive differences for men and women in work life, development, and patterns of vocational participation. For example, the woman's main role is that of a homemaker, which is dynamic yet orderly and developmental. Zytowski also perceives that vocational participation of women will cause a departure for them from their main role in life. He concludes his postulates by stating that selected factors are responsible for a pattern of vocational participation for men and women. Interestingly, both Psathas[35] and Zytowski[52] focus on the homemaker's role as the primary one in the occupational life of a woman.

It appears that the difficulty with developing a theory uniquely for women relates to the ever-changing role of women.[30,52] Fitzgerald and Crites[9] support this contention and continue by stating that women form a much more heterogeneous group than men with regard to life-career patterns. These factors do make the formulating of a relevant theory difficult, but the lack of a theory for women does not mean that established theories of career development are of no value. All individuals, regardless of sex, share the basic human need for self-fulfillment through meaningful work.[9] In other words, theories can provide a practical means of viewing career development of women. Fitzgerald and Crites believe that these theories can apply in some degree to everyone. Super[48] suggests that the general concepts of career development are applicable to women if modifications are made to provide for the childbearing role. Therefore, it seems appropriate at this time to apply selected aspects of the career development theories to women.

CAREER DEVELOPMENT: NOT POSSIBLE IN NURSING?

Career development in nursing can be evaluated using Super's theory and incorporating Murphy and Burck's renewal stage. For example, the stage of utmost importance to the new graduate nurse is the stage of establishment. This stage includes employment with a commitment to that particular choice. The final occupational choice is accepted as the one that provides the best opportunities to meet the individual's goals and expectations. Another stage of career development that is applicable is the renewal stage. To reiterate, the renewal stage, as defined by Murphy and

Burck,[28] relates to the midlife career changes persons may experience between the ages of 35 and 45. Individuals reconsider occupational goals and plans and decide either to rededicate themselves to the original goals or to move in other directions with a midlife change. During the maintenance stage, as identified by Super,[48] individuals attempt to continue or improve their occupational situation.

Keough,[22] in her editorial "The Need for Nursing Career Development," defines a career development program for nurses. It is a program where goals are set, needs are identified, counseling and guidance are available, plans are implemented, and activities are evaluated in order to revise plans as needed. This approach resembles the components of Super's last three stages because of its focus on behavior and action. In both processes, the person must become actively involved in career development and not just verbally communicate the intent of behavior. Otherwise no advancement can be made toward the achievement of the individual's desired career goals. Theoretically, I have adapted Super's vocational stages to nursing via Keough's defined system of organization. But does career development exist within nursing?

There is evidence within the literature that career development does not exist. It does not appear in nursing because nurses cannot move through the vocational development phases of establishment into a satisfactory position within the maintenance stage. Nurses can secure entry-level employment, but they do not develop stable positions, so retention becomes a problem. Hospitals are having trouble retaining registered nurses.[7,10,11,34] Parker and Drew[31] and Colavecchio,[4] using similar terms, tie this inability to retain nurses to inadequate staffing, poor hours, low status, limited recognition, and changing assignments.

Surveys conducted by Donovan,[7] Gulack,[15] and Wandelt, Pierce, and Widdowson[51] support certain factors identified by Colavecchio. These factors of discontent can be grouped into three categories: substance or content of the job itself, working conditions, and organizational factors. The major source of dissatisfaction in relation to job content is that of a quantitative overload.[51] Nurses identify the high patient-staff ratios, the volume of paperwork, and the intense time pressure to complete work as components of this overload phenomenon. Pines and Maslach[33] contend that it is the overload that leads to burnout rather than the intense interpersonal nature of the work.

The second major issue contributing to the nurses' dissatisfaction stems from concerns about their working conditions. Nurses are concerned about (1) the variable schedules, long hours, and floating from unit to unit; (2) the insufficiency of fringe benefits; (3) the problems of interacting with a support staff of questionable competence; and (4) compensation.[7,15,51]

The third source of discontent among nurses relates to organizational factors.[7,15,51] The specific factors were the lack of support and recognition from both hospital administration and medical staff. Nurses were also dissatisfied with the lack of recognition they received for their professional competence, the lack of input into the job, and the need for improved nurse-physician relations.[5] Another factor was the inability to advance within the system due to the flat organizational structure. As it exists, the organizational structure offers the professional very few possibilities for promotion and upward mobility.

Thus when disenchantment occurs, the nurse moves to another job or another occupational choice, or withdraws. National League for Nursing statistics[29] reported in the *Journal of Advanced Nursing* support this changing of jobs or withdrawal from the system. Data show an increase in the proportion of nursing graduates employed in nonnurse positions as the years since graduation increased. After 5 years, 1% of the graduates were in nonnurse occupations, whereas 6% were in those types of positions after 10 years. There was also a sizable shift from full-time work to part-time employment. For example, 1 year after graduation 85% of the graduates worked full-time and 5% worked part-time; 10 years after graduation the percentages were 37% full-time and 22% part-time.

Data collected by Donovan[7] convey a similar picture. Two of every five nurses drop out of the job market at some point in time. Other statistics from Donovan's article support a declining job stability within the profession. Nurses in the 45-and-older age bracket have stayed in each of their jobs for at least 7 years, whereas nurses in the 25-to-34-year-old age bracket have held each of their jobs for approximately 2.5 years.[7]

Although burnout has been given as a reason for increased mobility and temporary or permanent withdrawal, Kleinknecht and Hefferin[23] indicate that indecision about professional goals is also an important factor. Limited opportunities for professional development and the inability to determine and direct one's own future produce turnover and a low sense of achievement. Now the problem of nurses not focusing on career development goals is complicated by a nurse shortage and budget constraints. Administrators have to float or relocate nurses from specialty area to specialty area to provide patient care or to maintain financial solvency. These moves are made without considering the interests, goals, or experiences of the nursing staff involved. Price and Randolph[34] contend that this scenario makes career development unrealistic.

Two other factors are relevant in considering the lack of career development for individuals within nursing. Nursing is still predominantly a female occupation, although the number of males is increasing.[41] But with nursing's being female oriented, certain behaviors associated with women are bound to exist within the profession. Mahoney[24] contends that women do not plan. Consequently they do not think about employment-related possibilities. Similarly, Brink[2] believes that men are more able to differentiate between job requirements and career requirements and so are able to protect their career goals better than women. She continues by stating that males are socialized early to assert career priorities, while women remain job oriented. In addition, women seem less inclined to apply the term *career* to their work.[2,6,11] Nurses do not think in terms of a planned series of steps of development or advancement. Friss[10] also examines this idea in relation to the individual nurse. Nurses are not geographically mobile; they tend to fashion their careers around local labor markets. Carr[3] relates this lack of planning to the system. He believes that nothing exists within the system to allow talent and ability to be used at higher levels.

Mahoney[24] comments on another attitude common to women that, if prevalent, would suggest that it would be extremely difficult to operate in nursing and have a career development orientation. She contends that women do not look beyond the expectations of employment when they choose their occupations. Hudek[19] writes that a career should be concerned with issues that go beyond the work world. Several nurse authors unknowingly have applied these attitudes about employment to nursing. In a statement that could be related to Mahoney's, Masson[25] says that nurses today believe that the early appeal of nursing as a career eludes them. Friss[10] again comments on the relationship of nursing or nurses to a career: Nurses have minimal career aspirations, and those who want to develop a paying work career do not enter nursing.

Other reasons for this short-term orientation to work are presented by Donley.[6] Generally nursing has not been viewed by parents as a career, as exemplified by the statement, "It's good preparation for marriage." Subsequently nurses themselves view nursing as a temporary job. Nursing is also viewed as an occupation that is easy to enter and to leave without being demoted.

Rankin[36] and Ellis and Hartley,[8] in separate writings, identify other factors not evident in the nursing profession that are important aspects of career development. These include a mentoring system with dominance, support for risk taking, and a noncompetitive environment. In addition, nurses do not set professional priorities, ask pertinent questions, or follow up in actions.

Nursing continues to be challenged by the lack of planning, which is critical to career development. As Keough[22] points out, staffing crises occur frequently because vacancies exist. However, the major deterrent to career development in nursing is nurses' inability to identify strengths and to plan and create opportunities, all of which enhance their vocational positions. This factor is a main contributor to the high rate of staff turnover and professional dropout.[12] Thus, because nurses cannot change or choose not to change those unpleasant aspects that exist in their work situation, they are driven out of their positions and the profession. They do not advance through the maintenance stage of Super's career development theory *or* remain within the profession.

CAREER DEVELOPMENT IS POSSIBLE IN NURSING

There are opportunities within nursing to assist new graduates in securing appropriate positions. Reres[37] and Smith[41] present the idea of an appraisal tool that helps nurses recognize their goals, skills, and personal needs. Furthermore, this process is usable in attaining a position compatible with one's lifestyle, talents, and goals. Reres[37] approaches this idea from a benefits perspective, noting that it allows the nurse to maximize and realize the rewards of the system. The knowledge of one's own skills allows the nurse to view opportunities for advancement more positively. Similarly, Hefferin and Kleinknecht[16] have developed an assessment of work-related preferences for certain kinds of nursing activity, the Nursing Career Preference Inventory (NCPI). This assessment is to assist individual nurses in identifying their personal patterns of nursing work interests or preferences and determining the primary nursing practice areas and the hospital-based nursing role positions that most often reflect the identified work interest patterns. Although the instrument is based on an inpatient health care setting, the results may be useful to nurses in other traditional and nontraditional settings when assessing their career goals. Sears[38] writes in "Developing a Career through Nursing" that changes in nursing and the work environment call for an increase in attention to career development. With this in mind, she has developed a brief and practical guide for nurses to assist them in planning a positive career direction. Through a process of self-evaluation, nurses examine their personal value system and lifestyle, their strengths and weaknesses, and their access to role models and mentors.

Super[48] states that persons within the stabilization phase are secure and comfortable. Nurses are becoming more comfortable psychologically within the profession. Smoyak[42] reports that nurses value one another more than they did 10 years ago. For example, nurses are seeking each other out for consultation, are acknowledging one another, and are more positive with regard to what they have to offer.

Another aspect of either the establishment or the maintenance stage relates to financial gains. Granted, nurses have not made major gains financially, but one point needs to be reinforced. The economic motivations of women and men are not different. But even though this difference does not exist, Smoyak[42] and Osipow[30] argue that discrimination with respect to pay between genders still exists. Smoyak does contend that this discrimination is being countered by activity-oriented women.

Once an individual has secured a position, decision making and goal setting can be used to formulate a career path that points to future opportunities and advancement. Of importance within Super's maintenance stage and Murphy and Burck's renewal stage are not only goal setting and decision making but also the availability of informational resources. Smith[41] comments on the variety of resources accessible to nurses: counselors, career planning literature, university courses, continuing education offerings, and personnel and staff development offices. Specifically to address the issue of professional career development, the nursing department of Mount Sinai Hospital in New York City established the Nurse Career Counseling Services. According to Vezina,[50] the nurse career counselors assist the nursing staff by providing counseling and guidance on pertinent career development issues.

Other aspects of career development are evident within nursing. Smoyak[42] perceives that nurses' interest in one another's development has created an "upsurge of mentorships." Rankin[36] has identified having a mentor as one of the contributing factors for career success as well as personal and professional goal attainment and actualization. She identifies the stages of the mentoring relationship as exploration, initiation, early development, working, and closure. Although aspects of mentorship are present within nursing, Rankin writes of its slow development.

Smith[41] believes that the entire profession is active in career development, not just the individual nurses. An example is the presence of courses within nursing programs to assist students in formulating their career plans. Jarczewski[20] in "The Career Plan: A Luxury Item?" presents the format for a career planning unit of a trends course offered in the final semester of a nursing program. Content of the unit includes the selected concepts of professionalism, career planning, and management of various roles of career nurses. Similarly, Miller, Shortridge, Woodside, and Gutjahr[27] report on an elective for nursing students on career planning and professional development. Following a format like the career planning unit discussed by Jarczewski, this elective offers additional content that helps students with developing insight into the reality of the work world and developing communication techniques. Faculty members can also promote the career planning of their students in a different way. Faculty members who maintain their clinical skills act as role models for students. Smith[41] perceives that this clinical orientation reinforces for the students the reality of a hospital career commitment. Blanchard[1] argues that when graduating nursing students do not have a realistic view of the work situation, this leads to dissatisfaction and turnover, which is a major inhibiting factor in the promotion of nursing as a career.

Sossong and associates[43] describe how managers who recognized the significance of staff nurses to patient care were able to create a stimulating environment for career development. The program provided nurses with the opportunities to advance professionally and financially within their area of choice. With the staff nurse as the center of the RN Career Opportunities Program, the career options branch into the areas of nursing management, education, practice, or research. Each of the these work options is influenced by the nurse's interests, goals, and desires. With most career advancement options requiring national certification or advanced degrees, the administration has worked to provide opportunities to attain these.[43] Subsequently, advancement to the next higher position is based on position availability, performance, educational degrees, and recommendations by superiors. Thus career opportunity programs do exist within medical centers to assist in the professional development of nurses.

Other examples of the profession's commitment to career development exist. Kleinknecht and Hefferin[23] explain the open and closed models for career development. The open system includes all appropriate persons in assessing and planning the individual's career with the knowledge that all benefit. But the focus of the closed system is to prepare the individual for one particular position within the organization. Kleinknecht and Hefferin discuss the similarities and differences of the systems. Both models focus on the nurse who is currently employed within the primary organization, believe that all persons are interested in the career chosen, and are relevant for any identified nurse occupational group. The major difference is the breadth and depth of the career paths available. The closed system looks primarily at opportunities within the employing organization, while the open system allows for consideration of opportunities outside of the organization as well. But regardless of whether the system is open or closed, models are operating to provide opportunities to learn new skills and meet the requirements for newly established positions—positions that offer the nurse a choice for professional development and advancement. Shaffer and Moody[39] view models as a means of keeping nurses out of the traps that can occur at certain job levels.

In her article on staff development, Sovie[44] presents a systematic approach to hospital career development. It includes the aspects of professional identification, professional maturation, and professional mastery. Within each of these components, Sovie identifies activities or behaviors to be accomplished. Specifically for nurses to move toward professional maturation, they must master their job functions, display meritorious performance with clinical competence, and formulate a psychological contract with the employing organization. On completion of these tasks and others, one is eligible for development and eventual career advancement.

Another option for nurses within the Sovie model[44] is an approach to assist those who may not choose to progress through professional identification, professional maturation, and professional mastery. A nurse may consciously decide to stay in the first or second component. Sovie believes that the individual should be given every opportunity possible to make this career decision and retain the perception of a valuable professional. Sovie,[45] in the second article of a two-part series, perceives that the career model she has identified is applicable to other hospital nursing careers, not just to nurses providing patient care.

Shaffer and Moody[39] and Kleinknecht and Hefferin[23] write in separate articles of the career development approach that is operating within selected units of the Veterans Administration nursing service in the United States. Kleinknecht and Hefferin present the major elements as orientation to career development, self-assessment techniques, and program implementation sessions. During the orientation, the nursing career facilitator presents the focus of the program, the career opportunities available within the system, and the experiences offered through the program to help nurses advance. Then selected tools are completed in order to gain pertinent information about the nurse's past experiences, interests, strengths, and professional goals. In the third component, the nurse is involved with a facilitator in individualized counseling sessions. During these sessions, the nurses gain insight into their qualifications, potential interests, and career opportunities.[23]

Some evidence of the aspects of career development does exist within nursing. Programs have been developed to help nurses evaluate their own interests, goals, and values. These approaches also provide activities to ensure advancement and career fulfillment. They can provide a means to meet the particular needs of the individual and the agency, while expanding the talent and achievement aims of the current nursing work force.[23]

WHAT IS CLEAR: THE NEED FOR CAREER DEVELOPMENT IN NURSING

Whether or not career development exists within nursing is truly debatable, but the need to promote career development for nurses is not. Sovie[44] reports that 35 of 41 studies identified professional recognition, career mobility, and advancement opportunities as professional needs of nurses. Nurses in health care settings do want more career opportunities. But most important, the individual nurse will not be the only one to profit from career development; the profession will as well. Smith[41] contends that through careful career planning, the profession can meet the demands of nurse utilization within the health care system.

Individuals who are professionally alive understand that they continually need new skills to do their jobs.[26] In addition to having a willingness to acquire new skills, nurses who are career-minded become involved in professional organizations.[26,40] These opportunities assist nurses in increasing their knowledge of content and relevant issues and their skills. An added benefit of professional organizations is the networking. Hudek[19] believes that networking is an important tool for career development. It facilitates self-promotion and the sharing of ideas and opinions.

Sovie[45] believes that career-oriented nurses cannot exist within an organizational system in which they are on the bottom rung of the ladder. Thus to secure and retain those persons in the positions for which they chose nursing—nursing practice—career development must be a realistic possibility within the profession.

I believe that the individual nurse, as well as the profession, should possess a true commitment to career development. Nurses need to be knowledgeable of their own interests, values, and aspirations. Abilities and skills need to be realized, and individuals need to take responsibility for their own actions. Nurses need to feel confident in taking risks and seeking out opportunities for employment and/or advancement.

Professionally, career development models like Sovie's[44,45] and Kleinknecht and Hefferin's[23] need to be applied to a variety of nursing settings. Other career models need to be generated. More staff educators should be involved in career development experiences with nurses of differing educational and work backgrounds. One strategy that needs to be enhanced is the process of mentoring. Within the workplace, individuals should be invited to codevelop a plan to mutually assist each other in their own professional development. Rankin[36] suggests creating a mentoring packet that would include a philosophical statement on mentoring, and the purpose, role functions, and tasks of each person. Time would be built in to allow individuals to work together to develop and succeed with their proposed plan.

Other assessment tools and strategies need to be devised and tested, with the results being communicated in professional publications. Nurses need to read these materials and put the ideas and strategies into practice. It is only through application of these tools, strategies, and models that the ones most appropriate to nursing can emerge.

In closing, nursing service and nursing education must work together on career development. They can work to change the individual nurse's current view of nursing as a haphazard series of jobs. Both can help a nurse to see nursing realistically and as a challenging, interesting, and rewarding profession. Both can be vehicles to discuss ethical issues, personal values, and trends to assist nurses to evaluate their own career development. But of utmost importance is the fact that education and service can provide opportunities for career planning. Nursing has much to offer its practitioners, but career development with the involvement of nursing education and service must be part of nursing's future.

REFERENCES

1. Blanchard, S. L. (1983). The discontinuity between school and practice. *Nursing Management, 14*(4), 41.
2. Brink, P. J. (1988). The difference between a job and a career [Editorial]. *Western Journal of Nursing Research, 10*(1), 5-6.
3. Carr, A. (1980). Promotion: Family vis-à-vis career. *Nursing Mirror, 150*(11), 14.
4. Colavecchio, R. (1982). Direct patient care: A viable career choice? *Journal of Nursing Administration, 12*(7), 17-22.
5. Davis, D. A., Hagen, N., & Stroug, J. (1962). Occupational choice of twelve-year-olds. *Personnel and Guidance Journal, 40*(7), 628-629.
6. Donley, R. (1984/85). Nursing careerists. *Imprint, 32*(5), 9-11.
7. Donovan, L. (1980). What nurses want (and what they're getting). *RN, 43*(4), 22-30.
8. Ellis, J., & Hartley, C. (1991). Motivating yourself and others. In J. Ellis & C. Hartley (Eds.), *Managing and coordinating nursing care.* Philadelphia: J. B. Lippincott.
9. Fitzgerald, L. F., & Crites, J. O. (1980). Toward a career psychology of women: What do we know? What do we need to know? *Journal of Counseling Psychology, 27*(1), 44-62.
10. Friss, L. (1981). An expanded conceptualization of job satisfaction and career style. *Nursing Leadership, 4*(4), 13-22.
11. Gardner, D. (1992). Career commitment in nursing. *Journal of Professional Nursing, 8*(3), 155-160.
12. Gibson, L. W., & Dewhirst, H. D. (1986). Using career paths to maximize nursing resources. *Health Care Management, 11*(2), 73-82.
13. Ginzberg, E. (1972). Toward a theory of occupational choice: A restatement. *Vocational Guidance Quarterly, 20*(3), 169-176.
14. Ginzberg, E., Ginsburg, S. W., Axelrad, S., & Herma, J. L. (1951). *Occupational choice: An approach to a general theory.* New York: Columbia University Press.
15. Gulack, R. (1982). Why not fit the job to the nurse? *RN, 45*(5), 27-39.
16. Hefferin, E. A., & Kleinknecht, M. K. (1986). Development of the nursing career preference inventory. *Nursing Research, 35*(1), 44-48.
17. Henning, M., & Jardin, A. (1978). *The managerial woman.* New York: Pocket Books.

18. Hollender, J. (1967). Development of a realistic vocational choice. *Journal of Counseling Psychology, 14*(4), 314-318.

19. Hudek, K. (1990). Nursing: Make it a career. *Canadian Nurse, 86*(2), 18-19.

20. Jarczewski, P. H. (1986). The career plan: A luxury item? *Nursing Success Today, 3*(10), 6-10.

21. Kelso, G. I. (1975). The influence of stage of leaving school on vocational maturity and realism of vocational choice. *Journal of Vocational Behavior, 7*(2), 29-39.

22. Keough, G. (1977). The need for nursing career development. *Journal of Continuing Education in Nursing, 8*(3), 5-8.

23. Kleinknecht, M. K., & Hefferin, E. A. (1982). Assisting nurses toward professional growth: A career development model. *Journal of Nursing Administration, 12*(7-8), 30-35.

24. Mahoney, M. E. (1981, October 24). *Part-time for a life-time: The limits facing most working women.* Presentation given at Wellesley College.

25. Masson, V. (1982). Nursing: Healing in a feminine mode. *Journal of Nursing Administration, 11*(10), 20-25.

26. McBride, A. B. (1985). Orchestrating a career. *Nursing Outlook, 33*(5), 244-247.

27. Miller, M. M., Shortridge, L. A., Woodside, D. J., & Gutjahr, C. (1984). Career planning and professional development. *Nurse Educator, 9*(3), 40-42.

28. Murphy, P. P., & Burck, H. D. (1976). Career development of men at mid-life. *Journal of Vocational Behavior, 9*(3), 337-343.

29. National League for Nursing. (1979). Summary report on American nurse career pattern study: Baccalaureate degree nurses ten years after graduation. *Journal of Advanced Nursing, 4*(6), 687-692.

30. Osipow, S. (1983). *Theories of career development* (3rd ed.). Englewood Cliffs, N.J.: Prentice Hall.

31. Parker, J. E., & Drew, K. F. (1982). Women, work and health. *Occupational Health Nursing, 30*(7), 27-38.

32. Patterson, L. E. (1973). Girls' careers—expression of identity. *Vocational Guidance Quarterly, 21*(4), 268-275.

33. Pines, A. M., & Maslach, C. (1978). Characteristics of staff burnout in mental health settings. *Hospital and Community Psychiatry, 29*(4), 233-238.

34. Price, J. L., & Randolph, G. (1984). Career trajectory in nursing: The Randice approach. *Nursing Success Today, 1*(2), 21-25.

35. Psathas, G. (1968). Toward a theory of occupational choice for women. *Sociology and Social Research, 52*(2), 253-268.

36. Rankin, E. A. (1991). Mentor, mentee, mentoring: Building career development relationships. *Nursing Connections, 4*(4), 49-57.

37. Reres, M. (1979). Self-assessment and career choice. *Imprint, 26*(3), 13-16.

38. Sears, H. J. (1991). Developing a career through nursing. *Nursing Standard, 6*(13-14), 32-33.

39. Shaffer, M. K., & Moody, Y. K. (1980). A model for career development. *Journal of Nursing Education, 19*(8), 42-47.

40. Sharkey, C. J. (1988). Decide to manage your career. *American Journal of Nursing, 88*(1), 105-106.

41. Smith, M. M. (1982). Career development in nursing: An individual and professional responsibility. *Nursing Outlook, 30*(2), 128-131.

42. Smoyak, S. A. (1982). Women/nurses in 1982: How are we doing? *Occupational Health Nursing, 30*(7), 9-13.

43. Sossong, A., Benson, M., Ballesteros, P., Dauphinee, S., Dolley, P., Garrick, E., Gray, P., Couch, D., Miller, P., Pollard, A., & Smith, C. (1987). An expanding universe: Professional career opportunities. *Nursing Management, 18*(2), 46-48.

44. Sovie, M. D. (1982). Fostering professional nursing careers in hospitals: The role of staff development: Part 1. *Journal of Nursing Administration, 12*(12), 5-10.

45. Sovie, M. D. (1983). Fostering professional nursing careers in hospitals: The role of staff development: Part 2. *Journal of Nursing Administration, 13*(1), 30-35.

46. Super, D. E. (1963). Vocational development in adolescence and early adulthood: Tasks and behaviors. In D. E. Super, R. Stavishevsky, N. Matlin, & J. P. Jordaan (Eds.), *Career development: Self concept theory* (Research Monograph No. 4). New York: College Entrance Examination Board.

47. Super, D. E. (1980). A life-span, life space approach to career development. *Journal of Vocational Behavior, 16*(3), 282-285.

48. Super, D. E. (1984). Career and life development. In D. Brown & L. Brooks (Eds.), *Career choice and development* (pp. 210-234). San Francisco: Jossey-Bass.

49. Tiedeman, D. V. (1968). Decision and vocational development: A paradigm and its implications. In D. G. Zytowski (Ed.), *Vocational behavior* (pp. 207-224). New York: Holt, Rinehart and Winston.

50. Vezina, M. L. (1986). A new approach to professional development nurse career counseling. *Journal of Nursing Staff Development, 2*(1), 38-39.

51. Wandelt, M. A., Pierce, P. M., & Widdowson, R. R. (1981). Why nurses leave nursing and what can be done about it. *American Journal of Nursing, 81*(1), 72-77.

52. Zytowski, D. G. (1969). Toward a theory of career development for women. *Personnel and Guidance Journal, 47*(7), 660-664.

CHAPTER 75

Viewpoints

Nursing's quest for professionalism

BARBARA BRODIE

The movement to professionalize nursing—its practice and practitioners—has been important to every generation of nurses. Each generation has, in its respective ways, struggled to change nursing's image and status from that of a female domestic service to that of a scientifically based human care service freed of gender qualifications. An analysis of this pursuit of professionalism reveals that although its roots can be found in the writings of the founders of United States nursing, the quest is marked by distinct stages, each characterized by different claims for being a profession and by diversity among leaders as to the strategies and actions necessary to advance the process. Significant to the analysis is the role that others, predominantly physicians, have played in the movement. Also significant is the fact that, although the quest for professionalism is frequently portrayed as beneficial and necessary for society and the discipline, evidence suggests that the movement has not benefited all nurses equally.

STAGE 1: PROFESSION AS A DOMESTIC ART, 1870 TO 1890

The genesis of organized nursing in the United States was, in large measure, a by-product of a reform movement to reorganize hospitals and systematize the care of their patients. Spearheaded by socially active women committed to ameliorating the deplorable conditions found in city hospitals of the 1870s, a movement was begun to refashion hospitals from social warehouses for the poor into institutions of true refuge.[21] To rid hospitals of their filth, chaos, and foul atmosphere, and to address indifference toward and neglect of patients, the reformers had to upgrade the hospital work force. To find the type of workers needed, they turned to an emerging and available group—female domestic servants. The reformers hoped that among this group they might attract "daughters of clergymen, professional men and farmers—those with a true missionary spirit—[who would be] intelligent, women of small means who would be offered an adequate support while learning a profession."[22]

The reformers, many of whom had servants in their homes, believed that if given the proper rigorous training, female domestics could not only handle the hard labor necessary to cleanse the physical environment but would also bring a degree of respectability to the hospital. In addition, provided with a little nursing knowledge and some basic skills, these domestics could be trained to observe patients and to follow physicians' prescriptions and the directions of the hospital director.

Many from the available pool of semieducated women seeking employment in the era were enticed into the apprenticeship nursing programs initiated by hospitals. Promised that they would be taught how to be proficient in caring for private paying patients, pupil nurses submitted to strictly disciplined training regimens that tested physical stamina and shaped character. The moral character of a pupil was considered to be as important to the dignity of her position as the knowledge and skills she brought to the patient's bedside. Lacking moral credibility, she could not be trusted in a family's household nor could she share in what was then perceived to be the physician's awesome powers over life and death.

The authoritarian apprenticeship system of training—with its rigid hierarchical structure, consisting of directors, physicians, and superintendents of nursing directing the pupil work force—proved so effective in reforming institutional care of the sick that it was quickly adopted by scores of hospitals. Over time, nursing superintendents, while endorsing some of the beliefs of the initial reformers, began to redefine nursing and to question some of the existing training methods. Perceiving an image of nursing different from that of the reformers, these nursing leaders began to develop new occupational aspirations and a new occupational identity—one closer to a professional model.

STAGE 2: PROFESSION AS A RELIGIOUS CALLING, 1890 TO 1920

The view of nurses as domestic servants and of nursing as a domestic art requiring minimal skills was gradually rejected by nursing leaders, who initiated steps to change these perceptions. In the spirit of Florence Nightingale's life and writings, choosing to be a nurse began to be portrayed as a calling or a response to a higher being. Nursing was seen as a way to fulfill a special ministry dedicated to the intelligent care of the sick. As a ministry or vocation, the character of nursing took on additional moral attributes, for in serving others the nurse cast a moral influence over her patients that possessed therapeutic overtones. Pupil nurses were now exhorted to be dutiful, loyal, obedient, courageous, and reliable because "it is what a nurse is in herself and what comes out of herself, out of what she is . . . that exercises a religious influence over her patients," aiding them in their recovery.[7]

The attitudes behind the historical fact that women had traditionally served as servants and untrained nurses for centuries were also reshaped to emphasize the nurse's special womanliness. The unique feminine temperament, with its inherent powers of insight and intuition, it was argued, provided women with special wisdom, talents, and abilities to serve as nurses. Nursing, in its commitment to the care of the sick, was truly in the sphere of women's social responsibility.[18]

This redefined view of nurses, with its new emphasis on the intellectual demands and caring skills involved in modern nursing, allowed leaders to begin to portray nursing as a profession, a profession in the image of the traditional professions—divinity, medicine, and law—whose mission was to serve mankind in unique ways.

This new breed of nurses provided expert services for ill patients more in fulfillment of their sacred duty than as an employment opportunity. Nurses were exhorted to be selfless in performing their duty to society,

which had granted them the privilege of tending to the ill. Adelaide Nutting,[18] a pioneer nursing educator, captured this sentiment in a 1912 graduation address when she informed the graduates that the "world expects us to respond unfailing to the call of duty, to stay at our posts while strength holds us, to give our best effort in unstinted measure, and with self-forgetful devotion, and to surrender [our] personal desires and interests to the claims of duty."

The declaration by some leaders that nursing was a profession did not, however, assure the occupation of this status. Nursing leaders recognized that the achievement of the professionalization of nursing would require sustained effort and time. To reach this goal, nursing pioneers chose to follow the path of medical reformers who, at the turn of the century, were in the midst of improving medicine by upgrading medical education and of attaining legal licensure for competent physicians.[23]

In 1893, at the World's Fair in Chicago, a group of educators were invited by Isabel Hampton, superintendent of nurses at Johns Hopkins, to attend an educational program. Various papers outlining the problems inherent in, and ways of improving, nurses' training generated a commitment from the group to organize as the American Society of Superintendents of Training Schools for Nurses (renamed the National League for Nursing Education in 1912 and later, in 1952, the National League for Nursing). From the beginning the group knew that it faced the formidable task of gaining control of nursing education. Due to the positive gains accruing to hospitals from having an intelligent, healthy, and dedicated pupil work force willing to provide patient care, to attend to running the hospitals, and to work 12-hour days for little money, hundreds of hospital training programs had been spawned by the 1890s. In many of these institutions, nursing service activities consumed all of the pupils' time and energy. Little attention was paid to educating prospective nurses beyond that knowledge needed to complete the activities required by the hospital sponsors. As daunting as the task of reform appeared, the superintendents argued that it must be undertaken, for without adequate education, nurses could not fulfill their professional ministry.

Changing state of medical and nursing knowledge

Scientific knowledge about the etiology, diagnosis, and treatment of disease was at a nascent stage at the time that the first three Nightingale-modeled schools opened in 1873; but ensuing discoveries in microbiology, pharmacology, pathology, and physiology would propel medicine into a new age. Many of the physicians teaching pupil nurses, however, remained rooted in the nineteenth-century concept of diseases. This view of medicine, referred to as nosology, categorized diseases by symptoms, which were then specially treated. The knowledge nurses needed to provide care for these physicians' patients centered, to a great degree, on the principles of ventilation, cleanliness, dietetics, materia medica, and the orderly care of the sick and sickroom—concepts Nightingale[17] wrote of in 1859 when she instructed women in ways of providing care for their ill family members. Lacking textbooks, pupils slavishly memorized physicians' preferred nursing procedures, drug use, and dietetic orders.[20]

By the turn of the century, however, changes in medicine, particularly surgery, demanded that nurses be knowledgeable in the developing medical therapies. To teach this new information, physicians and nurses wrote nursing textbooks. In the 1890s two major architects of nursing, Lavinia Dock[8] and Isabel Hampton,[14] wrote several books that incorporated elements of science and ethics into nursing's expanding disciplinary knowledge.

The publication in 1907 of the first volume of Lavinia Dock and Adelaide Nutting's engrossing account of the historical origins of nursing provided the fledgling profession with a sense of legitimacy and heritage. The next three volumes, which covered the origins of modern professional nursing in countries around the globe, strengthened the sense of pride that nurses in the United States and other countries were feeling about the universality of the movement to create a modern profession.[10]

Other signs of professional growth included the creation of the Nurses' Associated Alumnae in 1887 (renamed the American Nurses Association in 1911) and the initiation of nursing journals (*Trained Nurse* in 1888 and *American Journal of Nursing* in 1900). Both actions, directed toward helping graduate nurses organize and remain informed about important issues pertinent to the field, also revealed that different opinions existed among leaders on how the group should attain professional status. Graduate nurses, their training already behind them, noted that they failed to benefit from the raising of educational standards sought by educators. Of more critical concern to the graduate nurses was competition from untrained women who claimed to be nurses and who threatened the graduates' fragile hold on private duty employment. The graduate nurses needed substantial pragmatic, rather than theoretical, support in their bid to practice as professionals.

The early journals covered legal as well as educational issues. For example, in the first issue of *American Journal of Nursing,* Lavinia Dock's article[4] "What We Might Expect from the Law" set into motion the process by which nurses, through their state groups, attained legal sanction to function as registered nurses. The first registration laws, enacted in 1903 in North Carolina, New Jersey, Virginia, and New York, would establish state boards of nursing with powers to accredit programs and, through examinations, to approve future graduate nurses.

The protracted struggle faced by superintendents in managing hospitals and in training students convinced educational leaders that graduate education was essential to the profession. In 1899 a course in hospital economy, sponsored by the society of superintendents, was begun at Teachers College, Columbia University. From this course would grow a world renowned department of nursing and health (chaired in the beginning by the first professor of nursing, Adelaide Nutting) that would produce generations of superintendents, educators, and researchers committed to the advancement of the profession.[6]

Developing image of nursing

In addition to fostering private duty and hospital nursing, nurses, at the century's turn, initiated new health services, roles, and organizations. Public health nursing, notably led by Lillian Wald, became a driving force in bringing nursing care and health education to citizens in cities and rural communities. Numbering almost 3000 nurses in 1912, the National Organization for Public Health Nursing (with its journal, *Public Health Nursing*) focused its efforts on preparing nurses to bring health care to the community.[4] The field of nurse anesthetists was also developed and organized as a specialty group in 1931.[2] These fields, which generated specialized knowledge, skills, and patient responsibilities, broadened the parameters of nursing.

Other actions, on a smaller scale, that helped shape and strengthen nurses' sense of professionalism during this period included their wise use of uniforms, school caps, and pins to establish a public image of a private duty trained nurse. A nurse attired in a bright white starched uniform and her school's cap and pin became the public symbol of a trained registered nurse. So sensitive were nurses to the symbolic value of the uniform that the wearing of it was restricted solely to time spent at the patient's bedside. Outdoor capes were worn to protect the uniform in transit to and from patients' homes.[12]

The Florence Nightingale pledge, an idealized nursing version of the Hippocratic oath, was developed in 1893 because nursing educators believed that nursing needed an ethical focus.[15] This oath, used at graduations for over 70 years, reminded graduates of the solemnity of their vocation and of both their ethical responsibilities to patients and their loyalty to physicians. Among similar views expressed by nurses of the era, this simplistic oath served as their primary ethical guideline.

The forces that initiated and sustained the first hospital and nursing reform movements began to wane during the 1910s, while advances in medical sciences and technology accelerated. Hospitals, viewed in the 1880s as refuges for individuals lacking a competent caring family, were evolving into agencies of efficient scientific healing. Nurses, both students and graduates, began to view nursing not as a sacred calling but as a vocational choice. Although nurses continued to feel a sense of duty toward patients, they now also valued themselves as important to the care of ill patients and to the advancement of health in the community.

STAGE 3: PROFESSION AS A SKILLED DISCIPLINE, 1920 TO 1940

Reflective of the public's growing belief in the effectiveness of medicine as practiced in hospitals to ameliorate diseases and illnesses was the increase in the number, size, and services of hospitals. In 1922, 7370 hospitals, with a total bed capacity of 813,926, offered specialty services in pediatrics, maternity, tuberculosis, mental disorders, cancer, contagious diseases, orthopedic defects, and disorders of the eye, ear, nose, and throat. Flocking to use the new services, patients spent over 53 million days in general hospitals in 1922, the equivalent of 1 day for every two members of the population.[25]

Medical advances

Hospital nursing services, still staffed by student nurses, worked diligently to keep pace with advances in medicine and surgery. Such events as the discovery of insulin in 1922 by Canadian physicians Banting and Best and the advances in physiological surgery pio-

neered by Alexis Carrel of the Rockefeller Institute revolutionized the treatment of diabetes and vascular surgery, respectively.[11] These and additional discoveries radically altered the practice of nursing. Functions formerly performed by physicians, such as monitoring patients receiving blood and other intravenous solutions, became nursing functions and, as such, required nurses knowledgeable in physiology. The quest for competently trained nurses became crucial not only to nursing but also to hospitals charged with the responsibility of caring for patients undergoing new medical procedures.

New nursing strategies

How nursing should develop into a true profession for the twentieth century was a frequent topic of debate among nursing personnel in this period. Using criteria developed by Abraham Flexner in 1915 to define the characteristics of a profession, some argued that nursing fulfilled three of Flexner's characteristics: (1) the possession of special knowledge as distinguished from mere skills, (2) the use of knowledge beyond academics and theory, with practical applications for the betterment of others, and (3) a responsiveness to the needs of society rather than to the sole advancement of nurses.[3] It was acknowledged, however, that nursing had not yet attained the level of intellectualism that indicated a highly specialized discipline, nor did it have the ability to generate through research new patient care knowledge.

Endorsing the first generation of educators' belief that professional status for nursing could only be attained through upgrading the standards of nursing education, current leaders intensified their efforts. Two large-scale studies, supported in part by philanthropic groups and nursing organizations and focusing on nursing education and practice, documented the limitations of nursing education and how these limitations affected the graduate nurses' ability to find employment and provide care.[5,13] The results of these studies led to National League for Nursing Education curriculum guidelines that were used by nursing superintendents across the country to upgrade nursing programs.

As committed as educators were to the goal of improving nursing education, differing views of where this professional education should reside surfaced in the 1920s. The majority of nurses believed that improved hospital-based diploma education, with its rich clinical resources, offered the best background. Others argued, however, that hospitals were service institutions incapable of educating a professional nurse. Only when nursing was incorporated into institutions of higher education, the collegiate group argued, could nurses be prepared to assume the responsibilities of a profession. Following this belief, the group dedicated its efforts to establishing university-based programs, and, in 1932, the Association of Collegiate Schools of Nursing was formed to support the growth of baccalaureate programs and the initiation of master's and doctoral education.[21]

Improved nursing knowledge

One of the tangible benefits of collegiate education was the improvement in the quality and dissemination of knowledge. Textbooks, a major indicator of the state of nursing knowledge, were now either coauthored by nurses and physicians or authored solely by nurses in every clinical area. The nursing content presented reflected a broader understanding of both the basic and social sciences. Aspects of psychology and sociology were incorporated into the rationale of nursing care, as was the latest information in pharmacology. The recognition that hospitals had become diversified and complex, and that the management of resources and people had been added to the role of supervising nurses, led to new nursing literature in the area of management and efficiency.

Nursing research studies, another indicator of the field's development, appeared in the literature by the 1920s. The studies, focused primarily on educational or staffing problems, remained rudimentary during this era, but the research path had been opened for future nurses to follow.[23]

Physicians' role in nursing education

Although physicians were vocal in their belief that nurses were being overeducated, the increased acceptance by medicine of internships and residencies beginning in the 1920s changed the relationship of nurses and physicians. Armed with the newest information from medical school, young physicians joined nurses in learning how to provide patient care. Working as a team they had ample opportunities to assess the strengths and limitations of each profession, and for nurses the experience provided a level of in-service education not available anywhere else. This last factor was of particular importance to registered nurses, as many hospitals during the economic depression of the 1930s closed their training programs and began employing graduates to staff their patient wards.

Plight of private duty nurses

Private duty nurses during this era experienced drastic changes in where, how, and when they were able to practice. Improvements in guarding the public's health through sanitary and educational measures had eliminated these nurses' major sources of employment. Instead of suffering from typhoid fever, which promised 3 weeks of employment for private duty nurses, patients with medical and surgical problems entered hospitals, where they were cared for by student nurses. Competition for the few remaining private patients left many registered nurses unable to earn a living or keep current with the new medical therapeutics. Even when hospitals began to employ registered nurses for staff positions, the older nurses, especially graduates of small hospital programs, were rarely hired because of their inability to provide competent care for patients and to manage the administrative tasks required by the hospitals.[16]

The American Nurses Association (ANA), under president Janet Geister, a strong advocate for private duty nurses, devised several measures such as creating state association employment registries to help these displaced nurses. But these efforts proved unsuccessful.[19] What graduate nurses needed were educational opportunities to upgrade their knowledge and skills. The educators of the era, unfortunately, were committed solely to improving the educational programs for student nurses.

STAGE 4: PROFESSION AS A POOL OF EXPERT MANAGERS, 1940 TO 1960

Changes brought about in the 1940s and 1950s by World War II and the postwar era significantly changed the relationship of nurses to patients. The war stripped hospitals of their staff; as a result, nursing students, aides, and Red Cross volunteers, under the direction of registered nurses, became the patients' direct care givers. Postwar conditions only intensified the situation. Fueled by a severe shortage of nurses and a growing population desiring hospital care and possessing health insurance to pay for it, staff nurses were forced to formally adopt a team approach to nursing. Instead of providing bedside care, registered nurses managed the unit and coordinated patient care assignments.

An increase in federal funding, especially Hill-Burton funds, led to a rapid expansion in the size and services of hospitals. As the complexities of managing the hospital infrastructure and the patients' medical care mounted, many traditional patient care responsibilities began to slip from the domain of nursing. Housekeeping and dietary duties were assumed by newly created autonomous departments, although when these and other support services were minimally staffed over weekends, they reverted back to the domain of nursing. This fragmentation of patient care and the shifting boundaries of what constituted professional nursing confused and frustrated nurses.

Adding to their dilemma was the fact that nurses lacked control over their practice. Trained to believe that the most sacred value in the professional ideology of nursing was the welfare of the individual patient, nurses found that if they remained at the patient's bedside they were penalized. The tangible rewards of nursing—higher salaries, recognition, authority, esteem, and deference—were reserved not for clinical nurses but for those who could and would assume the role of a manager or administrator.

STAGE 5: PROFESSION AS A POOL OF EXPERT CLINICIANS, 1960 TO ?

The social and intellectual ferment that characterized the 1960s touched nursing in ways that changed its practice, organizations, and education. Advances in medical sciences and technology began to alter radically the responsibilities of nurses. Medical and surgical subspecialties required new types of high-technology units, such as coronary and neonatal units. To manage the innovative and complex therapeutic regimens in these units, physicians demanded the services of graduate nurses. Eager to return to caring for patients, nurses quickly joined forces with physicians. Acting under medical protocols, nurses assumed responsibilities for diagnostic and curative actions that proved nurses indispensable to these units. In addition, their expanded clinical prowess began dismantling the long-held image of nurses as handmaidens of physicians.

The clinical specialization of nurses also led to diversification in nursing's organizations. The ANA, which had represented all nurses, was replaced by multiple organizations. These new organizations, responding to the special interests of their members, offered continuing education programs, developed standards of practice, and began a certification process. These activities indicated a significant growth in the independence of graduate nurses and a new level of professionalization for nursing.

The complexity of operating a nursing service department altered dramatically the relationship of nursing service and nursing education. Since their founding in 1873, nursing service and education had resided in one unit, under one director. By the 1960s, however, service and education each operated as separate entities charged with different responsibilities. Patient care was now in the hands of graduate nurses, and nursing departments moved to develop resources essential to the recruitment and retention of a professional staff.

Professional and technical education

Federal funding granted to schools to ease the nursing shortage in the 1960s was especially beneficial to the developing associated arts, baccalaureate, and master's programs. The shift away from diploma education, bitterly fought by proponents of hospital schools, was intensified by the 1965 ANA position paper[1] on nursing education. The paper acknowledged differences in levels of patient care and argued that entry to professional practice should be at the baccalaureate level and entry to technical practice at the associate arts level. Because of this move, the term *professional* took on intellectual and emotional overtones that are still present today. Again, as in the past, the quest for higher educational standards was viewed by many nurses as divisive because of its exclusionary dimensions. Those without a baccalaureate degree feared that being categorized as technical nurses demeaned the quality of their education and threatened their economic livelihood.

While the movement that transformed the clinical domain of nursing at the patient's bedside was underway, academicians were concurrently attempting to conceptualize nursing into theoretical models and to create a nursing diagnostic language. These activities were initiated to clarify the caring component of nursing, a component that many feared was being lost in the medicalization of nursing.

TODAY'S QUEST

Many activities currently under way are extensions of previous generations' search for a professional status for the discipline and its practitioners. But whether or not nursing has entered a new stage of professionalism is impossible to determine at this point of time. What is clear is that contemporary nursing is viewed as being dominated by the experience of change. The speed of technological and medical innovation, the erosion of traditional values, and the lack of unity in nursing are often cited as evidence that we live in a world radically different from that of the past, and that the past can therefore be ignored. This is a superficial assessment that denies the field of nursing knowledge that is crucial to its movement into the future.

Some of the questions generated from this study need to be addressed by today's leaders. They include the following: (1) Should clinical specialization continue as on-the-job training, or should formalized residency-like programs be developed? And if developed, should these programs be degree granting or sponsored by the specialty organizations? (2) Has the time come for nursing education and service to reunite, and if so, what are the benefits and limitations of unification? (3) Are there differences in degrees of professionalism expected for associate arts and baccalaureate graduates, and if so, what are their characteristics? (4) Has nursing's role in the technological transformation of patient care been adequate? Should nursing research address technological issues?

Analysis of nursing's quest for professionalism reveals that the educational standards for practitioners have increased over the decades and that much of nursing's current claim to professionalism is based on mastery of medical knowledge and skills. It also reveals that the price of professionalism must be borne by the discipline and the individual practitioner. How successful nursing will be in achieving the level of professionalism required for the twenty-first century will be determined by many factors, not the least of which is how well the lessons from the past are learned.

REFERENCES

1. American Nurses Association. (1965). First position paper on education for nursing. *American Journal of Nursing, 65*(12), 106.
2. Bankart, M. (1989). *Watchful care: History of America's nurse anesthetists.* New York: Continuum.
3. Brown, E. L. (1940). *Nursing as a profession.* New York: Russell Sage Foundation.
4. Buhler-Wilkerson, K. (1989). *False dawn: The rise and decline of public health nursing, 1900-1930.* New York: Garland.
5. Burgess, M. A. (1928). *Nurses, patients, and pocketbooks: Report of a study on the economics of nursing.* New York: Committee on the Grading of Nursing Schools.
6. Christy, T. (1969). *Cornerstone for nursing education: History of nursing education of Teachers College, Columbia University, 1899-1947.* New York: Teachers College, Columbia University Press.
7. Cook, E. (1913). *Life of Florence Nightingale: Volume 2* (p. 201). London: Macmillan.
8. Dock, L. (1890). *Materia medica for nurses.* New York: G.P. Putnam's Sons.
9. Dock, L. (1901). What we might expect from the law. *American Journal of Nursing, 1*(1), 8.
10. Dock, L., & Nutting, M. A. (1907). *History of nursing.* New York: G. P. Putnam's Sons.
11. Duffy, J. (1979). *The healers: A history of American medicine.* Urbana, Ill: University of Illinois Press.
12. Eldredge, A. (1907). Common things in nursing. *American Journal of Nursing, 7*(2), 62.
13. Goldmark, J. (1923). *Nursing and nursing education in the United States: A report of the committee for the study of nursing education.* New York: Macmillan.
14. Hampton, I. (1898). *Nursing: Its principles and practice.* Cleveland: E. C. Koechert.
15. Kalisch, P., & Kalisch, B. (1978). *The advance of American nursing.* Boston: Little, Brown.
16. Melosh, B. (1982). *The physician's hand: Work culture and conflict in American nursing.* Philadelphia: Temple University Press.
17. Nightingale, F. (1969). *Notes on nursing.* New York: Dover Publications.
18. Nutting, M. A. (1926). *A sound economic basis for schools of nursing* (p. 200). New York: G.P. Putnam's Sons.
19. Reverby, S. (1983). Something besides waiting: The politics of private duty nursing in the depression. In E. Lagemann (Ed.), *Nursing history: New perspectives, new possibility* (pp. 133-156). New York: Teachers College, Columbia University Press.
20. Reverby, S. (1987). *Ordered to care: the dilemma of American nursing, 1850-1945,* (pp. 1-21). New York: Cambridge University Press.
21. Robert, M. (1954). *American nursing: History and interpretation.* New York: Macmillan.
22. Scott, A. (1991). *Natural allies: Women's associations in American history.* Urbana, Ill: University of Illinois Press.
23. Simmonds, L., & Henderson, V. (1964). *Nursing research: A survey and assessment.* New York: Meredith.
24. Starr, P. (1982). *The social transformation of American medicine.* New York: Basic Books.
25. Stevens, R. (1989). *In sickness and in wealth* (p. 109). New York: Basic Books.

CHAPTER 76

Strategies for changing nursing's image

ROSEMARY DONLEY, MARY JEAN FLAHERTY

Although the nursing shortage of the 1980s appears to be under control, the poor public image of nursing that emerged as an explanatory factor in the shortage continues to be troublesome. This chapter will examine the impact of image on the recruitment, employment, and retention of nurses borrowing concepts from provided by the U.S. Health and Human Services' Secretary's Commission on Nursing.[44] This framework will permit us to examine contemporary images from the viewpoint of significant publics—lay persons, prospective students, practicing nurses, and their administrative and medical colleagues—and provide the vehicle for describing what is and what can be.

RECRUITMENT

Historically, nursing schools have enrolled single white female students. Today data from national studies[13] show that a larger percentage of women are attending college. However, interest in health careers seems to be shifting toward medicine and away from nursing. In 1968 freshmen women aspiring to nursing outnumbered future physicians 3:1. In the fall of 1986 more college women wanted careers in medicine.[18] Interestingly, although the longitudinal research of Austin, Champion, and Tzeng[4] says that gender no longer explains career aspirations or college majors, the majority of nursing students are women. That gender differences persist in nursing but not in other health fields means that public perceptions about women can easily become image problems for nursing. Today, problems specific to the job, the marketplace, and professional and social situations that have filled nursing journals are common themes in the evolving women's literature.[9,11] There are, however, some differences. One difference lies in attribution or the historical explanation given for the problem. Traditionally nursing has traced its difficulties to medical and hospital dominance. Liberation meant freeing nursing education and practice from these controls. Feminists have rooted the problem more deeply in social structures. Cleland[12] has related nursing's problems to the historical problems of women—alienation from sources of power. This theme was reiterated 20 years later by Mason, Backer, and Georges,[33] who described marginalization as the professional dilemma of wanting to provide care in an environment that values efficiency and high technology. Another difference flows from the lack of consensus about the form and the shape of nursing's image and symbols. Paul[37] sees it this way: "Nurses . . . have worn caps of powerlessness, decorated with bands of fear." Newton[36] presents a provocative minority view for the therapeutic importance of the "gentle sister" image. Holt[19] suggests that we are sending mixed messages by substituting PhD or Ms. for RN:

It is no longer permissible to travel incognito. It is time we conveyed clearly what nursing practice is, what nursing research is, what difference nurses can make in the future of health care in our nation, and what changes are needed to make those differences possible. We must be visible in our own work setting, in the political arena, and on the national scene.

When Krantzler[25] studied advertisements in the *Journal of the American Medical Association* and the *American Journal of Nursing,* he found that physicians exchanged their symbols (white coats and stethoscopes) for business suits, emerging as senior consultants and entrepreneurs. Nurses gave up their caps for white coats and stethoscopes. Webster[45] reminds nurses that the public gave value-oriented meanings to the white uniform. Curran[14] acknowledges that nurses ignored the symbolic power of the uniform when they opted for street clothes. Little[30] compares the taking off of the uniform to the "strip tease."

Another illustration of the search for symbolic identity comes from the report of the American Hospital Association (AHA) Special Committee on Nursing[2] that questioned whether or not the word *nurse* reflected professional responsibilities and duties.

Unlike modern feminists who joke about baking cookies, nurses are ambivalent about personal and professional symbols. If nurses present themselves as caring, compassionate persons, they risk being perceived as weak and powerless. If they take on medical (masculine) symbols, they lose touch with their tradition and adopt the symbols of an oppressive system. The media contribute to and reflect this ambivalence. For example, when interest in nursing among college freshmen fell from 8.4% in 1983 to 4% in 1987,[3] analysts said that nursing was no longer attractive to career-oriented young women. When there was a resurgence in the number of applicants, waiting lists were reported, the number of graduates rose, and 100 new nursing programs were proposed, the U.S. economy was credited for the renewed interest in nursing.[35]

It can be argued that the nursing community should "lighten up" because the media have no influence on the self-concept of the practicing nurse:

The best image of nursing is reality. If enough real nurses practice professionally with competence and caring, if they create, direct and/or practice in innovative settings that provide needed care to patients, if they are risk-takers not afraid to develop or assume "different" roles in health care, if with research they find answers to better patient care . . . if they simply demonstrate the existing diversity in nursing, there will be like-minded men and women who will see nursing as a worthwhile career opportunity.[22]

However, the media may influence the opinions of future recruits and shape the attitudes of the general public. Media portrayals of nursing range from the heroic and scientific nursing footage in *Movietonenews*,[41] to a nurse accepting a cash tip from a patient in "Murder, She Wrote," to the nurses in the *Playboy* centerfold,[16] or the sexpot, silly student nurses in the "Nightingales" series. Nurses' work can be glorified as valuable and desirable for women; it can be routinized; it can be glossed over as irrelevant to the script; or it can be a colorful backdrop for the sexual exploitation of women and the perpetuation of sexual stereotypes.[15,32] That nurses take media intrusion into their image seriously is evidenced by their documentation of these negative portrayals, the outcry against the "Nightingales" series of 1988 to 1989, and the boycotting of its sponsors.[15,32] That nurses lack power and

symbolic consensus about their work is evident. When the "Nightingales" series was canceled, some nursing leaders wanted to improve the series because "the show is all we have going for us."[17] Most analysts agree that media nurses who appear as dumb, silly sexpots or battle-axes are the greatest obstacle to the accurate portrayal of nurses.[6,32,38,40]

However, other sources of information about nursing leave much to be desired. It seems that persons who know nurses can sift through stereotypes. Lippman and Ponton,[29] who obtained a 54% response rate from a survey of 1000 faculty members in 19 northeastern universities, found that the faculty had a more positive view of nursing than is presented in the media. Common stereotypes of the nurse as "angel of mercy" or "good mother" were disappearing. Nurses were seen as educated, autonomous, compassionate, vital in health care, peers on campus, and scholarly. However, when Kaler, Levy, and Schall[21] asked 110 people in a shopping mall to compare professionals, nurses received high scores for nurturant and feminine traits. They were viewed as cooperative, most concerned about others, and significantly warmer than other professionals. On a scale measuring academic preparation, nurses fell below doctors, lawyers, teachers, and clergy, but above secretaries and homemakers. When Smith[39] analyzed a representative sample of 27 books used in health courses in 50 states, she found 427 descriptions about what nurses do, where nurses work, and what education nurses receive. She also reported that the 12 nursing roles identified in the texts were not linked with descriptions of contemporary practice. Most frequently nurses were described as assisting the doctor, reinforcing Bishop's contention[5] that the public thinks that nurses do what they are told by physicians. Smith[39] also found that a balanced view of nurses could be obtained if a person read all 27 books! Most schools required one text. Another illustration of the difficulty of finding the real nurse comes from the 1984 NBC 10-minute health sequences in which psychologists, registered dietitians, pharmacists, doctors, and safety control experts made health presentations. Although the word *nurse* was used in describing the potential for school nurses to identify vision problems, nursing was not represented in the series. An information booklet sent to 250,000 people made no reference to the nursing profession. Later, when 300 nurses and nursing students were surveyed, all respondents perceived a need to include accurate, detailed information about nurses' roles in health promotion. However, only one viewer noted the absence of nurses and no one suggested the inclusion of nurses in the series.[43] While cause and effect relationships cannot be demonstrated between media presentation of nursing and the size and quality of the nursing student body, public education can be employed to inform about contemporary nursing practice.

IMAGE AS A FACTOR IN EMPLOYMENT

The effects of self-images and public images in the workplace are complex and contradictory. People who look to the workplace for explanations of cyclical nursing shortages are intrigued by the seemingly insatiable demand of hospitals, nursing homes, and home care settings for registered nurses. The U.S. Congress, poised to increase significantly the federal budget for nursing, placed special emphasis on the workplace in its revision of the Nurse Education Act of 1988. Schools of nursing and health care institutions have been encouraged by grant programs to develop and test new schedules, salary and benefit programs, and innovations in the scope and division of work. Private foundations have sponsored demonstration projects to entice hospitals to reform their nursing services.[42] In market economies, high demand produces a greater supply and/or raises the price for the desired commodity. However, the high demand for nurses has not resulted in higher salaries, increased status or satisfaction, control of entry into the field, or influence over professional standards. An American Nurses Association survey[20] of 3500 nurses found dissatisfaction with: levels of support from nurse administrators (76%); salaries (70%); availability of help when a patient needs extra care (70%); registered-nurse-to-patient ratios (67%); value given to the importance of nurse membership on the health team (60%); and work schedules (50%). When nurses in this study were asked to identify what was bad about nursing, they cited child care facilities (78%), levels of support from hospital administrators (66%) and nurse administrators (65%), salary (52%), and benefits (42%). The AHA Special Committee on Nursing[2] identified the following complaints: 14-hour industrial positions, task-oriented functions, lack of support staff, complex technology, severity of patients' illnesses, and documentation of environmental hazards. In the nursing workplace, increased demand seems to bring with it greater dissatisfaction. Image problems seem to intensify in periods during which need or demand for nursing services gives the profession high visibility. Expressed another way, the nursing community does not seem to be able to capitalize on its demand cycles.

Image problems in employment can be discussed under four headings: differentiation, substitution, autonomy, and status. When the National Commission on Nursing Implementation Project[34] described the tendency to ignore differences in age, experience, education, or specialty preparation in assigning clinical responsibilities, they addressed the undifferentiated practice of nursing. Failure to differentiate between nurses touches the root of the image problem. While law defines the practice of licensed nurses and sets limits on unlicensed health care workers, there are few legal distinctions between the job expectations of 2-, 3-, and 4-year registered nurses and 1-year practical or vocational nurses. Failure to differentiate, especially in hospital-based nursing practice, is encouraged by the dazzling array of educational choices in nursing (the 2-, 3-, 4-, 5-, and 6-year curriculums) and the generalized meaning of the term *registered nurse*. However, when a nurse is a nurse is a nurse, there is disparity between clinical authority and responsibility, confusion about identity and scope of practice, and a blurring of the image of the registered nurse. The traditional failure of hospitals to distinguish between members of its nurse force is intensified during periods of shortage. Failure to differentiate contributes to the levels of dissatisfaction that nurses experience during these periods.

Closely related to the problem of differentiation is the problem of substitution. Substitution is the use of nurses to carry out the work of other health professionals (dietitians and pharmacists) and ancillary personnel (housekeepers, ward clerks, and messengers). The effects of this cost containment strategy are overwork, a blurring of nursing roles, and an impression that nursing practice lacks boundaries and identity.

Autonomy is the third area to be examined in our study of image in the workplace. The findings of the American Academy of Nursing's magnet hospital study team,[1] who revisited selected magnet hospitals during the nursing shortage, show that autonomy in clinical nursing judgments, control of nursing practice and conditions of work, and participation in governance are critical factors in professional self-image.[23,24] When nurses lack autonomy in the workplace, the work of nursing is undervalued and unrecognized.

Status is closely linked to autonomy. Nurses are frequently perceived in relationship to others in the health care hierarchy. This parochial view holds that nursing status is rooted in the mission and authority of the hospital and its medical staff. Deriving importance from the status of another negates the professional image of individual nurses and the status of the profession itself. When the public status of nursing is denied, there is less interest in naming nurses to positions of influence in the worlds of policy, finance, and business. The media assign a limited place to nurses outside the hospital when they describe nurses who sit at business or policy tables as ex- or former nurses.

Although the women's movement has raised the sights of many women, too many nurses bring an early closure to their careers. Limited visibility in boardrooms,[27] and the tendency within the profession to see head nursing, a deanship, or a nursing vice presidency as the end of the rainbow also conspire against personal and professional actualization. In a study of 386 nurse executives, Krugman[26] found that early socialization and the climate of their institutions influenced nursing's occupational self-image. Boyle[7] found that the 42 nurse educators she studied did not buy into the monastic-military ethos of nursing or socialize students into "doctor-nurse" games or other passive aggressive behaviors. It must be recognized that the image of nursing is not an egocentric preoccupation. If nursing is successful in improving its status in the workplace, there will be political and financial consequences for organized medicine, the hospital industry, and the system of health care service delivery.

RETENTION

What can be said about the image of a profession where the work is frustrating, hours are uncertain, rewards are few, recognition is limited, and salaries are poor? Who stays in a field that can be described in such negative terms—the entrapped, the ignorant, or the holy? The members of the Health and Human Services Secretary's Commission on Nursing[44] phrased the question about attrition and retention in this manner: Why, in the face of an ever-increasing number of graduates from schools of nursing, is there an insufficient number of nurses to meet the demands of the workplace? The expected answer was that nurses leave the work force shortly after they enter it. However, Department of Labor statistics, which show the percentage of employed nurses to be the highest among traditionally female work forces, cast doubt on the "attrition hypothesis" and stimulated a comprehensive

look at the expectations of employing agencies. The so-called demand factor has been discussed earlier in this chapter. The commission found the nursing shortage to be the result of overdemand for nursing services rather than the result of undersupply or attrition from the work force. The commission concluded that many nurses were overextended, underutilized, and assigned inappropriate responsibilities and duties. The historic failure of nursing to organize its work and the expectation that nurses would substitute for or complement the work of professional and technical health workers contributed to the contextual backdrop for the critical nursing shortage in the mid-1980s. Changes in health care financing also contributed to the shortage. When the majority of third-party insurance companies followed the cost containment principles of prospective payment and the use of diagnostic-related groupings as the unit of reimbursement, hospitals responded by shortening the period of inpatient care. Patients were hospitalized for the most acute phases of illness or the most intensive part of their therapy. As a consequence of these factors, demand for nurses became so constant that a worldwide shortage of nurses ensued. As a consequence of this analysis, attention turned away from schools of nursing to the design of work, conditions in the workplace, and the deployment of the nursing staff.

Another significant dimension important to the understanding of retention is nursing's compensation and benefit structure. Admittedly nurses are a bargain.[28] While starting staff-level salaries were estimated in 1992 to range between $22,800 (Seattle) and $39,395 (San Francisco), the national average for staff nurses was $34,462 and for licensed practical nurses was $21,877. However, nurses with 10 years of experience do not fare as well.[8] Salary compression characterizes the economic underpinnings of nursing practice. This is interesting because workers in highly technical industries are paid for what they know. Usually employers also pay for experience and reward those who have seniority in the industry. The hospital environment has not considered education, experience, or "knowledge acquired through practice" as something to be valued or rewarded. Feminine imagery, expectations, and responsibility have resulted in limited earning power and restricted professional advancement. Buscherhof and Seymour[10] think that nurses face salary depression because their work is associated with housewifely and nurturing skills rather than with technical or specialized knowledge. Nurses may not be taken seriously as careerists because society considers the work of nursing to be preparatory for more important work, marriage, and motherhood. A significant portion of the nursing work force is employed part-time and receives few benefits,[2] further contributing to the depression of salaries and to the image of nurses as "seasonal" workers. It is possible to blame the victims or minimize the demands placed on women in the work force.[31] However, the real culprit behind salary compression and depression is a social reality—the system of health care financing. The current configuration of health care financing does not enable the public to choose nurse providers as they choose medical or institutional providers. Reimbursement policies deny qualified nurse-midwives, nurse practitioners, and nurse clinicians the status of providers. Within institutions, nursing service is most frequently "packaged" with charges for room and board. This particular accounting practice hides the professional and specialized nature of nursing practice and perpetuates the image of nurses as homemakers and caretakers. Until a major reorganization of the third-party payer system is achieved and nurses are recognized as contributors to the health care delivery system, adjustments to salary and compensation for hospital and nursing home nurses will be merely cosmetic.

The story of the image of nursing is very much like the story of Cinderella. When the real image of nurses is acknowledged, the reflecting mirror of power and greed that has distorted nursing's image will be broken.

REFERENCES

1. American Academy of Nursing. (1983). *Magnet hospitals: Attraction and retention of professional nurses.* Kansas City, Mo: American Nurses Association.
2. American Hospital Association. (1988). *Report to the special committee on nursing.* Chicago: Author.
3. Astin, A., Korn, W., & Green, K. (1987). *The American freshmen: Twenty year trends.* Los Angeles: Higher Education Research Institute.
4. Austin, J. K., Champion, V. L., & Tzeng, O. C. S. (1985). Cross-cultural comparison of nursing image. *International Journal of Nursing Studies, 22*(3), 231.
5. Bishop, B. (1987). Don't wait to be asked [Editorial]. *Maternal-Child Nursing, 12,* 85.
6. Bohn, V. L. (1986). The image of nurses in television. *Nursing Success Today, 3*(2), 20.
7. Boyle, C. W. (1990). *Who perpetuates sex role socialization? The changing image of the professional nurse educator from traditional to cycle-breaking: A qualitative interview study.* Unpublished dissertation, University of Massachusetts.
8. Brider, P. (1992). Salary gains slow as more RNs seek full-time benefits. *American Journal of Nursing, 92*(3), 34-40.
9. Bunting, S., & Campbell, J. (1990). Feminism and nursing: Historical perspectives. *Advances in Nursing Science, 12*(4), 11-24.
10. Buscherhof, J. R., & Seymour, E. (1990). On my own terms: The redefinition of success in nursing. *Image: The Journal of Nursing Scholarship, 22*(2), 84-88.
11. Chinn, P. L., & Wheeler, C. E. (1985). Feminism and nursing. *Nursing Outlook, 33*(2), 74-77.
12. Cleland, V. (1971). Sex discrimination: Nursing's most pervasive problem. *American Journal of Nursing, 71,* 1542.
13. College enrollment by racial and ethnic group. (1992, March 18). *Chronicle of Higher Education,* p. A35.
14. Curran, C. (1984). Seeing ourselves as others see us. *Today's O.R. Nurse, 6*(18), 23.
15. Curtin, L. L. (1990). Nurses: Playgirls on the boob tube. *Nursing Management, 21*(5), 7-8.
16. Dains, J. E. (Ed.). (1984). Nurses' image: An act of betrayal. *Journal of Emergency Nursing, 10*(3), 20A-21A.
17. Final word: On snatching defeat from the arms of victory. (1989). *Nursing and Health Care, 10*(6), 346.
18. Green, K. C. (1987). The educational "pipeline" in nursing. *Journal of Professional Nursing, 3*(4), 247.
19. Holt, F. M. (1989). Speak with clarity and pride to improve the image of nursing. *Clinical Nurse Specialist, 3*(3), 126-127.
20. Huey, F. L., & Hartley, S. (1988). What keeps nurses in nursing: 3,500 nurses tell their stories. *American Journal of Nursing, 88*(2), 181-188.
21. Kaler, S. R., Levy, D. A., & Schall, M. (1989). Stereotypes of professional roles. *Image: The Journal of Nursing Scholarship, 21*(2), 85-89.
22. Kelly, L. (1989). Image, niceness and the illusion of quality. *Nursing Outlook, 37*(6), 259.
23. Kramer, M., & Schmalenberg, C. (1988). Magnet hospitals: Part I. *Journal of Nursing Administration, 18*(1), 13.
24. Kramer, M., & Schmalenberg, C. (1988). Magnet hospitals: Part II. *Journal of Nursing Administration, 18*(2), 11.
25. Krantzler, N. J. (1986). Media images of physicians and nurses in the United States. *Social Sciences and Medicine, 22*(9), 933.
26. Krugman, M. E. (1990). Nurse executive role socialization and occupational image. *Nursing and Health Care, 11*(10), 526-530.
27. Kusserow, R. P. (1988). *Management advisory report: Nurse participation in hospital decision making—potential impact on the nursing shortage.* Washington, D.C.: U.S. Department of Health and Human Services, Office of Inspector General, Office of Analysis and Inspections.
28. Landers, R. K. (1988, March 25). What is causing the nursing shortage? [Editorial]. *Research reports.* Washington, D.C.: Congressional Quarterly.
29. Lippman, D. T., & Ponton, K. S. (1989). Nursing's image on the university campus. *Nursing Outlook, 37*(7), 24-27.
30. Little, D. (1984). The "strip tease" of nurse symbols or nurse dress codes: No code. *Imprint, 31,* 49.
31. Lynaugh, J. E., & Fagin, C. M. (1988). Nursing comes of age. *Image: The Journal of Nursing Scholarship, 20*(4), 184-189.
32. Mallinson, M. D. (1989). NBC's tinsel handmaidens. NBC TV's Nightingales. *American Journal of Nursing, 89*(4), 453.
33. Mason, D. J., Backer, B. A., & Georges, C. A. (1991). Toward a feminist model for the political empowerment of nurses. *Image: The Journal of Nursing Scholarship, 23*(2), 72-77.
34. National Commission on Nursing Implementation Project. (1987). *Timeline for transition into the future nursing education system for two categories of nurse and characteristics of profes-*

sional and technical nurses of the future and their educational program. Milwaukee: Author.

35. News: BSN schools see graduations gaining, more men choosing nursing careers. (1992, June). *American Journal of Nursing, 84,* 88.

36. Newton, L. (1980). A vindication of the gentle sister: Comment on "the fractured image." In S. Spicker & S. Gadow (Eds.), *Nursing images and ideas: Opening dialogue with the humanities* (pp. 34-41). New York: Springer.

37. Paul, S. A. (1991). Remodeling the image of nursing: A powerful tool for clinical specialists. *Clinical Nurse Specialist, 5*(3), 156-158.

38. Siegel, F. A. (1985). Lights, camera, action! The nurse's image in theater and film. *Nursing Success Today, 2*(8), 20.

39. Smith, M. K. (1989). What high school texts say about nursing. *Nursing Outlook, 37*(1), 28-30.

40. Smith, S. J. (1985). Nursing's public image: What they see versus what you know. *California Nurse, 81*(4), 8.

41. Stevens, S. Y. (1990). Sale of the century: Images of nursing in the Movietonenews during World War II. *Advances in Nursing Science, 12*(4), 44-52.

42. Taft, S. R., & Stearns, J. E. (1991). Organizational change toward a nursing agenda: A framework from the strengthening hospital nursing program. *Journal of Nursing Administration, 21*(2), 12-21.

43. Turnbull, E. (1986). Nurses respond to NBC over "accurate portrayals." *Nursing Success Today, 3*(6), 4-13.

44. U.S. Department of Health and Human Services. (1988). *Secretary's Commission on Nursing: Interim report.* Washington, D.C.: Author.

45. Webster, M. L. (1985). Professional style: An update. *Nursing Life, 5*(2), 63.

CHAPTER 77

Feminism

The new look in nursing

CAROLE A. SHEA

What goes around, comes around. And the latest *ism* to come around nursing is *feminism.* Yes, feminism is once again a hot topic in nursing. However, this time around, the instigating force is not the women's movement itself, nor nursing's reaction (both pro and con) to the women's movement. This time the impetus for taking a fresh look at the connections between feminism and nursing is coming from within the profession and from events in the larger society—that is, from ideologies of nursing, economic realities of the health care scene, and personal politics of gender relations in everyday life.

IDEOLOGIES
Caring

An ideology has profound and far-reaching effects when it permeates a discipline. Such is the case in nursing with the ideology of caring. This ideology seeks to promote the artful (versus scientific) practice of nursing.[10] It defines the lived experience of nursing by concentrating on characteristics that are usually associated with femininity: subjectivity, intuitive thinking, holism, spirituality, and moral aesthetics.

Caring has always been regarded as the essence of nursing, but its essence was not critically examined until the 1980s. Benner and her colleagues[4] may be credited for their seminal work on the primacy of caring in nursing as "central to human expertise, to curing, and to healing."[4] In keeping with phenomenological and feminist approaches, they focused on understanding the lived experience of nurses and their patients by having nurses tell their own stories about what it is like to be a nurse and how they know what really matters to people. These powerful stories, called paradigm cases, illuminated nursing expertise and gave a framework and credibility to caring as the essential ingredient of nurses.

The resurgence of interest in the ideology of caring has swept through nursing within a relatively short period of time. Caring has been conceptualized and researched as a human trait, a moral imperative, an affect, an interpersonal interaction, and a therapeutic intervention.[23] The burgeoning literature describes how the ideology of caring is used to define nursing care, evaluate patient outcomes, set agendas for research, guide curriculum development, and determine the profession's goals. The ideology of caring is reflected in modes of inquiry and research, conceptual models for education and practice, and programs for personal and professional growth. Whole conferences are designed around caring, with proceedings published by mainstream nursing organizations.[10] While debate continues about caring—the significance of its various conceptualizations and its relevance for practice[23]—the ideology of caring has a sustaining presence in nursing practice, education, and research.

The rediscovery of caring as nursing's historical bedrock and *raison d'être* dovetails neatly with the current discourse on feminism in nursing.[26] Feminism, the feminist perspective, and feminists are also enjoying a new currency in nursing. The fascination with feminism has been sparked in part by the inevitable links between the caring ideology and nursing as a woman's profession; and in part by the tone of the feminist discourse, which has become "kinder and gentler." The appeal of this *soft feminism* (as Venner Farley coined the term) is much broader and more persuasive to nursing than that of the activist feminism of the 1960s and 1970s.

Revisiting feminism

The origins of modern feminism are grounded in the first wave of the women's movement in the nineteenth century.[7] In those early days, gender was the foundation of all programs to advance the cause of women. The principal goal was to obtain equal rights through suffrage. In addition to the rights and prerogatives accorded to men, women sought a revaluing of their distinct nature and abilities. Nursing served as one vehicle for women to obtain education, provide a valuable service, and engage in organized social reform. Many of the early nursing leaders espoused feminist views and were active in the women's movement.[29]

However, once the right to vote became a reality, feminism and nursing parted ways. With victory for women's suffrage, feminism emerged as an ideology devoted to women's rights and their rightful place in society. The underlying theme of the women's movement at this time was that "women are equal to men." The movement shifted into high gear to do battle on all fronts of the male power structure. It ignored the needs and desires of those women who failed to confront the gender hierarchy or refused to abandon traditional roles. Nursing, entrenched in a patriarchal hospital system established in Nightingale's days, became disenfranchised by the women's movement. Feminist leaders were more interested in pursuing equal opportunities for women and men in law, medicine, politics, finance, and the ministry. However, faced with fierce resistance from the prevailing power structure and lacking a unifying theme to attract the majority support of women, the women's movement gradually became dormant.[7]

The second wave of the women's movement came on the scene in the 1960s. This time women's place in society was reexamined but women's work was still devalued.[25] Some nursing leaders joined the radical feminists, hoping to tap into the movement's angry energy to reform nursing and the movement itself from within.[18] For a brief time feminists and nurses did become united in the communal spirit of the early 1970s. Wilma Scott Heide, a nurse, was a president of the National Organization for Women (NOW). She inspired nurses to form Nurses NOW to exercise their political clout as a critical mass within the health care system. But this unity between feminism and nursing was also short-lived. The failure of the passage of the Equal Rights Amendment and the declining influence of NOW and other, radical feminist groups stalled the second wave of the women's movement. The feminists who had concentrated on gender-based equality issues did not take up the cause of nursing with much enthusiasm. Although there was some overlap in their agenda for equal rights and nursing's agenda for autonomy as a profession, the most notable issue of agreement was the right to equal pay for comparable work.[19] The strongest impediment to a closer working relationship was nursing's aversion to the radical philosophy and militant tactics that characterized this branch of the women's movement. However, seeds of feminism from the branch that nurtured the uniqueness in women began to germinate in nursing.

Applying feminist ideology

Today's feminism is drawn from theoretical perspectives that stress the differences rather than the similarities between genders. The goal of this type of feminism is twofold: (1) respect for the unique contribution women make to society and (2) recognition that women have distinctive ways of knowing, seeing, and being in the world that are not deficient or deviant when compared to men's ways.[6] The keystones to this feminist perspective are connectedness, valuing relationships, and social responsibility as described in *Women's Ways of Knowing*[3] and *In a Different Voice*.[12] This perspective does not deny the effects of female socialization in the prevailing patriarchial society. Rather, there is acknowledgment that the behaviors women exhibit are cultural, not merely biological, and as such, understandable and acceptable as responses to systematic oppression. In fact, they may be essential alternatives for survival in a male-dominated culture that is oriented toward individuality, competition, and aggression.

Feminist arguments along these lines have an intrinsic appeal to nurses (97% women), who are acutely aware of their differences—both personal and professional—from physicians (70% men). Feminist nurses have sought to have those differences reframed as positive assets, instead of being berated by radical feminists for engaging in "women's work" and submitting to the entrenched inequities of the health care system.[37] In their workplace, nurses have experienced countless effects of enforced subordination and sexual stereotyping.[13,25] Within the nursing profession, efforts to redress their lack of autonomy and power have met with very limited success. In society at large they have endured dismissive attitudes of a public that clings to the notion that nursing is "natural and maternal" or that subscribes to the "angel of mercy" myth. Within their private self, nurses have suffered self-disparagement for participating in a low-status profession and continuing to play doctor-nurse games from a one-down position. Therefore, feminist theories that reflect an enlightened understanding of nursing's historical development and compassion for those nurses awakening to a new awareness of their professional self are gaining acceptance and acclaim within the mainstream of nursing.[22]

Here are some examples of how feminism is influencing nursing practice, education, and research in new ways.

Practice. Many consider the "nursing process" to be sacrosanct, so embedded in standard nursing practice that it is taken for granted. However, Kobert and Folan[21] propose that the nursing process is incompatible with holistic nursing practice, because the nursing process is derived from the scientific method, uses linear thinking, and reduces the patient to component parts. They suggest that taking a "feminine world view that is reflective, relational and organismic" will enable nurses to practice in a way that is congruent with their holistic beliefs. Conversely, Smith[32] argues that use of the nursing process allows the nurse to become involved in caring for people, not curing disease. She purports that the nursing process is both a philosophy (people-centered) and a method (the way to express nursing ideologies). These authors draw on the links between caring and feminism to discuss their ideas about how to make the ideology of caring congruent with feminist-influenced nursing practice.

Education. Nursing educators are beginning to view the "uneasy alliance" between feminism and nursing[37] as a thing of the past. Hedin and Donovan[17] describe the characteristics of a feminist model that advocates nursing education as a "freeing process." Such a program is egalitarian; less hierarchical; empowering; concerned with relatedness, context, and wholeness; integrative and inclusive; ethical; moral; and process, as well as outcome, oriented. Boughn[5] takes another approach by suggesting that nursing students should participate in a women's health course that seeks to instill attitudes and behaviors that are vital for nurses as providers and consumers of health care. The course curriculum is comprised of a body of knowledge related to women's health and strategies to increase self-awareness, independence, and risk taking. Caring for self is linked to caring for others through the concept of empowerment. Boughn reports that students who participated in this course expressed increased identity with other women, self-worth, and motivation to engage in professional activism.

Research. In the area of theory development and research, the feminist perspective has really taken hold. Duffy[8] has specified criteria for feminist research: the principal investigator is a woman; the methods are interactional or nonhierarchical; the study potentially helps the subjects; the focus is the experience of women; the purpose is to study women; feminist literature is included in the references; and nonsexist language and the words *feminist* and *feminism* are used in the report. Parker and McFarlane[27] applied Duffy's criteria to their study of the effects of physical abuse during pregnancy on maternal-child outcomes. They found that applying feminist principles to their research was an empowering process to them as researchers and to their subjects. Anderson[1] also discusses the value of the feminist principles in conducting her phenomenological study with women who have diabetes. Her subjects' requests for information about their illness during the study interview posed a dilemma for the researcher, until the context of the field interview was construed as a means to equalize power between the interviewer and interviewee.

Research studies conducted according to feminist principles do not fit the mold of the traditional experimental model of objective science and are often criticized in reference to their reliability and validity. To counteract these criticisms, Hall and Stevens[15] suggest that there are standards of scientific rigor that nurse investigators can apply in planning and evaluating their research. To determine the adequacy of their studies, investigators should examine their research questions, designs, and findings in terms of the following dimensions: reflexivity, credibility, rapport, coherence, complexity, consensus, relevance, honestly, mutuality, naming, and relationality.

These are just a few of the ways in which the ideology of caring and the feminist perspective are becoming interwoven throughout nursing practice, education, and research.

ECONOMIC REALITIES

At a time when nurses could be contemplating the rewards of putting an empowering ideology into practice, they must respond to multiple pressures engendered by the economic crisis in America's health care system.[13,22] Taking time to discover hidden strengths, internalize feminist values, practice empowerment strategies, let go of silence and invisibility, and express their expertise in providing nursing care is a luxury few nurses can afford. Competition with assistive personnel for employment, allocation of scarce resources, ethical dilemmas, continuing conflicts with physicians over autonomy and clinical decision making, role strain related to family demands and personal needs—these are only a few of the issues that put nurses to the test and threaten to produce a crisis of confidence in newly acquired feminist principles.

However, there are several forces operating in the society at large that may serve to advance the cause of nursing during these unsettled times. Simply put, from an economic standpoint, women's business is "Big Business,"[2] and nursing, a women's occupation, is by definition women's business. Women's business is connected to feminism and nursing in several direct and indirect ways. Three areas have particular relevance to this discussion: (1) women's health, (2) science and research agendas, and (3) public media.

Women's health

Women are the major purchasers of health care services, and they constitute the largest group of consumers of health care. With a long lifespan, they seem certain to remain a large, active constituency of purchasers and consumers in the health care system in the coming decades. In addition, women comprise the largest majority of health care professionals and other care givers.

Health planners and policymakers have long recognized that women control the spending of health care dollars by making decisions about seeking medical care and treating illness when their family members are sick. Health care administrators and manufacturers have learned to expect women to be savvy consumers. Therefore, the marketing of health care and health care products is directed toward women, further enhancing women's purchasing power in this major industry.

Women used to be reluctant to seek care for their own health problems; but today's woman is more health conscious and better informed. Women are also known to be cost conscious and to look for good value for their health care dollar. They are receptive to receiving care from nurse practitioners, nurse-midwives, and other nurses practicing in advanced roles. Consequently, despite major declines in nursing enrollments in the 1980s, graduate nursing programs are now functioning at maximum capacity to educate more nurses for advanced practice in order to meet the demand for services. This in turn is leading to the delivery of more women-to-women (nurses-to-consumers) services with a focus on health promotion and disease prevention. These events, essentially women-driven, have the potential of making major shifts in what constitutes health care, who will provide which services, and what will be the health outcomes.

Another aspect of women's health as big business concerns the medicalization of various conditions experienced by women. The best examples involve conditions that commonly occur in the middle years of life, such as menopause,[28] infertility,[31] eating disorders,[38] family violence,[24] and depression.[33] Feminists believe that culture, social roles, economic situations, and the oppressive structure of society have at least as much influence on women's health and illness as biomedical factors.[30] They have particularly criticized the medicalization of normal physiological processes in women, such as menopause and osteoporosis. For example, physicians and drug companies are advocating aggressive treatment with estrogen and calcium replacement therapy for these "medical conditions" despite controversial evidence regarding the long-term effects and benefits of these treatments. These practices are costly in many ways to women, and ultimately to society, and they may be actually harmful to women's health.

As the Baby Boom generation moves into maturity, it is expected that more products will be developed for this growing segment of the population. Some will undoubtedly fill legitimate health needs; others will be marketed to promote youth and beauty, those obsessive ideals of our ageist and sexist society. The danger is that products will be developed that will play on women's unwarranted fears of aging and disability.[30] A tragic example is the promotion of breast implants. Women had silently endured disease, pain, and disfigurement as a result of breast implants. Then a few went public with evidence of their suffering. Their shocking revelations and the subsequent stonewalling by governmental officials who refused to conduct a thorough investigation should serve as a reminder that neither the health care industry nor the government has women's best interests at heart. Nurses will play an increasingly important role in educating the woman consumer to make enlightened choices about the benefits of such medical "progress."

One outcome of all this attention to women's health needs is that many providers are learning through personal encounters to take women seriously, that women as knowledgeable purchasers and consumers of health care will not be ignored or patronized. This has implications for the training of professionals and the conduct of the nurse-patient relationship, as well as the nurse-doctor and doctor-patient relationships. Nursing schools are teaching their students feminist approaches to empower the nurse and the patient. Some medical schools are beginning to teach communication skills and the humanitarian approach as effective means for their students to manage the doctor-patient relationship. Yet to come are sustained opportunities for nurses and doctors to learn with and from each other, and from empowered patients.

Science and research agendas

The public is generally unaware that women have been systematically excluded from the ranks of senior scientists and funded scientific endeavors. The "old boys" network has operated to shut out women from positions in academia where most scientific breakthroughs take place and to deny grants for funded research at the university and federal levels. There are some notable exceptions—for instance, the preeminent geneticist Barbara McClintock. However, women scientists have been forced to remain at the margins of the organized scientific enterprise because they lacked the opportunities for training, professional socialization, mentoring, and financial support built into the system for men scientists.[20] In terms of research, the lack of studies that include women as subjects or that focus on women's issues was so drastic that the federal government was forced to *mandate* that women must be included in studies that receive federal funding.

Feminists are not content with having more women serve as subjects in traditional research projects, or with having more studies about women. The question is not simply, What about women in science? The question is, What about feminism in science?[16] Feminist scientists are examining the whole premise on which science is based, the philosophy and methodology of Western science that guides the scientific process from the research question to the published report. And it is here that nurses who are close to women's issues, who are familiar with subjective, relational, inductive thought and qualitative methods, are coming together with feminists in nursing and other disciplines to develop a new science on common ground.

Signs of progress are on the horizon. Bernadette Healey, MD, was the first woman director of the National Institutes of Health, a position of great power and prestige. One of her first acts was to initiate a large program to study breast cancer, which claims the lives of one in nine women—obviously a high priority for feminist nurses and all women. In 1992 the National Center for Nursing Research achieved the status of a full institute among the other National Institutes of Health. This event has significance in terms of giving nursing an equal status with other programs of research, a higher priority for funding, additional resources and support for nursing researchers, and greater access to study populations.

On the supply side, the number of graduates from nursing doctoral programs has increased dramatically. Many of these schools encourage a feminist perspective within the curriculum as well as in the dissertations that cap the student's scholarly pursuit. The literature is filled with these innovative analyses of women's lived experience. As published nursing doctoral studies and the work of feminist scientists move into the realm of the nurse's workplace, this new knowledge base promises to revolutionize the ways nurses think, feel, and give care.

Public media

While nursing publications are a useful resource and source of pride to nurses, they have not yet captured the public's attention in the same way that the *New England Journal of Medicine* has, frequently making the evening news headlines. But nursing itself has become a best-seller in academic circles and even with the public at large. In no small measure this has come about because of the connection between the feminists' concern about the broader issue of women's place in the world and nurses as the prototype of those who do women's work in a male-oriented society.

Reverby's *Ordered to Care: The Dilemma of American Nursing*[29] led the way with her revisionist historical analysis of nursing. This was followed by Gordon's *Prisoners of Men's Dreams*,[14] which was written in the context of the nursing shortage and economic boom times of the 1980s. Gordon describes what happens when nurses adopt men's values toward themselves and their work and conspire with men to keep themselves and their work invisible. These works do not flatter nursing, but they portray an empathetic picture of the difficulties nurses face and the reasons why it is worth the effort to make nurses' strengths and contributions more visible to the public and other professions. Because the authors are not nurses (one is a social scientist and the other is a journalist), their ideas reach a wider audience. This may be a fact of their professional socialization that fosters public dissemination of their own work. It is also a measure of their skills in translating a scholarly work on complex issues into language that is captivating and understandable to the public. Both authors are excellent role models for nurses.

PERSONAL POLITICS

Is there any woman in the United States who does not know who Anita Hill is and what she did for women? For that matter is there any man? A new discourse on women, feminism, and nursing has begun—thanks to Anita Hill and her courage in speaking about a truth all women have experienced and her fortitude in withstanding the vicious, misogynistic attacks by the congressional committee broadcast on national television during Clarence Thomas's confirmation hearing as a Supreme Court judge. Her dignified, clear testimony sensitized women and men to issues in the workplace that had never been discussed in public before. For many women it caused a flood of painful memories. For others it was an energizing force that empowered them to speak out and say, "No more!" It is too soon to know, but in years to come this signature event may be regarded as *the* moment at which women examined the personal politics of their life and took charge of their workplace.

Anita Hill's legacy to people in the United States is demonstrated by the surge of interest in and popularity of books written by women about women and women's issues. These books were already in the works or even published, but the publicity generated by Hill's testimony caused editors, talk show hosts, and conference planners to take a more indepth look at writings that deal with feminism and women's concerns.[11] The following are just a few of the many: Faludi's *Backlash: The Undeclared War against American Women;*[9] Steinem's *Revolution from Within: A Book of Self-Esteem;*[34] Tannen's *You Just Don't Understand: Women and Men in Conversation;*[36] and Wolf's *The Beauty Myth: How Images of Beauty Are Used Against Women.*[39] Bestsellers, prime-time TV speakers, college campus stars, and the cover of *Time*[11] magazine—all have a message for the American people about women and their lived experience.

With the nation's attention directed toward women and their issues, how can nursing reap some of the benefits? Given that the third wave of the women's movement is just around the corner,[35] what will nursing's contribution be?

Here are some predictions:

1. One thing is clear. The strategy of "one for all and all for one" does not work in nursing. This goes against conventional wisdom in nursing,[22] but it is substantiated by history. Given their historical background, nursing and nurses are too diverse to speak as a group with one voice. Furthermore, they are not "joiners' in the classic sense. For example, only about 10% of all nurses belong to the American Nurses Association. Nurses value their differences and their individuality. Capitalizing on their strengths—the ability to know what really matters (caring) and the one-to-one relationship—a better strategy would be "getting to know you, getting to know all about you." Nurses have the knowledge and skills to establish meaningful relationships that are goal directed. Learning to express one's deepest thoughts and feelings is easier in familiar one-to-one situations. If each nurse shared her or his passionate conviction about feminism and nursing with one family member, one friend, one co-worker, and one community member, pretty soon the message would reach the powers that be, and various changes would take place. There might be divergence in setting the agenda at the top levels, but there would be *many* nurses to press their concerns and interests, not just a few nursing leaders. With so many nurses sharing similar ideologies of caring and feminism, a consensus for action could be achieved.

2. Nurses are getting ready to express themselves in public. Letters to the editor in professional journals and daily newspapers are on the increase. And nurses have stories to tell that the public wants and needs to hear. How long will it be before nurses begin to publish their own stories, rather than tell them to researchers? Where is the Perri Klass (a pediatrician who publishes "doctor stories" in the popular press) of nursing? Again, the strategy might be to turn inward, to keep a journal for personal consumption, at first; then to share the journal with a trusted colleague; then to schedule readings of the journal in a work group formed to develop writing skills . . . and so it goes.

3. The need for good public role models is desperate. Nurses can completely redo their interior life; they can rearrange their immediate surroundings; but lasting, dramatic changes will take place only when society changes, too. The

main vehicle for change in American society is television. The public has come to expect that images of "real life" appear on television. Nursing needs another "China Beach" series—updated and reflective of what nurses really do, and how they think and feel. Nursing also needs a presence in other public venues. Nursing needs the Women in the Military Service Memorial so that all Americans can recognize and admire nursing's patriotic contribution. Nursing needs humor, not the kind that denigrates, but the kind that lets nurses have fun with their foibles and laugh with others at themselves. In order for these things to happen, some nurses will have to devote their full attention to "nonnursing things" such as writing scripts, performing on the stage, taking photographs, developing artwork, and making feature-length films and documentaries featuring nurses. Fortunately, there is nursing talent to take on these creative projects, and some have done so already. Those nurses need to come out of the closet so that their achievements can be openly applauded.

4. Nursing needs to care for its young. They are not only the hope for the future; they hold the keys to the present. Today's nurses are the products of at least two waves of the women's movement, whether they acknowledge that fact or not. They do not come to nursing with the same baggage as those who were born before 1960. They may still need some guidance from experienced clinicians and educators about who they are and where they are going. But they have much to teach organized nursing. Applying feminist principles, socialization into nursing has to change toward becoming a more empathic, nonhierarchical, mutually beneficial process. There must be tolerance of different learning styles and cultural values, reflecting the diversity of the population of nursing. Many nurses today bemoan the lack of a mentor. Mentoring, a product of the "old boys" system, may not be nearly as effective as "caring." If nurses truly were to care for other nurses, they would be putting their feminist principles into practice. And if that were to happen, the world would indeed be a better place.

REFERENCES

1. Anderson, J. M. (1991). Reflexivity in fieldwork: Toward a feminist epistemology. *Image: The Journal of Nursing Scholarship, 23*(2), 115-118.
2. Barclay, L., Andre, C. A., & Glover, P. A. (1989). Women's business: The challenge of childbirth. *Midwifery, 5*(3), 122-133.
3. Belenky, M. F., Clinchy, B. M., Goldberger, N. R., & Tarule, J. M. (1986). *Women's ways of knowing: The development of self, voice, and mind.* New York: Basic Books.
4. Benner, P., & Wrubel, J. (1988). *The primacy of caring: Stress and coping in health and illness.* Menlo Park, Calif: Addison-Wesley.
5. Boughn, S. (1991). A women's health course with a feminist perspective: Learning to care for and empower ourselves. *Nursing and Health Care, 12*(2), 76-80.
6. Bunting, S., & Cambell, J. C. (1990). Feminism and nursing: Historical perspective. *Advances in Nursing Science, 12*(4), 11-24.
7. Cott, N. F. (1987). *The grounding of modern feminism.* New Haven, Conn: Yale University Press.
8. Duffy, M. (1985). A critique of research: A feminist perspective. *Health Care for Women International, 6,* 341-352.
9. Faludi, S. (1991). *Backlash: The undeclared war against American women.* New York: Crown.
10. Gaut, D. A. (Ed.). (1992). *The presence of caring in nursing.* New York: National League for Nursing Press.
11. Gibbs, N. (1992, March 9). The war against feminism. *Time,* p. 50.
12. Gilligan, C. (1982). *In a different voice: Psychological theory and women's development.* Cambridge, Mass: Harvard University Press.
13. Gordon, S. (1988, July 10). The crisis in caring. *Boston Globe Magazine,* p. 22.
14. Gordon, S. (1991). *Prisoners of men's dreams: Striking out for a new feminine future.* Boston: Little, Brown.
15. Hall, J. M., & Stevens, P. E. (1991). Rigor in feminist research. *Advances in Nursing Science, 13*(3), 16-29.
16. Harding, S. (1986). *The science question in feminism.* Ithaca, N.Y.: Cornell University Press.
17. Hedin, B. A., & Donovan, J. (1989). A feminist perspective on nursing education. *Nurse Educator, 14*(4), 8-13.
18. Heide, W. S. (1982). Feminist activism in nursing and health care. In J. Muff (Ed.), *Socialization, sexism, and stereotyping: Women's issues in nursing.* St Louis: Mosby.
19. Holcomb, B. (1988). Nurses fight back. *MS, 16*(12), 72-78.
20. Keller, E. F. (1985). *Reflections on gender and science.* New Haven, Conn: Yale University Press.
21. Kobert, L., & Folan, M. (1990). Coming of age in nursing: Rethinking the philosophies behind holism and nursing process. *Nursing and Health Care, 11*(6), 308-312.
22. Mason, D. J., Backer, B. A., & Georges, C. A. (1991). Toward a feminist model for the political empowerment of nurses. *Image: The Journal of Nursing Scholarship, 23*(2), 72-77.
23. Morse, J. M. (1990). Concepts of caring and caring as a concept. *Advances in Nursing Science, 13*(1), 1-14.
24. Moss, V. A. (1991). Battered women and the myth of masochism. *Journal of Psychosocial Nursing, 29*(7), 18-23.
25. Muff, J. (Ed.). (1982). *Socialization, sexism, and stereotyping: Women's issues in nursing.* St Louis: Mosby.
26. Neil, R. M., & Watts, R. (Eds.). (1991). *Caring and nursing: Exploration in feminist perspectives.* New York: National League for Nursing Press.
27. Parker, B., & McFarlane, J. (1991). Feminist theory and nursing: An empowerment model for research. *Advances in Nursing Science, 13*(3), 59-67.

28. Quinn, A. A. (1991). Menopause: Plight or passage? *NAACOG's Clinical Issues in Perinatal and Women's Health Nursing, 2*(3), 304-311.

29. Reverby, S. (1987). *Ordered to care: The dilemma of American nursing 1850 to 1945.* New York: Cambridge University Press.

30. Sampselle, C. M. (1990). The influence of feminist philosophy on nursing practice. *Image: The Journal of Nursing Scholarship, 22*(4), 243-7.

31. Shattuck, J. C., & Schwarz, K. K. (1991). Walking the line between feminism and infertility: Implications for nursing, medicine and patient care. *Health Care for Women International, 12*(3), 331-339.

32. Smith, P. (1991). The nursing process: Raising the profile of emotional care in nurse training. *Journal of Advanced Nursing, 16,* 74-81.

33. Steen, M. (1991). Historical perspectives on women and mental illness and prevention of depression in women, using a feminist framework. *Journal of Mental Health Nursing, 12*(4), 359-374.

34. Steinem, G. (1992). *Revolution from within: A book of self-esteem.* Boston: Little, Brown.

35. Strohmeyer, S. (1992, September 14). Vermont women prepare for "third wave of feminism." *Valley News,* pp. 1, 6.

36. Tannen, D. (1990). *You just don't understand: Women and men in conversation.* New York: William Morrow.

37. Vance, C., Talbott, S., McBride, A., & Mason, D. (1985). An uneasy alliance: Nursing and the women's movement. *Nursing Outlook, 33,* 281-285.

38. White, J. H. (1991). Feminism, eating, and mental health. *Advances in Nursing Science, 13*(3), 68-80.

39. Wolf, N. (1991). *The beauty myth: How images of beauty are used against women.* New York: William Morrow.

CHAPTER 78

Collaboration between nurses and physicians

What is it? Does it exist?

JUDITH G. BAGGS

COLLABORATION BETWEEN NURSES AND PHYSICIANS: WHAT IS IT?

According to my office dictionary,[61] to collaborate is to "work jointly with others or together," from the Latin *collaborare,* "to labor together." Indeed, this is the heart of the meaning of collaboration as we use it in nursing to describe a type of working relationship we value with physicians. But working together is not specific enough as a definition. Working together could mean working in parallel, without communicating or planning together, or simply working in the same geographical area.

In a review of the construct of collaboration, Schmitt and I[7] found these critical attributes for collaboration in the nursing literature: sharing in planning, decision making, problem solving, goal setting, and responsibility; working together cooperatively; coordinating; and communicating openly. We used a conceptual model developed by Thomas[60] to help us develop a definition that could be operationalized and measured for research.

Thomas proposed that collaboration is a form of handling interpersonal interactions that combines cooperativeness, or concern for the other's interests, and assertiveness, or concern for one's own interests. Based on the critical attributes and the Thomas model, the definition of collaboration that we developed is as follows: "nurses and physicians cooperatively working together, sharing responsibility for solving problems and making decisions to formulate and carry out plans for patient care."[7] A similar, although more clinical and less conceptual, definition has recently been adopted by the Congress of Nursing Practice.[42]

But does collaboration mean the same thing to physicians as it does to nurses? The construct of collaboration is addressed more often by the nursing profession than by medicine. Evidence for this assertion may be found in the primary library indices for the professions. *The Cumulative Index to Nursing and Allied Health Literature* (CINAHL) has had a subject heading called "collaboration" since 1989. In the volume covering 1991, that heading has more than a full page of citations. *Index Medicus* does not use "collaboration" as a subject heading; rather, one must look under "interprofessional relations" or "patient care team." Both those headings also are in CINAHL.

Most of the literature about collaboration between physicians and nurses is written by nurses,* or by nurses and physicians together.[2,19,36] Some physicians have written about the construct. Occasionally physicians even use the term *collaboration* in their titles.[43]

In other articles physicians discuss collaboration, although they do not indicate that it is the major focus of their interest. For example, in 1990, Stein, Watts, and Howell[57] updated Stein's classic article[56] on the "doctor-nurse game," noting that the earlier relationship between the professions has changed. In their view, nurses now are more highly educated and have a defined area of expertise, functioning more as autonomous health professionals. In the past, nurses could only have input by convincing physicians that they, the physicians, had initiated any decision making themselves.[56]

Acknowledgments: I thank Madeline H. Schmitt, RN, PhD, FAAN, and Nancy Wells, RN, DNSc, who reviewed this manuscript and offered helpful suggestions.

*References 1, 4, 8, 9, 16, 20, 32, 34, 37, 40, 41, 55, 58, 62.

Stein and colleagues[57] characterize the new relationship between physicians and nurses as one of "mutual interdependency." They cite movement toward collaboration and collegiality, with a less hierarchical and more open relationship than in the past. They indicate the possible positive and negative aspects of this new relationship but are generally approving of the direction it is taking. They appear to be speaking of collaboration with a definition comparable to the term used in the nursing literature.

Despite this evidence of comparability of definition, there is also evidence of differences in meaning or implications of collaboration for the two professions. Styles[58] noted that physicians often feel threatened when nurses discuss collaboration. They see the process as one of invasion of their position of authority and power. Indeed, a secondary definition of collaboration is "to cooperate with an agency or instrumentality with which one is not immediately connected."[61] The physicians' sense of a collapsing hierarchy, presumably caused by physicians collaborating with nurses, is noted by Stein and colleagues[57] in their description of the negative aspects of collaboration, a loss of the security of the old hierarchy and the potential for competition and disputes. Indeed, the movement toward interdisciplinary team care, a construct related to collaboration, has been described in part as a move by nurses to make interprofessional relations more egalitarian and less hierarchical.[10]

Physicians who were comfortable with the older caste-like system,[63] where nurses were subordinate, are not likely to welcome collaboration in practice.[11,49] Their ultimate fears are reflected in the title of a presentation by the administrator of a hospital management group,[25] "Changing Roles in the '90s: Will RNs Manage MDs?" Nurses, too, may feel threatened by increased responsibility and accountability in a mode of collaboration.[12,50]

For nurses to fulfill the assertive aspect of collaboration, they will need to assume accountability and increased authority in practice areas. The different perceptions held by nurses and physicians regarding areas appropriate for an increase in nursing authority are suggested in a recent research article by Katzman.[30] She asked nurses and physicians from a Southwestern general hospital to rate their agreement—on a scale of 1 (disagree) to 5 (agree)—with statements that certain specific nursing roles, functions, and behaviors reflect the current status of nursing authority. She then asked them to rate the same behaviors in an ideal situation.

The area of greatest difference between ratings from nurses and physicians in the current situation concerned nurses not serving primarily as physician assistants, where the nurses' mean score was 3.85 and the physicians' was 2.53. In the ideal ratings the greatest difference concerned nurses' having equal say with physicians in health policy making; the nurses' mean score was 4.46, while the physicians' was 2.2. Some of the areas of greatest disagreement concerned nursing care, with physicians according nurses less authority both in current and ideal situations. In an ideal situation nurses rated their authority to decide standards of nursing care at 4.59, while physicians gave it 3.24; in determination of nursing care for patients, the nurses' rating was 4.64, while the physicians' was 3.31. Perhaps in other settings and with other groups of providers some of these differences would diminish, but these disagreements about nursing authority suggest that we have to expect difficulties in moving to more collaboration in practice.

There is research evidence for different interpretations or observations of collaboration. In a medical intensive care unit (MICU), staff nurses and medical residents were given the same definition of collaboration and asked to report how much collaboration was involved in making decisions about individual patients. The correlation between their reports of amount of collaboration in making decisions was only $r = .10$ $(p = .10)$.[6]

An earlier study involved interviews of administrators in medicine and nursing about interdisciplinary team care. The goals expressed by each profession for team care differed. Physicians expected nurses to act as physician extenders, while nurses expected to use their knowledge to direct patient care.[59] Although there was agreement about the definition of a team (people with differing expertise working together to provide patient care), there was conflict about leadership and authority in decision making and concern about territory.

The definitions of collaboration appear similar for the professions of nursing and medicine, but there are differences in the implications of the term for each. Not too surprisingly, the loss of power by physicians and the gain in power by nurses that are inherent in collaboration in practice lead the two professions to approach such a move differently. Nurses and physicians also may observe or interpret interactions differently in assessing how collaborative they were. The meanings or connotations of the term go beyond its definition or denotation and may differ between professions.

COLLABORATION BETWEEN NURSES AND PHYSICIANS: DOES IT EXIST?

One of the first groups to promote the notion of collaboration between physicians and nurses in practice was the National Joint Practice Commission (NJPC), which was established in 1971 "to make recommendations concerning the roles of the physician and the nurse in providing high quality health care."[45] The commission, founded by the American Medical Association and the American Nurses Association, was composed of equal numbers of physicians and nurses. They set forth five guidelines for the development of what they termed joint or collaborative practice: establishment of a joint practice committee, primary nursing, encouragement of nurses' individual clinical decision making, integrated patient records, and joint patient care record reviews. Several model collaborative practice units were established implementing these five guidelines for practice. Although data obtained were primarily subjective opinions of participants, increased quality of care, patient satisfaction, and nursing job satisfaction were reported.[16,18,45]

Now, about 20 years after these guidelines were developed, many of them have been implemented in various institutions, particularly primary nursing and integrated patient records. Does their implementation mean that collaborative practice is a reality? Work by Prescott and associates[49] suggests that we are not yet at that point. In a study reported in 1985, they used the Thomas model to classify the modes of handling disagreements reported by nurses and physicians in acute care settings. They found that only 14% of the physicians and 7% of the nurses reported using collaborative problem solving; the primary mode used by both providers was competition.

Further analyses of data from the same study suggested that the staff nurse role in clinical decision making about patient care is, at best, interdependent rather than truly collaborative, with physicians accepting nurses' input but handling final decision making themselves in most situations.[50] The nurses in the study were generally satisfied with this arrangement, provided that they believed their input was listened to and valued by physicians. Many of the nurses did not want more responsibility for decision making. Physicians were only willing to cede to nursing decisions considered unimportant. In fact, they did not view the nurses as making decisions at all. This is less the new collaborative mode promoted in nursing and more the older doctor-nurse game, with the change that nurses now may openly make suggestions.

Prescott believes that we have not gone far enough toward collaboration, despite many nurses' satisfaction with the status quo. She sees collaboration as important in the development of professional practice and financially in the management of hospital care.[48,50,51] Professional practice is enhanced by nurses who have independence in some decision making, for example, in decisions about administering analgesics for headache or changing diets as tolerated. Enabling nurses to make some decisions frees them from wasted and expensive time spent looking or waiting for physicians. Such decision making supports the assertive aspect of collaboration.

Prescott and her coauthors[51] note the importance of collaboration as a way of improving patient outcomes. There are a number of empirical studies that support such a belief. Studies based in long-term care have demonstrated interdisciplinary care leads to a slower rate of deterioration in chronic diabetics[23,53] and lower mortality.[52] Outcomes of collaboration in acute care hospital general units include lower costs[34] and increased patient satisfaction.[35] In intensive care units (ICUs), investigators have found better-than-predicted mortality,[33,44] a decreased risk of death or readmission to the ICU,[6] and evidence of nurse satisfaction and retention.[5,44]

Collaboration between nurses and physicians may also support improved bioethical decision making in health care. Nurses' closeness to and communications with patients[38] and their support for patient autonomy[15,46,47,66] make their inclusion in ethical decision making important. Nurses tend to use a style of decision making that identifies the importance of personal relationships, while physicians are more concerned with rights and rules.[27] The combination of perspectives may enrich ethical decision making.

But in ethical decision making, too, there is evidence of a lack of collaboration. Researchers in several studies have demonstrated nurse-physician differences about how aggressively to treat patients.[22,24,64] In three recent studies, nurses perceived ethical decision making as a problematic area in their interactions with physicians.[21,26,29]

Collaboration in practice is not yet a reality for most nurses. Obstacles to collaborative practice come from both the nursing and medical professions. In some of the areas where we would most expect to find collaborative practice, it is missing, for example, in primary care teams of nurse practitioners and physicians where the nurses are highly educated in their area of practice. Lamb and Napodano[36] audiotaped interactions between team members on two teams. They found that only 23% of the interactions qualified as collaborative, although the providers rated themselves as collaborating 59% of the time. More recently McLain—who says, "The research literature is strikingly devoid of studies that have demonstrated the actual existence of collaborative practice as a predominant pattern between nurses and physicians"[40]—found that both physicians and nurses promoted distorted communication and nonmeaningful interactions that blocked collaboration.[40,41]

Critical care nurses have identified collaboration with physicians as their most important professional issue.[28] In our study, both ICU nurses and residents reported collaboration in decision making at a mean level that was closer to the high than the low end of the scale. For both, collaboration was significantly associated with satisfaction with the decision making process. However, the lack of a significant correlation between the nurses' and residents' scores and the stronger association between collaboration and satisfaction for nurses than for residents suggest that the two groups may have been talking about a different construct.[5,6]

Many writers have asserted the importance of collaboration. Some continue to develop new models to promote it. One recent example is a special care unit in Cleveland, developed for the treatment of the chronically critically ill.[13,14] In this unit, a nursing case management model using protocols for common patient problems, such as ventilator weaning, has decreased costs using a less hierarchical, more collaborative interdisciplinary approach to care. Care is organized around the patient, not around a physician team leader.

Another idea that has been proposed to improve physician-nurse collaboration is to begin with nursing and medical students, implementing elements into the curriculum so that they learn together from the beginning.[31,39,54,65] Model programs recently have been described at New York University[8] and Mount Sinai.[3] Such programs could assist the two professions to have a better idea of each other's roles, supporting cooperation and promoting respect for assertion of the individual professional perspective in patient care situations.

There is support both conceptually and empirically for collaboration in practice between nurses and physicians, and there are examples of it. Some writers believe that collaboration is already occurring in practice, particularly in ICUs;[2] but there is still work to be done in understanding and promoting collaboration in practice. On the whole, collaboration is not the usual mode of practice today.

REFERENCES

1. Alt-White, A. C., Charns, M., & Strayer, R. (1983). Personal, organizational and managerial factors related to nurse-physician collaboration. *Nursing Administration Quarterly, 8,* 8-18.
2. Ames, A., & Perrin, J. M. (1980). Collaborative practice: The joining of two professions. *Journal of the Tennessee Medical Association, 73,* 557-560.
3. Anvaripour, P. L., Jacobson, L., Schweiger, J., & Weissman, G. K. (1991). Physician-nurse collegiality in the medical school curriculum. *Mount Sinai Journal of Medicine, 58*(1), 91-94.
4. Aradine, C. R., & Pridham, K. F. (1973). Model for collaboration. *Nursing Outlook, 21,* 655-657.
5. Baggs, J. G., & Ryan, S. A. (1990). Intensive care unit nurse-physician collaboration and nurse satisfaction. *Nursing Economic$, 8,* 386-392.
6. Baggs, J. G., Ryan, S. A., Phelps, C. E., Richeson, J. F., & Johnson, J. E. (1992). The association between interdisciplinary collaboration and patient outcomes in medical intensive care. *Heart and Lung, 21,* 18-24.
7. Baggs, J. G., & Schmitt, M. H. (1988). Collaboration between nurses and physicians. *Image: The Journal of Nursing Scholarship, 20,* 145-149.
8. Barnum, B. J. (1991). At New York University, the Division of Nursing develops a model for nursing and medical school collaboration. *Nursing and Health Care, 11*(2), 89-90.
9. Bradford, R. (1989). Obstacles to collaborative practice. *Nursing Management, 20,*(4), 72I, 72L, 72M, 72P.
10. Brown, T. (1982). An historical view of health care teams. In G. J. Agich (Ed.), *Responsibility in health care* (pp. 3-21). Dordrecht, Holland: D. Reidel.
11. Campbell-Heider, N., & Pollock, D. (1987). Barriers to physician-nurse collegiality. *Social Science and Medicine, 25,* 421-425.
12. Cape, L. S. (1986). Collaborative practice models and structures. In D. A. England (Ed.), *Collaboration in nursing* (pp. 13-26). Rockville, Md: Aspen.
13. Daly, B. J., Phelps, C., & Rudy, E. B. (1991). A nurse-managed special care unit. *Journal of Nursing Administration, 21*(7-8), 31-38.
14. Daly, B. J., Rudy, E. B., Thompson, K. S., & Happ, M. B. (1991). Development of a special care unit for chronically critically ill patients. *Heart and Lung, 20,* 45-51.
15. Davis, A. J., & Jameton, A. (1987). Nursing and medical student attitudes toward nursing disclosure of information to patients: A pilot study. *Journal of Advanced Nursing, 12,* 691-698.
16. Devereux, P. M. (1981, May). Essential elements of nurse-physician collaboration. *Journal of Nursing Administration, 11,* 19-23.
17. Devereux, P. M. (1981, June). Does joint practice work? *Journal of Nursing Administration, 11,* 39-43.
18. Devereux, P. M. (1981, September). Nurse/physician collaboration: Nursing practice considerations. *Journal of Nursing Administration, 11,* 37-39.

19. Dunbar, S., & Bryan-Brown, C. (1988). Collaborative practice. In J. Boller (Ed.), *1988 International conference book* (pp. 153-154). Newport Beach, Calif: American Association of Critical-Care Nurses.

20. England, D. A. (1986). *Collaboration in nursing.* Rockville, Md: Aspen.

21. Erlen, J. A., & Frost, B. (1991). Nurses' perceptions of powerlessness in influencing ethical decisions. *Western Journal of Nursing Research, 13,* 397-407.

22. Farber, N. J., Weiner, J. L., Boyer, E. G., Green, W. P., Diamond, M. P., & Copare, I. M. (1985). Cardiopulmonary resuscitation values and decisions. *Medical Care, 23,* 1391-1398.

23. Feiger, S. M., & Schmitt, M. H. (1979). Collegiality in interdisciplinary health teams. *Social Science and Medicine, 13A,* 217-229.

24. Frampton, M. W., & Mayewski, R. J. (1987). Physicians' and nurses' attitudes toward withholding treatment in a community hospital. *Journal of General Internal Medicine, 2,* 394-399.

25. Gamble, S. W. (1989, November 20). Changing roles in the '90s: Will RNs manage MDs? *Hospitals,* p.42-44.

26. Gramelspacher, G. P., Howell, J. D., & Young, M. J. (1986). Perceptions of ethical problems by nurses and doctors. *Archives of Internal Medicine, 146,* 577-578.

27. Haddad, A. M. (1991). The nurse/physician relationship and ethical decision making. *AORN Journal, 53,* 151-156.

28. Hartwell, J. L., & Lavandero, R. (1991). What's important to critical care nurses. *Focus on Critical Care, 18,* 364-371.

29. Holly, C. (1989). Critical care nurses' participation in ethical decision making. *Journal of the New York State Nurses Association, 20*(4), 9-12.

30. Katzman, E. M. (1989). Nurses' and physicians' perceptions of nursing authority. *Journal of Professional Nursing, 5,* 208-214.

31. Kenneth, H. Y. (1969). Medical and nursing students learn together. *Nursing Outlook, 17,* 46-49.

32. Kerfoot, K. (1989). Nurse/physician collaboration: A cost/quality issue for the nurse manager. *Nursing Economic$, 7,* 335-338.

33. Knaus, W. A., Draper, E. A., Wagner, D. P., & Zimmerman, J. E. (1986). An evaluation of outcome from intensive care in major medical centers. *Annals of Internal Medicine, 104,* 410-418.

34. Koerner, B., & Armstrong, D. (1984). Collaborative practice cuts cost of patient care: Study. *Hospitals, 58*(10), 52-54.

35. Koerner, B. L., Cohen, J. R., & Armstrong, D. M. (1985). Collaborative practice and patient satisfaction. *Evaluation and the Health Professions, 8,* 299-321.

36. Lamb, G. S., & Napodano, R. J. (1984). Physician-nurse practitioner interaction patterns in primary care practices. *American Journal of Public Health, 74,* 26-29.

37. Lewis, F. M. (1991). Consultation and collaboration among health care providers. In S. B. Baird, R. McCorkle, & M. Grant (Eds.), *Cancer nursing: A comprehensive textbook* (pp.957-964). Philadelphia: W. B. Saunders.

38. Luce, J. M. (1990). Ethical principles in critical care. *Journal of the American Medical Association, 263,* 696-700.

39. Mason, E., & Parascandola, J. (1972). Preparing tomorrow's health care team. *Nursing Outlook, 20,* 728-731.

40. McLain, B. R. (1988). Collaborative practice: A critical theory perspective. *Research in Nursing and Health, 11,* 391-398.

41. McLain, B. R. (1988). Collaborative practice: The nurse practitioner's role in its success or failure. *Nurse Practitioner, 13*(5), 31-38.

42. McLoughlin, S. (1992). Congress of Nursing Practice meets. *American Nurse, 24*(3), 18, 23.

43. Michelson, E. L. (1988). The challenge of nurse-physician collaborative practices: Improved patient care provision and outcomes. *Heart and Lung, 17,* 390-391.

44. Mitchell, P. H., Armstrong, S., Simpson, T. F., & Lentz, M. (1989). AACN demonstration project. *Heart and Lung, 18,* 219-237.

45. National Joint Practice Commission. (1981). *Guidelines for establishing joint or collaborative practice in hospitals.* Chicago: Author.

46. Ott, B. B., & Nieswiadomy, R. M. (1991). Support of patient autonomy in the do not resuscitate decision. *Heart and Lung, 20,* 66-72.

47. Ouslander, J. G., Tymchuk, A. J., & Rahbar, B. (1989). Health care decisions among elderly long-term care residents and their potential proxies. *Archives of Internal Medicine, 149,* 1367-1372.

48. Prescott, P. A. (1989). Shortage of professional nursing practice: A reframing of the shortage problem. *Heart and Lung, 18,* 436-443.

49. Prescott, P. A., & Bowen, S. A. (1985). Physician-nurse relationships. *Annals of Internal Medicine, 103,* 127-133.

50. Prescott, P. A., Dennis, K. E., & Jacox, A. K. (1987). Clinical decision making of staff nurses. *Image: The Journal of Nursing Scholarship, 19,* 56-62.

51. Prescott, P. A., Phillips, C. Y., Ryan, J. W., & Thompson, K. O. (1991). Changing how nurses spend their time. *Image: The Journal of Nursing Scholarship, 23,* 23-28.

52. Rubenstein, L. Z., Josephson, K. R., Wieland, G. D., English, P. A., Sayre, J. A., & Kane, R. L. (1984). Effectiveness of a geriatric evaluation unit. *New England Journal of Medicine, 311,* 1664-1670.

53. Schmitt, M. H., Watson, N. M., Feiger, S. H., & Williams, T. F. (1981). Conceptualizing and measuring outcomes of interdisciplinary team care for a group of long-term, chronically ill, institutionalized patients. In J. E. Bachman (Ed.), *Interdisciplinary health care: Proceedings of the third annual conference on interdisciplinary team care* (pp.169-181). Kalamazoo, Mich: Center for Human Services, Western Michigan University.

54. Shumaker, D., & Goss, V. (1980). Toward collaboration: One small step. *Nursing and Health Care, 1*(11), 183-185.

55. Steel, J. E. (1986). *Issues in collaborative practice.* Orlando, Fla: Grune and Stratton.

56. Stein, L. I. (1967). The doctor-nurse game. *Archives of General Psychiatry, 16,* 638-642.

57. Stein, L. I., Watts, D. T., & Howell, T. (1990). The doctor-nurse game revisited. *New England Journal of Medicine, 322,* 546-549.

58. Styles, M. M. (1984). Reflections on collaboration and unification. *Image: The Journal of Nursing Scholarship, 16,* 21-23.

59. Temkin-Greener, H. (1983). Interprofessional perspectives on teamwork in health care: A case study. *Milbank Memorial Fund Quarterly, 61,* 641-658.

60. Thomas, K. (1976). Conflict and conflict management. In M. D. Dunnette (Ed.), *Handbook of industrial and organizational psychology* (pp.889-935). Chicago: Rand McNally College Publishing.

61. *Webster's Ninth New Collegiate Dictionary.* (1989). Springfield, Mass: Merriam-Webster.

62. Weiss, S. J., & Davis, H. P. (1985). Validity and reliability of the collaborative practice scales. *Nursing Research, 34,* 299-305.

63. Wesson, A. F. (1966). Hospital ideology and communication between ward personnel. In R. Scott & E. Volkhart (Eds.), *Medical care* (pp.458-475). New York: Wiley.

64. Wolff, M. L., Smolen, S., & Ferrara, L. (1985). Treatment decisions in a skilled-nursing facility. *Journal of the American Geriatrics Society, 33,* 440-445.

65. Yeaworth, R., & Mims, F. (1973). Interdisciplinary education as an influence system. *Nursing Outlook, 21,* 1973.

66. Zorb, S. L., & Stevens, J. B. (1990). Contemporary bioethical issues in critical care. *Nursing Clinics of North America, 2,* 515-520.

CHAPTER 79

Multidisciplinary community-based education and practice

CYNTHIA L. LENZ

Multidisciplinary community-based education and practice is a concept that means very different things to different people. The definition and description of the concept offered here have been developed through the thoughts and experiences of many, over time, and after immersion in a multidisciplinary project. Years of focused activity in multidisciplinary community-based environments and experience with the W.K. Kellogg Foundation provided the experiential learning that brought the concept to its current stage of development.

This chapter offers insight on multidisciplinary community-based education and practice, clearly from a nursing perspective. It offers a lived experience that continues. Participation in multidisciplinary community-based education and practice projects has proved to be the most challenging, mind-expanding, and rewarding experience imaginable.

DEFINITION OF TERMS

The definition offered for multidisciplinary community-based education and practice is complex and must be broken down into its constituent and supporting parts.

Multidisciplinary

The term *multidisciplinary* indicates more than one professional discipline. This implies a notion of "team" and "collaboration." Collaboration enhances the likelihood of positive outcomes, offers an increased likelihood of a more cost-effective health care delivery system, and potentially provides a superior mode of operation and decision making than does professional isolation.

More subtleties exist when a multidisciplinary approach is applied to education and practice. Areas of professional overlap are likely to exist between providers on the team, but each discipline brings a particular set of strengths and a unique body of knowledge and skills. In a successful multidisciplinary team there is mutual respect, equity in power, and shared decision making. Often lines that demarcate realms of responsibility and control are blurred, and a process of decision making and conflict resolution equitable to all involved is critical.

Optimally, multidisciplinary decision making must abandon traditional areas of control and focus on the outcome. Recognition of the individual(s) best suited to meet the challenges of the task is critical in decision making in a collaborative professional partnership. Cost effectiveness should be considered in decision making, given the paucity of resources available in health care and education.

Leadership of the multidisciplinary team must shift according to the situation and be based upon knowledge and skills, not traditionally assigned tasks. Depending upon the need, the nurse, social worker, physical therapist, physician, or other provider may emerge as the leader. Strong communication and group facilitation skills are often required of the leader. At times, technical or specific discipline-based knowledge will determine the appropriate leader, and leadership shifts within the team in response to the dynamic situations encountered.

Theoretically, an employer-employee relationship may be collaborative and embrace these ideas; but in reality, collaboration is much more likely to occur in a true partnership. The hiring and firing power of the employer creates an imbalance of power that prohibits collaboration in any but the most rudimentary manner. Associations of professionals, each dependent upon the other, promote collaboration, even when faced with societally defined status inequalities.

Community-based

The concept of the term *community-based* is complex, which leads to great divergence in its meanings. For the purpose of this chapter, community-based means integrated into the community, immersed in the community, part of the fabric of the community. Community-based means that the practice or educational entity is inseparable from the community, yet maintaining identity. The community fabric includes the community-based education and service. Community-based is *not* outreach. It is *not* superimposing an entity upon a community. Community-based is more simply translated into "the community, *we*" versus "the community, *they*."

The addition of the terms *education* and *practice* to *multidisciplinary* and *community-based* creates issues and ideas that are often controversial, sometimes explosive, and rarely easy. Simply, community-based education and practice occurs in the community. The faculty, students, and their families live, work, and go to school in the community. The community is home.

Practice

Community-based practice is that which is unique and responsive to the specific community. The community-based practice evolves with the community, and they should be supportive of each other.

Community-based practices incorporate the broad community needs into their professional and personal realms of responsibility. Resources available to the practitioner are mobilized to meet the needs of the community. In return, the community takes on the care of the practitioner. This broadens the professional realm of responsibility to all aspects of the community life; it is no longer restricted to only the health care arena.

An example of a community-responsive practice decision is the provision of services at times that are tailored to meet the needs of the patients. For instance, a practice serving poor employed families with school-aged children must be willing to provide services at times when family members are not working. Minimum or near minimum wage earners are rarely free to rearrange their work schedules to accommodate pursuit of health care. The children's absence from school will place an additional burden on an already-disadvantaged group. When such factors are not considered, health care needs go unmet, treatment for ill-

ness is sought only at advanced stages, prevention is completely out of the question, and patient teaching and promotion of self care is hopeless.

An example of this concept could include the willingness of the health care provider to serve on the school board or other public office or to utilize contacts at the local university to assist a local agency with writing a grant for needy families.

Education

Multidisciplinary community-based education, along with faculty practice, integrates all these concepts into one whole. Education comes out of the proverbial ivory tower. The community is recognized as a major force, an asset, and a decision maker with input into curricular content and setting institutional priorities.

Faculty members practice, provide service, teach, and live in the community. The community assumes responsibility for "Community 101" through "Community 999 + ." The community, through exposure of its participating members, will become even more effective as the result of the increased knowledge base.

Health care and instruction are developed to incorporate community resources and consider community needs. Community-based education enriches the community as well as the academic program. The resources of the university at large are available to the community for solving problems.

Community-based education provides role models for the youth of the community, brings resources of the educational institution, and provides a valuable addition to the infrastructure of the community. In return, the educational institution gains a learning environment for its students that cannot be produced in a simulation or laboratory. The educational system gains an entire community of teachers. Students gain a true-to-life learning environment.

Community-based education is a partnership that requires collaboration. Collaboration can only occur in a balance of power or control. It requires trust that exists and grows as experiences reinforce this important aspect of relationships. There must be an acceptance of each other's weaknesses and a willingness to engage in complementary behaviors to support each other and to function as partners.

The community-university partnership can be likened to the health care provider-patient relationship in the area of control and influence. The reality of these situations is that the client and the community hold the ultimate power. Diagnosis and prescriptive treatment plans have no influence if compliance to the treatment regimen does not occur. Lifestyle or more dramatic alternations in daily living patterns will rarely occur unless the patient is engaged as a partner.

The most powerful, dependable, and effective resource available is self-help. Communities, families, and individual patients must be solicited as partners to realize the greatest influence and long-term effectiveness. Power and influence are given, not demanded or taken.

WHY CHANGE?

Our health care delivery system is sick. Our country spends more on health care per capita than any other country and records significantly worse health indicators than other westernized countries. In 1950 we spent a billion dollars monthly on health care. In 1988 we spent a billion and a half dollars *daily*. The gross national product devoted to health care has increased from 4.4% in 1950 to nearly 12% in 1990.[5] An estimated 37 million people in the United States lack access to health care, yet 20% to 30% of all medical procedures are unjustified, and $20 of every $100 expended goes to unnecessary paperwork. In our country, we offer the very best in technological medical care and the very worst in our ability to offer coordinated, personalized, comprehensive family-based primary care that is accessible and cost effective. Availability of resources (money) may purchase a new heart but cannot buy a personal health care provider who knows you and your family over time. Problems exist because health professionals are caught in the knowledge trap of reductionism. The relationship between professionals' knowledge base and the problems of society is very precarious. In many cases the knowledge is of no use at all.[4]

The state of our health care system indicates that education and practice are failing miserably in meeting the health needs of the American public. A major change is needed. A new type of health worker and health care system is needed for the future. Multidisciplinary community-based education and practice presents the best hope for change in the system.

Professional role of the nurse

In multidisciplinary community-based education and practice, the nurse must operationalize two main roles. These roles are provider and educator. These roles are often complementary but at times cause conflict. The demands and needed skill mix for the two roles are not duplicative.

The role of the nurse as a community health care provider is fettered with contradictions and real and imagined constraints. Yet, the community-based health care system can be one of the most rewarding and influential environments in which a nurse can practice.

The role of the nurse educator is primarily to educate the next generation of nurses. How and where this is done will have an unalterable impact on the professionals of the future and on the health care delivery system of our country. Educators are rooted in the practice arena of professional nursing and remain inextricably connected to what occurs there. Success, or failure, is bound to the results realized through the future practice of students after graduation.

Nurses hold the key to holistic, comprehensive care. Allegiance to individualized, family-centered care and patient empowerment is pervasive in the nursing heritage. Nurses explore the roles of other providers and learn to mobilize others to complement the nursing role. The nursing profession has embraced the patient advocacy role and enjoys a sense of intimacy and trust experienced by no other group. Self-care and education to promote understanding is a continual goal of nearly all nursing interactions. Nursing possesses the knowledge and skills to fully realize these community-based provider roles.

However, a number of factors exist that serve as barriers to community-based education and practice. These barriers prevent nursing from fully realizing its goals and from experiencing the full potential the professional role offers.

Nursing education focuses on the tertiary care arena. The nurse develops a professional identity closely connected and tied to the tertiary care environment. The public image of the nurse reflects this. Students are told that they must practice in the hospital to gain needed skills, they are immersed in the high-technology environment of the hospital, and they are exposed to faculty role models that socialize the aspiring student into the tertiary care environment.

The hospital is the environment that provides the least recognition for the patient's and nurse's power and control. Hospitals today are driven by revenue generation. Physicians admit patients, drive the treatment regimen, and continue to hold the control, power, and influence. Nursing, along with housekeeping, dietary, and physical plant, is a nonrevenue cost center of the hospital. Vital nursing services continue to be hidden from patients as part of the room rate.

Nurses do have power in the hospital. Due to the great numbers of nurses, viability of the hospital can be threatened if we unite. Yet, this environment fosters our division, creates subsets among us, encourages development of unit-based subcultures, and generally "divides and conquers." This environment limits our influence in the public and political power structures and significantly lessens our ability to control ourselves, our profession, and our practice.

Technological, hospital-based care is an important facet of the nursing profession. Yet, less than 20% of health care occurs in the hospital environment. Like medical training, 80% of nursing education occurs in the restrictive hospital environment. During the depression years, nurses became captives of the hospital environment. The advent of antibiotics and the incorporation of technology from the space age have extended the captivity. Our roots are in the community, delivering direct services to the public, working in partnership with other providers, and receiving direct reimbursement.

The opportunity to regain any of our historical roots exists in the health system reform underway in our country. The profession of nursing has a pivotal and influential place in nearly every reform proposal. Multidisciplinary community-based service provides the vehicle for nursing to make the contribution it is capable of making. Nursing can model the concept of community and patient empowerment and be the leader in teaching self-care and self-efficacy.

Nursing must use its knowledge, value system, and unique expertise to become a responsible provider, willing to invest and to take on a professional role. We must model shared decision making and partnership, and recognize the power of patients. Nursing can keep high-technology practices to complement its professional services, but it must reintegrate patient care foundations and influence policy to enable these community-based goals to become a reality.

Barriers facing professional nurses. Several barriers exist that compromise the full realization of the potential nursing offers. These barriers impact acutely upon practice outside the tertiary care environment. These factors are artificially classified as internal to the profession and external to the profession; however, the two are in reality inseparable.

Internal Practice Barriers. Several internal factors exist that continue to compromise the profession's ability to fully realize its potential. This chapter does not offer a comprehensive listing or discussion of factors, but serves only to identify and communicate some of the major issues.

Systems skill is one major constraining factor for the nursing profession. Few nurses possess the skills needed to effectively operate in the systems of health care. These skills cover one-to-one relationships with other providers in the state, national, and international arenas. These skills include communication in a systems environment, knowledge of the system, power and control, finance, and politics. Nursing programs include these concepts and develop beginning knowledge but fail in development of usable skills. The educational focus continues to be on technical skill development. The practicing nurse is likewise constrained in the development of these skills. Day-to-day responsibilities focus upon meeting immediate and relentless needs of others. Rather than attempting to influence the system, we become more and more internally focused as we strive to meet daily demands.

One specific example of systems skill is political action. Token political activism may be presented in the senior year during an immersion experience in a clinical practicum. Consequently, the nursing students rarely develop into the political activists. Few grasp the notion that holding power and influence in these arenas is one of the most effective ways we can operationalize patient advocacy. Nursing socialization continues to perceive power and influence as negatives and define their uses in primarily negative terms.

Additional internal factors include oppression and its resulting behaviors. Nursing as a profession suffers from the negative connotations of femaleness and a perception of inferiority. Many factors contribute to this phenomenon, but the reality is that nursing exhibits typical behavior patterns of an oppressed societal group. These characteristics do not facilitate openness and resolutions of interpersonal problems.

Oppressed groups develop when a system exists that allows selected access to services, rewards, benefits, and privileges of the society. This access is granted based on membership in a particular group. Those excluded by the dominant group develop a parallel society based on the oppression.[3] Common characteristics of oppression include low self-esteem, acceptance of the identity that society assigns, identification with the dominant group, suffering from the "blame the victim" syndrome, social isolation from the mainstream, depression as a result of anger turned against self, and little access to the institutions of the society.[2] Partnerships and collaboration are difficult to build and maintain in this situation.

External Practice Barriers. A number of factors that are primarily external to the profession also serve to compromise our ability and success in a partnership. Practice and reimbursement laws, male dominance, socialization of males in our society, and the societal definition of physician practice as all-powerful serve as constraining forces. Physician practice is defined in law as all-encompassing, as legislative control of medical practice does not exist. The profession of medicine is charged with regulation. However, nurse practice is defined in an explicit and exclusionary manner, with legislative definition of practice and associated legislative policing functions.

Reimbursement for services becomes a major and volatile issue in the nonhospital setting. National and state reimbursement laws present nearly unconquerable obstacles for the nurse desiring to offer direct nursing care to the public. Many nurses operate closet practices and resort to a "cooperative" relationship with a physician to circumvent the system. Nurses buy physician billing services in order to obtain access to reimbursement, use presigned prescription pads, and practice in many other hostile and humiliating circumstances in order to realize their goal of direct delivery. These practices continue in the face of extensive research that supports the viability and rationality of nurse-managed care. These approaches, which are designed to circumvent the obstacles and manage the system, devalue nursing and necessitate add-on costs, causing further deterioration of the cost effectiveness of the system. These factors erode the environment needed to create partnerships and they keep nursing practice on the fringes of the mainstream.

Nurses must gain all the rights, privileges, and respect of professional practice. This independence must be realized before nursing can compromise in a partnership. Nurses must establish value independently so as to be recognized for the value they bring to a partnership. Without access to reimbursement and the skills to use the option, nurses will continue to be perceived as cost burdens, their services always vulnerable to replacement by options perceived as cheaper or simply to omission.

Nursing practice also faces directly the public and popular image of the health care provider. The physician is portrayed as the "knight in shining armor" who rides in to save the day, and nurses are "air-headed blondes" or "battle-axes." Images of both professional groups serve to create obstacles that sap our energies and hinder our performance. These public images mislead prospective students, create the need to unlearn, and constrain our contributions. Many times the role and services provided by the nurse are subsumed in the minds of the public under medicine. Nurses, in sync with their socialized humility, rarely act to bring their contributions to the forefront and to correct the inaccurate images held by the public. Nursing continues to suffer from false and misconstrued public images of dependency, lack of intellectual challenge in the profession, and moral questionability.

Examples of other external factors include restrictive practice laws, uninsurability of nurse providers, and the unavailability of economic resources for nurse professionals desiring independent practice.

Barriers for the Educator. The nurse educator faces similar and additional barriers that limit the ability to engage in collaborative practice and that compromise those persons in the academic arena. Nurse educators possess the general characteristics of the practice group and are likewise in need of skill development.

The academic arena poses special problems for all professional groups. In the community of academicians, professional programs face some level of disdain. Professional programs are regarded by this society of academic purists as less than pure. Nursing's societal image as a less-than-intellectually-rigorous pursuit serves to add barriers for the nurse educator.

Academia does not recognize practice for the professional as it does performance for the musician. Scholarly performance is judged on the most rigorous of standards for the practice professions. Practice for nurses in the academic environment falls into the service area, which of the tripart mission of the university (teaching, research, and service) is the least valued by the academia. Nurses must practice to remain professionally current, yet cannot afford to practice given the low value placed on practice by their academic colleagues. Nurse faculty meet the rigor of academia and are judged by universitywide norms for promotion and tenure.

An example of this phenomenon was recently experienced and was associated with planning for a university honors program. An assumption of the committee was that nursing could not possibly participate in an honors program. Nursing on this campus competes more successfully for external funds (grants) than *any* academic unit. Nursing faculty are more widely published than any other group, have the third-largest graduate program, and participate across all committee and governance structures of the university. Still, the perception of nursing as a "nonhonors" profession persists.

Physician-nurse issues

Most literature written on the topic of multidisciplinary activities in the health care arena focuses on the dyad of nursing and medicine, although experiences are broader than this dyad and include public and allied health, business, education, counseling, and sociology-anthropology. The nursing-medicine dyad is repeatedly the focus of the greatest number of problems and presents the most difficult resolutions. The frequency of the conflicts and the intensity of the problems often become overwhelming; at times the conflicts are irreconcilable. Too frequently the resolution becomes a win-lose situation instead of the desired win-win outcome. This is true even with two highly committed parties or groups. Other professions make very valuable contributions to this partnership. In this experience, the public and allied health profession especially served as a binding agent for the multidisciplinary team and catalyzed efforts leading to resolution. The presence of others in the team has actually been referred to as "glue" on occasion.

A number of areas provide the backdrop for these collisions. Some are controllable and can be managed by learnable skills and behavior modification; others, it seems, are more difficult to resolve.

Models of Education. In the professional arena, nurses and physicians work together daily. Given this, it is amazing that the professional groups know so little of each other. Nursing faculty know little of the curricular content of the medical students, and the physician faculty know little of nursing. Faculty in these schools rarely collaborate on instructional delivery even though students are educated on the same campus and in the same health care facilities. The expertise of one group is rarely brought to the other.

A simple example of this comes from the multidisciplinary experiences related to the curriculum analysis for development of common course content. Physical assessment, taught to beginning medical students, was for all practical purposes identical to that taught to undergraduate nursing students. An analysis of the syllabi of both disciplines and of the faculty's class guides and notes confirmed this conclusion. The faculty team found that both groups utilized identical texts and accompanying videotapes.

Conflicting values often cause some of the most emotional and difficult problems between groups or individuals. One fundamental area of value conflict between nursing and medicine is found in the educational model of nursing versus the apprenticeship model of medicine.

Medical education is built upon the apprenticeship model. Medical school faculty define their roles through the practice approach, with the education of students incidental to practice. This approach is reinforced by revenue generation from the delivery of services that provides income to the individual faculty member and to the school through the practice plan. Funding agencies or institutions further reinforce the apprenticeship model through a number of actions. For example, budgets are devised based upon major revenue production and provision of multiple and elaborate practice support facilities. The apprenticeship model is dependent upon a large number of patients, so that the few required patient experiences are "calculated" guesses based on the practice profile. Proficiency in processing patients (speed) is a learned outcome, and it is clearly indicated that the number of encounters in a given time period becomes an indicator of performance and achievement for the medical student or resident. This system, in itself, is not necessarily good or bad, but it is presented as a major difference in the culture of the profession (versus that of nursing) and it builds a point of incompatibility between nursing education and medical education.

Nursing, on the other hand, is fully entrenched in the educational model. Nursing schools infrequently have a practice environment for faculty, and even more rare is the utilization of the entrepreneurial model. Educationally based nursing practices are generally nursing clinics offering direct nursing services to a chosen patient population group. These practices exist to provide operational models of direct public access to nursing care and to support the educational program. Client groups are cultivated and scheduled to meet the learning needs of the students rather than the population's health needs. Nursing centers generally receive support *from* the school, rather than producing excess revenue *to* (support) the school. One result of this situation is that few nursing faculty and subsequently few students possess the skills necessary to be successful in the open-market environment with direct delivery of nursing care.

Socialization. Socialization of the student is a major role of the professional school. The shaping of professional behaviors, values, beliefs, and mores forms the structure of the professional society. Socialization serves to bind groups together and creates common identity. The society supports social-professional needs of its members. The challenge facing multidisciplinary programs is to develop a society of multidisciplinary health care providers, retain the valuable parts of the pure professional identity, and incorporate the community as a partner.

The society of medicine is very strong in the practice setting. Medical students begin their socialization into the profession of medicine early. Medicine has different academic calendars, has practice plans when none exist for others in the academic world, has special funding arrangements, requires a higher staff-faculty ratio and higher faculty-student ratio, and so on. In general, medicine probably both consciously and unconsciously sets itself apart at every opportunity.

Nursing, on the other hand, is defined by law. The bounds of general practice and advanced practice are articulated and circumscribed. These legislated bounds continually face and restrict the evolution of the profession. However, nursing is one of the few professions that has any concrete provisions in the law that clearly define the right to practice. Most health professionals exist in the gray bounds of delegated authority and rights without clear statutory authority. Many overlap or duplicate the purview of medicine and are consequently controlled by the medical practice laws and the medical profession. The fact that nursing exists by statutory rights, as opposed to delegated privilege, is likely one of the fundamental sources of problems and conflict between the professions. A stage is set for legal and professional conflict in the practice setting between nursing and medicine. Other professional groups have experienced their success on the relative fringes of the legislative arena without as much practice overlap and through their subsequent dependent relationship with the medical profession.

The equivalent society of nursing exists, but it is much less strong and united in its identity. Consequently the existence of the society and its value go unrecognized. The value systems reinforced by nursing and education revolve around service above self and patient advocacy. Much of the socialization of nurses is aimed at behaviors of compliance and service and does not include empowerment of nurses and self-efficacy.

The relatively weak socialization of nurses facilitates the division of nursing ranks, allows our primary allegiances to be pledged to diverse groups, and fails to provide a consolidating force for the profession. Strengthening this area will strengthen the profession.

Strength of the society will allow nurses to realize their potential to influence the health care delivery system in our country. This is especially important given the emergent nature of this system. Clarity of the society and success in our socialization of the nursing rank and file will allow us to remain bonded together as a profession in the face of potentially divisive forces and during times of internal and external strife. Socialization seems to be a key factor in the empowerment and mobilization of the nursing profession.

From theory into practice: moving into the community

Moving from the traditional setting into the multidisciplinary community-based practice and education environment is a monumental task. Longstanding traditions are difficult to violate, and individuals who have been socialized into the system truly believe in the merits of existing, tried and "proved" approaches. Few, if any, consciously decide to resist the alternative, and many intellectually believe in the alternative. However, traditions die slowly, and, particularly in times of threat and difficulties, we tend to return to the familiar, which is traditional tertiary care settings.

Moving the educational program into the community poses a great threat to the educator. This move places faculty and students in unfamiliar environments, where they have relatively little control and relatively little power. They are outsiders, at least in the beginning. In this move the faculty member has left the familiarity of the campus and has relinquished the control and relative safety that the educational institution provides. The faculty member in the community leaves the academic culture that has nurtured the professional growth and development of faculty for centuries.

The complexities of multidisciplinary education and practice have been extensively discussed. The addition of the community adds complexity that nearly defies description. The number of factors and influences that come to bear upon the professions, the individuals, and the educational institutions compound the issues exponentially. The community faces similar phenomena with the addition of the university and its educational programs.

The community brings to the partnership great expertise and perhaps the greatest motivation of all—the lack of access and the effects of rapidly rising health care delivery costs. The ultimate success of these efforts will be gauged by the increased access to health care by people in the community. The community is the customer we must strive to serve.

One significant piece of multidisciplinary community-based education and practice is the education of health provider faculty and students by the community. Together, the community, faculty, practitioners, and students can design a new plan for the delivery of health care that will meet the challenges of today and tomorrow. New paradigms often emerge from individuals outside the existing system. Outsiders have little to lose and a great deal to gain. They are more successful at innovation because they are relatively uncontaminated by the professional and educational systems to frame their reality. Truly innovative ideas are often too threatening for those directly affected or displaced by a new paradigm. This concept is much like Columbus proposing that the world was round, not flat. He had little to lose and much to gain and was not burdened by the scientific theory of the day. Many revolutionary ideas have been born in this manner. A great asset of the multidisciplinary approach is that community partnership in the fullest can serve to ensure community support and acceptance.

The community offers us an opportunity to break down the stereotypes of our professional groups, and the community has an opportunity to break down our stereotypes of them. Health professionals will gain firsthand knowledge about those served and their expectations of us. Providers will learn what the community is willing to do to improve its health, learn the role of shared decision making with patients, and unlearn prescriptive modes of behavior. Students will benefit from hands-on exposure to the community. The community will learn what the students have in their hearts—their goals, aspirations, and dreams. Hopefully the community and faculty will nurture these idealistic notions. The community will learn what it is that attracts providers and keeps them enthusiastic, involved, and feeling satisfied.

The community offers tremendous resources to be mobilized to address the health education and health care access problems. Community lay workers can greatly extend the efforts of the health care delivery team. Community individuals, working with the health professionals and carrying the knowledge into the community, can be extenders and serve as the eyes and ears of the professionals. This group can also serve to educate the professionals about the community—its culture, the norms, and informal and formal decision makers—and generally work to facilitate the goals of the project. The community people directly attached to the partnership serve as interpreters to assist the rest of the community in recognizing the value of the partnership and to pull greater numbers into the ranks of supporters and participants.

If this seems complicated, it is. Yet the potential to reach otherwise unattainable goals exists with this partnership. Talent, resources, and untapped power and influence exist for both parties in the partnership, and everyone wins and is better off together than going it alone. Plans will be reality based, and systems usable and acceptable to the consumers of the services.

The following short story by Lawrence Wheeler is provided in an effort to capture the importance of the community in this partnership:

Once upon a time a committee was formed to design a house for an elephant. The committee included an architect, interior designer, engineer, sociologist, and psychologist. The elephant was not on the committee.

The five professionals met and elected the architect as their chairman. His firm was paying the engineer's salary, and the consulting fees of the other experts, which of course made him the natural leader of the group.

At their fourth meeting they agreed it was time to get at the essentials. The architect asked just two things: "How much money can the elephant spend?" and "What does the site look like?"

The engineer said that precast concrete was the ideal material for elephant houses.

The psychologist and the sociologist together said, "How many elephants are going to live in this house?" . . . It turned out that one elephant was a psychological problem, but two or more were a sociological matter. The group finally agreed that though one elephant was buying the house, he might eventually marry. Each consultant could, therefore, take a legitimate interest in the problem.

The interior designer asked, "What do elephants do when they're at home?"

"They lean against things," said the engineer. "We'll need strong walls."

"They eat a lot," said the psychologist. "You'll want a big dining room . . . and they like the color green."

"As a sociological matter," said the sociologist, "I can tell you that they mate standing up. You'll need high ceilings."

So they built the elephant his house. It had precast concrete walls, high ceilings, and a large dining area. It was painted green to remind him of the jungle. And it was completed for only 15% over the original estimate.

The elephant then was called to review the house. He told the committee he always ate outdoors, so he had no use for the dining room. He never leaned against anything, because he had lived in circus tents for years and knew that walls fall down when you lean on them. The girl he planned to marry hated green, and so did he. They were very urban elephants.

And the sociologist was wrong too . . . they didn't stand up. So the high ceilings merely produced echoes that greatly annoyed the elephant's sensitive hearing. The elephant refused to buy or move into the house.[1]

THE BOTTOM LINE

The final question to be answered related to multidisciplinary community-based practice and education is, Is it worth it? The answer comes from those involved and from the recipients of the efforts. Those who pay the tab will need some say as well.

The bottom line is yet to be seen. At a minimum, if faced with failure, some valuable insights into what will not work will be gained. To date, experiences are concurrently joyful and positive, and pure misery. These projects test the absolute extremes of personal and professional bounds for all participants.

We are, however, experiencing successes. Mind-sets are changing. Curriculums outside the projects are changing as a result of the project activities. Sacred cows are being threatened and their validity questioned. However, the costs, especially to individuals extensively involved, are phenomenal. Perhaps naively, we expect the ramifications of this effort to extend far beyond the bounds of the university and our region. We are banking on having an impact on the grander system.

Personally, my answer would be a resounding *yes,* it is a success. The benefits to the nursing profession alone are worth the effort. Successes already realized in the nursing faculty of this school, the resulting impact on our core curriculums, and the great benefits already realized by our communities offset the costs. The projects provide us with the resources and expertise to pursue a dream. This dream has grown from a vague notion and desire to serve and develop community involvement into a much grander project. This fact is reward in itself. We have stretched our bounds and have grown dramatically. The costs, however, are significant. Many in our profession would give anything to have the opportunity to pursue their ideals as we have had through these projects.

It has been said that the costs are high. I think it is too early to tell. It seems we will have to wait for years to realize the fruits or failures of our efforts. We will have to wait to see if the elephant will live in the house that we are laboring to design and build.

REFERENCES

1. Klien, J. T. (1990). *Interdisciplinarity history, theory and practice.* Detroit: Wayne State University Press.
2. Kornblum, W. (1991). Who is the underclass? Contrasting approaches, a grave problem. *Dissent,* pp. 202-211.
3. Reynolds, A. L., & Pope, R. L. (1991). The complexities of diversity: Exploring multiple oppressions. *Journal of Counseling and Development, 70,* 174-179.
4. Richards, R. W., Grace, H. K., & Henry, R. C. (1991). *Community partnerships: A Kellogg initiative in health professions education.* Battle Creek, Mich: W. K. Kellogg Foundation.
5. VanBuren, M. (1991). Health professions education: Toward improved health care. *International Journal of the W. K. Kellogg Foundation, 2*(2), 7-10.

CHAPTER 80

Nursing in Russia

Impact of recent political changes

LINDA S. SMITH

UPHEAVAL IN RUSSIA

The Independent Republic of the Russian Federation became reality on December 25, 1991, but on January 2, 1992, restrictions were lifted and prices on most commodities skyrocketed.[16] Life in Russia is a constant fight for minimal existence. Amid rumors of imposed government rationing, chronic shortages are worsening due to panic buying and hoarding of bread and other staples. Bread and milk prices increased 400%.[33] As years' worth of savings disappear, Russians have taken to borrowing and begging. Inflation increases daily, and medical workers, including nurses, are often last in line to be paid for their work (L. Svirenko, personal communication, May 7, 1992). On February 4, 1992, doctors blocked Moscow traffic and closed down hospitals, demanding higher wages.[10] In April 1992, Russian nurses and physicians staged a slowdown, cutting nonemergency care and threatening a full-scale strike if their demands for better salary and working conditions were not met.[26]

Russian unemployment has soared. In 1992, unemployment increased to at least 15%—a jump from 3 to 11 million.[6] As with unemployment, destructive inflation levels and budget deficits rise. To hold inflation in check, money and credit need stability, but the Russian parliament and Russia's independent central bank continue to print the nearly worthless rubles.[2] Escape may be the only answer. Nine million Russians have applied to the U.S. embassy in Moscow for exit visas (D. Black, personal communication, January 1991).

Production and distribution of food in Russia is problematic. Soil erosion in southern Russia has meant decreased grain yields that have changed Russia from a major grain exporter (from 1909 to 1913, 30% of the world's grain came from Russia) to a country desperate for food aid. Russians are only able to get 7 or 8 bushels of wheat per acre (yields in Kansas are as high as 60 bushels per acre).[39]

Food aid is forthcoming, but not without conditions. Top finance officials from the world's seven richest countries will be approving the $24 billion financial aid package to Russia *only* if Russia can stabilize its currency and continue to make painful economic and political reforms.[29] (To help Russia's chances for aid relief, Yeltsin has agreed to cut, by the year 2003, Russia's nuclear forces to one third their 1992 status.)

One important step toward stabilization was made on July 1, 1992, when Russia created a single official value for the ruble.[28] The ruble's nonconvertibility has been a major obstacle to Russia's global economy integration. Rubles could not purchase foreign services or products because rubles were not accepted by the world bank and strict laws prohibited rubles beyond Russian borders. Until rubles are convertible and transferable, Russians will be unable to purchase medical supplies and pharmaceuticals.

RUSSIA'S DISORDERED HEALTH CARE SYSTEM

Though former Soviet Union territory has 1.2 million doctors[21] and 3.5 million nurses, Russian health care is deteriorating. By U.S. standards, the present system is poor. Hospital equipment is obsolete. Hospital buildings are old and in need of repair. Many hospitals lack cleaning supplies needed for proper sanitation. They are dirty, dark, and cold.[7,14,16,19] Only about 3% to 4% of Russia's gross national product (GNP) is devoted to the health care industry (compared with 11% to 13% in the United States). Traditionally, resources that would have been spent on social programs were funneled into the military.[21]

In Moscow alone, and considered to be related to poor sanitation, there have been 120,000 new tuberculosis (TB) cases and 700 cases of diphtheria.[7] Outside of cities, few homes have plumbing.[14] Almost 75% of the former Soviet Union territory is considered polluted. Almost one half of all rural hospitals and clinics have no sewage connections, 80% are without hot water, and 17% are without piped water at all. Copper and nickel industries have left some of the highest lung cancer rates in the world.[5]

Medical and dental offices lack autoclave equipment for proper sterilization—only 33% of all hospitals have sterilization equipment[1] (P. Moffat, personal communication, June 22, 1992). Instruments may simply be dipped into an alcohol solution. (Vodka is sometimes used when straight alcohol is unavailable. Vodka is also considered to be the most used pain remedy in Russia.) Essential anesthetics, antibiotics, and analgesics may also be unavailable. Highly technical equipment such as computerized axial tomography (CAT) scanners, dialysis machines, patient-controlled analgesia (PCA) pumps, and computerized data systems are rare. For example, only six CAT scanners existed for the entire Moscow population district of 9 million[19] and 9 out of 10 Russians needing kidney dialysis were told there was no room for them. Due to these severe shortages, Russian doctors and nurses must ration medicines and equipment, "playing God" as they decide who will live and who will die.[4]

For decades we would not ask and never knew. The *isms* of communism, isolationism, and McCarthyism kept everyone from knowing the life and work of our Russian nursing colleagues. Nurses of the former Soviet Union were hidden from us and from themselves. In fear and paranoia, our ignorance grew.

Now, for the first time in decades, icy iron curtains have lifted—allowing us opportunities to work with, watch, learn from, and embrace the Russians who share our beloved nursing profession.

NURSING IN RUSSIA

By its very nature, nursing is political. As the international women's movement makes progress, so does the profession of nursing, and so does and will nursing in Russia. As in the West, nursing in Russia is female dominated; approximately 97% of all practicing Russian nurses are women. The word for "nurse" in Rus-

sian means medical sister. As sisters, nurses work with common goals and a common purpose. As women, nurses become more politically and professionally assertive. Nurses can no longer "ask permission" to participate in the vital health care decisions being made at the bedside or at the highest levels of government policy making. Nurses *are* and *must be* participants—first, because nurses endure gender bias and oppression as women and nurses, and second, because nurses care for the women and children victims of ill-conceived social policies.

Nurses protest the allocation of scarce resources for weapons when social programs are underfunded or forgotten. Nurses continuously strive to change laws and regulations that strangle their power and rights—keeping them from delivering quality, cost-effective health care. Internationally, in all aspects of practice, nurses are a powerful health force. Nursing's role is to help governments understand that the health of a nation is an extremely cost-effective means toward national social and economic security.

In the United States, nurses have fought hard for rights to influence nursing practice. U.S. nurses are educated by nurses, governed by nurses, and supervised by nurses. U.S. nurses write nursing journals, nursing texts, and nursing newsletters. U.S. nurses formulate, implement, and evaluate nursing standards of care, job descriptions, and practice parameters. U.S. nurses create licensing requirements for new and continued nursing registration. But do Russian nurses have similar experiences? *Nyet!*

A changing political climate in Russia contributes to these problems of power and control. Many military and communist managers, fearing the loss of prestige and privilege, are fighting against change. Therefore, Russian health care is bureaucratic, conservative, and stagnant.[11]

Currently Russian nurses are not allowed independent practice and have little or no input as to their patients' care. They are frustrated, for they believe themselves to be qualified, not as assistants, but as equal and valuable health care partners.[19] Russian physicians govern nursing practice. Trained with a 6-year inclusive undergraduate and graduate education, Russian physicians continue to protect this privilege related to the oppression of nurse by doctor and nurse by society. These physician powers will not be readily relinquished. They will need to be taken, if not by actual force, then through well-organized and sophisticated political activism on the part of Russian nurses.

Better Russian nursing education and improved testing and standards of care will *not*, alone, be the answer. Actually, these efforts may serve only to increase the perceived threat—focusing only on the nurse and away from the real problem of an oppressive social system. The only solution to the discrimination against nurses and women in Russia is activism and unification.

Oppressed Russian women

Russian women work (50.8% of all workers are female), but they earn 30% less than Russian men and hold lower career positions. Their pensions are lower because they have worked at lower-paying jobs. Though 67% of all physicians are female, female physicians often do not hold positions of authority,[13] and in medical specialties such as surgery, physicians are mostly male.[14]

In addition to a full outside-the-home workweek, Russian women also must spend 40 hours per week on child care and household chores (Russian men rarely participate in these tasks). Russian women who work evening and night shifts, such as nurses on 24-hour rotations, face child care dilemmas. Most child care facilities only operate during the day. This is a particularly serious problem for Russian mothers because nearly one in two Russian marriages ends in divorce and child custody is almost always granted to the mother.[13]

Due to food shortages and hoarding, Russian women must endure long hours of waiting in endless lines. And it is no surprise that alcoholism is getting worse in Russia, especially for women. During the past 2 years, Russian women have been drinking vodka at almost the same rate as men.[23]

Women's childbearing rights have also been affected by present economic problems. Abortion is legal and widely practiced but can be expensive. Birth control pills, when available, cost 350 to 1000 rubles per month, and condoms are inferior and scarce. Even so, Russian families are small, usually with one or two children. Russian women have recently achieved one victory. Russian law has changed to allow women a year and a half of paid maternity leave and an additional 18 months of unpaid leave. Russian nurses express pride in this breakthrough.[35]

The enlightened, united cry of women leaders in the former Soviet Union is, "Democracy without women isn't democracy!"[24] Russian women understand the need for women's research efforts and studies. However, recent political changes in Russia have been mixed blessings for Russian women. Under communist rule, a mandated percentage of legislative officers were female. Now, that proportion has dropped significantly due to free elections. Women who do hold power, however, are vocal and progressive regarding important issues affecting Russian women. Of course, new freedoms have helped.[24]

Oppressed Russian nurses

With the rate of exchange at 135 rubles per U.S. dollar (July 1992), a nurse's salary at 1500 to 3000 rubles per month is a disgrace; a pound of coffee costs 325 rubles (R. Reach, personal communication, July 14, 1992). Physicians are also poorly paid (earning lower salaries than bus drivers, lawyers, or construction workers),[8] but they earn approximately twice as much as nurses.[11] Russian nurses can and do work overtime to supplement meager salaries, but there are only small salary increments for increased experience levels. Russian nursing's best and brightest often leave nursing and become physicians.

On interpersonal and societal levels, nurses and physicians are not recognized as coprofessionals. On top of receiving only a poverty-level salary, Russian nurses must work long difficult hours under poor conditions. A typical Russian nurse cares for approximately 30 patients at a time. One group of physicians accused the nurses they worked with of too frequently questioning medical orders. "Nurses complain too much about their duties," one physician said. In addition to patient care duties, nursing responsibilities include washing dishes, floors, walls, and equipment.[19] Latinis-Bridges and Clancy[14] explained that nurses were considered too unimportant to speak with foreign visitors. It is no wonder that Russian nurses want independence from physicians.

At a recent meeting with the health ministry of the Russian federation, Larisa Svirenko, president of the newly formed First Independent Nurses' Association, outlined the benefits of nurses controlling their own profession. Svirenko recommended that with additional nursing education, nurses should function as nurse educators. Unfortunately, directly following these recommendations, Svirenko's position was eliminated. A report of Svirenko's recommendations will, however, soon be considered by the Committee on Health Practices to the Supreme Soviet of the Russian Federation (R. Reach, personal communication, June 29, 1992).

REFORM
Perestroika and Glasnost

Russian president Boris Yeltsin[33] proclaimed there would be no turning back for Russian reform. Yeltsin was determined as he spoke to the U.S. Congress, saying, "I've told my fellow countrymen—I will not go back on the reforms. It is impossible to topple Yeltsin in Russia. I will not say uncle before I make the reforms, even in the face of obstacles."[9] Though Yeltsin's approval rating in Russia is low and only half of the Russians want him to keep moving, no other person has been identified to take his place. Yeltsin is, therefore, reasonably secure.[31]

With Yeltsin's election (the first time Russian citizens elected a president by democratic ballot), Russian people demonstrated a commitment to change.[12] Perestroika (the restructuring of a nation) held the promise of a new birth, in which improved social conditions were the reform goals. It was hoped that perestroika would prioritize funding for child care and maternal-child medical centers, as well as for an honest and open appraisal of women's problems.[13,30] These goals have yet to be realized.

Glasnost promised Russians the freedom to think and communicate. With glasnost in mind, Yeltsin[38] promised a new era of free communication and honesty. But power struggles continue in Russia over who controls that communication. Economic chaos has forced newspapers and publishing houses to bend toward government-imposed boundaries (government subsidies are essential to turning out products when there are little or no other financial resources).[22] *Meditsinskaya Sestra,* once Russia's only nursing magazine and the world's largest-circulating nursing journal, is no longer available. Furthermore, glasnost has not reduced the intense Russian espionage activities that continue internationally and at home.[27] Glasnost has, however, "freely" exposed the political, economic, and social difficulties of life in Russia.

The Commonwealth of Independent States (CIS) can produce only 15% to 20% of needed medical supplies. Broken equipment cannot be fixed or replaced. Clean syringes are precious. One 950-bed Russian hospital received one or two clean needles per day for a 6-month period. Aware of this dilemma, the ministry sent instructions on how to sterilize and reuse disposable needles. Hepatitis B and human immunodeficiency virus (HIV) are spread as syringes and needles are repeatedly reused (parents are afraid to have children immunized due to the risk of infection from unsterile needles).[7] Syringe shortages are likely to increase the number of confirmed acquired immunodeficiency syndrome (AIDS) cases (from 2000 to 5000).[1]

Frances Petrick,[19] president of the U.S.-Russian Nurse Exchange Consortium, explained:

One nurse told me that [in] the hospital she works in—a 1200-bed hospital—one of the nurses there inadvertently and unknowingly had given AIDS to 15 children by injecting them with a dirty needle. Needles, unfortunately must be used over and over and over again and they [nurses] have to make a choice between not giving the medicine or the chance that they could be transferring some kind of infectious disease.

For years, Russians received free medical care. Now as their health care system collapses, they may be forced to pay, and few Russians have the money to do so.[25] Special privileges in health care services were always awarded to academic, military, or government officials or to those who could bribe their way to the front of the line.[11,21,32] Not only does it require a great amount of time and effort to find medical treatment but also patients are generally on their own in securing whatever medicines they need.[11] Very simple problems are inoperable and potentially fatal. But until recently, Russia imported most of its pharmaceuticals and medical supplies (65% to 70%) from East Germany, Hungary, and Poland.[34] Now these sources want hard currency for their products. To compound this problem, three pharmaceutical plants in Russia have been closed down due to a lack of quality control[34] (P. Moffat, personal communication, June 22, 1992).

Health care facilities have been forced to borrow money from banks in order to pay for medical supplies, salaries, and food. Now it is 10 times more expensive to feed a patient for one day[34] and ambulances are idle because of the shortage and expense of gasoline.

Due in part to these problems, medical facilities in Moscow have begun to establish a private-pay system. This translates into higher patient costs but better salaries and better equipment. Additionally, health care insurance is being introduced into the private sector and state-funded insurance for the poor and elderly is being piloted. The goal of implementing an insurance program is to attract health care financing beyond the government's chronic underfunding.[21] A few experiments in privatization of dental clinics, hospitals, and physical therapy clinics are also taking place, and a few state-owned hospitals have been sold into private ownership.[34]

Changes for nursing in Russia

Nursing education. Though recent job market changes for nurses changed the age and education levels of new enrollees, nursing students in Russia are still very young. Currently, Russian students enter nursing school at age 16 or 17 after high school graduation (high school consists of 10 years of education) (P. Moffat, personal communication, February 5, 1992; R. Reach, personal communication, June 29, 1992).

The standard for nursing education in Russia is a 2-year program inclusive of clinical rotations in pediatrics, obstetrics, surgical, medical, and psychiatric units. Enrollees are primarily new high school graduates. However, because of the severe shortage of nurses in Russia, a few nursing programs continue to admit students after the eighth or ninth grade. If a student has a high school education, the length of time needed to complete the nursing program of study is 2 years. If the student is admitted after the eighth or ninth grade, it will take an additional year of study (high school–level science and math courses are integrated into the first year). It is generally considered by the Russian nursing and medical communities to be unwise to admit students who have not completed high school.

Currently, there exist two nursing programs (with potential for two more) that give experienced nurses an additional 2 years of preparation (a kind of "2 + 2" arrangement). To date, these programs are in Moscow. Unfortunately, it seems that there is no position open for nurses to teach in nursing schools, so the graduates of these advanced programs will be applying their additional skills and education clinically. This is unfortunate because American and Russian nurses have lobbied hard for the position of nurse educator within nursing schools. It was agreed in 1990 to 1991 that graduates of these advanced nursing studies programs could and would be the future nursing faculty. This has not come about as yet. Russian physicians continue to hold (almost exclusively) positions as faculty and administrators of nursing programs. Therefore, students and graduates of these advanced preparation nursing programs do not know what the result of their additional education will be. They truly believe, however, that the extra two years will be helpful to them somehow.

In Russia, the best and brightest Russian nurses are strongly encouraged economically and socially to become physicians or dentists (economically because of the low salaries paid to nurses and the heavy work burdens Russian nurses must endure). Until 1991, there was no other formal education available for nurses.

Of further interest is an intermediate medical position known as a *feldsher*. A *feldsher* is a kind of doctors' assistant. He or she is not a nurse but assumes a role not unlike that of American physician assistants. *Feldshers* may prescribe some medications, do minor suturing, ride in ambulances, and so on. This Russian *feldsher* position usually requires 3 years of study.

Russian nursing classes are small, with 10 to 15 students. Students attend classes in chemistry, anatomy and physiology, microbiology, nursing ethics and discipline, general care fundamentals, obstetrics, and psychiatric care. Examinations measuring competence, with practice and written components, are administered after each course. A new idea has emerged that patients can demand service. Therefore, study also includes legal aspects of practice. Malpractice insurance has also recently been introduced. Approximately half to two thirds of students' time is spent administering nursing care in clinics and hospitals (P. Moffat, personal communication, February 5, 1992). Costs of nursing education are covered by the government. Interestingly, nursing students learn to apply medicinal leeches for the treatment of cardiac disorders such as angina and venous stasis, migraine headaches, blood clots, and reconnected tissues. Hirudo medicinalis, the leech used, produces valuable chemicals that produce the effects of anticoagulation, vasodilation, and anesthesia.[37] At the time of graduation, nurses receive a school diploma and license (R. Reach, personal communication, July 19, 1992).

A recent change for nursing students takes place immediately after graduation. With a tighter job market, new nurses are not assigned but rather must secure a position independent of the government (R. Reach, personal communication, July 14, 1992). Russia also has a system of mandatory continuing education for nurses. Every 5 years, nurses must enroll in refresher courses lasting from 3 to 6 months.[35]

As a department of the medical university, a new 4-year nursing program began in Moscow in September 1991. It is hoped that this program will provide higher education for nursing faculty. Sixty students were admitted, but unfortunately 75% of these enrollees were new nursing graduates without experience (R. Reach, personal communication, June 29, 1992).

Nursing practice. Russian nursing, it is said, includes doing whatever needs to be done. Though patient care is a priority, nurses also must fold and sew sponges. Nurses wash, dry, and repowder surgical gloves;[3] wash floors and dishes; clean equipment; sterilize supplies; prepare meals; and sort and dispense medications. Separate nurses are assigned to treatments and medications.[35] Most Russian nurses wear lab coats over street clothes and shoes, and don tall white caps. Beyond this "uniform," however, nurses usually work without benefit of personal protective equipment, and the nurse-patient ratio is often as high as (or higher than) 1:30. Usually patients remain hospitalized for long periods of time (most hospital stays last 7 to 14 days for minor treatments and over 30 days for major problems). Typically, a nurse spends 90 minutes each way on travel to and from work. Thus, to diminish wasted time and expense, a nurse may choose to work 24-hour shifts. Russian nurses are busy and have little time to provide psychological comfort to patients.[18]

Nursing in clinics has similar problems. In the community, doctors may see patients in their homes, or patients may go to polyclinics. Each polyclinic, with one nurse and one doctor, serves 180,000 people. Here nurses do health screenings, immunizations, and documentation of prescribed treatment.[35]

Nursing organizations. On April 27, 1992, in the city of Moscow, the first association of medical nurses was registered. Larisa Svirenko was named as president and Lena Paritskaya[25] as vice president. Assistance in the organization and foundation of this association was rendered by the international fund of social support. The first goal of this Russian nursing association is to change the work load for nurses from 30 patients to 5 or 6 patients each. (Recently there has been unemployment for nurses related to the closing of hospitals and oversupply of physicians.) Though the nursing supply has improved, government mandates now maintain the 1:30 ratio (R. Reach, personal communication, June 29, 1992). The second goal of the association is to prove the need for better medical equipment that will help nurses work efficiently. And the third goal is to prove the need for a government position that is supportive of nursing and responsive to nursing's needs.

The first meeting of this new organization was held on June 26, 1992, with 170 nursing leaders in attendance. This 2-hour Moscow conference explained the need and mission of the organization. Experienced nurses from all specialties are eligible for membership. Individual dues are 100 rubles (R. Reach, personal communication, June 29, 1992).

East-West collaboration

What we will learn. Russians are known for their wonderful warmth and hospitality toward guests.[30] Westerners, however, know little about them and can learn much. Many Western nurses lack the knowledge our Russian colleagues have regarding holistic, homeopathic health care. Russian nurses understand the art and science of massage therapy, contactless massage, acupuncture, and acupressure. With advanced training, they perform these techniques to promote patient relaxation and as noninvasive pain remedies. Russian nurses have truly learned to treat with their hands.

What we will teach. Russian nurses have watched their Western counterparts in awe. They admire the professional autonomy and teamwork displayed—physicians and nurses collaborating with mutual respect. Russian nurses are hungry to apply nursing process concepts to care planning and case management.

It has been noted that in Russia nursing and medical attitudes toward dying patients are far different from those held in the West. Russian patients are not informed if they are dying; nurses and physicians tend to fear and avoid the terminally ill. Therefore, psychosocial concepts—as well as grief and crisis resolution—need to be shared.[35] Sharing will also take place regarding infection control standards and sophisticated assessment and intervention procedures performed without the aid of complex technology.

Russian nurses need information regarding the following:

- Western systems of nursing licensure
- Methods of health care funding
- University education that provides nurses with advanced knowledge, degrees, and research skills
- Nurse-friendly hospital models
- Legal and ethical aspects of nursing
- Teaching methods in nursing that support and encourage thought and creativity
- Media promotion techniques such as writing and speaking that will improve nurses' political and public image
- Journalistic writing skills to help Russian nurses write and publish nationally and internationally, thereby promoting unity, friendship, and knowledge sharing
- Formulation and implementation of career ladder programs

- Nursing curriculums that recognize the diversity of the human spirit as well as complexities of the nursing profession
- Nursing practice acts, nursing boards, and nursing organizations that define and promote quality nursing care

Russians desperately need medical supplies, including the following:

- Acetaminophen and aspirin
- Antibiotics, anesthetics, and analgesics
- Insulin
- Baby formulas, children's vitamins, and vaccines
- Bandaging material
- Condoms
- Gloves and glass syringes
- Supplies for the operating room

Systematic problem solving via nursing diagnosis and the nursing process is often taken for granted in the West but may be an unfamiliar and exciting tool for Russian nurses. This tool, in conjunction with assertiveness training, patient advocacy concepts, and political savvy, will dramatically change the way Russian nurses practice. Frustrated Russian nurses, like Russian women in general, are desperate for new hope and vision. Therefore, when an environment can be created that strengthens and supports an improved sense of self-worth, Russian nurses will be ready and able to meet their profession's political and economic future.[24]

Aid-to-Russia controversy. From 1990 to 1992, approximately $50 billion in foreign aid to Russia disappeared, and about $20 billion in gold and hard currencies, in the hands of former communist officials, has been lost. As the Russian economy disintegrates, a thriving black market gains power and scope.[40] Though President Bush granted "most favored nation" status to Russia,[31] inflation and loss of control over Russian money and credit have created huge government deficits.

The proposed 1992 $24 billion aid package was only a small portion of what was needed to aid Russian people and prevent self-destruction of Yeltsin's reform programs. U.S. president George Bush proposed that $12 billion of this aid would come from the United States. But with only $1 billion of federal money allocated toward confronting urban problems (joblessness, powerlessness, disease, and despair), U.S. mayors are angry. How can the United States justify foreign aid spending when such a desperate need for help exists within U.S. borders[17]—especially when that aid is perceived as helping only a privileged few?

However, aiding Russian democracy was identified by Bush as the most important foreign policy issue of our time.[9] Can we turn our backs on the Russia that has made a choice for freedom and democracy for its people?

"Why don't you give us some medicines?" Yeltsin[33] repeated twice during a June 14, 1992, television interview with Leslie Stahl. "You're a rich country! There is no medicine to treat the mother of Yeltsin. She's in a hospital room with 10 other patients. I had to bring her medicine from Moscow—and she's the mother of a president!"

Nurse-to-nurse efforts. Nurses will help. In August 1992, the U.S.-Russian Nurse Exchange Consortium again had an opportunity to send a large shipment of medical aid to Russia. Larisa Svirenko personally oversees receipt and distribution of these supplies to the Russian people (especially children) in greatest need. *Truly, who would be better than a nurse and president of a nursing association for such an important task?*

In addition to making these direct shipments of medical supplies and pharmaceuticals, Western nurses have a responsibility to share their lives, their homes, their knowledge, and their love for nursing with Russian colleagues. This is the goal of the U.S.-Russian Nurse Exchange Consortium—to improve democracy, peace efforts, and ultimately patient care through collaboration. As the international language of caring, the goals of nurses everywhere are the same—helping patients achieve the highest possible wellness levels. To this end, all nursing interventions are unified.

Here lies hope and promise for the future of Russian nursing—but there is much work yet to be done. Russian nurses are ready for reform. They are ready to speak against an oppressive social system that negates their potential as women *and* health care professionals. They want liberty and control over their own destiny, and they believe strongly that people-to-people sharing will help them accomplish this end. Optimism thus prevails.[15]

The economic and social growth potential of nurses is and will be dependent upon changes in the Russian health care system. Russian nursing is ready to make this happen—with a little help from their Western friends.

REFERENCES

1. Corwin, J. (1990). Soviet medicine. *US News and World Report, 109*(14), 16.

2. Corwin, J. (1992). The tug of war over the ruble. *US News and World Report, 112*(11), 45.

3. Creedon, C. M. (1991). Nursing glasnost: Treating burn victims in the Soviet Union. *Today's OR Nurse, 13*(2), 32-35.

4. Ensor, D. (Journalist-reporter). (1992, April 26). Financial aid to Russia. *ABC World News Sunday* [Television news].

5. Feshbach, M., & Friendly, A. (1992, April 25). Rubbishing of a superpower. *Economist,* pp. 99-100.

6. Greenhouse, S. (1992, March 31). UN agency sees Russia's jobless soaring to 11 million this year. *New York Times,* p. A6.

7. Hartman, A. (1992, February 25). Life or death for Russian children. *New York Times,* p. A21.

8. Hofheinz, P. (1992). Who can afford what in Moscow. *Fortune, 125*(8), 15.

9. Hume, B. (Journalist-reporter). (1992, June 17). Yeltsin speaks to Congress. *ABC World News Tonight* [Television news].

10. Jennings, P. (Anchorman). (1992, February 4). Russian doctors block Moscow traffic. *ABC World News Tonight* [Television news].

11. Kinsey, D. V. (1989). Nursing and health care in the USSR. *Nursing Outlook, 37*(3), 120-122.

12. Kostikov, V. (1991, July). Boris Yeltsin's political victory. *Soviet Life,* pp. 2-4.

13. Koval, V. (1989, March). Working women: Common problems. *Soviet Life,* pp. 24-25.

14. Latinis-Bridges, B., & Clancy, B. J. (1988). An American perception of Soviet health care. *The Kansas Nurse, 63*(3), 1-2.

15. Marshal, T. (1991, September 24). Winter: Soviet food supplies questionable. *Los Angeles Times,* pp. H1, H4.

16. Monisov, A. A. (1992). Public health assessment—Russian Federation. *Journal of the American Medical Association, 267*(10), 1323-1324.

17. Nation's mayors attack federal aid to Russia. (1992, June 21). *The Journal Times* (Racine, Wis; AP), p. 7A.

18. Pehlivanian, E., & Campbell, M. E. (Producers and directors). (1992). *Nursing—the East and West* [Film documentary]. Minneapolis: Pelicamp Productions.

19. Petrick, F., Bratton, M., Doyle, M. A., & Reach, R. (1991). United in caring—the Soviet experience. *ADvancing Clinical Care, 6*(3), 24-28.

20. Pfister-Nelson, V. (1990). A firsthand look at the Soviet health care system. *American Association for Respiratory Care Times, 14*(1), 42-47.

21. Robbins, A., Caper, P., & Rowland, D. (1990). Financing medical care in the new Soviet economy. *Journal of the American Medical Association, 264*(9), 1097-1098.

22. Robbins, C. A. (1992). For Izvestia, a familiar and ominous story. *US News and World Report, 113*(4), 11.

23. Rosenberg, N. D. (1992, June 25). Russians tour treatment centers. *Milwaukee Journal,* pp. B1-B3.

24. Ross, J., & Searing, S. E. (1992). Women's studies take on Russian flavor. *Wingspread The Journal, 14*(2), 1, 8-9.

25. Russian doctors, ambulance medics strike. (1992, April 24). *The Journal Times* (Racine, Wis; AP), p. 12C.

26. Russian nurses and physicians. (1992). *American Journal of Nursing, 92*(7), 9.

27. Russians still spying. (1992, April 21). *The Journal Times* (Racine, Wis; AP), p. 8A.

28. Russia's problems mount. (1992, July 2). *The Journal Times* (Racine, Wis; AP), p. 10C.

29. Sawyer, F. (Anchorman). (1992, April 26). Top financial officials consider Russian aid package. *ABC World News Sunday* [Television news].

30. Smith, H. (1990, October 28). The Russian character. *The New York Times Magazine,* pp. 31-33, 60, 62, 71.

31. Smith, H. (Commentator-consultant). (1992, June 19). Are things going to get better in Russia? *Washington Week in Review* [Television PBS broadcast].

32. Stahl, L. (Journalist-reporter). (1992, May 17). Heart to heart. *CBS News 60 Minutes* [Television news magazine].

33. Stahl, L. (Journalist-reporter). (1992, June 14). Yeltsin interview. *CBS News 60 Minutes* [Television news magazine].

34. Svirenko, L. (1992, February 10). *Society and health care crisis in the former Soviet Union: The Racine connection.* Paper presented at the Wingspread Symposium, The Johnson Foundation, Inc., Racine, Wis.

35. Trevelyan, J. (1990). Soviet sisters. *Nursing Times, 86*(22), 16-17.

36. Trevelyan, J. (1991). Bringing hope. *Nursing Times, 87*(3), 16-17.

37. Truax, S. (1991, March). Misunderstood and repulsive, leeches prove medical value. *Compass Readings,* pp. 68-70.

38. Yeltsin POW revelations raise more questions than answers. (1992, June 18). *The Journal Times* (Racine, Wis; AP), p. 2A.

39. Yeltsin visits US heartland. (1992, June 19). *The Journal Times* (Racine, Wis; AP), p. 2A.

40. Zuckerman, M. B. (1992). The rubles just don't add up. *US News and World Report, 112*(16), 80.

PART TEN

ROLE CONFLICT

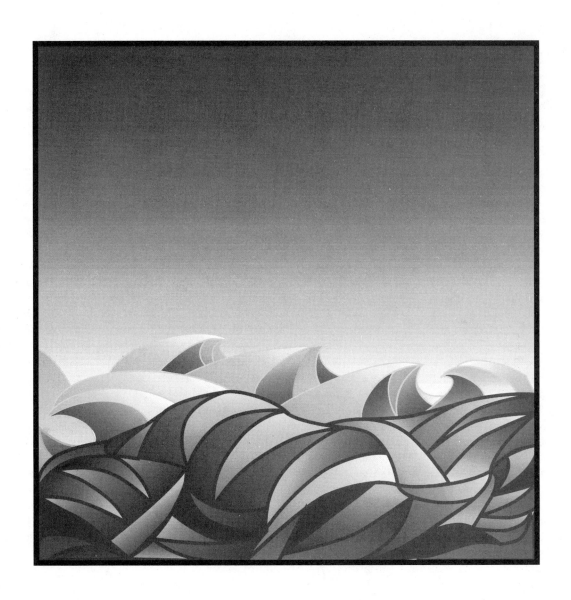

Choosing our conflicts

JOANNE COMI McCLOSKEY, HELEN KENNEDY GRACE

Throughout this book, the conflicts experienced by nurses are frequently identified as contributory to diminishing the influence of the profession. Some are conflicts within nursing: turf battles among organizations, the distance of nursing leadership and education from the concerns at the practice level, disagreements over educational preparation for nursing, and the vying of specialty groups against one another. At the same time, there are conflicts experienced by nurses that come from without: disagreements with physicians and conflicts with administrators, policymakers, and other health care professionals. Some would say that we need to choose our conflicts and our conflict resolution strategies more carefully—sometimes we need to take up and confront the conflict; other times we need to avoid the conflict. This section is about some of the conflicts that nurses experience and some strategies for dealing with them.

Addressing the issue of nursing organizations, Partridge in the debate chapter poses the question, Can there be one nursing organization? Representing approximately 200,000 of the more than 1 million registered nurses in the United States, the American Nurses Association (ANA) is one of the largest professional organizations in the world. Yet nursing has several dozen other professional organizations that compete with the ANA for membership and recognition. Partridge reviews the issue of consolidation of nursing organizations that has been discussed at varying times since 1924. Early on, territorial boundaries were established between the ANA and the National League for Nursing (NLN) making the ANA responsible for practice and professional employment issues and the NLN responsible for nursing service and educational issues. Over the years, there has been considerable blurring of these divisions of turf. And in recent years, the proliferation of specialty organizations serves as a threat to

both the ANA and the NLN, resulting in increased collaboration between these two major organizations. Partridge's list of the national specialty organizations shows that they number more than 80. The strength of the specialty organizations can be noted in the 74,000 members of the American Association of Critical Care Nurses and the 47,000 members of the Association of Operating Room Nurses. The National Federation of Specialty Nursing Organizations (NFSNO) was formed in 1973 and now has a combined membership equal to the ANA's. To counter the likelihood of the NFSNO's becoming an organization separate from the ANA, the Nursing Organization Liaison Forum (NOLF) was created as a part of the ANA in 1983. These organizations have held parallel meetings every year since, each seeking to represent specialty groups in nursing. While the number of nursing organizations is not decreasing, these and other cooperative efforts represent a form of consolidation. Noting the obstacles, Partridge concludes that consolidation is important for the survival of the nursing profession.

Moving from the macrolevel of the profession to the microlevel of practice, Mauksch addresses the need for support and recognition of the staff nurse. In a thoughtful chapter, he examines the concept of abandonment as it applies to the bedside nurse. Focusing on hospital nursing, he points out that anonymity and powerlessness are associated with bureaucratically structured positions. The education of beginning nurses, which emphasizes professional status and individual responsibility, does not prepare one for the minimal power and anonymity of the staff nurse position. The result is that nurses feel betrayed and unappreciated upon confronting the real situation. Mauksch discusses several changes during the past few years that have intensified the sense of abandonment felt by the staff nurse. These include increased patient care demands with no additional support for the nurse; the increasing differentiation between the nursing intelligentsia and the grass roots nurses; changes in the organizational structure whereby the director of nursing becomes a vice president and moves up into institution management but away from staff nurses; the acceptance of feminism and a sensitivity to the issues of equality that have made the physician's approval less rewarding and less acceptable and, in turn, have decreased the physician's tendency to express appreciation; and perhaps most important, the fact that the daily routine of hospitals facing the increasing demands of technology and cost containment emphasizes more and more the subordinate and technical dimensions of care at the expense of activities that are unique to nursing. It is no wonder, asserts Mauksch, that bedside nurses feel that "real" nursing has been abandoned. According to Mauksch, neither the bureaucratic model of the hospital nor the individualism model of the educational institution is right for the bedside nurse. Structural changes are needed that promote a system of collective teamwork and group accountability. All nurses, grass roots and others, will find this chapter very helpful in explaining the complex and subtle conflicts experienced by the staff nurse.

Conflict is a form of stress. In the next chapter, Gardner Huber discusses the many sources of job stress for nurses and its unfortunate consequences of dissatisfaction, turnover, and poor performance. This chapter includes a review of much of the relevant literature on the subject of stress. Research instruments in the areas of stress, conflict, hardiness, and burnout are identified. As demonstrated in this chapter, these topics have been frequently addressed and studied in nursing. Gardner Huber summarizes some of the sources of stress for nurses and outlines possible strategies for stress reduction and coping. Clarity and direction for the nursing profession would help, she says, to decrease the stress levels of individual nurses. The research has identified the sources and the consequences of stress. Now we need to work on ways to reduce or manage the stress.

A specific conflict is examined in the next chapter, that of nurses versus physician assistants (PAs). As more and more physician assistants appear on the health care scene, their relationship to nurses is of greater concern. Fowkes and Mentink do an excellent job of informing us of the facts about PAs and then discussing issues and challenges. Physician assistant programs began in the 1960s, around the same time

that nurse practitioner programs began. Today, more than 20,000 physician assistants have graduated from 55 programs and practice in multiple settings. PAs come from a variety of disciplines and many have bachelor's or graduate degrees upon program entry. Increasingly, there are more women PAs. The authors compare and contrast the roles of physician assistant and nurse practitioner. They discuss areas of conflict, which include issues associated with gender, competition for salaries or jobs, and confusion about professional policies or laws. In some areas the two groups are working collaboratively to support the common interests of both. The authors point out that physician assistants are well established and urge their continuing collaborative arrangements with nurses to share skills and perspectives.

Collaboration is taken up as the solution of choice in the next chapter. Coining the phrase "nurses' voice" to describe the unique perspective and contribution that nurses bring to patient care, Pike urges nurses to choose colleagueship over silence. Pike's review of the external and internal forces that have silenced nurses' voice sounds similar to Gardner Huber's review of sources of nurses' stress. These constraints, says Pike, have inflicted wounds on nurses' professional self-esteem. Rather than acting out the appealing victim role and remaining silent and blaming physicians, Pike urges nurses to speak out, to define themselves as colleagues. The taking up of the conflict requires, she says, an understanding of the uniqueness of nursing, a breadth of clinical experience, a language to communicate to others the nature of nursing, and an understanding of the constraints imposed on nurses. Using two case studies, she illustrates that nurses' silences have significant implications for patient care as well as for nurses' role and satisfaction. This is a thought-provoking and important chapter. All nurses should read and act upon it.

The case for conflict as a positive force is taken up strongly by Johnson in the next chapter. Nurses, she says, traditionally the least powerful group of providers in health care, are particularly vulnerable to the conflicts that accompany change and adaptation. She states that nursing's traditional response to conflict—prevention at all costs—is nonproductive and not acceptable in today's health care environment. Nursing must confront and manage its conflicts if we are to benefit from the many changes taking place. Johnson presents an overview of conflict dynamics from a nursing perspective and then discusses issues related to the management of conflict. She supports her view that nurses need to be more skilled in confrontation and conflict management with an excellent overview of the literature and research in the area. She also discusses how important it is for nurses to develop the skills needed to acquire and use power. Power, she says, influences outcomes by limiting the management strategies available to participants of conflict. Collaboration is not possible when the power differences between individuals or groups are great. She concludes that the current crisis in health care provides nursing with an opportunity to move to a more equal partnership. To do so, however, requires that nurses confront and manage conflict. Are we ready?

More conflict from women nurses in Brazil would be welcomed by the authors of the international chapter in this section. The history of nursing in Brazil is outlined within the context of the history of the country. The authors show that nursing in Brazil was born linked to the domestic and undervalued activities of women. Early training schools for nurses had stiff prerequisites, such as the requirements of a foreign language, that excluded women of lower classes. While some nurses in Brazil today have university education, most health care is provided by a lesser-trained or untrained work force. The poor have no access to formal health care and rely, much as they did in the past, on mystical practices and healers. The history of nursing is linked to the history of women in all cultures. In Brazil the submissive status of women has shaped and severely handicapped the nursing profession. The authors challenge nurses in Brazil to refuse to accept their submissive role as natural. In Pike's terms, they need to find their nurses' voice. The chapter and challenge have relevance to nurses in many countries.

Throughout the world, nurses must identify and then work to minimize and manage the various conflicts. Ignoring the conflicts and doing nothing is no longer an option. Collaboration is a real possibility but requires certain skills and power bases. Having or not having conflicts is a choice we all should make. Choosing our conflicts wisely will more the profession ahead.

CHAPTER 81

Debate

Can there be one nursing organization?

REBECCA PARTRIDGE

Representing about 200,000 out of the 1 million registered nurses in the United States, the American Nurses Association (ANA) is one of the largest professional organizations in the world. With the consolidation of the ANA and other organizations, nursing could have not only the largest professional organization in the world but also, and more importantly, the most powerful health-oriented professional organization in the world.

This chapter presents a historical review and discussion of the present situation regarding the development of nursing organizations. It is intended to serve as an aid in the current debate on the changing structure and identity of national nursing organizations.

THE EARLY DEVELOPMENT OF NURSING ORGANIZATIONS

Alumnae associations were the first formal organizations established by nurses. The first of these societies was started by graduates of the Bellevue training school for nurses in 1889, and many others were started in the years that followed.[5] Because of the nature of the training school environment and the apprenticeship model, a strong sense of rivalry among schools developed and was maintained.

Hospital-operated training schools successfully inculcated in their students an ardent loyalty to their home institution, a loyalty that persisted throughout a graduate's career.[2] The symbol of this institutional loyalty, the wearing of a cap signifying one's school persisted in many areas of the country until very recently. School loyalty and the "singular objective of promoting their own schools"[5] kept the focus of the alumnae associations narrow and their impact minimal. Even more important, the rivalry provoked by this myopic loyalty to one's school militated against collective action among alumnae societies.[5]

In 1893 nursing leaders began to recognize the need to cooperate on a national level to solve two major problems: the "lack of standardization in nurse training as well as the need for laws to protect the public from poorly trained nurses."[5] Although these problems are inextricably linked, the leaders of nursing formed two separate organizations to seek remedies for them.

The American Society of Superintendents of Training Schools for Nurses was created in 1893 to develop and implement a universal standard for training. This organization was the precursor to the National League for Nursing Education (NLNE) and, finally, the National League for Nursing (NLN), which still exists today as the officially recognized accrediting body for nursing education programs (Fig. 81-1).

Protecting the public from ill-prepared nurses through the enactment of licensure laws became the task of the second nationally based organization, the Nurses' Associated Alumnae, which was started in 1897. This organization was later to become what we now know as the ANA. Ironically, these first two national organizations were started by many of the same nursing leaders. It was at this point that issues of nursing education and practice were first dichotomized. This initial split was to grow wider and deeper in the years to come. Ashley[2] contends in the following statement that the decision to form two organizations instead of one was a critical error nursing has yet to remedy.

With the control of education in the hands of one organization and the control of practice in the hands of the other, gaps in communication were inevitable. The lack of concerted

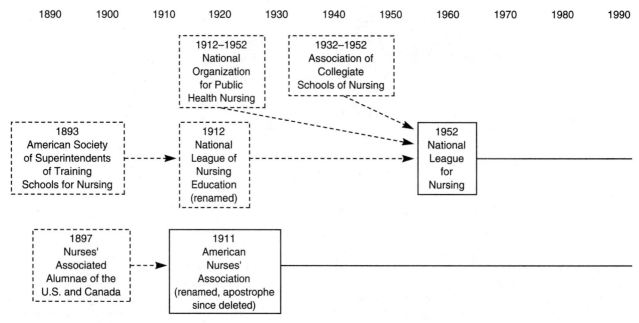

Fig. 81-1. The growth and development of nursing organizations in the United States.

action by both educators and practitioners created serious problems, as future decades were to prove. With this separation of functions, the foundation was laid for continuing lack of unity accompanied by conflicts and misunderstandings. The two separate organizations still exist today, and so do the conflicts and the misunderstandings.

EARLY PROPOSALS FOR CONSOLIDATION

In 1924 the NLNE and the ANA, along with the National Organization for Public Health Nursing, first discussed the advantages of consolidation, but they decided to remain separate organizations. Again in 1939 consolidation was considered when the ANA formed a special committee to consider the formation of one national nursing organization. But World War II intervened, and the pursuit of one organization was not renewed until 1946, when the ANA contracted with Raymond Rich Associates to conduct a study of the six existing national nursing organizations:

- American Nurses Association
- National League for Nursing Education (became the NLN)
- National Organization for Public Health Nursing (merged with the NLN)

- Association of Collegiate Schools of Nursing (merged with the NLN)
- National Association of Colored Graduate Nurses (dissolved and joined that ANA)
- American Association of Industrial Nurses (remained independent)

The Rich report[17] identified three issues dividing these organizations: membership of nonnurses, devotion to special interests, and program emphasis. Although special interests and program emphasis were matters of concern, the membership and participation of nonnurses was the pivotal issue, and this fact was reflected in the nature of the two plans Rich proposed. The first plan called for the creation of a single nursing organization, the American Nursing Association, and conferred full membership privileges on nonnurse participants.

The second plan recommended the establishment of two nursing organizations with linkage provided by a national nursing center. One of these organizations would include only nurses; the other would include nurses and nonnurses among the membership.

It is perplexing to note that the ANA provided the impetus for the consolidation study conducted by Rich Associates, and then rejected the recommendation to unite. However, it is clear from the following statements, made at the 1947 convention, that the ANA strongly desired the organizational strength consolidation would provide. "You agree you want a united front organization for nursing. You want a strong, vital organization representing all of the nurses. You want to eliminate duplication, overlapping . . ."[3] But the delegates also wanted the ANA to "remain the national organization representing all graduate professional nurses and [to] retain its status in an expanded form in any unified action which may be undertaken."[16]

In addition to the desire of the ANA to retain its identity, the issue of nonnurse participation was a major obstacle to the consolidation efforts. The plan for one organization proposed by Rich included full membership privileges for nonnurses, and this would have made it impossible for the new organization to be a member of the International Council of Nurses.

To remedy this problem, the ANA suggested the establishment of one nursing organization that would limit the participation of nonnurses, nursing service agencies, and schools of nursing to advisory forums. "ANA's recommendation was not acceptable to the representatives of the other five nursing organizations who argued that such a proposal would hinder the execution of vital nursing-related activities requiring full participation of nonnurse groups."[5] The consolidation effort was not a complete failure, however, as it was successful in combining the six nationally based nursing organizations into three: the NLN, the ANA, and the American Association of Industrial Nurses (AAIN).

An attempt at coordinating the endeavors of the ANA and the new NLN was made for the purpose of identifying appropriate domains for the two organizations.

According to Chairman Pearl McIver, the joint coordinating committee attempted to assign "those functions which should be the sole responsibility of the members of a profession" to the American Nurses Association and "those functions which the members of any profession should share with the consumers of their product and allied professional workers" to the National League for Nursing.[5]

The territorial boundaries were defined by assigning practice and professional employment issues to the ANA, and nursing service and educational matters to the NLN. As pointed out earlier, the division between practice issues and educational issues is nebulous and to an extent artificial. The many areas of overlap fostered competition and rivalry in the years that followed.

For example, the ANA has periodically sought to expand its organizational boundaries by co-opting tasks previously performed by the NLN. A recent example of this behavior is the ANA credentialing study. The study was conducted in response to a resolution passed by the 1974 House of Delegates that called for the ANA "to move with all deliberate speed to establish a system of accreditation of basic, graduate, and continuing education programs in nursing."[5]

This action was, not surprisingly, perceived by the NLN as a blatant and offensive invasion of its organizational domain. The NLN was invited to cosponsor the study. But this invitation by the ANA was primarily designed to offer the NLN the opportunity to share the financial burden of funding the study rather than to actively participate in it, as the actual study was to be contracted out to an independent research group.

PROLIFERATION OF SPECIALTY ORGANIZATIONS

During the first half of this century, medicine and nursing relied on general practitioners. In 1934 only 15% of physicians were specialists. By 1960 the trend toward specialization was well established, with 63% of physicians limiting the scope of their practice.[7]

This shift toward specialization occurred in nursing as well, but precise statistics on the volume of specialty nurses are not available. The most dramatic evidence reflecting the trend toward specialization in nursing is the establishment of numerous organizations with a particular clinical focus.

Starting in the 1960s, many specialty nursing organizations have been created to address dozens of emerging specialties. The current roster of national specialty nursing organizations[1] follows:

- Alpha Tau Delta National Fraternity for Professional Nurses
- American Academy of Ambulatory Nursing Administration
- American Academy of Nurse Practitioners
- American Academy of Nursing
- American Assembly for Men in Nursing
- American Association of Colleges of Nursing
- American Association of Critical Care Nurses
- American Association for the History of Nursing
- American Association of Legal Nurse Consultants
- American Association of Neuroscience Nurses
- American Association of Nurse Anesthetists

- American Association of Nurse Attorneys
- American Association of Occupational Health Nurses
- American Association of Office Nurses
- American Association of Spinal Cord Injury Nurses
- American Cancer Society, Section on Nursing/Patient Care
- American College of Nurse-Midwives
- American Heart Association, Council on CV Nursing
- American Holistic Nurses' Association
- American Hospital Association
- American Nephrology Nurses' Association
- American Nurses' Foundation
- American Organization of Nurse Executives
- American Psychiatric Nurses' Association
- American Society of Ophthalmic Registered Nurses
- American Society of Plastic & Reconstructive Surgical Nurses, Inc.
- American Society of Post Anesthesia Nurses
- American Thoracic Society, Section on Nursing
- American Urological Association Allied, Inc.
- Association for the Care of Children's Health
- Association of Community Health Nursing Educators
- Association of Nurses in AIDS Care
- Association of Operating Room Nurses
- Association of Pediatric Oncology Nurses
- Association for Practitioners in Infection Control
- Association of Rehabilitation Nurses
- Dermatology Nurses' Association
- Drug and Alcohol Nursing Association, Inc.
- Emergency Nurses' Association
- Federation for Accessible Nursing Education and Licensure
- Frontier Nursing Service
- Intravenous Nurses' Society, Inc.
- National Alliance of Nurse Practitioners
- National Association of Directors of Nursing Administration in Long Term Care
- National Association for Health Care Recruitment
- National Association of Hispanic Nurses
- National Association of Neonatal Nurses
- National Association of Nurse Practitioners in Reproductive Health
- National Association of Orthopaedic Nurses, Inc.
- National Association of Pediatric Nurse Associates and Practitioners
- National Association of Physician Nurses
- National Association for Practical Nurse Education and Service
- National Association of School Nurses, Inc.
- National Black Nurses' Association, Inc.
- National Consortium of Chemical Dependency Nurses
- National Federation of Licensed Practical Nurses
- National Federation of Specialty Nursing Organizations
- National Flight Nurses' Association
- National Gerontological Nursing Association
- National League for Nursing
- National Nurses in Business Association
- National Nurses' Society on Addictions
- National Nursing Staff Development Organization
- National Organization for Associate Degree Nursing
- National Organization of Nurse Practitioner Faculties
- National Organization of World War Nurses
- National Student Nurses' Association
- North American Nursing Diagnosis Association
- Nurse Consultants Association, Inc.
- Nurse Healers–Professional Associates
- Nurses Association of the American College of Obstetricians and Gynecologists
- Nurses' Christian Fellowship
- Nurses' Educational Funds, Inc.
- Nurses' Environmental Health Watch
- Nurses' House, Inc.
- Nurses' Organization of the Veterans' Administration
- Nursing Network on Violence Against Women
- Oncology Nursing Society
- Respiratory Nursing Society
- Retired Army Nurse Corps Association
- Sigma Theta Tau International
- Society for Education & Research in Psychiatric–Mental Health Nursing
- Society of Gastroenterology Nurses & Associates
- Society of Otorhinolaryngology & Head/Neck Nurses
- Society for Pediatric Nurses
- Society for Peripheral Vascular Nursing
- Society for Retired Air Force Nurses
- Transcultural Nursing Society

This roster does not include all organizational entities that address specialty practice issues. For example, the following subdivisions within the ANA are devoted to specific domains in nursing:

- Center for Credentialing Services
- Center for Ethics & Human Rights
- Center for Labor Relations
- Congress on Nursing Economics
- Congress on Nursing Practice
- Division of Governmental Affairs
- Division of Practice, Economics & Policy

Although the ANA has always had a section concerned with practice issues, the organization has clearly devoted most of its energies toward the following two objectives, which transcend the boundaries of clinical specialization:

1. Increasing the minimum education of professional nurses to the baccalaureate level (commonly referred to as the entry-into-practice issue)
2. Increasing wages and promoting better working conditions for nurses (the union activity known as the economic and general welfare program)

Both of these major objectives undertaken by the ANA have resulted in predictable internal conflict and membership losses in the 1960s and 1970s. However, things seem to be stabilizing. No longer does the mere mention of a baccalaureate education requirement cause heated debate. Most nurses agree that this level of education is both necessary and inevitable for the future of nursing. A similar realization has occurred relative to the ANA's union activities. Although some nurses still view collective bargaining as a vaguely unprofessional and unsavory affair, most readily acknowledge the financial gains that have accrued as a result.

While the ANA was occupied with the universal issues of education and compensation, numerous organizations were created to address clinical issues in the growing number of nursing specialties. In the early 1970s, the rapid proliferation of independent specialty organizations led to the suggestion that they band together to address common issues. Donna Zschoche,[20] executive director of the American Association of Critical Care Nurses, called for a meeting of the first National Nurses' Congress, which later came to be known as the Federation of Nursing Specialty Organizations and ANA.

NATIONAL FEDERATION OF SPECIALTY NURSING ORGANIZATIONS

In 1973 the Federation of Specialty Nursing Organizations was formed. The designation of "specialty nursing organization" refers to a "national organization of which the majority of the voting members are RNs governed by an elected body with by-laws defining its purpose and function for improvement of health care, and a body of knowledge and skill in a defined area of clinical practice."[12] Shortly after its inception, the meetings of this group came to be officially known as the Federation of Nursing Specialty Organizations *and* ANA. The purpose of meeting was "not to take action or make decisions binding on the member organizations, but to discuss matters of common interest and concern."[11]

The federation began as, and remains, a loose affiliation of organizations with divergent interests. It began with no formal structure, bylaws, headquarters, staff, or officers. Within the political lexicon, this federation would more accurately be described as a confederation or coalition. This lack of structure precipitated an offer from outside the nursing profession. In 1975 the former staff of the National Commission for the Study of Nursing and Nursing Education made an offer to the federation. The impetus for the offer can be traced to recommendation number 17 in the commission's 1970 report[9] entitled *An Abstract for Action*:

The national nursing organizations (should) press forward in their current study of functions, structures, methods or representation, and interrelationships in order to determine: (*a*) Areas of overlap or duplication that could be eliminated, (*b*) Areas of need that are currently unmet, and (*c*) Areas or functions that could be transferred from one organization to another in the light of changing systems and practice.

The offer extended to the federation by the commission staff consisted of a proposal to

establish an ad hoc committee on planning, purposes, and structure for the organization along with funding from an outside agency interested in the further professionalization of nursing. To the surprise of the grantor, the proposal was rejected on the basis that this, somehow, might lead to a superorganization of nursing that would be more powerful than any of the participating groups including the American Nurses Association.[10]

Although the federation had rejected an offer of outside assistance that would have expedited the process of collaboration and planning, in 1977 a survey of member organizations revealed only modest progress had been made toward the goal of cooperative activity. Lysaught[10] summarizes their responses:

All felt that the current level of organization was essentially preliminary to more definitive progress on mutual goals. Six organizations felt that the group had already made significant strides toward presenting an effective voice of nursing on issues, whereas nine organizations felt that this had not yet been accomplished.

In the longitudinal 10-year follow-up on the recommendations of the National Commission for the Study of Nursing and Nursing Education, Lysaught[10] revealed in the monograph's title a sense of frustration over the continuing need for unity of action in nursing: *Action in Affirmation: Toward an Unambiguous Profession of Nursing.*

In 1983, after 10 years of meetings, the group, which had by then changed its name to the National Federation of Specialty Nursing Organizations (NFSNO), convened an educational workshop to consider long-range plans and possible incorporation (i.e., a legal action that would require the development of bylaws, structure, and goals). In an address by Margretta Styles,[18] the workshop participants were reminded that they were faced with four alternatives:

1. The federation could propose to broadly organize all of nursing so loosely and without direction that unity would not likely be achieved.
2. The federation could propose to broadly organize all nursing to provide unity, leadership, and direction; and therefore promote a competitive stance toward the ANA.
3. The federation could propose to focus specifically upon specialty practice issues and strive toward collaboration with the ANA.
4. The federation could delay action on long-range planning and continue with its current informal structure.

The NFSNO selected the fourth alternative. This delay allowed the NFSNO to consider the role of the ANA's new Nursing Organization Liaison Forum (NOLF). The forum was created as part of a major internal restructuring approved at the 1982 ANA convention. The first meeting of the ANA's Nursing Organization Liaison Forum took place in December 1983.[13]

The NFSNO and the NOLF have held parallel meetings in the subsequent years, each seeking to represent specialty interests within nursing. In January 1988 the NFSNO finally made the decision to incorporate, and this was accomplished a year later in the state of Illinois. It was hoped that incorporation might provide the mechanisms needed for this group to take actions and thereby refute the criticism that it was unneeded and powerless. This negative image was presented in a 1986 editorial,[14] which began as follows:

It is time for the NFSNO to disband—gracefully. . . . the Federation resembles a ladies' bridge club. All the members play the same game but oppose each other once in a while, each member takes a turn hosting the party and providing refreshments, and lots of information is exchanged. At the end of the game, plans are made to meet again.

In the meantime, the NOLF continues to meet and function in an advisory role to the ANA's board of directors. The NOLF concerns itself with national issues that concern most nurses, such as legislative action and health care policy reform. In contrast, the NFSNO is seen as focusing more on specialty practice issues. However, to the casual observer it seems that continuing both the NOLF and the NFSNO may be redundant and potentially divisive.

The challenge of achieving collaborative action with such a vast diversity among nursing organizations is great. The difference in size alone presents major obstacles. The ANA has 200,000 members through 53 state and regional associations. The NFSNO has 38 affiliating organizations ranging dramatically in size. There are 74,000 members in the American Association of Critical Care Nurses and 47,000 members in the Association of Operating Room Nurses; many specialty nursing organizations have only a few thousand members, and some have only a few hundred members. The combined membership of the NFSNO is about the same size as the ANA membership.[13]

INTERORGANIZATIONAL BEHAVIOR

It may be helpful at this point to examine the behavior of organizations from a theoretical perspective. Interorganizational behavior can be viewed as either competitive or cooperative. Competition implies that a sense of rivalry exists and that the weaker of the two may be eliminated. The three subtypes of cooperative behavior are bargaining, co-optation, and coalition. Bargaining refers to the negotiation of an agreement through the use of an exchange process. Co-optation is a method of absorbing some elements of one organization into another. And coalition refers to the temporary or partial alliance of two organizations for the purpose of achieving a common goal. To this spectrum of organizational behavior described by Thompson and McEwen,[19] I would like to add consolidation, which is the permanent and complete combination of two organizations, effectively blurring the singular identity previously held by each.

Nursing organizations have much in common and much to gain from consolidation. But there exists a high degree of hostility and distrust that must first be overcome.

Once conflict and hostility exist, we tend to develop supporting stereotypes that maintain the conflict. Thus each side exaggerates the differences that exist—and once the perception is established, only small actual differences are necessary to maintain the stereotype. This is facilitated by a decrease in intergroup communication that accompanies conflict. If forced to interact, each side listens only to its own representatives. Indeed, in the absence of any shared goals, communication tends to reinforce stereotypes, and relations to deteriorate further.[6]

Nursing organizations must continue their dialogue. Members of each should be encouraged to join the other organization, and common goals should be identified. Forming a coalition on important issues facing nursing could be the antecedent to a successful consolidation of organizations.

OBSTACLES TO CONSOLIDATION

There are, of course, areas of disagreement among nursing organizations, and these will continue to be obstacles to consolidation unless each side is willing to compromise. With thoughtful discussions and rational exchanges, an agreement could be reached that would allow organizations to unite for the benefit of all nurses and health care consumers.

A number of issues will require debate, discussion, and, ultimately, compromise before a consolidation can succeed. Some of these issues are the composition of membership, dues structure, union function, educational requirements for practice, and accreditation of educational programs.

Membership

The problem of who should be included among the membership remains. The ANA currently comprises only registered nurses (RNs). NLN members include lay and agency representatives in addition to licensed vocational nurses (LVNs) and registered nurses. Specialty organizations may include RNs, LVNs, and other categories of health care workers. A consolidated organization would best be served by a membership that included all nurses: RNs and LVNs. Nonnurses could participate through advisory councils without full

membership privileges. This type of action, the ANA giving up its RN-only stance and the NLN and other organizations relinquishing full membership for nonnurses, is a good example of how compromise might be achieved through the appropriate use of an exchange mechanism. Each participant in a compromise must be willing to give up something to ultimately gain through cooperative action.

Dues structure and union function

The ANA dues structure is relatively high and acts to limit membership. Many nurses argue that the tangible benefits derived from ANA membership are too few and, by contrast, the NLN and specialty organization dues appear quite reasonable.

In a consolidation, the memberships of all involved organizations (approximately 200,000 from the ANA and an equal number of nurses from other organizations) would combine to form a powerful unified body representing nursing. A new dues structure would have to be designed for the new organization, and it should be low enough to attract, rather than repel, new members. One method of restructuring dues to achieve this goal is to separate the economic and labor relations program (the union function of the ANA) from the other parts of the new organization and allow members to join the union component of the organization separately. In this way, dues could be reasonably priced and affordable to all nurses. Using this type of fee-for-service dues structure would relieve the nurse who is not working in a contract situation from the responsibility of financially supporting the economic and labor relations program, while those who enjoy the benefits of working under a contract would be responsible for paying the costs of negotiation and maintenance of their contracts.

Unionization is still a controversial issue in nursing. Using the fee-for-service mechanism described, the new consolidated organization could meet the needs of nurses who favor, as well as those who oppose, union activities in nursing. Nonnursing unions have repeatedly targeted nurses as a potential source of workers to bolster their declining memberships, and if nurses fail to defeat these recruitment attempts by nonnurse unions, nursing will be further weakened and fragmented.

Education and practice

The ANA has long advocated that nursing education take place within institutions of higher learning. This position validates associate degree and baccalaureate education for nursing, but it implicitly calls for phasing out of non-degree-granting programs (vocational and diploma). The NLN, however, continues to support four educational methods of entering nursing: vocational, diploma, associate degree, and baccalaureate.

In this college-oriented society, it is unjustifiable to continue to prepare nurses outside of institutions of higher learning. Not only is it unfair to the nursing student to be denied a degree after years of study, but it is also unfair to the health care consumer to be subject to a system of training that fosters nurse loyalty to an employing institution rather than professional accountability to patients.

The consolidation of the ANA and the NLN would require concessions on the part of the NLN. Undoubtedly, it would be required to abandon support of non-degree-granting nursing programs, but in return its accreditation functions could be preserved in the new organization.

The artificial hiatus between hospital-based acute care and community-based continuing care could be bridged by a merger of the ANA and the NLN. Historically, the ANA has usually represented the interests of nurses involved in acute care, whereas the joining of the NLNE with the National Organization for Public Health Nursing in 1952 incorporated the community nursing focus into the NLN.

With the rapidly escalating costs of acute health care and the increasing attention to prevention, the time is right for nursing to intervene by closing the gap between hospital and community-based care. A consolidation of the ANA and the NLN would bring together nursing leaders from hospital-based and community-based nursing services so that more effective nursing care could be provided in a variety of settings.

If nursing organizations fail to unite, it is quite possible for the "conflict to continue indefinitely with neither side able to gain the advantage, to the extent that both sides contribute to the ultimate loss of whatever values each was seeking to uphold."[8] It is for this reason, the potential loss of all that is important to both organizations, that nursing organizations must consolidate.

THE NEED FOR UNITY

Throughout its history, nursing has been represented by small, impotent groups primarily concerned with their own self-interest and self-preservation. Rather than worrying about individual organizational survival, nurses should concern themselves with their collective survival. Continued fragmentation will leave nursing vulnerable to the "circling opportunists . . . who do not recognize the nature of the nursing process . . . and seek to control it."[4]

The conflicts and misunderstandings among nursing organizations have periodically flared into open competition that has had a destructive effect on the profession as a whole. It is time that the organizations join together to work cooperatively. Nursing must put aside its relatively petty "internal struggles [that] have sapped its strength and energy" and defend itself against the "medical profession, health departments, education departments, [and] hospital associations" and labor unions that "relentlessly pursue their strategy to divide and conquer nursing."[15]

"In the 1890s, it was called esprit de corps; in the 1940s, a united front; in the 1960s, a spirit of oneness; and in the 1970s, collaborative action,"[5] and in the 1990s perhaps we shall call it unity, and finally succeed in achieving it through consolidation of the major groups in nursing—the ANA and the NFSNO. A century ago Edith Draper succinctly stated the prerequisite to our success: "To advance we must unite."[5]

REFERENCES

1. AJN's 1992 directory of nursing organizations. (1992). *American Journal of Nursing, 92,* 87.
2. Ashley, J. (1976). *Hospitals, paternalism and the role of the nurse* (p. 112). New York: Teachers College Press.
3. Densford, K. (1948). *Proceedings of the special sessions of the Advisory Council (1947-1948) and the House of Delegates (1947) of the American Nurses Association* (p. 159). New York: American Nurses Association.
4. Driscoll, V. (1973). Beware the circling opportunists. *Journal of the New York State Nurses Association, 4,* 5.
5. Flannagan, L. (1976). *One strong voice: The story of the American Nurses Association* (p. 26). Kansas City, Mo: American Nurses Association.
6. Hampton, D., Sumner, C., & Webber, R. (1973). *Organizational behavior and the practice of management* (p. 673). Glenview, Ill: Scott, Foresman & Co.
7. Kalisch, P. A., and Kalisch, B. J. (1979). *The advance of American nursing.* Boston: Little, Brown.
8. Klein, D. (1976). Some notes on the dynamics of resistance to change: The defender role. In W. B. Bennis, & K. D. Benne, R. Chin, & K. E. Corey (Eds.), *The planning of change* (3rd ed.). New York: Holt, Rinehart and Winston.
9. Lysaught, J. A. (1970). National Commission for the Study of Nursing and Nursing Education. In *An abstract for action.* New York: McGraw-Hill.
10. Lysaught, J. A. (1981). A longitudinal follow-up on the recommendations of the National Commission for the Study of Nursing and Nursing Education. In *Action in affirmation: Toward an unambiguous profession of nursing.* New York: McGraw-Hill.

11. Nursing Federation compares notes on certification and continuing education policies and procedures. (1974). *American Journal of Nursing, 74,* 416.

12. Nursing organizations adopt group name. (1973). *American Journal of Nursing, 73,* 1306.

13. McCarty, P. (1983, September). Federation for specialty groups studies incorporation proposal. *American Nurse, 15,* 3.

14. Palmer, P. N. (1986). The nursing profession does not need two federations. *AORN Journal, 43,* 784.

15. Powell, D. J. (1976). Nursing and politics: The struggles outside nursing's body politic. *Nursing Forum, 15,* 342.

16. *Proceedings of the special sessions of the Advisory Council (1947-1948) and the House of Delegates (1947) of the American Nurses Association.* (1948). New York: American Nurses Association.

17. Rich, R. (1946). Report on the structure of organized nursing. In *Proceeding of the Thirty-fifth Biennial Convention of the American Nurses Association, Vol I, House of Delegates.* New York: American Nurses Association.

18. Styles, M. (1983, June 24). *The anatomy of a profession.* Paper presented at the long-range planning committee workshop on future directions for the National Federation of Specialty Nursing Organizations, Pittsburgh, Pa.

19. Thompson, J. D., & McEwen, W. J. (1958). Organizational goals and environment. *American Sociological Review, 23,* 23.

20. Zschoche, D. (1972). Letter calling for a national nurses' congress. *Heart and Lung, 1,* 589.

CHAPTER 82

Viewpoints

Has the frontline nurse been abandoned?

HANS O. MAUKSCH

Many voices from nursing, medicine, and health care administration would answer the question, Has the frontline nurse been abandoned? with a resounding negative. Yet evidence has been accumulating during the last decade that demonstrates despair, rage, and frustration by nurses engaged in direct patient care. Beyond the voices of anger and abandonment there is evidence of the survival of dreams and of commitment to patients, to nursing, and to health care. In this chapter I chose to focus on the nurse's perception of abandonment. What people feel and experience and how they define their own reality influence their behavior more significantly than data assembled through laborious research that lacks sensitivity. Even rigorously validated data may not be meaningful to the population whose experiences they are supposed to reflect.

In examining subjective realities of significant groups, it must be acknowledged that in all social situations there may be—and probably is—more than one truth. These truths, which are all partially valid, need to be understood in order to grasp the meaning of each situation. From the point of view of sociopsychological search it is futile to look for what is true and what is false; for the behavioral sciences, truth is fundamentally a plural.

Nowhere are these general principles more evident than in the case of nursing. In a crowded field, working in close proximity, each group and profession has developed its own vantage point and brings its own priorities and values to the stage of daily work. This chapter is not merely a summary of assembled views and expressions but rather an effort to examine the nurse's perceived world as a system governed by a logical albeit subjective thought system.

Even the title of this chapter begs the question. Do the following pages merely try to answer the question with a yes, a no, or a maybe? Aren't the key questions linked to this population's perspectives and to the power of its perceived subjective reality? Whether the facts indicate that the frontline nurse has indeed been abandoned is less significant than the researcher's ability to analyze, to understand, and to explain the conditions—objective or subjective—that lead the nurses to feel abandoned if that is the finding. To examine the factors accounting for stress and frustrations typical of nurses employed by hospitals and other institutions requires an approach in which the observer takes on the perspectives of the grass roots nurse and accepts the relevance of those issues that the nurse claims to be significant.

This point of departure governs the interpretation of data and choice of methodology. This objective view of the subjective, experiential perception takes precedence over different views expressed by administrators, physicians, or researchers concerning changes in the last decade. Furthermore, the diminished homogeneity of the nursing population demands care and caution in assessing various views and the substructures in nursing from which these views have arisen. The splintering of the body of nursing beliefs and nursing values is possibly the most significant and most threatening working assumption of this chapter. The aim of this chapter is to synthesize the views of the practicing nurse while screening the nurse's voice through the spectroscope of institutional and professional conditions.

IMPLICATIONS OF THE INSTITUTIONAL ENVIRONMENT

We shall start with the implications of corporate employment by contrasting it with the conditions that would prevail for someone who functions as a fully accountable individual practitioner. The nurse in private practice enjoys more personal recognition, visibility, and individuality than the nurse who functions as a member of the staff of an institutional system or department (unless the private practice nurse is merely a substitute employee of an agency). A bureaucratically organized department rendering nursing care is, to a significant degree, collectively responsible. Although several dimensions of the abandonment problem will be examined in the following pages, a fundamental and causally significant factor has to be the difference between the attention paid to individually functioning and individually accountable practitioners and the quasi anonymity of those professionals who are part of organizational systems with collective accountability—a staffing pattern based on assumed substitutability of frontline practitioners.

The difference between the implications of individual and institutional functioning can be observed in other settings. The aura and power of physicians derives from the deliberate efforts to present the physician as an individually autonomous practitioner rather than to acknowledge him or her as a component of an institutional system.[6] Indeed, some medical departments have assumed bureaucratic organization and functions and have absorbed the consequences. Some of the consequences of institutionalized bureaucratization can be seen in organizations like the public health service or U.S. armed forces, in which one can observe the reduction of the physician's individuality and in which replacement, substitution, and transfer are the norm, with the concomitant reduced consideration of individual capabilities and preferences.

Having made the basic point that anonymity and powerlessness are associated with being the occupant of a bureaucratically structured position, we turn now to the case of nursing and to the nurse's socialization prior to assuming responsibilities at the grass roots level of practice. Unlike the novice in the armed forces and unlike the worker in an industrial bureaucracy, the new practitioner of nursing is not adequately prepared to function in an environment of substitutability, minimal power, and anonymity. On the contrary, most of the educational experiences of the nursing student emphasize professional status, individual responsibility,

and the symbolic importance of joining a profession. For the sake of nurses' mental health, it might be better to emphasize the reality of the nurse's position, even though such a change would exact a heavy cost for the profession.[8] Notwithstanding the nurse's capability, knowledge, and readiness, the image that seems to describe the real institutional environment within which the nurse functions resembles the image of the industrial worker whose accountability is limited, who can be moved and replaced, and whose expertise is perceived to be the result of situational training rather than of knowledge and inquiry.

COMPLICATING FACTORS

The nurse feels betrayed and unappreciated when confronting the reality of the work environment. Several developments in the past few years have actually intensified this sense of abandonment and frustration and have substantiated the grass roots nurse's belief that "nobody really understands what I am doing." One of the complicating forces results from the needs of the patient and the growing complexity of patient care.[4] As more and more detailed knowledge has been identified, a growing number of specialists have fleeting contacts with the patient. The patient, who may be overwhelmed by so many different people and so much new information, increasingly looks to the nurse as the source of information and reassurance, and as the integrator of diverse and confusing stimuli. To serve as the interpreter of complex events requires, minimally, a sense of security and a sense of being supported. The employment conditions described previously are not conducive to providing a feeling of being trusted and being respected. Under these adverse conditions, trying to meet the needs of the patient for knowledge and understanding becomes a fairly risky and stressful activity for the nurse rather than a morale-enhancing reaffirmation of the nurse's worth.

The second, more complex and divisive source of feelings of abandonment is an unintended consequence of some of the most desirable historical trends in the development of nursing. The transfer of the major site for nursing education from the hospital to the college campus and the emergence of increasing numbers of nurses with advanced degrees represent changes that the profession appropriately endorses and welcomes. Yet every gain exacts a price. The intelligentsia of the profession, an ever more important, influential group since the 1970s, is characterized by different cultural roots, different concerns, and by a different language than those applied to the grass roots–level nurse. This applies even to many staff nurses who have earned the baccalaureate. In the 1930s and 1940s the leaders and administrative chiefs in nursing had social and cultural origins that were similar to those of the frontline nurse. Presumably there was a sense of collective belonging, and the typical leader in nursing was someone with whom the staff nurse could identify.

The differences between the frontline nurse and the academically advanced nursing intelligentsia must be ascribed to attitudes and behaviors on both sides. It may be controversial to assert that among nurses with advanced academic degrees there is little sense of identification with the grass roots nurse and that even highly motivated programs of research and action appear as if they were done "for them" rather than done "for us." Similarly, grass roots nurses look with some suspicion at the fancy language and the emphasis on research and abstraction that leave them wondering whether they have allies and colleagues in academia or whether they serve primarily as objects of study or, worse yet, sympathy.

As the differentiation between the practicing nurse and the nursing intelligentsia has intensified, we can apply the notion of abandonment even more appropriately. It has been shown that a frontline nurse looks to his or her colleague with advanced degrees as to one who models and demonstrates the contributions of research to daily practice and who shows that all of this knowledge can be applied to a unified pattern of action. The word *sympathy* was emphasized earlier because it points to a pervasive and very significant experiential deficit identified by many grass roots nurses. A recognition of real worth cannot occur without an acknowledgment of equality. Charity, no matter how well intended and how much motivated by sympathy and caring, implies a difference in social status. Indeed, an act of charity creates inequality and social distinction while participation and sharing need not do that. It does not matter whether such inequality was intended by those who wield the symbolic or structural power. Deprivation gives rise to additional perception of deprivation. Those who have relationships with nurses in frontline roles have to be sensitive to the risk of triggering a perception of inequality, regardless of intent.

Another similar yet also profoundly different source of feeling abandoned and frustrated has to be associated with changes in the organizational structure of the hospital.[4] Fifty years ago nurses working directly with patients became part of a nursing service department headed by a director of nursing. This organizational pattern and its label conveys a message of inequality and of subservience to a departmental authority structure, to management, to the physician, and above all to the administrator of nursing. This subservience was intensified because people in deprived situations have greater need for identifiable leadership and for symbols of the existence of nurturing and support.[1] The director of nursing was that role model and visible leader, and someone who spoke for nursing, although there may have been major differences between what was said and what was done. These images of the director of nursing have changed, although nurses' needs remain consistent. In recent years the chief of nursing has become increasingly involved in the complexity of hospital management and issues of organizational efficiency. The director of nursing became redefined as a vice president within the hospital management structure. Now the title changed and the director *of* nursing became vice president *for* nursing; it might not even be that specific. Superficially it seemed that the status of nursing was being elevated by nursing's becoming part of top-level institutional management. Yet the emotional and role needs of the staff members paid a heavy price. The nursing executive became much less visible and, regardless of real intent, appeared to the staff nurse to have abandoned nursing by joining the administrative elite.

That these changes were defined as abandonment has been shown in several studies of nursing morale and of recruitment and turnover.[7,8] The functions of nursing by their very nature seem to require more support and recognition than tasks in other professions.[3] The reality of a diminished social affirmation of importance has accentuated nurses' needs for support and leadership. This phenomenon is intensified by an additional event that, paradoxically, constitutes a highly desirable development yet exacts a further high price from the frontline nurse.

The deference that characterized the behavior of nurses vis-à-vis physicians and that females generally displayed toward males was expected and accepted 40 years ago. In those days the staff nurse gained satisfaction and symbolic rewards from approval and appreciation given to her by a physician. The nurse thought that proximity to the physician provided an advantage over nursing administrators and nursing educators. The latter had little access to the pat on the head that is the physician's patriarchal gesture of approval.

There was a delicate balance between the gratification gained from physician recognition and the benefits derived from the structure of nursing leadership. The slowly spreading acceptance of feminism and of sensitivity to issues of equality has made the physician's traditional form of approval less rewarding and less acceptable, and has subtly diminished the physician's tendency to express appreciation in the traditional, patronizing way. The rays of sunlight emanating from the physician's aura may have lost much of their luster, yet the comparable warmth and glow derived from the nurturance offered by the director of nursing also diminished by escaping behind the clouds of the management system. The grass roots-level nurse thus experiences several layers of abandonment. Not only have the secondary sources of reward and recognition been severely diminished, but the very processes that everyone else sees as progress (i.e., modern technology and feminist consciousness) have exacted a heavy price from the staff nurse.[5] No wonder nurses say, "No one understands my situation." Indeed, these powerful subtleties are really not understood by many.

How occupants of social roles and institutional positions are treated by others and how close they are perceived to be to "center stage" depend very much on the perspectives and interests of other actors. This is particularly true if these others wield a certain amount of power, and it is even more true if the institution is a composite of widely differing vantage points, interests, and cultures. These conditions prevail in the typical U.S. hospital and have a specifically complicating consequence for nurses. Nursing happens to be placed where the processes of medicine, management, and nursing and patient desires converge. Each of the major participants in the processes of institutional functioning and patient care provision sees the nurse differently in worth, as well as in scope of function. Nursing is caught in a competitive struggle for domain and for control over its own activities. That the perspective of others does not coincide with that of the nurse at the front lines of care should not be surprising. It is better to acknowledge divergent priorities than to use patronizing benevolence as a substitute for real understanding.

It is not surprising that physicians prefer to work with nurses who follow orders without questioning them and who acknowledge the physician's power and prerogatives as evidence of wisdom and the natural order.[6] It is equally understandable that the hospital management team finds it advantageous to see the nurse as a substitutable occupant of personnel slots who can be moved according to staffing needs and reassigned without considering specialization, team effectiveness, or the prerequisites of professional control over one's own practice. Yet the nurse is frequently placed in the position of serving as confidant for the patient, as interpreter, and as advocate in negotiating with those people who come and go hurriedly and leave their decisions on charts and policies. Such inconsistency in role expectations cannot help but produce stress and disillusionment. This has been particularly true in recent years, when the one source of symbolic and real support—the director of nursing—has become more remote and suspected of having divided loyalties.

Additional impetus for feeling that one has landed on a blind and forgotten spur away from the main line arises from the images, reputations, and prestige distribution that is conveyed by word of mouth, professional publications, and the media. The researcher, the teacher, and, generally, the academically oriented nurse appear in the limelight. The grass roots nurse would not begrudge such attention if it did not occur at the expense of recognition of direct nursing care and if the direct care nurse could enjoy recognizable benefits derived from the accumulation of impressive knowledge and the delivery of sophisticated practice.

The paradox that seems to exact from the grass roots nurse the byproducts and indirect costs of apparent progress intensifies if one examines the glorified advances in the technology of patient care and what they mean for nursing. The record is mixed. The technology needed by the intensive care nurse has added tactical strength to the nursing side of the nurse-physician interaction. Conversely, most of the technology of primary patient care has placed limits on nursing judgments and has made the health care practitioner a functionary whose work is controlled by the dictum of technological apparatus. One should not forget that the growth of technology was not accompanied by a reassessment of the labor force and that the management and monitoring of instruments compete with those activities that are generally seen as the core of direct patient-oriented nursing.

Notwithstanding changing technology in patient care and resulting changes in the demand on nursing time, nursing skills, and nursing knowledge, many nurses feel that the plans for the deployment of nurses essentially have not changed. A comparison of charts of patients with similar diseases in 1945 and 1985 would show that the number of medical orders and procedures and the complexity of intervention have risen dramatically. Time of hospitalization has been reduced dramatically, so the periods of heavy demand on nursing effort occur much more continuously and intensively. There is less per-patient nursing time available, notwithstanding the increased needs of the patient and the range of intervention indicated. Almost always the medical orders, as shown on the chart, will be carried out before those activities that are the most challenging and most central to modern concepts in nursing. The nurse in the 1990s increasingly feels frustrated by being forced to execute tasks initiated by others at the expense of those activities that are properly and exclusively nursing.

It is not surprising that the grass roots–level nurse concludes that "real" nursing has been abandoned, at least the opportunity to place priority on practicing the core of what is unique to nursing. It is not surprising that many nurses rank their identity as conveyors of nursing functions as being less worthy, less significant, and less consequential than their role as agents for medical or management directives. Their daily reality emphasizes the subordinate and the technical dimensions of the nurse's functions, thus contradicting painfully the lessons learned in the school of nursing. Unfulfilled expectations are much more frustrating and destructive than experiences anticipated without the distortions of rose-colored glasses.

Being forced to accomplish delegated tasks that typically are a matter of record emphasizes the significance of medical and management directives. Not only is the nurse not able to provide many of the nursing functions that are nursing's own, but those functions are frequently not recorded and are subject to judgment rather than to rules. This imbalance explains much of the conviction of nurses across the country that they are understaffed and misused. The objective observer has to concur with the reality of inadequate staffing in most institutions. Furthermore, the observer cannot help but wonder whether the nurses' feeling so keenly about inadequate staffing derives partly from the obstacles to rescuing the actual nursing components from the mix of each day's pressures. Increased staffing may indeed provide some opportunities for doing more and for doing it better. Yet the question remains whether the current structure and organization will ever affirm the importance of the functions that are unique to nursing and also the importance of the nurse's membership in the health care team.

It may be difficult for administrators to appreciate fully the intensity and the focus of the frustration and the sense of undue burdens that characterize the feelings of nurses. On the whole those feelings are not a reaction to "working too hard." There are two themes that must be heard clearly and must be distinguished from the notion of mere complaints of overwork: "I can't provide all the care to which the patient is entitled" and—even more pervasively—"Everything I have to do as an adjunct to the physician and to others prevents me from really providing nursing as it should be."

If this explanation of nurses' feelings is understood, it will not come as a surprise that nurses consider the use of the so-called contract nurse to be demeaning and destructive rather than being a welcome help, as many administrators believe it should be interpreted. For most frontline nurses, knowledge about the patient and commitment to the patient's nursing needs supersede concern with tasks per se. The contract nurse shares neither familiarity nor commitment to the patient with regular staff nurses. Most nurses feel that the contract nurse creates additional work and additional stress; the contract nurse needs interpretation, assistance, and a tolerant link, which is normally what strangers require to function in a new environment.

THE NEED FOR A BETTER MODEL

Earlier the conflict between two models of the nursing presence was mentioned. One, emanating from educational socialization, stresses the "professional" client-oriented perception of the nurse as an autonomous, fully accountable, decision-making functionary. The other pattern, a byproduct of actual employment, presents the quasi-industrial model of a labor force with personnel slots to be filled and with the occupants of these positions being replaceable and movable. Many morale and performance problems derive from this dualism. Worse yet, neither model seems to fit the nurse's experience and satisfy the grass roots–level nurse's felt needs for satisfying and secure working conditions. Interpreting comments, reactions, and themes of interviews leads one to conclude that the actual experience of the grass roots–level nurse resembles neither model but rather approximates an organizational reality resembling the social structure of a symphony orchestra or a football team. These social models combine a group of individually skilled and specialized performers who demonstrate a deliberate interdependence. The orchestra and the football team alike succeed not solely because of the individual artistry of team members but because of the cooperation characterized by mutual respect and skilled anticipation of collectively supported behaviors. Placing the effort of the whole team ahead of individual achievement frequently offers the real key to the team's success. In addition to the high level of individual capabilities that are required, the skills and attitudes required for the success of the collectivity are paramount.

The application of this model to nursing becomes more persuasive after examining other approaches. Neither the authoritarian, bureaucratic system nor unbridled individualism satisfies the sophisticated understanding of most bedside nurses. Structural changes are desperately needed that combine more effective individual involvement by nurses with a system of collective, group-based accountability.

Exemplifying the general thrust of this need are the pervasive comments about head nurses.[2] In group interviews, professional nurses as much as nurses' aides voiced their concern about needed support for the head nurse. They ranked the strengthening of the head nurse position and the concomitant need for the head nurse to be educated and supported as the single most important area of change. The support and the recognition accorded to the head nurse appear to be viewed as indicators of the value and dignity given to the work of the grass roots–level nurse. The empowerment of the head nurse and the recognition of the head nurse's importance are reassuring to all members of the team since their own sense of respect and acceptance is reflected in and measured by the place of the head nurse in the scheme of the system.

Among the most pervasive indicators of respect is the acknowledgment of the head nurse's position as one that requires effort, time, and concern. In institutions in which the head nurse is expected to carry a full patient load and squeeze managing responsibilities into the remaining time or into off-duty hours, the staff nurses and the nursing assistants uniformly conclude that nursing is not competitive in the hierarchy of respected jobs. Sensitivity to the symbols of recognition is intensified by some of the characteristics of the occupants of nursing positions and by their organizational positioning. A study by Mauksch[3] revealed a high level of need for succor combined with an even more pronounced need to avoid blame-producing situations. Recognizing that the need to receive nurturing support is among the most important for nurses, one can easily see that organizational practices that feature rewards, recognition, and active support are directly related to the nurturant and caring themes characteristic of nursing functions.

This constellation of needs makes the current institutional placement of the frontline nurse a dramatic paradox. Any effort to deliberately minimize a supportive structure could only place the nurse at the interface of medical authority, administrative authority, nursing authority, and patient demands. Nurses feel that they are exposed to the risk of being blamed and held responsible without having the backing of institutional authority or support. This type of exposure also gives rise to the phenomenon called "dumping," which is usually associated with the expectation that some functionaries, because of their image of commitment, will be willing to absorb extraneous tasks that have been neglected by others.[2]

The perception that "nobody understands" easily changes during low-morale and high-stress periods to "nobody cares," culminating in the belief that "nobody thinks it is worthwhile to understand." Almost all of the researchers who have tried to elicit the worldview of the grass roots–level nurse agree about the dominant thrust of their results. Nurses in the front ranks feel deprived if they are not recognized as individuals, if they are not involved in the development and modification of policies, and if they cannot find a willing ear to listen seriously. They demand to be accorded dignity. To be devalued, discounted, and trivialized is tantamount to being abandoned. These issues are linked to matters of dignity and courtesy, such as being known by name, being treated as a competent practitioner, and receiving credit for sharing through action and concern in the drama of care. On a different level, the practicing nurse wants to receive the recognition that the total range of nursing competence far exceeds the mere implementation of medical orders; the nurse wants to invest in the well-being of patients but also in the stability and effectiveness of the team. Being frequently pulled to another patient care unit is experienced as an amputation from a delicately balanced system. Pulling diminishes the opportunity to gain satisfaction in rendering comprehensive, high-quality nursing care. The arbitrary moving of nurses is perceived to be a denial of the crucial importance of the nursing team and of the special competence of the nurse. Pulling does not nurture the team because it disrupts the system of mutual support and reciprocity of function. It is a recurring experience of nursing researchers to observe that, although other issues may be mentioned more frequently, none is protested with as much feeling and fervor as pulling.

CONCLUSION

In these pages the questions of existence and worth as they affect the frontline nurse have been explored. It was emphasized that a distinction should be made between abandonment as an objectively demonstrable and measurable condition and abandonment as a pervasively felt perception of working realities. It was further suggested that abandonment is frequently conveyed through organizational restraint or neglect of functions unique to nursing. Lack of dignity and respect characterizing one's professional interactions is a destructive, devaluing experience. Most of the changes proposed to improve the situation are administratively feasible and require only modest financial outlays. Fostering customs of courtesy, face-to-face respect, and recognition of the importance of participation is not difficult to implement if the current power wielders, be they the medical staff or the administrative hierarchy or even nursing management, are willing to acknowledge that giving respect and dignity does not diminish their own status. A system based on mutual respect will benefit all participants and, according to some suggestive data, may actually improve the quality of the product.

Every working person needs a degree of control commensurate with responsibility and accountability. Hardly any position in the repertoire of human work demonstrates so wide a gap between expectations and responsibility, on one hand, and institutionalized control over conditions of work, on the other hand. To feel included, the nurse must be a participant in the making of policies and regulations, and the formulation of objectives. To be in control of the conditions of work, the nurse should be free from the notion that nurses must absorb whatever others dish out. Assertiveness should stem from the right to ensure quality and should not be labeled a quasi-militant display of insubordination.

REFERENCES

1. Ashley, J. (1976). *Hospitals, paternalism and the role of the nurse.* New York: Columbia University Press.
2. Corley, M. C., & Mauksch, H. O. (1988). Registered nurses, gender and commitment. In A. Statham, E. M. Miller, & H. O. Mauksch (Eds.), *The worth of women's work: A qualitative synthesis.* Albany, N.Y.: State University of New York Press.
3. Mauksch, H. O. (1963). Becoming a nurse: A selective view. In J. K. Skipper, Jr., & R. Leonard (Eds.), *Social interaction and patient care.* Philadelphia: J. B. Lippincott.
4. Mauksch, H. O. (1973). Ideology, interaction and patient care. *Social Science and Medicine, 7,* 817.
5. Morgan, A., & McCann, J. M. (1983). Problems in nurse-physician relationships. *Nursing Administration Quarterly, 7,* 1.
6. Prescott, P., & Bowen, S. A. (1985). Physician-nurse relationships. *Annals of Internal Medicine, 103,* 127.
7. Wandelt, M. A. (1980). Work conditions cause nurses to leave. *American Nurse, 12*(10), 5.
8. Wandelt, M. A., Pierce, P. M., & Widdowson, R. R. (1981). Why nurses leave nursing and what can be done about it. *American Journal of Nursing, 1,* 72.

CHAPTER 83

What are the sources of stress for nurses?

DIANE GARDNER HUBER

"If job stress were a justification for worker's compensation claims, then we would all be eligible for worker's comp." The personnel director of a Midwestern community hospital once told me that this was the reply given to a staff nurse who had called to inquire about the potential for worker's compensation benefits due to stress. Stress predominates within work environments generally within our society. In nursing, as a part of a dynamic and rapidly changing health care system, stress is an occupational hazard. High levels of work-related stress are thought to affect nurses' health, job satisfaction, absenteeism, and turnover, and patient welfare.[49] The profession of nursing, then, has a stake in assessing and diagnosing the sources of job stress as a foundation for planning, implementing, and evaluating strategies to manage occupational stress among nurses. It is probably safe to assume that stress will never be eradicated; rather, the goal needs to be to successfully cope with and harness the stress and the stressors.

SOURCES OF STRESS

Stress can and does arise from many sources. Because stress is an occupational concern for nurses and a managerial concern generally, the related literature is extensive. For a more detailed discussion of the theoretical and empirical bases of much of this literature, see Hardy and Conway,[23] Hinshaw and Atwood,[26] and Lyon and Werner.[36] The purpose of this chapter is to briefly highlight the relevant literature and history related to the sources of stress in nursing and to present a perspective on the present status and on future directions for nursing.

At the most fundamental level the sources of stress arise from either the individual worker or the work environment. The individual sources of stress can be either external or internal. A useful distinction can be made between stress deriving from an individual's personality or personal family situation and that arising from the work environment. For example, an individual's personality or personal characteristics may not "fit" in a given work situation (external or situational origin).[18] The individual may carry internal personal or family conflicts over into the work environment (internal origin). The need to balance multiple life roles also may create personal stress; this is related to the concepts of intrapersonal conflict and women's careers.[15,20]

Contrasted with the individual sources are the stresses derived from the work itself or the specific work environment. Scholars have long recognized the stress related to nursing's work: being at the bedside around the clock to assist patients through their experiences of illness and hospitalization.[38,59] Multiple and often conflicting demands[19] and the role of the nurse[13] have been identified as sources of stress. A debate has raged about whether or not special care areas or certain kinds of nursing specialties have more stress.[16,21,25,37,50,56]

Organizational theorists have examined hospitals and health care organizations as environments whose contexts contain elements that may help or hinder the work of nursing.[43] Stress is seen as varying with other organizational variables such as job satisfaction, turnover, productivity, and group cohesion[10,26,27] as well as with other structural, procedural, and contextual factors.[34,42] Examples might include administrative support of nurses and nursing, quality of nursing leadership, interprofessional turf battles, constantly changing technology, or organizational restructuring.

The sources of stress identified by McGrath[46] include the physical and technical environment, the social medium or patterns of interpersonal relations, and the focal person under consideration. Leatt and

Schneck[35] conceptualized the sources of stress as falling into two major categories: role-based situations and task-based situations. From their review of the literature on nursing staff turnover, stress, and satisfaction, Hinshaw and Atwood[26] identified the following categories of stressors: the physical work environment; professional-bureaucratic role conflict; role strain and tensions from multiple expectations; management, communication patterns, and leadership style of nursing administration; staffing and work load problems; negative patient outcomes; communications with physicians; lack of participation in policy and practice decisions; and inadequate knowledge and skills for role functions. Huckabay and Jagla[30] categorized the 16 stressors in intensive care unit (ICU) nursing as falling into four classes: interpersonal communication, knowledge base, environmental, and patient care. Data from a stress audit on 1800 ICU nurses indicated agreement on the following factors in the ICU as causing the most stress: conflict with other health care providers, inadequate staffing patterns, lack of support in dealing with death and dying, inadequate work space and other inefficient factors in the physical work environment, and unresponsive nursing leadership.[4] Table 83-1 summarizes and categorizes the sources of stress. Suggested strategies to manage the sources of stress are also identified.

DEFINITION OF STRESS

The theoretical basis for a discussion of stress in nursing has its foundation in Selye's general stress theory.[54] Selye[54,55] saw stress as a nonspecific state that comprises a variety of induced changes in the human biological system. Stress is a syndrome reflected by characteristic symptoms. After delineating the biological manifestations of stress, the concept then was applied to social-psychological states. McGrath[46] saw stress as something that happens when persons interact with their environment and are presented with a demand, constraint, or opportunity for behavior. Stress has been considered to be cognitively mediated and assigned a positive or negative perception by the individual.[3,8,10] Within nursing research, stress has been seen as a stimulus, a response, or a transaction.[36] Job stress involves "disquieting influences" and those demands encountered within the roles and functions of employment.[26] Levels that are too high or too low have been seen as decreasing individual productivity.[5,10,26] The

consequences of very high job stress in nursing have been identified as "burnout."[3,44,56]

ROLE THEORY

Derived from the behavioral science literature, role theory[58] represents a collection of concepts and formulations that predict how actors will perform in a given role or under what circumstances certain types of behavior can be expected.[11] Using a systems framework, the concepts of role stress and role strain have been borrowed from other fields such as physics, engineering, biochemistry, and endocrinology[24] and linked to stress in social systems.[22,48] Hardy[22] identified a role stress typology generated from research on role occupants who had difficulties with role expectations, the location of the role in the social structure, the inadequate resources of role occupants, and the social context. Seven classes, with definitions, were identified: role ambiguity, role conflict, role incongruity, role overload, role underload, role overqualification, and role underqualification.

According to Hardy and Hardy,[24] role stress is external to a role occupant and is a social structural condition in which role obligations are vague, irritating, difficult, conflicting, or impossible to meet. Role strain is a subjective state of emotional arousal in response to the external conditions of social stress. Other theories related to an understanding of role stress and strain are symbolic interaction,[24,31,58] social structural role theory,[24,47,51] and social exchange theory.[6,12,29] An extensive treatment of role stress and role strain can be found in Hardy and Hardy[24] and Conway.[11]

ORGANIZATIONAL BEHAVIOR

Another approach to analyzing sources of stress in nursing has evolved from the analysis of the behavior of individuals in organizations. Two levels have been addressed. Organizational psychologists have focused on how individuals behave and make decisions given certain organizational characteristics or contextual factors operant in the environment. The focus is on the individual decision maker. Organizational sociologists have focused on how aspects of organizations influence the structure and functioning of the group and/or individual members. The focus is on the contextual variables. Calkin's view[9] is that organizations and their environments provide a major contingency for the social behavior of the members.

Table 83-1 Summary of the sources of stress for nurses and some suggested strategies for stress management

Source of stress	Suggested strategies
Individual worker	
Personality fit	Screening and selective hiring
	Personal self-awareness
	Coaching and performance appraisal
Personal-family situation	Counseling and support to resolve inner conflicts and to improve coping ability
Balancing multiple life roles	Flexible scheduling
	Child care-eldercare benefits
	Counseling
	Career planning
	Exercise; relaxation; imagery
Work environment	
Role of the nurse	
Caring for the sick and dying; negative patient outcomes	Stress management programs
	Administrative and social support; support groups
	Respite
Multiple, conflicting role demands	Administrative leadership for role clarification
	Negotiation and delegation skills
Professional-bureaucratic role conflict	Conflict management and negotiation skills
Inadequate knowledge or skills to fulfill role functions	In-service education and continuing education benefits
	Coaching and counseling
Communications and interpersonal relationships	
Interprofessional turf battles	Communication and negotiation skills
	Conflict mediation and management strategies
	Administrative support
Social support and interpersonal relationship patterns	Analysis of organizational culture
	Establishment of open and honest communication patterns
	Development of work group teamwork
Communication patterns	Analysis and support for positive, open communications and atmosphere of trust
Conflict with other health care workers; "the doctor-nurse game"	Conflict management and negotiation skills
	Constructive confrontation
	Grievance handling
	Mutual respect
Verbal abuse	Improvement of self-esteem
	Improvement of organizational attitudes and collaboration
	Assertiveness
Administrative support for nursing	
Quality of leadership; leadership styles; leadership responsiveness	Leadership training
	Administrative support
	Culture management
	Development of morale
Quality of management	Management training and support
	Role models of performance under stress
	Management of infrastructure
Amount and type of participation in policy and practice decisions	Shared governance; decentralization
	Continuous quality improvement
	Delegation to work group teams
	Control over practice

Continued.

Table 83-1 – cont'd. Summary of the sources of stress for nurses and some suggested strategies for stress management

Source of stress	Suggested strategies
Environmental change	
Constantly changing technology	Adaptation of technology for nursing efficiency
	In-service education
Organizational restructuring	Administrative support
	Participation by nurses
	Visible benefits to nurses or increased satisfiers
Physical work environment	
Inadequate work space	Structural changes
Inefficient factors in physical work environment	Structural and functional changes to adapt space
	Technology and work processes to fill nursing's work needs
	Computer technology and resources for nursing
Task-based situations	
Staffing	Analysis of patient classification systems and resource allocation decisions
	Determination of staff mix
Work load	Analysis of staffing
	Resource allocation
	Care modality and human resources deployment decisions
	Delegation skills

MEASUREMENT

It is entirely possible that stress is a curvilinear variable, that each nurse has a personal stress curve over which performance rises initially but then, past a certain limit of tolerance, falls.[1] If so, then certain measurement techniques would be more valid and predictive than others. It is difficult to operationalize job stress due to the lack of conceptual clarity and lack of agreement on its definition. Measures have been located for stress, conflict, hardiness, and burnout. See Tables 83-2 through 83-4 for a listing of some identified measures of these concepts.

RECENT CHANGES

How the issue of role conflict has changed in focus can be traced through its treatment in *Current Issues in Nursing*. The emphasis was on reality shock or education-service disjunctiveness in the first edition.[39] In the second edition,[40] the focus was on conflict within nursing itself: between professional organizations and between groups of nurses. The focus of the third edition[41] was on the conflicts within nursing that are identified as contributing to a decrease in the influence of the profession. Certainly the literature has been extensive. In 1987 Lyon and Werner[36] reported that 976 stress-related articles had appeared in nursing

journals since 1956. Of the research conducted by nurses and published from 1974 to 1984, they identified 82 studies for analysis. Researchers at the American Hospital Association[2] found 619 citations between 1975 and 1987 using the descriptors "burnout" and "stress" in connection with turnover.

Within nursing, the role theory and organizational psychology streams have been manifested in the literature on physician-nurse conflicts,[28,57] reality shock,[32,33] burnout,[3,56] and hardiness.[45,53,60] The concepts addressed in this literature include professionalism, conflict, and professional-bureaucratic role conflict. In the research-based literature in nursing, job satisfaction and turnover have been the main variables of interest.[27,34,42,52,61] Using a causal modeling approach with sociological variables, these studies have resulted in similar findings about the effect of an acute care organization on individual nurse employees.

Job satisfaction is a major predictor of anticipated turnover or intent to stay or leave, and anticipated turnover or intent to stay or leave is a major predictor of actual turnover.[25] Hinshaw and Atwood[26] included job-related stress as a variable. They suggested that job stress was mediated by job satisfaction, and they later found that job stress had no direct effect on anticipated turnover but only influenced job satisfaction. They viewed job stress as an individual factor in the second

Table 83-2 Measures of stress

Author	Date	Instrument of measurement	Measurement aspect
Baily, Steffen, and Grout	1980	Stress audit	Stressors and satisfiers of ICU nurses
Gray-Toft and Anderson	1981a	Nursing stress scale	Frequency and major sources of stress experienced by nurses in hospital units: physical, psychological, and social environment including conflict
Gray-Toft and Anderson	1981b		
Hinshaw, Smeltzer, and Atwood	1987	Baily and Claus's job stress scale	Job stresses such as complex and numerous decisions inherent in patient care, professional-bureaucratic role conflict, and multiple care expectations
Huckabay and Jagla	1979	Questionnaire of stressful factors in the ICU	Four main categories of stressful events: interpersonal communications, knowledge base, environmental, and patient care
Norbeck	1985		
Koch, Gmelch, Tung, and Swent	1982	Administrative stress index (ASI)	Comprehensive measure of job-related stress: role-based, conflict-mediating, task-based, and boundary-spanning stress
Leatt and Schneck	1980	Stress questions (head nurse)	Sources and frequency of stress: patient-based, role-based, task ambiguity, staff movement, and physician-based stress
Zeitlin	1985	Coping inventory	A general coping measure of adaptive behavior

Modified from Bailey, J. T., Steffen, S. M., & Grout, J. W. (1980). The stress audit: Identifying the stressors of ICU nursing. *Journal of Nursing Education, 19*(6), 15-25; Gray-Toft, P., & Anderson, J. G. (1981). Stress among hospital nursing staff: Its causes and effects. *Social Science and Medicine, 15A,* 539-647; Gray-Toft, P., & Anderson, J. G. (1981). The nursing stress scale: Development of an instrument. *Journal of Behavioral Assessment, 3*(1), 11-23; Hinshaw, A. S., Smeltzer, C. H., & Atwood, J. R. (1987). Innovative retention strategies for nursing staff. *Journal of Nursing Administration, 17*(6), 8-16; Huckabay, L. M. D., & Jagla, B. (1979). Nurses' stress factors in the intensive care unit. *Journal of Nursing Administration, 9*(2), 21-26; Norbeck, J. S. (1985). Perceived job stress, job satisfaction, and psychological symptoms in critical care nurse. *Research in Nursing and Health, 8,* 253-259; Koch, J. L., Gmelch, W., Tung, R., & Swent, B. (1982). Job stress among school administrators: Factual dimensions and differential effects. *Journal of Applied Psychology, 67*(4), 493-499; Leatt, P., & Schneck, R. (1980). Differences in stress perceived by head nurses across nursing specialties in hospitals. *Journal of Advanced Nursing, 5,* 31-46; and Zeitlin, S. (1985). *Coping inventory: A measure of adaptive behavior.* Bensonville, Il: Scholastic Testing Service.

stage of the five-stage causal ordering of variables related to turnover.[27] Norbeck[49] found that perceived stress in critical care nursing was related to job satisfaction and psychological symptoms. Job satisfaction affects turnover,[19,52] and psychological symptoms are likely to impair performance.[49] One result of this literature stream was recommendations for nurse retention and job satisfaction strategies, covering primary nursing and all registered nurse staffing, as ways to reduce turnover and control a nursing shortage.[17]

Of the long list of work-related stressors, some may be reduced by augmenting the coping and adaptive ability of nurses. For personality hardiness, the only direct application or intervention appears to be to increase nurses' awareness. The literature review revealed a role for nurse managers in caring for the psychological needs of the staff. The use of counseling, support groups, and stress management programs have been advocated. Some stressors might be reduced by making

structural or organizational changes.[49] Suggested strategies have included advocating adequate staffing, correcting problems in the physical environment, and reducing communication problems for nurses. The institutional environment component of the American Hospital Association's retention model[2] included internal factors related to organizational structure, patient care variables, support services, and patterns of nursing care. The study concluded that individual-directed remedies have some positive aspects but produce only temporary, cosmetic benefits because they do not alter the sources of stress. Institutional remedies, if based on staff input, focus on altering a malfunctioning system. The internal barriers identified by the Pew-Robert Wood Johnson grantees included the following: inadequate nursing resources, nursing practice deficits, insufficient departmental support services, unmet compensation needs, nursing-medical staff relations, lack of nursing management participation in hospital-wide

Table 83-3 Measures of conflict

Author	Date	Instrument of measurement	Measurement aspect
Corwin	1961	Image of nursing scale	Bureaucratic and professional components of nursing role
Snyder	1982		conceptualization
Gardner	1992	Perceived conflict scale	Four aspects of perceived job conflict: intrapersonal, interpersonal, intergroup-support services, and intergroup-other departments
Landstrom, Biordi, and Gillies	1989	Semistructured interview schedule	Task-oriented and benefit-oriented valuation of organizational inducements
Marvick	1954	Inducement valuation scale	
Rahim	1983	Rahim organizational conflict inventory (ROCI)	Three aspects of organizational conflict: intrapersonal, intragroup, and intergroup
Thomas	1975	Thomas-Kilman conflict mode instrument	Five modes of handling conflict: competing, collaborating, compromising, avoiding, and accommodating
Tilden, Nelson, and May	1990	Interpersonal relations index (IPRI)	Three aspects of interpersonal relations: social support, reciprocity, and conflict

Modified from Corwin, R. G. (1961). The professional employee: A study of conflict in nursing roles. *American Journal of Sociology, 66,* 614-615; Snyder, D. J. (1982). New baccalaureate graduates' perceptions of organizational conflict. *Nursing Research, 31*(5), 300-305; Gardner, D. L. (1992). Conflict and retention of new graduate nurses. *Western Journal of Nursing Research, 14*(1), 76-85; Landstrom, G. L., Biordi, D. L., & Gillies, D. A. (1989). The emotional and behavioral process of staff nurse turnover. *Journal of Nursing Administration, 19*(9), 23-28; Marvick, D. (1954). *Career perspectives in a bureaucratic setting.* Ann Arbor: University of Michigan Press; Rahim, M. A. (1983). *Rahim organizational conflict inventories: Experimental edition.* Palo Alto, Calif: Consulting Psychologists Press; Thomas, K. (1975). Conflict and conflict management. In M. D. Dunnette (Ed.), *The handbook of industrial and organizational psychology.* Chicago: Rand McNally College Publishing; Tilden, V. P., Nelson, C. A., & May, B. A. (1990). The IPR Inventory: Development and Psychometric Characteristics. *Nursing Research, 39*(6), 337-343; and Tilden, V. P., Nelson, C. A., & May, B. A. (1990). Use of qualitative methods to enhance content validity. *Nursing Research, 39*(3), 172-175.

Table 83-4 Measures of hardiness and burnout

Author	Date	Instrument of measurement	Measurement aspect
Jones	1980	Staff burnout scale for health professionals (SBS-HP)	Assessment of burnout and work stress in terms of cognitive, affective, behavioral, and psychophysiological reactions
Kobasa	1979	Hardiness inventory (HI)	Three aspects of hardiness: control, commitment, and challenge
Maslach and Jackson	1981	Maslach burnout inventory	Three aspects of experienced burnout: emotional exhaustion, depersonalization, and reduced personal accomplishment
Pollock and Duffy	1990	Health-related hardiness scale (HRHS)	Three aspects of health-related hardiness: control, commitment, and challenge

Modified from Jones, J. W. (1980). *The staff burnout scale for health professionals (SBS-HP).* Park Ridge, Il: London House; Kabasa, S. C. (1979). Stressful life events, personality, and health: An inquiry into hardiness. *Journal of Personality and Social Psychology, 37*(1), 1-11; Maslach, C., & Jackson, S. E. (1981). The measurement of experienced burnout. *Journal of Occupational Behavior, 2,* 99-113; and Pollock, S. E., & Duffy, M. E. (1990). The health-related hardiness scale: Development and psychometric analysis. *Nursing Research, 39*(4), 218-222.

decision making, and job dissatisfaction.[14] Changing staffing patterns, shifting work loads, and negotiating staff assignments have been proposed as mechanisms for reducing job stress, as have using the satisfiers in the setting and altering of structural and environmental aspects such as by implementing primary nursing.[26,44,61] The most current focus of work environment reformation is on changing the organization as a system.

FUTURE DIRECTIONS

Stress is an undisputed aspect of the work of nursing. Research has documented its presence and some of the sources from which it is derived. The hypothesis that higher perceived job stress is related to decreased job satisfaction and increased psychological symptoms has an empirical basis.[27,41] Conflict also appears to be related to decreased job satisfaction.[16] These findings have been applied to investigations of turnover and retention in nursing.

Health care delivery systems are experiencing an era of turbulence and change. Partially due to economic considerations and a knowledge-technology explosion, the present context is marked by uncertainty, stress, and a lack of clarity of roles. Generalized stress is an inevitable manifestation of massive organizational changes. Cost containment drives sweeping organizational restructuring. Differentiated practice and the use of nurse extenders are implemented as ways to change staffing patterns and shift work loads. Total quality management or continuous quality improvement (TQM-CQI) programs are implemented to improve organizational systems.

However, changes of this magnitude require new ways of thinking and of doing. Stress, the more global response, arises from the practical reality of how people respond to the specific workplace conflicts derived from little clarity, much uncertainty, and role overlaps. Turf battles can be predicted during restructuring. Delegation disarticulation or discomfort can be predicted during the implementation of new care giver roles and responsibilities. Teamwork and collaboration may be very new ways of operating when TQM-CQI programs begin.

While we know something about the sources of stress for nurses, we know less about how to manage their work-related stress. What we know about managing work-related stress in nursing does not lend itself readily to a prescription for action. Suggested institutional remedies need to be based on staff input and include climate changes, worker preparation, reduction of paperwork, and worker participation in decisions.[2] Nurses voice the need for work load relief,[7] yet specific directions on how to administer nursing care delivery systems under conditions of stress and change are missing. It is easy to prescribe the "remedies" for work stress as administrative awareness, staff development, and staff empowerment. It is much more difficult to achieve these goals and to know that they will thereby improve nursing productivity.

If so much is changing so rapidly, would clarity and direction from the profession help? Can we clear up the confusing number of levels and roles in nursing care delivery? If the profession would decide what is the work of nursing and who should do it, and set a standard for roles and responsibilities, then the debates about preparation and deployment could more easily be resolved. Let's not ignore the nursing research already available to indicate what satisfies and motivates nurses. To clear up the confusion about roles within nursing seems to be the necessary first step to reducing stress in nursing.

Once nursing determines nursing care workers' roles and preparation, this vision can be articulated and integrated within organizational systems. In acute care institutions, the goal of patient care primarily involves the work of nursing since patients are admitted to a hospital when they cannot care for themselves. Thus the stress generated by systems restructuring may be diminished if nursing personnel are clear about their roles and can therefore concentrate on negotiation, culture, conflict management, and collaboration instead of fighting turf battles and resisting the art of delegation.

If stress is part of the work environment in nursing, then nurses need to pay attention to positive actions that will manage the stress and the conflicts that generate the stress. Let's start with the fundamental basis of nursing: What is our work and who should do it? The basic task is formidable but possible. Let's clear up the roles and responsibilities. The best response in uncertain times is clarity of direction.

REFERENCES

1. Al-Assaf, A. F. (1992). Executive stress: An ounce of prevention. *Nursing Management, 23*(8), 69-72.
2. American Hospital Association. (1989). A model for hospital nurse retention: New findings. *Nursing Economic$, 7(6), 324-331.*
3. Bailey, J. T. (1980). Stress and stress management: An overview. *Journal of Nursing Education, 19*(6), 5-8.
4. Bailey, J. T., Steffen, S. M., & Grout, J. W. (1980). The stress audit: Identifying the stressors of ICU nursing. *Journal of Nursing Education, 19*(6), 15-25.
5. Benson, H., & Allen, R. L. (1980). How much stress is too much? *Harvard Business Review, 58*(5), 86-92.
6. Blau, P. M. (1964). *Exchange and power in social life.* New York: John Wiley and Sons.
7. Blegen, M. A., Gardner, D. L., & McCloskey, J. C. (1992). Who helps you with your work? Survey results. *American Journal of Nursing, 92*(1), 26-31.
8. Broverman, D. M., & Lazarus, R. S. (1958). Individual differences in task performance under conditions of cognitive interference. *Journal of Personality, 26,* 94-105.
9. Calkin, J. D. (1988). The effects of organizational structure on role behavior. In M. Hardy & M. Conway (Eds.), *Role theory: Perspectives for health professionals* (pp. 133-158). New York: Appleton and Lange.
10. Cleland, V. S. (1965). The effect of stress on performance. *Nursing Research, 14,* 292-298.
11. Conway, M. (1988). Theoretical approaches to the study of roles. In M. Hardy & M. Conway (Eds.), *Role theory: Perspectives for health professionals* (pp. 63-72). New York: Appleton and Lange.
12. Cook, K. S. (1987). *Social exchange theory.* Beverly Hills, Calif: Sage Publications.

13. Dewe, P. J. (1987). Identifying the causes of nurses' stress: A survey of New Zealand nurses. *Work and Stress, 1*(1), 15-24.

14. Donaho, B. A., & Kohles, M. K. (1992). *Strengthening hospital nursing: A program to improve patient care.* St. Petersburg, Fla: The Pew Charitable Trusts/Robert Wood Johnson Foundation/ Strengthening Hospital Nursing Program.

15. Gardner, D. L. (1992). Career commitment in nursing. *Journal of Professional Nursing, 8*(3), 155-160.

16. Gardner, D. L. (1992). Conflict and retention of new graduate nurses. *Western Journal of Nursing Research, 14*(1), 76-85.

17. Gardner, K. (1991). A summary of findings of a five-year comparison study of primary and team nursing. *Nursing Research, 40*(2), 113-117.

18. Getzels, J. W. (1958). Administration as a social process. In A. W. Halpin (Ed.), *Administrative theory in education* (pp. 150-165). Chicago: University of Chicago Press.

19. Gray-Toft, P., & Anderson, J. G. (1981). Stress among hospital nursing staff: Its causes and effects. *Social Science and Medicine, 15A,* 539-647.

20. Greenhaus, J. H., & Kopelman, R. E. (1981). Conflict between work and nonwork roles: Implications for the career planning process. *Human Resource Planning, 4*(1), 1-10.

21. Hardin, S. B. (1990). Nursing occupational distress. In J. C. McCloskey & H. K. Grace (Eds.), *Current issues in nursing* (pp. 490-494). St Louis: Mosby.

22. Hardy, M. E. (1978). Role stress and role strain. In M. E. Hardy & M. E. Conway (Eds.), *Role theory: Perspectives for health professionals.* Norwalk, Conn: Appleton-Century-Crofts.

23. Hardy, M. E., & Conway, M. E. (1988). *Role theory: Perspectives for health professionals* (2nd ed.). Norwalk, Conn: Appleton and Lange.

24. Hardy, M. E., & Hardy, W. L. (1988). Role stress and role strain. In M. Hardy & M. Conway (Eds.), *Role theory: Perspectives for health professionals* (pp. 159-239). New York: Appleton and Lange.

25. Hinshaw, A. S. (1989). Programs of nursing research for nursing administration. In B. Henry, C. Arndt, M. Di Vincenti, & A. Marriner-Tomey (Eds.), *Dimensions of nursing administration* (pp. 251-266). Boston: Blackwell Scientific Publications.

26. Hinshaw, A. S., & Atwood, J. R. (1983). Nursing staff turnover, stress, and satisfaction: Models, measures, and management. In H. H. Werley & J. J. Fitzpatrick (Eds.), *Annual review of nursing research* (pp. 133-153). New York: Springer Publications.

27. Hinshaw, A. S., Smeltzer, C. H., & Atwood, J. R. (1987). Innovative retention strategies for nursing staff. *Journal of Nursing Administration, 17*(6), 8-16.

28. Hodes, J. R., & Van Crombrugghe, P. (1990). Nurse-physician relationships. *Nursing Management, 21*(7), 73-75.

29. Homans, G. C. (1974). *Social behavior: Its elementary forms* (rev. ed.). New York: Harcourt, Brace, and World.

30. Huckabay, L. M. D., & Jagla, B. (1979). Nurses' stress factors in the intensive care unit. *Journal of Nursing Administration, 9*(2), 21-26.

31. Joas, H. (1985). *G.H. Mead.* Cambridge, Mass: Cambridge University Press.

32. Kramer, M. (1974). *Reality shock: Why nurses leave nursing.* St Louis: Mosby.

33. Kramer, M., & Schmalenberg, C. (1977). *Path to biculturalism.* Wakefield, Mass: Contemporary Publishing.

34. Landstrom, G. L., Biordi, D. L., & Gillies, D. A. (1989). The emotional and behavioral process of staff nurse turnover. *Journal of Nursing Administration, 19*(9), 23-28.

35. Leatt, P., & Schneck, R. (1980). Differences in stress perceived by head nurses across nursing specialties in hospitals. *Journal of Advanced Nursing, 5,* 31-46.

36. Lyon, B. L., & Werner, J. S. (1987). Stress. In J. J. Fitzpatrick & R. L. Taunton (Eds.), *Annual review of nursing research* (pp. 3-22). New York: Springer Publications.

37. Maloney, J. P. (1982). Job stress and its consequences on a group of intensive and nonintensive care nurses. *Advances in Nursing Science, 4*(2), 31-42.

38. Mauksch, H. O. (1966). The organizational context of nursing practice. In F. Davis (Ed.), *The nursing profession: Five sociological essays* (pp. 109-137). New York: John Wiley and Sons.

39. McCloskey, J. C., & Grace, H. K. (1981). Overcoming the sources of conflict. In J. C. McCloskey & H. K. Grace (Eds.), *Current issues in nursing* (pp. 619-621). Boston: Blackwell Scientific Publications.

40. McCloskey, J. C., & Grace, H. K. (1985). Overcoming the sources of conflict. In J. C. McCloskey & H. K. Grace (Eds.), *Current issues in nursing* (pp. 875-876). Boston: Blackwell Scientific Publications.

41. McCloskey, J. C., & Grace, H. K. (1990). Conflicts within nursing. In J. C. McCloskey & H. K. Grace (Eds.), *Current issues in nursing* (pp. 472-474). St Louis: Mosby.

42. McCloskey, J. C., & McCain, B. E. (1987). Satisfaction, commitment, and professionalism of newly employed nurses. *Image: The Journal of Nursing Scholarship, 19,* 20-24.

43. McClure, M., Poulin, M., Sovie, M., & Wandelt, M. (1983). *Magnet hospitals: Attraction and retention of professional nurses.* Kansas City, Mo: American Nurses Association.

44. McConnell, E. (1979). Burnout and the critical care nurse. *Critical Care Update, 6,* 5-14.

45. McCranie, E., Lambert, V., & Lambert, C. (1987). Work stress, hardiness, and burnout among hospital staff nurses. *Nursing Research, 36,* 374-378.

46. McGrath, J. E. (1976). Stress and behavior in organizations. In M. D. Dunnette (Ed.), *Handbook of industrial and organizational psychology* (pp. 1351-1395). Chicago: Rand McNally College Publishing.

47. Merton, R. K. (1968). *Social theory and social structure* (rev. ed.). New York: Free Press.

48. Miller, J. (1971). The nature of living systems. *Behavioral Science, 16,* 278.

49. Norbeck, J. S. (1985). Perceived job stress, job satisfaction, and psychological symptoms in critical care nursing. *Research in Nursing and Health, 8,* 253-259.

50. Norbeck, J. S. (1985). Types and sources of social support for managing job stress in critical care nursing. *Nursing Research, 34*(4), 225-230.

51. Parsons, T. (1951). *The social system.* New York: Free Press.

52. Price, J. L., & Mueller, C. W. (1981). *Professional turnover: The case of nurses.* New York: Spectrum Books.

53. Rich, V. L., & Rich, A. R. (1987). Personality hardiness and burnout in female staff nurses. *Image: The Journal of Nursing Scholarship, 19,* 63-66.

54. Selye, H. (1965). *The stress of life.* Toronto: McGraw-Hill.

55. Selye, H. (1976). *Stress in health and disease.* Boston: Butterworth.

56. Stehle, J. L. (1981). Critical care nursing stress: The findings revisited. *Nursing Research, 30,* 182-186.

57. Stein, L. I., Watts, D. T., & Howell, T. (1990). The doctor-nurse game revisited. *New England Journal of Medicine, 322*(8), 546-549.

58. Thomas, E. J., & Biddle, B. J. (1966). Basic concepts for classifying the phenomena of role. In B. J. Biddle & E. J. Thomas (Eds.), *Role theory: Concepts and research* (pp. 23-45). New York: John Wiley and Sons.

59. Volicer, B. J., & Burns, M. W. (1977). Preexisting correlates of hospital stress. *Nursing Research, 26*(6), 408-415.

60. Wagnild, G., & Young, H. M. (1991). Another look at hardiness. *Image: The Journal of Nursing Scholarship, 23*(4), 257-259.

61. Weisman, C. S., Alexander, C. S., & Chase, G. (1981). Determinants of hospital staff nurse turnover. *Medical Care, 19*(4), 431-443.

CHAPTER 84

Nurses and physician assistants

Issues and challenges

VIRGINIA KLINER FOWKES, JANET MENTINK

The concept of the profession of physician assistant (PA) began in the mid-1960s as a response to widespread concern about the geographical and specialty maldistribution of health personnel, particularly physicians. There was a recognized need to improve access to primary care services for medically underserved rural and urban populations. The first training of PAs began at Duke University in 1965 when Eugene A. Stead, MD, initiated a 2-year program with three ex-military corpsmen. Oddly enough, this followed a collaborative project with a member of the nursing faculty, Thelma Ingles, in the late 1950s and early 1960s in the training of nurse practitioners (NPs) through the master's program at Duke. The National League for Nursing denied accreditation for the program on three different occasions, suggesting that the assumption of medical tasks by nurses was inappropriate and potentially dangerous.[2] Without accreditation, nurse practitioner training was discontinued. Unfortunately, considerable acrimony occurred between medical and nursing leaders as a result of these decisions. As another source of clinically experienced personnel, Dr. Stead then turned his attention to corpsmen who were returning from the Vietnam War and were interested in civilian roles in health care.

Dr. Stead's vision of a new role in primary care was shared by other medical and nursing leaders at the time. Their intent was to recruit individuals with patient care experience and train them in the skills necessary to practice primary care in rural settings or settings with medically underserved populations. NP programs began to develop shortly thereafter.

PHYSICIAN ASSISTANTS
Education

Through the Health Resources Administration, Bureau of Health Manpower, the federal government provided funding for most of the initial PA training programs. The federal program did not restrict training to medical schools. Rather, to provide closer ties with ambulatory settings, programs were encouraged to offer the required basic and clinical sciences in other academic settings.

Today, there are 55 PA programs offering a variety of academic options and different approaches to clinical training. The majority of programs (82%) are part of a university or 4-year college. Other programs are sponsored by 2-year colleges (11%), the military (6%), and a hospital (2%). The majority of programs (67%) award a baccalaureate degree; five programs (9%) award a master's degree; and the remaining award a certificate and/or an associate degree.[6]

The typical program is 24 months in length and includes instruction in basic and behavioral-social science; physical assessment and clinical medicine; and supervised clinical rotations, clerkships, and preceptorships. All programs teach pharmacology, with an average of 66 hours. Basic science courses include anatomy, physiology, microbiology, biochemistry, nutrition, and epidemiology. Behavioral social sciences typically include content about psychosocial aspects of care, health promotion, medical ethics, professional role development, human sexuality, health care systems, and multicultural needs, among other topics. Following this background, PA programs provide instruction in interviewing skills, patient education, and basic counseling techniques. Clinical instruction takes place in a variety of primary care specialties including family medicine, general internal medicine, obstetrics and gynecology, pediatrics, and geriatrics. Most of the primary care training is conducted in hospital outpatient clinics, community clinics, private physician practices, or other ambulatory settings where PAs learn to care for clients of all ages. Most PA programs in the Western states have preceptorships based in community outpatient or office practice settings where students receive almost all of their clinical training. The preceptorships are often located in medically underserved areas. The programs utilize a multidisciplinary faculty including PAs, MDs, basic and social scientists, and NPs.

Background

All PA programs build on students' individual academic and prior health care experiences. Well over half of the students entering programs in the class of 1991 were over 27 years of age. Approximately half have bachelor's, master's, or higher degrees upon program entry. Others have associate degrees or other academic preparation. The vast majority have had health care experience prior to program entry, with a mean of 4.5 years.[6] PAs may have clinical backgrounds as nurses, emergency medical technicians, physical or respiratory therapists, pharmacists, laboratory technicians, or health aids, or in other similar occupations.

There are regional differences in both the background characteristics and training of PAs. For example, students in the Central and Western states tend to be older and to have more health care experience than students in other areas.[3,6] And, as mentioned earlier, most programs in the Western states utilize community-based ambulatory settings, as opposed to hospital inpatient areas, for the majority of clinical training.

The number of women entering PA programs has increased steadily, with a mean enrollment for the past 8 years of 62%.[6] A 1988 national survey reported that 22% of entering PAs were ethnic minorities. A study conducted at the same time of PA program graduates in California reported 30% minorities. Most of this group reported using a language other than English—usually Spanish—with their clients, and over one third of this group reported speaking Spanish with fluency.[3]

National certification and state licensure

All PAs take national board examinations administered by the National Commission on the Certification of Physician Assistants in collaboration with the National Board of Medical Examiners. The examination is a rigorous one with both written comprehensive and clinical practicum components. To maintain national certification, PAs take a recertifying examination every 6 years. Most states accept satisfactory completion of the national board examination as qualification for PA licensure. Some states have well-defined licensing procedures, and in others the process is more flexible, taking the form of a registry or list of practitioners. State laws also vary in the provisions for PA practice. Most allow a broad range of functions in any setting of health care.[5]

The method of supervision of PAs by physicians takes different forms. Examples include one-to-one review of patient care; regular review of chart notes; remote supervision by telephone when the PA seeks consultation; and protocols or standardized procedures, where physicians and PAs establish in writing the procedures and plans necessary for the care of specific client problems.

Current roles

The PA functions as a member of the health care team. There are more than 20,000 PAs practicing in this country. In 1990 the American Academy of Physician Assistants (AAPA) conducted a survey of its 12,000 members and received a 97.5% response. PAs practice in a variety of specialties. Almost two thirds (64.4%) practice in primary care, including family practice, internal medicine, obstetrics and gynecology, and pediatrics. Others are in surgery (18.4%), emergency medicine (7.9%), orthopedics (7.1%), occupational medicine (4.2%), psychiatry (1.4%), or other subspecialties (6.0%).[1]

The practice settings of PAs also vary. The vast majority (70%) practice in outpatient settings, with group practice attracting the greatest numbers (Fig. 84-1). Of all PAs, 15% are employed in population areas of 10,000 or less and 7.5% are in areas of 5000 or less.

A profession is sometimes defined as a unique body of knowledge, tasks, skills, or responsibilities. The PA profession overlaps with other professions, particularly that of physicians. The PA both substitutes for and augments services customarily performed by physicians. She or he can substitute for the physician by

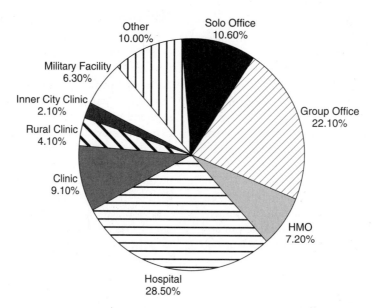

Fig. 84-1. Practice settings of physician assistants. (*From the American Academy of Physician Assistants, 1992. Used with permission.*)

performing routine care, such as health maintenance, and allowing the physician more time for complex problems; the PA can see the same types of clients as the physician and thus expand the numbers of clients receiving care in the practice setting; and/or the PA can substitute for the on-site presence of the physician in a setting such as a nursing home, client home, or remote rural clinic. The PA augments physician services in several ways. The PA's clinical background may offer new services to the practice. For example, a PA who was formerly a nutritionist can bring new knowledge and services in counseling to a practice. Or a male physician's hiring of a female PA who has special interests in women's health may attract more women to the practice. In both of these examples, PAs make possible more health education for clients.

There are both nonnegotiable and negotiable aspects of the PA role. Nonnegotiable is the fact that all PAs function under the supervision of physicians. The PA profession is dependent upon the laws and regulations that govern practice and define the PA's relationship to the physician. However, the PA performs services independently or interdependently with the health care team. In other words, the PA has an independent role within a dependent practice.[7]

The negotiable aspects of the PA role are numerous. PAs can influence their duties and responsibilities. For example, they may negotiate their own practice pref-erences. They may function as coordinators with clinical and management tasks interspersed, or as case managers for a particular group of clients.

A role delineation study conducted by the AAPA in 1935 found that there were distinct differences in practice characteristics among PAs in the various specialties. However, they identified the following nine clusters of activities that were common to PAs in practice across specialty lines: (1) gathering data, (2) seeing common problems and diseases, (3) conducting laboratory and diagnostics studies, (4) performing management activities, (5) performing surgical procedures, (6) managing emergency situations, (7) conducting health promotion and disease prevention activities, (8) prescribing medications, and (9) using interpersonal skills in patient education and counseling.[7]

PHYSICIAN ASSISTANTS AND NURSE PRACTITIONERS
Similarities and differences

A few years after the PA movement began, schools of nursing began to develop nurse practitioner programs. NPs are discussed in Chapter 3. PAs are often compared with NPs, and it is useful to understand the similarities and differences between these two groups of professionals who often practice in the same settings. With regard to similarities, both the PA and NP professions were established in the mid- to late 1960s by their medicine and nursing counterparts in response to the needs for more primary care services. Studies have documented that both PAs and NPs increase access to care in rural areas and for underserved populations; they provide high-quality care; they decrease costs of medical care to employers and society; and they provide care that is generally satisfying to patients, particularly in the interpersonal aspects of care.[8]

Many settings employ both PAs and NPs, posting the same job descriptions for both and utilizing the same mechanism for physician collaboration and supervision. Thus the functions of PAs and NPs within the same specialty (e.g., family practice) and in the same setting may be very similar. Other similarities can be noted in the goals of some programs, particularly those targeting underserved populations, and in components of curriculums (e.g., management of patients with chronic disease or skills in taking a patient history or performing a physical examination). These similarities are more obvious within a given specialty, such as between a primary care PA and a family NP.

There are also numerous differences between and within these professions, which include differences in practitioner backgrounds and educational, legal, professional, and political considerations. With regard to background, NPs are licensed registered nurses, whereas PAs enter training with a variety of backgrounds, some being nurses. The educational preparation of PAs was developed initially by physicians, and most training programs have been established within, or with strong attachments to, medical schools. The majority of programs provide baccalaureate degrees. Clinical training is similar to that of medical students, consisting of rotating clerkships combined with clinical didactic courses. On the other hand, educational programs for NPs were developed, for the most part, within schools of nursing. While there are very few certificate programs remaining, the majority of NP education occurs at the master's level. NP students build on their skills in advanced nursing practice. The National Organization of Nurse Practitioner Faculties (NONPF) has developed guidelines for curriculums in several domains that include components in research and administration and that set a useful national standard. This document recommends multiple pathways for attaining skills and advanced degree prerequisites.[9]

There has been considerable discussion about differences in the educational preparation of PAs and NPs. One common, somewhat confusing, reference describes PA education as the "medical model" and NP education as the "nursing model." A careful examination of curriculums for both types of programs reveals many similarities in content. For example, although different labels may be used, such as "behavioral science" in PA programs and "psychosocial studies" in NP programs, the emphasis within both of these components includes the development of sensitive skills in taking histories from clients, formulating plans, conducting education, and advocating empowerment. Unique to a master's program, whether PA or NP, is a research component. A nursing program includes nursing theory, whereas PA programs do not. Also, PA programs tend to have a multidisciplinary faculty, while in most NP programs the majority of didactic and most clinical training is conducted by nursing faculty.

There are obvious differences in specialty training programs within and across disciplines. There are accredited programs for PAs—in such areas as primary care, women's health, or neonatal or surgical specialties—that differ in content. Similarly, there are numerous NP program specialties (e.g., family, adult, obstetrics-gynecology, pediatrics, and geriatrics.

Each discipline has its own educational organization, accrediting body, and certification procedures. The Association of Physician Assistant Programs (APAP) is the organization of PA educational programs. The Committee on Allied Health Education and Accreditation (CAHEA) of the American Medical Association is the agency responsible for accrediting PA programs. The American Nurses Credentialing Center sponsors examinations in several specialties for NP national certification. However, states vary considerably in licensure requirements for NP practice. For example, California does not require national certification for practice.

There are legal differences in licensure requirements, reimbursement, and state practice acts. While these factors differ substantially from state to state, generally speaking, PAs practice under some provision of the states' medical practice acts and under the direct supervision of physicians. NPs, on the other hand, practice under nursing licensure and provisions made in nurse practice acts. Provisions are made for collaborative practice where the functions of nursing practice and medical practice overlap.

Professional differences are important to recognize. NPs identify with their nursing backgrounds. Each discipline also has its own professional organizations. For PAs, the most widely recognized is the American Academy of Physician Assistants; for NPs, there are multiple national organizations in the various specialties, all of which have representatives to the National Alliance of Nurse Practitioners.

Finally, there are political differences, generated by the disparate origins and unfortunate beginnings in antagonism and conflict between organized medicine and nursing as well as by the assumptions of the educational programs. Political differences are accentuated locally where there is competition for employment sites or regarding state legislative issues, such as privileges for practice, reimbursement, or prescribing. Even within the PA or NP discipline these sensitivities exist. An awareness of these sensitivities is critical in working with PAs and NPs in the same setting. Acknowledging similarities where they exist (e.g., in goals or purposes) and respecting differences are necessary parts of any collaborative efforts.

In some regions, such as California, there is evidence of educational and professional collaboration between the two disciplines.[4] For nearly a decade the California council on NP and PA programs, an organization of all NP and PA program directors, met regularly to pursue common political interests toward improving legislation. Practicing PAs and NPs have developed local professional organizations for purposes of continuing education, peer support, and local political strength. Recently the PA and NP state professional organizations agreed to exchange and publish information in each other's newsletters. Another example of collaboration is the professional journal *Clinician Review*. Cofounded by a group of PAs and NPs, the journal's editorial board comprises representatives of both groups.

Areas of role conflict

Nurses obviously may be employed in any of the settings in which PAs practice—the most common being hospitals. The interaction between nurses and PAs in settings of common practice is that of parallel figures in either patient care or an assisting function. Legally, the PA is an agent of the physician. She or he may be ordering procedures, treatments, or prescriptions on behalf of the physician. Nurses, then, interact with the PA much as they would with the physician, as comembers of the health care team. Periodically there is conflict in the intersection of their roles. The conflict may be the result of personalities, unclear institutional policies or state regulation and practice acts, or a misunderstanding of roles due to previous bias or lack of exposure. Where role conflict occurs, it can be related to issues associated with gender, competition for salaries or jobs, or confusion about local or state professional policies or laws.

Gender issues

The number of women entering the PA profession has increased substantially. There were no women PAs in 1967, and in recent years they represent a majority of PA student enrollment and graduate practitioners. The PA movement evolved along with a national women's movement characterized by many women reentering careers or broadening their career options. However, for the first decade the PA profession was dominated by men. Thus both subtle and overt male-female issues are evident as their roles intersect. More subtle are issues about style. For example, the PA profession has its roots in medicine, a profession still dominated by men. Men tend to be more comfortable working or leading in a solo style. Women more typically have learned a participatory, collaborative style in work and decision making. Such differences in style may create conflict when male PAs interact with female nurses in the care and management of patients. Perhaps as the gender gaps lessen in these health professions, such perceptions will be mitigated.

A more specific issue concerns salary differences. Some nurses resent the fact that PAs earn higher salaries. Since salary scales for any profession vary considerably—based on geographical location, number of hours, on-call hours, amount of experience, amount of responsibility assumed in the practice, and other factors—issues about salary have been difficult to study.

In medicine and the PA profession, it is known that salaries for men have been and continue to be higher than salaries for women. However, it is unclear whether this relates to a choice by women to work fewer hours or to actual gender discrimination. Salary discrepancies appear to have lessened as nurses have organized and advanced their issues and achieved recognition within hospital systems.

Competition issues. Competition is usually the issue underpinning arguments against increased utilization of PAs. This issue is often veiled in arguments about concerns for patient safety or quality of care. When this occurs, the issues are often muddled and not substantiated by good data. Competition between professional interests can be manifested in many ways, such as in work settings or policies.

Because PAs and NPs are often hired in the same settings, either group of professionals may find themselves competing for jobs. This is particularly an issue if an area is dominated by one group, jobs are limited, and the other professional group seeks employment. Physicians and employers who indicate strong preference for one group over another usually do so because they are familiar with one and not the other. In settings where PAs and NPs have been trained together with common goals, a sense of mutual respect develops and competition is not a professional issue.[4]

The reimbursement system for health care services has contributed to competition between PAs and NPs with a confusing array of policies. For example, the federal Medicare program developed separate policies for the reimbursement of PAs and NPs. There is also unevenness in the policies of individual states toward PAs and NPs in the implementation of Medicaid programs.

Issues of local or state policy. The introduction of a new type of health professional or someone new to the role in an established health care system generates uncertainty and confusion unless there are clear policies within the institution and state practice acts. Both PAs and NPs have suffered from lack of policies that facilitate their practices. This creates confusion for nurses. For example, in one state, the nurse practice act specifies that nurses are to take orders from physicians, dentists, podiatrists, or clinical psychologists. Nurses who function in hospitals have thus questioned the authority of PAs to give orders. A number of states have clarified the issue by having attorneys general issue opinions about state regulations supporting PAs giving orders. In one state, the nurse practice act was revised and no longer lists the individual professions from which nurses can take orders.

Some nurses, particularly those in hospitals, view PAs as inhibiting their communication with physicians. PAs act as agents of the physician. Where there are good communications between the PA, nurse, and physician, and clearly defined protocols and institutional policies, these problems are less likely to occur.

Challenges

PAs are well established in our nation's health care system. PAs and nurses share common goals in the prevention of disease and the caring for and curing of patients. In many regions, one group of nurses, that of nurse practitioners, has recognized this and developed collaborative relationships where common professional needs and interests are evident. Hopefully conditions of mutual respect among these health professions will continue to be fostered by each profession's acknowledging and valuing the different perspectives and skills that the other can contribute to the health care team.

REFERENCES

1. American Academy of Physician Assistants. (1990). *General census data survey on physician assistants.* Unpublished survey.
2. Bliss, A., & Cohen, E. D. (1977). *The new health professionals: Nurse practitioners and physician assistants.* Germantown, Md: Aspen Systems.
3. Fowkes, V., & McKay, D. (1990). A profile of California's physician assistants. *Western Journal of Medicine, 153,* 328-329.
4. Fowkes, V., O'Hara-Devereaux, M., & Andrus, L. H. (1979, October). A cooperative education program for nurse practitioners/physician assistants. *Journal of Medical Education, 54,* 781-787.
5. Gara, N. (1989, July-August). State laws for physician assistants. *Journal of the American Academy of Physician Assistants, 2,* 303-313.
6. Oliver, D. (1991, May). *Seventh annual report on physician assistant educational programs in the United States, 1990-91* (p. 46). Alexandria, Va: Association of Physician Assistant Programs.
7. Schaft, G., & Cawley, J. (1987). *The physician assistant in a changing health care environment.* Rockville, Md: Aspen.
8. U.S. Congress, Office of Technology Assessment. (1986, December). *Nurse practitioners, physician assistants, and certified nurse-midwives: A policy analysis* (OTA-HCS-37). Washington, D.C.: U.S. Government Printing Office.
9. Zimmer, P. A., Brykczynski, K., Martin, A. C., Newberry, Y. G., Price, M. J., & Warren, B. (1992). *Advanced nursing practice: Nurse practitioner curriculum guidelines.* Unpublished final report by the National Organization of Nurse Practitioner Faculties, Education Committee.

CHAPTER 85

Entering collegial relationships

The demise of nurse as victim

ADELE W. PIKE

Scholars of women's development have observed a uniqueness in women's ways of thinking, of knowing, of relating to others, and of being.[4,8,12] They refer to this uniqueness as "women's voice." Their metaphor of voice is borrowed here and applied to nurses. "Nurses' voice" thus refers to the unique perspectives and contributions nurses bring to patient care. Disturbingly, this voice is often silent in acute care settings. That this voice is frequently inaudible is seriously demoralizing to nurses. For patients the consequences are more grievous, as the silence denies them the integration of the nursing perspective into the care they receive.

The factors involved in silencing—in censoring—nurses affect the way nurses define their professional self-concept, often leading them to perceive themselves as helpless victims. Most of the factors arose from cultural and sociological mores that, despite being outdated and no longer applicable in present day health care, are deeply etched in memory. Despite the persistence of their legend, the power of these traditions to silence nurses should be rendered invalid.

For this to occur, nurses must appreciate that they are now presented with opportunities for choice—the choice to remain silent or to become equal colleagues in the health care team. This chapter presents an analysis of the factors that suppress nurses' voice and of the significance of the choice nurses make with regard to making their voices heard. In discussing the implica-

tions of this choice, critical incidents[5] depicting patients and families facing ethical dilemmas will be used in order to contrast two divergent outcomes that result from the different ways in which nurses choose to exercise their voice.

SILENCING OF VOICE

Numerous forces affect nurses' voice. Many of them are external, such as the historical role of nurse as handmaiden, the hierarchical structure of health care organizations, the perceived authority and directives of physicians, hospital policy, and the threat of disciplinary or legal action. Equally plentiful are internal constraints. Characteristics such as role confusion, lack of professional confidence, timidity, fear, insecurity, or sense of inferiority lead nurses to choose silence as often as external forces impose silence on them.[15,23]

The internal and external constraints that silence nurses are deeply rooted in history, and their influence is pervasive. They have evolved as integral aspects of the socialization of health care providers and the organization of health care systems. So tightly woven are these constraints in the fabric of health care delivery that their influence has been mistakenly accepted as fact and they have been blindly accorded the authority to define who nurses are and what nurses do.[15,23]

These internal and external constraints inflict wounds on nurses' professional self-esteem. These wounds deepen and expand the innate capacity for self-doubt that nurses, like all individuals, have. Having been wounded, nurses experience great difficulty believing in their own capacity to contribute to patient care as autonomous, vital, and equal professionals. Their ambitions and aspirations are stifled. Their vision

The critical incidents published in this paper initially appeared in: Pike, A. W. (1991). Moral outrage and moral discourse in nurse-physician collaboration. *Journal of Professional Nursing, 7*(6), 351-363. Used with permission.

The author wishes to acknowledge the assistance of Jane Corrigan Wandel, RN, MS, in the preparation of this chapter.

grows myopic, and they fail to recognize opportunities for self-advancement. Such an inclination establishes a pattern in which nurses perceive themselves as inferior and unable to change their lot.[18]

This poor professional self-concept sabotages any possibility of collaboration between nurses and other care providers, as it identifies nurses as embattled victims and customarily marks physicians as their antagonists. Such a relationship urges an adversarial stance in which the victims place the onus of responsibility for the problematical relationship on their perceived aggressors rather than accepting responsibility and accountability for who they are and what they want to be.[18]

The stance of victimization is very seductive. There are many incentives for maintaining the role of victim. Victims are perceived as innocent, and by assigning the locus of their control to external forces they avoid responsibility and accountability. Victims are spared the stresses of change, because in the matrix of victimization it is the oppressor who must change in order for the victim's condition to be improved.[6,18]

There can be no argument that, in the past, nurses were the victims of oppression and were made to suffer the subjugation of physicians and hospital administration. They had no choice but to be exploited as conveniences. Today nurses must grapple with the memory of this exploitation. While the memory exerts a dangerously powerful influence, described earlier in terms of internal and external constraints, present-day nurses have more opportunities for choice. The maturation of the profession and advances in nursing education, administration, practice, and research are unraveling the traditional socialization of health care providers and the culture of health care organizations. Consequently nurses have, with increasing frequency, a choice. They can either carry the historical baggage of past injustice and let it define their professional self as victim; or they can leave the baggage behind and move on to define themselves as equal members of the health care team.[6,18]

This choice is not easy given the unconscious incentives to remain a victim.[6] Defining oneself as an equal colleague means being responsible and accountable—stressful, difficult, and frightening burdens. Being equal means overcoming self-doubt and timidity. It requires relentless effort to overcome the internal and external constraints that inhibit the voice, the aspirations, and the talents of nurses. While the choice is difficult, silence is an unacceptable alternative.

BEING A COLLEAGUE

Part of the difficulty for nurses in defining themselves as colleagues of other health professionals, particularly physicians, is that so little is known about how best to operationalize the role.[2,14,17,19,20] Equal colleagueship with physicians involves entering into a collaborative relationship that is characterized by mutual trust and respect and an understanding of the perspectives each partner contributes. Collaboration involves a bond, a union, a depth of caring about one another and the relationship. The colleagueship this breeds obliges individuals to put aside the feelings of interprofessional competition and antagonism that are rooted in history, so that the work and expertise of all participants may be integrated and patient care maximized.[2,3,15,22]

Colleagues openly acknowledge that they share a common goal: the health and comfort of patients in their care. They recognize their interdependence and, accordingly, share responsibility and accountability for patient outcomes. Collegial relationships are safe. Each participant accepts the other as someone who is well-intentioned and trying to do his or her best. When conflict arises, it is addressed at its source and not escalated up a hierarchical chain of authority.[2,10,16]

Colleagueship has many characteristics of a caring relationship, as defined by the ethic of care (M.C. Cooper, personal communication, 1992). As colleagues, individuals attend to each other's growth and development, protect each other from belittlement, and enhance each other's professional dignity.[7,11,13,21]

Incorporating the concept of colleague into one's professional identity is a developmental process that requires critical self-reflection. In order to collaborate with another, a nurse must understand and value the unique perspective nursing offers. Being a colleague requires a breadth of clinical experience that solidifies professional confidence. Nurses who define themselves as colleagues must develop a language that allows them to articulate their unique perspective to nonnurses so that that perspective will be apprehended. This definition of professional self also requires the maturity to recognize the incentives to remain victimized, and to reflect on how one might be seduced by them. Additionally one must understand the historical and cultural roots of the internal and external constraints imposed on nurses and appreciate that their influence can quickly subjugate nurses at a time when there is more opportunity for advancement than ever before. Nurses who choose to define themselves as colleagues must overcome these constraints and learn to manage their backward pull.

Operationalizing the concept of professional self as equal colleague frees nurses from the internal constraints that contribute to the silencing of their voice. Once the influence of these internal forces is curtailed, nurses can question, challenge, and overcome external constraints. Colleagueship is difficult work fraught with anxiety, confusion, and frustration; but it is also a very fruitful enterprise offering tremendous promise and benefits to both nurses and patients.[15]

CONSEQUENCES OF CHOICE

The way in which nurses choose to construe their professional selves has significant implications for patient care, as well as for nurses' role and satisfaction. The consequences of their choice are particularly dramatic in the care of patients and families in the throes of ethical uncertainty. Consider the following critical incident involving Mr. S. This incident describes a dilemma not unfamiliar to nurses, and it leaves powerful images of morally unacceptable care.

Mr. S. was a 72-year-old man admitted to the hospital from a nursing home. The reason for this admission was failure to thrive and a severe infection. On admission he was frail, cachectic, and minimally responsive, with vital signs of: temperature 101.8F, heart rate 160 beats per minute in atrial fibrillation (AF), respiratory rate of 28 breaths per minute, and an unstable blood pressure. His blood tests suggested severe dehydration.

Mr. S.'s peripheral veins were small and fragile, and repeated attempts to start an intravenous [IV] line in his arms were unsuccessful. A line was finally established in his foot, and IV fluids and antibiotics were begun.

Long before his admission, Mr. S. had made it known that he did not want "heroic measures" taken to prolong his life in the event of a grave illness. It was documented and well known that "Do Not Resuscitate" (DNR) applied in his case.

We were unable to determine the source of his infection. Even gentle attempts to provide hydration exacerbated his congestive heart failure and AF. His kidneys failed, and his lungs, damaged by years of smoking, were barely able to meet the increased demands of his illness. It seemed clear that Mr. S. was dying. His nurses worked to minimize any pain or distress he might suffer during his terminal illness.

On his fourth hospital day, Mr. S.'s IV infiltrated and another peripheral IV line could not be placed. On the following day, the physicians involved in Mr. S.'s care felt obligated to establish a central IV line, since, in the absence of peripheral IV access, Mr. S. was not receiving any fluid or antibiotics. At the time, no one openly questioned this decision, despite the fact that his nurses considered such an invasive, aggressive intervention to be wrong in the context of Mr. S.'s illness and wishes.

During the central line insertion Mr. S. suffered a pneumothorax, and an emergency chest tube was inserted. At this point he exhibited notable signs of pain and discomfort, which had been absent during the earlier days of his admission.

Mr. S.'s family was called, and they were distressed that invasive interventions had been carried out. They requested that no further aggressive treatment be used in his care.

Mr. S. was given oxygen and morphine for comfort. He died less than 2 days later, but continued to show signs of respiratory distress throughout this period.

The nursing staff agonized over the pain and suffering he experienced. We began to place blame, and among ourselves talked of the callousness, aggressiveness, and insensitivity of physicians . . . of their ability "only to cure, not to care." We felt anger, frustration, pain, remorse, and guilt.

The story of Mr. S. is a story of moral failure and moral outrage that resulted in large measure, from the silencing of nurses' voice. Mr. S.'s nurses encountered a moral dilemma as they cared for him. The dilemma was whether to place a central line and continue hydration or to forgo the line and allow him to die. Faced with this dilemma, the nurses used moral reasoning—theoretical, experiential, and contextual—to reach a decision about how to respond to Mr. S.'s predicament. They saw Mr. S. as being at the end of his life and wanted to prevent his pain and suffering.

Mr. S.'s physicians, faced with the same dilemma, reached a different decision. Tragically there was no discourse, and the authority and directives of the physicians upstaged the nurses' plan. The physicians' action was seen as unquestionable, and this perception served as a constraint to the nurses who had legitimate concerns about Mr. S.'s suffering. The physicians' response effectively (but unnecessarily) censored the nursing perspective.

It is true that the physicians acted in an authoritative manner and never solicited nursing advice. But they had accomplices in censorship. The nurses caring for Mr. S. chose to be silent: "no one openly questioned this decision." The words used by the nurse reporting this incident suggest the unspoken thoughts that she and her peers were disturbed, even horrified, by the physicians' decision. Yet no nurse spoke up.

The nurses responded to their silencing with moral outrage. An emotional response to the inability to carry out moral choices or decisions, moral outrage is characterized by demoralizing frustration, anger, disgust, and a sense of powerlessness.[15] The nurses were furious about the moral failure of Mr. S.'s care, yet they only blamed the physicians, failing to recognize their contribution to this tragedy. Had any one of Mr. S.'s nurses defined herself as an equal colleague, instead of as a helpless victim, nurses' voice would have been heard, moral outrage would have been averted, and moral discourse would have ensued. In the end, Mr. S. most likely would have received more morally appropriate care.

In contrast, the following case of Mrs. H. illustrates the morally acceptable care that resulted from a nurse's choice to see herself as an integral and equal colleague of physicians.

Mrs. H. had been a healthy, active 65-year-old woman until she suffered massive intracerebral bleeding. She showed severe neurological impairment, with only occasional and minimal responses to noxious stimuli. The prognosis for neurological recovery was grim. Mrs. H. had prepared a handwritten statement 2 years before at the time of her husband's death from cancer. It was a request that her life not be sustained in the event of an irreversible illness or injury. A photocopy of this statement hung on the bulletin board in her room.

Mrs. H.'s children, however, expressed their desire to pursue every treatment possible. They were adamant that they wanted their mother resuscitated in the event of a cardiac arrest. Mrs. H's physician felt obliged to comply with her children's wishes. I understood and respected his feeling of obligation, but found it morally conflicting. I suspect he did also.

Mrs. H. was deteriorating daily. Aggressive, invasive care continued. I had to leave the room more than once during invasive procedures due to the assaultive nature of the treatments. I saw them [as being] clearly in opposition to Mrs. H.'s wishes.

I spoke with her children and physician each day. Although I could see and appreciate the agony each was experiencing in light of the massive ethical issues facing them, it was if were all speaking different dialects of the same language. We needed a three-way conversation to help us understand the perspectives each of us brought to the situation.

I arranged a conference during which the patient's family, [the] physician, and I reviewed Mrs. H.'s condition, prognosis, and elaborated care plan options. Her family spoke of their grief, and their feelings that they would be abandoning their mother if invasive treatments were discontinued. The physician and I explained that we believed that pursuing a less invasive plan did not constitute abandonment, and that their mother never would be abandoned. We discussed how we could provide care for her in accordance with her wishes, and what the specifics of that care would be. In the end Mrs. H.'s family decided to change the aim of care and focus on keeping her comfortable until she died.

This is a difficult and poignant story. There was clearly a dilemma, and clearly conflict. At an earlier point in her professional development, Mrs. H.'s nurse might have taken on the role of helpless victim and remained silent. The conflict would have simmered and bred moral outrage. Instead this nurse chose to see herself as an equal colleague, thereby accepting responsibility and accountability for her moral obligation to facilitate discourse among all involved parties. In doing so she not only avoided her own moral outrage but also transformed the meaning of the situation from conflict to miscommunication. Her actions prompted a discussion that allowed all perspectives to be integrated into Mrs. H.'s care. Her exercise of nurses' voice changed the nature of care for this patient, making it more consistent with the patient's wishes and comfortable for her family.

CONCLUSION

These critical incidents strongly suggest that the choice a nurse makes about how she defines her professional self affects not only her morale but also the nature of care patients receive. When a nurse identifies herself as the victim of deeply rooted internal and external constraints, she increases the probability that her voice will be silenced. The stance of victimization can lead to feelings of moral outrage and denies patients the benefits of the nursing perspective. However, when a nurse makes the choice to envision herself as a colleague, participating in patient care as an equal, she seizes opportunities for professional fulfillment while affording patients the benefits of integrated care.

The responsibility and accountability for defining oneself as a colleague resides in individual nurses. Perhaps it does not seem fair that nurses—because they have inherited internal and external constraints to their professional identity, autonomy, and aspirations—now have to rescue themselves from subjugation. Perhaps it would seem fairer if those whose predecessors had exploited nurses made concessions. Fairness aside, history shows that members of dominant groups do not, in general, offer restitution to those whom they have exploited.[18] While growing numbers of physicians are to be commended for enlightened attitudes and behaviors, nurses will only grow increasingly frustrated by waiting for past injustices to be repaid.

While the issue of fairness will always linger, it is, ironically, fortunate that compensation is not forthcoming. For the possibility of compensation keeps the responsibility for collegiality with physicians and leads to the familiar slogan among nurses, "we're ready to be colleagues just as soon as the doctors change." Making colleagueship dependent on changes among physicians maintains nurses as victims; it asks nonnurses to exercise nurses' voice. The only one who can declare herself an equal colleague is the individual nurse, and to do so she must emancipate herself from internal and external constraints.

Nurses' choice to define themselves as colleagues, as full-fledged vital members of the health care team, holds great moral significance for nursing and for patient care. In making this choice, nurses take the opportunity to overcome subjugation and to assume a stance of empowerment. By defining themselves as equal colleagues, nurses initiate a move on their own behalf and on behalf of their patients to make their voice audible.[6] Such a professional self-concept is a prerequisite for, as well as a driving force in, the development of collaborative relationships with physicians and other health care providers. Collaboration unifies the contributions of all those involved in patient care, making that care more efficient, effective, and comprehensive.[1,9,15,17] By choosing to make their voices heard, nurses afford patients not only the advantages of the nursing perspective but also the full benefit of integrated care. The promise this holds for advancing the care delivered to patients and families cannot be underestimated.

REFERENCES

1. Aiken, L. H. (1990). Charting the future of hospital nursing. *Image: The Journal of Nursing Scholarship, 22*(2), 72-78.
2. Alpert, H. B., Goldman, L. D., Kilroy, C. M., & Pike, A. W. (1992). 7 Gryzmish: Toward an understanding of collaboration. *Nursing Clinics of North America, 27*(1), 47-59.
3. Aradine, C. R., & Pridham, K. F. (1973). Model for collaboration. *Nursing Outlook, 21*(10), 655-657.
4. Belenky, M. F., Clinchy, B. M., Goldberger, N. R., & Tarule, J. M. (1986). *Women's ways of knowing.* Boston: Basic Books.
5. Benner, P. (1984). *From novice to expert.* Menlo Park, Calif: Addison-Wesley.
6. Cooper, M. C. (1991). Response to moral outrage and moral discourse in nurse-physician collaboration. *Journal of Professional Nursing, 7*(6), 362-363.
7. Gadnow, S. A. (1985). Nurse and patient: The caring relationship. In A. H. Bishop & J. R. Scudder (Eds.), *Caring, curing, coping: Nurse-physician-patient relationships.* University, Ala.: University of Alabama Press.
8. Gilligan, C. (1982). *In a different voice.* Cambridge, Mass: Harvard University Press.
9. Knaus, W. A., Draper, E. A., Wagner, D. P., & Zimmerman, J. E. (1986). An evaluation of outcome from intensive care in major medical centers. *Annals of Internal Medicine, 104*(3), 410-418.
10. Mangiardi, J. R., & Pellegrino, E. D. (1992). Collegiality: What is it? *Bulletin of the New York Academy of Medicine, 68*(2), 292-296.
11. Mayeroff, M. (1971). *On caring.* New York: HarperCollins.
12. Miller, J. B. (1976). *Toward a new psychology of women.* Boston: Beacon Press.
13. Noddings, N. (1984). *Caring: A feminine approach to ethics and moral education.* Los Angeles: University of California Press.
14. Petro, J. A. (1992). Collegiality in history. *Bulletin of the New York Academy of Medicine, 68*(2), 286-291.
15. Pike, A. W. (1991). Moral outrage and moral discourse in nurse-physician collaboration. *Journal of Professional Nursing, 7*(6), 351-363.
16. Pike, A. W., McHugh, M., Canney, K., Miller, N., Reilly, P., & Seibert, C. P. (1993). A new architecture for quality assurance: Nurse-physician collaboration. *Journal of Nursing Care Quality, 7*(3), 1-8.
17. Prescott, P. A., & Bowen, S. A. (1985). Physician-nurse relationships. *Annals of Internal Medicine, 103*(127), 127-133.
18. Steele, S. (1990). *The content of our character.* New York: St. Martin's Press.
19. Stein, L. I. (1967). The doctor-nurse game. *Archives of General Psychiatry, 16*(6), 699-703.
20. Stein, L. I., Watts, D. T., & Howell, T. (1990). The doctor-nurse game revisited. *New England Journal of Medicine, 322*(8), 546-549.
21. Watson, J. (1988). *Nursing: Human science and human care.* New York: National League for Nursing.
22. Weiss, S. J., & Davis, H. P. (1985). Validity and reliability of the collaborative practice scales. *Nursing Research, 34*(5), 299-305.
23. Yarling, R. R., & McElmurry, B. J. (1986). The moral foundation of nursing. *Advances in Nursing Science, 8*(2), 63-73.

CHAPTER 86

Conflict and nursing professionalization

MARION JOHNSON

Conflict has been, and continues to be, a pervasive force affecting nursing's professional development. Longstanding conflicts about educational preparation for nurses and nurse-physician relationships are receiving renewed attention as nursing roles expand. Strategies to increase nurse autonomy and nurse satisfaction, such as differentiated practice and collaborative practice, require that these conflicts be addressed. New conflicts are being created as the health care system adapts to a rapidly changing environment. Cost containment, competition, and restructuring of health care organizations have given rise to (1) conflict created by differences in economic and professional values, that is, the need to economize versus the commitment to professional behavior,[2,33] and (2) conflict created by competition between and among professionals and corporate executives as roles are redefined and power redistributed.[2] As the largest but traditionally least powerful group of workers in health care, nursing is particularly vulnerable to the conflicts that accompany change and adaptation. How nursing responds to current conflicts within the profession and with other health care professions may well determine nursing's role in tomorrow's health care system.

Nursing's traditional response to conflict — prevention at all costs[3] — is nonproductive in today's health care setting. Many of today's conflicts, if prevented or avoided, can produce results that are dysfunctional for the individual, the organization, the profession, and the consumer. Neither nursing, health care organizations, nor the consumer will benefit if conflicts about the allocation of increasingly scarce resources, health care values, the expanding role of the professional nurse, the appropriate educational preparation for new roles, or the reallocation of power within the health care system are avoided. It has become increasingly important for nursing to confront and manage both its internal and external conflicts if nursing is to benefit from the changes taking place in health care.

The effective management of conflict requires an understanding of the dynamics of conflict and an appreciation of the benefits that can be derived from conflict. Although much has been written about conflict management, there is less information about the potential benefits of conflict for nursing or how conflict dynamics apply to the conflicts experienced by the profession and by individual nurses. Understanding is also hampered by the overabundance of theoretical perspectives on conflict and the paucity of empirical data.[4] This chapter will present an overview of conflict dynamics from a nursing perspective, with an emphasis on conditions that predispose to conflict and potential benefits of conflict, and will conclude with a discussion of issues related to the management of nursing conflicts.

CONFLICT DYNAMICS AND NURSING

Conflict can be viewed as a process developing over time and having predictable dynamics. Each conflict episode can be envisioned as consisting of five stages that need not proceed sequentially. The stages of a conflict episode are latent conflict (conditions), perceived conflict (cognition), felt conflict (affect), manifest conflict (behavior), and conflict aftermath (outcomes).[28] Conflict can also be analyzed in relation to the context in which it occurs. This perspective focuses on the structural and contextual factors that predispose to conflict and influence the way in which conflict is managed. Contextual factors can include predispositions or usual responses to conflict, social or environmental pressures, incentives to manage conflict, and rules and procedures that govern conflict management.[41] Combining these perspectives can provide a model (Fig. 86-1)

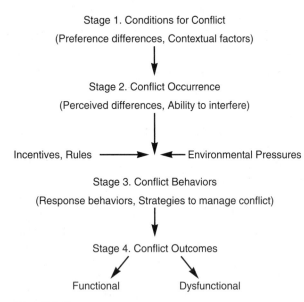

Fig. 86-1. Conflict and nursing professionalization.

for describing intergroup and organizational conflict and for analyzing current conditions that contribute to nursing conflicts.

Conflict conditions

Preference differences can occur when members of a group disagree about goals, values, facts, or methods of achieving goals. Work conflicts experienced by new graduates have been shown to arise from differences between practice values in the work setting and practice values learned in the educational setting.[21,38] Differences have also been demonstrated between values held by nurse administrators and faculty teaching nursing administration.[42] Additionally, the diversity of educational programs preparing nurses may promote different value sets among nurse practitioners. In a study of preferences of workers in a psychiatric hospital, findings showed a high level of conflicting preferences among nurses and demonstrated little homogeneity in values among nurses as a group.[14] These types of conflict serve to highlight the fact that nurses as a group do not possess strong, discipline-specific values.

As hospitals become increasingly business oriented, value conflicts can occur between the humanistic values long held by service-oriented organizations and health care professionals and the cost-effective, product-oriented values of business.[33] The potential also exists for value conflicts between nurse administrators oriented to business values and responsible for organizational goals, and clinical nurses oriented to holistic patient care and responsible for individual patient outcomes. As the way in which health care organizations conduct business changes, nurses are having to analyze how professional and business values can be clarified to manage conflicts and promote goal agreement.

Common task and resource dependencies that require coordination are correlated with higher levels of organizational conflict.[43,48] When a high degree of task dependency is coupled with differences in power and autonomy, the potential for conflict is increased. For example, client care requires the interaction of multiple health care professionals, but differences in power between physicians and nurses have traditionally resulted in nurses' using accommodating rather than cooperative responses. Nursing has a history of dependency on physician practice that has created a relationship characterized by a "pattern of physician dominance and nurse deference, with increasing conflict between the two groups."[29] As the knowledge base of nursing practice has developed, both the profession and individual nurses have sought increased autonomy and expanded roles—actions that augment existing role conflicts between nurses and physicians.

Differences within nursing and with other health professionals about the allocation of scarce financial and human resources continue to be potential sources of conflict for nurse administrators. Because nursing comprises the largest group of workers in most health care organizations, it is the group most vulnerable when organizational resources decline. Changes in nursing care delivery structures to contain costs and use fewer registered nurses are forcing nursing to redefine professional practice roles, often adding to the already-existing role conflicts in nursing.

Complex organizations characterized by nonuniform tasks, high levels of specialization and differentiation, and a high degree of interdependency experience higher levels of conflict.[10,12,15,27] Health care organizations, although characterized by task variability, have traditionally used formalized rules and procedures to control nursing practice—methods that can produce conflict in settings that rely on the application of professional knowlege to provide personalized services. Conflicts can arise between the policies of the organization and the actions of individual nurses as they interact with clients and other professionals. The use of practice standards rather than rules and procedures to control quality can decrease the potential for this type of conflict while increasing the autonomous practice of nurses.

The rapid growth in technology use and the expansion of nursing knowledge have fostered nursing specialization and provided additional opportunities for conflict; for example, conflicts are precipitated when nurses are expected to float to a unit in which nursing knowledge and skills differ.[40] Additionally, high degrees of horizontal and vertical differentiation continue to exist in health care organizations and in nursing departments despite trends toward decentralization. Either type of differentiation can be a source of role ambiguity, role conflict, and conflict about the allocation of authority and power—conflicts common in nursing. Differentiation can also make it more difficult to adjust to changing roles, as with the introduction of nurse case managers in acute care settings. Creation of these positions provides opportunities for vertical role conflicts within nursing and lateral role conflicts with other professionals who view case management as part of their role.

Varied degrees of conflict can be expected to occur as traditionally hierarchical nursing departments decentralize decision making. Studies indicate that decentralized decision making is related to increased conflict.[48] Decentralization, in addition to altering roles, increases the number of individuals involved in decision making with the possibility that group members will become more aware of their differences. However, the long-term effects of this conflict can be positive if members are allowed to clarify their values and can agree on goals that are acceptable to all. Decentralization also has the potential to decrease conflict if it results in less complex units and departments. For example, having all workers on a unit responsible to the nurse manager reduces opportunities for interdepartmental conflicts. Despite the potential for precipitating conflict, decentralization of authority as well as responsibility can be an effective, long-term method for resolving conflicts about the goals, functions, and roles of nursing.

Conflict occurrence

Changes taking place in the health care system have been used to highlight conditions that predispose to conflicts involving nursing. However, these conditions alone will not produce conflict; perceived differences and the ability to interfere must be present for a conflict episode to develop. A conflict occurrence begins when group members perceive interpersonal differ-

ences about issues important to them. It is not necessary that actual differences exist; it is the perception of differences that initiates the conflict. In addition to perceived differences, conflict requires the opportunity to interfere with the goals or actions of others; one participant's actions must be able to interfere with the desired outcomes of the other participant.[4]

Conflict behaviors

Conflict behaviors include expressions of affect as well as the actions employed by individuals or groups in response to perceived differences. Behaviors commonly identified in the literature include avoidance, accommodation, competition, compromise, collaboration, and unilateral action. It is generally suggested that the response be chosen to match the conflict situation. However, research suggests that nurse managers in various settings tend to reuse the same strategy rather than adjust behavior to the situation.[3,23,47] In general, nurse managers in these studies used avoidance and compromise behaviors more frequently than managers in other disciplines;[3] these are behaviors often used when power differences exist between the conflict participants.

Conflict outcomes

Outcomes of conflict can be functional or dysfunctional for individuals and organizations. The result will depend on the type of issue, the structural components of the situation, and the strategies chosen to manage the conflict. Of these, the most critical is how the conflict is managed.[12]

Because functional outcomes have not always been recognized, management interventions continue to be influenced by past orientations to conflict. The traditionalist philosophy dominant in organizational thought until the mid-1940s viewed conflict as a destructive force that interfered with the ideal organizational climate of stability and harmony.[13] Emphasis was placed on preventing, eliminating, or suppressing conflict. The human relations school of thought, prominent in the late 1940s and early 1950s, recognized the existence of conflict but continued to assign it a negative role in organizations.[13] Emphasis was placed on resolving conflict. For both of these positions, conflict represented a management failure. For the traditionalist, conflict was a failure in planning and controlling; for the behavioralist, conflict was a failure of leadership.[27] For both, conflict was seen as an organizational liability rather than a potential for benefit.

By the 1960s a more positive view of organizational conflict began to emerge. It was suggested that conflict could increase group cohesion and group morale,[19] improve work relations,[18] and motivate group members[43]—effects that should promote individual and group productivity. The interactionist view of conflict proposed by Robbins[31] was a radical departure from previous approaches to organizational conflict. Robbins identified conflict as a necessary component of organizational growth and placed emphasis on using conflict as a resource. Today the idea that conflict can promote creativity and produce change, important prerequisites of organizational growth, has gained increased recognition.[10,30] More effective problem solving has been identified as another constructive function of conflict.[34,35] By allowing divergent interests and beliefs to emerge, conflict can force decision makers to define the problem, examine conflicting opinions, and ideally arrive at more creative solutions.

Although benefits of conflict are now recognized, there is little empirical evidence supporting this perspective. One study[8] that looked at conflict in hospitals found benefits consistent with those described in the literature. Conflict was found to stimulate innovation and change, motivate individuals and groups to resolve differences, and promote the most efficient reallocation of resources.

Strategies chosen to manage conflict strongly influence the outcomes, making it important to know how nurse managers view conflict outcomes. If they perceive conflict as having functional outcomes, they are more likely to seek management strategies that will produce these outcomes. Both positive and negative effects of conflict were identified by nurse administrators in a study by Myrtle and Glogow.[26] Positive outcomes of conflict were identified in 51% of the responses; however, the negative aspects of conflict were higher (176 responses) than the positive aspects (167 responses) when considering the effect on people rather than on task. The positive "people" outcomes identified in the study included increased self-awareness, individual growth, release of tension, increased motivation, team building, and increased participation and group interaction. The positive "task" outcomes were increased task achievement and improved problem resolution.

A descriptive study[17] examining nurse administrators' perceptions of the benefits of conflict in the context of individual and organizational characteristics produced similar findings. The sample included nurse administrators in top management positions in schools of nursing in institutions of higher education (deans) and departments of nursing in teaching hospitals (directors). Questionnaires were mailed to 834 nurse administrators and 480 usable questionnaires were returned, for a response rate of 57.5%.

A summated rating scale was used to examine nurse administrators' perceptions of the benefits of conflict in their work settings. The scale was designed to measure five potential functions of conflict identified in the literature:

1. A unifying function measured as increased group cohesion
2. A group-preserving function measured as the prevention of accumulated hostility
3. An integrative function measured as group stability
4. A growth function measured as innovation, creativity, and change
5. A problem-solving function measured as improved problem solving

Four items, also derived from the literature, were used to measure each function. All items were written as positive statements—for example, increases trust among members, prevents the accumulation of hostility, promotes accomodation between groups. Four choices were provided for each item: strongly agree, agree, disagree, and strongly disagree.

Respondents chose the "agree" and "disagree" categories more frequently than the "strongly agree" and "strongly disagree" categories; therefore, the categories were collapsed and the results are presented as "agree" or "disagree" (Table 86-1). Only one function—the unifying function—had a higher percentage of responses in the "disagree" category, and this occurred only with deans. The "disagree" category was chosen, for all functions, more frequently by deans than by directors. When t-tests were used to test for significant differences in the responses of deans and directors, the differences were statistically significant ($p < .05$) for all the functions except the preserving function.

Other variables measured in this study may account for these differences. Agreement with the functions of conflict was found to be significantly greater ($p < .01$) in organizations with over 100 staff members, predominantly hospitals ($n = 210$) rather than colleges ($n = 6$), and if the administrator indicated a high degree of decisional autonomy in her or his position ($p < .05$). Autonomy was rated higher by directors (74% high or very high) than by deans (48% high or very high).

Table 86-1 Perceptions of benefits of conflict

Function	Deans*		Directors		Both groups	
	Percentage agree	Percentage disagree	Percentage agree	Percentage disagree	Percentage agree	Percentage disagree
Unifying	43	57	57	43	50	50
Group preserving	55	45	59	41	57	43
Integrative	55	45	68	32	61.5	38.5
Growth	56	44	72	28	64	36
Problem solving	74	26	80	20	77	23

*Deans, $n = 259$; directors, $n = 221$; both groups, $n = 480$.

The findings of this study indicate that these administrators view outcomes of conflict related to growth and problem solving positively. These functions are, to a large extent, dependent on the creative, innovative, and analytical skills of staff. There was less agreement with the preserving and unifying functions of conflict, functions that are more dependent on interpersonal relationships. The findings are consistent with those of Myrtle and Glogow[26] in their study of nurse administrators' perceptions of conflict outcomes. This would suggest the need for nurse administrators to be aware of the potentially negative effects of conflict on group relations when selecting management strategies.

ISSUES IN THE MANAGEMENT OF NURSING CONFLICTS

Conflict can be a positive force for nursing if it is used to foster growth-producing change in the profession and in the organizations in which nurses work. However, nurses must manage conflict effectively to realize these benefits. Effective management requires an analysis of the issues involved and the situational components that assist or impede conflict resolution. This will allow the manager to select the behavioral strategies and/or structural interventions most appropriate for the situation.[40] Effective management also requires a positive attitude toward conflict. Recognizing the potential benefits to be gained from conflict can encourage nurses to develop management behaviors that foster positive outcomes. Conversely, recognizing the potential for destructive outcomes can alert nurses to outcomes that require careful monitoring when a conflict occurs.

Identifying the type of issue in a conflict situation is important for achieving positive outcomes because conflicts about values and ends are more divisive than conflicts about means. Values are deeply held beliefs less likely to be amenable to negotiation. When value differences are suspected, value clarification techniques will help to identify the differences and may allow participants to recognize that values can differ without being incompatible.[33] Incompatible values can often be managed by downgrading the conflict, that is, defining it as a problem in means rather than ends.[44] For example, well-defined criteria about admissions to an intensive care unit can be developed more readily if the decisions about admissions are defined as priority problems rather than value problems. When value conflicts cannot be downgraded or resolved, agreements must be reached about how the group will continue to function or action be taken even though it may fragment the group temporarily. The current trend to differentiate practice roles on the basis of educational preparation is one method of handling the entry-into-practice issue without resolving underlying value differences about nursing education.

A potentially destructive value difference confronting nursing is that between system values and professional values. Nursing continues to embody the values of caring, while the settings in which most nurses work value efficiency and technical care.[24] The result is frustration, defeat, and anxiety as nurses attempt to function in two different spheres, one of which—the system—is considered superior. Unless nursing is willing to abandon its values of caring, these values must be integrated into the health care system; and the responsibility to do this rests largely with nursing.[24]

The ability to recognize the potential for conflict is important for effective management. Understanding conditions that predispose to conflict makes it possible to predict likely conflicts. Conflicts often difficult to recognize are those that become institutionalized in an organization in the form of attitudes, beliefs, rituals, and other aspects of organizational culture.[25] These cultural patterns repress conflict by providing members with an accepted means of handling conflicting interests. The underlying conflicts become apparent only if rituals are analyzed or organizational roles changed. Management of institutionalized conflict, as with other institutionalized behaviors, requires changes in organizational structures or roles.

The essential role of power in conflict presents one of the more difficult issues in the management of nursing conflict. "Power is the medium through which conflicts of interest are ultimately resolved. Power influences who gets what, when, and how."[25] Historically, nursing power has been less than that of medicine or administration. As health care organizations realign their structures, nurse administrators have moved into executive positions; but changes in title may not be accompanied by increases in power and authority. Nurse executives who continue to feel overpowered in work relationships often experience work-related stress[5] and are unable to lead their department effectively.[32] For nursing to benefit from changes in the health care system, it is essential for nurse executives to develop the skills needed to acquire and use power.[32]

Although important, increasing executive power only is not sufficient for empowering nursing. Nurses at all levels must have the positional and decisional power necessary to control their own practice if nursing is to gain professional autonomy. Nursing's political interaction with medicine depends on its ability to speak with one voice, an ability that has been impeded by schisms between nurses of different levels.[39] Despite recent efforts to increase nurse autonomy, staff nurses continue to have little or no positional power[6,9] and their expert power is limited if their expertise is easily replaced.[45] However, a number of factors have positive implications for increasing staff nurse power. First is the nursing shortage that has focused attention on the value of nurses in health care.[16] Second is the continued recognition of the need to increase nurse autonomy as evidenced in the immense body of literature on empowerment, decentralization, and shared governance. And last, but of great importance, is the American Nurses Association bylaws change that provides for the inclusion of four staff nurses on its board of directors.[11]

Power also influences outcomes by limiting the management strategies available to participants of a conflict. Collaboration is the most effective strategy for managing conflict to achieve long-term benefits. However, collaboration is rarely used when there is a wide difference in power between the groups involved. Compromise and accommodation, strategies frequently used by nurses, are the most frequently occurring responses when differences in power allow one group to predominate. Power disparity has been a major impediment to collaboration between nursing and medicine, but the differences in power are diminishing as nurses become more adept at identifying and using their sources of power.[1,7,20,22,36,39]

CONCLUSION

The current crisis in health care provides an opportunity for nursing to move from dependent to autonomous and mutually interdependent roles with other health care professionals. To do so, nurses must confront and manage conflicts that have plagued nursing's professional development. The penalty for failure to do so may be great, not only for individual nurses and the profession, but for the clients they serve. As Aaronson[1] so aptly stated, "If nursing is willing to take the risks it has been socialized to avoid, . . . society might have a real choice in health care."

REFERENCES

1. Aaronson, L. S. (1989). A challenge for nursing: Reviewing a historic competition. *Nursing Outlook, 37,* 274-279.
2. Aydelotte, M. K. (1987). The nurse executive in 2000 AD: Role and functions. In M. Johnson (Ed.), *Series on nursing administration* (Vol. 1, pp. 2-13). Menlo Park, Calif: Addison-Wesley.
3. Barton, A. (1991). Conflict resolution by nurse managers. *Nursing Management, 22*(5), 83-86.
4. Blalock, H. M. (1989). *Power and conflict toward a general theory.* Newbury Park, Calif: Sage.
5. Brown, C. H., & Schultz, P. R. (1991). Outcomes of power development in work relationships. *Journal of Nursing Administration, 21*(2), 35-39.
6. Chandler, G. (1991). Creating an environment to empower nurses. *Nursing Management, 22*(8), 20-23.
7. Chavigny, K. H. (1988). Coalition building between medicine and nursing. *Nursing Economic$ 6,* 179-204.
8. Cochran, D. S., Schnake, M., & Earl, R. (1983). Effect of organizational size on conflict frequency and location in hospitals. *Journal of Management Studies, 20,* 441-451.
9. Corley, M. C., & Mauksch, H. O. (1988). Registered nurses, gender and commitment. In A. Atratham, E. M. Miller, & H. O. Mauksch (Eds.), *The worth of women's work: A qualitative analysis* (pp. 135-149). Albany, N.Y.: State University of New York Press.
10. Daft, R. L. (1989). *Organization theory and design* (3rd ed.). New York: West.
11. Delegates remodel ANA as a "lean machine" with more staff nurses in the driver's seat. (1989). *American Journal of Nursing, 89,* 1228.
12. Gibson, J. L., Ivancevich, J. M., & Donnelly, J. H. (1991). *Organizations behavior—structure—processes* (7th ed.). Homewood, Ill: Irwin.
13. Gray, J. L., & Starke, F. A. (1980). *Organizational behavior: Concepts and applications.* Columbus, Ohio: Merrill.

14. Guy, M. E. (1984). An interorganizational analysis of interdisciplinary conflict in a psychiatric hospital. *Administration in Mental Health, 12*(1), 45-64.

15. Guy, M. E. (1986). Interdisciplinary conflict and organizational complexity. *Hospital and Health Services Administration, 31*(1), 111-121.

16. Inside track, changing roles in the '90s: Will RNs manage MDs? (1989, November 20). *Hospitals*, pp. 42-44.

17. Johnson, M. (1986). *Nurse administrators' perceptions of the utility of conflict as related to personal and organizational characteristics.* Unpublished doctoral thesis, University of Iowa, Iowa City.

18. Julian, J. W., Bishop, D. W., & Fiedler, F. E. (1966). Quasi-therapeutic effects of intergroup competition. *Journal of Personality and Social Psychology, 3,* 321-327.

19. Katz, D., & Kahn, R. L. (1966). *The social psychology of organizations.* New York: John Wiley.

20. Koerner, B. L., Cohen, J. R., & Armstrong, D. M. (1986). Professional behavior in collaborative practice. *Journal of Nursing Administration, 16*(10), 39-43.

21. Kramer, M. (1974). *Reality shock: Why nurses leave nursing.* St Louis: Mosby.

22. Mariano, C. (1989). The case for interdisciplinary collaboration. *Nursing Outlook, 37,* 285-288.

23. Marriner, A. (1982). Comparing strategies and their use: Managing conflict. *Nursing Management, 13*(6), 29-31.

24. Mason, D. J., Backer, B. A., & Georges, C. A. (1991). Toward a feminist model for the political empowerment of nurses. *Image: The Journal of Nursing Scholarship, 23,* 72-76.

25. Morgan, G. (1986). *Images of organizations.* Beverly Hills, Calif: Sage.

26. Myrtle, R. C., Glogow, E. (1978). How nursing administrators view conflict. *Nursing Research, 2,* 103-106.

27. Perrow, C. (1979). *Complex organizations: A critical essay* (2nd ed.). Glenview, Ill: Scott, Foresman.

28. Pondy, L. R. (1967). Organizational conflict: Concepts and models. *Administrative Science Quarterly, 12,* 296-320.

29. Prescott, P., & Bowne, S. A. (1985). Physician-nurse relationships. *Annals of Internal Medicine, 103,* 127-133.

30. Rahem, M. A. (1986). *Managing conflict in organizations.* New York: Praeger.

31. Robbins, S. P. (1974). *Managing organizational conflict: A nontraditional approach.* Englewood Cliffs, N.J.: Prentice Hall.

32. Rotkovitch, R. (1989). The power of the nurse executive. In B. Henry, C. Arndt, M. DiVincenti, & A. Marriner-Tomey (Eds.), *Dimensions of nursing administration theory, research, education, practice* (pp. 195-203). Boston: Blackwell Scientific Publications.

33. Scalzi, C. C., & Nazarey, P. (1989). Value conflicts in nursing administration. In B. Henry, C. Ardnt, M. DiVincenti, & A. Marriner-Tomey (Eds.), *Dimensions of nursing administration theory, research, education, practice* (pp. 583-591). Boston: Blackwell Scientific Publications.

34. Schwenk, C. R., & Thomas, H. (1983). Effects of conflicting analyses on managerial decision-making: A laboratory experiment. *Decision Science, 14,* 467-480.

35. Sexton, D. L. (1980). Organizational conflict: A creative or destructive force. *Nursing Leadership, 3*(3), 16-21.

36. Smeltzer, C. H. (1991). The art of negotiation: An everyday experience. *Journal of Nursing Administration, 21*(7-8), 26-30.

37. Smith, C. G. (1985). Women, nurses, power conflict: Competition and cooperative approaches. In R. R. Weiczorch (Ed.), *Power, politics and policy in nursing* (pp. 58-63). New York: Springer.

38. Snyder, D. L. (1982). New baccalaureate graduates' perceptions of organizational conflict. *Nursing Research, 31,* 300-305.

39. Stein, L. I., Watts, D. T., & Howell, T. (1990). The doctor-nurse game revisited. *New England Journal of Medicine, 322,* 546-549.

40. Strader, M. (1992). Conflict management. In P. Decker & E. Sullivan (Eds.), *Nursing administration: A micro/macro approach for effective nurse executives* (pp. 549-568). Norwalk, Conn: Appleton and Lange.

41. Thomas, K. W. (1976). Conflict and conflict management. In M. Dunnette (Ed.), *The handbook of industrial organizational psychology* (pp. 889-935). Chicago: Rand McNally.

42. Ulrich, B. T. (1987). Value differences between practicing nurse executives and graduate educators. *Nursing Economic$, 5,* 287-291.

43. Walton, R. E., & Dutton, J. M. (1969). The management of interdepartmental conflict: A model and a review. *Administrative Science Quarterly, 14,* 73-84.

44. Wax, J. (1986). Solving ethical problems. *AORN Journal, 43,* 608-612.

45. Weins, A. G. (1990). Expanded nurse autonomy: Models for small rural hospitals. *Journal of Nursing Administration, 20*(12), 15-22.

46. Woodtli, A. (1987). Conflict: Insights before intervention. *Nurse Educator, 12,* 22-26.

47. Woodtli, A. (1987). Deans of nursing: Perceived sources of conflict and conflict handling modes. *Journal of Nursing Education, 26,* 272-277.

48. Zey-Ferrell, M. (1979). *Dimensions of organizations.* Santa Monica, Calif: Goodyear.

CHAPTER 87

Traditional roles for women and the impact on nursing services in Brazil

ROSENI ROSANGELA CHOMPRÉ, ANAMARIA VAZ de ASSIS MEDINA,
MARIA AUXILIADORA C. CHRISTOFARO

Throughout much of the history of mankind the work of women, considered by many societies as essential for the production of food and survival, was invisible. Women's work was done behind the conspicuous activities of the highest levels of popes and kings, wars and discovery, tyranny and defeat, as told in official history. Women, through their work, wove the true screen of history that is still to receive the attention due it.[6]

Given this picture, it may be noted that the longer any society lives in a given situation, the less urgent or conflicting that situation appears. It comes to be regarded more as a condition than a contradiction or problem. In the case of women, the nonalteration of the division of labor during so many centuries and in different geographical spaces made reproduction and the care of people within and without the context of the family their unquestioned responsibility.[4] This activity consolidates itself as a traditional role of woman carried out within the domestic sphere. Due to their biological capabilities of gestation, delivery, and breast-feeding, women extend their actions of nutrition and care to other families and communities in the roles of midwives, faith healers, healers, and wet nurses.

Gestation and breast-feeding, especially, create relations between women and the concepts understood in certain periods, societies, or social groups as limiting factors to their insertion in production and public space. As an example, the reduction of mobility, common during the phases of gestation, delivery, and breast-feeding, is seen in many societies as a "loss," inhibiting women from taking on certain roles and functions.

The hegemonic assumption that the family is the nuclear basis of organization, harmony, security, and development, both economically and morally, is intrinsically linked to women; to be "mother," "wife," and "housewife" becomes socially part of the function of procreation, strengthening the ideal model in which the home becomes the power domain of women.

Besides the role of reproduction and care, women also carry out the role of educator, transmitting beliefs, values, and knowledge about social dynamics and the functioning of the body. Even as women hold the function of perpetuating values and traditions, the very evolution of society exerts an influence over these traditions, so as to change them. It must not be forgotten that there are complex interrelations between differentiated movements and tendencies at the heart of society that determine the coexistence of prevailing, residual, and emerging values. It is in this permanent process of change that there occurs the alteration of the traditional roles of women.

The passing from acceptance of the so-called feminine condition to an analysis of the problems of women only became relevant, in the course of history, when three basic factors appeared simultaneously. The first factor is a reality perceived by society as inadequate and unacceptable, that is, the status of women in society as a whole, and male domination. The second factor is the existence of proposals to solve the questions considered problematic, and the third is the moment or political climate favorable for change.

These factors are at the root of the history of nursing in Brazil because of the strong link of the history of women with a significant repercussion of their traditional roles on the evolution of Brazilian nursing in the country as a whole.

WOMEN AND THE HISTORY OF NURSING IN BRAZIL
Earliest roots of nursing

In order to analyze the evolution of nursing in Brazil, it is necessary to look at the different stages of the development of Brazilian society and, within society, the development of women.

The origins of Brazil, as a Western country, are linked to the European trade expansion beginning in the fifteenth century.

The native culture of the precoloneal period continues today to be marginalized and discounted in the power structure and organization of Brazilian society, both in its values and in its social, political, and economic parameters.

Concurrent with the process of exploration of the natural resources of the new land, the process of "civilizing" the inhabitants—the so-called Indians—was carried out through the invasion and massacre of tribes, Jesuit catechism, and enslavement of Indians and Africans. This resulted in the imposition of Portuguese culture and domination in a comprehensive way throughout all the territory.

The issue of participation of women in this expansion is only gradually being revealed. The point of view of distinguished historians was usually more concerned with the conquests than with the colonial settlements. This left the impression that, in this great period of navigational exploration, there were in the world only a few women, mostly of the nobility (Isabel I of Spain; Catherine of Austria, wife to Dom João III of Portugal; and Elizabeth I of England, for example).

However, when the subject of colonizing the new land was raised, the effort of women rose in importance, given the traditional social roles relating to them. This was due to the fact that effective colonization was based on the formation of the family, which in joint work and with functions divided between its members, would do the work of production and reproduction.

Mixing with native women in the new lands was considerably more common among the Portuguese than it was among other peoples. In addition, the mother country made an effort in various ways to send local women to the colonies to establish families so as to lay down their habits and customs, which included the dominant language and religion.

While the men opened new horizons, fought the natives, and advanced into new areas looking for Eldorados, the women usually produced food, adminis-

tered the goods and properties, had children, and then, very often, fought hard for their own survival and that of their children.[5]

In order to get white women and send them to the new territories, the methods utilized included everything from recruiting volunteers to kidnapping and permanent removal, involving direct trafficking.

Besides the presence of Portuguese and native women in the colonization of Brazil, the large-scale production activities of the plantation demanded the incorporation of large numbers of workers, made up of enslaved and transported Africans.

In the setting up of Brazilian society, women of different ethnic origins became the object of commercial stimulus to the reproduction and occupation of land, together with the wish to spread the Roman Catholic faith. Each ethnic group contributed its knowledge and specific cultural baggage in shaping the Brazilian nation.

Portuguese women came from two classes: the noble or rich families and the lower classes. Given the social concern with the division of goods and properties through inheritance, noble women were limited to the domestic arena or religious institutions. Keeping up the traditions of the home country in general, the rich Portuguese women only left their homes accompanied by male relatives for religious ceremonies or were restricted to convents. This same treatment of women, transported to Brazil, would result in the kind of family made up of a "taciturn father, obedient mother and withdrawn children," referred to in the famous phrase by Capistrano de Abreu.[1]

The lower-class women, on the other hand, made up the great majority and included the poor Portuguese, the half-caste, the freed African slave, and the slave. Many documents of the colonial period show them as unchaste women or libertines. But the great concern of this social group was truly their survival and that of their children. The high mortality rate of men and the instability of the relations between the sexes must not be forgotten. Due to the circumstances at that time, most of the families were mother-centered.

Although they were the largest segment of the female population, the values, beliefs and modus vivendi of the lower class did not shape the predominant ideals of Brazilian society in terms of the roles of women. It was always the poorest who took on the responsibility of feeding, caring for and educating the children, caring for the sick, handling and administering medicine, assisting in delivery, and feeding the children of other women, together with all the activities of cleaning. These activities would determine the informal process of health care, carried out by midwives, faith healers, and those who cared for the dying and the dead.

Institutionalization of health care and formal training

Given the nature of the work of women, they were accredited to join the work force when health care was institutionalized. However, as this care was organized institutionally, it was not these women from the lower classes who would take on the nursing procedures in the hospitals. Given the living conditions and social organization at that time, the services were institutionalized under the responsibility of nuns, who came mainly from the higher classes.

The first health institutions in Brazil were the Santas Casas de Misericordia (Holy Houses of Mercy), which had been planned by the Portuguese monarchy from the earliest days of colonization. The first one in Brazil was the Santa Casa de Santos, established in 1543. In spite of the almost immediate establishment of hospitals in Brazil after the arrival of the Portuguese (1500), there is no reference to any kind of systematic health care available to slaves and other lower classes. This was true until the second half of the nineteenth century. Therefore, while nobility and the high classes were cared for by doctors from Portugal, the other social layers were cared for by the same poor women, very often considered transgressors against the dominant social norms and carrying out volunteer work. For Germano,[3] nursing in Brazil can trace its beginning to this context and virtually kept the same profile until the period of the so-called Old Republic, or up to 1930. From the early eighteenth century, the doctor became involved in a more active way with activities related to reproduction and women's health. He invaded rituals that were lived in an exclusively feminine community, as for example the moment of delivery, when knowledge transmitted from mother to daughter brought together the pregnant woman, the midwife, and others (women friends and neighbors) in a warm meeting of public and private spheres.

It may be emphasized, therefore, that nursing as a social practice in Brazil is linked to domestic activities and the empirical practice of mothers, nuns, slaves, and even those seen as prostitutes. Silva,[7] in his study on medicine and nursing in the precapitalist period, states that these origins result in a lack of prestige for the

continuing work in this field of knowledge, since it is seen as mere common sense.

In 1808 the royal family migrated to Brazil, fleeing the invasion of Portugal by French troops. They moved first to Bahia and later to Rio de Janeiro. This event, added to the opening of the ports to friendly nations, helped in the process of political, economic, and social transformation in Brazil in the nineteenth century. These changes stimulated other commercial links, especially with England, which demanded a new urban structure, mainly in the ports. In the same year of 1808 the first educational course of surgery, anatomy, and obstetrics was created in Bahia.

In 1832 the medical-surgical academies of Rio de Janeiro and Bahia were called schools or faculties of medicine, and a specific course for midwives was created. During the second half of the nineteenth century other faculties of medicine appeared, often created with midwifery, pharmacy, and dentistry courses. In 1854 a new statute for the schools of medicine was approved, in which prerequisites were established for the courses of obstetrics, pharmacy, and "cirurgioes boticarios" (surgeons who could also mix their own medicines) as "annexes" to the medical courses, again concentrated in Bahia and Rio de Janeiro. Only in 1890 was the first course for midwives established in the state of São Paulo.

The continuation and consolidation of the agricultural and exporting model meant that the imperial government that was established after independence from Portugal (1822) had to set up strategies of social action. Among these was health care, since endemic diseases such as yellow fever, smallpox, and plague threatened commercial relations with other countries. Among the measures adopted, priority was given to action directed at collective diseases and a system of sanitary vigilance was established for the control of endemic diseases and hygiene in the cities. These measures meant new demands on health care at that time, including that carried out by women. This work was now done inside the hospitals and would later become nursing services.

The first nursing school in Brazil was created in 1890 as part of the Hospital Nacional de Alienados of Rio de Janeiro. Since the beginning, the institutionalized training of nurses involved several prerequisites to enroll. It was necessary, for example, to know a foreign language (French or English), as well as arithmetic and geometry. Previously, these had been relevant to male courses at pregraduate level, available only to people of the social elite. Even in the teaching for women of the upper class, handicrafts was substituted for geometry.

As a result, demands would not allow entry in the courses of nursing by women of lower classes, who continued to carry out a significant part of the formal and informal health action.

Besides this characteristic, it is important to highlight another, which is also relevant. Although efforts were made to include community health content based on the control of endemic diseases and other public health problems, the institutionalized training of nurses was done in the hospital setting and remained disconnected from the health needs of most of the population.

Modern nursing

So-called modern nursing, along the lines of the Nightingale system, was established in Brazil through English professionals recruited to organize the nursing services of the Hospital of the Foreigners' Association in Rio de Janeiro in 1892.

The beginning of the twentieth century saw the expansion of institutions for the training of nurses with the creation of the School of Nursing of the Hospital Samaritano (1901) and the School for Midwives (1902).

At the turn of the century there was also a serious crisis in commercial relations resulting from, among other causes, the reappearance of yellow fever in the main ports. The threat of having trading countries cut their relations with Brazil led the government to define tough measures for the control and eradication of endemic diseases, with the obvious consequences on health activities. Working on an emergency contract basis for the government, the sanitary agent Oswaldo Cruz defined a very comprehensive program for the control of endemic diseases. This increased the demand for specialized nursing labor in order to carry out the Oswaldo Cruz Plan. In spite of the existence of institutions responsible for the training of health professionals, the greater part of the nursing work force, even at this time, did not have systematic training.

In order to respond to the lack in both quality and quantity of this work force, international cooperation was invited in order to organize a model of training considered adequate. This resulted in the setting up of the school of nursing by the National Department of Public Health in 1922. In 1926 this institution became the Ana Nery School of Nursing, which was a "model school" for the establishment of other schools in the country. Although the training was originally proposed

as a strategy for collective health actions within the Oswaldo Cruz Plan, once again hospital care came to predominate in the training of nurses as a result of the methodology adopted in the teaching.

The continuity of the institutionalization and expansion of higher education nursing courses (currently about 100) did not eliminate the use of unqualified labor, which even today is the wide base of the work force. On the other hand, the hospital has been kept as the main place for the practice of the nurses.

Nowadays nursing is done by four distinct categories, according to levels of qualification. The "nurse," representing about 10% of nursing personnel, has university training (a minimum of 4 years beyond high school). The "technical nurse" and the "nursing auxiliary" make up approximately 30% of nursing professionals, and they have high school or equivalent training. The fourth category of "nursing attendants, helpers, and health auxiliaries" makes up 60% of the total, and its members have no specific training. The greater part of them have only 4 years of basic schooling. In all these categories, women make up about 97% of the work force. Their efforts not only represent work by women but reflect the very depreciative nature of "women's work" in Brazilian society.

CONCLUSION

In Brazil as in other parts of the world, access to all levels of schooling was limited for women, and this was particularly true with regard to university training. Adding the usual discrimination to this, the greater presence of women is in socially undervalued professions, such as nursing and education.

A large part of the population does not have access to health services. The poor continue to be left to the resources of informal care, carried out even today by housewives, midwives, faith healers, and healers. These practices are often associated with mystical values and esoteric prescriptions, which are deeply ingrained in Brazilian culture.

Social recognition of these practices is reinforced by their affective connotation and the sense of belonging to a group, which is generally missing in formal health care institutions. But, as in these institutions, informal health care also seeks to meet the demands of allopathic therapy presented by the population and predominant as the healing model. Therefore teas, potions, bottled homemade medicine, and ointments mix with prayers and medicine from the drugstore.

In spite of the importance of women, both in terms of quality and quantity in producing health and nursing services in the country, it must be highlighted that women and nursing care have been held back by many government policies of protection of family, maternity, and infancy. Among these policies, we further emphasize those that are meant to control pregnancy, delivery, and the neonatal period, and family planning, which are meant to control the woman's body. Therefore, by being the subjects and objects of formal and informal health care, the "docile bodies" of women[2] are transformed into productive, reproductive, consuming bodies, perpetuating a culture that, in spite of this, very often excludes them.

In the sphere of the health institutions and professions, this exclusion is even clearer in nursing, which is looked down on as women's work that has become institutionalized. It is clear, therefore, that nursing in Brazil is not only influenced by the traditional roles of women in society, but it has also incorporated and accepted them as inherent and necessary, derived from a conceptual framework of feminine submission.

In Brazilian society the submissive status of women has already begun to advance insofar as relevant issues are being raised and changes have begun. However, in the sphere of nursing this status is seen as a "natural" state of affairs and is not, therefore, something that has to be overcome.

REFERENCES

1. Abreu, C. (1934). *Capitulos de historia colonial* [Chapters from colonial history], 1500-1800. Rio de Janeiro: Briguiet.
2. Foucault, M. (1984). *Vigiar e punir: Nascimento da prisao* [Watching and punishing: The birth of prison]. (3rd ed.). Petrópolis: Vozes.
3. Germano, R. N. (1983). *Educacao e ideologia da enfermagem no Brasil* [Education and nursing ideology in Brazil]. São Paulo: Cortez.
4. Medina, Anamaria Vaz de Assis. (1991, April-June). Questoes e direitos relativos a mulher nas Constituicoes do Brasil e de Minas Gerais [Issues and rights relating to the woman in the fundamental laws in Brazil and Minas Gerais State]. *Revista de Informacao Legislativa*, 28(110), 181-198.
5. Medina, Anamaria Vaz de Assis. (1992). *Que faziam as mulheres portuguesas enquanto estavam a ver navios?* [What did the Portuguese women do while they watched the ships?]. Unpublished manuscript.
6. Miles, R. (1989). *A historia do mundo pela mulher.* [The woman's world history]. Rio de Janeiro: Livros Tecnicos e Cientificos, Editora Ltda. and Casa-Maria Editorial.
7. Silva, G. B. (1986). *Enfermagem profissional: Analise critica* [Professional nursing: A critical analysis]. São Paulo: Cortez.

PART ELEVEN

CULTURAL DIVERSITY

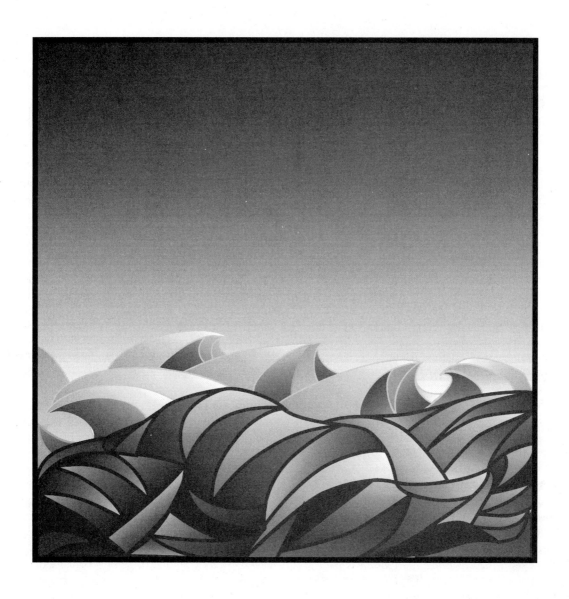

Addressing the imbalances

JOANNE COMI McCLOSKEY, HELEN KENNEDY GRACE

Throughout this book, the plight of nurses has been detailed. Nursing as a profession has faced many of the challenges common to the experience of underserved groups in this country. Because of this common experience, it might be assumed that nursing would be welcoming, receptive, and encouraging of inclusion of a broad cross section of underrepresented groups at all levels of the profession. Nursing, throughout its history both in the United States and in other parts of the world, has been a vehicle for upward social class mobility. Despite the low pay and less than desirable working conditions, nursing is an occupation that has been an "acceptable" field for women world over. But nursing, not unlike other oppressed groups, is more restrictive and exclusionary than other mainstream fields. This section provides an overview of the multifaceted dimensions of the difficulty the profession has had in dealing with cultural diversity.

In the opening debate chapter, Brink poses the question, How much cultural diversity can we tolerate in nursing? According to the evidence she provides, the answer is a resounding "very little." Starting with the educational content of nursing programs, she notes that only a few programs in the country have developed major content related to cultural diversity. In many programs, cultural diversity is addressed as a curricular strand. The danger in this is that faculty are unprepared in this area and unlikely to place proper emphasis upon the subject in an integrated teaching approach. The lack of textbooks related to the area and the reluctance of publishers to support such texts are further indication that insufficient attention is paid to the topic. Also, the relative lack of attention to cultural diversity in the field is evidenced by the small numbers of students who are from underrepresented groups. Not surprisingly, faculty and clinical nursing staff are similarly unrepresentative of the broader population.

Furuta and Lipson address in greater depth issues related to cultural diversity in the student body. Noting that there has been little change in the percentages of minority students admitted to nursing programs despite more dramatic shifts in the distribution of minorities in the general population, the authors propose a number of steps needed to address these imbalances: (1) develop minority applicant pools; (2) create orientation and preceptorship programs; (3) personalize recruitment efforts; (4) formalize nontraditional admissions criteria; (5) enroll a cohort of minority students; (6) create a culturally sensitive learning environment; (7) mainstream student services; and (8) recruit minority faculty. This article concludes with an admonition to the nursing profession: "Ultimately the issue is not about affirmative action or even the improvement of cultural diversity in the student body but about nursing's own humanity."

The challenge of overcoming biases related to "unpopular patients" is addressed by Kus. Patients with low social value (the aged as contrasted with the young), those of low moral worth (prostitutes as contrasted with priests), the stigmatized (homosexuals), those who are perceived to be responsible for their ill health, those who are frightening, those who behave negatively (hypochondriacs), and those with whom the nurse feels incompetent are likely to fall into the category of "unpopular." Lack of recognition of the problems posed by unpopular patients is likely to have negative consequences both for the patients and the nurse dealing with such patients. Kus proposes a number of steps to combat these negative outcomes. A first step is to admit negative feelings toward patients; another is to examine negativity factors that can be changed either by the patient or in the nurse's response. Prisoners are provided as an example of patients that are generally regarded as unpopular. Kus challenges nurses to fight for prison reform and concludes as follows: "A nurse is always a nurse. Our clients are all humanity. . . . Nursing is for me a radical social activism designed to protect the dignity of *all* humans. . . . The mistreatment of fellow humans should rekindle a fire in every nurse . . . that will not stop until every human on earth is treated with true dignity." This is the true challenge for nurses in addressing cultural diversity.

Returning to the issues related to the composition of the nursing profession, the next two chapters address approaches to redressing imbalances related to minorities and men in the field. Castiglia first notes the inconsistency of the use of terminology related to minorities in our continuing tendencies to sort people out, but she then goes on to address the imbalances within the profession as reflective of the broader society. Not only are there problems in the percentages of minority groups entering the profession but also there is evidence that these imbalances become compounded the higher the level of education. This has profound implications for the future in that if the numbers of minorities attaining graduate degrees continue to be small, the numbers of minorities in faculty and leadership positions in nursing who would be recruiters, role models, and mentors to increase the percentages will remain inadequate. Federal, state, and local support, counseling and tutorial services, and encouragement of organizations that form support networks for nurses in minority groups are approaches that are suggested. Halloran and Welton address the question of why there aren't more men in nursing. Four contributing factors are offered: (1) historical links between nursing and the struggle to bring down social barriers that excluded women from participating in the nondomestic economy; (2) military policy that has dictated that men participate in times of war as soldiers and not as part of the nursing corps; (3) the economy and the lack of incentives for males to enter nursing because of the low salary levels; and (4) sex-role stereotyping that has defined nursing as women's work. Given the large numbers of women now entering traditionally male-oriented fields, it is imperative that this imbalance

within nursing be addressed. The American Assembly for Men in Nursing is actively involved in the encouragement of men to enter the nursing field and the uniting of men within the profession. But the challenge to the profession as a whole is that of actively opening up the profession and consciously recruiting and nurturing a more diverse nursing work force.

In the final chapter in this section, Meleis and Aly shift the focus away from nursing per se to the broad consideration of women's health as a major area of concern internationally. Noting that most of the concern for women's health is traditionally focused on reproduction, the authors challenge nursing to adopt a broader perspective. Women's health issues in this broader perspective are defined as the following: (1) eating disorders and nutritional problems; (2) infections; (3) violence against women; (4) reproductive health; and (5) occupational health. The development of health care programs that incorporate women's perspectives and the use of strategies to empower women are advocated. Nurses joining with women and women's organizations around the world can be a powerful force for change in addressing the health care needs of women.

As nurses struggle to attain greater equity in the health care arena, the profession must consciously address the imbalances in representativeness of nurses related to the general population. Increased numbers of African-Americans, Hispanics and Latinos, Native Americans, and men are absolutely essential if nursing is to be a significant force in improving the health of people in the United States, and indeed around the world. As nursing educational programs seek to develop an international perspective, they must examine their efforts within the context of the communities in which they practice and address questions of similarity of composition between their student bodies and the populations with which they work in their clinical practicum experiences. If we do not address these imbalances, our language related to concerns for the patients whom we serve is hollow and our actions do not match our rhetoric.

CHAPTER 88

Debate

Cultural diversity in nursing

How much can we tolerate?

PAMELA J. BRINK

When nurses talk about cultural diversity, they often mean something like: "Cultural diversity is how to assess the cultural variable." This definition implies that cultural diversity constitutes a data base from which to derive a nursing diagnosis. One of the basic meanings of cultural diversity in nursing has to do with cultural diversity content in basic nursing education. A second meaning refers to the racial, national, and ethnic diversity of the nursing school student body. Beyond that, cultural diversity also can mean the racial, national, and ethnic diversity of the faculty, or of the staff and administration in clinical settings. In this text, cultural diversity also includes the issue of men in nursing (see Chapter 92). The answer to the question, How much cultural diversity can nursing tolerate? will differ depending on the particular type of cultural diversity referred to.

CULTURAL DIVERSITY CONTENT IN THE CURRICULUM

In the 1960s the division of nursing provided traineeships to nurses interested in doctoral study in anthropology (among other fields) for the express purpose of producing nurses doctorally prepared in anthropological theory and methods. The basic concept these nurses brought back to nursing was that of cultural diversity. Most were trained in cultural anthropology and some in biological anthropology, but all were convinced of the need to include cultural as well as biological diversity in nursing's armamentarium of knowledge. A number of textbooks were written in the 1970s and 1980s to provide students and faculty with an introduction to the issue.[1-19] Today literature on cultural diversity is found primarily in chapters of clinical texts, and some articles also appear in professional nursing journals.

Beliefs about the importance of cultural diversity in the curriculum

Some schools of nursing (notably the University of Washington at Seattle; the University of California, San Francisco; and the University of Miami) have developed cultural diversity as a major component of the curriculum and devote prerequisite and required courses to the topic. In these schools not only is introductory anthropology a prerequisite to nursing but some form of medical anthropology or transcultural nursing also is part of the undergraduate curriculum. And, at the graduate level, students can specialize in transcultural or international nursing.

In other schools of nursing, cultural diversity is not considered a major part of the curriculum. Anthropology is not required and the only cultural diversity content occurs in introductory sociology courses that address the sociocultural problems of American ethnic groups. In these schools an advanced course in sociology (even medical sociology) is not considered necessary.

The predominant American belief system appears to view cultural diversity as a relatively unimportant subject for study. I can just hear some of my colleagues saying, "I think cultural diversity is very important, and I stress to all my students that they must assess the cultural variable!" My rejoinder would be, "Good! Then on your list of curricular priorities, of what students absolutely *must* know to graduate from your school, where do you place cultural diversity? In the top 10? In the top 20? The top 30?" Then I would ask, "Other than demanding that your student assess the cultural variable, how do you assist them to learn how to do that in your clinical setting? Please tell me, step by step, what you do." Although some faculty would be able to describe specific teaching techniques, most would not.

How cultural diversity should be taught

Opinions differ as to how cultural diversity should be taught. Nurses trained in anthropology believe that both an introductory course in anthropology and an upper-division course in cultural or medical anthropology are necessary to teach the concepts of cultural relativity and biological diversity. These nurses argue that students need to understand not only how beliefs and values affect customary patterns of behavior and social mores, but also how evolution, gene pools, and environmental isolation have produced specialized biological variations that affect health and illness, and how differing economies (from horticulture and herding to a cash economy) create certain disease patterns and curing techniques that are relevant to the cultural group. Consequently, nurse anthropologists are concerned that nursing students learn about varying human populations and their health and nursing problems, not just about health problems in their own particular communities. Cultural diversity is developed as a global theme, making it important to expose students to the world as much as to their own country.

Some schools of nursing incorporate only medical anthropology as a required or elective course, whereas others rely on introductory sociology or medical sociology to provide cultural diversity content. Sociology and anthropology, however, are separate fields in the United States, each providing different content. The theory and methods of one discipline do not substitute for the theory and methods of the other. Both content areas are important components of nursing education.

To what degree is cultural diversity actually taught?

In many schools of nursing, perhaps because it was once required by the National League for Nursing (NLN) for accreditation, cultural diversity content remains as a strand in the formal written curriculum. In reality, however, cultural diversity content is frequently ignored. Faculty often are unprepared to teach this content, passing their ignorance on to their students.

In other schools of nursing, faculty who are prepared to teach the content area are not asked to do so or to advise other faculty on related lecture content. In still other schools of nursing, cultural diversity is treated as an important curricular component, which is taught by competent, knowledgeable members of the faculty and for which students are held accountable.

Opinions differ as to whether cultural diversity is best taught through incorporation into existing courses or in separate courses. Both approaches have advantages and disadvantages. When approached as a curricular strand, cultural diversity is in danger of never being taught. For any curricular strand, someone must be able to teach the content at each level, monitor the progress of that strand, and monitor students' increasing facility with that content. In addition, lectures on cultural diversity by themselves are not sufficient. The student must be able to apply that knowledge in the clinical setting. Culturally relevant assessments and interventions cannot be supervised and evaluated by faculty who are not themselves specialists or perhaps not even knowledgeable in this area.

When cultural diversity is taught in separate courses, responsibility for the students' level of knowledge clearly falls on the individual teaching the course. The instructor is expected to be conversant with the content, and all students presumably are uniformly exposed to this content in any given term. Application of this knowledge to clinical problems, however, remains problematic. Formal course work can provide the necessary knowledge base from which to develop culturally relevant skills, but faculty who cannot apply cultural content will impede skill development in their students.

Evidence of lack of cultural diversity content in the curriculum

American nurses know very little about cultural diversity and are not taught much about the topic. Evidence supporting this claim is easy to find.

One indicator of professional interest in a topic is the number of books in the area. Many of the textbooks mentioned previously are out of print, primarily because schools of nursing failed to adopt them. U.S. publishers are now reluctant to publish books on cultural diversity for nursing simply because they have not sold well in the past. Why didn't the books sell? Aside from the subject's not being taught at all, the number of courses targeted toward cultural diversity may well have been insufficient to support the texts.

Alternatively, faculty members teaching cultural diversity as curricular strand may have been unable to agree on a single text that could be used throughout the curriculum. A third possibility is that faculty relied on clinical texts featuring a chapter on cultural diversity. So one can surmise, based on the lack of cultural diversity textbooks presently available, that nurses' knowledge of cultural diversity gained from basic nursing education is very limited.

One difficulty involved in writing a nursing textbook on cultural diversity is determining what content to emphasize. The texts that have survived use the "cookbook" approach to nursing the culturally different client: "This is a black client; this is how to nurse him;" or "This is a Mexican-American client, and this is how to nurse her;" or "This is an Asian client who needs to be assessed for 1, 2, and 3. Then intervene in 2, 3, and 4." These books are much more popular than texts that provide theories of cultural diversity and allow the student to make the application to the particular client. Apparently nurses prefer formula nursing.

The problem is that in cultural diversity the emphasis should be on diversity rather than homogeneity. Nurses who have studied anthropology have discovered that there is more diversity within than across cultures and that once they try to pin down an individual in terms of cultural differences they find culture to be ephemeral. Although nurses may seek guidelines and rules to work from and generalizations to increase nursing efficiency, anthropology cannot provide such shortcut strategies. It is easy to become frustrated, therefore, with the entire concept of cultural diversity because it is so difficult to pin down. Cultural diversity remains elusive without a theoretical framework. Theories provide the base from which each nurse can develop an assessment tool that will generate for each client cultural rules and regulations that are inviolate and those that are nice but not mandatory. In other words, once the nurse is able to sort out the important rules for the client's behavior, a determination can be made about appropriate nursing care.

One of the difficulties of developing nursing care strategies is that there are so few nursing diagnoses on cultural diversity. As a result, there are even fewer nursing interventions. The lack of nursing diagnoses and interventions that reflect cultural diversity content is another indication of nursing's seeming lack of interest in this area.

Proposed remedies

One remedy for the existing weaknesses is to prepare all faculty to teach cultural diversity content in both lecture and clinical settings. Not everyone needs to be a nurse anthropologist, nor does everyone need to have a doctoral degree in transcultural nursing; however, exposing every nursing faculty member to this content through continuing education courses could increase both their enthusiasm and their knowledge about this important area of nursing. Another remedy could be to designate at least one member of the faculty as a transcultural nursing authority, to be held responsible for developing and teaching the cultural diversity content in the curriculum. That individual would have as much credence as the critical care specialist and would be given as much respect for her or his particular knowledge base as for that of any other clinical area. Such faculty members would need advanced preparation to teach this content if they had not received training in anthropology or transcultural nursing previously. Continuing education courses and workshops on cultural diversity could be developed to prepare those individuals.

Cultural diversity content can be presented to students in a number of ways. The two most frequently used approaches have been to develop required or elective courses in the basic curriculum or to weave a curricular strand that runs through all courses. In addition, students can be deliberately given clinical placements in culturally diverse neighborhoods and be required to include cultural diagnoses and interventions in their care plans. For schools of nursing that are not in culturally diverse neighborhoods, appropriate clinical placements might require busing students out of the local area. For example, a school in Iowa might send its students to Chicago, Minneapolis, or Kansas City, or provide for optional study-abroad experiences. Some undergraduate students have negotiated for experiences on American Indian reservations, clinics in migrant workers' camps, a year of study in Nigeria, and so on. Another alternative is to invite students or clients from other cultures or ethnic groups to talk to students about their experiences with health and illness at home. If every clinical course had a panel of experts (clients from different ethnic and cultural backgrounds) who talked about their experience with that particular clinical area, allowing for student-client interaction and questions afterward, at least some exposure to cultural diversity could be achieved. In addition, the expert panel approach may be less costly than sending students away.

All these solutions need support from the designated head of the school or department of nursing. Cultural diversity will not be taught if the dean or department chair does not think it is important. Conversely, cultural diversity will be taught and taught well if made a priority by the chief executive officer. Just as in any other organizational structure, the leader both sets the tone of the school or department and strongly influences faculty response. The decision on cultural diversity, as any other decision, has budgetary implications.

CULTURAL DIVERSITY IN THE STUDENT BODY

A second major area of cultural diversity is the diversity of the student population. For the most part, faculties prefer a homogeneous student body. Homogeneity makes the task of teaching easier. One can better determine the appropriate content, pace, clinical experiences, examinations, and level of reading assignments when students share common backgrounds and ability levels. Indeed, one duty of selection committees is to provide a fairly homogeneous student group. Too much diversity impedes efficiency as ranges of content, pace, experience, and readings must expand to take into account a broader range of student abilities and backgrounds. When faculty have been accustomed to teaching students with a mean grade point average (GPA) of 3.5, they will complain bitterly when the mean GPA drops to 3.0. If faculty complain that it is harder to teach a fairly homogeneous group with a lower mean GPA, how much more will they complain when a lower mean GPA occurs in conjunction with an increase in heterogeneity and a wider range of abilities? How many faculty prefer not to teach foreign students to whom English is a second language because "they take too much time"? And time is indeed the issue, especially when classes are large, teacher-student contact hours are long, and faculty are pressed into other duties besides teaching. An added hardship is the expectation that students from other cultures will graduate with their peers rather than progressing more slowly through the program.

But a culturally diverse student population, although requiring more faculty time and effort, provides a breadth of experience for the American student who may not have had prior exposure to other cultures. Associating with people different from themselves exposes students to different values and beliefs and provides them with the chance to know, like, and learn to respect people with diametrically opposed views and customs. Because American nurses are working more and more alongside nurses from other countries, it seems sensible to have them learn alongside students from other countries. In fact, international students can be used as informants about differential cultural beliefs, values, and health care practices, thus offering an educational resource not otherwise available. If this experience is valued, it will be given time and effort; if not, faculty will continue to complain of excess work loads.

One of the major tenets of Branch and Paxton's book[3] was that the ethnically diverse population of the United States deserves to be nursed by people who are not just knowledgeable about the special problems of particular subgroups but are themselves members of those groups. Branch and Paxton made a plea for more schools and departments to "open their doors wider"* to ethnic students of color and provide them with the chance for a nursing education even if it takes them longer to complete the program.

Although Branch and Paxton were referring specifically to the highly visible disadvantaged ethnic populations in the United States, their plea is easily extended to disadvantaged students from developing countries. Schools of nursing might consider sponsoring one student a year from a disadvantaged U.S. minority group or a Third World country to increase cultural awareness of students and faculty. Such sponsorship might be affected through institutional linkages, sister schools, or church affiliations. Students and faculty might raise the money for tuition and fees by providing services through fee-for-service nursing clinics. If a culturally diverse student body is desired, means of achieving that goal can be found.

CULTURAL DIVERSITY OF THE FACULTY

A third, rarely discussed, area of cultural diversity is the need for culturally diverse faculty to teach nursing students. This diversity can be achieved simply by hiring qualified faculty from American ethnic groups (an

---

*This concept derives from Boston University's seminal program of the early 1960s ODWIN (Opening the Doors Wider in Nursing).

expedient approach), by recruiting faculty from other countries, or by seeking out faculty who have extensive experience with or knowledge of other cultures and countries. All three approaches would enhance the quality of the educational experience.

There are educationally prepared and doctorally trained "ethnic nurses of color" (in Branch and Paxton[3] terminology) competing for faculty positions. I still believe that when two applicants are equally qualified, the ethnic person of color should be given a slight edge in hiring to increase the numbers of culturally diverse faculty. When an ethnic minority nurse is available to lecture to students but is ineligible for a permanent faculty position (for whatever reasons), that nurse's expertise and experience should be used in whatever way possible. The relationship with the school may be formalized through the use of the "lecturer" title. Here, the sought-for expertise is in the form of nursing diagnoses and interventions specific to that individual's experience. These nurses would not be expected to teach courses on medical anthropology or transcultural nursing but rather would serve as guest lecturers for the cultural diversity strand in the curriculum.

A second resource for cultural diversity content is faculty members who have been Fulbright scholars, Peace Corps volunteers, missionaries, or World Health Organization employees, or who have conducted research on American, Third World, or other national populations. These faculty need to be part of the cultural diversity pool of expertise developed to lecture on cultural diversity content to provide clinical examples from their experience. The wealth of experience provided by our own faculties is frequently wasted.

A third resource for cultural diversity content is faculty from other schools of nursing around the world. There are a variety of ways to solicit their lecture services on a temporary or permanent basis. Formal university linkages can facilitate faculty and student exchanges for varying periods of time. Foreign faculty who come to a U.S. university to complete requirements for a degree can serve as faculty lecturers during that time. If these faculty were to provide an occasional lecture in every course during the period of the stay, each student in the school would have at least one contact with a person from that country. A lecture beginning with, "In my country, when a person has an automobile accident . . ." could finish with a reconstruction of emergency services, orthopedics, or surgery. A lecture beginning, "In my country, when a woman becomes pregnant . . ." could move through household and family customs, compare traditional birthing methods to those of the Western health care delivery system, and provide anecdotal data from personal experiences with childbirth. Other lectures might begin, "In my country, nursing administrators are . . ." or "nurses become faculty by . . ." The ideas for such lectures are limited only by one's imagination.

Nurses from other countries also frequently visit the United States on an informal basis. Many would be delighted to deliver a lecture for a small honorarium. Any school interested in having guest lecture by a foreign nurse can contact the International Council of Nurses or the World Health Organization for information.

Increasingly, the cultural diversity of the faculty will expand the range of cultural experiences to which students are exposed. Such expansion of cultural experiences is not merely desirable but necessary. How can nurses care for culturally, ethnically, and nationally diverse patients with any sense of familiarity if they have never met anyone from that or a similar culture?

Unfortunately, several barriers make such faculty expansion difficult to accomplish. All faculty members of schools of nursing are required to hold a valid state license to practice nursing. This requirement is held as sacred by those who do not want foreign nurses in their schools. The requirement of licensure is upheld by state boards of nursing to prevent unscrupulous, poorly trained nurses from practicing bad nursing. Some nurses believe that faculty from Third World countries are so lacking in technological familiarity that they have nothing to offer our students. Others see European nurse researchers as conducting simplistic research with little to offer advanced U.S. students. For these reasons, nurse faculty and deans are hesitant to invite foreign nurses to their schools, and they support rigid state board regulations that prevent these nurses from teaching in the United States. I believe these practices and excuses should change.

CULTURAL DIVERSITY OF THE CLINICAL STAFF

The last area of cultural diversity I want to mention is rarely discussed in the literature. For some reason the cultural mix of staff in clinical settings is rarely seen as an educational advantage for students. Yet many clinical agencies are staffed by nurses from other countries who could provide clinical preceptorships in cultural content. When students present their cases, these nurses could offer valuable advice on cultural differences, particularly if the patient is from the same country as the nurse. Third World physicians, who frequently come to the Untied States for residencies, could be tapped as resources for the health beliefs and practices in their own countries. Very little use is made of foreign staff members' expertise about their own countries. Our profession relies on educational degrees to validate an individual's expertise, giving little credence to experience as an avenue to such expertise. Yet many nationals in the United States have clinical experiences that could enhance students' learning.

Again, however, a culturally homogeneous staff is often easier to work with. Faculty understand staff members who share their background and experience and speak the same language. Working with staff of another country is time-consuming and beset with communication problems. These difficulties in themselves are worthy of discussion; entire clinical conferences could be devoted to this issue. Patients are confronted with these cultural variations daily, yet no one talks about them. How does the American patient cope with nursing and medical staff from different countries who may have different expectations of the patient? How do students learn from foreign nationals? What is common and what is different? Again, such discussion assumes a knowledgeable moderator. And knowledge can come from experience as well as from short in-service courses.

Cultural diversity of clinical staff is not a choice but a reality. Nurses' abilities to work with a culturally diverse staff could be enhanced by exposing them to such environments as students. A knowledgeable teacher will lead discussions about the difficulties of working with people from different cultures and strategies for overcoming those difficulties. For example, foreign nurses are expected to make all the adjustments, and rather rapidly, with few American nurses seeking them out for what they can give.

WHAT MORE IS NEEDED?

American nurses need to respect cultural diversity in all four areas: educational content, students, faculty, and clinical staff. This respect can be demonstrated in a variety of ways other than those already described. First and foremost, state boards of nursing can improve nursing's relationship with other countries by relaxing the rules and regulations for foreign students, enabling them to obtain temporary licensure. This temporary

licensure could be extended as a courtesy to foreign nurse faculty who come to the United States to teach for brief periods. So long as they are employed as faculty, they could be granted a license to practice. In both instances, these nurses should work in U.S. institutions to learn how things are done and to take with them a better notion of what American nursing is really like. American nursing would not be contributing to the "brain drain" by mandating that foreign nurses have a regular license but would instead acknowledge that their presence, although temporary, is still valuable.

Second, American nurses can present more papers at conferences abroad and bring back with them the work done by other nurses to share with their students. Conversely, when an international conference is held near a school, faculty may find some of the participants willing to stay on an extra day or two to talk to their students.

In addition, nursing journals from other countries can be placed regularly on reading lists. U.S. nurses tend to read and refer to only their own journals, even though nurses in other countries are conducting valuable research in important areas. Reading foreign journals should be reciprocal—nurses in other countries are expected to keep up with research in the United States.

Not only can we read journals from other countries, but we can include more cultural diversity content in American nursing journals. Editors, however, need to know that American nurses want to read about health and nursing issues in other countries and cultures. Otherwise editors will continue to reject manuscripts on the advice of reviewers who say that the content is of no interest to American nurses.

Perhaps one of the easiest ways of including cultural diversity content in journal articles is to begin by identifying the cultural diversity of our research populations. We are becoming much more sophisticated in our appreciation of gender differences in our sociocultural and physiological research. It is time we became more sophisticated in the cultural and ethnic differences in our samples. When we describe our samples, when we make comparisons based upon demographic variables, we need to include ethnicity as a consistent variable. As we become more familiar with this form of reporting we become impatient with those who do not include this content.

Finally, work groups or open forums at international meetings can facilitate exchange programs and linkages among faculties. Schools looking for particular persons with specific expertise can advertise through these organizations and interview applicants at meetings. Schools desiring to form linkages can advertise their particular interests at meetings. Such an open exchange of interest would be exciting and refreshing. European schools of nursing are beginning to request Fulbright scholars on a regular basis, seeking particular expertise for their new programs. American nurses need to know both that Fulbright awards exist and that several exchange programs are available for nurses.

The United States' greatness rests in its enormous cultural diversity, its tolerance for a wide variety of ways of doing things. American nurses also can benefit from this diversity. Rather than seeking uniformity, homogeneity, and efficiency, cultural diversity in educational content, student populations, faculty, and clinical settings can be used to advantage.

Schools of nursing may have to allocate specific funds at the expense of other needs until cultural diversity is an accepted part of nursing education. To nourish cultural diversity, nurses will have to focus on it, give it attention, and make it work. Without this attention, cultural diversity will remain a dream rather than a goal and will never be a reality.

Cultural diversity does not happen peacefully, without struggle and strain. The United States has had numerous difficulties in coming to terms with its diverse population, in ensuring everyone the same freedoms and same opportunities. How then can we in nursing expect that our efforts to promote cultural diversity will go smoothly? Without conflict or pain, change and growth remain unattainable.

REFERENCES

1. Bauwens, E. E. (Ed.). (1978). *The anthropology of health.* St Louis: Mosby.
2. Boyle, J. S., & Andrews, M. M. (1989). *Transcultural concepts in nursing care.* Boston: Scott, Foresman.
3. Branch, M. F., & Paxton, P. P. (Eds.). (1976). *Providing safe nursing care for ethnic people of color.* New York: Appleton-Century-Crofts.
4. Brink, P. J. (Ed.). (1990). *Transcultural nursing: A book of readings.* Prospect Heights, Ill: Waveland Press.
5. Brownlee, A. T. (1978). *Community, culture and care: A cross-cultural guide for health workers.* St Louis: Mosby.
6. Clark, A. L. (Ed.). (1978). *Culture, childbearing, health professionals.* Philadelphia: F. A. Davis.
7. Dobson, S. (1991). *Transcultural nursing.* London: Scutari Press.
8. Henderson, G., & Primeaux, M. (Eds.). (1981). *Transcultural health care.* Menlo Park, Calif: Addison-Wesley.
9. Holden, P., & Littlewood, J. (Eds.). (1991). *Anthropology and nursing.* London: Routledge.
10. Kay, M. A. (1982). *Anthropology of human birth.* Philadelphia: F. A. Davis.
11. Leininger, M. (1970). *Nursing and anthropology: Two worlds to blend.* New York: John Wiley and Sons.
12. Leininger, M. (Ed.). (1978). *Transcultural nursing: Concepts, theories, and practices.* New York: John Wiley and Sons.
13. Mangay-Maglacas, A., & Pizurki, H. (1981). *The traditional birth attendant in seven countries.* Geneva: World Health Organization.
14. Martinez, R. A. (1978). *Hispanic culture and health care.* St Louis: Mosby.
15. Morse, J. M. (Ed.). (1989). *Cross-cultural nursing: Anthropological approaches to nursing research.* New York: Gordon and Breach Science Publishers.
16. Orque, M. S., Bloch, B., & Monrroy, L. S. A. (1983). *Ethnic nursing care: A multicultural approach.* Toronto: Mosby.
17. Spector, R. E. (1979). *Cultural diversity in health and illness.* New York: Appleton-Century-Crofts.
18. Todd, H. F., & Ruffini, J. L. (Eds.). (1969). *Teaching medical anthropology: Model courses for graduate and undergraduate instruction,* (Society for Medical Anthropology Special Publication No. 1). Washington, D.C.: American Anthropological Association.
19. Waxler-Morrison, N., Anderson, J., & Richardson, E. (Eds.). (1990). *Cross-cultural caring: A handbook for health professionals in western Canada.* Vancouver: University of British Columbia Press.

CHAPTER 89

Viewpoints

Cultural diversity in the student body revisited

BETTY S. FURUTA, JULIENE G. LIPSON

Twenty years ago students in American schools of nursing were predominantly young, white, middle-class women. Today nursing is much the same. Although there are slightly more minority students, their numbers remain small. The multicultural expansion that has taken place in so many other areas of society has not occurred in nursing. Branch[3] has characterized the problem as follows: "It is safe to say that the momentum of the 1960s and early 1970s has almost disappeared. Ethnic recruitment and retention programs have dropped in number and intensity. . . . This mood in nursing echoes the mood in the nation as a whole and it is a dismal prospect for both." The reason for Branch's discouragement can be seen in the data. Over the past dozen years, from 1978 to 1990, admissions of African-Americans to basic registered nurse (RN) programs increased only 3.8%; that of Hispanics, 1.5%; that of Asians, 1.7%; and that of Native Americans, 0.7%.[8,9] In 1990, the most recent year for which data are available, approximately 11.1% of all students admitted to the basic nursing programs were African-American; 3.2%, Hispanic; 3.0%, Asian; and 0.6%, Native American.[9] Of the number of RNs estimated to be employed in nursing, 4.0% were African-American; 2.7%, Asian; 1.4%, Hispanic; and 0.4%, Native American.[11]

These are not encouraging figures. What increases there have been are small, and the numbers of minority nurses are not proportional to the size of their respective population groups. This is in spite of a demographic shift in the United States that forecasts that by the year 2000 one of every three Americans will be a member of an ethnic minority. It is important to understand why there are so few nurses from the underrepresented groups and what can be done to encourage their participation—important for the profession, its practitioners, and its patients. Unless nursing can draw from those whom it serves, it risks not benefiting the changing society of which it is a part.

Although applications to RN programs have begun to increase, recruiting qualified ethnic students remains a challenge. Restoring effective recruitment efforts, instituting change where needed, and introducing new strategies have not been easy to accomplish, but some important lessons have been learned from the past.

DEVELOP A MINORITY APPLICANT POOL

Historically, generalized recruitment has failed to yield robust numbers of minority students. There simply is not a reservoir of prospective applicants waiting to be admitted into the profession. Schools must aggressively develop their own applicant pools—for example, by creating a consortium of schools in a cooperative recruitment effort.

Structuring and maintaining linkages with schools and programs that have the potential for providing prospective applicants over time permits a "pipeline" to exist between these schools and schools of nursing, a pipeline that can provide a relatively steady stream of applicants. A pipeline also enables the institution to track the student's course of study and, after matriculation, their academic progress. Recruitment of a school's own minority students into graduate study, at either the master's or doctoral level, is made easier, as well.

To establish a pipeline, nursing schools should establish formal or semiformal arrangements that oblige them to sponsor recruitment activities on a regular basis. Such activities might include giving scheduled recruitment presentations, inviting potential students to audit classes, offering regular counseling sessions with an assigned advisor to provide specialized help, and participating in preadmission or remediation courses. As able students are identified, they should be placed into the institutional pipeline, ideally with an assigned advisor to provide guidance.

CREATE ORIENTATION AND PRECEPTORSHIP PROGRAMS

Precollege and summer transition programs can do much to prepare entering students for the rigors of nursing education. Such programs provide an opportunity to foster necessary learning skills and to make clear the support services that are available to students, as well as to familiarize the students with the expectations of the school and its academic environment.[6]

An example is a university school that invites prospective students to visit the campus as part of an outreach program designed to introduce promising students from traditionally underrepresented groups to the nursing workplace and the academic environment. This same school offers undergraduates the opportunity to compete for one of several 10-week minority student summer research residencies. Students are awarded a modest stipend, mentored by recognized nursing faculty researches, and integrated into the research team during their residency. This model effectively immerses students in the intricacies of nursing research, which constitutes a major focus of graduate study. For preprofessional students who want to learn more about professional nursing and its specialty areas, there is also a 6-week summer program. The commonality among these efforts is piquing the interest of academically able minority students early in their careers by directly engaging them in the complex array of nursing activities that require advanced educational preparation.

Another approach is to create specific preceptorship programs that involve nurses in some advanced facet of the profession. Formal preceptorship and mentorship programs for doctoral students from underrepresented groups can be instituted that include dissertation-year funding and eventual postdoctoral fellowships to prepare them for research and academic careers. In addition to the obvious pedagogical benefits that accrue from such relationships, these doctoral nurses would learn to present research papers at conferences, write grant proposals, and undergo the rigors of external peer review, all of which are invaluable experiences. Taking advantage of occasions to publicize such preceptorships in the media not only recognizes the accomplishments of these students but also tacitly holds faculty accountable for helping them succeed.

The careful assignment of a faculty advisor in such programs is crucial. It is the advisor who helps create the social support for students that makes them feel welcome in a new environment. The advisor can also introduce minority students to one another and direct them to ethnic organizations on campus. These advisor positions are sufficiently important that fewer advisees should be assigned to those faculty that fill them so as to allow those faculty members the additional time that inevitably is required to function as advisor and advocate.

PERSONALIZE THE RECRUITMENT EFFORT

Sustained personal contact with prospective applicants, wherever one might find them, does make a difference. Not surprisingly, many matriculated students reveal that their reason for choosing to enroll at a particular institution was personal contact with either an enrolled student, a faculty member, or a member of the alumni. Students make the best recruiters, especially if they themselves are from ethnic minority groups. Every qualified minority student who has expressed interest in the health sciences and professions should be regarded as a prospective nursing student. At a minimum, that person should be personally contacted and provided information on current application deadlines and assistance with admission requirements.

It has been learned that more individually tailored approaches are needed. Although recruiters discuss topics that are germane to any student—such as program planning, class schedules, and part-time study—ethnic applicants may have other concerns that are as important. For instance, the attitude and receptiveness of the school toward the ethnic student may be of concern, or the potential financial burden to the family or student. Even the perceived benefit of the degree in terms of student goals may be questioned. These concerns are legitimate and are as specific as the needs of the individual. The recruiter should be prepared to answer them or help find the answers.

Recruiting qualified minority graduate students requires not only personal but competitive effort, since they are likely to be highly sought after. This might mean—for students at the master's and, even more so, the doctoral level—subsidizing prospective students' travel and per diem costs to visit the campus to meet potential faculty mentors and matriculated students. Nursing schools might even be able to provide honorariums and special recognition for those persons who have successfully recruited and mentored prospective ethnic applicants.

FORMALIZE NONTRADITIONAL ADMISSIONS CRITERIA

Applicants from underrepresented groups who are socioeconomically disadvantaged, especially those with weak educational preparation, typically score lower on standardized tests and may apply with marginal grade point averages. Such traditional indicators of academic achievement and capability are not always predictive of the academic success of minority students.[2] Variables other than scores on traditional tests (with their susceptibility to cultural bias) are needed to predict how minority students will fare in school. Carefully screened and given the opportunity to succeed, many do well in higher education. The supplemental criteria by which to evaluate these applicants are already requested by most nursing schools; examples are employment record, including promotions; evidence of leadership and/or creative behavior, wherever it may have been demonstrated; and a personal interview to validate or clarify ambiguous details or elicit other supporting information.

Although not intended for use as a nontraditional evaluation of applicants, the concept of "hardiness" seems applicable and may hold promise as a predictor of a person's educational success. Kobasa, Maddi, and Hahn[6] characterize hardiness as *control* (the belief that occurrences in one's life can be controlled), *commitment* (the ability to feel deeply involved in or committed to the activities of one's life), and *challenge* (the anticipation of change as an exciting opportunity for further development). There has been no systematic data collected on the utilization of hardiness as an admissions criterion. Rather, some experienced admissions reviewers concur that, when the qualifications of minority applicants are wanting, they search for precisely those behaviors described as hardiness that might surmount deficiencies identified by conventional

criteria. Aggressive but reasonable risk taking with minority nurses who have nontraditional credentials can have salutary outcomes, and institutions should adapt their norms, knowing that the quest for excellence need not be compromised.

A school's commitment to cultural diversity should also be shown in its willingness to admit applicants for whom English is a second language and whose culture, habits, and appearance may differ from that of other students. If much of their schooling was obtained elsewhere, immigrants can be faced with difficult admissions problems, especially if English is their second language. They may score poorly because of language problems or the unfamiliar construction of tests (e.g., multiple-choice questions). There also may be difficulties due to a different mode of reasoning and conceptualization, a lack of knowledge in certain required subjects such as the social and behavioral sciences, and an emphasis on interpersonal skills unfamiliar to them.

The challenge to admissions committees is to stipulate what the nontraditional criteria are and then to formally standardize how they will be considered in lieu of grade point averages and traditional test scores. A profile can be developed of minority applicants who have a reasonable chance of succeeding, including those for whom English is a second language. This profile would be determined by a review of the applications and the academic and clinical performance of students for whom the school has acted affirmatively in the past. Such data would provide qualitative support for a decision to admit into nursing when, by traditional indicators, an applicant's quantitative profile is marginal.

ENROLL A COHORT OF MINORITY STUDENTS

Even after admission, the underrepresented student is in a minority, with few, if any, peers. Pettigrew[10] has characterized this situation as the "solo phenomenon." It can be felt by anyone who is in a minority or thought to be different, and it can be a lonely experience, for there is little or no opportunity to be with one's peers. Self-consciously visible, the individual cannot assume the anonymity of the group, as those in the majority can. With a cohort of minority students which Pettigrew suggests should be approximately 20% of the student body, the expression of one's ethnic identity may even be threatened as with—for example—an international student who lacks the opportunity to converse in one's own language or a minority student who is unable to share an ethnic insight. The presence of such a "critical mass" can provide not only necessary peer support but also cross-cultural learning for students in both the majority and minority cultures. Without it, the attrition of ethnic students is much more likely, particularly when they are so few in number to begin with. Rather than endure the continual tension that accompanies self-consciousness and the constant maintenance of one's ethnic identity, students may opt to leave school altogether.

Isolation and self-consciousness can also be moderated by deliberately clustering underrepresented students in the same class or session for one or two appropriate courses. Such grouping can offer necessary peer support and provides ethnic students with an opportunity to engage one another directly on substantive nursing content and learn about its cultural relevance. Sustained and supervised small group studying can also alleviate a sense of being alone.

A companion to the solo experience is "tokenism," which occurs when an institution makes a minimal but visible gesture of compliance to a policy or practice. In affirmative action, a consequence of tokenism is the persistent questioning, usually not verbalized either by the ethnic student or others, as to whether admission was earned on academic merit or represents institutional tokenism. Being ethnically identifiable, even outstanding students may occasionally wonder during the course of their education whether or not they are tokens. Students in the majority may raise the same question and unfairly deny minority students recognition of their achievement. Clustering can mitigate this perception of the presence of tokenism.

CREATE A CULTURALLY SENSITIVE LEARNING ENVIRONMENT

That a diverse student body and inclusion of cultural content in a nursing curriculum are mutually enhancing has been recognized since the mid-1970s. One project that sought to increase the enrollment of students from underrepresented groups, for example, soon broadened its mission to encourage faculty to improve their cultural knowledge and awareness for more effective teaching. But progress in the last two decades has been uneven, and nursing education still emphasizes the dominant culture.

Administration and faculty both can play a critical role in building a diverse student body and maintaining a culturally sensitive environment. There should be a willingness on the part of faculty, for example, to modify ineffective teaching and evaluation methods and to explore their own racial attitudes.[12] Black faculty and staff models can be a critical factor in the retention of black students, yet this fact is not always recognized by their white colleagues.[1] If what is perceived as bias, cultural naiveté, or entrenched ethnocentrism in insensitive faculty members is repeatedly encountered, minority students are apt to withdraw from nursing school. With little diversity among faculty and students, misinformation and misunderstanding about various ethnicities may result in stereotyping.

Ethnic and immigrant students can enrich the experiences of their peers by helping them understand what they have observed, read about, or inadvertently overlooked, and by offering practical suggestions. Minority faculty members, argues Harvey,[5] also enhance the learning experience of all students, both in serving as role models for the students in the minority and in the sharing of their scholarship—and even their very presence—with students in the majority. This experience allows the meaning of cultural differences to come alive and be consensually validated.

MAINSTREAM STUDENT SERVICES

Increased minority and ethnic student enrollment and the retention of these students are the measures of success. It is important, therefore, that programs and academic services for these students be integral to the institution. With worthy intent, schools in the 1960s and 1970s frequently created separate services for underrepresented students that paralleled existing ones on campus. Yet they were susceptible to being identified as remediation centers for poorly prepared affirmative action students. Majority faculty and students also tended not to accept any responsibility for assisting underrepresented students when it was perceived that a special service and staff existed for that purpose. Furthermore, these services usually were funded by federal and/or state grants that were vulnerable to political and economic vicissitudes and arbitrary deadlines. When funding terminated, so did the service.

It is better to integrate minorities within the mainstream of services (e.g., learning resources center, counseling service, and financial aid office) that have been established for all students. Support services should be identified as being offered to all and not stigmatized as available only for certain groups; otherwise, students may be made to feel more separate, not less.

Family responsibilities and problems in adjustment can jeopardize the success of minority students just as surely as any academic difficulty. Past experience has shown that minority students need more financial assistance earlier in their education and for longer periods than do other students. Financial services, too, should be mainstreamed to normalize their use by minority students.

Continuing students can socialize new students into the institution and offer friendly support and advice in an unfamiliar setting. Such an arrangement can be voluntary or encouraged through a structured course for which credit is assigned, perhaps as single-unit independent study that is graded as pass-fail. In addition to requiring that students meet regularly with one another, the course may also require a group seminar once or twice during the term. Students would be obliged to develop learning objectives that relate to their arrangement as a basis for learning about cultural diversity.

RECRUIT MINORITY FACULTY

Increasing cultural diversity in the student body is made more difficult by its absence among faculty. A homogeneous faculty tends to perpetuate its own kind, and this needs to change. Nurse educators need to be recruited from underrepresented groups and their development nurtured once they are appointed.[4] Yet there are pitfalls in the quest to increase minority faculty. An institution may find it easier to hire underrepresented faculty into a clinical or other nontenured position, which does not require the rigor of an academic-ladder appointment. Since such positions are apt to be funded by grants or other less stable resources, these appointments are vulnerable to termination.

Besides customary assignments and responsibilities, ethnic faculty may also inherit some tasks that others do not, such as being assigned as an advisor to most, if not all, minority students; being appointed the ethnic member to committees; and being asked to serve as the institution's ethnic representative at events. Faculty can become overburdened with such visible public responsibilities and resentful that there are not colleagues who can share them. As a result, the ethnic faculty member may be less productive in the traditional areas of academic responsibility—teaching, research, and professional or community service. These, too, are important criteria for tenure and may put the overburdened faculty member at risk. The net result can be the loss of minority faculty.

Of course, nursing schools should groom their best and brightest minority doctoral students and postdoctoral fellows for faculty careers. But this will take time, and schools must learn to compete in the marketplace for doctorally prepared ethnic faculty. Such people are already highly recruited or in well-established positions. The courtship will require time, energy, resources, imagination, persistence, and luck. Some university administrations have set aside academic-ladder positions for which departments can compete only by recruiting top ethnic faculty. Salary savings from unfilled positions can also be used to support recruitment efforts. Ideally, minority members already on the faculty will have the mentorship of a senior colleague who can provide guidance for structuring scholarly work and assignments so as to ensure the productivity necessary for promotion.

CONCLUSION

Nursing education needs to make a stronger effort to represent the kaleidoscope of American society in its student body. But recruiting adequate numbers of diverse students is not enough. Administrators must actively commit their schools to nurturing minority students so that they can complete their program and contribute to the profession. This means providing a genuine institutional commitment to cultural diversity, a curriculum that includes cultural content in nursing care, and a culturally diverse presence among faculty. Nursing cannot solve the problems of society in general, and it will continue to feel those problems, itself, in the admission of students.

Nursing, however, can provide a model for itself to increase opportunities for students from underrepresented groups and to do so aggressively as it approaches the twenty-first century. Nursing has a moral and professional obligation to reaffirm its commitment to the education of minority students from all parts of society. Unless it does so, nursing risks becoming isolated from the communities it seeks to serve. Ultimately the issue is not about affirmative action or even the improvement of cultural diversity in the student body but about nursing's own humanity. It needs to attend to this moral imperative; otherwise, both the profession and those excluded from it will suffer.

REFERENCES

1. Allen, M. E., Nunley, J. C., & Scott-Warner, M. (1988). Recruitment and retention of black students in baccalaureate nursing programs. *Journal of Nursing Education, 27,* 107-116.
2. Boyle, K. K. (1986). Predicting the success of minority students in a baccalaureate nursing program. *Journal of Nursing Education, 25,* 186-192.
3. Branch, M. F. (1985). Ethnicity and cultural diversity in the nursing profession. In J. C. McCloskey & H. K. Grace (Eds.), *Current issues in nursing* (2nd ed., pp. 935-939). Boston: Blackwell Scientific Publications.
4. Furuta, B. (1992). Nursing faculty: Weavers of the dream. In Division of Nursing, Office of Minority Health, *Caring for the emerging minority: Creating a new diversity in nurse leadership* (pp. 61-75). Bethesda, Md: U.S. Department of Health and Human Services.
5. Harvey, W. B. (1988, January 22). Where are the black faculty members? *Chronicle of Higher Education,* p. 96.
6. Jones, S. H. (1992). Improving retention and graduation rates for black students in nursing education: A developmental model. *Nursing Outlook, 40,* 78-85.
7. Kobasa, S., Maddi, S., & Hahn, S. (1982). Hardiness and health: A prospective inquiry. *Journal of Personality and Social Psychology, 42,* 168-177.
8. National League for Nursing. (1990). *Nursing student census, 1989* (Pub. No. 19-2291). New York: Author.
9. National League for Nursing. (1991). *Nursing datasource, 1991: Vol. 1. Trends in contemporary nursing education* (Pub. No. 19-2420). New York: Author.
10. Pettigrew, T. (1984, February). *Proceedings of a colloquium on affirmative action in higher education: The second decade.* San Francisco: University of California.
11. U.S. Department of Health and Human Services, Division of Nursing. (1990, June). *The registered nurse population: Findings from the national sample survey of registered nurses, March 1988.* (NTIS No. PB91-145391). Rockville, Md: Author.
12. Wong, S., & Wong, J. (1982). Problems in teaching ethnic minority nursing students. *Journal of Advanced Nursing, 7,* 255-259.

CHAPTER 90

Nurses and unpopular clients

ROBERT J. KUS

Once a visitor watched Mother Theresa, founder of the Missionaries of Charity, care for a dying street person. Because the dying person was dirty, smelly, and had open lesions, the visitor turned to Mother Theresa and said, "I wouldn't do what you do for all the money in the world." Mother Theresa turned to him and said, "I wouldn't either!"

Few of us in nursing would dare compare our sanctity with that of Mother Theresa, yet I believe most of us would agree that our own motivation for caring for clients cannot be explained by money alone. For one thing, no amount of money could adequately compensate us for doing what we do. But more important, most of us in nursing see our work as transcending ordinary toil; it is, rather, a reflection of the human spirit, spirituality at its very best.

All nurses at some time have patients they do not like. Such encounters often make life miserable for the nurse and can actually harm the patient. Understanding the nature of unpopularity in clients can help nurses recognize the roots of their feelings and combat negative behaviors in themselves that can be harmful for patients they do not like. This will improve their own mental health as well as the care of their patients.

This chapter, then, examines the concept of unpopularity as it refers to nurses' patients, identifies the roots of unpopularity, and offers some ideas on how to prevent our negative views of clients from becoming destructive to ourselves and to them. Finally, one unpopular, vulnerable, and mistreated population in our society will be examined—prisoners—and some suggestions will be made concerning how nurses can intervene as nurses and citizens to combat the everyday antihuman treatment that prisoners endure.

THE CONCEPT OF UNPOPULARITY

Popularity comes from the Latin word *populus,* meaning "people." It refers to the state of something being liked or accepted by the population at large. *Unpopularity,* then, refers to a person, place, or thing being seen as not likable or acceptable by most people. When we say patients are unpopular, it is important to note that there is nothing intrinsic to any patient making that person unpopular or popular. Unpopularity can only exist when an external evaluation is placed on a person, place, or thing by people, in this case by nurses. Another important point is that there is often broad agreement among nurses about who is unpopular, whereas at other times defining a patient as unpopular is specific to a single nurse. An example of the former would be clients who are obnoxious toward nurses; an example of the latter is the client who looks like a nurse's despised ex-spouse.

THE ROOTS OF UNPOPULARITY

Why are some patients unpopular with nurses? This section explores some of the roots of unpopularity.

Low social value. Some persons are seen by nurses and other helping professionals as having less social value than others. This has been well documented by sociologists Glaser and Strauss,[1] among others. Social value is determined by demographic characteristics such as age, marital status, income, and the like. For example, a 98-year-old person is often seen as having less social value than a 20-year-old person. As a result, the heroic measures used to save the 20-year-old will often be withheld from the 98-year-old. Likewise, married persons—especially those with small children—are often seen as having higher social worth than single persons or married persons with no children. Nurses, being human, often see clients with low social value as being less desirable—unpopular—than those with high social value.

Low moral worth. Sometimes nurses classify persons as moral or immoral. Those deemed to be immoral become unpopular and thus may receive inferior nursing care to those deemed to be moral. For example, nurses may see a prostitute as immoral and a priest as moral because of the moral implications of their careers. Or the nurse may define clients who use physical violence to discipline their children as immoral. In short, when a client behaves in ways that go against our own value systems, we may define that person as immoral and unpopular.

Unchosen stigmata. Certain persons carry with them one or more stigmata that they did not choose, which make them unpopular with large numbers of people. Examples of such stigmata include gay or lesbian sexual orientation, gender (either male or female), and race or ethnicity. If the nurse is antimale or antiblack, chances are that male or black patients will be unpopular with that nurse.

"Own fault" diagnoses. Sometimes the root of unpopularity is the medical diagnosis the patient carries. If nurses perceive the disease or condition to be the result of behaviors chosen by the clients, they often find such patients unpopular. Typical examples of such patients are alcoholics, heavy smokers who have lung cancer, adults who contracted acquired immunodeficiency syndrome (AIDS) from having unsafe sex or from needles contaminated with human immunodeficiency virus (HIV), and suicidal patients. Often nurses want to care for "innocent" persons who "deserve" their care rather than those whom they feel are "getting what they deserve."

Fear-causing conditions. Some patients' behaviors or medical diagnoses are frightening to nurses, which makes such patients unpopular. The person with a highly contagious, incurable disease or the violent patient are two common examples. Fear of contracting a disease, however, is often a cover-up for bigotry, as when a truly homophobic nurse claims that a fear of catching the disease is the reason for refusing to care for a gay man with AIDS.

Clients who behave negatively. In addition to violent clients who frighten nurses, certain clients behave in ways that are generally perceived by nurses to be negative. These include clients who are seen as un-

grateful, "spoiled brats," hostile, staff-splitters, manipulators, eager to sue, constant complainers, and noncompliant. In addition, people who seem to be "professional patients" (hypochondriacs) and those who overuse their call lights are often unpopular with many nurses.

Incompetence on the nurse's part. Sometimes clients are unpopular with nurses simply because the nurses do not feel competent to care for them. It is frightening and dangerous to care for clients about whom you know little. For example, child-health nurses floated to a coronary care unit might see their new clients as having needs far beyond their ability to meet.

THE CONSEQUENCES OF UNPOPULARITY

When clients are defined as unpopular by their nurses, there are potential consequences for both clients and nurses. For nurses, caring for unpopular patients may lead to job dissatisfaction, which, in turn, may lead to diminished health—physical, mental, and spiritual. Nurses may increasingly call in sick; suffer from insomnia, anorexia, or other compulsive behaviors; withdraw from their peers; criticize the profession or the institution; or exhibit a lack of energy on the job. If nurses begin to put all or most of their patients in the unpopular category—as might nurses who cannot find work in their field of expertise—quitting the job or the profession might result.

Nurses may also take out their negative feelings toward unpopular patients by engaging in behaviors based on hostility or frustration. They can withhold pain medications, ignore call lights, act cool and detached instead of warm and sensitive, ignore basic psychosocial needs, and turn other staff against such patients. These behaviors harm the unpopular patient, certainly, yet they also may harm the nurse. For example, although it might give the nurse immediate gratification to get back at an obnoxious patient, in the long run it might (and should) produce feelings of guilt. On the other hand, wise nurses may engage in hyperpositive behaviors toward their unpopular clients to counteract their inclinations to treat them unkindly.

COMBATING NEGATIVE EFFECTS OF UNPOPULARITY

Because defining certain clients as unpopular often leads to negative feelings and behavior on the part of the nurse, and because this labeling often leads to negative nursing behavior directed toward such clients, it is wise to explore how nurses can minimize these negatives.

First, nurses need to admit to their negative feelings toward certain clients. They need to identify those patients who make them feel uncomfortable, angry, self-righteous, and the like. Second, they need to make a list of unpopular patients. Writing down the characteristics of such patients is most helpful, as this will help nurses identify more easily the categories that emerge. Nurses should analyze this list to determine exactly what it is about such patients that makes them unpopular. In other words, what are the "negativity generators." Negativity generators will be defined here as those client characteristics that generate negative feelings in nurses and, therefore, make such clients unpopular. Are they skin color? Religion? Obnoxious or seductive behavior? Legal status, as in the case of prisoners?

After examining the categories of persons on their lists, nurses can ask themselves whether the negativity generators are changeable or unchangeable. Negativity generators are considered unchangeable if the client has no control over their existence. These would include such characteristics as gender (transsexuals excluded), race, ethnicity, sexual orientation, age, and often various disease conditions such as cerebral palsy. Likewise, the client may have done something in the past and received a label that generates negative feelings in the nurse. Examples of these include heavy smokers who now have lung cancer or prisoners. Although prisoners may have been responsible for doing something negative that led to their being incarcerated, they are not able to change their current status.

In contrast to the unchangeable generators, there are two types that are clearly changeable. One type includes characteristics that nurses would usually be reluctant to try to change. Examples of these include religion or marital status. A second type is characteristics that nurses generally feel require nursing intervention to change to make the client a more fulfilled person. Examples of these would be behaviors that are nonassertive, manipulative, seductive, violent, hostile, noncompliant, or generally obnoxious.

Third, nurses must examine how they treat those clients they see as unpopular. Do they give such patients less time than they do other patients? Do they avoid them? Talk negatively about them to other staff? Withhold pain medication? Neglect their psychosocial needs? If nurses find that they care for each client in a caring, sensitive, and professional manner no matter what the circumstances, then they need go no further. But if nurses realize they are treating certain patients negatively either directly (e.g., by withholding pain medication or by being unfriendly) or indirectly (e.g., by turning other staff against them or by allowing staff to treat such patients negatively), they must then make a decision to change any negative behaviors in which they are engaging toward unpopular clients. This requires reminding themselves of the lofty nursing ideals that all humans, by virtue of their humanity, are worthy of total respect, care, and compassion regardless of their various life circumstances or past or present behaviors.

If nurses find that their negative patient list includes people who have unchangeable personal characteristics, nurses can do one of three things: (1) stay clear of such patients, (2) change their attitudes, or (3) keep their attitudes but change any behavior that would reflect their negativity toward the client.

Staying clear of such patients is a relatively straightforward prospect. A nurse who cannot stand children might quit a hospital job on a pediatric unit to become a medical nurse, or a psychiatric nurse might leave a medical-surgical unit to work in a mental health center. Changing negative attitudes is more difficult. It requires work and a great willingness to change. If nurses find they are antiwhite or antigay, for example, they must be willing to confront white people or gay people to change their feelings. If they cannot change, they must simply adopt the third strategy of keeping their attitudes but changing any negative behaviors they may use toward such clients.

If nurses find their unpopular patient list is composed of persons whose negativity generators are changeable, they need to ask themselves whether helping the client to change these characteristics is ethical or not. For example, a person's religion is usually not something a nurse tries to change unless it is a cult generally seen as dangerous by society at large. On the other hand, if a client has a pattern of violence or seductive behavior, the nurse would be helping the patient by encouraging such a change in behavior. Such change would not only eliminate negativity on the part of the nurse, it would also benefit the patient in the long run.

Fourth, nurses can combat the negative effects of unpopularity in patients by seeing nursing as a way of life, not merely a job having relevance when the nurse is on duty. When nurses do this, they not only focus on their particular patients or believe in taking action only in their work setting, but also see themselves and their profession as holding the key to radically changing negative actions toward all humans, in all settings, at all times. Thus, no policy that degrades any human is deemed outside the province of nursing. Let us look at one such example.

THE PRISONER AND NURSING

Having read this far, most nurses, I am sure, feel pretty confident that they are not too far off the mark in treating all patients with the dignity they deserve simply because of their humanity. After all, nurses are pretty decent folk. Those readers who have identified some clients whom they have treated negatively are probably willing to change.

But before becoming too smug and complacent, we nurses need to ask ourselves some difficult questions. One is, when are we nurses? Only when officially on duty or at all times? If we answer only when on duty, then we may indeed pat ourselves on the back if we strive to treat all patients, even the most unpopular ones, with great compassion, sensitivity, and care. On the other hand, if we see ourselves as being nurses at all times, then we will be less smug.

The second question we must ask is, who are our clients? If we believe our clients are only those persons to whom we are legally responsible while on duty, then we probably can be comfortable in examining our care. On the other hand, if we believe that all humanity is our client, then we have to realize that nursing has just begun to be practiced.

The third question is, what is nursing? For some nurses it is traditional functions such as one-to-one counseling, patient teaching, and performing technical procedures. For others it is a radical social activism designed to elevate humanity to its highest level by eliminating the suffering of *all* humans and destroying the roots of suffering of *all* humans. I believe nurses must make every attempt to ensure that the Golden Rule—"Do unto others as you would have them do unto you"—be followed for *all* humans, not just those who are popular.

This brings us to prisoners. No persons in our society are more vulnerable to the hatred and truly dark, punitive side of human nature. Nurses are certainly not immune; they have been shown to be followers, rather than leaders, in prison reform and the general treatment of prisoners.

But talking about prisoners often generates intense feelings in some individuals. Many argue that prisoners "deserve" to be punished. Thus they are not merely content to see police, prison guards, judges, and others mistreat prisoners; they often encourage it. Nurses have proved time and again to be a reflection of the larger society—followers rather than leaders or social activists.

From my perspective, all actions that counteract the Golden Rule are acts of antilove. All antilove acts are against the dignity of humanity. All acts against human dignity are morally wrong. All such acts are, then, against the very core of nursing. And as long as such acts continue, nurses must fight to eliminate them.

So it is not okay to chain human beings to beds. It is not okay to parade human beings around hospitals or anywhere else in identifiable prison garb and chains and handcuffs. It is not okay to allow prisoners to be raped. It is not okay to lock persons up in prisons *as they exist today*.

If nurses believe these things are violations of human dignity, what can they do? They can oppose all policies that permit prisoners to be chained to beds or paraded around in prison garb and chains. These disgusting practices offend the sensibilities of any person who has an ounce of decency. True, there must be a way to prevent escape or, more accurately, to prevent police from harming prisoners under the guise of "preventing attempted escape." But could we not invent a device to be worn under clothing that would prevent a person from running? Could we not have nonuniformed guards by clients' beds instead of chaining them to a bed? Of course we can. The question is not whether we can but whether we value human life and human dignity enough to do so.

Nurses need to fight for prison reform, or rather for the elimination of virtually all prisons except for a limited number to house those who are truly dangerous. Some people need to be out of society. But they do not need to be treated like rabid animals as they are today, and certainly they do not need to be confined in the antihuman institutions that many prisons are today. Prison architecture and programs must be designed to provide the prisoner with the highest quality of life possible. It seems to me that being locked away from loved ones, denied basic freedoms, stigmatized for life, and forced to associate with people who have devoted much of their lives to degrading human beings—judges, probation and parole officers, police, prison guards, and the like—is truly enough punishment. Nurses must also fight against the rape of prisoners, most of whom are males, just as hard as they fight against the rape of nonincarcerated females. To do otherwise is incredibly sexist.

From my perspective, a nurse is always a nurse. Our clients are all humanity. However, although all people are our clients in a moral sense, those who suffer—especially the disadvantaged—deserve our most fervent and compassionate attention. And nursing is for me a radical social activism designed to protect the dignity of *all* humans and destroy *all* things that lead to a person's mental, physical, and spiritual distress. The mistreatment of fellow humans should rekindle a fire in every nurse, a fire born of rage and fervor, a fire that will rock the very foundations of our profession in a radical social activism that will not stop until every human on earth is treated with true dignity.

REFERENCES

1. Glaser, B. G., & Strauss, A. L. (1968). *Time for Dying*. Chicago: Aldine.

CHAPTER 91

Increasing the pool of minority students

PATRICIA T. CASTIGLIA

The very fact that we must identify persons as minority members in our society as we approach the twenty-first century is in opposition to our early roots as a nation. Why do we still feel compelled, after generations, to attach prefixes to designate certain Americans, such as African-Americans and Mexican-Americans? It is interesting to note that other groups have not been so identified, as they have been assimilated. We do not usually say "Albanian-Americans," for example. A complete discussion of this issue is beyond the scope of this chapter, but it is an important issue that should be recognized and discussed as a basis for actions the nursing profession must take to increase the pool of minority students.

MINORITY REPRESENTATION IN NURSING

Nursing can no longer sustain itself without incorporating, to a greater extent, diverse minority groups into the profession. Interwoven with the issues related to minorities in nursing are a number of issues that reflect societal views toward women, toward subcultures of our society, and toward demographic changes that have occurred over time. Although the number of men in nursing has increased, the profession remains a predominantly female profession (approximately 96%). Therefore, gender socialization has played and continues to play a major role in both the continuation and the development of nursing. Stereotypes related to gender, as well as to ethnicity, cannot be artificially separated when examining the past, present, and future considerations of minorities in nursing.

Basic influences when selecting a career relate to one's beliefs about oneself. Where do I belong or fit? What is an acceptable career from the viewpoint of my family and my social group? Where can I find personal fulfillment? Financial reward? Advancement? Security? Ability to be mobile, yet permanence in a career?

The estimated registered professional nurse population in 1988 was 2,033,032. Of this number, 91.7% were white (non-Hispanic), 3.6% were black (non-Hispanic), 2.3% were Asian–Pacific Islander, 0.4% were American Indian–Alaskan Native, 1.3% were Hispanic, and 0.7% were of unknown heritage.[17] Between 1984 and 1988, the total number of professional nurses with a minority background remained the same, with about one half of these nurses being black. During this same time period, a modest increase in the number of men in nursing occurred (3.0% to 3.3%). And during the same period, graduates from basic nursing educational programs became somewhat older. In 1984, 20% of all graduates were under 30 years old, and in 1988 this had decreased to 15.6%.[17]

These figures must be related to what is occurring in nursing education. Obvious questions to be investigated include: Are members of minority groups attracted into nursing? Do they successfully complete programs of study? Do they remain in the profession? Why should we be concerned about the representation, or rather the lack of representation, of significant numbers of minorities in nursing? What directions should we pursue?

CURRENT STATUS OF MINORITIES IN NURSING EDUCATION PROGRAMS

Nursing is not unique among the professions, which have traditionally attracted predominantly white students. This has persisted despite efforts at equal opportunities for the culturally diverse segments of American society. It is indeed incongruous when one considers Hodgkinson's 1985 study[11] of demographic trends and the impact these trends will have on our educational system. The Hodgkinson study concludes that by the year 2000, one in every three citizens will be nonwhite. Harris[10] predicts that one third to one half of all students will be students of color by the twenty-first century.

During the 1980s declining enrollments in nursing education programs encouraged schools to actively pursue minority candidates. The Nurse Training Act of 1964 and subsequent revisions provided special funding to increase the number of disadvantaged and minority students in schools of nursing. In 1965 the Sealantic fund (Rockefeller Brother's fund) began sponsoring a program in nursing education for disadvantaged students. This project emphasized recruitment, counseling, summer enrichment programs, and financial assistance. The American Nurses Association (ANA) minority fellowship program and the Kellogg fellows program are other examples of attempts not only to improve numbers of minority nurses but to assist minority nurses to advance in the profession.

The National Student Nurses' Association developed the Breakthrough to Nursing project in 1963, which focused on recruiting minorities into the nursing profession. Federal funding for this project was obtained in 1971 and again in 1974. The Breakthrough project has emphasized the establishment of one-to-one relationships with prospective candidates. The program also includes a planned tutoring-advocacy-counseling component.[5] Despite this 25-year effort in nursing, the racial-ethnic composition in nursing education programs remained the same as the figures reported for all higher education students in 1988, with the number of blacks being marginally higher in nursing. The number of blacks was just under 10% for all students, and in nursing blacks represented 11.4%. In 1990 Carter[6] reported increases in American Indian, Hispanic, and black students in 2-year institutions, while there were more Asian-Americans enrolled in 4-year institutions.

The tracking of nursing students by the National League for Nursing (NLN) clearly illustrates that the minority composition of nursing students varies across geographical areas of the country. For example, the largest percentage of black graduates, 12.3%, is found in both the North Atlantic and Southern regions; while most Hispanic, Asian, and American Indian students are found in the west.[13] In addition, the NLN report found that more Hispanics and American Indians graduated from licensed practical nurse and licensed vocational nurse (LPN-LVN) programs than from registered nurse (RN) programs. Men continue to represent only a small minority in nursing; and since the recruitment efforts in nursing focus on ethnic minorities, it is expected that this representation will continue. However, while the national average for male enrollment in nursing is 7% to 9%, once again geographical areas vary. In West Texas, for example, males constitute anywhere from 15% to 18% of the student nursing enrollment. It may be that the increased enrollment of males in this area is a reflection of males viewing nursing as a route upward in the social and economic structure, the acceptance in this community of males in a predominantly female profession, or the great need for nurses in this area.

Statistics related to minority enrollment in nursing programs become of even greater concern when considered in relation to the enrollment in specific types of nursing programs. For example, at the baccalaureate level Hispanics constitute 2.9% of the total enrollment, but at the master's and doctoral levels their enrollment is only 1.7% each. Although blacks generally represent the largest minority in nursing, it is worth noting that of all black nursing students, 8.8% are enrolled in generic baccalaureate programs; 7.4%, in RN baccalaureate programs; 5.2%, in master's programs; 4.3%, in doctoral programs; and only 1 of 14 postdoctoral students was black.[3]

Factors influencing the need to change minority ratios

A persistent decline in the number of young people eligible for college admission is documented nationwide. Concurrently there has been an increase in the number of older students, those over 25 years old, who are interested in pursuing college careers including nursing.

Applications to nursing programs have recovered from the 1980s slump. This is due to the compounded impact of the nursing shortage, a lack of access to health care for many Americans, an aging population, a shift to an emphasis on primary community health care, cost containment efforts by hospitals (including the use of diagnostic-related groups), and a movement to break down barriers between the health professions through expanded reimbursement by Medicaid, Medicare, and third-party insurers for specifically prepared nurses. These factors have forced the health care system to upgrade salaries and benefits for nurses. When adequate financial reimbursement occurs in a profession, members of that profession develop an increased sense of self-esteem and colleagues in other professions develop an increased respect. The waiting lists for admission to many schools of nursing attest to the increased attractiveness of the nursing profession today. Unfortunately, adequate remuneration has not extended to areas of need beyond hospital settings. Public health nursing salaries, school nursing salaries, and salaries in extended care facilities still lag. This is a serious manifestation of the blatant lack of provision for quality health care to the poor, to rural and urban underserved and underinsured citizens, and to minority populations, and particularly a diminished commitment to health promotion and disease prevention activities.

The question of quality in nursing practice continues to be a factor that must be carefully considered. In the past, nursing schools were tempted to make exceptions to admissions requirements in order to maintain programs through sustained enrollments. Now the pendulum may swing toward admitting only the most highly qualified applicant in relation to quantitative measures such as American College Test (ACT) scores, Scholastic Aptitude Test (SAT) scores, or grade point average (GPA). Because of the increased applicant pool, admissions committees may be tempted to fill classes with only the "best" students as measured by traditional criteria. If efforts are not made on elementary, middle, and high school levels to better prepare minority students, we may find that our equal opportunity access has been thwarted. Most admissions evaluations cannot accommodate all minimally prepared applicants, so admissions committees seek to select the students with the most potential for success.[4] If this is carried to the extreme, minority students may suffer because they will not be afforded the opportunity to attempt to succeed.

Traditionally, minority students have been classified as high-risk students because they often experience higher attrition rates than white students. The most frequently used criteria upon which admission to nursing is based include high school GPA, high school rank, interviews, health data, college GPA, ACT assessment scores, SAT scores, and autobiographical essays. There have been a number of conflicting studies regarding the usefulness of these criteria for the prediction of success in a nursing program. Dell and Halpin[8] recommended the use of high school GPA, SAT scores, and NLN scores as effective for use with all ethnic groups. The Boyle study[4] found that the ACT score was the strongest and most effective predictor of state board examination achievement and of the final GPA. Entering GPA

was the only variable that was found to account for program completion, but it did not accurately predict program dropouts. The higher the entering GPA, however, the greater the likelihood of program completion. The predictive power for blacks was less than for other minorities, but an earlier investigator, Schwirian,[16] maintained that less than 50% of attrition is really related to academic difficulty and that attrition may rather be due to greater social and economic disadvantages. A study by Schmidt, Pearlman, and Hunter[15] sought to evaluate the validity and fairness of employment and educational tests for Hispanic Americans. The results of this study indicate that there is strong evidence that the tests are neither differentially valid for, nor unfair to, Hispanics. The validity and slope differences were found to be due to chance, as reported in an earlier study of blacks.

In recent years, women have been attracted to professions other than the traditional occupations of nursing and teaching. The attractiveness of the nursing profession has been enhanced by the development of new and expanded roles in nursing. These new roles are characterized by increased autonomy and by increased appreciation and recognition from the public and from professional colleagues.

High school students today have a broad range of career choices. The American Association of Colleges of Nursing (AACN) report[2] dealing with enrollment management found that a large percentage of students cited nursing as a career objective and that parents exerted the most influence on student career choice. When students were asked why they had an interest in nursing, they cited the following desires: (1) to help others, (2) to work directly with people, and (3) to work with life-and-death situations. The reasons they lacked interest in nursing were related to the requirements to (1) work in high-pressure situations, (2) work in stressful situations, and (3) work different shifts. Parental goals for their children were reported as follows: (1) to be financially secure, (2) to do rewarding work, and (3) to have time to spend with family. These items were rated number 11, 2, and 10 respectively by parents in relation to the nursing profession.[2]

The Hispanic student in nursing

The term *Hispanic* covers the Spanish, Mexican-Americans, Puerto Ricans, and those of Cuban descent. The greatest numbers in the United States are Mexican-American (Chicanos). A study by Vasquez[18] found that sex-role restrictions and low socioeconomic status rather than culture or language partially accounted for the relatively low number of Chicanas (Mexican-American women) in postsecondary education. Chicanas are no different from other people in wanting education as a means to socioeconomic mobility and independence. Unfortunately, Mexican-American women, who are often the first in their families to attend college, experience dissonance in relation to their expected role in Mexican-American society as wife, mother, and subservient person to the male; all of these factors exert an influence to diminish professional career expectations. Mexican-American students unfortunately are often steered into taking non college preparatory courses in high school. This may be promulgated by the family as a means of keeping women in less demanding work, which in turn is perceived as having a less negative impact on the woman's traditional role. Such advice from family members may be reinforced by educators who often stereotype Mexican-American students as unable to prepare for more challenging careers. Most Mexican-American students need financial assistance, as their parents are generally unable to contribute as much to their education as Anglo-American parents can.[18] Therefore they generally rely heavily on scholarships and work-study programs and, to a lesser extent, on loans. Because of the difference in cultures and the difficulty in acculturation, many of these minority students feel more comfortable in smaller colleges or community colleges. Support systems such as associations and organizations that can recognize, promote, and reinforce cultural values are important for student adjustment regardless of the size of the educational setting.

Financial difficulty and uncomfortableness in the setting, while problematic, are not the primary factors for leaving educational programs. A study by Cope and Hannah[7] found that the motivation to finish college was influenced in great measure by the family's emotional support of the student. This may be a comforting fact to relay to parents who fear "losing" their child when she or he pursues higher education. Since parents do influence their child's choice of a career, some reassurance from an individual's ethnic group—such as continued inclusion in family and community activities—has been found to be a necessary positive component of adjustment and success in college. This finding may reassure Mexican-American parents of their continued important role. In fact several researchers, including Ramirez and Castaneda,[14] have found that participating in two or more cultures may provide

for a more flexible adjustment. It would appear to be self-evident that Hispanic students, like other students, would tend to persist in their education when their parents have higher educations and when parental occupations result in higher incomes. Low family income, for many students, results in their dropping out of school. Since Mexican-American families generally have lower incomes, and either larger or extended families to absorb the income, their children are at risk for attrition. Therefore efforts must persist to obtain scholarships and grants to attempt to alleviate some of this pressure. In 1991 the Department of Health and Human Services instituted a new scholarship program called Scholarships for Disadvantaged Students (SDS). These scholarships recognize that the concept of being disadvantaged is not necessarily tied to ethnicity alone but rather is tied to socioeconomic factors including deficits in a particular school district's ability to offer enriched programs for students.

The black student in nursing

Nursing education has historically provided one of the few avenues for black women to acquire a respected profession. However, for many years that education was primarily obtained in black hospitals and colleges. Early graduates worked only with blacks. As the profession of nursing evolved, an elitist system developed in which most white schools had racial quotas. An early effort to recruit black nursing students was stimulated during World War II by the Cadet Nurse Corps program. Today the emphasis is on attracting black and other minority students, not to fill quotas, but to develop a cohort of professional nurses who better represent the general population.

Between 1976 and 1982 the National Advisory Committee on Black Higher Education and Black Colleges and Universities studied the admission and retention problems of black students at seven predominantly white universities. Although this committee no longer exists, the problem it faced, the retention of black baccalaureate nursing students, persists.[1]

Black students, like other minority students, often have had a poor secondary education. Their self-esteem has been low and the university has generally been perceived as hostile. Not only have high school counselors failed in encouraging black students to pursue higher education but, additionally, university counselors have not been able to effectively thwart the feelings of loneliness and alienation that black students frequently experience. Inadequate financial aid has been found to be a barrier to both the admission and the retention of black nursing students.[1]

Graduate nursing education and the minority student

Graduate education in nursing continues to grow, as indicated by an 8.1% increase in master's graduates from 1989 to 1990. In addition, the number of doctoral programs rose to 50 in 1990.[12] The expansion of advanced educational preparation in nursing is related to increased specialization in the practice arena necessitating increased preparation in terms of the complexity and competency needed to administer quality nursing care and to pursue relevant research.

Funding for students to attend graduate programs is always subject to the legislators' awareness of the importance of and need for such funding. Federal monies distributed as a result of the Nursing Education Act are primarily allocated for nurses pursuing advanced preparation as nurse practitioners, nurse-midwives, nurse anesthetists, and advanced clinical specialists.

As in undergraduate education, geographical differences exist, with the largest number of graduate minority students found in the South and the smallest number in the West.[12] Almost two thirds of all master's graduates prepare for advanced clinical practice, 9% prepare for administration, and 12% prepare for teaching. Of those nurses prepared at the graduate level, 14.2% are members of minority groups: almost 7% are black, 3% are Hispanic, 4% are Asian, and 1% are American Indian. The number of those who actually complete graduate programs is somewhat lower.[12]

Between 1989 and 1990, the number of nursing doctoral degrees awarded dropped from 324 to 295. The National League for Nursing[12] speculates that this may be due to increased numbers of part-time students, decreased funding for dissertation research, and a lack of doctorally prepared faculty to work with students. Minority enrollment in doctoral programs has been reported as 1.1% or less for American Indians or Alaskan Natives, 1.7% for Hispanics, and 4.3% for blacks. All minority groups are represented by lower percentages at the graduate level as opposed to those at the baccalaureate level. This is in contrast to the white students, who increase in percentage at the graduate level. Whites account for 81.9% of all baccalaureate students and increase to 86.1% of all master's and 83.0% of all doctoral students. It should be noted that at the doctoral level 2.6% (more than Hispanics and

Asian or Pacific Islanders) are nonresident alien students and 5.3% are of unknown heritage.[3]

What do these data mean? It is obvious that the numbers of minority students seeking higher education in nursing are not representative of the general population, especially in the case of Hispanics. Therefore these nurses are not able to move within the profession to positions of leadership and power. Why does this happen? Once again a variety of factors interact. The following interpretation is a premise for those of Hispanic origin. Because of the low economic status of most Mexican-American families, when the student completes the basic nursing program, she or he is expected to go to work immediately, often the day after graduation, to contribute to the family's finances. In more than one instance, the graduate is expected to put the next child through college. In addition, at this stage in their lives, marriage and child rearing become a focus. The Mexican-American family culture frowns on leaving children at day-care centers or in the care of non-family members. In addition, the basic cultural value of the dominant male figure often overrides a career drive. In other words, the nurse resumes life in a culture that generally does not encourage advanced preparation. Survival of the family unit is the primary motivator. This is not to judge that value but rather to acknowledge that it exists and that it may be a factor that discourages minority nurses from pursuing graduate education.

STRATEGIES TO IMPROVE THE ETHNIC MIX IN NURSING

If demographic trends persist, there will be an increase in Hispanic and Asian populations and a modest growth in the black population.[13] Mexican-Americans comprise the second largest minority group in the United States and can be found not only in the Southwest but in urban areas throughout the United States. Therefore, increasing representation of these minority groups must be a priority. As these populations grow, there will be an increased need for nurses who can relate to, understand, and be accepted by the community. An important role will be in assisting people who have been deprived of access to health care to participate in the existing health care system and in molding the future health care system to be responsive to their needs.

In order to accomplish this, federal, state, and local financial support must be available. Inequities in public education must be addressed. Local public school boards must direct resources toward the goal of quality educational opportunities for all children. Poor school tax districts must receive assistance from the state.

At the postsecondary level, institutions must provide counseling and tutorial services as well as financial aid. The composition of nursing facilities must reflect an ethnic mix not just for token representation, or to reflect a specific community, but to become a living model of diversity in collaboration—a model that stresses competence, academic ability, caring, and true equality. Potential minority faculty members must be identified as early as possible in their academic careers and supported in their efforts to obtain graduate degrees. In one possible system, they could pay back the institution's financial support through a committed service period. These young faculty members, like all junior faculty, must be nurtured through a mentoring program. They have the potential to serve as role models for minority students and, in time, can serve as mentors themselves.

In recent years there have been philosophical discussions about whether or not there should be organizations for minorities in nursing, such as the Hispanic Nurses' Association or the National Black Nurses' Association (NBNA). It would appear that these organizations provide support and networking for minority nurses who may not be able to take advantage of opportunities in the major nursing organizations because of their small numbers. Therefore, until such time as the minority nurses themselves feel that a need no longer exists, local chapters of these organizations should be encouraged. Professional nursing success is necessary to advance in the profession. Professional nursing success can be interpreted as psychological success whereby an internalized goal includes ego involvement. Psychological success increases self-esteem and strengthens a commitment.[9] A supportive social network is a means of minimizing threats to one's sense of self-worth and fostering career enhancement.

At present there is a greater proportion of black faculty members in nursing as contrasted with their representation in all other colleges. There is a smaller percentage, however, of all other minority groups in nursing as contrasted with all other colleges. Regional population differences exist, with more blacks in the South and more Asians and Hispanics in the West. Associate programs appear to have more faculty diversity.[13] This may be related to the minimal aca-

demic credential of a bachelor's degree required to teach in an associate degree program. Additionally, fewer than 8% of the chief administrators of nursing programs are designated as members of a minority group.[13] These figures are similar for all nursing administrative positions.

Nursing education has a direct responsibility to educate practitioners for the future. The demographics of the United States have changed. Spanish has become a second language for many parts of the country, and we must educate to meet these changes.

SUMMARY

Access to health care must be improved. All health care professionals must be better utilized, and economics will guide much of the needed reform. When an analysis of nursing student populations does not coincide with the demographics of the general population, nurse educators must take steps to ameliorate that situation. Suggestions for strategies have been explored, and conscious recognition of the problem can move nursing forward so that minorities are appropriately represented in our faculties and student bodies.

REFERENCES

1. Allen, M. E., Nunley, J. C., & Scott-Warner, M. (1988). Recruitment and retention of black students in baccalaureate nursing programs. *Journal of Nursing Education, 27*(3), 107-116.
2. American Association of Colleges of Nursing. (1990). *Enrollment management for programs in nursing education* (Pub. No. 19-2419). Washington, D.C.: Author.
3. American Association of Colleges of Nursing. (1992). *1991-1992 enrollment and graduations in baccalaureate and graduate programs in nursing* (Pub. No. 91-92-1). Washington, D.C.: Author.
4. Boyle, K. K. (1986). Predicting the success of minority students in a baccalaureate nursing program. *Journal of Nursing Education, 25*(5), 186-192.
5. Carnegie, M. E. (1988). Breakthrough to nursing: Twenty-five years of involvement. *Imprint, 35*(2), 55-56, 59.
6. Carter, D. J. (1990). Racial and ethnic trends in college participation: 1976-1988. *Research Briefs* (American Council on Education), *1*(3).
7. Cope, R. G., & Hannah, W. (1975). *Revolving college doors: The causes and consequences of dropping out, stopping out, and transferring.* New York: Wiley-Interscience.
8. Dell, M., & Halpin, G. (1984). Predictors of success in nursing school and on state board examinations in a predominantly black baccalaureate nursing program. *Journal of Nursing Education, 23*(4), 147-150.
9. Hall, D. T. (1976). *Careers in organizations.* Pacific Palisades, Calif: Goodyear.

10. Harris, R. L. (1990). Recruiting Afro-Americans into the graduate school pipeline. *Perspectives, 28*(1), 6, 11-12.

11. Hodgkinson, H. L. (1985). *All one system: Demographics of education, kindergarten through graduate school.* Washington, D.C.: Institute for Educational Leadership.

12. National League for Nursing. (1991). *Nursing data review (1991)* (Pub. No. 19-2419). New York: Author.

13. National League for Nursing. (1991). *Nursing datasource: Vol. 3. Leaders in the making: Graduate education in nursing* (Pub. No. 19-2422). New York: Author.

14. Ramirez, M., III, & Castaneda, O. (1974). *Cultural democracy, bicognitive development and education.* New York: Academic Press.

15. Schmidt, F. L., Pearlman, K., & Hunter, J. E. (1980). The validity and fairness of employment and educational tests for Hispanic Americans: A review and analysis. *Personnel Psychology, 33*(4), 704-724.

16. Schwirian, P. (1977). *Prediction of successful nursing performance: Part 2. Admission practices, evaluation strategies and performance prediction among schools of nursing* (HEW Pub. No. HRA 77-27). Washington, D.C.: U.S. Government Printing Office.

17. U.S. Department of Health and Human Services. (1990). *The registered nurse population: Findings from the national sample survey of registered nurses, March 1988.* Washington, D.C.: Author.

18. Vasquez, M. J. T. (1982). Confronting barriers to the participation of Mexican-American women in higher education. *Hispanic Journal of Behavioral Success, 4*(2), 147-165.

CHAPTER 92

Why aren't there more men in nursing?

EDWARD J. HALLORAN, JOHN M. WELTON

There were approximately 67,626 men nurses in the United States in 1988, which represented 3.3% of the country's 2,033,032 registered nurses (Table 92-1). Although the proportion remains insignificant, the number of nurses who are men continues to increase at a rate exceeding the growth rate for all nurses. In 1984 the proportion was 3.0% of all nurses—that represents a 4-year growth rate of 18%, compared with a growth rate of 7% for all nurses.[1]

Four issues emerge that explain the paucity of American men in nursing. History, economics, the military, and sex-role stereotyping have all weighed heavily against nursing as a career choice for American men. Paradoxically, the issues that have constrained the entry of men into nursing can also serve as an impetus for change. Only ignorance and complacency prevent more active recruitment of men into nursing. In this chapter we will attempt to deal with the ignorance. Only the readers can act on complacency.

HISTORY

Florence Nightingale's achievement in establishing modern nursing was remarkable for two reasons: she established the science of nursing, and she overcame extreme societal pressure for women to conform to Victorian mores that segregated the sexes. Nightingale confronted, and successfully overcame, social barriers that excluded women of class from participating in nondomestic economic activity.

Nightingale equated "nursing" with "female" for several reasons. Her pre-Crimean search for a career in helping the sick took her through Europe, where religious and lay sisters had a long tradition of caring for those suffering from illness. Nightingale was greatly influenced by this. Victorian women of privilege had no opportunity for meaningful contribution beyond the home in English society. Her essay "Cassandra,"[31] written just before her Kaiserworth nurse training, details and laments the role of high-class women in Victorian society. She was determined to care for the sick and accepted a post as a hospital matron. The British war with Russia intervened. She organized and led a group of 38 women (independently organized but sanctioned by the British government) to the Crimea to nurse the wounded. But she was stymied by the military and medical bureaucracy, which was controlled by men. The men caring for the wounded were neglectful or unfit for other duty. Nightingale, due to her perseverance and her independence from the military, was able to reform the barrack hospital at Scutari and significantly reduce the hospital mortality rate. One strategy she seemed to use to ensure the success of nursing was to organize the school separately from the hospital (as was the first nursing school at St. Thomas Hospital) and limit the school's enrollees to women. In promoting a separate organization for the nursing school, Nightingale defined nurses as female and used societal prohibitions on integrating the sexes to maintain independence for nurses. Describing nursing as a field for women accomplished two of Nightingale's objectives: to create an opportunity for women outside the home and to have a measure of independence from men in the medical-hospital bureaucracy. These matters are thoroughly covered by Nightingale in "Subsidiary Notes as to the Introduction of Female Nursing in to Military Hospitals."[30]

On Nightingale's return from the Crimea in 1856, Queen Victoria asked the heroine what she wanted as a favor from the monarch of a grateful nation. While other British subjects may have requested title, Nightingale asked for a commission to investigate the causes of morbidity and mortality among army troops. Her intent was to institute reforms to prevent recurrence of

Table 92-1 Men in nursing

Year	Total number of nurses	Number of male nurses	Percentage
1910	83,327	5,819	6.98
1920	149,128	5,464	3.66
1930	294,189	5,452	1.85
1940	369,287	8,072	2.19
1950	374,584	9,613	2.57
1960	504,000	4,587	0.91
1970	1,127,657	14,625	1.30
1980	1,615,846	44,237	2.74
1984	1,887,697	57,199	3.03
1988	2,033,032	67,626	3.33

Modified from American Nurses Association. (1942-1988). *Facts about nursing*. Kansas City, Mo: Author.

the unsanitary conditions that had nearly defeated the army. Nightingale's testimony written for the Commission to Examine the Sanitary State of the British Army and her written comments on the commission report were privately published in 1858 as *Notes on Matters Affecting the Health, Efficiency and Hospital Administration of the British Army*.[27] Two other books soon followed: *Notes on Nursing*[29] and *Notes on Hospitals*.[28]

Another British sanitary and hospital reformer, and a rival of Miss Nightingale, was John Simon, a London public health official and surgeon on the staff of St. Thomas Hospital. A lesser-known accomplishment of Simon was the formation of an experimental, volunteer field hospital assembled, shipped, and installed in Bingen on the Rhine, Germany, in 1870 during the Franco-Prussian War. Only male nurses were hired to staff the hospital, and all of the latest in sanitary science was used to ensure that the experimental hospital would be a success. According to Lambert, Simon's biographer, and reports in the *Times* of London, Listerian methods were used and the mortality rates among the troops were kept abnormally low.

Men nurses distinguished themselves both during America's Civil War (1861 to 1865) and again in Germany. Yet few accounts document these achievements. Walt Whitman[39] wrote a small volume describing his nursing efforts during the Civil War. Mr. Romeo Galleuga, a head nurse in Simon's experimental hospital, also wrote a moving account of his and his colleagues nursing ministrations during the Franco-Prussian War, in a letter to the *Times* of London printed September 23, 1870.

In the nearly 1000 years before Nightingale, men played a predominate role in organized nursing in Western society. Among the earliest nurses were the Knights Hospitalers of St. John of Jerusalem who established a hospital in 1065 for pilgrims to the Holy Land. Throughout their turbulent history these nurses served and protected Europeans in the environs of the Mediterranean Sea from their base, first in Jerusalem, later in Rhodes, most prominently in Malta (where they became known as the Knights of Malta), and now headquartered in Rome.[4,16,21] Branches of the Knights of St. John of Jerusalem organized and staffed voluntary ambulance services in the United Kingdom, Australia, New Zealand, and Canada. The most prominent American branch of these European religious orders of men nurses is the Alexian Brothers, now based in Elk Grove Village, Illinois, who own four hospitals and for 25 years operated a nursing school for men in Chicago.[20] In Europe the tradition of these orders accounts for a higher proportion of men among nurses—in the United Kingdom, 10%, and in Belgium and the Netherlands, 15%.

The Mills School of Nursing for Men at Bellevue Hospital in New York was established 10 years after the first American nursing school graduated its first nurse. The school was founded on the premise that men as well as women could provide care. The men were the earliest graduates of nursing schools in this country and were educated for the same reasons as the women nurses. To quote Nightingale, they were to "place patients in the best possible condition for nature to act favorably upon them."[29]

Technological advances in anesthesia and infection control shifted nursing care from the home to the hospital. Care in the home was provided in the main by families, and to some extent by graduate nurses, and care in the hospital was increasingly provided by students and graduate nurses. Conflict emerged during the first few decades of organized nursing over whether the objective of nurse training was the education of students or the provision of service for patients.[17] The service orientation prevailed, due largely to the training schools' loss of independence from hospitals. American nursing schools in the Nightingale tradition were run by women nurses who had no more inclination to train men than did men's professions to train women. Specialty institutions providing care to the mentally ill actively recruited men into their training programs. This early division of labor was consistent with the social prejudice against women caring for male patients

with urological disorders. Thus concern for quality patient care for selected categories of patients led to the
only involvement of men in post-Nightingale nursing.

THE MILITARY

A major cause of the relative dearth of men in nursing
was the demands of the military. During World War I it
was apparent that available nurses could not meet the
needs of both civilian and military patients. Because
men were combatants in the war, the major recruitment of nurses during that period involved women. In
1918 alone there was a 25% increase in the entrants in
American nursing schools.[18] Even men who were nursing students at the time were vulnerable to the draft
and participated in the war as soldiers in the trenches
rather than as nurses. The U.S. Army Nurse Corps,
which was established in 1901, specifically excluded
men. Kalish and Kalish[18] wrote, "The effect of the war
and of selective service was practically to wipe out the
enrollment of men in schools of nursing."

The situation for men during World War I remained
identical at the outbreak of World War II. Men who
were nurses found themselves bearing arms and driving earth movers rather than caring for the sick and
injured.[35] Men in nursing were very well served by
Leroy Craig, RN, director of the school of nursing for
men in Pennsylvania Hospital, Department of Mental
and Nervous Diseases. Concerned about the possible
repetition of events that affected male nurses during
World War I, Craig and other men at the 1940 American Nurses Association (ANA) convention petitioned
for recognition. The following January the ANA board
of directors created the "Men Nurses" section of the
ANA. The initial objectives of this section were the
improvement of patient care, but soon the concerns
gravitated toward the treatment of men nurses in the
military and the inadequate salaries for nurses.

Another nurse, Luther Christman, as a 1939 graduate of the Pennsylvania Hospital school of nursing for
men, found that he could not enlist in the Army Nurse
Corps at the outset of World War II. Men nurses were
not even given priority enrollment in medical corpsmen schools because their knowledge often intimidated less well educated teachers. Christman enlisted
in the merchant marine as a medical corpsman and
then petitioned the ranking Army medical officer for
appointment to the Army Nurse Corps and assignment
to the front, where women (and nurses) were not assigned. His request was rejected in a terse letter from

the general. Christman sent his correspondence with
the general to all members of the U.S. Senate and to
two thirds of the House of Representatives. The stir
Christman created subsided only after the Allies won
the Battle of the Bulge, obviating the need to draft
women nurses.

According to Olga Benderoff, Chief Nurse of the
Fourth General Hospital, who served in the South Pacific during World War II, Army nurses received less
pay than their counterparts of equal rank in the medical corps. She remembers receiving a substantial pay
raise while serving in New Guinea. Frances Payne Bolton was responsible for the raise, having introduced
Congressional legislation giving Army nurses pay parity with other Army officers.

For nearly all of its 12-year history the ANA's Men
Nurses' section was concerned with equal treatment
and adequate salaries for men and women nurses in the
U.S. Armed Forces. Equal treatment did not become a
reality during the life of the Men Nurses' section, but
the men were sufficiently involved in the mainstream
of the professional nursing organization that they did
not disappear, as they had shortly after World War I.
The ANA reorganized in 1952, and the Men Nurses'
section, in support of the reorganization, voted itself
out of existence. Edward Lyon became the first registered nurse commissioned as a reserve officer in the
Army Nurse Corps on October 6, 1955. The legislation
facilitating his commission was again introduced by the
representative from Ohio, Frances Payne Bolton. More
than a decade later men were given the first commissions as regular officers in the Army Nurse Corps. During the conflict in Vietnam, more than 500 men nurses
were drafted and provided commissions in the Military
Nurse Corps, and, at last, they cared for the injured as
registered nurses.

Paradoxically, the role of the military is now quite
positive. More than 30% of the registered nurses in the
Military Nurse Corps are men. Many of the more recent
male recruits to the nursing profession are former medics and corpsmen who saw, and see, men nurses on
active duty. The military is the only place that a nurse
can stand across the operating room table from a surgeon and outrank her or him.

THE ECONOMY

Another major force having an impact on men in the
nursing profession was the economy. After World War
I, the number of men admitted to nursing schools was

slow to increase. During the 1920s the salaries for nurses were not competitive with those for teachers, union laborers, or municipal workers. Most graduate nurses worked in private duty, a particularly unstable source of income. As a consequence, in a growing economy, there was no economic incentive for a man to become a nurse. The number of male recruits to nursing increased considerably during the Depression. Nursing school became one of the few places in which an education could be obtained along with room, board, and a small stipend. The pattern of specialization established earlier continued. Men tended to be admitted to training programs in hospitals that specialized in the care of mental illness. But because American nurses at the entry level were generalists, all of them had to have experience in the care of maternity patients, children, and acutely ill adults in general hospitals.

The low salary levels for nurses between World War II and 1970 continued to discourage men from entering nursing, as America was in the midst of a growth economy. A turning point was the passage of Medicare legislation (1966), which infused new money into hospitals. Salaries for high-demand positions began to rise and entry-level nurse salaries increased. Secondary effects of the post-Medicare increase in money for health care have been increases in the number of nurses being trained and the number of nurses in the work force. Since the oil embargo of 1973, economic cycles have produced intermittent unemployment and loss of job security. Both the salary changes and a depressed economy in manufacturing and in government employment produced the economic conditions necessary to increase the rate of men entering nursing. The prospective payment system and decreased availability of nurses is likely to contribute to increased wages and therefore contribute to increased enrollment of men, if the number of men in nursing serves as an index of economic well-being of nurses. However, the general economic prosperity experienced during the late 1980s has slowed the high rate of growth in men entering nursing. The growth rate for 1977 to 1980 was 63%, and half that, 29%, since then.

Economic effects are also paradoxical. Economic forces that repel men from nursing also keep women in the profession. Neither women's pay nor investments in women's educational programs have reached parity with men's pay and investment in their educational programs. In general, it still seems acceptable to pay women 59 cents for every dollar earned by a man. Similarly, there is not much investment in educating women except, of course, as women enter fields in which men predominate. Molly Yard, former president of the National Organization for Women, stated in a speech at the Cleveland City Club that the admission of women into law, medical, business, and theological schools is related less to fundamental changes and beliefs about women than to the receipt of federal funds to comply with Title 9 of the Civil Rights Act. Those places that have a long history of educating women—schools of nursing, social work, education, and library science—are all experiencing economic difficulties.

In contrast, the costs of legal, business, and medical education have skyrocketed. Support for medical education now comes from patient charges through the hospital, federal grant funds, tuition, and state subsidies. These economic realities are the only plausible explanation for the concern over fluctuating nursing school enrollments and intermittent nurse shortages.

The per-graduate registered nurse education expense in the United States is actually shrinking at an alarming rate. As hospitals have taken diploma nursing schools out of service, the dollar expenditures for capital (school of nursing building and expenses of operating it) administrative overhead and the low student-faculty ratio (1 faculty member to 3.9 students for diploma programs, versus 1 faculty member to 6.3 students for associate degree programs) have evaporated. More than 540 such hospital schools have been closed since 1965.[36] Local governments have replaced hospital schools with community college programs (605 associate degree schools have been added since 1965). Associate degree programs graduated 57 students per school in 1984. Diploma programs graduated 35 per school during the same year.[36] There are many controversial issues surrounding this shift in education from hospital to community college about which nurses do not agree. Yet all those familiar with contemporary patient care would agree that more, not less, money should be spent on the education of tomorrow's nurse. This lack of investment in the education of the nurse seems to me to be fundamentally related to the absence of much investment in the education of women. If women are to be well educated in our present society, they must now enter a field that was once the exclusive domain of men. For the health and well-being of all, greater investments must be made in the education of nurses in order for them to meet demands reasonably placed on them as society proceeds toward the economic, epidemiological, and demographic realities to occur in our aging society in the early decades of the next century.

When salary benefits and working conditions for nurses become competitive economically, then nurses will have achieved their appropriate valuation. Such valuation may not necessarily mean much more money for women, but rather a redistribution, or even less money for men. Another, perhaps even more desirable, redistribution process can involve the development of a national health scheme that would cut the disparity between the incomes of doctors and nurses, now at a 5:1 ratio, and at the same time lower the cost of health care and provide greater access to care. When such revaluation occurs, there will be a noticeable shift in the gender mix of nurses. The 97% female ratio in the United States can be compared with that in other countries such as the Cameroon in equatorial Africa, where half the nurses are men. The economic disincentives mentioned do not exist there.

The effects of economic gender bias are pervasive. Women nurses must take the lead in redressing economic wrongs because men nurses cannot claim gender discrimination even if they are affected by wage discrimination. Nurse executive salaries have been ample by any measure, save one. Men in similar executive positions, with equal or less responsibility as compared to the chief nurse (for example, the chief of staff or the chief financial officer), earn half again as much money. The annual salary surveys reported in *Hospitals, Journal of the American Hospital Association,* and *Modern Healthcare* graphically illustrate this point. In the case of the nurse executive, the market external to the hospital is most often invoked to establish starting salaries under the premise that "you can't make more than the nursing director at Mass General." Because the wage is established using women nurse executives as the reference point, the wage tends to be less than that of their male co-workers.

Three women nurses who have sought and won redress for gender bias are Rozella Schlotfeldt, Ada Jacox, and Virginia Cleland. At some personal expense (Schlotfeldt, for example, was chastised by her university president) and at the urging of the American Nurses Association, these determined women, all university professors, filed a sex discrimination complaint against their universities and the Teachers Insurance and Annuity Association (TIAA) for paying women less than men in monthly retirement income benefits. TIAA justified the practice by arguing that women live longer. Schlotfeldt, anticipating their response, argued that differential benefits were not paid to African-Americans, who actuarially had even shorter life spans.

Retirement benefits are now equal for men and women, black or white.

NURSING AS WOMEN'S WORK

In our culture most people see human behavioral characteristics as being either feminine or masculine. Women who display masculine characteristics and men who display feminine characteristics are seen as being unusual. Cultural tolerance of these aberrations varies with gender. The young woman who acts like a tomboy is more acceptable than the young man who acts like a sissy. It is no wonder that nursing, a profession Nightingale and other Victorians identified as being feminine, is not even considered a possibility for most boys.[26] These sex-role stereotypes are common throughout life but tend to moderate somewhat with age. Cultural predispositions tend to reinforce sex-role stereotypes and are partly responsible for the relative scarcity of men in nursing and for the age of those men who do enter the nursing profession.[15] Holtzclaw[14] concluded that men who succeed in nursing are apt to be better accepted if they retain attributes associated with masculinity.

Nuttall,[32] in a study of British nursing, expressed concern that half of the top posts in nursing within the national health service were held by men. The most recent figures indicate that men occupy 50.3% of the top administrative positions but represent only 8.6% of all nurses.[13] When Nuttall examined the council of the Royal College of Nursing, she found that 15 of the 31 elected members were men. Nuttall suggested that women nurses were giving away these leadership positions to men. If both men and women agree on appropriate leadership qualities and they seem to be consistent with masculine characteristics, then men nurses exhibiting these traits will continue to be identified by nurses as leaders.

The picture in the United States is complicated by a rigid educational hierarchy among registered nurses. In America, unlike Britain, nurses in top posts tend to have experience and graduate educational qualifications as prerequisites. The paucity of American men in nursing, educated at those levels, may prevent a repetition of the British situation Nuttall describes. London[23] urges caution. She proposes that the male power base in British nursing thrusts men into administrative and executive positions. She writes, "A large proportion of men at the top [of nursing] would tend to be self-perpetuating. Once this domination was established, it

Table 92-2 Percentage of men admitted to schools of nursing

Year	1978	1981	1984	1985	1986	1988	1989
Diploma	5.3	5.6	5.1	5.9	5.3	6.8	9.2
Associate	6.8	7.9	8.0	6.5	7.1	7.6	8.6
Baccalaureate	5.7	6.2	7.3	6.4	5.9	7.1	6.7
Total admissions	6.3	7.3	7.0	6.3	6.6	7.3	8.2
Total graduations	5.5	5.8	5.8	5.7	5.5	5.7	5.7

Modified from National League of Nursing. (1993). *Nursing data review.* New York: Author.

would be very difficult for women to regain leadership roles." Dingwall[8] suggests that male domination in British nursing is related to the rise of "scientific nursing and scientific management." Dingwall warns that this perceived impersonal and scientific approach to nursing that is ascribed to men is neither socially desirable nor in the best interests of the patient. London and Dingwall delineate an obvious anxiety about men in British nursing.

Austin[2] takes a more extreme position. She suggests that nursing "is bound up with a female and feminine input. Caring and ministering encompass activities and attitudes that within a pretty well world-wide cultural understanding are thought to be only, or at any rate better, served by women." Austin[3] essentially rejects male nursing: "while the feminine bedside imagery matched nursing's professional ideology, masculine nursing ideology today is out of step with the continuing predominance of feminine nursing imagery." London and Austin perpetuate the myth that nursing is a woman's profession that directly links feminine gender traits with the profession and practice.

Sex-role measures have traditionally identified gender characteristics as bipolar and unidimensional. A person was scored as either masculine or feminine on a continuum. More recent measures, though, conceptualize sex-role characteristics as independent dimensions.[5,12] From this perspective, a person can exhibit both masculine and feminine traits. Individuals who score high on both masculinity and femininity are labeled psychologically androgynous. Low scores on either trait are labeled as sex-role stereotyped. Galbraith[11] suggests that individuals who exhibit both strong masculine and feminine traits are more able to cope with the complexities of modern life.

Minnigerode and others[24] investigated psychological androgyny in graduate and undergraduate nursing students. These students identified the ideal nurse as having high feminine and high masculine traits. This sample is not representative of nursing attitudes in general but supports the idea that nursing transcends traditional sex-role stereotyping. The authors write, "the ideal nurse in this study was described not as stereotypically feminine but as someone capable of displaying both feminine characteristics (i.e., warmth, understanding, gentleness, helpfulness, kindness) and characteristics considered masculine (i.e., independence, competitiveness, self-confidence, decision making).[24] Rossi,[37] Holtzclaw,[14] and Pontin[34] report similar results and support the perception of nursing as representing the best of both genders.

A noteworthy finding of the Holtzclaw study[14] was that men and women nurses are highly supportive of their sons and daughters entering the nursing profession. Research on men in nursing indicates that most men nurses have been influenced by a living role model who encouraged their entry into the nursing profession.[7,14] Most men nurses could identify a nurse (woman or man)—frequently a spouse, other close relative, or co-worker—who encouraged them to study nursing.

Holtzclaw could find no logical reason for the gender disparity of modern nursing.[14] In the past, nursing was one of the few professions that women could enter because women were barred from other fields of endeavor. The past several years have seen changes in opportunities for women entering nontraditional fields. Women are now choosing and succeeding in accounting, engineering, and law as well as a wide range of previously male-dominated occupations. This creates an interesting dilemma whereby there are fewer women entering nursing. Table 92-2 outlines the increase of male admissions to nursing schools from 6.3% in 1978 to 8.2% in 1989. If nursing's gender balance were more representative of the population, we could effectively double the number of nurses. Yet graduations of men from nursing schools lag admissions, suggesting that the climate in nursing schools is not an entirely welcoming one for men.[22] These two problems will shrink the pool of graduate nurses in the years to come.

Men have much to offer the profession. Studies indicate that they are older and have had other career experiences before entering nursing.[6,11,40] Egeland and Brown[10] surveyed men nurses in Oregon and found that they were mostly married (74%) and had been employed in nursing for 8 years. The authors also found that most men nurses were employed in staff positions (60.5%) as opposed to administrative positions (18%). Men also have staying power. Dwight and Staunton[9] report that 85% of men entering the profession remain permanently, contrasted with 35% of women who remain.

Kanter[19] proposed a theory that explains some of the problems faced by gender minorities. She poses a concept called critical mass. This theory suggests that small minorities encounter increasing resistance as they increase their percentage within the work force until a critical mass of 20% to 40% is reached. Ott[33] used this theory to study men in nursing and women in law enforcement in the Netherlands. The theory was supported in the law enforcement group—women tended to see increasing resistance to their presence. Men in nursing found greater acceptance in increasing numbers, though. The authors pose that women, and women nurses specifically, are willing to share their domain with men. This is encouraging in light of the previously noted comments that resist attempts by men to be an active and integral part of the profession.

We are faced with a challenge. Traditional nursing ideals have shunned men, but women are actively pursuing other fields rather than entering nursing. This leaves few options for cultivating new nurses. The idea of nursing as women's work is paradoxical. Both men and women have something to contribute and men represent an untapped resource. If society (of which nurses are part) can reject bias and traditions, we may find a more prosperous and well-rounded profession.

ORGANIZED NURSING AND MEN

The number and proportion of men in nursing can change just as the number and proportion of women in traditionally men's professions has changed. There is, however, no corollary application of Title 9 of the Civil Rights Act barring gender discrimination against men in nursing. Clearly, Title 9 was the definitive action that made a place for women in professional schools. Can

and/or should nursing schools apply Title 9 spirit and logic to the problem of fewer men in nursing than women? While we believe that action can and should be taken to address the imbalance, we don't believe that most nurses think gender imbalance is a problem. If a problem were perceived, then action of the following type would be more evident:

1. Actively advertise nursing as a career that appeals to men; job security, pay, promotional opportunity, flexibility, and retirement (pension availability) are career attributes that appeal to men
2. Treat men as men like to be treated; ask around (focus groups—no spouses or male offspring) if you don't know what this means
3. Hire role models to recruit men to nursing programs; emphasize the historic contribution of men in nursing
4. Sensitize women in nursing to special needs of men
5. Promote nursing as an excellent way to enter related fields such as hospital management, medicine, and dentistry; ambition is a trait thought beneficial for men
6. Reestablish the men nurses section in the American Nurses Association and professional nursing schools predominantly for men
7. Promote diversity in all endeavors—variety *is* the spice of life

Implementing a few of these suggestions may help all nurses to improve their economic valuation.

AMERICAN ASSEMBLY FOR MEN IN NURSING

One way to increase the proportion of men nurses in America is for men nurses to be visible and to support nursing as a satisfying and rewarding profession. To achieve visibility, Dennis Martin of Michigan organized the American Assembly for Men in Nursing (AAMN) in 1971. The independent group of nurses, formerly known as the National Male Nurse Association, has several hundred members in nearly every state of the union. The objectives of the organization were restated in 1981 when the association was renamed:

1. Men and boys in the United States are encouraged to become nurses and join together with all nurses in strengthening and humanizing health care for Americans.

2. Men who are now nurses are encouraged to grow professionally and to demonstrate to each other and to society the increasing contributions made by men within the nursing profession.

3. The American Assembly for Men in Nursing intends that its members be full participants in the nursing profession and its organizations and use this association to achieve the limited goals just stated.

The work of the AAMN is carried on by voluntary officers who both organize and conduct an annual meeting and who work through local chapters located in Atlanta, Philadelphia, Chicago, Indianapolis, Los Angeles, San Francisco, New York, Cleveland, North Carolina, Florida, and Tennessee.*

There have been two court cases of interest to men in nursing. The first was a Supreme Court decision in which the majority opinion was issued by Justice Sandra Day O'Connor. The case involved the Mississippi Women's University practice of limiting enrollment to women and denying otherwise-qualified men the right to enroll for credits in its school of nursing. Speaking for the court, Justice O'Connor held that the practice was in violation of the equal protection clause of the Fourteenth Amendment. O'Connor[25] wrote, "Rather than compensate for discriminatory barriers faced by women, Mississippi Women's University policy of excluding men from admission to its School of Nursing tends to perpetuate the stereotype of nursing as an exclusively women's job." She also wrote, "Although the test for determining the validity of a gender-based classification is straightforward, it must be applied free of fixed notions concerning the roles and abilities of males and females."

In the second case, *Backus v. Baptist Medical Center,* nurse Gregory Backus was rejected in his repeated attempts to obtain employment in the Baptist Medical Center obstetrical and gynecological unit. After being refused this position, he resigned from the hospital and, in October of 1979, sued Baptist Medical center, charging discrimination based on sex. A lower court agreed with the Baptist Medical Center's position that having a male nurse work in the obstetrical unit violated the patients' right of privacy. On appeal to the U.S. Court of Appeals for the Eighth Circuit, the judge refused to hear the case because Backus had quit his

job at the Baptist Medical Center voluntarily. It is not clear how the case would have been decided had the court not determined that the point was moot. Trandel-Korenchuk and Trandel-Korenchuk[38] point out that the court did not condone an outright ban of male nurses but supported the hospital's policy of restrictions only on the labor and delivery ward.

In light of both these cases and the issues they represent, the American Assembly for Men in Nursing has developed a position statement on the role that gender should play in the nursing profession in terms of entry into nursing education programs and access to employment in nursing. Members of the AAMN believe that "Every professional nurse position and every nursing educational opportunity shall be equally available to those meeting the entry qualifications regardless of gender."

The argument is not that the wholesale addition of men nurses will make the nursing profession a better one. In fact, past sex-role stereotyping has funneled a disproportionate number of highly intelligent, well-motivated women into nursing. Men in nursing may contribute to a decrease in the economic bias associated with women's work and women's education. Increasing the number of men nurses will, however, make the profession different. The difference will enable our patients to experience a fuller range of professional interventions for their human response to actual or potential health problems. Men nurses are not the answer to all the problems of the nursing profession, but their presence in greater numbers may well be a barometer of the economic value that society affords nurses. If men in nursing are that barometer, then recent trends in men's enrollment indicate that society is moving forward too slowly in it economic valuation of nurses.

REFERENCES

1. American Nurses Association. (1942, 1957, 1960, 1961, 1962-63, 1964, 1966, 1972-73, 1982-83, 1984-85, 1986-87, 1992). *Facts about nursing.* Kansas City, Mo: Author.
2. Austin, R. (1977). Sex and gender in the future of nursing, Part 1. *Nursing Times, 73*(34), 113-116.
3. Austin, R. (1977). Sex and gender in the future of nursing, Part 2. *Nursing Times, 73*(35), 117-119.
4. Bedford, W. K. R., & Holbeche, R. (1902). *The Order of the Hospital of St. John of Jerusalem being a history of the English Hospitalers of St. John, their rise and progress.* London: F. E. Robinson.
5. Bem, S. L. (1974, April). The measurement of psychological androgyny. *Journal of Consulting and Clinical Psychology, 42,* 155-162.
6. Brock, R. (1988). Men in nursing: Part of the solution to the nursing shortage. *Nurse, 1*(2), 1, 3.

---

*For information, write to the following address: AAMN, P.O. Box 31753, Independence, OH 44131.

7. Brown, R., & Stones, R. (1973). *The male nurse. Occasional papers on social administration, Number 52.* London: Social Administration Research Trust at the London School of Economics.

8. Dingwall, R. (1979). The place of men in nursing. In M. M. Colledge & D. Jones (Eds.), *Readings in nursing.* London: Churchill Livingstone.

9. Dwight, D., & Staunton, V. (1989). Marketing nursing to men. *Nursing Management, 20*(6), 74.

10. Egeland, J., & Brown, J. (1989). Men in nursing: Their fields of employment, preferred fields of practice, and role strain. *Health Services Research, 24*(5), 693-707.

11. Galbraith, M. (1991). Attracting men to nursing: What will they find important in their career? *Journal of Nursing Education, 30*(4), 182-186.

12. Heilbrun, A. B., Jr. (1976). Measurement of masculine and feminine sex role identities as independent dimension. *Journal of Consulting and Clinical Psychology, 44,* 183-190.

13. Holmes, P. (1987). Men in nursing: Man appeal. *Nursing Times, 83*(20), 24-27.

14. Holtzclaw, B. J. (1981). The man in nursing: Relations between sex-type perceptions and locus of control. *Dissertation Abstracts International.* University Microfilms (No. 81-16, 752).

15. Hudson, H. (1974). *Source book: Nursing personnel* (DHEW Pub. No. HRA 75-43). Washington, D.C.: Department of Health, Education and Welfare.

16. Hume, E. E. (1940). *Medical work of the Knight Hospitalers of St. John of Jerusalem.* Baltimore: Johns Hopkins Press.

17. *The Johns Hopkins Hospital: Hospital construction and organization: Five essays relating to the construction, organization and management of hospitals.* (1875). New York: William Wood.

18. Kalish, P., & Kalish, B. J. (1978). *The advance of American nursing* (2nd ed.). Boston: Little, Brown.

19. Kanter, R. M. (1977). *Men and women of the corporation.* New York: Basic Books.

20. Kauffman, C. J. (1976). *The history of the Alexian Brothers: Vol. 1. Tamers of death, Vol. 2. The ministry of healing.* New York: Seabury Press.

21. Kingsley, R. G. (1918). *The Order of St. John of Jerusalem (past and present).* London: Skeffington and Son (Reprinted 1978, New York AMS Press)

22. Kippenbrock, T., & May, F. (1986). *Attrition among men students in nursing programs.* Proceedings of the Indiana University School of Nursing Research Colloquium.

23. London, F. (1987). Should men be actively recruited into nursing? *Nursing Administration Quarterly, 12*(1), 75-81.

24. Minnigerode, F. A., Kayer-Jones, J. S., & Garcia, G. (1978). Masculinity and femininity in nursing. *Nursing Research, 27,* 299-302.

25. Mississippi University for Women v. Hogan, 458 U.S. 718 (1982).

26. Nemerowicz, G. (1979). *Children's perceptions of gender and work roles.* New York: Praeger.

27. Nightingale, F. (1858). *Notes on matters affecting the health, efficiency and hospital administration of the British army.* London: Harrison and Sons.

28. Nightingale, F. (1859). *Notes on hospitals.* London: John W. Parker and Sons.

29. Nightingale, F. (1860). *Notes on nursing.* London: Harrison.

30. Nightingale, F. (1954). Subsidiary notes as to the introduction of female nursing into military hospitals. In L. R. Seymer (Ed.), *Selected writings of Florence Nightingale.* New York: Macmillan.

31. Nightingale, F. (1979). Cassandra. In M. Start (Ed.), *Cassandra.* Old Westbury, N.Y.: Feminist Press.

32. Nuttall, P. (1983). British nursing: Beginning of a power struggle. *Nursing Outlook, 31*(3), 184.

33. Ott, E. M. (1989). Effects of the male-female ratio at work: Policewomen and male nurses. *Psychology of Women Quarterly, 13*(1), 41-57.

34. Pontin, D. J. T. (1988). The use of profile similarity indices and the Bem sex role inventory in determining the sex role characterization of a group of male and female nurses. *Journal of Advanced Nursing, 13*(6), 768-774.

35. Rose, J. (1947). Men nurses in the military service. *American Journal of Nursing, 47*(3), 146-148.

36. Rosenfeld, P. (1986). *Nursing student census with policy implications: 1985.* New York: National League for Nursing.

37. Rossi, A. (1964). Equality between the sexes: An immodest proposal. *Daedalus, 93,* 607.

38. Trandel-Korenchuk, K. M., & Trandel-Korenchuk, D.M. (1981). Legal forum: Restrictions on male nurse employment in obstetric care. *Nursing Administration Quarterly, 6,* 87-90.

39. Whitman, W. (1875). *Memoranda during the war.* Boston: Applewood Books.

40. Williams, R. A. (1973). Characteristics of male baccalaureate students who selected nursing as a career. *Nursing Research, 22,* 520-525.

CHAPTER 93

Women's health

A global perspective

AFAF I. MELEIS, FERIAL A. M. ALY

The purpose of this chapter is to discuss global issues related to women's health. Several universal issues were selected for presentation to provide a context for understanding health care for women and to challenge the readers to identify potential threats to quality care. In addition, principles that have been proposed for the development and implementation of a viable and comprehensive health care system for women are identified and discussed. There is no intent here to capture the situation and health experience of women in all parts of the world, nor is it possible to address all the contextual contingencies needed for addressing women's health. Rather, the intent is to provide a framework for understanding the neglect that women have encountered in all aspects of their lives, including health care. Furthermore, our aim is to provide those who have been committed to health care for women with support in their attempt to provide quality health care for women. Finally, our goal is to raise the readers' consciousness of women's health needs beyond the United States. We fully realize that women's health issues cannot be understood in isolation from the specific sociocultural context of women's situation; however, by highlighting some universals, perhaps we can underscore the need for global cooperation in taking a more coherent and coordinated approach to providing affordable and quality health care for women.

There are certain contextual patterns that are global. There is a universal tendency to define women by their marital status and there is an overall pressure to conform to certain global expectations that are considered normative and ideal. Women are expected to attach themselves to a father, a brother, a husband, or a son. Although the intensity and the quality of this normative ideal differs from one country to another, from one culture to another, and from one class to another, there is a general agreement that young girls are socialized to prepare themselves for spousal and maternal roles. These expectations decrease the potential for promoting and supporting educational or career goals and increase the potential for status and power issues.

Similarly, there is a global focus on reproductive health and on reducing women's health concerns to the reproductive aspects of their life cycle. The focus on physical reproduction, as opposed to socially productive tasks of women, tends to decrease the potential for understanding and attending to the critical needs of women throughout the life cycle and beyond conceiving and delivering a healthy baby.[24] The focus on reproductive aspects of women's health also tends to take reproductive issues out of context and render the results unsatisfactory for both planners and recipients of health care. Family planning programs that focus on birth control are good examples of how an important issue in women's lives that is bound to the family and society is reduced to the question of birth control methods. This in turn tends to decrease the potential success of these programs. McFarland[19] reviewed the literature on development theory and women and made the following assertion:

In the population policy and reproductive rights area, women's perspective has been ignored. Planners have had little understanding of women's mixed responses to family planning. The role of children as workers, old age security, and property inheritors has been ignored, as well as the fact that all or most of the birth control methods are unsafe or unsatisfactory.

Questions and studies about family planning inspired by such an approach, that is, one with a focus on women as defective reproductive beings, tend to center on (1) why women are unable to plan the size of their families and the spacing of their children (that is, what is wrong with them?); (2) mortality and morbidity related to reproduction; (3) why women are not capable of taking advantage of the great services provided by the ministries of health in the various countries; and (4) how it is that all of the grant money that is being allocated for these purposes appears not to be effective in halting the frightening growth in the population of the world. These kinds of questions do not address the ways in which women are constrained from using the services provided, nor do they address the parts played by other important variables (such as roles, societal expectations, and spousal demands) that may be far more compelling in influencing women's options, choices, and decisions. In addition, a large percentage of women are neither pregnant nor in the process of childbearing, and a focus on reproductive health ignores other equally—if not more significant—health issues that women confront.

Another universal trend centers on women's caregiving roles. Women tend to be the care givers in most regions of the world. They are expected to be either the primary or the sole care providers for children, spouses, parents, and the elderly in their families, and they are expected to teach sound health practices to future generations. In addition, they are expected to provide similar care-giving services and education to their spouses' extended families. These responsibilities are additive in nature instead of being substitutive, the result of which is overload and limited time, energy, and resources to attend to their own personal needs. This continues to be true whether women are working inside or outside the household and whether their work is visible and acknowledged or invisible and unacknowledged.

However, most of women's work is invisible and devalued. Women work extended hours as spouses and mothers and are labeled nonworking women or housewives. Or they are the farmers who carry the major bulk of domestic work and are paid minimally for it. They also tend to be the nurses, teachers, and clerical workers, for which their income is incongruent with their worth and their work. The no- or low-income positions bring with them limited resources, a lack of regulatory policies to protect women as laborers, and inadequate enforcement of their rights. Furthermore, in many countries women's contributions are falsely reflected in labor statistics[27] because of the invisible nature of their work, that, in turn, makes their contributions even more invisible. Invisibility brings with it neglect, neglect breeds abuse, and abuse renders women more vulnerable and powerless. The cycle then continues, with more violence against women.

Women also have other invisible roles that consume their time and energy and are equally ignored. An example is women's work in facilitating health care for family members. Women are consistently expected to be the first gatekeepers to preventive, promotive, and curative health care; they are the key providing access to, and utilization of, health care for others in the family and the community.[22]

In spite of the apparent involvement of women in productive work in or outside the house, and in spite of their needs for "development" and for better compensation, development programs have focused primarily on men. These programs are designed to make men's lives easier by developing the technology to support their work, whether that work is farm work or sales work. Even when development programs have considered women, they have tended to label their work as craftwork, which means that it is extra and not as central to a country's economy as other forms of productive work.[19] There is a growing discomfort with development programs in general because of the lack of clarity of their missions. Questions such as Development of what, for whom, by whom, and for whose benefit? need to be carefully and ethically debated. Exploitation of resources and labor in developing countries for the benefit of "first world" white males is being questioned and debated in developing and developed countries.

ILLNESS EXPERIENCES AND RESPONSES

Within this context, we would like to describe and discuss some aspects of women's health related to the experience of and response to illness. In addition to the communicable diseases and other illnesses shared by both sexes, there are a number of illnesses and injuries that are primarily associated with women.[29] These nonreproductive health problems are less likely to be detected and treated because of the narrow framework used in considering health care for women, which is due to the lack of awareness of both the recipients and providers regarding the extent of women's health care needs and their need for comprehensive care. By and large, women are either not aware of such health care needs; or they are aware but tend to ignore these needs because of their demanding role responsibilities, work load, and other care-giving activities; or they have been prevented from seeking health care and from maintaining their health by limited resources and structural constraints. Personal health hazards that make women more vulnerable thus remain obscured until the women show symptoms related to reproductive health, which makes their illness situation more legitimate. Or women seek health care later than they should, after their work becomes affected. Education of women in many countries influences women's chances to obtain better jobs and affects women's lifestyle and health practices.[27]

We have selected only five aspects of women's health to discuss here.

Eating disorders and nutritional problems

In developing countries, there are at least 1 million people who consume fewer calories than needed; women make up the bulk of this population. Similarly, the death rate for the female child is higher than that for the male in some parts of the world such as India and Egypt. One reason for this is society-imposed eating conditions that increase the probability of nutritional deficiencies in women—"they eat last and least."[37,38]

For example, in one country a study of intrafamilial sex bias in the allocation of food and health care showed that among children the caloric consumption was on average 16% higher for boys than for girls. This was reflected in a significantly higher prevalence of malnutrition among the female children— 11% of them being severely malnourished compared with 5% of the male children.[37] Moreover, girls start work early as helpers in household chores. Accordingly, the increased energy needs and deficient caloric intake affect girls' weights and heights. In addition, many of these girls start their reproductive life early, which drains more of their energy reserves, leading to pregnancy-related complications. These nutritionally deficient women will give birth to children with low birth weight, to start the vicious cycle again.[38]

Nutritional anemias in women warrant special emphasis. Nutritional anemias are due to metabolic defects, hemorrhage, or chronic blood loss. However, they are also due to deficiencies in the diet that restrict the formation of new blood cells. Shortage of iron, folate, or B_{12} in the diet can all contribute to anemia. Anemia occurs more commonly in women because of dietary restriction and increased iron needs during re-

productive years. It has been estimated that 47% of all women and 59% of all pregnant women in developing countries are anemic.[6]

Another nutritional deficiency of importance affecting these women is rickets. Rachitic osteomalacia and contracted pelvis—a condition that still occurs in developing countries—is almost extinct in the more economically advantaged countries. The same story is repeated in many other nutritional deficiency conditions that are aggravated by the maternal depletion syndrome. Studies have shown that poor nutritional status can lead to low–birth weight babies, unfavorable reproductive history, obstetrical complications, and increased susceptibility to infection.[6] Similar nutritional status is manifested in more economically advantaged countries, where they are labeled eating disorders. Examples are obesity, bulimia, and anorexia nervosa. These eating disorders can only be adequately understood when considered within the context of societal expectations of women and the myths surrounding women's figures and weight.

Infections

Infections and reinfections of the female organs are numerous, widespread, increasing, and continuing to be ignored. They are caused by viruses, yeasts, bacteria, and other agents that are acquired through poor hygiene around the menstrual period; through sexual intercourse, childbirth, or abortion; or through the use of intrauterine devices (IUDs). These last were introduced to help planners control family size and to help women gain control over their lives. However, limited long-term, careful research resulted in the creation of another menace to women's health and a threat to the quality of their lives; more infections resulted or were aggravated by the IUDs.

These genital infections, besides their effect on the general health of the female, affect the reproductive health by causing infertility or by forming the basis for later ectopic pregnancies and other problems such as low birth weights and congenital anomalies. Pelvic inflammatory disease (PID), which involves fallopian tubes and/or ovaries and uterus, follows genital infection, particularly gonorrhea. In many developing countries, endemic diseases such as schistosomiasis and filariasis weaken tubal tissue and make it more vulnerable to secondary infection, and may also affect the incidence of PID.

These genital infections are of serious consequence and may lead to infertility. It is estimated that 10% to

17% of all women who suffer from genital inflammatory disease become infertile because of blockage of fallopian tubes. In addition, in Central and West Africa it was estimated that 30% or more of these genital infections not only affect the women but also the offspring, with effects ranging from low birth weight to congenital deformity to death of the coming baby.[6]

Women are also prone to communicable diseases that are acquired through their care-giving activities for the sick members of their families. Also, during their household duties they are exposed to many unsanitary conditions that put them at risk. Predisposition to diseases is counteracted by resistance, but this is compromised by malnutrition and complications of pregnancy.

Violence against women

The lower status of women in the family in many cultures makes them more liable to violence.[30] In some communities and nations, manliness and machismo tend to support a system in which the wife and the child are considered property of the men in the family; such systems condone "disciplinary" actions through all forms of abuse. In wars and other upheavals, women are usually very susceptible to violence. For example, there are many chilling historical accounts of violence to, and abuse and rape of, women in the Pakistan-Bangladesh war, during the coup against Salvador Allende in Chile, and in the Persian Gulf war. The newspaper stories in the United States included incidents of women in the military being abused by their colleagues and superiors. These women were afraid to discuss their abuse. Reporting of violent incidents is minimal for fear that exposure will bring dishonor to the woman and her family and for fear of reprisal.

Female circumcision is a practice that is carried out in some societies and is considered by many to be a form of violence. There are three types of circumcisions: clitoridectomy, excision, and infibulation. According to the type, either the clitoris only is excised; or the clitoris and the labia minora are excised; or the clitoris, the labia minora, and the labia majora are excised and are stitched together causing scar tissue.[15] All forms of female circumcision are done to diminish or prevent the sexual arousal of the female as a method of preserving her chastity before marriage. It is related to beliefs of purification and is called "Tahara," which means purification. It is reinforced by aggressive structural components in societies and by the matriarchal side of families.[2,14]

The origin of this custom is obscure. It is not a part of Islamic doctrine, but it is a part of the definition of rites of passage for women in many parts of Africa and the Middle East. This practice was alleged to have been based on religious practices, but it is now known beyond a doubt that this is not the case.[1] Female circumcision is against the law in most communities in the world but is still practiced, usually under unhealthy conditions, without anesthesia, and by practitioners who range from traditional birth attendants to so-called gypsies to health care providers. All forms of female circumcision have serious implications for female personal health in the form of shock, hemorrhage, infection, urine retention, and injury. There are still cases in the hospital records of developing countries of young girls being admitted in shock as a result of postcircumcision bleeding.[35]

There are many other aftereffects of this practice, such as the psychological trauma for young girls. The effect on the women's sex life is tremendously profound and shapes their view of sexuality and of their participation in the sexual encounter. These women are even blamed for their husbands' drug use, since it is claimed that men use drugs in order to derive sexual satisfaction from the "surgically mutilated frigid wives." Moreover, some of these extended circumcisions may have an effect on the process of childbirth, causing injuries and bleeding during labor. Contrary to popular belief, the custom of circumcision is carefully guided and supported by women in the family. Although men may condone it, they are not the ones who keep it in practice.

Circumcision is not the only form of violence against women. More compelling and more significant from the women's perspective are the laws that condone and support domestic violence under the pretense of men's obligation to preserve face or honor against women's so-called insubordination, infidelities, or freedoms. Women also consider the lack of regulatory laws to protect their rights in socially unequal societies and in systems that condone colonialism and patriarchy as aggressive acts that are invariably ignored. Nor are the West or the "developed" countries immune from other forms of "circumcision" or "vaginal mutilation." Young women are socialized to deny early sexual abuse experiences (molestation and rape) in favor of adopting more sanctioned and socially acceptable roles that mirror purification and normative expectations. The influence of these experiences on women's mental health is well documented.[4,25,31,42]

Reproductive health

Reproductive health and maternity form an important aspect of women's health and are considered an element of primary health care, especially as they relate to maternal-child health. Also, women usually enter the health care system for reproductive care. In a number of countries, maternal mortality rates remain at alarmingly high levels, as does the low nutritional status of women throughout their reproductive cycles.[9,40] It has been estimated that there are at least half a million maternal deaths in the world per year that are preventable.[39] This maternal mortality is not evenly distributed in different parts of the world—for example, women in Bangladesh face a risk of dying 400 times greater than that of women in Scandinavia, and 50 times greater than that of women in Portugal. The maternal mortality rate is as high as 900:100,000 in some countries of the world, compared with a rate below 10:100,000 in developed countries.[39] Moreover, according to a survey in India between 1974 and 1979, for each maternal death there were 16.5 illnesses related to pregnancy, childbirth, and the puerperium. Many authorities believe these figures to be underestimated.[39]

The factors behind the immense difference in the effects of childbirth in developing versus developed countries have been widely examined. Some of them are health service factors, while others are socioeconomic and medical; there are also reproductive factors that include pregnancy before reaching 18 years of age, pregnancy after age 35, pregnancy of more than four children, and less than 2 years between pregnancies.[9]

It has been estimated that the number of maternal deaths would decline by over 20% if the first through the fifth births were confined to women from 20 through 39 years of age.[39] In addition, these changes would reduce the total number of births, lowering the general fertility rate by 25%.[33] The number of maternal deaths would drop by one third. The number of maternal deaths would decline even further if there were no births after age 35, or beyond the fourth child.[18,28] Women having more than four children are at risk; this is known as a grand multigravida. Different studies have shown that primigravidas have slightly higher mortality rates, which decrease during the second deliveries and start rising again after the third, increasing with the number of pregnancies and the lack of adequate spacing between pregnancies. Not only parity and age, but also intervals between births, have an effect on maternal mortality. In Bangladesh and Indonesia, for example, the highest death rates are found in women under the age of 20 with three or more children.[7,34] There are, however, limited studies that have examined the effect of birth intervals independent of age and parity.[33]

The other factor affecting reproductive health of women and their general health is age at marriage. Early marriage is a norm in many parts of the world; and for some, puberty marks a milestone for marriage. For example, in Bangladesh two thirds of all women aged 19 or younger are already married;[3] and in Afghanistan, Malawi, Mali, Nepal, North Yemen, and Egypt more than one half of all women who are 19 or younger are married.[11] In the Middle East, South Asia, and parts of Africa, marriages arranged by families are often between adolescent girls and considerably older men. These conditions increase women's risk of morbidity and mortality and decrease women's options for education and employment. In turn, decreased options may influence women's awareness of their health needs and their access to quality health care. Developed countries are not immune to adolescent pregnancy. In the United States, adolescent pregnancy has been linked to low birth weight and maternal complications.[41] However, the availability of health care resources in the high-income countries acts as a buffer against these complications.

Abortion is an important factor that also affects women's health in general. Abortion is considered illegal in most of the Christian and Islamic doctrines and is viewed as a defiance of God's will. Religious law forbids the killing of innocent children, yet innocent mothers who are trying to exercise control over their own bodies become the victims. Induced abortions, which are unregulated because of restrictive laws, expose women to another set of major risks. This is particularly problematic. In the majority of developing countries, abortion is illegal but is the most widely used method of fertility regulation. It is estimated that 35 million to 55 million pregnancies worldwide are terminated through induced abortion.[5] Infection, hemorrhage, and trauma are quite common. Tetanus is a serious danger accompanying criminal abortion. Its effect on the procedure, even if that procedure spares the woman's life, seriously affects her fertility and personal health later.

Even in those developing countries where laws are liberal, as in India, lack of facilities renders legal abortion unobtainable for most women; therefore, women resort to ways of ending their unwanted pregnancies that increase their health risks. Such ways include introducing plant stems or foreign bodies into the uterus through the vaginal canal, or herbal pastes prepared by the herbalist.

Recently, developing countries have been watching the struggle of the United States as it attempts to resolve the issues surrounding abortion in a way that addresses and encompasses the rights of women and the rights of their unborn children. Limiting and regulating conception is considered a woman's problem in most of the world. Even when methods are developed to help women decrease the health problems related to reproduction, these methods are not carefully developed and monitored. Safety of contraceptive methods has been assumed more than proved, and not until recently have these methods been investigated through longitudinal research studies. As a result, a number of methods have been withdrawn from the market, after having been used for decades, because of new discoveries related to adverse long-term effects on women's health. For example, the relationship between smoking and contraceptive pills has promoted the issuance of new warnings.[27] The interaction between contraceptives and other major lifestyle factors has been largely ignored.

Occupational health

Women are equally exposed to the occurrence of health hazards as are men, whether in developed or developing countries. Some conditions, however, make women more vulnerable. For example, women's work at home exposes them to hazards that have been overlooked because women's work is either invisible (housework, farm work) or devalued (clerical work, domestic work, hospital work). Lane and Meleis[16] reported that farmers' wives fall off roofs or are exposed to unwarranted illnesses and diseases while attending to their daily roles and responsibilities such as scooping manure with their bare hands.

Agricultural workers exposed to chemicals used in pesticides are at risk for cancer, and pregnant women tend to suffer additional consequences that affect the health of their children. They may suffer from pregnancy complications such as miscarriage, and/or their babies may show birth defects. This occurs more often in developing countries, where overspraying by untrained workers takes place and wearing of protective clothing is largely unknown. The toxic effect of the chemicals is passed to the infants through the mother's milk. In addition, the effects of anesthetic gases that cause higher incidence of miscarriage, congenital defects, and infertility among nurses working in the operating room have been inadequately studied and poorly regulated.[8]

Women are also more vulnerable to overwork as an occupational hazard.[12] Working women take care of their households and children in addition to their full-time jobs outside the household. The "double day," or second shift phenomenon,[13] in which there is a combination of economic and family responsibilities, results in fatigue and predisposes women to mental health problems. A 1988 study analyzed 2.3 billion women (92% of the world's female population) in an effort to determine and score their social status.[27] Five aspects were included: health, education, employment, marriage and children, and equality. Fifty-one of the 99 countries included in the study fell into the lowest third of the ranking. The results further indicated that 60% of all women and girls in the world live under conditions that threaten their health, deny them a chance for childbearing, limit their educational attainment, restrict their economic participation, and fail to guarantee them equal rights and freedom from oppression.

One of the interesting findings is that the number of births is related to the status score. In countries with higher scores, indicating a higher status for women, the pregnancy rate is lower as compared to the rate in countries with poor or lower ranking in social status. The number of births in the countries with high ranking ("very good" to "good" categories) averages two per woman, while it is four or above in the "poor," "very poor," and "extremely poor" countries.

Better education and work that produces financial remuneration increase women's options and resources, and enhance their power base. However, women seem to be disenfranchised even as they attempt to exercise these options. Sons are favored over daughters for education. Even when they enter the educational sector, girls get less time to study; and in some countries, their education is terminated at puberty under the false pretense of preserving their honor and their chastity. Education and employment, key in women's health, are both related to resources and to a level of consciousness. A unique situation is that, as health care providers, women often constitute a majority. Available statistics suggest that in most countries the labor force in the formal health system tends to be predominantly female. But here again, women tend to feel underpaid, holding the less prestigious jobs rather than those with status and decision-making power.

Women also constitute the majority of the volunteers in hospitals, clinics, and other community health organizations. The unique predominance of women in the health care system makes them a major target of importance in primary health care (PHC). It is also the woman who is expected to be the health provider and educator in the family. She is the one who teaches sound health practices to the future generations, creates a home environment conducive to better health through factors such as clean water and nutrition, and ensures that the children are immunized and cared for during the crucial years of their lives. A good share of the essential elements of PHC fall almost exclusively into the woman's domain at the family level.[36]

The woman's role as primary health provider could be enhanced by considering this role within the totality of her daily life experiences. For example, it is recommended that women who live in rural areas boil drinking water; the implications of this seemingly simple act, which are far-reaching for an already-overburdened woman, must be considered. To boil water, women have to carry water receptacles for long distances, search for and obtain burning fuel, and use different containers for boiling and for storing the water. Another example is breast-feeding. Breast-feeding for prolonged periods of time (2 years) has been proved to result in healthier babies, less time spent by women on sick children, and less money spent on formula.[40] It also has a contraceptive effect (although this is questionable because of factors such as length of feeding and amount of milk). However, breast-feeding for a prolonged time has also been related to an increased likelihood of the woman's becoming anemic.

WOMEN'S HEALTH: A CHANGING AGENDA

To enhance women's health globally, health care programs should be established within a framework that acknowledges women's perspective, experiences, and context. The context of the totality of women's daily situations and daily experiences and role responsibilities as women themselves see them need to be captured, described, and carefully integrated into health care plans.[21] It is through such an approach that groups of women who are most vulnerable to health risks may be identified and that appropriate resources that are more congruent with their needs may be developed.[32] To do these things, health care researchers, planners, and providers need to think of ways in which

the women's different voices can be heard. Gaps in knowledge related to women's situations should become a top priority. The ways in which women tend to integrate their roles on a daily basis and the patterns of management of the complex and intricate aspects of each of their daily roles need to be uncovered and addressed.[20,23] Special attention should be given to how women perceive and enact their roles as providers, mothers, care givers, spouses, daughters, and workers, and to such experiences as render them vulnerable. Vulnerability is defined as "the process or state of persons being unprotected or open to damage in their interactions with a challenging or threatening environment."[10] A focus on women's roles, integrations, and vulnerabilities could help to identify women's critical needs.

Strategies are needed for the development of nursing therapeutics to empower women. A focus on empowerment is holistic, encompassing, and potentially fruitful. Empowerment does not just include increased understanding of women and their problems or enhancing their education; more importantly, it means providing them with resources and a social structure that support them in carrying out their various roles. It also means providing them with accessible services. Health service accessibility includes cost, convenience, and compatibility. Cost involves not only the cost of the service but the cost of transportation to the service for the mother and/or child. The convenience of the service, including the time schedule, should be compatible with the scheme of the mother's life. Women cannot easily leave their day-to-day chores and responsibilities. Compatibility of services includes compatibility with the woman's beliefs, her preferences, and her habits. The most outstanding example of incompatibility would be the discomfort of some women in dealing with an unfamiliar male health provider. In this respect, the use and upgrading of already-existing services, such as traditional birth attendants, can be of great benefit. Careful analysis and consideration of laws that put women at risk, and of the gaps between the spirit of the law and its implementation should be a context for any discourse related to women's health; examples of relevant laws are those that govern age requirements for marriage, leaves of absence for domestic workers, and working with hazardous materials. Discourse about laws related to such issues as female circumcision should be handled within sociocultural and historical contexts. To have a viable women's health program, women need to think both locally and globally. The development of a united front is the single most powerful strategy to improve women's status and situation, which in turn could have a profound effect on women's health. Examples of the effects of a united front are the United Nations Decade of Women that started in 1975 in Mexico City and ended in 1985 at the world conference in Nairobi, and the review of accomplishments that occurred in Copenhagen in 1980. These brought women together from around the world to address women's issues.[26] These international meetings were powerful in enabling women to initiate more local changes.

Involvement of women's organizations at different levels in the upgrading of women's health has been continuously suggested. This approach has been followed in some parts of the world and proved to be effective—for example, in Indonesia. Involvement of other sectors of the community in programs to ensure better health for women is mandatory. Participation by members of the grass roots in each community should be promoted. The framework to guide women's health care should attempt to capture all the work that is defined as non-work and thus goes unreported, undocumented, unrewarded, and unregulated. Therefore, a crucial role for governments is providing priority social support for women in all their roles, instead of relying on the informal social support of their extended families.[17]

Finally, a commitment to women's health is needed at all levels to advance the development of policies to protect and promote it. Action agendas similar to those provided by the U.S. National Council for International Health[24] are significant in providing local frameworks. However, policies and international aid programs that are developed without careful consideration of the diversity of women and without recognition of their critical needs and the extensiveness of their tasks and responsibilities ignore their contributions, stifle their potential, and decrease the likelihood of their long and active participation.

REFERENCES

1. Ahoyo, V., & Kaamel, A. (1987, April 6-10). *Islam in the face of traditional practices affecting mothers and children*. Report on the regional seminar on traditional practices affecting the health of women and children in Africa, p. 70. Addis Ababa, Ethiopia: International African Committee on Traditional Practices Affecting the Health of Women and Children.

2. Baasher, T., Bannerman, R., Rushwan, H., & Sharas, I. (Eds.). (1982). *Traditional practices affecting the health of women and children: Female circumcision, childhood marriage, nutritional taboos*. Background papers to the WHO seminar, Technical Publications, 2(2). Alexandria, Egypt: World Health Organization.

3. Bangladesh Ministry of Health and Population Control. (1978). *Bangladesh fertility survey (1975-1976)*. Dacca, Bangladesh: Author.

4. Bickerton, D., Hall, R., & Williams, A. L. (1991). Women's experiences of sexual abuse in childhood. *Public Health, 105,* 447-453.

5. Blair, P. (1980). *Programming for women's health*. Report prepared for the office of women's development of the U.S. agency for international development. (Unpublished report).

6. Bruce, J. (1981). Women oriented health care: New Hampshire feminist health center. *Studies in Family Planning, 12*(10), 353-363.

7. Chen, L. C., Geshe, M. C., Ahmed, S., Chowdhury, A. I., & Mosely, W. H. (1974). Maternal mortality in rural Bangladesh. *Studies in Family Planning, 5,* 334-341.

8. Datta, K. K., Sharma, R. S., Razack, P. M. A., Ghosh, T. K., & Arora, R. R. (1980). Morbidity pattern amongst rural pregnant women in Alwar, Rajasthan—a cohort study. *Health and Population Perspectives and Issues, 3,* 282-292.

9. *Family planning programs, healthier mothers and children through family planning* (Population information program, Series 1, No. 27). (1984, May-June). Baltimore: Johns Hopkins University.

10. Hall, J. M., Stevens, P. E., & Meleis, A. I. (1992). Experiences of women clerical workers in patient care areas. *Journal of Nursing Administration, 22*(5), 11-17.

11. Hassan, E. O. (1988). *Safe motherhood—efforts and the role of professional societies in Egypt*. Paper presented at the World Health Organization workshop "Role of Obstetricians and Gynecologists in Promoting Women's Health and Safe Motherhood." Alexandria, Egypt: World Health Organization.

12. Hibbard, J. H., & Pope, R. P. (1991). Effect of domestic and occupational roles on morbidity and mortality. *Social Science and Medicine, 32*(7), 805-811.

13. Hochchild, A. R. (1989). *Second shift: Working parents and the revolution at home*. New York: Viking.

14. Kaamel, A. (1987, April). *Activities against female circumcision in Egypt*. Reports on the regional seminar on traditional practices affecting the health of women and children in Africa. Addis Ababa, Ethiopia: International African Committee on Traditional Practices Affecting the Health of Women and Children.

15. Koso-Thomas, O. (1987, April 6-10). *Female circumcision and related hazards*. Reports on the regional seminar on traditional practices affecting the health of women and children in Africa, p. 65. Addis Ababa, Ethiopia: International African Committee on Traditional Practices Affecting the Health of Women and Children.

16. Lane, S., & Meleis, A. I. (1991). Roles, work, health perceptions and health resources of women: A study in an Egyptian delta hamlet. *Social Science and Medicine, 33*(10), 1197-1128.

17. Leonard, A. (Ed.). (1989). *Seeds: Supporting women's work in the Third World*. New York: Feminist Press.

18. Maine, D. (1982). *Family planning, its impact on the health of the women & children*. New York: Columbia University Press.

19. McFarland, J. (1988). The construction of women and development theory: A review essay. *Review of Canadian Sociology and Anthropology, 25,* 299-308.

20. Meleis, A. I., & Bernal, P. (in review). The paradoxical world of "muchacha de por dia" in Colombia. *Social Science and Medicine.*

21. Meleis, A. I., Kulig, J., Arruda, E. N., & Beckman, A. (1990). Maternal role of women in clerical jobs in southern Brazil: Stress

and satisfaction. *Health Care for Women International, 11,* 369-382.

22. Meleis, A. I., & Rogers, S. (1987). Women in transition: Being versus becoming or being and becoming. *Health Care for Women International, 8,* 199-217.

23. Meleis, A. I., & Stevens, P. E. (1992). Women in clerical jobs: Spousal role satisfaction, stress and coping. *Women and Health, 18*(1), 23-40.

24. National Council for International Health. (1991). *Women's health—The action agenda.* The 18th Annual International Health Conference of the National Council for International Health, Arlington, Va.

25. Orbach, I. (1986). The insolvable problem as a determinant in the dynamics of suicide behavior in children. *Journal of American Psychotherapy, 40,* 511-520.

26. Pietila, H., & Vickers, J. (1990). *Making women matter: The role of the United Nations.* London: Zed.

27. Population Crisis Committee. (1988). In S. Kemp, M. Barberis, & C. Lasher (Eds.), *Country ranking of the status of women: Poor, powerless, and pregnant.* (Population Briefing Paper No. 20). Washington, D.C.: Author.

28. Rochat, R. (1979). Effect of declining fertility on maternal and infant mortality. In W. P. McCreevey & A. Shelfield (Eds.), *Guatemala: Development and population* (Working Paper No. 4, pp. 21-43). Washington, D.C.: Battele Population.

29. Rodin, J., & Ickovics, J. R. (1990). Review and research agenda as we approach the 21st century. *American Psychologist, 45*(9), 1018-1033.

30. Russo, N. F. (1990). Overview: Forging research priorities for women's mental health. *American Psychologist, 45*(3), 369-373.

31. Scott, K. D. (1992). Childhood sexual abuse: Impact on a community's mental health status. *Child Abuse and Neglect, 16,* 285-295.

32. Stevens, P. E., Hall, J. M., & Meleis, A. I. (1992). Examining vulnerability of women clerical workers from five ethnic/racial groups. *Western Journal of Nursing Research, 14*(6), 754-774.

33. Trussell, J., & Pebley, A. R. (1984). *The impact of family planning programs on infant, child and maternal mortality.* Unpublished manuscript, World Bank Staff Working Paper.

34. Williams, I. I. (1973). Some observation on maternal mortality in Jamaica. *West Indian Medical Journal, 22*(1), 1-14.

35. World Health Organization. (1979). *Traditional practices affecting the health of women and children: Female circumcision, childhood marriage, nutritional taboos, etc.* (Technical Pub. No. 2). Geneva: Author.

36. World Health Organization. (1982). Report of the second WHO consultation on women as providers of health care, Geneva, August 16-20. Unpublished WHO document HMD/82.10.

37. World Health Organization. (1984). Report on women, health and development activities in WHO's programs 1982-1983. Unpublished WHO document LHG/84.1.

38. World Health Organization. (1985). Report on women's health and development. Report by the Director General, WHO Offset Publication, No. 90. Geneva: Author.

39. World Health Organization. (1986). Maternal mortality: Helping women off the road to death. *WHO Chronicle, 40*(5), 175-183.

40. World Health Organization. (1991). *Strengthening maternal and child health programs through PHC* (WHO Regional Office for the Eastern Mediterranean, Technical Pub. No. 18). Alexandria, Egypt: Author.

41. Zambrana, R. E. (1988). A research agenda on issues affecting poor and minority women: A model for understanding their health needs. *Women and Health, 12*(3-4), 137-160.

42. Zimmerman, J. K. (1991). Crossing the desert alone: An etiologic model of female adolescent suicidality. *Women and Therapy, 11*(3-4), 223-240.

PART TWELVE

ETHICS

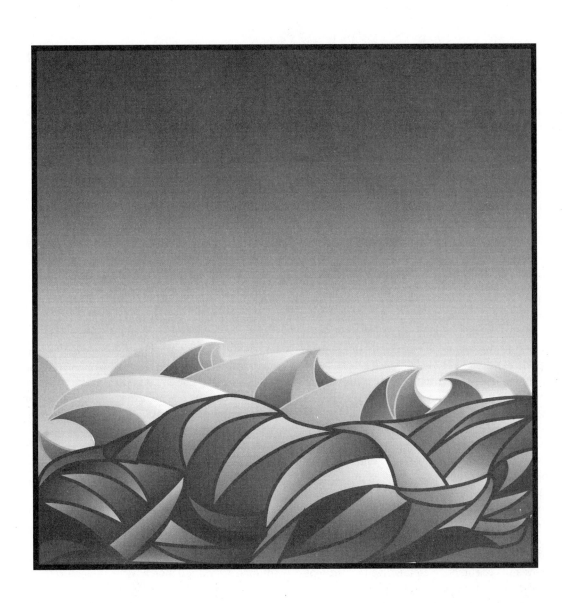

Ethics of caring decisions

JOANNE COMI McCLOSKEY, HELEN KENNEDY GRACE

As life-saving technology grows, as more people live longer, as resources become stretched, as society and its health care needs become more complex, there are more decisions that must be made about who gets what. Throughout this volume, underlying much of the content and discussion, has been a theme of ethical decision making. In this important last section, the topic of ethics is addressed in more detail.

One way to deal with problems of equity in health care services is rationing. In the debate chapter, Fry presents an overview of three types of rationing: market, implicit, and explicit. As these have not proved successful in reducing health care costs, a new strategy related to age is being explored by policymakers. Fry presents the arguments for and against limiting services for the elderly. Each side of the debate has merit and leaves one wondering what to do. What Fry would do is refocus the discussion on caring as the central goal of health care. She reviews a number of caring strategies. She believes that if models of caring, rather than curing, were used to plan for the distribution of health care resources, then a discussion about rationing targeting the elderly would not occur.

The topic of rationing is continued in the first viewpoint chapter. Capuzzi gives an overview of the process of developing the controversial Oregon Health Plan that increases access to health services by eliminating those that are nonessential. The decision-making process involved three stages: prioritization, resource allocation, and implementation. At each stage she lists those involved and discusses the ethical decisions they had to make. Nurses and consumers were involved in all steps of the process, as well as legislators, physicians, and other health professionals. Seventeen service categories were identified and 709 condition-treatment pairs were prioritized. The implementation and evaluation phases are in process. Readers will find the chapter interesting

for a number of reasons. It provides information on the Oregon plan, is an excellent example of collective decision making, and illustrates the many challenges and ethical concerns involved in any health care reform.

Each of the next four chapters discusses the ethics of care delivery to a particular population. In the first of these, Malloy addresses the complex and difficult issues related to indigent care. During the Great Society of the 1960s, Medicare and Medicaid legislation were passed to provide access for all. Paradoxically, this encouraged corporations—observing that public financing of health care could be profitable—to enter the health care market. But corporations do not want to serve the poor who have no insurance. This trend, Malloy says, combined with federal budget cutbacks, has eroded indigent accessibility to health care. Nearly 40 million Americans have no health insurance and many more have inadequate insurance. Malloy reduces the debate about indigent care to two basic questions: Who receives care? and Who pays? The ethical dilemma, she says, is one of social responsibility versus individual responsibility. She says that a radical departure from the medical model is needed for solutions to the indigent care problems. Noting that nurses have traditionally championed the cause of health care for the poor and vulnerable, she calls for a "modern-day Lillian Wald, a mover and a shaker of purse strings and conscience." She suggests nursing intervention in three areas: policy formulation, innovative demonstration projects, and educational curriculums.

The continuing rise in the numbers of patients with human immunodeficiency virus–acquired immunodeficiency syndrome (HIV/AIDS) constitutes a further challenge to nurses' concerns for humane care for all people. In this chapter, Forrester outlines the world-wide problem and then discusses ethical challenges for nurses. He points out that health care professionals also participate in the stigmatization of persons with HIV/AIDS. Nurses, he says, should reject and counteract social stereotypes, assess personal values and risks more accurately, and identify their responsibilities in providing care that demonstrates value for the autonomy of the person with HIV/AIDS. Helping actions include hearing about current therapies and risks, sharing information in a sensitive and truthful way, conducting research, and engaging in clarification of values. Forrester points out that since 1982 the American Nurses Association (ANA) has adopted 22 policies and position statements related to HIV/AIDS. All of them say that nurses need to deliver care to all persons without prejudicial behavior. Forrester concludes that an appropriate nursing response to the AIDS epidemic should have three objectives: (1) to prevent HIV infection, (2) to provide care for those already infected, and (3) to participate in national and international efforts to fight HIV/AIDS and its associated stigma.

The next population discussed is children. Child abuse is a major concern for nurses working with children and families. Cowen's chapter on this important and growing problem is informative. She presents an overview of four types of child abuse—physical abuse, neglect, sexual abuse, and emotional abuse—and lists physical and behavioral indicators of each. A model of child maltreatment by Garbarino and several assessment tools are available to help nurses recognize a child abuse situation. Cowen discusses what to do if one suspects child abuse. She points out that nurses are often perceived by the family as being helpful and less threatening than others. Cowen says that this is a multifaceted problem that requires multidisciplinary efforts. Nurses must understand the current problems and the ethical, legal, and social ramifications of child abuse to play a leadership role in this area.

Shifting to a discussion of ethical dilemmas associated with reproductive technology, Olshansky focuses on the nurse's role in helping patients to maintain their "personhood" while undergoing the impersonal interventions associated with that technology. Reproductive technology includes in vitro fertilization, artificial insemination, gamete intrafallopian transfer, oocyte donation, frozen embryo transfer, and surrogate mothering. Personhood refers to the individual's sense of self as an autonomous being. Personhood can be enhanced or decreased as a result of using reproductive technology. Olshansky discusses the issues of choice and control. She points out that only women who can pay or who are below a certain age are eligible for certain

treatments. The concept of choice becomes intertwined with that of control and the meaning of parenthood in our society. The nurse has responsibility for counseling patients so that they are informed and knowledgeable and can make appropriate decisions for themselves.

As the previous discussion illustrates, technology in health care has changed the way we do things but has created complex ethical dilemmas. The next chapter, by Thompson, Amos, and Graves, focuses on the ethics associated with using technology. They divide health care technology into three categories: biomedical, information, and knowledge. Knowledge technology entails the use of computers to generate new knowledge. Creation of knowledge technology, or expert systems, holds the promise of assisting nurses in clinical management but presents unique ethical concerns. The authors give examples of systems and outline several ethical questions that need to be addressed. Cost-benefit issues in establishing expert knowledge systems in clinical practice are explored by the authors. Additional benefits result when an expert system lies on top of a clinical nursing information system. The authors conclude that the costs of technology are high and say that nurses and computer companies must develop approaches that cost less. The advent of inexpensive microcomputers presents a major opportunity for nursing.

Knowing the legal boundaries and mandates are a part of ethical decision making. As of December 1991, U.S. federal law mandates that health care facilities inform patients of their rights to have a living will or durable power of attorney for health care. These "advance directives" are legal mechanisms to support decision making by others when one is no longer able to make those decisions. Kjervik says that the right to refuse treatment is the corollary of the right to consent to treatment. She discusses the types of advance directives and reviews the ethical principles on which these legal mechanisms are based. She discusses four objections to advance directives and refutes each. She outlines the nursing role in the use of advance directives. Nurses cannot assist a patient to examine values without self-reflection and decision making about their own views of life and death. Nurses, she says, "should recognize the variety of 'right' answers available to patients, . . . should recognize their equalities and inequalities with patients, and should become comfortable with their own irrational sides." Nurses, she points out, often have skills in developing trusting relationships with patients that can be used as a model for other health professionals as they attempt to improve their communication with patients.

Faced with the same situation, some people act one way, others act another. Carpenter's interesting chapter entitled "Tutor or Tyrant?" gives a helpful perspective on the causes of ethical and unethical behavior. She says that when individuals interpret events as educative (tutorial), they have many behavior options to choose from and ethical choice is possible. When, however, the events are interpreted as dictatorial (tyrannical), then behavior options are limited and the outcome is likely to be unethical. Carpenter first reviews traditional and recent theories of ethics. The traditional view of women as morally inferior has been challenged by Carol Gilligan. Carpenter warns us, however, against setting up a new unhelpful dualism between the traditional male justice view and the newer female caring view. She also points out that tyrants are not always external forces. She discusses three within nursing: tyranny of emotions, tyranny of metaphors and images, and tyranny of habit. Carpenter challenges nursing to examine several assumptions. For example, the profession's replacement of the metaphor of handmaiden with that of advocate has brought some needed changes. But is the new metaphor itself limiting? She also challenges the notion that ethics concerns only the dramatic. She gives numerous examples of how nurses confront important ethical decisions every day and make these decisions based on habit rather than informed choice. The chapter challenges nurses to think about internal barriers and to dismantle the barriers as a step toward change.

When ethical issues are viewed across cultures, new issues emerge. In the final chapter, Holleran raises the controversial question of whether or not ethical standards should vary throughout the world. She notes some key concerns and encourages nurses to become informed and speak out against ethical abuses. The export of outdated drugs and drugs not yet certified as safe, and the promotion and aggressive sale of nonessential drugs are questionable practices. The promotion of commercially prepared baby formula is another practice of concern to many. Policies regarding AIDS testing, questionable practices associated with organ transplants, and the jailing of health workers because they have provided emergency care to political dissidents are all areas of concern for nurses. Holleran's chapter demonstrates that the ethical implications of a particular topic are often viewed differently in different parts of the world. The answers, she says, are not easy but involve broadening our awareness, respecting our differences, and engaging in discussions about our concerns. The International Council of Nurses (ICN) Code for Nurses offers broad guidelines that can be adapted by national nursing associations for specific needs.

As the chapters in this book have demonstrated, the issues confronting nurses throughout the world are complex. Maintaining a focus on the needs of people for health care services and the responsibility of nurses to see that equitable services are provided for all is a major challenge as we move closer to the next century.

CHAPTER 94

Debate

Do we have health care rationing?

SARA T. FRY

It is not surprising that health care costs have risen sharply in recent years. The growth of medical knowledge, development of new technologies, public demands and expectations concerning health issues, and other matters have helped create a spiraling escalation of private and public costs for available health care services. In 1989, approximately $550 billion was spent on health care, and it is projected that by the year 2000, this amount may triple to 1.5 trillion.[3] Given these costs, questions are being raised by economists, legislators, consumers, and ethicists about the benefits of such care. At issue are the appropriate amounts of government spending for health care, restrictions for some health care services, and the ethical implications of health care rationing strategies.

It is generally believed that the ethical implications of various actions and their alternatives should be considered before choosing a course of action and putting it into practice.[1] Therefore it is appropriate, if not prudent, that the ethical implications of various cost containment measures in health care be considered before limitations on government spending for health care are decided and some health care goods are rationed. Whenever a decision is made that some persons will receive an available but scarce medical resource that cannot be provided to everyone who needs it, a rationing decision is made.[1] A cautious approach to these matters is very important because limiting health care resources often has serious implications for the health professions as well as for the consumer.

In this chapter, several methods of rationing health care will be presented. The pros and cons of health care rationing, in general, will be discussed, and the ethical implications of various rationing strategies will be described. A proposal for the provision of nursing care under conditions of rationing will also be considered.

The goal of this chapter is to emphasize how rationing strategies pose significant challenges to professional ethics. Rationing of health care resources has the potential to dramatically affect how nurses, in particular, view their professional responsibilities as mandated by society.

CURRENT RATIONING STRATEGIES

It is widely understood that current cost containment measures in health care use a mixture of rationing methods that affect access to health care.[11] These methods influence either the behavior of the consumer (market rationing), the behavior of the health professional (implicit rationing), or the administration of health care services (explicit rationing).

Market rationing

In the market system before the 1950s, health care was rationed by consumer ability to pay for services, the availability and distribution of medical personnel and services, and professional decisions about the allocation of professional services.[10] This was essentially a fee-for-service system that was gradually eroded by social forces resulting from the rapid rise in medical knowledge and technology and government subsidy of health care. The market system then slowly shifted to a system dominated by a variety of third-party payments for health care services. As the new system grew, however, availability of health resources to all consumers became a genuine problem. Other methods for rationing health care were needed.

Cost sharing for health care, in the form of coinsurance and deductibles, is a method that promised to help alleviate the problem of resource availability. Its initial success as a method of rationing indicated that consumers tend to use health care services more wisely if they share in the cost. The result, of course, would be reduced utilization of services, depending on the specific cost-sharing arrangements agreed to, and the economic status of the persons involved.

Unfortunately, in living up to its promise to reduce utilization of services, cost sharing reduces medical consultation for less serious problems or for those conditions that can be treated more adequately if appraised early. It is also recognized as a method that differentially affects low-income rather than high-income groups and results in inequities in the distribution of health care.[11] Although it is not the best of rationing strategies and not the most popular method among consumers, it remains a feature of many health care programs.

Implicit rationing

Implicit rationing is another method that is frequently used in limiting health resources. Its aim is to set limits on providers' decisions without interfering with clinical judgments for individual consumers. In other words, health professionals rather than health administrators make decisions about allocations of professional time and resources among client populations. When limitations on provider decisions occur, they are imposed by capitation payments for clients, limitations on available hospital beds, limitations on available specialists, and, in some cases, fixed budgets for health care resources. This method is most often seen with prepaid health care or group practice such as health maintenance organizations (HMOs).

Implicit rationing is initially attractive to practitioners because their clinical judgments are supposedly not hampered by outside forces. Providers are simply encouraged, through various incentives, to be conservative in their use of health resources. These incentives, however, may exert a strong influence on the clinical practitioner. It is well known that if professionals on contract with HMOs or prepaid group practice overuse available resources for clients, they may be dropped from employment with the organization.[9]

This method of rationing also carries certain disadvantages for the consumer. For example, the way in which health professionals allocate their time can always be influenced by personal tastes and by professional interests. If individual practitioners spend more time with disorders or ailments of greater interest than others, an unjust distribution of professional resources for all persons may result. Furthermore, as long as practitioners do not overutilize resources, it is unlikely that their use of resources will ever be questioned. It is a rationing method that allows the individual practitioner to work at a comfortable and leisurely pace or to give disproportionate time to some patients in comparison to others.[11] Obviously, implicit rationing can be exploited by health care professionals and may lead to inequities in the distribution of health care. However, it is a rationing strategy that is firmly established in the U.S. health care system.

Explicit rationing

As an alternative to market rationing and implicit rationing, explicit rationing is frequently employed as a cost containment method and a means to limit resource consumption. Explicit rationing involves administrative decisions about coverage within health care plans, the limitation of health care visits including specific resources or procedures, and, also, the setting of required intervals between certain services.[11]

This method is used in federally supported health programs such as Medicare, and in some private and nonprofit health insurance programs. It is well liked by health administrators because it allows direct control over health care allocations. It is not as well liked by health care practitioners because administrative control of health care decisions often interferes with clinician decision making and professional autonomy. As a result, practitioners often seek ways to "beat the system" or otherwise manipulate the administrative rules regulating the allocation of health resources including the use of themselves.

This method of rationing also has the undesirable side effect of overlooking individual consumer health needs. Administrative decisions on resource allocations are typically made on the basis of aggregate data about health care needs, consumption, and available resources. By setting limits on the amount of available health resources, this kind of decision making acts against individual health needs and usurps provider decisions about individual care. These undesirable effects are especially pronounced when explicit rationing strategies are used in limiting health care resources to the elderly.

RATIONING HEALTH CARE AND THE ELDERLY

Given the fact that market, implicit, and explicit rationing strategies have done little to reduce health care costs or reduce resource consumption during the past 50 years, new strategies are being explored. The most provocative of these strategies target certain segments of the population for reduced health care attention and resource consumption because of the high costs of providing them with care. The elderly is one such population group that has received a great deal of attention in recent years whenever the topic of rationing health care has been discussed. Should explicit rationing of health care resources really start with wide-scale restrictions of resources for the elderly? Is age a criterion for the use of certain health care resources?

Pro argument

The elderly should be targeted for health care rationing for several reasons. First, it is inevitable, given the high cost of providing the elderly with needed health care. According to Callahan,[2] the cost of health care for the elderly who are in their last year of life amounts to about 1% of the gross national product (GNP) each year. Their needs in the last year of life usually require the use of costly technology, and the length of time that care is needed is often protracted. All of this amounts to enormous amounts of money spent in trying to forestall death—money that could have been used to prevent health care problems in younger populations.

Second, the number of people over 65 years of age in the United States is rapidly increasing, and this trend is expected to continue over the next 20 years.[14] Indeed, the elderly over 85 years of age comprise the most rapidly growing age group in our society today.[5] Given the high rate of consumption of health care resources by the elderly, this means that depletion of health care resources will occur at a rapid rate over a very short period of time. It is imperative that some limitations on health care consumption be implemented to make sure that those in their 30s and 40s will have necessary health care services when they become elderly.

Third, the elderly should not expect to receive some health care resources after a certain age. As argued by Callahan,[2] the proper role of the elderly in society is to care for the young and future generations, and *not* to concentrate on their own welfare. After all, it is possible to live out a meaningful old age that is limited in time and in health care support—in other words, to live "a natural life span." This is a view of the life cycle that supports health as a wholeness of the body combined with the wholeness of a human life. It sees the life cycle as being followed by a "a tolerable death" that occurs at that stage at which one's moral obligations have been discharged, the majority of life possibilities have been fulfilled, and it will not seem offensive to others if one dies.[2] Death is then viewed as a sad but relatively acceptable event that occurs when life possibilities have, on the whole, been fulfilled. This is a view of aging that focuses on the ends and meaning of aging and promotes individual acceptance of one's mortality.

Fourth, rationing health care to the elderly would support a needed change in the goals and aims of medicine and nursing. No longer would the goal be to cure the elderly person of underlying disease or to extend life. The goal would be to provide an honorable and viable life in later years and to provide humane, sensitive care appropriate to the special needs and dignity of the aged person. This would allow changes in medical and nursing education that would focus on supportive care and the needs of the elderly and dying patient rather than on saving lives at all costs.

Last, if rationing strategies are *not* targeted toward some age groups, then deciding who gets what health care resources may be done in an ad hoc, situation-dependent manner that will, in the long run, seem unfair to all health care consumers rather than just to the elderly. If restrictions on available resources based on age are made in advance, then expectations will change over time and the system will not seem unfair as long as all others who are the same age experience the same restrictions. Using age as a criterion is a fair approach that recognizes that high levels of resources are being expended with little hope of benefit in caring for the elderly.

For these reasons, health care resources for the elderly should be rationed. It is reasonable, just, and pragmatic.

Con argument

Health care rationing strategies should *not* target the elderly for the following reasons.

First, age should not be a criterion for the use of certain health care services. Resource allocation decisions should be based solely on need and not age. Age-based decision making will inevitably disadvantage the healthy elderly. If one has taken care of one's health, exercised, eaten the right foods, lived moderately, and so forth, one should expect no restrictions on health care resources if a major health care crisis should be experienced in later years. In fact, a healthy 70-year-old person might do better if treated than an unhealthy 50-year-old suffering from the same disorder. If a certain treatment has been shown to benefit a condition, it should be available to the person who has need of that treatment regardless of the person's age.

Second, the elderly have contributed more to society than younger members of society. Because they have a longer working history and have made significant contributions to the harmony and stability of society, they are actually more deserving of treatment while they are elderly than those who have not contributed as much. If rationing must occur, it should be targeted toward younger members of society rather than the elderly because the young have not contributed very much to the accumulation of health care resources.

Third, health care rationing strategies should be aimed at restriction of very costly technologies used in providing health care to all age groups and not restriction of resources for use by the elderly. Many very costly technologies have low benefits or are used in treatments for individuals who have little potential to contribute to society, even with the treatment. These technologies should be targeted for rationing schemes, and not the elderly.

Fourth, rationing of resources for the elderly is potentially disrespectful to our older members of society and may characterize our society as inhumane. Most societies throughout the world honor the older member and support special responsibilities toward older citizens. If our country treated the elderly differently, it would lower our moral standing among all countries and would cause others to regard the United States as an undesirable place to live. It might also discourage younger citizens from contributing much to society if they do not see themselves as reaping some special benefits from their contributions as they become older.

Last, health professionals would find it extremely difficult to limit health care resources for the elderly given their codes of professional ethics. Physicians and nurses are mandated to provide care to individuals regardless of religion, culture, race, economic circumstances, or the nature of the disease. If age were introduced as a criterion for receiving health care services, health professionals would find this discriminatory and contradictory to their ethical obligations.

They would refuse to limit resources for the elderly and the rationing strategy would not work.

For these reasons, health care rationing strategies should not be targeted toward the elderly in our society.

AN ALTERNATIVE TO RATIONING RESOURCES FOR THE ELDERLY

What is needed in any consideration of reducing health care costs is a refocusing on the goals and aims of health care. As Callahan[3] points out, the disciplines of medicine and nursing must refocus their efforts away from the cure of disease and the extension of nonmeaningful life for any person. Instead, they should focus on *caring* as the central goal of health care. It is the ideal of caring that promises to unite the health professions in their efforts to resolve ethical dilemmas posed by cost containment measures and health care rationing strategies.

A number of caring-focused approaches are beginning to appear in the health care literature. Gadow,[6] for example, argues that the value of caring provides a foundation for a professional ethic that will protect and enhance the human dignity of patients receiving health care services. Viewing caring in the nurse-patient relationship as a commitment to certain ends for the patient, Gadow analyzes existential caring as demonstrated in the actions of truth telling and touch. By telling the truth to a patient, the nurse assists the patient in assessing both the subjective and the objective realities in illness and in making choices based on the unique meaning of the illness experience for that patient. Through touch, the patient is affirmed as a person rather than an object, and the value of caring as the basis for nursing actions is communicated.

This approach identifies a moral foundation for a professional ethic that is supported by others.[4,7,8,12] Caring is viewed as a natural state of human existence and as one way in which individuals relate to the world and other human beings. Caring is also viewed as occurring in society to serve human needs. As an ideal for health care professionals, caring actually gains moral significance when it is formally adopted by those who have responsibility to serve the needs of others.

Another model of caring with important implications for health care practices under rationing strategies is Watson's model[15] of human care. In this model, "caring calls for a philosophy of moral commitment toward protecting human dignity and preserving humanity." Caring is a value and an attitude that eventually manifests itself in concrete acts. But caring is also an ideal that transcends the act of caring to influence collective acts of the professional group. Such human caring is transcribed into a philosophy of action and is based on moral notions of needs and considerations for the welfare of others.

Pellegrino[13] offers a third approach to human caring that focuses on the relationship between care giver and care receiver and promises to enhance the carrying out of moral obligations to vulnerable individuals in the health care system. Four senses of care are essential to Pellegrino's approach. The first sense is care as compassion, or being concerned for another person. This is a feeling, a sharing of someone's experience of illness and pain, or just being touched by the plight of another person. To care in this sense is to see the ill individual not only as the object of our ministrations but also as a fellow human.

The second sense of caring is doing for others what they cannot do for themselves. This type of caring entails assisting the individual with activities of daily living that are compromised by illness. It is the type of caring that nurses have traditionally been recognized for, but that is in danger of being lost during the nursing shortage.

The third sense of caring is caring for the health problem experienced by the patient. It includes inviting the patient to transfer responsibility for and anxiety about what is wrong to the care giver. It is a type of caring that assures that knowledge and skill will be directed to the patient's problem. It also recognizes that patient anxiety needs a specialized type of caring that is best provided by the professional care giver.

The fourth sense of caring is to take care, or to carry out the necessary procedures (personal and technical) in patient care with conscientious attention to detail and with perfection. Not entirely separable from the third sense of caring, it is what most professionals understand as "competence."

When joined together, the above four senses of caring comprise a moral obligation for the health professional. Such caring is not an option that can be exercised or interpreted idiosyncratically within the health care system. As Pellegrino[13] claims, the moral obligation to care in this manner is created by the special human relationship that brings together the one who needs assistance (or is ill) and the one who offers to help. It requires an understanding of the professional ethic as something that attends to the concept of caring in the broad sense and that makes caring a strong moral obligation between care giver and care receiver.

These approaches to caring can assist in refocusing the aims and goals of health care toward more equitable and judicious uses of health care resources without the employment of rationing strategies. They provide an acceptable alternative to rationing aimed at the elderly and are more consistent with professional obligations toward members of society. Indeed, if the aims and goals of the health professions were changed, rationing might not even be viewed as an acceptable way to contain health care costs.

SUMMARY

Since market, implicit, and explicit rationing strategies have not proved successful in reducing health care costs or resource consumption during the past 50 years, an age-based rationing strategy is being explored. This strategy is aimed at the elderly and will limit their access to some health care resources after certain ages have been attained. Arguments in favor of this rationing scheme emphasize: the high cost of providing care, especially in the last year of life; the increasing numbers of elderly citizens who expect costly health care services; faulty expectations of the elderly geared toward their own welfare rather than toward the care and sustenance of the young; support for changes in the aims and goals of providing health care; and the fact that it is a more equitable method of reducing health care costs than ad hoc decision making.

Arguments against rationing of resources for the elderly emphasize: the unfairness of limiting health care access for one age group in society; the fact that the elderly are entitled to all health care resources because they have already contributed more than younger groups in society; the idea that rationing should be aimed at the technologies and their costs rather than at a population group; the belief that targeting the elderly is disrespectful and may have serious political and cultural implications for our society; and the belief that rationing strategies are contrary to codes of professional ethics and hard to implement.

As an alternative to rationing health care resource consumption by the elderly, it is proposed that the health professionals refocus their aims toward caring rather than cure and its associated high costs. If models of caring were used in planning for the distribution of health care resources, then discussion of a rationing strategy aimed at the elderly might be moot.

REFERENCES

1. Beauchamp, T. L., & Childress, F. F. (1989). *Principles of biomedical ethics* (3rd ed.). New York: Oxford University Press.
2. Callahan, D. (1987). *Setting limits: Medical goals in an aging society.* New York: Simon and Schuster.
3. Callahan, D. (1990). *What kind of life? The limits of medical progress.* New York: Simon and Schuster.
4. Cooper, C. C. (1988). Covenantal relationships: Grounding for the nursing ethic. *Advances in Nursing Science, 10*(4), 48-59.
5. Davis, K. (1986). Aging and the health-care system: Economic and structural issues. *Daedalus, 115,* 234-235.
6. Gadow, S. (1985). Nurse and patient: The caring relationship. In A. H. Bishop & J. R. Scudder (Eds.), *Caring, curing, coping: Nurse, physician, patient relationships* (pp. 31-43). Birmingham: University of Alabama Press.
7. Griffin, A. P. (1983). A philosophical analysis of caring in nursing. *Journal of Advanced Nursing, 8,* 289-295.
8. Huggins, E. A., & Sclazi, C. C. (1988). Limitations and alternatives: Ethical practice theory in nursing. *Advances in Nursing Science, 10*(4), 43-47.
9. Luft, H. S. (1982). Health maintenance organizations and the rationing of medical care. *Milbank Memorial Fund Quarterly, 60,* 268-306.
10. Mechanic, D. (1980). Rationing of medical care and the preservation of clinical judgment. *Journal of Family Practice, 11,* 431-433.
11. Mechanic, D. (1985). Cost containment and the quality of medical care: Rationing strategies in an era of constrained cost. *Milbank Memorial Fund Quarterly, 63,* 453-475.
12. Packard, J. S., & Ferrara, M. (1988). In search of the moral foundation of nursing. *Advances in Nursing Science, 10*(4), 60-71.
13. Pellegrino, E. D. (1985). The caring ethic: The relation of physician to patient. In A. H. Bishop & J. R. Scudder (Eds.), *Caring, curing, coping: Nurse, physician, patient relationships* (pp. 8-30). Birmingham: University of Alabama Press.
14. Bureau of the Census. (1984). *Current population reports. Series P-25. No. 952. Projections of the population of the United States by age, sex, and race: 1983-2080.* Washington, D.C.: U.S. Government Printing Office.
15. Watson, J. (1985). *Nursing: Human science and human care.* Norwalk, Conn: Appleton-Century-Crofts.

CHAPTER 95

Viewpoints

The Oregon model of decision making and its implications for nursing practice

CECELIA CAPUZZI

Health care reform is a major political topic in the United States. Currently 40 bills on the topic have been introduced in Congress, with more expected by the end of the year.[4] States are also implementing reforms.

Because health care is considered a common good, its distribution and financing becomes an ethical issue.[5] It also is an ethical issue because "one can appeal to moral considerations for taking each of two opposing courses of action."[2] In other words, there may be no one right way of dealing with current health care problems. If access is given for all health care services to all individuals, cost will be a burden; on the other hand, if access is limited to certain individuals or to certain health services, some may suffer.

To get beyond an ethical dilemma, decisions have to be made. This raises the question of *what* decisions should be made, *who* should make them, and *how* they should be made.

The tradition in the United States has been for privately financed health care decisions to be left to the marketplace, in which consumers indicate their preferences or values. For publicly financed health care, decisions are made in the legislative and administrative arenas. In the former situation, marketplace decision making has not worked well, because those who participate frequently lack the knowledge to make free choices. In addition, their choices are usually limited by the providers' prescriptions. In the latter situation, health care decisions are made by a limited number of players, and the effects are often implicit. Over time, there has been a recognition that a nonmarket decision-making process is needed to shape both the

privately and publicly financed health care systems, a process that involves the entire community.[6]

In 1983, a President's Commission for the Study of Ethical Problems in Medicine and Biomedical and Behavioral Research published a report on securing access to health care. In this report, the commission[9] stated, "there is a felt obligation to ensure that some level of health services is available to all." Furthermore, the commission avowed that a basic level of care was a societal obligation, not just a governmental responsibility. The commission suggested that decisions about health care should involve experts in health care, economists, and the public. In 1989, Oregon legitimized a nonmarket decision-making process with enactment of the Oregon Health Plan.

THE OREGON HEALTH PLAN

The enactment of the Oregon Health Plan was driven by the increasing numbers of people who were uninsured and by rising costs.[7] In addition, policymakers were dissatisfied with the then current process for making health care resource decisions. There was the realization that legislators and administrators were implicitly rationing health care each time a health care allocation decision was made. The Oregon Health Plan changed the decision-making process so that explicit policy outcomes would be derived with input from a broader array of individuals.

With nine planning principles as a guide (see the box on p. 712), three bills were enacted during the 1989 legislature. Senate Bill (SB) 27 expanded the numbers of

---

PRINCIPLES GUIDING THE OREGON HEALTH PLAN

1. Allocations for health care must be part of a broader allocation policy which recognizes that health can only be maintained if investments in a number of related areas are balanced.
2. The resource allocations policy must include a mechanism to establish clear accountability for the allocation decisions themselves and for their consequences.
3. There must be universal access for the state's citizens to a basic level of health care.
4. It is the obligation of society to provide sufficient resources to finance a basic level of care for those who cannot pay for it themselves.
5. There must be a process to determine what constitutes a "basic" level of care.
6. The criteria used in this process must be publicly debated, must reflect social values, and must consider the common good of society.
7. The health care distribution system must offer incentives to use those services and procedures which are effective and appropriate rather than those which are of marginal or unproven benefit.
8. The distribution system must avoid creating incentives for overtreatment.
9. Funding must be explicit and the system must be economically sustainable.

From Kitzhaber, J. (1990). *The Oregon basic health services act.* Salem, Ore: Oregon Senate.

SUMMARY OF SENATE BILL 27

1. Provide medical assistance to those in need whose family income is below the federal poverty level.
2. Establish a Health Services Commission (HSC) which will develop a list of health services ranked by priority (with certain exemptions).
3. Submit a report on the list ranked by priority, from the most important to the least important, representing the comparative benefits of each service to the entire population to be served to the Joint Legislative Committee on Health Care and to the Governor the following session.
4. Conduct public hearings prior to making the report.
5. Solicit testimony and information from advocates for seniors; handicapped persons; mental health services consumers; low-income Oregonians; and providers of health care including but not limited to physicians licensed to practice medicine, dentists, oral surgeons, chiropractors, naturopaths, hospitals, clinics, pharmacists, nurses, and allied health professionals.
6. Solicit public involvement in a community meeting process.
7. Obtain an actuarial report to determine rates necessary to cover the costs of services.
8. Provide services offered under prepaid managed care contracts when feasible.

From Oregon 65th Legislative Assembly. (1989). *Senate Bill 27.* Salem, Ore: Author.

---

people covered by Medicaid by increasing eligibility to 100% of the federal poverty level (FPL). A summary of SB 27 is outlined in a box above. Senate Bill 935 required all businesses, including small businesses, to offer health insurance to their employees and dependents, or contribute to a state insurance pool by 1994; and Senate Bill 534 mandated that the state establish a high-risk insurance pool. The benefits for the latter two bills would be derived from the prioritized list of health services that governed Medicaid.

In 1991, three additional bills were enacted to expand access and contain cost; these also became part of the Oregon health plan. Senate Bill 44 expanded the jurisdiction of SB 27 to cover services for the aged, blind, and disabled; House Bill (HB) 1076 suggested further insurance reforms for small businesses; and HB 1077 established a health resource commission to develop alternatives to the certificate of need process.

HEALTH CARE DECISION MAKING IN OREGON
The legislative-administrative decision-making model

Prior to the enactment of SB 27, a legislative-administrative decision-making model was used in Oregon (Fig. 95-1). Authority for deciding who would get publicly sponsored health services rested solely with the legislature and the state Medicaid agency operating within the federal guidelines. Health care providers, and the public and special interest groups advised on health care issues, but the ultimate decisions were made by legislators and administrators. There were no guarantees that these decision makers would listen to the input.

The decision-making process under the legislative-administrative model involved (1) proposing health care decisions through legislation or administrative rule making; (2) inviting testimony from health pro-

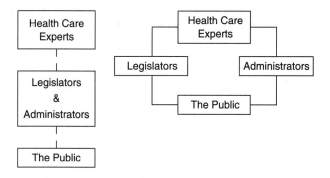

Fig. 95-1. A comparison of the Legislative-Administrative Decision-Making Model and the Oregon Decision-Making Model.

fessionals, the public, and special interest groups; and (3) ultimately having the legislature or administrators make a decision either to accept the originally proposed law or rule, to accept an amended version, or not to adopt the proposal.

In Oregon, there have been four types of decisions to finance and distribute Medicaid resources: (1) define (or redefine) *eligibility*; (2) change the *list of specific services* provided; (3) change *reimbursement to providers*; and (4) improve *productivity* at a given level of expenditure.[5]

The Oregon decision-making model

Senate Bill 27 introduced a new model for decision making by broadening *who* had decision-making authority, redefining the decision-making *process,* and changing the *types* of decisions that could be made. In essence, the legislation created a four-part decision-making model that included health care experts, the public and special interest groups, legislators, and administrators.

The decision-making process now involved three stages—a prioritization stage, a resource allocation stage, and an implementation stage—with the four groups of decision makers involved in each phase with varying degrees of authority (see the box above). In addition, SB 27 mandated that no longer would eligibility change, nor would provider reimbursement be altered. Everyone at or below 100% of the FPL would be entitled to a basic set of health services. If resources fell short of expectations, the number of services provided would be decreased. Although service reduction decisions had been used with the legislative-administrative model, under the new process services would be eliminated because they were deemed by health experts and

---

DECISION MAKERS AND DECISION-MAKING STAGES IN THE OREGON PLAN

Stage 1: Prioritization
Decision makers—Health Services Commission (health care experts and consumers)
Public hearings—Health care experts, Consumers
Community meetings—Consumers
Values survey—Consumers
Panels—Health care experts

Stage 2: Resource allocation
Decision makers—Legislators
Public hearings—Health Services Commission
—Health care experts
—Consumers
—Administrators
—Special interest groups

Stage 3: Implementation
Decision makers—Administrators
Rule-making hearings—Health care experts
—Consumers
—Special interest groups

---

the public to have a lower priority than those retained. The health services required to be offered to businesses and high-risk individuals would be those also provided to Medicaid recipients from the prioritized list.

ETHICS, POLICY, AND THE OREGON HEALTH PLAN

Aroskar[1] indicates that politics and ethics are integrally intertwined in the health policy arena. Furthermore, she suggests four areas of concern that need to be addressed before decisions are made: (1) the choice of policy goals that maximize certain values and minimize others; (2) the definition of the targets of change and how they are involved in the process; (3) the means chosen to implement the policy; and (4) the direct and indirect consequences of the proposed policy. Callahan[3] outlines four categories of ethical problems potentially raised by the Oregon plan: (1) its moral context and political setting; (2) its formal and explicit goals; (3) its means of achieving those goals; and (4) its practical implementation, including possible unintended consequences.

Within the moral and political context, one needs to look at the past and current situation with Medicaid funding and the provision of health care to the poor.[3] One specific criticism of the Oregon plan was that it "amounts to a futile tinkering with a fundamentally defective system."[6] In light of this criticism, even before the enactment of the Oregon Health Plan, individual nurses and groups of nurses had to make the decision of whether or not it was morally prudent to participate in the process outlined by SB 27. By participating, were better policy options being neglected? Again, the interaction of politics and ethics emerged. While most nurses believe that universal access to health care is needed, pragmatically, the chance of this occurring in the near future seemed remote. Is it better to support this current proposal, rather than wait for years until a more ideal policy is feasible?

To further evaluate this concern, attention needed to be given to goals, process, and outcomes specifically with reference to access, costs, and quality. Were the goals right? Would this plan increase access to health care for more Oregonians and would the costs of such a plan be distributed so that the burdens to various groups would be fair? Was the proposed process fair? Was a broad array of individuals included in the decision-making process? Was the process for prioritizing just? Other questions included, Were the potential outcomes of this process likely to produce more harm, or was this harm outweighed by the good that might occur? and, Would the plan compromise the quality of health care to a morally indefensible position?

Individual nurses, including myself, and nurses representing different organizations debated these issues. I ultimately decided that the plan was ethically sound. I believed that the goal to expand access for all Oregonians was a just decision despite the knowledge that not all health care services would continue to be provided. I also thought that prevention might now be provided, since SB 27 cited these services and also suggested that those medical treatments that were less effective be deemphasized. I believe that it is unethical not to provide services that can prevent individuals from becoming sick. I also knew that the criticism that the Oregon plan was solely focusing on the poor was incorrect, as SB 935 and SB 534 had been enacted. Last, I did not think that the plan precluded further health care reform that would move Oregon toward a more ideal policy in the future. Other nurses made the same decision to support the proposed plan and began to participate in the new decision-making process.

PRIORITIZATION
An authority for nursing

As cited earlier, the enactment of the Oregon Health Plan altered the group that comprised the decision makers, the process to be used to make health care decisions, and the types of policy decisions that could be made. It was during the first stage of the decision-making process, the prioritization stage, that the major authority was given to health professionals.

The decision-making responsibility for the prioritization of health services was given to the newly appointed Health Services Commission. The composition of the HSC included seven health professionals—one of whom was a public health nurse—and four consumers. (The other health professionals were five physicians—one each from pediatrics, general medicine, family practice, obstetrics or women's health care, and osteopathy—and a social services professional).

The mandated nursing position gave nurses authority to sit at the policy-making table and to have a voice in shaping health policy. It was a momentous occasion; it also was an onerous occasion, as nurses now had the burden of weighing the ethical ramifications of health care decisions.

The data collection phase

The HSC had two major tasks. The first was to collect technical and values data, and the second was to develop a prioritized list of health services. SB 27 directed the HSC to obtain technical data from health experts and values data from the public. Three methods for utilizing the health experts were initiated: (1) a review of the research literature, (2) testimony of health professionals at public hearings, and (3) participation by panels of health experts giving input on the benefits and duration of specific treatments.

The essence of the public testimony from nurse experts focused on (1) the need to consider the broader category of health services, not just medical services; and (2) the need for health promotion and disease prevention services. Nurses cited situations that their clients encountered and advocated a more just and equitable system.

Nurse practitioners were participants on the expert panels and were asked to evaluate treatments for specific health conditions. They were asked to estimate the probable outcomes of treatments for specific conditions in terms of levels of well-being (e.g., full recovery, or condition improved but not cured). These data were later used in a net benefit formula to develop the list of prioritized health services. The nurse practitioners also illustrated where the commission was limiting input by narrowly defining the questions. For example, the conditions and treatments identified for evaluation were obtained from the *International Classification of Diseases* (9th revision) and the *Physician's Current Procedural Terminology* (4th edition) texts that did not include health-promoting and prevention activities. These comments raised awareness of the fact that to develop a fair package of health services, consideration should be given to services that private-paying patients often were entitled to or frequently paid themselves.

Although these were the structured situations in which health expertise was sought, in actuality, input was given throughout the prioritization stage. When the HSC was evaluating case management as a service, there was testimony suggesting that this service be used to limit access; other spoke of its role in coordinating care. Two commissioners—the public health nurse and a consumer—asked for feedback from nursing experts. At a later time, nurses and other health professionals advised the commission on the content of preventive services.

Each time that input was given, nurses had to weigh the effect of their information on the prioritization process, for the promotion of one service had the implication that others would be given lesser priority. In turn, this ultimately affected the services that would be provided to citizens.

The values data were obtained from consumers through participation in community meetings, testimony at the public hearings, and input from a telephone survey of 1000 randomly selected consumers. I believed that nurses as consumer advocates had an ethical obligation to facilitate public participation; otherwise the entire decision-making process was morally flawed. The prime area where we could facilitate public input was that of the community meeting process whereby citizens expressed their values regarding health care.

Several nurses besides myself were members of the Oregon Health Decisions' Advisory Board for implementing the community meeting process. We developed the process so that the meetings were presented at an appropriate language level; we also insisted that interpreters be present for those for whom English was a second language or who were hearing impaired. We also made arrangements for transportation and child care services during all meetings. Last, information about the community meetings was placed in local newspapers, announced on the radio, and placed in social service and health agency offices. Financial and time constraints prevented taking the community meeting process to specific sites where more of the underrepresented lived (e.g., homes for the aged and Head Start centers).

Although there were criticisms about the representation of consumers at the meetings, the opportunity for consumer input was available. Meetings were held in 33 of the 36 counties in Oregon with more than 1000 citizens attending. Out of these meetings, 13 community values* were identified, and these later influenced the prioritization process. Many of the values were those also espoused by nurses.

The ranking of health services

The second step of the prioritization stage was to develop the prioritized list of health services. SB 27 was not specific on how this prioritization should occur, so the HSC decided to try several approaches.[8]

Early in the process, the HSC decided that data on effectiveness of treatments could not be evaluated without considering the condition for which the treatment was prescribed. Thus all technical data were based on specific condition-treatment pairs (e.g., appendicitis-appendectomy).

The first method used to develop a prioritized list of services employed a cost-benefit formula with a quality-of-life factor, but the results were not satisfactory. This formula did not incorporate the community values data; additionally, some services such as education were not paired with a particular disease condition and comparable outcome data could not be gathered.

After several modifications of the formula, the commission decided to try an alternative method. Utilizing the community values and values data presented at public hearings, the commission created 17 service categories (see the box on p. 716) and then ranked each category according to priority. Next, each condition-treatment pair was placed under one of the categories; then, each condition-treatment pair was prioritized within its category using the results produced by the net benefits component of the formula (Net benefit = [outcomes × probabilities with treatment] −

---

*The community values were as follows: prevention, quality of life, cost effectiveness, ability to function, equity, effectiveness of treatment, benefit for many, mental health and chemical dependency, personal choice, community compassion, impact on society, length of life, and personal responsibility.

HEALTH SERVICE CATEGORIES

1. Acute Fatal, treatment prevents death with full recovery
2. Maternity Care, including most disorders of the newborn
3. Acute Fatal, treatment prevents death without full recovery
4. Preventive Care for Children
5. Chronic Fatal, treatment improves life span and quality of life
6. Reproductive Services
7. Comfort Care
8. Preventive Dental Care
9. Proven Effective Preventive Care for Adults
10. Acute Nonfatal, treatment causes return to previous health state
11. Chronic Nonfatal, one-time treatment improves quality of life
12. Acute Nonfatal, treatment without return to previous health state
13. Chronic Nonfatal, repetitive treatment improves quality of life
14. Acute Nonfatal, treatment expedites recovery of self-limiting conditions
15. Infertility Services
16. Less Effective Preventive Care for Adults
17. Fatal or Nonfatal, treatment causes minimal or no improvement in quality of life

From Oregon Health Services Commission. (1991). *Prioritization of health services, A report to the governor and legislature.* (pp. G11-G12.) Salem, Ore: Author.

[outcomes × probabilities without treatment]). The outcome data were provided by the health experts and the benefits data were obtained from the individual responses of consumers on the quality-of-life survey. Last, a draft list of prioritized health services was produced and the commission members used professional judgment and their perceptions of the community values to rerank any items that were thought to be in the wrong position.

With each step of the ranking process the commissioners, including those who were health professionals, used their expertise to make their decisions. Moreover, the commission meetings were open to the public and other input was accepted with each deliberation.

Although the HSC was not directed to determine what constituted a basic health care package, they thought that they had an obligation to indicate what services they deemed important. The commission decided that all services listed in the first 9 categories

were "essential" and that all services listed in categories 10 through 13 were "very important." The services in the remaining four categories were valuable to some individuals but were significantly less cost effective or beneficial. The HSC finished its work with a prioritized list of 709 condition-treatment pairs. Finally, actuarial data were attached to each health service indicating the cost of providing that care.

Ethical concerns

There were three major ethical criticisms that related to the prioritization process. The first asserted that health providers should not be involved in allocation decisions; health providers were patient advocates and should leave the rationing decisions to the legislators.[6] I disagreed with this concept, as I believe that health professionals are daily confronted with allocation decisions for their patients; furthermore, I believe that nurses and other health professionals have an ethical obligation to lend their knowledge about patient conditions and health care benefits to shaping a better system.

The second criticism focused on allowing the public to have input; it was thought that "the plan may seriously corrupt community spirit by legitimizing a mean-spirited attitude toward the poor."[6] Again, I disagreed with this idea. I believe it is important to involve the public in decisions that affect them; moreover, I had confidence that as they heard more of the facts, they would express values that considered all of society.

The third concern was with the prioritization process itself. Many believed that ranking health services was too complex.[6] I strongly believe that we as a society are going to have to grapple with this complex issue and that the time to begin is now. I think that because the process allowed for both scientific data and values data, the prioritization process was feasible. I also thought that the outcomes would be no worse than the irrational decisions that are currently made in the legislative arena. In addition, I see this process as evolving with new scientific and values information being added in the future.

THE RESOURCE ALLOCATION AND IMPLEMENTATION STAGES
The resource allocation stage

During the second stage of the decision-making process, the authority switched to the legislators. Although legislators were not allowed to alter the prioritized list that was submitted by the HSC, these policymakers determined the funding levels for the Medicaid program; thus ultimately they decided which services would be part of the basic package of health services that would be offered under publicly sponsored programs. These decisions may also set the direction for shaping future private insurance programs; it is too early to ascertain this outcome.

Since the public and health care professionals had set the prioritized list, even if the funding was less than optimum, these groups were guaranteed that the services that they thought were of the highest priority would be maintained. And as before the enactment of SB 27, citizens and health providers could lobby legislators for additional funding.

The implementation stage

During the third stage, in which the Medicaid agency develops agreements with managed-care groups, the decision-making authority shifts to agency administrators. And as in the pre-SB27 decision-making model, health providers, and the public can still advise administrators who are shaping how the services will be provided and by whom. Currently, this stage is underway.

Ethical concerns

The fourth area for ethical consideration mentioned by Aroskar[1] and Callahan[3] was that of the long-term consequences of the policy decision. Are there inequalities in outcome and are they justifiable?

It is too soon to say whether Oregonians are better or worse off, since the provision of a basic set of health services has yet to be implemented. Nurses should continue to monitor the policy and begin to collect data to determine the impact on the health of clients.

In summary, the Oregon plan altered the decision-making process for health care, expanding the authority to health professionals—including nurses—and the public. With this authority came ethical responsibilities. Each decision throughout the process has ethical implications about the fairness of access, costs, and quality of health care for many Oregonians.

REFERENCES

1. Aroskar, M. A. (1987). The interface of ethics and politics in nursing. *Nursing Outlook, 35*(6), 268-272.
2. Beauchamp, T. L., & Childress, J. F. (1983). *Principles of biomedical ethics.* New York: Oxford University Press.
3. Callahan, D. (1991). The Oregon initiative: Ethics and priority setting. *Health Matrix, 1,* 157-170.
4. Ewelt, B. (1992, May). What's happening in Washington? *Network News, 4,* 2-3.
5. Garland, M. J. (1991). Setting health care priorities in Oregon. *Health Matrix, The Journal of W-Medicine, 1*(2), 139-156.
6. Garland, M. J. (1992). Rationing in public: Oregon's priority setting methodology. In M. A. Strosberg, J. M. Wiener, R. Baker, & I. A. Fein (Eds.), *Rationing America's medical care: The Oregon plan and beyond* (pp. 37-57). Washington, D.C.: Brookings Institution.
7. Kitzhaber, J. (1991, August). *The Oregon solution.* Presentation at the 1991 Conference on Health Care. Portland, Ore.
8. Oregon Health Services Commission. (1991). *Prioritization of health services. A report to the governor and legislature.* Salem, Ore: Author.
9. President's Commission for the Study of Ethical Problems in Medicine and Biomedical and Behavioral Research. (1983). *Securing access to health care.* Washington, D.C.: U.S. Government Printing Office.

CHAPTER 96

Indigent care

CATHERINE MALLOY

From Lillian Wald's work on Henry Street a century ago to contemporary models of nurse-managed health care services, nurses have responded to our most vulnerable populations. Medically indigent individuals are vulnerable and are increasing in number as a result of the growing population of uninsured and underinsured citizens. Vulnerable populations are composed of young and old, of rural and urban residents, of white and minority people. The common characteristic they possess is that they are poor and lack access to even essential health care services. The nation's 2 million nurses, as care givers in a myriad of settings, experience firsthand the breakdown of the health care system.

How does American society balance humanitarian values with cost containment in creating a just health care policy? How are questions of equitable access and quality considered in a fiscally conservative environment? Can a just society permit the creation of a two-tiered system of health care: one for the "haves" and one for the "have nots"?

Ethical questions of care for the medically indigent are embedded in the social-political system and the organization of health care delivery in the United States. While it is generally agreed that our health care system was founded on the premise that quality care should be available to all without discrimination or rationing, actual practice is often at odds with this belief. Since a society is judged by how it cares for its most vulnerable members, the principle of social justice is particularly relevant in considering the problem of indigent care.

Providing health care for indigent patients has been a persistent problem throughout the history of American health care. However,

the obligation to aid the sick and afflicted is ubiquitous in the code of ethics. The medical profession is appropriately pledged to promote high quality health care for all people.

Likewise, the mission statements of most hospitals contain similar commitments.[33]

Access to health care as a basic right of the citizen is an assumption supported by professional nurses. In fact, access to health care is viewed as a social contract as illustrated in the American Nurses Association[3] social policy statement. Why is it then that there are more and more reports of people being turned away from hospitals because of an inability to pay—the new "dumping syndrome"? Why is it that some physicians refuse to treat Medicaid and even Medicare patients?[16] A study of physician involvement with uninsured patients using a representative sample of nonfederal patient care physicians revealed marked variations in physician involvement with uninsured patients according to specialty class, employment status, and other practice characteristics. The study found that the proportion of the average physician's patients who were uninsured was substantially below estimates of the proportion of the general population that was uninsured. These results suggest that people without coverage face serious access problems.[7]

Indigent care, with its inherent questions of access and financing, has become a serious social problem and ethical dilemma. Aydelotte[5] noted that an ethical dilemma emerges when a society perceives its resources to be limited. In the case of indigent care, the dilemma emerges from the competing pressures of the need to provide essential health care services and the need to control costs. Nurses must understand the social, political, economic, and practice issues involved in the problem to become part of the solution.

FROM THE GREAT SOCIETY TO CORPORATIZATION TO DISARRAY

During the Great Society of the 1960s, health care policy focused on providing accessible, quality health care for all. The passage of Medicare and Medicaid legislation in 1966, and programs for mothers, infants, children, and other categorical populations, reflected the social value of ensuring adequate health care to all.[20]

However, 5 years after Medicare and Medicaid, expenditures had increased from 5.2% of the gross national product (GNP) in 1965 to 6.6% of the GNP in 1970.[9] Furthermore, public expenditures for total health care rose dramatically from 26% to 37%.[26] Ironically, the passage of Medicare and Medicaid had opened a Pandora's box. For those clever enough to see that public financing could be profitable, a revolutionary era was born: the corporate transformation of American health care delivery. Thus Medicare and Medicaid, which were enacted to increase access to health care, paradoxically resulted in the penetration of health care markets by corporate conglomerates.[26]

The implications of corporatization are particularly ominous for indigent health care. Corporations will not locate their hospitals in areas with large Medicare and Medicaid populations. Also, decreasing reimbursement for Medicare and Medicaid recipients have serious consequences for those hospitals serving large numbers of poor and uninsured. A study on Medicaid shortfalls and unreimbursed hospital care for the poor revealed that Medicaid shortfalls ($4.2 billion) and unsponsored care ($8.9 billion) accounted for $13.1 billion in unreimbursed hospital costs in 1989. Most of the recent growth in unreimbursed hospital costs for the poor has been caused by rising Medicaid shortfalls rather than increases in unsponsored care.[10] Hultman[14] studied the effects of hospital ownership, location, and Medicare's prospective payment system (PPS) on inpatient uncompensated care. Results suggested that not-for-profit and investor-owned hospitals are becoming more similar in levels of uncompensated care. Further, the study revealed that PPS has had a negative effect on rural hospital profitability.

The shift from retrospective to prospective payment combined with federal budget cutbacks has further eroded indigent accessibility to health care. Exacerbating the problem are socioeconomic changes. The economy has changed from an industrial model to one dominated by service with a rise in part-time labor and businesses unable to provide insurance benefits.[11] Nearly 40 million Americans have no health insurance.[8] These individuals do not seek care because of their inability to pay. However, when situations occur in which they must obtain care, they will get into the

health care system, and someone will have to pay.[13] Continuing increases in the national debt and ominous predictions of a depleted Medicare fund by the end of the 1990s make cost containment a matter of the highest concern.

Cost containment has led to serious cutbacks in federal and state programs for the indigent. Further, policies of the Reagan administration that promoted antiregulatory approaches to a free market in health care lessened responsibility of the government for people's health.[24] The 1980s ushered in a "competition versus regulation" health care policy as the key to cost containment.[22] However, the 1990 census reveals striking changes in the demographics of the United States that will profoundly influence cost containment. The largest foreign-born population in history, a shrinking middle class, increases in poverty whereby nearly a fifth of all children are poor, increasing racial and ethnic diversity, and a rise in the elderly provide evidence of stratification of U.S. society. It is likely that these changes will result in new demands for health care services. It is also unlikely that competition versus regulation will work.

FALLING THROUGH THE CRACKS: WHERE IS THE SAFETY NET?

Medically indigent people are those who have no public or private insurance and who cannot afford to pay for health care out of pocket. "The number of uncompensated care patients—the medically indigent—has almost doubled from an estimated 25 million to 40 million in the past 10 years."[34] According to the American Hospital Association[2] report on care for the indigent, the best indicator of medical indigence is whether or not a person is insured. Medically indigent patients are composed of three groups: the nonworking uninsured, the medically uninsurable, and the employed uninsured.[36] In 1983, approximately 15% of all Americans— 35 million people—lacked health insurance coverage.[15] Recent figures suggest the number ranges from 37 to 40 million. Whitman and associates[35] reported that the

common thread that binds the working poor together most tightly is the absence of health insurance. . . . Two out of three poor workers, representing more than 9 million Americans and their dependents, have no employer or union subsidized health insurance.

Almost 65% of the uninsured are working adults or their dependents, including 4.1 million uninsured dependents of insured working adults.[2] According to

Moccia and Mason,[21] 15.2% of the population is struggling financially. A dramatic increase in the numbers of poor families headed by women has given rise to the "feminization of poverty." Almost 40% of all poor are children; in fact, poverty affects blacks, Hispanics, other minorities, and women disproportionately.[21] Tragically, reports abound of elderly individuals who have their life's savings depleted because of an illness requiring long-term care. The spouse and patient often end up indigent, having to choose between food, heat, and medicines.[31]

Many Americans hold distorted perceptions of the medically indigent. Inner-city welfare poor represent only a small fraction of the United States' poor. The working poor tend to be low-wage, semieducated people who work in agriculture and the private sector. The working poor are a group with whom the public can identify, and their numbers have swollen tremendously. Surprisingly, the numbers of poor adults who work have increased by 52% in the last decade to include 7 million Americans.[35]

Other uninsured are newly unemployed workers and their families who have lost their insurance benefits. Health insurance loss because of job layoff has become a more serious problem than anyone anticipated. Those already ill or disabled for whom finding insurance at an affordable rate is impossible are also included in the indigent group.[20]

Attention must also be directed to special population groups that have increased since the 1980s. The homeless, the mentally and physically disabled, and acquired immunodeficiency syndrome (AIDS) victims are particularly vulnerable to the inequities of the present health care system. Lack of primary health care has cost this country a great deal both in lives lost and in loss of productivity.[4]

A QUESTION OF PRIORITIES

The major barriers to accessing health care are lack of insurance, inadequate insurance, or a longstanding or catastrophic illness, all having financial implications. Corporate restructuring of health care has further excluded the underinsured from care. McCarthy[19] reported that the competitive market produced many desirable results but cautioned that competition and cost containment measures were placing "increasing numbers of uninsured in serious jeopardy." It seems clear that the corporatization trend is unlikely to benefit the medically indigent. For-profit organizations find little incentive to assume responsibility for care of the uninsured. In assessing the competitive environment, Kuder[17] reported that since Medicaid rates were below the usual physician fees, there was a "disincentive for physicians to treat the poor with the same standard of care as for patients who pay higher fees."

All traditional ways of financing care for indigents have been eroded as competition among providers has increased. In the past, care may have been subsidized by taxes, by governmental health insurance or welfare programs (Medicare and Medicaid), by cost shifting from insured patients, or by charitable donations. The prospective payment system eliminated cost shifting. The Reagan administration reduced programs. Medicare and Medicaid recipients cannot always access care because of inadequate coverage, and some providers refuse to treat patients on the Medicare or Medicaid program. It is easy to see that current policy does not address continuity or comprehensiveness of care.

HEALTH AND POVERTY

The relationship between poverty and health status has been well documented. Because of lack of insurance and lack of funds for medical care, people do not seek care until it is "too late, leading to complications that require more and longer care."[15] Those who are poor or near poor have a higher prevalence of infant mortality, chronic diseases, and disability.[20] Throughout life, poverty exposes the poor to more health risks. Poor people get sick more often, have more serious complications, take longer to recover, and are less likely to regain their full level of functioning.[21]

Often the magnitude of social disability is as much a result of social definitions, inadequate coping skills in dealing with the illness and the treatment regimen, and deficient problem-solving capacities as it is a result of the illness as such.[20]

Indigent patients often feel powerless in the system. Preoccupation with securing the basic necessities of life (food and shelter) precludes a future-oriented approach to their health. Consequently, they tend to seek help only when in pain or experiencing acute illness. Providers face numerous challenges in caring for indigent patients including structural barriers and contextual barriers. Communication between providers and patients often falls short because of inadequate sharing of information and a power asymmetry.[32]

THE ETHICAL DILEMMA: WHO PAYS?

The Medicaid program is often misunderstood. While people generally believe that Medicaid is the major source of financing of medical care for the poor, in reality, it covers less than 40% of the poor population. In fact, Medicaid has become more of a supplemental insurance for individuals receiving Medicare. Only one quarter of Medicaid's expenditures paid for medical care for the poor in 1984.[2] In 1982, more than one third of the uninsured— 11.6 million people—were below the poverty line but still did not qualify for Medicaid. Two thirds of the uninsured population had incomes below 200% of the poverty levels.[20] Almost a decade later, this trend persists.

Responsibility: Public or private

Approaches to improving access to care have been instituted, but not as comprehensive and coordinated national policy. National health insurance legislation has failed to date, probably because of public resistance to tax increases and the influence of special interest groups.

Innovative models at the state and local level independent of federal action include the creation of high-risk pools or expanded Medicaid coverage. Other approaches include grouping employees of small businesses into insurer pools or multiple employer trusts (MET) as a shared risk concept. Some states provide primary health care coverage for children.[28] Efforts to require employer-sponsored health insurance coverage have fallen on hard times. Some recommend rationing care to those who are able and willing to pay as a way to meet health care costs.[1] Fuchs[12] noted that, like it or not, health care rationing is already occurring, and that the real questions seem to be, Who will ration? and What will be rationed?

Barriers to public action are many. A Gallup poll reported that 62% of adults felt that it was the government's responsibility to pay for the health care of the poor. When asked to specify the level of government that was responsible, 37% indicated that it was the federal government's responsibility; 15% judged it to be a state government responsibility; and 6% indicated that it was a local government responsibility. Of those responding, 69% reported that they would be willing to pay higher taxes for indigent care.[27] However, many people with adequate health care insurance fear that more taxes will result if indigent care is addressed. Some analysts believe that the public cannot afford additional taxes or increased insurance premiums and

will not support measures likely to have those consequences. Basically the debate comes down to two questions. Who receives care? Who pays?

The dilemma

In a culture of contradictions and competing values, an ethical dilemma emerges. The American ideal of self-reliance and rugged individualism is in opposition to the realities of the indigent problem. Perhaps the dilemma is best expressed in the context of social responsibility versus individual responsibility or, stated another way, access and quality versus rationing.

Veatch[30] holds that defining health care as a product in typical economic terms is unacceptable if a society affirms health care to be a right. A society professing humanitarian values should not treat health care as a market commodity to be regarded as any other product in a competitive arena. This would not be consistent with the ethical codes of nursing and medicine that have always included the patient's right to care.

Should a society offer its citizens equal opportunity in the pursuit of personal-social goals and equitable access in an increasingly complex society? Should a just society tolerate escalating levels of poverty and hunger and increasing numbers of persons without adequate care? People hold to the belief that a middle-class lifestyle is available for anyone who works hard enough to get it. The indigent problem suggests that that conviction simply is not true.

ACCESSIBLE AND EQUITABLE CARE: NURSING STRATEGIES

Current approaches in health care are failing to provide access and quality care for all. Perhaps the strategies that have been implemented to restructure the health care system rely too heavily on high technology and on the illness model with the physician as provider. A radical departure from the medical model may provide alternative solutions to some of the indigent care problems. Primary care is the most economical safety net we can implement.

Efforts led by the American Nurses Association to address issues of access to care have culminated in a formal proposal in 1991, Nursing's Agenda for Health Care Reform.[4] The agenda calls for a restructured health care system with essential health care services available to all citizens in the United States financed through public-private partnerships. This plan would provide coverage for the poor, the indigent who now fall through the cracks. Nurses have demonstrated the ability to dramatically impact the cost and effectiveness of care in a variety of settings. In fact, nurses are increasing access to care by providing cost-effective services outside the traditional health care system. Nurses are strategically positioned to create such a change. From the early days of nursing to the present, nurses have been the architects of creative practice arrangements to meet the health care needs of the poor and the vulnerable while promoting their well-being. What is needed now is a modern-day Lillian Wald, a mover and a shaker of purse strings and conscience. Nurses as a collective force can create a Waldian composite to expand their contribution to the pressing problem of indigent care.

Three major approaches for nursing intervention are suggested: (1) developing a role in policy formulation, (2) designing innovative indigent care projects, and (3) redesigning educational curriculums.

Policy formulation

Attention will need to be centered on shaping public policy and increasing the knowledge of the public about the indigent care issue. Nursing's contribution to health care policy can be made through research and practice. Legislation to provide direct Medicaid reimbursement to nurse practitioners, clinical nurse specialists, and certified nurse-midwives to meet the needs of the underserved and uninsured should be promoted.

Nurses should be documenting issues related to access, services provided, and advantages of health promotion services as cost containment measures. Research should be conducted regarding the health needs, practices, coping mechanisms, and environment of the poor.[21] Nurses can serve as advocates for the medically indigent by presenting this research to legislators and the public.

The socialization of nurses should emphasize the nurse's role in policy formulation. Nursing skills must include assertive decision making, political skills, coalition building, and advocacy. Nurses should be actively involved in policy formulation at every level: local, regional, state, and national. A solution to the health care crisis will require a coordinated effort, with all levels of government, private and philanthropic sectors, third-party payers, employers, consumers, and providers working together. Nursing can take a leadership role in articulating Nursing's Agenda for Health Care Reform to these publics. The agenda[4] is formulated around several basic principles:

- Access to essential health services (a core of care available to all)
- Primary health care services
- Consumer focus
- Consumer access to a full range of providers at convenient sites
- Consumer responsibility for their own care in partnership with providers
- Focus on preventive care
- Efficient use of resources
- Financing by private and public sources
- Mechanisms to protect against catastrophic costs

Designing innovative projects

It is time for nurses to take a bold step in creating nurse models for indigent care. Healthy People 2000[29] provides clear goals for a healthier America. Nurses can develop comprehensive care projects as demonstrations of compassionate and dignified care. Such projects can integrate preventive and therapeutic services and coordinate resource management. Nurse-managed clinics can serve as models of case management demonstrating effectiveness and cost-efficiency and continuity of service.[18] These projects that are targeted to the homeless, elderly, and other underserved groups need to be showcased to illustrate to the public what nurses can do as part of the solution.

Blancett[6] reported on the common risk factors of the indigent. The most frequently recorded risk factors were smoking, alcohol consumption, obesity, lack of prenatal care, and street drug use. Clearly these risk factors call for lifestyle modification. The nurse has a role in assisting indigent patients to decrease risk factors through health promotion activities. Improvement of self-care practices—developing more effective ways of coping, maintaining function, and preventing disability—will positively affect the ultimate cost of health care for indigents. Currently, the federal government spends only 3% of the budget on health promotion. Perhaps a policy shift from illness care to prevention would be more cost effective in the long term.

The crisis in indigent health care presents an opportunity for nurses to take adversity and turn it into advantage. At a time when the health care system is strained, when predictions of economic disaster loom everywhere, nurses can improve access, promote quality, and demonstrate cost savings. An excellent opportunity awaits nurses in the competitive arena. By establishing partnerships with indigents, nurses can take an active part in changing the community's use of resources. Efforts toward self-care will empower the indigents to reframe their own definition of health care. An example of what nurses can do to address the indigent care dilemma is a project designed by Ridenour[23] to meet the health needs of the uninsured by marketing services to the uninsured, to employers, and to the responsible units of federal and state government.

Redesigning nursing curriculums

A report of the Pew Health Professions Commission,[25] *Healthy America: Practitioners for 2005,* challenges the nation's health professional schools to develop programs that are responsive to the changing health care needs of Americans. The commission believes that schools have a responsibility to shape the values and the direction of the health care system. Inherent in this would be a restructuring of basic attitudes regarding the patient-provider interface. The new professional must get closer to patients and their families and understand why they behave as they do, particularly when they are under stress. New models of teaching and learning will need to be developed to meet the Pew recommendations. Existing licensure and accreditation requirements act as barriers to some of the recommended innovations. Thus nurse educators need to develop mechanisms to work with their boards of nursing and with the National League for Nursing in designing revitalized educational models. Additionally, funding sources to support new models of education will need to be identified. Health outcomes should be the ultimate focus of educational preparation. Educational reform, as postulated by the Pew Commission, should produce more effective and humane practitioners.

The nursing profession has the opportunity to show how nurses can make a difference. By using the guidelines of *Healthy People 2000, Nursing's Agenda for Health Care Reform,* and the Pew Health Professions report, *Healthy America: Practitioners for 2005,* the nursing profession will evolve a system of education and practice that will respond to a changing world and will, by its direction, include all people so that indigency will no longer be a concept of inadequate health care. To do less would not be in keeping with the profession's heritage.

REFERENCES

1. Aaron, H., & Schwartz, W. (1990). Rationing health care: The choices before us. *Science, 247* (4941), 418-422.
2. American Hospital Association. (1986). *Cost and compassion: Recommendations for avoiding a crisis in care for the medically indigent.* Report of the special committee on care for the indigent. Chicago: Author.
3. American Nurses Association. (1980). *Nursing: A social policy statement.* Kansas City, Mo: Author.
4. American Nurses Association. (1991). *Nursing's agenda for health care reform.* Kansas City, Mo: Author.
5. Aydelotte, M. K. (1985). Catastrophic, long term, and indigent care. In J. C. McCloskey & H. K. Grace (Eds.), *Current issues in nursing* (2nd ed.). Boston: Blackwell Scientific Publications.
6. Blancett, S. S. (1987). Health care for low income. *Journal of Nursing Administration, 17*(12), 18, 31, 44.
7. Blumenthal, D., & Rizzo, J. A. (1990). Who cares for uninsured persons? A study of physicians and their patients who lack health insurance. *Medical Care, 29*(6), 502-520.
8. Caper, P. (1989). Solving the medical care dilemma. *New England Journal of Medicine, 318,* 1535-1536.
9. Feldstein, P. (1988). *Health care economics.* New York: John Wiley and Sons.
10. Fraser, I., Narcoss, J., & Kralovec, P. (1991, Winter). Medicaid shortfalls and total unreimbursed care for the poor, 1980-1989. *Inquiry, 28*(4), 385-392.
11. Freedman, S., Klepper, B., Duncan, P., & Bell, S. (1988). Coverage of the uninsured and underinsured: A proposal for school enrollment–based family health insurance. *New England Journal of Medicine, 318,* 843-846.
12. Fuchs, V. (1990). The health sector's share of the gross national product. *Science, 247*(4942), 534-538.
13. Gold, A. R. (1989, July 30). The struggle to make do without health insurance. *New York Times,* pp. 1, 11.
14. Hultman, C. I. (1991, December). Uncompensated care before and after prospective payment: The role of hospital location and ownership. *Health Services Research, 26*(5), 613-622.
15. Jones, K., & Kilpatrick, K. (1986). State strategies for financing indigent care. *Nursing Economic$, 4*(2), 61-65.
16. Kirkman-Liff, B. L. (1985). Refusal of care: Evidence from Arizona. *Health Affairs, 4*(4), 15-24.
17. Kuder, J. M. (1986). No miracle remedies in sight for financing health care for the poor. *Henry Ford Hospital Medical Journal, 34*(4), 252-256.
18. Malloy, C., Christ, M., & Hohloch, F. (1990). The homeless: Social isolates. *Journal of Community Health Nursing, 7*(1), 25-36.
19. McCarthy, C. M. (1988). Financing indigent care: Short and long-term strategies. *Journal of the American Medical Association, 259*(1), 75.
20. Mechanic, D. (1986). Health care for the poor: Some policy alternatives. *Journal of Family Practice, 22*(3), 283-289.
21. Moccia, P., & Mason, D. J. (1986). Poverty trends: Implications for nursing. *Nursing Outlook, 34*(1), 20-24.
22. Nutter, D. O. (1984). Access to care and the evolution of corporate, for profit medicine. *New England Journal of Medicine, 311*(14), 917-919.
23. Ridenour, N. (1988, January 29). *A community approach to providing quality health care for the uninsured.* Paper presented at the meeting of the American Academy of Nursing, Atlanta, Georgia.
24. Roemer, R. (1988). The right to health care—gains and gaps. *American Journal of Public Health, 78*(3), 241-246.
25. Shugars, D. A., O'Neil, E. H., & Bader, J. C. (Eds.). (1991). *Healthy America: Practitioners for 2005, an agenda.* Durham, N.C.: Pew Health Professions Commission.
26. Starr, P. (1982). *The transformation of American medicine.* New York: Basic Books.

27. Steiber, S. (1987, October 5). Indigent care: Public wants government to pay. *Hospitals,* p. 152.

28. Udow, M., Smith, V., & Mason, M. (1991). *American Journal of Diseases of Children, 145*(5), 579-580.

29. U.S. Department of Health and Human Services. (1991). *Healthy people 2000: National health promotion and disease prevention objective 1991.* Washington, D.C.: U.S. Government Printing Office.

30. Veatch, R. M. (1983). Ethical dilemmas of for-profit enterprise in health care. In B. H. Gray (Ed.), *The new health care for profit.* Washington, D.C.: National Academy Press.

31. Vehara, E. S., Geron, S., & Beeman, S. K. (1986). *Gerontologist, 26*(1), 48-55.

32. Ventres, W., & Gordon, P. (1990, Winter). Communication strategies in caring for the underserved. *Journal of Health Care for Poor and Underserved, 1*(3), 305-314.

33. Weems, W. L. (1987). Medical care for the indigent. *Journal of Mississippi State Medical Association, 28*(8), 218, 220.

34. Weis, D. (1987). Speaking out: Who are the working poor? *American Journal of Nursing, 87*(11), 1451-1453.

35. Whitman, D., Thornton, J., Shapiro, J. P., Witkins, G., & Hawkins, S. L. (1988, January 11). America's hidden poor. *US News and World Report,* pp. 18-24.

36. Wilensky, G. R. (1987). Viable strategies for dealing with the uninsured. *Health Affairs, 6*(1), 33-46.

CHAPTER 97

The evolving HIV-AIDS pandemic

A study in stigmatization and its ethical challenges for nursing

DAVID ANTHONY FORRESTER

The greatest challenge in putting pen to paper about HIV/AIDS is to ponder the imponderable.

On June 5, 1981, the Centers for Disease Control reported the occurrence of *Pneumocystis carinii* pneumonia in five previously healthy, sexually active, gay men in Los Angeles. Thus began the brief history of acquired immunodeficiency syndrome (AIDS). For little more than a single decade, the human immunodeficiency virus (HIV) that causes AIDS has precipitated a worldwide pandemic unprecedented in modern history. The evolving HIV-AIDS pandemic will likely remain our greatest worldwide public health challenge well into the twenty-first century.

As of May 31, 1991, the Centers for Disease Control had reported 179,136 cases of AIDS among Americans. Of these, more than 113,000 (63%) of the victims are reported to have died. AIDS currently ranks as the second leading cause of death among men 25 to 44 years of age and is one of the five leading causes of death among women 15 to 44 years of age in the United States.[10]

The World Health Organization[32] estimates that between 8 and 10 million adults and 1 million children worldwide are HIV infected. By the year 2000, between 40 and 100 million persons will be infected with HIV. More than 90% of these HIV-infected persons will reside in developing countries in sub-Saharan Africa, South and Southeast Asia, Latin America, and the Carribean. Additionally, mothers or both parents of more than 10 million children will have died from HIV-AIDS during the 1990s. Thus the HIV-AIDS pandemic is a vastly complex, global phenomenon with extraordinary social, cultural, economic, and political dimensions and impact.

The universal fear and hysteria that AIDS has engendered is unprecedented in contemporary society. The profound scope of the HIV-AIDS pandemic forces all segments of society to reexamine their values and address many troublesome ethical issues. Nurses are no exception. Many of these issues are born out of the unique epidemiological features of this illness and the pervasive social stigma associated with those afflicted with it. From a nursing perspective, this stigma may be viewed as being as much a part of the pathology of AIDS as the virus itself.

Exploring some of the factors contributing to the stigmatization of persons with HIV-AIDS may be helpful in formulating an understanding of the ethical challenges that nurses must address as this pandemic continues to evolve. Some of these challenges relate to safeguarding the personal autonomy of persons with HIV-AIDS, ethical issues inherent in current methods of HIV-AIDS treatment and research, and nurses' personal and professional values.

STIGMATIZATION OF PERSONS WITH HIV-AIDS

It may be considered an accident of history that AIDS was discovered in the gay community of the United

States. AIDS could just as easily have been discovered in a number of other countries. Had it been discovered in Africa, for example, it might have been known as a heterosexual disease that, because it is sexually transmitted, also affects gay men. Thus the unfortunate, worldwide, and false impression that AIDS is a "gay" disease might not have come about.[25] Unfortunately, the history of this illness cannot be rewritten and the social and cultural meanings of AIDS continue to contribute to widespread stigmatization of persons with HIV-AIDS, frequently resulting in discrimination.

Undoubtedly, one of the most serious threats that person with HIV-AIDS face is the powerful social stigma associated with being HIV infected or actually having AIDS. AIDS has so far had its greatest impact on already socially stigmatized groups including gay and bisexual men, intravenous drug users, and prostitutes.[8,9] The indigent and black and Hispanic racial minorities are also disproportionately affected.[19] Persons with HIV-AIDS have lost jobs and insurance benefits and have even occasionally been denied educational opportunities and medical care.[26]

During the social crisis of a pandemic, further stigmatization of already disenfranchised groups serves to project that which is feared (e.g., fears of contagion, immorality, and mortality) on those outside the mainstream of society. This occurs at great expense to the disenfranchised groups and results in their being in the double bind of being stigmatized individuals with a stigmatized life-threatening illness.

As a result of the stigma associated with AIDS, persons with HIV-AIDS frequently encounter discrimination. Like other forms of discrimination, HIV-AIDS discrimination is "the unfair treatment of individuals based upon irrational fears and prejudices about groups."[28] The resulting mentality of "us" versus "them" is potentially very costly to society as a whole. Because they fear discrimination, stigmatized groups, whether HIV infected or not, may naturally be less willing to come forward and participate voluntarily in society's efforts to control the spread of HIV.

HIV-AIDS engenders much fear and apprehension. For many people, including some health care providers, "AIDS carries with it all the connotations of sin" and images of an illicit disease associated with illicit behavior.[24] Two important aspects of "AIDS fear" are the fear of disease and fear of social disorder.[28]

Far more complex than the obvious and possibly realistic fear of contagion, fear of HIV infection and AIDS as an illness is compounded by a number of factors. First, human sexuality and, more specifically, homosexuality and bisexuality are issues about which many members of society are uncomfortable and ill-informed. A second factor is society's ambivalence regarding mental illness. As treatment modalities improve and life expectancy lengthens for persons with HIV-AIDS, it is likely that we will see greatly increased numbers of HIV-demented people. These individuals will make increased physical and fiscal demands on existing and future mental health care systems and other social resources. Finally, a third factor contributing to the fear of AIDS as an illness is its incurable and invariably fatal prognosis. The fear of death is primal and pervasive, even among health care providers. In fact, health practitioners' personal fears regarding mortality may be particularly exacerbated by a fatal illness affecting large numbers of young, previously healthy people—in other words, people very much like themselves.

The fear of social disorder, relative to the evolving HIV-AIDS pandemic, stems from the attrition of persons with HIV-AIDS from the work force, removing their economic contributions from society. This is further compounded by their acutely increased needs for public support for medical care, food, and housing.

Historically, focusing social panic onto such stigmatized groups has resulted in scapegoating and isolation. For example, in an effort to control the spread of sexually transmitted diseases (STDs), 30,000 prostitutes were isolated during World War I. In spite of the restriction of these individuals' civil liberties, the incidence of STDs increased dramatically during this period.[7] Similarly, as a result of fear during World War II, the U.S. Supreme Court upheld the incarceration of Japanese-Americans.[28]

During the 1980s, many similarly extreme measures were proposed, such as mandatory HIV testing, mandatory disclosure of HIV status, and even mandatory quarantine of persons with AIDS. Gratefully, these prescriptions have generally been rejected on the basis of their clearly being counterproductive. Few individuals who believed that they had been exposed to HIV through risk-taking behavior would voluntarily come forward. In effect, such measures would simply serve to drive HIV-AIDS "underground" and would surely thwart responsible public health efforts such as screening, counseling, and education to prevent the further spread of this deadly virus.

ETHICAL CHALLENGES FOR NURSES

As members of society, health care professionals also participate in the stigmatization of persons with HIV-AIDS. Numerous research studies have documented negative attitudes of physicians and nurses toward gay men, intravenous drug users, and persons with HIV-AIDS in general.* Such attitudes may be based on practitioners' opinions about patients' personal attributes, lifestyle, or personal worth. Whatever their origins, such attitudes engender social prejudice from which discrimination emerges.

The complex phenomenon of HIV-AIDS stigma, in itself, poses major personal and professional challenges to nurses who wish to provide persons with HIV-AIDS with optimal, sensitive health care. Understanding the social etiology of HIV-AIDS stigma should assist nurses in (1) rejecting and counteracting social stereotypes, (2) assessing personal values and risks more accurately, and (3) identifying their professional responsibilities in providing health care that demonstrates value for the personal autonomy of persons with HIV-AIDS.

Personal autonomy

Decision making regarding what constitutes appropriate medical treatment is the right of the individual.[22] The ethical challenge of respecting the autonomy of persons with HIV-AIDS in decision making is complicated, however, by many factors. For example, HIV-AIDS raises special considerations regarding personal autonomy because of the high incidence of either primary HIV infection of the brain or secondary opportunistic infections resulting in dementia or other mental impairment. Persons with HIV-AIDS are often unable to participate in decision making when decisions need to be made.

Nurses have an ethical obligation to assist HIV-infected individuals in making health care decisions early in the course of their illness. Advance directives such as a "durable power of attorney for health care" (DPAHC) should be discussed with persons with HIV-AIDS and their families in a frank and thoughtful way. These documents allow individuals to indicate treatment preferences and designate a surrogate decision maker before becoming incapacitated. Proxy decision makers are particularly helpful in planning care for many gay men who wish to have their life partner

rather than a "legally" sanctioned family member make decisions on their behalf. As knowledgeable practitioners, nurses have a responsibility to anticipate the need for advance directives and initiate discussion of such documents with HIV-infected individuals.

Other ethical challenges confront health practitioners when the expectations and treatment preferences of persons with HIV-AIDS or their proxy decision makers are inconsistent with those of the health team. For example, one study[29] of patients with AIDS indicated that a sample of gay men, although generally well educated about AIDS, significantly overestimated their chances of surviving intensive care treatment for *Pneumocystis carinii* pneumonia (PCP). Of this sample ($n = 118$), 55% wanted mechanical ventilation and 46% wanted cardiopulmonary resuscitation. Such unrealistic expectations seriously impair patients' ability to accurately evaluate the risk-benefit ratio in care planning and, thus, their ability to give truly informed consent.[22]

Medical and nursing paternalism is very tempting in such instances. However, paternalism by definition, even though altruistically motivated in such cases, negates the ethical principle of personal autonomy. Nurses are ethically obliged to be knowledgeable regarding currently available therapies and their potential risks and benefits for persons with HIV-AIDS. Furthermore, nurses have a moral responsibility to share this information in a way that is sensitive, supportive, and truthful.

HIV-AIDS treatment

Nursing recognizes an ethical obligation to provide care for persons with HIV-AIDS.[1,2] To meet this obligation nurse faculty and practicing nurses have an ethical responsibility to be sufficiently knowledgeable regarding HIV-AIDS to (1) overcome their fears and personal prejudices, (2) prevent transmission of HIV through occupational exposure, and (3) provide competent, safe, quality care. The nursing profession, therefore, has a responsibility to assist nurses in meeting these objectives.

This decade should see a marked increase in efforts to further educate nurses and the public about HIV-AIDS. These efforts may best be carried out through nursing's various academic curriculums and professional associations. Just as there is no segment of society unaffected by HIV-AIDS, neither is there an area of specialization in nursing that is not directly affected

---

*References 6, 11, 14, 16, 18, 20, 22, 23, 29, 32, 33.

by this pandemic. Nurses have a responsibility to seek out educational opportunities regarding HIV-AIDS. It is incumbent upon all of nursing's academic programs and specialty associations to develop, implement, and evaluate HIV-AIDS educational programming for nursing students, practicing nurses, and consumers of nursing services.

HIV-AIDS research

To date, relatively few scientific nursing research studies regarding HIV-AIDS have been published.[15,16,18,23] Nurse researchers have an obligation to consider the potential impact of HIV-AIDS on our national and international health. Furthermore, nurses should identify areas in which they might contribute individual or collaborative research efforts. Interdisciplinary studies should be undertaken that will result in valuable nursing contributions to the growing body of knowledge about HIV-AIDS.

As nurses become increasingly involved in scientific study regarding AIDS and persons who are HIV infected, many ethical dilemmas emerge. Research involving highly stigmatized groups at risk for discrimination brings into view ethical issues involving the rights of persons with HIV-AIDS to privacy, anonymity, and confidentiality. For example, how heavily does the individual's right to privacy weigh in the balance against the potential social good of HIV-AIDS research? And given the communal nature of inpatient care facilities and our age of computer-stored (and therefore easily accessible) patient records, how can research participants be *guaranteed* anonymity or confidentiality? Also, since it is generally agreed that intrusions into privacy in clinical care and research require informed consent from participants, how can the participation of HIV-demented individuals be ethically obtained? Finally, do the findings of scientific inquiry hold potential threats of harm either to persons with HIV-AIDS directly or to future public policy regarding HIV-AIDS?

The personal and social risks to persons with HIV-AIDS agreeing to participate in AIDS-related research are obviously quite high. Study participants must be fully informed about how research data are to be collected, used, and stored, and who will have access to it.[12] Researchers and clinicians must (1) faithfully adhere to published guidelines for research involving persons with HIV-AIDS, (2) minimize intrusions in participants' privacy, (3) assure anonymity whenever possible, (4) take necessary precautions to ensure con-

fidentiality, and (5) carefully consider the potential influence of study findings on the lives of persons with HIV-AIDS and the course of public policy.[12]

Personal and professional values

Holistic health care for persons with HIV-AIDS requires that nurses gain insight into their opinions, attitudes, and values. For example, nurses typically place high value on health and health-seeking behaviors in patients. Persons with HIV-AIDS who continue to use intravenous drugs or who continue to engage in high-risk sexual activity are often perceived as non-health seeking and therefore potentially pose a substantial challenge to nurses attempting to provide nonjudgmental care.[16] Such conflicting values are almost sure to result in ineffective nurse-patient relationships. To effectively counter this, nurses must engage in a process of values clarification. This process fosters personal and professional growth; it takes place through frank discussion of values conflicts and through such activities as participation in ethics committees and organized educational programs regarding persons with HIV-AIDS.[13]

Excellent health care for persons with HIV-AIDS is characterized by open interpersonal communication and social support. Effective care for persons with HIV-AIDS, as with *all* patients, requires an accepting, nonjudgmental approach by competent health professionals. Such practitioners are unencumbered by unrealistic fears of contagion or unfair personal prejudice.

Since 1982, the American Nurses Association (ANA) has adopted 22 policies and position statements related to HIV-AIDS. The ANA[1-5] offers guidance regarding personal risk, social prejudice, and moral responsibility. "Nursing is resolute in its perspective that care should be delivered without prejudice, and it makes no allowance for the use of the patient's personal attributes or socioeconomic status or the nature of the health problem as grounds for discrimination."[2] Nursing's code of professional ethics insists that "the need for health care is universal, transcending all national, ethnic, racial, religious, cultural, political, educational, economic, developmental, personality, role, and sexual differences. Nursing care is delivered without prejudicial behavior."[1]

At least one important conclusion can be drawn from these statements with regard to persons with HIV-AIDS. Personal attributes of patients and the social aspects of their illness are to be used only for their benefit in individualizing their care, not to their detriment.[17]

CONCLUSION

The history of the HIV-AIDS pandemic remains an open, largely unwritten book. HIV-AIDS has touched the personal and professional lives of most nurses worldwide. Nurses must be active participants in an organized global response to the profound ethical challenges that HIV-AIDS poses in the coming century. An appropriate nursing response to the evolving HIV-AIDS pandemic should have three main objectives: (1) to prevent HIV infection, (2) to provide care for those already HIV infected, and (3) to participate in national and international efforts to fight HIV-AIDS and its associated stigma.

First, to prevent HIV infection, we must base our actions on a sound epidemiological understanding of HIV-AIDS. From this knowledge, we derive the concept that the proper focus of prevention is *behavior*, not "risk group" membership or HIV antibody status. Information and education are essential but not enough. Only if we as nurses make ourselves available in a supportive social role will prevention truly have a fair chance of success.

The second objective is to ensure that all persons with HIV-AIDS receive humane care of a quality at least equal to that provided for people suffering from other diseases, and to provide comprehensive support and services to all who are HIV infected. Implicit in this goal are the responsibilities that all nurses share to (1) avail ourselves of accurate, up-to-date information pertaining to the occupational risks, epidemiology, and treatment of HIV-AIDS; (2) act in accordance with this knowledge both in our personal and professional lives; and (3) model appropriate behaviors to educate professional colleagues and the public about HIV-AIDS.

The third objective is nurse participation in national and international efforts to fight HIV-AIDS and its associated stigma. As litigation in the courts and debate in legislative bodies proliferates regarding the civil liberties of persons with HIV-AIDS, nurses must be active participants, providing their peers and the public with appropriate education and leadership. "Nurses, as health professionals, have an obligation to engage in the ensuing national [and international] debate about AIDS health policy issues in an informed manner."[22] We must continue to be a knowledgeable and vocal force in future decision making regarding such issues as international travel, HIV-AIDS in prisons, the neuropsychiatric aspects of HIV infection, and HIV-AIDS in the workplace.

The HIV-AIDS pandemic clearly poses some of the most compelling ethical challenges imaginable for nurses. Some of these challenges are unique to HIV-AIDS; some are common to other serious illnesses as well. The ethical issues raised by HIV-AIDS are amplified by the urgency associated with the rapidly evolving pandemic and the complex psychological, political, legal, and social problems it engenders. For this and future generations of nurses, the ultimate challenge of HIV-AIDS will be to provide sensitive, compassionate care while balancing individual rights and liberties against the duty to protect the public health.

REFERENCES

1. American Nurses Association. (1985). *Code for nurses with interpretive statements*. Kansas City, Mo: Author.
2. American Nurses Association, Committee on Ethics. (1986). *Statement regarding risk versus responsibility in providing nursing care*. Kansas City, Mo: Author.
3. American Nurses Association, Committee on Ethics. (1991). *Position statement on HIV testing*. Kansas City, Mo: Author.
4. American Nurses Association, Committee on Ethics. (1991). *Position statement on personnel policies and HIV in the workplace*. Kansas City, Mo: Author.
5. American Nurses Association, Committee on Ethics. (1991). *Position statement on post-exposure programs in the event of occupational exposure to HIV/HBV*. Kansas City, Mo: Author.
6. Bernstein, C. A., Rabkin, J. G., & Wolland, H. (1990). Medical and dental students' attitudes about the AIDS epidemic. *Academic Medicine, 65,* 458-460.
7. Brandt, A. M. (1986). AIDS: From social history to social policy. *Law, Medicine, and Health Care, 14,* 231-242.
8. Centers for Disease Control. (1988). Pneumocystis pneumonia—Los Angeles. *Morbidity and Mortality Weekly Report, 30,* 250-253.
9. Center for Disease Control. (1988). Quarterly report to the domestic policy council on the prevalence and rate of spread of HIV and AIDS in the United States. *Morbidity and Mortality Weekly Report, 37,* 223-227.
10. Centers for Disease Control. (1991). The HIV/AIDS epidemic: The first 10 years. *Morbidity and Mortality Weekly Report, 40,* 357-369.
11. Currey, C. J., Johnson, M., & Ogden, B. (1990). Willingness of health-professions students to treat patients with AIDS. *Academic Medicine, 65,* 472-474.
12. Durham, J. D. (1987). The ethical dimensions of AIDS. In J. D. Durham & F. L. Cohen (Eds.), *The person with AIDS: Nursing perspectives* (pp. 229-252). New York: Springer.
13. Farrell, B. (1987). AIDS patients: Values in conflict. *Critical Care Nursing Quarterly, 10,* 74-85.
14. Feldman, T. B., Bell, R. A., Stephenson, J. J., & Purifoy, F. E. (1990). Attitudes of medical school faculty and students toward acquired immunodeficiency syndrome. *Academic Medicine, 65,* 464-466.
15. Forrester, D. A. (1990). AIDS-related risk factors, medical diagnosis, do-not-resuscitate orders and aggressiveness of nursing care. *Nursing Research, 39,* 350-354.
16. Forrester, D. A., & Murphy, P. A. (1992). Registered nurses' attitudes toward patients with AIDS and AIDS-related risk factors. *Journal of Advanced Nursing, 17,* 1260-66.

17. Fowler, M. D. M. (1988). Acquired immunodeficiency syndrome and refusal to provide care. *Heart and Lung, 17,* 213-215.

18. Goldenberg, D., & Laschinger, H. (1991). Attitudes and normative beliefs of nursing students as predictors of intended care behaviors with AIDS patients: A test of the Ajzen-Fishbein theory of reasoned action. *Journal of Nursing Education, 30,* 119-126.

19. Jakush, J. (1987). AIDS: The disease and its implications for dentistry. *Journal of the American Dental Association, 115,* 395-403.

20. Kelly, J .A., St. Lawrence, J. S., Hood, H. V., Smith, S., & Cook, D. J. (1988). Nurses' attitudes toward AIDS. *Journal of Continuing Education in Nursing, 19,* 78-83.

21. Kelly, J. A., St. Lawrence, J. S., Smith, S., Hood, H. V., & Cook, D. J. (1987). Stigmatization of AIDS patients by physicians. *American Journal of Public Health, 77,* 789-791.

22. Koenig, B. A. (1988). Ethical and legal issues in the AIDS epidemic. In A. Lewis (Ed.), *Nursing care of the person with AIDS/ARC* (pp. 287-305). Rockville, Md: Aspen.

23. Larson, E. (1988). Nursing research and AIDS. *Nursing Research, 37,* 60-62.

24. Loewy, E. H., & Smith, S. J. (1986). Duty to treat AIDS patients clouded by fears. *Medical Ethics Advisor, 2,* 29-40.

25. Mann, J. (1988, July 15). *Global aspect of AIDS.* Paper presented at AIDS/ARC Update, University of California at San Francisco.

26. New York City Commission on Human Rights. (1986). *Report on discrimination against people with AIDS* (November 1983 through April 1986). New York: Author.

27. Oermann, M. H., & Gignac, D. (1991). Knowledge and attitudes about AIDS among Canadian nursing students: Educational implications. *Journal of Nursing Education, 30,* 217-221.

28. Schulman, D. I. (1988). AIDS discrimination: Its nature, meaning and function. *AIDS and the Law Symposium Nova Law Review, 12,* 1113-1140.

29. Steinbrook, R., Lo, B., Moulton, J., Saika, G., Hollander, H., & Volberding, P. A. (1986). Preferences of homosexual men with AIDS for life-sustaining treatment. *New England Journal of Medicine, 314,* 457-460.

30. Tesch, B. J., Simpson, D. E., & Kirby, B. D. (1990). Medical and nursing students' attitudes about AIDS issues. *Academic Medicine, 65,* 467-469.

31. Wachter, R. M., Cooke, M., Hopewell, P. C., & Luce, J. M. (1988). Attitudes of medical residents regarding intensive care for patients with the acquired immunodeficiency syndrome. *Archives of Internal Medicine, 148,* 149-152.

32. World Health Organization. (1991). *In point of fact.* Geneva: Author.

CHAPTER 98

Child abuse

What is nursing's role?

PERLE SLAVIK COWEN

We are not only our brother's keeper, we are also the keeper of our brother's children.

FREDRIC WERTHAM

The first legal intervention in a case involving child abuse occurred in the United States in 1874. Ironically, the case was brought to the public's attention by the American Society for the Prevention of Cruelty to Animals (SPCA) and involved a child who was malnourished, regularly beaten, and kept in rags by her adoptive parents. At that time, protective services for Mary Ellen Wilson could only be invoked on the basis that she belonged to the animal kingdom and was therefore entitled to protection.[26]

Today, all states have requirements for reporting maltreatment of children.[29] Most states mandate that nurses report child abuse; others encourage or authorize them to do so. For nurses to fulfill their professional, legal, and moral responsibility in reporting suspected child abuse and neglect, they must have knowledge of the indicators that are manifested before, during, and after the occurrence of child abuse. Early recognition and intervention with high-risk families is fundamental to treatment, and primary prevention is the ultimate goal of those involved in the well-being of children and their families. Nurses are the most prevalent group of providers to have early, direct contact with families, placing them in a strategic position for early assessment and treatment of child abuse.[10] Their roles as autonomous practitioners, child and family advocates, and members of multidisciplinary teams require them to demonstrate an understanding of the current problems and issues in child abuse, including ethical, legal, and social ramifications.

BACKGROUND

Dr. Henry Kempe coined the term *battered child syndrome* in 1962 to describe a "clinical condition in young children who have received serious physical abuse, generally from a parent or foster parent."[28] This description was further delineated in 1974 when Congress passed Public Law 93-247, which defines child abuse and neglect as "the physical or mental injury, sexual abuse, negligent treatment or maltreatment of a child under the age of eighteen by a person who is responsible for the child's welfare under the circumstances which indicate that the child's health or welfare is harmed or threatened thereby."[11] This general definition actually encompasses four distinct types of child abuse: physical abuse, neglect, sexual abuse, and emotional abuse (Table 98-1). Traditionally, there has been a singular approach to assessing, diagnosing, and treating each of these types of child abuse. However, current clinical thinking suggests that abused children are likely to be subjected to multiple forms of maltreatment.[9]

Child abuse is a complex, destructive phenomenon that cuts across all sectors of society. The results of the annual 50-state survey indicate that 2.6 million cases of child abuse were reported in 1991, up 6.2% from

Table 98-1 Types of child abuse

Type	Definition	Characteristics
Physical abuse	Nonaccidental injury of a child	Physical injury is typically at variance with the history given of it, and suffered by a child as the result of the acts or omissions of a person responsible for the care of the child; repeated patterns of physical punishment with short- or long-term effects
Neglect	Failure to provide a child with basic necessities of life when financially able to do so or when offered financial or other reasonable means to do so	Child is not provided with adequate food, clothing, shelter, supervision, assistance, hygiene, or medical care
Sexual abuse	Use of a child for sexual purposes including incest, rape, molestation, prostitution, or pornography	The perpetrator is usually someone in the child's family or known to the child; nonabusing parent or other family members often aware of the abuse
Emotional abuse	Nonphysical, often verbal, assault on a child, usually critical, demeaning, and emotionally devastating	Parent or other adult blames, belittles, rejects child, or persistently demonstrates lack of concern for the child's welfare

1990.[15] The distribution of these cases was as follows: 26% physical abuse, 16% sexual abuse, 55% neglect, 8% emotional maltreatment, and 8% unspecified. The reported mortality rate was 1383, up 10.3% from 1990. There was an average of three to four deaths per day, with over 79% of the children being less than 5 years old at the time of their death and 54%, under age 1. These figures most likely represent the lowest estimate of the problem, as they depend upon the level of involvement of child protective services and the varying levels of comprehensive investigation of child mortality cases by local authorities, and upon classification variances among the states in reporting deaths due to child abuse.[36]

The economic and human costs of maltreatment in American society are astronomical. It is likely that billions of dollars are spent in treatment and social service costs and lost in lessened productivity for a generation of maltreated children.[12] The human costs include a litany of death, morbidity, and psychological tragedies. The emotional damage due to maltreatment lasts a lifetime for many of the victims.

Theoretical perspectives on the causes and correlates of child abuse are many and varied.[12] The inability of the single-dimension models to adequately address the known characteristics of child abuse has resulted in multidimensional models of child maltreatment. One attempt in this direction has been proposed by Garbarino[21, 22] in his ecological model of child maltreatment, which in turn derives from Bronfenbren-

ner's ecological model[7] of human development (Fig. 98-1).

The Garbarino model is a paradigm for examining the complex interactions among parental and child characteristics, intra- and extrafamilial stressors, and the social and cultural systems that affect families. The model offers a framework for considering available forms of support and resources in relation to a topology of four levels—individual, familial, social, and cultural.[27] In addition, the model provides a framework for understanding the relationships among stress, social support systems, and child maltreatment, thereby providing guidance for child abuse prevention efforts. According to Garbarino,[22] "It is the unmanageability of the stress which is the most crucial factor, and this unmanageability is a product of a mismatch between the level of stress and the availability and potency of social support."

THE NURSE'S ROLE IN ASSESSMENT OF AT-RISK PARENTS

Maternal-child nurses, pediatric nurses, visiting health nurses, emergency room nurses, and school nurses have the direct opportunity to identify "at-risk" families. Because of this, nurses should be aware of the high-risk indicators that signal potential child maltreatment. Of equal importance, they must have confidence in their assessment findings—confidence to take responsibility for translating their assessments into in-

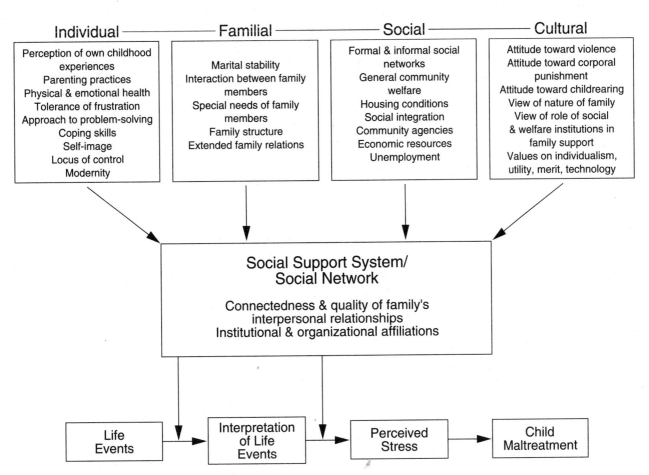

Fig. 98-1.   The ecological model of child maltreatment. *(From Howze, D.C., & Kitch, J.B. [1984]. Disentangling life events, stress and social support: Implications for the primary prevention of child abuse and neglect. Child Abuse & Neglect, 8[4], 401-9. Used with permission.)*

terventions that may involve a host of other specialties and agencies. Their role as advocate for the child and family is often the critical determinant of whether or not at-risk families are identified and receive the services they need.

The importance of early identification and intervention lies in its potential for reducing or preventing the occurrence of child abuse. Variables describing families at risk have been reported in the literature and can be classified into four separate domains according to sociocultural, family, caretaker, and child characteristics[21,22] (Table 98-2). Stress arising from these domains may be situational, acute, or chronic in nature.

While some variables within each domain may appear entrenched, there are two fundamental truisms to remember: (1) multifaceted problems require multidis-

ciplinary interventions (you are not in this alone); and (2) even slight remediation of stressors may change the individual's perception of those stressors (you are doing more good than you know). As nurses we not only offer valuable consultation on the physiological aspects of child abuse or neglect but we also provide information on such topics as parent-child interactions, a parent's ability to care for a child, and parenting stress levels.

Several tools are available to assist the nurse in assessing and evaluating at-risk families. However, it should be noted that, to date, research has not indicated that there are any factors that are present in all abusing parents and absent in all nonabusing parents.[45] The "Child Abuse Potential Inventory"[35] is a 160-item, client-administered screening device that

Table 98-2   Risk factors associated with child abuse

Sociocultural	Family	Caretaker	Child
Poverty, underemployment, economic stress	Marital discord and conflict	Psychological problems associated with being abused or rejected as a child (excessive hostility, anger, unhappiness, rigidity, distress, flattened affect)	Children 5 years of age or younger, particularly children less than 1 year of age
Lack of health care	Poor problem-solving abilities of caretakers	Fears, disturbances of affect, poor peer relationships, and other symptoms associated with victimization as a child	Teenagers, 15-17 years old, particularly boys
Lack of respite and crisis child care	Isolation from family and friends	Low self-esteem, poor motivation, poor impulse control, or limited social competencies	Twins
Inadequate support and educational services	Low rate of positive interaction among family members	Depression	Infants or children with feeding problems
Burden on one parent for child rearing, typically mother	Domestic violence	Limited coping skills	Children with significantly more major and minor health problems in the first year of life
Social or geographical isolation from relatives and friends		Limited financial and household management skills	Seriously ill newborns
Limited or unavailable prevention services in the community		Poor physical health	Preterm, low-birth weight, handicapped infants
Acceptance of corporal punishment of children		Stress-related symptoms that affect emotional or physical health	Children with subtle developmental abnormalities, such as attention deficits
Low priority for parenthood education and training programs		Substance abuse	A child engaged in protracted crying
Homelessness		Unrealistically high expectations of the child	
Depletion of economic resources in the community		Lack of knowledge of normal growth and development	
		Role reversal—expectations that the child will meet the caretaker's needs	

was determined to correctly classify 82.7% of the known abusive parents in a retrospective study. Abidin's "Parenting Stress Index"[1] consists of 101 items that measure the amount of stress experienced by the parent as a result of the parenting role, and it also includes a life stress scale. The Nursing Child Assessment by Satellite Training (NCAST) assessment tool consists of 73 items that were developed to evaluate critical features in parent-infant interaction.[6]

Browne[8] developed a 13-item checklist based on known risk factors and conducted a retrospective study involving a matched sample of 62 known abusing families and 124 nonabusing families. Nurse health visitors in conjunction with professional colleagues completed the checklist for both groups. Interestingly, while the tool could correctly classify 86% of the cases, the best predictor of child abuse was the health visitor's perception of whether the parent was indifferent, intolerant, or overanxious. The author concludes that perinatal screening for child abuse should have at least three stages: (1) perinatal screening for stressful social and demographic characteristics resulting in identification of a target group for further screening, (2) screening of the target group members at 3 to 6 months after birth for caregivers' perception of the newborn and their perceived parenting and life stress, and (3) assessment of the infant's attachment to the primary care giver and parental sensitivity to the infant's behavior at 9 to 12 months after birth.

THE NURSE'S ROLE IN RECOGNIZING CHILD ABUSE AND NEGLECT

Nurses who work with children and their families have a unique role in detecting child abuse and neglect, particularly with regard to physical and developmental manifestations in the child and the observed interaction patterns between the parents and the child. Nurses can often identify maltreatment during their initial physical examination of the child and/or their history interview with the child and the parents. Their background in child growth and development is superior to that of most social workers, and so it is their expertise that often forms the basis for questions that arise related to the child's behavior or the parent-child interaction patterns.

The physical indicators of child abuse and neglect may be mild to severe; however, they are usually readily observable to the experienced practitioner. Nurses are knowledgeable about the range of developmentally appropriate behavior expected of children, and they are quick to notice behaviors that fall outside of this range. Behavioral indicators of abuse may exist alone or may accompany physical indicators. They may appear as subtle clues that something is amiss, or they may raise questions that leave one with the "something is not right here" mind-set. The role of the informed inquisitor is absolutely fundamental to the assessment of child abuse and neglect.

The list of physical and behavioral indicators displayed in Table 98-3 is not intended to be exhaustive; many more indicators exist and can be included. Although a single indicator does not necessarily prove that child abuse or neglect is occurring, the repeated occurrence of an indicator, the presence of several indicators, or the appearance of serious injury or suspicious death should alert the nurse to the possibility of child abuse or neglect.

The involvement of the nurse is typically initiated because of the child's need for acute or preventive health care services. When it is necessary to interview the child concerning possible abuse or neglect, nurses must keep in mind that the child may be hurt, in pain, fearful, or confused and may have been warned not to say anything. Because children vary in their linguistic and interactive competence, it cannot be assumed that interviewing methods suitable for adults will work with children.[23] Additional factors that must be considered include the child's cognitive development, psychological competence, language development, level of socialization, and cultural background. In general, it is important to start with openness, a good basis in child development, and an empathetic approach. Basic techniques include the following: (1) use sentences with only three to five more words than the number of words in the child's average sentence, (2) use names rather than pronouns, (3) use the child's terms, (4) ask the child to repeat what you have said, (5) rephrase questions that the child does not understand, (6) avoid asking young children questions involving a time sequence, (7) do not respond to every answer with another question, and (8) be careful in interpreting responses to very specific questions, as children are apt to be very literal.[23]

The parents' behavior and attitudes and the history of the injury can offer valuable clues to the presence of child abuse and neglect and provide direction for interventions that address the family's needs (Table 98-4). In discussing suspicions of child abuse and neglect with the parents, the point of departure will most likely be the presenting problems of the child. The tone of the discussion should be professional, nonjudgmental, and supportive.

Some common guidelines include the following: (1) conduct the interview in private with everyone sitting down; (2) be professional, direct, and honest and never display anger, repugnance, or shock; (3) be attentive and supportive; (4) collect information and do not try to prove abuse or neglect by making accusations; (5) explain that you must make a referral to child protective services and explain the process; (6) document in detail your assessment of the child, your observations of the parents, and your conversation with the parents; and (7) make the referral.

Table 98-3 Physical and behavioral indicators of child abuse and neglect

Type of abuse	Physical indicators	Behavioral indicators
Physical abuse	**Unexplained bruises and welts** Located on eyes, mouth, lips, torso, buttocks, genitalia, thighs, and calves Injuries might be in shape of object used to produce them (e.g., sticks, belts, hairbrushes, buckles) Regularly appear after absence, weekend, or vacation **Unexplained burns** Pattern burns: suggest object used (e.g., iron, stove grate or electric burner); circular burns on feet, face, hands, chest, or buttocks suggest cigar or cigarette Immersion burns: have "socklike, glovelike, or donutlike" appearance from area's being immersed in very hot water or oil; typically arms, legs, or buttocks Friction burns: result from rope friction on legs, arms, neck, or torso **Unexplained fractures** Of skull, face, nose, or long bones Multiple or spiral fractures caused by twisting motion Shaft fractures from direct blows Fractures in various stages of healing **Unexplained lacerations or abrasions** To mouth, lips, gums, eyes, or genitals In various stages of healing Human bite marks of adult size **Intracranial, subdural, intraventricular, and intraocular hemorrhaging** Blows to head typically cause intracranial, subdural, and intraventricular hemorrhaging Whiplash shaken infant syndrome typically causes intracranial, subdural, and intraocular hemorrhaging Child presented nonresponsive or apneic **Disease that is resistant to treatment and signs and symptoms that change** Münchausen syndrome by proxy: illness is simulated or produced by parent or someone in parental role Acute symptoms abate when child is separated from perpetrator	Feels deserving of punishment Wary of adult contacts Apprehensive when other children cry Behavioral extremes: aggressiveness or withdrawal Frightened of parents Afraid to go home Reports injury by parents Vacant of frozen stare Lies very still while surveying surroundings Will not cry when approached by examiner Responds to questions in monosyllables Inappropriate or precocious maturity Manipulative behavior to get attention Capable of only superficial relationships Indiscriminately seeks affection Poor self-concept
Physical neglect	Underweight, poor growth pattern, or failure to thrive Consistent hunger, poor hygiene, or inappropriate dress Consistent lack of supervision, especially in dangerous activities for long periods Wasting of subcutaneous tissue Developmental delays Chronic malnutrition, or excessive intake of junk food Unattended physical problems or medical needs Abandonment Bald patches on scalp	Begging, or stealing food Extended stays at school (early arrival and late departure) Constant fatigue and listlessness Inappropriate affection seeking Assuming adult responsibilities States that there is no caretaker Stiff body; resists being held Apathy or watchful wariness Substance abuse and delinquency

Table 98-3 Physical and behavioral indicators of child abuse and neglect—Cont'd

Type of abuse	Physical indicators	Behavioral indicators
Sexual abuse	Difficulty in walking or sitting	Unwilling to change for gym
	Torn, stained, or bloody underclothing	Withdrawal, and fantasy
	Lacerations: vaginal or anal	Sophisticated sexual knowledge
	Reddened or traumatized genitals	Poor peer relationships
	Recurrent urinary tract infections	Change in school performance
	Poor sphincter tone	Insomnia
	Acquired sexually transmitted diseases	Sudden massive weight loss or gain
	Psychosomatic complaints	Delinquency or running away
	Pregnancy	Substance abuse
	Dramatic change in previously well managed chronic illness	Prostitution
		Aggression against self
		Suicide
Emotional abuse	Speech disorders	Habit disorders
	Lags in physical development	Conduct or learning disorders
	Failure to thrive	Neurotic traits or psychoneurotic reactions
	Physical developmental delays	Behavior extremes
		Cognitive developmental lags
		Attempted suicide

Modified from Heindl, C., Kroll, C., Salus, M., & Broadhurst, D. (1979). *The nurse's role in the prevention and treatment of child abuse and neglect* (p. 10). Washington, D.C.: U.S. Department of Health, Education and Welfare.

Table 98-4 Caretaker behavioral indicators of abuse present at admission

Unexplained injury	Caretakers can't explain the injury, their explanation of injury is vague or evasive, or their explanation is at variance with the child's actual injury
Alleged self-inflicted injury	Caretakers allege that a very young child deliberately injured himself or herself or was injured because he or she engaged in behavior inappropriate for the child's developmental level
Alleged third-party injury	Caretakers blame the child's injury on someone else, such as a neighbor, friend, or relative; a common allegation is that a sibling or another child caused the injury
Delay in seeking medical attention	Caretakers do not immediately obtain medical care for the child following injury
Discrepant history of injury	Caretakers' explanations of the child's injury conflict in terms of date, time, or cause; there is discrepancy between physical findings and the date of the injury, or the injury and the child's developmental level; parents' explanation of injury conflicts with the child's explanation of injury (if the child is verbal)

THE NURSE'S ROLE ON THE MULTIDISCIPLINARY TEAM

The multidisciplinary approach to diagnosing, evaluating, and planning the treatment of victims of child abuse and neglect has been widely advocated and adopted by hospitals and community-based protective service teams.[37] One of the primary purposes of this approach is to reduce the fragmentation of the service delivery system through coordination of professional activities both within and between agencies and organizations. Additional services typically include consultation, case management, and provision of current information concerning child abuse to other professionals or agencies.

The team is typically composed of representatives from nursing, pediatric medicine, psychology, psychiatry, social work, and child life, with each discipline providing a unique perspective and specialized interventions. Traditionally, the coordinator of these interventions has been the representative from pediatric medicine. However, the professional nurse is in a prime position in many instances to initiate, coordinate, and evaluate the multidisciplinary approach to the care of violent families.[10] Nurses are in a much less threatening position to elicit information because they are generally perceived by the family as being helpful rather than bureaucratic or authoritative. The case management that forms the basis of the multidisciplinary approach is an extension of the coordination and advocacy that is paramount to the nursing role. Clinical specialists with a background in maternal-child, pediatric, family, or community nursing are well suited to assume a leadership position in this area.

THE NURSE'S ROLE AS A MANDATORY REPORTER

Child abuse legislation in each state mandates the reporting of suspected child abuse and neglect and broadly sets forth the process through which reporting occurs. In general, these processes describe the conditions for reporting, who reports, and where reports are filed, and the legal protection afforded the reporter. Currently most states mandate that nurses report child abuse. However, because of the diversity in laws, particularly in regard to definitions, nurses should obtain a copy of their particular state's reporting statute and study its provisions carefully.

Typically, most state statutes require reports to be filed when there is "reason to believe" or "reasonable cause to suspect" that abuse or neglect may be occurring. While no state requires the reporter to have proof that abuse or neglect has occurred, most require that the report be made "in good faith."[34] To encourage reporting, all states provide at least qualified immunity or protection from legal liability for persons filing an abuse report.

Failure to report suspected child abuse or neglect may result in civil or criminal penalties. The basis for criminal liability varies among states, and some states impose criminal penalties regardless of whether the failure to report is deliberate or a case of negligence. Other state statutes base liability on a "knowing" or "willful" failure to report and may hold liable the reporter who suspects abuse or neglect, and knows the reporting requirement, yet deliberately refuses to file a report.[29] Regardless of the basis for this liability, the criminal charge for failure to report is generally a misdemeanor and the possible penalties for conviction are fines, imprisonment, or both.[3]

Civil liability can be brought for damages proximately caused by failure to report. The landmark case of civil liability for failure to report was a 1976 decision of the California Supreme Court, which held that a physician who fails to report suspected child abuse can be exposed to liability for subsequent injuries to the child on the theory of medical malpractice.[30] This case involved a California physician who failed to report the injuries of an 11-month-old child, which included a spiral fracture of her tibia and fibula, bruises over her entire back, superficial abrasions on other parts of her body, and an earlier, nondepressed linear skull fracture. Several months later the child sustained further injury and a different physician reported these injuries as suspected child abuse. Following this second incident, the minor brought an action against the initial examining physician for failure to diagnose the battered child syndrome properly and to report that diagnosis to the proper authorities. Under the law, a nurse having a similar opportunity to observe possible symptoms of child abuse would be equally liable for failure to report;[29] and in child abuse cases, a successful malpractice claim would not be covered by malpractice insurance.[3]

Record keeping or the documentation of evidence is vital, as it substantiates the basis for reasonable belief and provides the legal basis for state intervention on behalf of the child. Nursing history and daily charting are considered "germane to the diagnosis and treatment of the child" and therefore qualify as admissible during a court hearing. Entries should be recorded immediately following contact with the family, as they are admissible evidence only if they are recorded at or near the time of the event.[29] Documentation should reflect accuracy, timeliness, and objectivity and be devoid of "feelings" or conclusions that are made without documented evidence.

THE NURSE'S ROLE IN CHILD ABUSE PREVENTION

During the past two decades, increasing public concern about child abuse and neglect has resulted in the development of several approaches directed toward preventing its occurrence. Disappointment in the overall effectiveness of treatment strategies has contributed to the increased interest in prevention among practitioners. The availability of funding for prevention efforts has most certainly influenced the rapid development and dissemination of prevention techniques.[14] A wide range of child abuse prevention strategies are currently employed in programs around the country, many of which stem from Garbarino's multicausal ecological model.

Community-wide prevention efforts that are directed at each phase of the family life cycle, beginning with the prenatal period and continuing through a child's school years, have been identified as the most promising child abuse preventive interventions.[13] Two national research conferences on child abuse prevention, sponsored by the National Committee for the Prevention of Child Abuse, identified several key life cycle child abuse prevention approaches: (1) support programs for new parents, such as home health visitor and adolescent parenting programs; (2) parenting education programs; and (3) child care opportunities such as respite care services and crisis nurseries.[13]

Both home-based and center-based programs have demonstrated a wide range of positive client outcomes. Studies have identified gains that included (1) improved mother-infant bonding and maternal capacity to respond to the child's emotional needs;[2,16,17,38] (2) demonstrated ability to care for the child's physical and developmental needs;* (3) fewer subsequent unintended pregnancies;[5,33,39] (4) more consistent use of health care services and job training opportunities;[42] and (5) lower welfare use, higher school completion rates, and higher employment rates.[5,25,42] In identifying the types of parents most likely to benefit from these educational and supportive services, several investigators have noted particular success with young, relatively poor mothers[5,19,39] and with mothers who felt confident in their lives before enrolling in the program.[42]

A recent extensive study of the effectiveness of home health visitor programs reviewed randomized trials of prenatal and infancy home visitation programs for socially disadvantaged women and children.[40] The results of this study indicated that some home visitation programs were effective in (1) improving women's health-related behaviors during pregnancy, the birth weight and length of gestation of babies born to smokers and young adolescents, parents' interaction with their children, and children's developmental status; (2) reducing the incidence of child abuse and neglect, childhood behavioral problems, emergency department visits and hospitalizations for injury, and unintended subsequent pregnancies; and (3) increasing mothers' participation in the work force.[40]

The authors noted that home visitation programs with the greatest chances of success have the following three characteristics: (1) they are based either explicitly or implicitly on ecological models, (2) they are designed to address the ecology of the family during pregnancy and the early childbearing years with nurse home visitors who establish a therapeutic alliance with the families, and (3) they are targeted toward families at greater risk for maternal and child health problems by virtue of their poverty and lack of personal and social resources.[40]

A recent review evaluated studies that were undertaken from 1978 through 1988 and concluded that three primary issues must be addressed in future studies if we are to expand our knowledge of prevention. These were (1) formal evaluation of impact, including who benefited; (2) evaluation of change in the rate of occurrence; and (3) assessment of the efficacy of program interventions directed toward preventing child abuse versus their role in meeting broader societal needs.[18]

NURSING'S ROLE IN SPECIALTY TRACKS IN FAMILY ABUSE

Although a great deal of information related to child maltreatment has been compiled over the past 30 years, it is generally reported that academic training for professionals such as nurses, physicians, psychologists, attorneys, and social workers has not kept pace with the demands for expertise.[4,41,43] In response to the lack of university graduate programs in child abuse and neglect, the National Center on Child Abuse and Neglect (NCCAN) initiated a national effort to institutionalize interdisciplinary graduate training in child maltreatment.[20] In 1987, ten universities were selected by the NCCAN to receive $150,000 per year for 3 years to establish interdisciplinary graduate training programs in child abuse and neglect. The universities include Indiana University, New York University, Ohio State University, Temple University, University of California at San Diego, University of Michigan, University of Oklahoma, University of Pittsburgh, and University of South Carolina.

The training programs are designed for graduate and postgraduate students sufficiently trained in their own discipline to benefit from interdisciplinary education in child maltreatment. The programs have collaborated to achieve consistency in the didactic portion of the training and have reached a general consensus regarding the body of information that is necessary for professionals in the field of child maltreatment. All of the universities offer student stipend funds that range from $531 to $7000 per academic year, with an average stipend of $1959.[20] To date, a total of 418 students have

---

*References 17, 19, 24, 25, 31, 32, 39, 44.

graduated from this program, representing the following disciplines: social work ($n = 114$), psychology ($n = 97$), law ($n = 56$), medicine ($n = 36$), nursing ($n = 29$), education ($n = 20$), and combined others ($n = 66$).[20]

It is generally accepted that child maltreatment is a multifaceted problem that requires multidisciplinary efforts. Nursing—by virtue of the nature of the profession, the variety of its practice settings, and the sheer numbers of its practitioners—can provide leadership to these efforts.

REFERENCES

1. Abidin, R. R. (1990). *Parenting stress index.* Charlottesville, Va: Pediatric Psychology Press.
2. Affholter, D., Connell, D., & Nauta, M. (1983). Evaluation on the child and family resource program: Early evidence of parent-child interaction effects. *Evaluation Review, 7,* 65-79.
3. Allen, J., & Hollowell, E. (1990, June). Nurses & child abuse/neglect reporting: Duties, responsibilities, and issues. *Journal of Practical Nursing,* pp. 56-59.
4. Alpert, J., & Paulson, A. (1990). Graduate-level education and training in child sexual abuse. *Professional Psychology: Research and Practice, 21,* 366-371.
5. Badger, E. (1981). Effects of a parent education program on teenage mothers and their offspring. In K. G. Scott, T. Field, & E. Robertson (Eds.), *Teenage parents and their offspring.* New York: Grune and Stratton.
6. Barnard, K. E., & Bee, H. L. (1984). The assessment of parent-infant interaction by observation of feeding and teaching. In T. B. Brazelton & H. Als (Eds.), *Behavioral assessment of newborn infants* (pp. 199-218). Hillsdale, N.J.: Lawrence Erlbaum Associates.
7. Bronfenbrenner, U. (1977). Toward an experimental ecology of human development. *American Psychologist, 32,* 513-531.
8. Browne, K. (1989). The health visitor's role in screening for child abuse. *Health Visitor, 62,* 275-277.
9. Burgess, A., Hartman, C., & Kelley, S. (1990). Assessing child abuse: The TRIADS checklist. *Journal of Psychosocial Nursing and Mental Health Services, 28*(4), 6-8, 10-14.
10. Campbell, J., & Humphreys, J. (1984). *Nursing care of victims of family violence.* Reston, Va: Reston.
11. Child Abuse Prevention and Treatment Act of 1974, PL 93-247, *U.S. Statutes at Large, 88,* 4-8 (1974).
12. Cicchetti, D., & Carlson, V. (Eds.). (1989). *Child maltreatment: Theory and research on the causes and consequences of child abuse and neglect.* New York: Cambridge University Press.
13. Cohn, A. H. (1983). *An approach to preventing child abuse.* Chicago: National Committee for the Prevention of Child Abuse.
14. Daro, D. (1988). *Confronting child abuse: Research for effective program design.* New York: Free Press.
15. Daro, D., & McCurdy, K. (1992, April). *Current trends in child abuse reporting and fatalities: The results of the 1991 annual fifty state survey* (Working Paper No. 808). Chicago: NCPCA Publications.
16. Dickie, J., & Gerber, S. (1980). Training in social competence: The effects on mothers, fathers, and infants. *Child Development, 51,* 1248-1251.
17. Field, T., Widmayer, S., Stringer, S., & Ignatoff, E. (1980). Teen-age, lower-class, black mothers and their preterm infants: An intervention and developmental follow-up. *Child Development, 5,* 426-436.
18. Fink, A., & McCloskey, L. (1990). Moving child abuse and neglect prevention programs forward: Improving program evaluations. *Child Abuse and Neglect, 14,* 187-206.
19. Gabinet, L. (1979). Prevention of child abuse and neglect in an inner-city population: Vol. II. The program and the results. *Child Abuse and Neglect, 3,* 809-817.
20. Gallmeier, T., & Bonner, B. (1992). University-based interdisciplinary training in child abuse and neglect. *Child Abuse and Neglect, 16,* 513-521.
21. Garbarino, J. (1977). The human ecology of child maltreatment. *Journal of Marriage and the Family, 39,* 721-735.
22. Garbarino, J., & Sherman, D. (1980). High-risk neighborhoods and high-risk families: The human ecology of child maltreatment. *Child Development, 51,* 188-198.
23. Garbarino, J., Stott, F., & Faculty of Erikson Institute. (1989). *What children can tell us.* San Francisco: Jossey-Bass.
24. Gray, E. (1983). *Final report: Collaborative research of community and minority group action to prevent child abuse and neglect: Vol. 1. Perinatal interventions.* Chicago: National Committee for the Prevention of Child Abuse.
25. Gutelius, M., Kirsch, A., MacDonald, S., Brooks, M., & McErlean, T. (1977). Controlled study of child health supervision: Behavioral results. *Pediatrics, 60,* 294-304.
26. Helfer, R., & Kempe, R. (1987). *The battered child* (4th ed.). Chicago: University of Chicago Press.
27. Howze, D. C., & Kotch, J. B. (1984). Disentangling life events, stress, and social support: Implications for the primary prevention of child abuse and neglect. *Child Abuse and Neglect, 8,* 401-409.
28. Kempe, H., Silverman, F., Steele, B., Drogmeuller, W., & Silver, H. (1962). The battered-child syndrome. *Journal of the American Medical Association, 181,* 17-24.
29. Krietzer, M. (1981). Legal aspects of child abuse. *Nursing Clinics of North America, 16,* 149-160.
30. Landeros v. Flood, 17 Cal. 3d 399, 551 P. 2d 389, 131 Cal. Reptr. 69 (1976).
31. Larson, C. (1980). Efficacy of prenatal and postpartum home visits on child health and development. *Pediatrics, 66,* 191-197.
32. Love, J., Nauta, M., Coelen, C., Hewett, K., & Ruopp, R. (1976). *National home start evaluation: Final report, findings and implications.* Ypsilanti, Mich: High Scope Educational Research Foundation.
33. McAnarney, E., Roghmann, K., Adams, B., Tatlebaum, R., Kash, C., Coulter, M., Plume, M., & Charney, E. (1978). Obstetric, neonatal, and psychosocial outcome of pregnant adolescents. *Pediatrics, 61,* 2.
34. McKittrick, C. (1981). Child abuse: Recognition and reporting by health professionals. *Nursing Clinics of North America, 16,* 103-115.
35. Milner, J., Gold, R., & Wimberley, R. (1986). Prediction and explanation of child abuse: Cross-validation of the Child Abuse Potential Inventory. *Journal of Consulting and Clinical Psychology, 54,* 865-866.
36. Mitchel, L. (1987). *Child abuse and neglect fatalities: A review of the problem and strategies for reform.* Chicago: National Committee for the Prevention of Child Abuse.

37. National Center on Child Abuse and Treatment. (1975). *The community team approach to case management and prevention: Child abuse and neglect, the problem and its management* (Pub. No. OHD 75-30075). Washington, D.C.: U.S. Department of Health, Education and Welfare.

38. O'Connor, S., Vietze, K., Sherrod, K., Sandler, H., & Altemeier, W. (1980). Reduced incidence of parenting inadequacy following rooming-in. *Pediatrics, 66,* 176-182.

39. Olds, D., Chamberlin, R., & Tatlebaum, R. (1986). Preventing child abuse and neglect: A randomized trial of nurse home visitation. *Pediatrics, 78,* 65-78.

40. Olds, D. L., & Kitzman, H. (1990). Can home visitation improve the health of women and children at environmental risk? *Pediatrics, 86*(1), 108-116.

41. Polk, G., & Brown, B. (1988). Family violence: Development of a master's level specialty track in family abuse. *Journal of Psychosocial Nursing, 26,* 34-37.

42. Powell, D. (1986). Parent education and support programs. *Young Children,* pp. 47-53.

43. Sevel, F. (1989). Interprofessional approaches to public policy issues: Graduate program in child abuse and neglect. *Family and Community Health, 12,* 80-82.

44. Travers, J., Nauta, M., & Irwin, N. (1982). *The effects of a social program: Final report of the child and family resource program's infant and toddler component.* Cambridge, Mass: ABT Associates.

45. Wolfe, D. A. (1987). *Child abuse: Implications for child development and psychopathology.* Newbury Park, Calif: Sage Publications.

CHAPTER 99

Maintaining personhood in the context of assisted reproductive technology

ELLEN F. OLSHANSKY

In the past 15 years, there has been enormous growth in assisted reproductive technology (ART). In vitro fertilization (IVF) and artificial insemination are but two among many new technologies used to assist in reproduction. Other techniques are gamete intrafallopian transfer (GIFT), oocyte donation, and frozen embryo transfer, with newer technologies being developed. Surrogate mothering is also a technique used to achieve reproduction. These treatments offer hope for many infertile persons; at the same time, they pose great challenges not only for infertile persons but also for health care providers. For those who keenly feel the aching pain associated with infertility, this technology offers hope and the possibility of control over one's reproductive function. For others, however, this technology represents exploitation, immorality, and the possibility of loss of one's sense of self or "personhood." For health care providers, this technology challenges their skills in focusing on the persons for whom they care while effectively managing the technology.

The recent explosion in technological advances in infertility treatment, and in all medical treatment for that matter, creates a challenge to us, as nurses, to confront our obligation to care for persons who are receiving such technological interventions. The challenge is to help a patient to maintain his or her personhood while undergoing the highly impersonal interventions associated with technology. The central tension addressed in this chapter is as follows: Can technological interventions and promotion of one's personhood occur together? More specifically, can nurses promote personhood within the context of assisted reproductive technology?

The chapter is organized according to four major areas: (1) overview of ART, (2) the concept of personhood, (3) the influence of ART on a patient's personhood, and (4) the role of the nurse in promoting personhood within the context of ART. The intent of this chapter is to raise issues related to the humanistic, caring, and holistic nursing practice that occurs within the impersonal, compartmentalized context of the biomedical environment. The underlying question is whether such nursing practice is possible within such a context, or whether these two factors are mutually exclusive. I believe that it is possible to practice humanistic, caring, and holistic nursing within the technological environment. This practice occurs, however, through exploring and understanding as much as possible the person's experience in this technological environment.

OVERVIEW OF REPRODUCTIVE TECHNOLOGIES

A brief overview of the various current technological procedures used to assist reproduction serves as background information for the discussion that follows.

In vitro fertilization represents a method of conception in which the woman's fallopian tubes are bypassed. This procedure consists of medical hyperstimulation of the ovaries to produce several mature eggs, or follicles; the subsequent surgical retrieval of these eggs; and the fertilization of the retrieved eggs in a test tube by mixing the eggs and masturbated sperm from the woman's partner or from a donor. The resulting fertilized eggs, after undergoing a series of cell divisions, become embryos and are then transferred to the woman's uterus in the hope that a pregnancy will result.

Artificial insemination consists of collecting sperm from the male and inserting it into the woman's vagina, cervix, or uterus at the presumed time of ovulation. Sperm can be collected from the woman's husband or partner or from a known or anonymous donor. Various methods of artificial insemination exist.[12] Recently a more technologically sophisticated form of artificial insemination has become popular, involving the use of ultrasound and medical stimulation of the ovaries so that ovulation can be precisely timed and chances are greater that the woman will, in fact, ovulate. Sperm are washed in a special solution to improve motility and are inseminated into the woman's uterus.

Gamete intrafallopian transfer involves surgical retrieval of the egg or eggs and retrieval by masturbation of the partner's sperm. Both the sperm and the egg(s) are placed into the fallopian tube via laparoscopy in the hope that fertilization will occur in the tube and the resulting embryo will implant normally into the wall of the uterus.

The use of donor oocytes involves retrieving an egg or eggs from a known or anonymous donor who must undergo medical hyperstimulation of her ovaries. The recipient must also undergo hormonal therapy to ensure correct timing of her menstrual cycle so that her uterus is ready to accept a fertilized egg (fertilized by her partner's sperm or by donor sperm). In addition, the recipient must continue hormonal therapy for several weeks to ensure that her uterus can maintain the embryo until the placenta takes over this functioning. Frozen embryo transfer involves the freezing of embryos that have been created in a test tube, as described for IVF. These embryos can be frozen for an indefinite period of time, although the procedure is so new that no long-term studies exist regarding the impact of length of time of freezing. The embryos can then be transferred to the uterus of the woman (most likely the woman from whom the egg has been retrieved for fertilization and subsequent freezing).

Surrogate mothering is the process of artificially inseminating a woman, with the intent that she will carry the resulting conceptus to term and then, under contract, give up the baby for adoption by a couple with whom she has contracted. The couple usually consists of the sperm donor and his partner.

THE CONCEPT OF PERSONHOOD

Personhood refers to an individual's sense of self and identity as an autonomous being within a social context. This definition implies that one is independent but, at the same time, relates to and interacts with and thus is interdependent with others in one's social context or social world. This concept has its roots in Symbolic Interaction,[2] a social-psychological framework that postulates that persons are social beings, or actors, who interact with others within a social context and construct meaning through such interactions. One develops one's self through interactions with others and with oneself.[5] The social context is critical to the meanings attached to these interactions. Through the development of self and the construction of meaning and reality, one develops personhood.

The recent body of literature on caring in nursing[14] supports the notion of personhood as a concept of central importance to nursing. Nurses *care* for persons as medicine attempts to *cure* diseases. The person, rather than the disease or condition and its treatment, is attended to by the caring nurse. The nurse's work of assisting persons to function at as optimal a level as is possible for them is an integral aspect of nursing. Nurses must integrate an awareness of the social context when caring for persons. One instance in which the social context influences one's personhood is found in the biomedical context of assisted reproductive technology.

The concept of personhood in relation to infertility has been addressed previously. I have developed a program of research[7,8,9,10] focused on the human experience of infertility, specifically shedding light on how individuals' and couples' identities are constructed in the face of infertility. This concept of identity has been evolving in my work into the more encompassing idea of personhood, of which identity is a critical part.

THE INFLUENCE OF ASSISTED REPRODUCTIVE TECHNOLOGY ON ONE'S PERSONHOOD

The advances of ART have provided hope for many infertile persons and have successfully helped some to circumvent, or bypass, their infertility and conceive and bear children. In this respect, many infertility patients have regained their personhood by achieving parenthood, an important aspect in their constructed meanings of personhood. For others, however, their involvement with ART has exacerbated their tendency to take on infertility as a central identity, causing them to feel less autonomous and decreasing their personhood. Specifically, persons often internalize treatment failure to mean personal failure, a direct affront to their personhood.[11] In a sense, then, the risk of engaging in

ART in an attempt to achieve pregnancy and enhance one's sense of personhood is a diminished sense of personhood as one sees oneself as a personal failure.

Technology can also be a challenge to one's personhood if feminism is a strong part of one's definition of personhood. The women's movement and feminism have addressed the importance of choice, especially in relation to reproduction. The right of women to choose abortion is a prime example, and the potential loss of this choice in the current political climate poses a clear threat to a very basic right of women—the right to choose whether or not to bear a child. This concept also can be applied to infertile women, who represent the other end of the reproductive continuum in that they desperately want to bear a child but are unable to do so. These women also would like the right to choose. For them, techniques such as IVF represent the right to choose to bear a child, just as abortion represents the right of other women to choose not to bear a child.

The concept of choice related to high-technology infertility treatments is not quite so simple, however. Rothman[13] aptly addresses the issue of choice that actually becomes lack of choice in particular situations. She advances the view that technology does permit choice but questions whose choice this is, arguing that the medical practitioners rather than the patients are making those choices. She cites the example of physicians choosing to perform cesarean sections on women because of mild fetal distress apparent on the fetal heart monitor and asks whether this choice is actually appropriate.

One can raise the question of whether or not women truly are gaining more choice in the matter of fertility. When IVF and other techniques are prohibitively expensive, this choice may only be available to upper-middle-class women. Access to infertility treatment and specifically high-technology treatment is rarely available to poor women, although infertility does not limit itself to a particular socioeconomic status.

One can also question whether choice truly exists for all women when the medical profession often limits the criteria for eligibility for such choices, particularly with respect to certain high-technology procedures. Many IVF clinics have used 35 years as an age limit, although some are raising this limit to 40 and even 42 years. Single women or lesbian women are often excluded from the criteria, raising ethical and moral issues having to do with family values. These issues frequently reflect the views of the "gatekeepers" regarding choices people make and the values these gatekeepers have about those who are different. The concept of

choice, then, influences and is influenced by one's definition of personhood.

The concept of control is another idea central to one's view of feminism and personhood. Who controls women's bodies has long been a concern of the feminist and women's health movements. The area of reproductive control reflects this concern. With the advent of newer methods of contraception, particularly with oral contraceptives, women have gained a degree of control over their reproductive lives. However, issues of control over women's reproduction remain central. Important questions include the following: Who has control over reproduction, the providers or the recipients of such control? What are the consequences of such control (e.g., the side effects of oral contraceptives)? Under what conditions does such control exist (e.g., that of pharmaceutical experimentation with various contraceptive methods on women in Third World countries)?

It is clear that many infertile women view the new technologies as means of gaining more control over their reproductive functions, because they now feel that the possibility exists to achieve a pregnancy. This is crucial, since a common feeling verbalized among those experiencing infertility is that of being "out of control."[4]

Hubbard,[3] however, views the new technologies as means for the medical profession to gain more control over women's bodies. She views this as a greater threat than the benefits to a few individual infertile persons. Menning,[6] taking an opposing stance, clearly notes the value for infertile persons in terms of assisting them to gain more control over their own bodies. This debate elucidates the complexity of the issues surrounding reproductive controls, raising the issue of how one's personhood is influenced by reproductive technology.

THE ROLE OF THE NURSE IN PROMOTING PERSONHOOD WITHIN A TECHNOLOGICAL CONTEXT

A major aspect of nursing is to care for persons as they experience various health conditions. It is the person that is the focus of nursing care. A key component of caring for persons is to facilitate their sense of self, their identity, their abilities, and ultimately their personhood. The strong emphasis on disease within our biomedical system creates an atmosphere in which individuals lose their personhood and instead become patients. As patients, they represent organisms with varying degrees of potential for cure and, if not cure, for palliative treatment. However, the treatment (whether curative or palliative) often becomes internalized by patients and provides a reflection of their sense of self, particularly as successful or as failures. This can be seen in the biomedical context of assisted reproductive technology when persons have difficulty differentiating treatment failure from personal failure when interventions such as IVF are unsuccessful in assisting them to conceive and bear a child.[11] The nurse plays a key role in assisting infertility patients to maintain their sense of being persons rather than patients, particularly by helping them to maintain their personhood despite the outcome of the technological treatment.

One important area for nursing practice is assisting patients in the decision-making process. Nurses can help individuals or couples examine the options available to them and, in so doing, aid them in making decisions that are best for them. The decisions can include ending treatment and either adopting a child or choosing a child-free lifestyle, or aggressively pursuing any and all treatments available that provide even the slightest hope of conception. A very important aspect of counseling is helping patients to make decisions as they proceed with their infertility treatment(s). There may be a time when some patients want to stop treatment and "get on with their lives," a phrase commonly used by infertile persons in describing the desire to complete the very disruptive and stressful infertility treatments. The nurse counselor plays a key role in validating this desire and in assisting patients to realize their wish to stop treatment, while maintaining their personhood. An important role of the nurse counselor is to help patients to achieve good self-images and to view themselves as successful if they can come to some resolution regarding their infertility treatment.[9] For some, this resolution means stopping treatment, whereas for others it means attempting every possible treatment available to them, even if experimental. A sensitive, insightful counselor can help tremendously in this area.

Another important nursing function is to educate patients by making sure that they understand the procedures(s) they are choosing and by answering their questions. This will result in more informed consumers, possibly leading to increased consumer or patient control over their own decisions.

The counseling function of nursing is most apparent, because patients clearly are facing important, stressful, and difficult decisions with potentially significant consequences. Helping individuals or couples to understand the issues they are confronting and to put these issues into perspective is an essential role of counseling. The nurse can help couples assess their marital relationship, motivations for parenthood, and responses to infertility and its treatment.

Nursing research can contribute important data on the humanistic aspects of the use of reproductive technologies. More research is needed to investigate the human responses to high technology, the consequences of not conceiving despite the use of technology, and the experience of pregnancy that may result from such technology. In addition, research into the therapeutic aspect of nursing practice in relation to patients who choose high technology would provide important data for effective nursing interventions. With the help of well-designed research studies, nurses will be better able to provide caring, humanistic health care within a context of high technology.

REFERENCES

1. Benner, P., & Wrubel, J. (1989). *The primacy of caring: Stress and coping in health and illness.* Menlo Park, Calif: Addison-Wesley.
2. Blumer, H. (1969). *Symbolic interactionism: Perspective and method.* Englewood Cliffs, N.J.: Prentice Hall.
3. Hubbard, R. (1981). The case against in vitro fertilization. In H. Holmes, B. Hoskins, & M. Gross (Eds.), *The custom-made child?* Clifton, N.J.: Humana Press.
4. McCormick, T. M. (1980). Out of control: One aspect of infertility. *Journal of Obstetric, Gynecologic, and Neonatal Nursing, 9*(4), 205.
5. Mead, G. H. (1934). *Mind, self, and society* (Vol. 1). Chicago: University of Chicago Press.
6. Menning, B. E. (1981). In defense of in vitro fertilization. In H. Holmes, B. Hoskins, & M. Gross (Eds.), *The custom-made child?* Clifton, N.J.: Humana Press.
7. Olshansky, E. F. (1987). Identity of self as infertile: An example of theory-generating research. *Advances in Nursing Science, 9*(2), 54-63.
8. Olshansky, E. F. (1987). Infertility and its influence on women's career identities. *Health Care for Women International, 8*(2-3), 185-196.
9. Olshansky, E. F. (1988). Human responses to high technology infertility treatment: A grounded theory analysis. *Image: The Journal of Nursing Scholarship, 20*(3), 128.
10. Olshansky, E. F. (1990). Psychosocial implications of pregnancy after infertility. *NAACOG's Clinical Issues in Women's Health and Perinatal Nursing, 1*(3), 342-347.
11. Olshansky, E. F. (1992). Redefining the concepts of success and failure in infertility treatment. *NAACOG's Clinical Issues in Women's Health and Perinatal Nursing, 3*(2), 343-347.
12. Olshansky, E. F., & Sammons, L. N. (1985). Artificial insemination: An overview. *Journal of Obstetric, Gynecologic, and Neonatal Nursing, 14*(6s), 49.
13. Rothman, B. K. (1984). The meanings of choice in reproductive technology. In R. Arditti, R. D. Klein, & S. Minden (Eds.), *Test-tube women.* London: Pandora Press.
14. Watson, J. (1988). *Nursing: Human science and human care, a theory of nursing.* New York: National League for Nursing.

CHAPTER 100

Knowledge technology

Costs, benefits, and ethical considerations

CHERYL BAGLEY THOMPSON, LINDA K. AMOS, JUDITH R. GRAVES

Advances in technology over the last 50 years have been cited as the primary factor in the movement of the economy of the United States and the world. Nationwide in 1988, a total of $540 billion was spent for health, an amount greater than 11% of the gross national product.[11] Health care expenditures are projected to reach $1.5 trillion by the year 2000 — 15.0% of the gross national product.[9] Technology in health care has revolutionized the nature of care delivery and has significantly influenced cost, mechanisms of care delivery, and nature of health care benefits. Consumers of health care are demanding and expecting the highest quality of health care and technology at an ever-accelerating rate.

The issues of quality of care, access to care, cost of health services, and allocation of scarce resources have been before us for several years. They remain the priority issues for consumers and health care policymakers. Technological advances have created more complex dilemmas in each of the policy priority areas. Advances in biomedical and information technology have had significant influence on the ability to address major problems confronting health care providers today. New and complex challenges are confronted in the implementation, utilization, evaluation, and development of new technologies. At the same time, nurses strive to maintain and advance the basic core of their practice, which is focused on humane approaches to care and treatment of clients and their families.

The focus of this chapter is on a relatively new technology on the health care scene, knowledge technology. The purposes of this chapter are to (1) define and describe knowledge technology, contrasting it with the other two main types of health care technology, (2) describe the influence of this new technology on nursing practice and research and suggest a future based on such knowledge technology, (3) examine the ethical implications of knowledge technology, and (4) examine the costs and benefits of a future with knowledge technology.

BIOMEDICAL TECHNOLOGY

Health care technology can be grouped into three major categories: biomedical, information, and knowledge. Biomedical technology conjures up the image of complex machines or implantable devices for use in the patient care setting. Artificial implants, diagnostic tests, transplantation of brain tissue to treat Parkinson's disease, and robot servants for people who are disabled are all examples of biomedical technology that are currently available or in the development process.

The trend in biomedical technology is toward less invasive equipment and techniques. Lithotripters, micropumps, and lasers are good examples of external devices employed to replace surgical interventions. On a larger scale, the computerized tomography (CT) scanner and magnetic resonance imager have provided greater ability to look inside the body, decreasing the need for exploratory surgery.

Biomedical technology is largely grounded in hardware and appliances involving data applications. It often utilizes signal processing, imaging, and modeling to computationally process discrete data into information. Biomedical technology may also be combined with information technology, as in systems used to assist paralyzed persons to walk.

Biomedical technology has had a significant impact on nursing practice. Nurses often assume the responsibility for monitoring data generated by these devices and frequently take responsibility for assessing the effectiveness of the equipment.

INFORMATION TECHNOLOGY

Information technology refers to hardware and software used to manage and process information. Information applications combine data so that meaning is stressed. The emphasis is on organization, storage, retrieval, and communication management rather than on computational processing. Information applications frequently employ database technology.

In the health care field, information systems are the primary information application. Information systems are usually named to indicate the discipline or function they serve. For example, hospital information systems support hospital functioning and manage information for financial and other operational objectives; nursing and medical information systems manage information required for clinical practice; and nursing management information systems support administrative functions such as staffing.

Information technology stores data and information needed to support practice or decision making. It can restructure and re-present the information in ways that are requested by and useful to the decision maker.

Nurses assume much of the responsibility for data entry and retrieval. Computerized information systems have for the most part been used to replace the paper chart, requisitions, and other forms of interdepartmental communication. Time savings for the nurse and increases in quality of documentation have been hypothesized as benefits of this new technology. Documentation of these savings has been difficult, however.[16]

KNOWLEDGE TECHNOLOGY

A great deal of electronic and mechanical gadgetry has been interposed between patient and nurse, influencing the technical practice of nursing. Minimal impact has been made, however, on the core of nursing practice. The caring and nurturing of persons in health and in illness has been little changed by technological advances. The potential for computers to be something other than another electromechanical contrivance interposed between nurse and patient or client does exist, however. Because computers process symbols, they facilitate a technology of mind, a knowledge technology. This technology entails the use of computer systems to transform information into knowledge and to generate new knowledge. The processing component of knowledge technology is analogous to the cognitive processing of information by practitioners to make clinical decisions.

The creation of expert systems is one implementation of knowledge technology that shows considerable promise in assisting nurses with clinical management problems. An expert system is a computer program that mimics the deductive or inductive reasoning of a human expert or the outcome of that reasoning process by making inferences from internalized facts and rules.[13] To wit, the expert system processes knowledge to produce decisions.

An expert system has two main components: (1) a knowledge base (versus a database) containing the knowledge (rules and heuristics) that an expert applies to data and information to solve a problem and (2) an inference engine, that is, a computer program that controls the use of the knowledge. Computer processing of expert and research knowledge captured in domain-specific knowledge bases can suggest how to apply and interpret nursing data and information so as to make better clinical nursing decisions.[8]

Debate continues over the functional requirements of an expert system. One school of thought believes that to be truly expert, the system must mimic the processes of the expert. The second perspective is that the expert system can utilize whatever methodology is effective in achieving a performance consistent with that of the expert. In this view, validity of the expert system is maintained even if the computer uses a unique reasoning pattern to arrive at the correct output.

Extraction of expert knowledge is the bottleneck in the construction of expert systems. Several methods are used to facilitate this process. The use of a statistical model of expert knowledge is often seen as a relatively simple method of knowledge engineering. In this approach, statistical models such as multiple regression or Bayesian reasoning are used to extract expertise from actual data rather than from an expert.

A second methodology is the use of neural networks. An artificial neural network processes data in a fashion similar to that of biological neural systems. The typical model calls for presenting inputs to a layer of "nodes" (the "neurons"), each of which processes its input and then forwards the result to multiple nodes in the following layer. Nodes in this layer repeat the process. There may be several such layers between the inputs and the final output. By adjusting the strength of the connections between the nodes, a process called training, it is possible to have the network learn a relationship between inputs and desired outputs (i.e., recommendations for actions, diagnoses, and so forth). Once trained, the network is then ready for use with inputs it has learned, and with new inputs that it has never seen before.

Though both statistical and neural network approaches are used to develop expert systems, obtaining domain-specific knowledge directly from a content expert remains the most common method of knowledge engineering. Specialty knowledge obtained from an expert includes private knowledge and usually consists largely of rules of thumb or heuristics about how to combine the facts to make correct decisions under varying conditions.[14] These heuristics are developed by the expert as experience and expertise in the domain are gained. It is hoped that mimicking this knowledge will allow the computer to possess expertise, or at least to function in a fashion consistent with an expert.

Specialty knowledge to be included in the knowledge base also encompasses public or published definitions, facts, and theories that are contained within textbooks and other references. To reproduce, clarify, and represent the private and public knowledge of the specialty expert is the central problem of expert system development.

EXAMPLE OF AN EXPERT SYSTEM FOR NURSING

An expert system to assist with the weaning of the uncomplicated coronary artery bypass graft (CABG) patient was developed by Hafey[7] as part of her masters' project. She identified the physiological parameters that impact patient weaning and hypothesized that weaning the uncomplicated CABG patient is solely a function of ventilation. In other words, these patients are appropriately diagnosed as having an impaired breathing pattern.[1]

The knowledge obtained from the expert for this system was not in the form of rules of thumb but rather in the form of physiological equations to be used to manage patient care. This knowledge was then transformed by the knowledge engineer into if-then rules that could be used in the reasoning process by the expert system. When the expert system is presented with patient values for ventilation parameters, it calculates a deviation from desired parameters and presents a recommended course of action based upon physiological principles governing ventilation.[7]

EXAMPLE OF A LITERATURE-BASED KNOWLEDGE-BUILDING SYSTEM

A second type of knowledge system is under development at the University of Utah by Graves. ARKS, an acronym for A Research-Knowledge System, is a program designed to build literature-based knowledge bases in a domain.[4] Graves believes that it is both possible and desirable to turn health-relevant libraries into databases of findings, instead of collections of document information as provided by bibliographical databases. By aggregating variables linked together in (quantitative) research with the nature and direction of the relationship, the stochastic significance, and the findings, causal or directional maps can be created. ARKS-generated maps can assist clinicians in design of treatment strategies, researchers in design of research protocols, and nurse theorists and students in the understanding of the definition and structure of nursing concepts.

The domain-specific databases that result from the use of ARKS are considered knowledge bases because they store related variables and describe the knowledge embedded within the relationship. In addition, ARKS processes the knowledge contained within the knowledge base and, by restructuring it, represents new knowledge within a field.[5]

ETHICAL CONSIDERATIONS

Both information technology and knowledge technology bring with them important ethical considerations. Ethical considerations for information technology are those posed by any electronic information system. These considerations include privacy and security of data, both of which have been extensively addressed by previous employers of information technology, such as business and banking.[3]

Users of knowledge technology within health care also face other unique ethical issues. Questions often asked regarding an expert system include: How expert *is* the expert system? If it is in fact expert, are there normative effects of it? Will use of the system become prescriptive for the average practitioner? Will some systems become so expert and accepted that it will be considered inappropriate or evidence of malpractice to reach decisions without consulting them? Will use of the system diminish the performance level of the human domain expert? Until we have actual systems in clinical situations for testing, answers to all but one of the questions must wait or rest on theory and philosophy.

The answer to the question of how expert an expert system is resides largely in the quality of the system's decisions and advice and the correctness of the reasoning techniques used.[14] Error can occur in the facts, in the logic, and perhaps in the method for dealing with uncertainty. In systems that model the reasoning process (not just the outcome), a particularly worrisome possibility is that the program may come up with the right answer, for the wrong reasons. Do we accept the right answer? In systems that do not model the reasoning process, do we accept right answers if we do not understand how the computer arrived at an answer?

Factual items included in the knowledge base must be verified from the research literature when possible. In addition, research documentation of the logic should be obtained. Because most research in nursing deals with simple relationships, rather than decisions, this latter requirement is not always met. A system such as ARKS may help to document decision logic by detailing research studies and producing maps of related variables.

One potentially major source of unreliability in the systems is the limitation of the logic form itself. When representing knowledge as rules and using Boolean combinations, it is very difficult, except in the simplest of situations, to represent all items of information that the expert actually considers in making a decision. Furthermore, all data items must be "known" for a proper recommendation to be made. However, clinical decisions are rarely made on complete information. Consequently, even when all conditions are met, the most important conditions represented, and the logic correct, the decision frame must be demonstrated in clinical practice to work reliably with different patients. This requires clinical testing with real patients against an expert decision standard. Systems that meet these requirements are labor intensive to build, test, and maintain. In addition, the more rapidly the knowledge of a domain is changing, the greater the demand for updating and reevaluation of the knowledge base.

What is an acceptable level of performance for a system and for the individual decisions within that system? Medical diagnostic systems can be expected to outperform experts, but accuracy will still remain considerably under 100%. Accuracy of a clinical management decision is much more difficult to measure than accuracy of diagnosis. Unlike a diagnosis, a clinical management decision is highly context dependent. That context includes at least the patient as a person, the surrounding environment, the patient's past experience, and previous treatments. Is clinical management of patient care needs too difficult a problem to model at all? Obviously, we do not think so; however, we are aware of our obligations as domain experts and informaticists building a system to ask the hard questions, to find the boundaries of the problem, and to explore the limits, benefits, and consequences of use of such systems.

COSTS AND BENEFITS

The costs of technology can be divided into the categories of development, capital acquisitions, maintenance, operational expenses, and equipment replacement. These categories vary considerably among the different types of biomedical, information, and knowledge technology, especially in the development phase. Expert system development, like other knowledge technology development, is costly. Knowledge acquisition—obtaining the knowledge from the source and getting the knowledge into the computer system—is extremely time-consuming.

Capital acquisition is often the largest budget item with the introduction of information or knowledge technology. Computer costs are continually decreasing, but represent a major investment because of the amount of hardware needed by a large health care institution. The competitive market in computer technology presently is to the advantage of the purchaser. Though this situation may change as technologies advance, standards are developed, and vendors leave the health care market.

Deployment of staff for maintenance and operation of the system is the most expensive component of technology after the initial capital purchase. The marginal costs of repeated or additional use of some technology offsets the initial capital purchase.[10] Thus the high cost of technology can be cut, without losing benefits, by increasing use, enhancing productivity, abandoning unnecessary and ineffective technology, and working to avoid duplicative acquisitions of high-cost equipment in settings or geographical areas where it can be shared.

Additional cost considerations follow the initial investment in information or knowledge systems. Equipment replacement must be anticipated but was cited as accounting for only 5% of the annual cost of technology in hospitals in 1986.[11] Allowances for space, security, and special furniture must be included in an initial budget. Continuing expenses for maintenance contracts, supplies, personnel, and upgrading also need to be considered. In addition, there may be hidden costs that are difficult to assess upon initial investment in a system.

Human resources are an additional cost factor to consider. Despite user-friendly computer interfaces, training for system users and availability of sophisticated programmers and technicians add considerably to the cost of any information system. A careful approach to the introduction of computer software is essential for staff acceptance. Time is necessary to allow adequate preparation of all staff before implementation.

Though knowledge technology is costly, there are benefits that may justify this expense. A benefit usually is defined as some measure of ultimate worth or value of a desired outcome. Benefits also can be defined as the effect expected or achieved as a result of utilizing technology. Tangible benefits are frequently specified in dollar equivalents, while intangible benefits refer to aspects of quality or effectiveness.

Tangible benefits from technology in health care delivery can be viewed in a number of ways. An obvious benefit is the reduction in cost resulting from fewer hospital days than would have been possible without technology. The number of days that someone with a chronic illness or disability is kept from work can be decreased by technology and counted in dollar equivalents. Another fiscal benefit could be the savings created when professional personnel are freed from tedious and time-consuming administrative tasks. A final but more difficult issue to address is the value placed on the lives that are prolonged because of modern technology.

Intangible benefits of technology often have greater appeal for most health professionals and consumers than do tangible benefits. In the practice area, technology can improve client services. At the very least, there should be an improvement in the quantity and quality of services and information. Expert systems do outperform nonexpert human clinicians, at least in the medical domain. If this relationship holds true in nursing, beneficial effects can be expected on decision making by novices and by nurses working outside of their usual area of expertise. Knowledge technology may also be useful for orientation and in-service education. In addition, it is possible that job satisfaction will increase because knowledge technology will provide opportunities for a greater span of knowledge and control over data and its uses. The outcome of this increase in nursing job satisfaction may be a reduction in turnover rates and an added cost savings.

Additional benefits result from the combination of information and knowledge technology. When knowledge technology (an expert system) lies on top of information technology (a clinical nursing information system [CNIS]) and obtains its data directly from electronic charting of nurses, the decision-making process is expedited. The computer does not need time off for breaks and is never busy with another patient. Consequently, it never forgets when a patient needs to be treated for pain or checked for the effectiveness of the last treatment. The computer can remind the nurse of these interventions, improving quality of care through even trivial and obvious decisions.

With an expert system lying on top of a CNIS, documentation of observations, care, and patient outcomes can be expected to improve significantly. More important, perhaps, is the fact that the information system can be used to gather the data needed to measure the incidence of findings and treatment outcomes under varying conditions. This process will allow statistical modeling of problems and generation of new knowledge.

A final benefit of knowledge technology is the potential for implementing new knowledge into practice more quickly; that is, it provides a direct effect on research utilization. Because the research that is used to document the system is filtered by a domain expert, some of the major obstacles to research utilization are overcome.[6] Linking of research findings to a clinical decision also assures relevance of the information to the practitioner.

IMPLICATIONS

After the costs and benefits of technology have been assessed, the question of how much technology we can afford must be addressed. This important question can be only partially answered through a cost-benefit analysis.[12] Since the major consequences of technology in health care delivery cannot be measured meaningfully in monetary terms alone, it is essential that some qualitative indication of the impact of technology also be assessed. Examples of indicators include quality of information, speed of decision making, personnel satisfaction, improved services, impact on quality of life for the clients, and advances through discovery of new knowledge.

The discussion thus far has focused on cost-benefit analyses of mainly physical rather than human issues. It is far more difficult to analyze the costs and benefits of saving or prolonging human lives through technology. The real question is, At what point is the cost of extensive information or human life too high? Commercial insurers already face the dilemma of how much they will pay for a life-saving procedure such as an organ transplant. If costs remain high, the time may come when certain medical interventions are available only to the rich. Small or rural hospitals may find the costs of installing and maintaining an information and clinical decision support system prohibitive and forgo the benefits to be obtained.

Consumers, providers, and policymakers are acutely aware of the crises in health care financing. All are concerned about cost effectiveness, efficiency, and new alternatives for health care delivery because of the unacceptable rate of growth in health care costs. Consequently, it is incumbent on nurses and computer companies to develop approaches to the use of knowledge technology that cost less and increase productivity while maintaining a high-quality product.[2]

CONCLUSION

There have been many criticisms of the possible dangers of a technological society, particularly those dealing with the loss of the human element. It is important to recognize, however, that human beings can assess information technology in the same way we have always assessed progress in our society, namely, through careful, critical, and imaginative analysis.

The dichotomy between caring and technology reflects a fear of technology. Nurses must view technology and humanism as complementary in their contribution to human welfare, and we must see ourselves as the agents capable of melding the two as we help drive the changes for the future.[15]

Technological and computer advances cannot be thought to provide answers to all things. No matter how sophisticated computer technology becomes, the question of individual use or abuse of the system will be the true limiting factor in its ability to provide for efficiency and quality benefits in our lives. Inappropriate use of technology cannot be afforded, either in humanitarian or in economic terms. When we consider the full range of implications of our modern technologies, we begin to realize the possible consequences of misuse or misinterpretation and the vast potential for good.

The information revolution in nursing and health care will provide us with an opportunity to better control our practice and activities in ways that were previously unknown. Nurses should view the advent of inexpensive and sophisticated microcomputers with complex capabilities as a major opportunity for nursing

to advance its knowledge base at a pace faster than ever thought possible. Without investing in the costs of technology, nursing and health care practices can become outdated in a short time. While the costs of initial investment in hardware and software, personnel, instruction, supplies, space, and ongoing maintenance may require considerable money, we cannot afford *not* to take advantage of this significant opportunity to mainstream nursing so that significant strides can be made in the quality of care delivered and the expansion of the knowledge base for the profession.

REFERENCES

1. Carpenito, L. (1992). *Nursing diagnosis: Application in clinical practice.* New York: J. B. Lippincott.
2. Edwardson, S. R. (1985). Measuring nursing productivity. *Nursing Economic$, 3*(1), 9-14.
3. Fernandez, E. B., Summers, R. C., & Wood, C. (1981). *Database security and integrity.* Reading, Mass: Addison-Wesley.
4. Graves, J. R. (1992). Software demonstration presented at the American Nurses Association convention, Las Vegas, Nevada.
5. Graves, J. R. (1990). A research-knowledge system (ARKS) for storing, managing, and modeling knowledge from the scientific literature. *Advances in Nursing Science, 13*(2), 34-35.
6. Graves, J. R., & Corcoran, S. (1988). Design of nursing information systems: Conceptual and practice elements. *Journal of Professional Nursing, 4*(3), 168-7.
7. Hafey, L. (1991). *An expert system for weaning postoperative coronary artery bypass graft patients requiring short-term ventilator support.* Unpublished master's project, University of Utah, Salt Lake City.
8. Hannah, K. J. (1988). Classification of decision-support systems. In M. J. Ball, K. J. Hannah, U. G. Jelger, & H. Peterson (Eds.), *Nursing informatics: Where caring and technology meet* (pp. 260-266). New York: Springer-Verlag.
9. Health Care Financing Administration, Office of the Actuary, Division of National Cost Estimates 1986-2000. (1987). National health expenditures. *Health Care Financing Review, 8*(4).
10. Jennett, B. (Ed.). (1986). *High technology medicine: Benefits and burdens.* New York: Oxford University Press.
11. Kabcenell, A. I., Barker, D. C., Weisfeld, V. D., Pomphrey, A., Cox, E., & Hollendonner, J. (Eds.). (1991). *Challenges in health care: A chartbook perspective 1991.* Princeton, N.J.: Robert Wood Johnson Foundation.
12. Keller, J. (Ed.). (1983). *Making resource allocation decisions based on policy analysis and program review.* Boulder, Colo: National Center for Higher Education Management Systems.
13. Negoita, C. V. (1985). *Expert systems and fuzzy systems.* Menlo Park, Calif: The Benjamin/Cummins Publishing Company, Inc.
14. Shortliffe, E. H. (Ed.). (1984). *Role-based expert systems.* Reading, Mass: Addison-Wesley.
15. Smith, G. R. (1988). The evolution of alternative delivery systems: What will be nursing's role? In *Nursing practice in the 21st century.* Kansas City, Mo: American Nurses' Foundation.
16. Staggers, N. (1988). Using computers in nursing: Documented benefits and needed studies. *Computers in Nursing, 6*(4), 164-260.

CHAPTER 101

Advance directives

Implications for nursing

DIANE K. KJERVIK

One of the fundamental values in the United States is an orientation toward individualism. Individual freedom is seen as the hallmark of a democratic political system. Soldiers have fought and died for freedom from governmental oppression and for freedom of the individual to say and do what is desired. The Bill of Rights in the U.S. Constitution assures the freedom to speak one's own mind and to associate with persons and groups with whom one wishes to associate, the right to practice one's own religion, and the right of privacy.

Concomitant with the orientation toward individual freedom is a corresponding right to make decisions about where one lives, what one does with one's property, and, in terms of health care, what one will allow to be done with one's body. As Justice Cardozo[14] stated, "Every human being of adult years and sound mind has a right to determine what shall be done with his own body; and a surgeon who performs an operation without his patient's consent commits an assault, for which he is liable in damages." The concept of informed consent has become widely accepted in health care and legal circles as the standard for entering into a patient–health care provider contract for services. Part of the reason for implementing informed consent in health care is to empower the patient by providing information about services to be given so that the patient is able to make a more meaningful choice among the options available.[9] With knowledge of the options presented in a clear and consistent fashion, the patient becomes aware of his or her ability to participate actively and with authority in the decision-making process. In this way the patient is empowered as an active participant in the health care decision-making process, and the power imbalance created by the lack of information is redressed.[8] A corollary of the right to consent to treat-

ment is the right to refuse treatment.[4] Advance directives in the health care context usually state what the patient does not want done and, in effect, refuses to have done. Nurses are in a position to influence patients and their families regarding the use of advance directives and to encourage patients to use this form of empowerment.

TYPES OF ADVANCE DIRECTIVES

Advance directives are legal mechanisms that enable a person to make decisions about financial arrangements or health care services before the occurrence of a situation in which the person is unable to make such decisions. Advance directives enhance individualism by providing a written document signed by the person that indicates what that person wants done under certain specified circumstances. When properly legally executed, these documents serve as a valid statement of the person's wishes and cannot be invalidated without compelling reasons.

Advance directives include those relating to financial affairs such as wills, trusts, representative payeeships, powers of attorney, and joint tenancy.[18] These financial advance directives provide that a substitute decision maker, such as a personal representative in the case of a will or a trustee in the case of a trust, is empowered to act on behalf of the person who executed the document. The purpose of articulating these wishes in advance is to ensure that the individual's wishes will be predominant, rather than the wishes of persons who are likely to receive direct benefit from the estate of the individual. These legal arrangements have been available for a considerable period of time to handle financial matters. Directives can also be given to a third party regarding care for oneself rather than one's property, such as those relating to health care: the living will and the durable power of attorney for health care.

The living will is a document that states that under certain circumstances, such as terminal illness, an individual prefers to have certain choices exercised on his or her behalf. The typical direction of the living will is that life-sustaining activities such as the provision of food, fluid, and cardiopulmonary respiration are to be withheld so that the person may die a peaceful death. Without this kind of direction, a hospital or independent health care provider would feel obligated to maintain life for fear of a lawsuit alleging wrongful death. The durable power of attorney for health care enables the person to name another person to be a substitute decision maker under the circumstances of impaired functioning on the part of the person executing the document. If the person is impaired to the point of being unable to decide what to do, then the substitute decision maker can do so. Most states have enacted laws that provide for the living will and durable power of attorney for health care.[1,2] However, their usefulness in assisting clinical decision making is not yet clear.

ETHICAL ASPECTS OF ADVANCE DIRECTIVES

While advance directives are legal mechanisms to support substitute decision making, ethical principles underlie the development of the statutes and the practice related to advance directives. The concept of autonomy, which is a fundamental ethical principle, is closely related to the freedom of the individual to choose what is to be done with his or her body. Likewise, as Faden and Beauchamp[5] have pointed out, the principles of justice and beneficence are also served by the implementation of informed consent. Caring for patients (beneficence) is manifest in the concern for the individual's decision-making capability and the importance placed on empowering the individual to be part of the decision-making process. To give patients a voice in what happens with their health care is a beneficent act that is respectful of varying human values and recognizes differences among human beings regarding life-and-death matters. Katz[8] discusses the history of silence between physicians and patients that has led to the doctrine of informed consent. Nurses and patients have not experienced the same degree of silence in relation to nursing care. This could be because

nursing care involves patient participation and discussion about the implementation of nursing tasks. In addition, nurses have long espoused the importance of mutuality between nurse and patient. The principle of justice is served by giving all individuals a fair share of attention to their wishes about the prolongation of their lives. Whether a person is rich or poor, African-American or Caucasian should make no difference in the decision about whether or not to end one's life. Deontologically, the rules to be served by advance directives are those relating to the freedom of the individual to choose what will be done with his or her own body and the value of the individual's life and death. Teleologically, the goal to be served is that of peaceful and dignified death for all patients within the health care system.

Empowerment is also an ethical concern when one considers the possibility of coerciveness on the part of a more powerful party in the decision-making process. Coercion or manipulation make the choice of less powerful individuals meaningless. Cooperation and conflict resolution among human beings are enhanced by empowering all persons in the relationship. In the case of advance directives for health care, empowerment of both nurse and patient is an ethical matter. If the nurse has far more power than the patient in the interactions, the decisions made by the patient are suspect as lacking autonomy. Therefore the patient must be empowered to speak his or her mind with the nurse as they discuss the decisions to be made. Responsible assertiveness is a communication technique that can assist and empower a client to speak. As Lange and Jakubowski[10] point out, "Responsible assertion means not deliberately using personal power to manipulatively overpower weaker people in conflict situations." Therefore the more powerful individual has the responsibility to encourage and teach assertive behavior to a less powerful person. An advance directive can strengthen the patient's ability to speak his or her own mind by providing a visible, concrete form of the statement of preference. The nurse, too, is empowered by advance directives, because information is made available to the nurse about the patient's orientation toward life and death. This information assists the nurse in implementing the nursing process.

The living will is a clear way of stating what the patient values at a point in time that is outside the framework of the time of crisis, that is, when a patient is admitted to a hospital or a nursing home. It is under the circumstances of these critical admissions to a health care facility that decisions often must be made by the staff and family of the patient without benefit of prior consideration and decision by the patient. Effective December 1991, federal law mandates that hospitals and other health care facilities inform patients of their rights under state law to have living wills and durable powers of attorney for health care.[12] While it is useful for incoming patients to be informed of these rights, the time of admission is not the most fruitful time for development of this thought- and emotion-provoking document. However, the federal mandate to agencies and health care workers raises their awareness of the importance of these documents to patients, families, and society, and the effect of this attitudinal change is presumably passed on to patients.

Another fundamental ethical issue underlying advance directives is the value placed by society on life. In *Cruzan v. Director, Missouri Department of Health,*[4] it became apparent that U.S. Supreme Court justices were divided on the importance that could be attached to life per se in relation to quality of life. The majority of the justices in the Cruzan case believed that life per se was worth preserving and that a state had the right to set the parameters for using advance directives. The minority opinion emphasized the quality of life and the right of an individual to determine when that quality of life had deteriorated to the point that intrusive measures were no longer justified.

Considerations of the quality of life must always address the question of who is to determine the quality of life. Living wills and durable powers of attorney for health care are premised upon the belief that the patient determines what quality of life means for himself or herself. Other individuals who are willing to be more paternalistic in their orientation say that the quality of life is to be determined by health care providers or the government. In reality, the quality of one's life can only clearly be ascertained by oneself based upon an evaluation of whatever criteria the individual decides constitute quality. One's values are a critical element in ascertaining the quality of one's life and can be evaluated by use of a values history such as that developed by the Center for Health Law and Ethics at the University of New Mexico.[1]

OBJECTIONS TO ADVANCE DIRECTIVES

Several arguments are raised in opposition to advance directives. The first is the paternalistic belief that the health care provider, usually a physician, knows what is best for the patient. This notion is being eroded by consumer activism and by other health care providers who are interested in sharing power with other members of the health care team and their patients. The designation of "patient" is even undergoing challenge and revision because of its emphasis on a one up–one down relationship between doctor and patient. As consumers become more active and interested in their own health care, they expect to be part of the decision-making process and ultimately to make their own decisions. Certainly there are rare cases in which individuals do not want to be bothered with decisions about their health care. However, these cases are becoming less frequent as consumers become more sophisticated about health care alternatives and therefore interested in asserting their own voice. One reason that they are interested in asserting their own voice is their experience with inadequate diagnostic and treatment decisions by health care providers that have resulted in injury to patients and corresponding large medical malpractice awards.

Another argument against living wills states that these directives do not reflect an incompetent patient's interests accurately. Because these documents are formulated when the person is competent and presumably has different interests, it is argued that later, when the person becomes incompetent, the best interests are served in entirely different ways than those that the patient long ago envisioned.[13] Following this line of reasoning, one's will and choice would have to be recorded continuously for a living will or any other form of advance directive to be considered valid. Contracts, wills, and trusts would all have to be invalidated because they are developed before the time that they are acted upon. Clearly, this is an absurd result that would create tremendous dysfunction in several areas of the law.

A third argument points to research that shows that patients are willing to grant their surrogates leeway in the way the living will is interpreted and do not expect strict adherence to the wishes they have stated in their living wills.[15] The response to this argument is that specifications as to areas of leeway and principles to be followed can be enumerated and, indeed, should be enumerated in the living will itself. Alternatively, the proxy decision maker acting under the durable power of attorney for health care can be instructed orally by the patient as to the leeway to be given. Decisions of the surrogate thus can reflect an accurate and full discussion with the patient.

Probably the most vociferous argument against living wills has been raised in legislative sessions in which opponents warn of a slippery slope between living wills and murder or genocide. This argument can be rebutted by the realization that the law examines carefully any coercion or manipulation involved in entering into this, as with any other, legal contract. Therefore, only documents that are the will of the patient are to be followed. No independent judgment by health care professionals that a given patient or a given group of patients should die would control the situation in which a living will was in effect. The law would not want to reach the absurd result that no contract or other legal document could be entered into if there were any possibility of coercion or manipulation. Ethical and legal rules must be adopted based on their ability to organize human behavior. These rules cannot be controlled by the fear of numerous possibilities of human evil. As far as coercion and manipulation go, not to allow a person to determine what will be done with his or her body during a terminal illness is a form of coercion in which the outside person decides that the life of another should be preserved at all costs.

ADVANCE DIRECTIVES IN RELATION TO NURSING PRACTICE

Nursing process can be enhanced by use of advance directives. As part of the assessment of the patient's goals in relation to severity of health care status, the nurse can discuss provisions that exist in the patient's living will or durable power of attorney for health care. Members of the health care team need to respond to provisions of the living will, so they need to understand the meaning of the document to the patient, and they need to understand what the law within their state requires for the document to be considered valid. In a much-publicized 1992 case in Texas, the patient and his family were distraught when the patient's living will was not followed by the facility because state law required that two physicians certify the patient as terminally ill and only one physician had done so.[6] Close work with the attorney for the facility is necessary to make the legal mandates clear to staff and administrators. A values history can give a picture of the patient's beliefs about such things as organ donation, respirators, and independent functioning. If the patient has no advance directive, discussion of personal values may help the patient to make a choice to execute a living will. Knowing the patient's belief about artificial exten-

sion of life, the nurse can plan and implement care that is respectful of the patient. Care can be evaluated according to standards developed by the patient in addition to those imposed from the outside that have to do with technical choices such as which antihypertensive drug to prescribe. If the patient chooses to have no heroic measures exercised, the nurse will be present to assist with comfort measures. Interventions in the direction of this goal rather than the goal of preserving life might create moral conflict for some nurses. In the future, nurses may be called upon to take a more active role in assisting with death.[7] Nursing must take an active part in the debate about aid in dying, since without doubt nurses will be called upon to play a close, active role in the process.

Nurses are moral agents who are responsible for their own conduct. As Theis[16] has noted, "To conceive of the nurse as one who simply follows directives without moral reflection concerning the treatment being rendered fails to recognize the moral status of the nurse as an individual with standards of personal conscience and professional ethics." The nurse cannot assist the patient to examine values without having a sense of his or her own values. Therefore part of the process of caring for the patient involves self-reflection and decision making about how one views one's own life and death. Nurses can act as role models for behaviors considered valuable for the patient to demonstrate, for example, by having their own living wills.[17] Since only around 9% of the public have executed their own living wills,[3] nurses' role modeling is especially important.

Patients who have advance directives demonstrate health-promoting behaviors. By stating values and preferences manifestly in writing, the patient shows the strength to be an active participant in the maintenance of health rather than a passive observer and recipient according to the preferences of others. In the process of preparing an advance directive, the patient imagines his or her own possible incapacitation. Through the use of this imagery, the patient is able to consider all alternatives, including the life-and-death options. The act of imagining and then creating a written statement of choice is strengthening to patients who often feel like victims in the health care setting.

Advance directives also act as preventive measures. As primary prevention in health care means the practice of health-promoting and disease-preventing behaviors, risk management in the law means preventing legal difficulties. Advance directives prevent legal problems in the future when the viewpoint of the patient may be at issue. Economically, respecting the patient's choice may reduce escalating health care costs by ruling out a number of expensive procedures. As Katz[8] suggests, "first patient opinions" may be less costly than "second medical opinions."

The encouragement of advance directives may also provide an opportunity for nurses to apply a relational ethic of care. Parker[11] describes this ethic as a process of sharing relational stories of care giving. This process is based upon reciprocity and interconnectedness among human beings. To talk with patients about their stories of the meaning of life and death to them assists them in making decisions about advance directives. Self-disclosure by the nurse enriches the process and contributes to mutual understanding and concern.

The relationship between the nurse and the patient is an important foundation upon which are based the realization of an ethic of care; the principles of justice, beneficence, and autonomy; and the legal goal of self-determination. Trust is imperative to this relationship and can be enhanced by the execution of advance directives. Katz[8] poses several assumptions that are part of a relationship of mutual trust in the context of informed consent:

1. There is no single right or wrong answer for how life, health and illness should be lived. Numerous treatment options exist and suffering can be alleviated in a variety of ways.

2. Health care providers and patients both have vulnerabilities and conflicting motivations, interests and expectations. Sameness of interests cannot be presumed; it must be confirmed in conversation.

3. Both parties relate to each other as equals and unequals. Professionals share professional expertise and patients their personal expertise. At the outset, neither knows what each can do for the other.

4. Human behavior contains both rational and irrational elements. These elements must be accepted in health care providers and patients. Incompetence should not be presumed for either when signs of irrationality appear.

The assumptions enumerated by Katz indicate that the physician must engage in dialogue with patients about health care choices, options, and decisions. While nurses do not demonstrate the silence referred to by Katz, the assumptions still are important for nurses to consider. Nurses should recognize the variety of "right" answers available to patients, should be aware of their own vulnerabilities and be able to discuss these with patients, should recognize their equalities and inequalities with patients, and should become comfortable with their own irrational sides. As Katz[8] states,

"Trust must be earned through conversation." It is in the face-to-face encounter with the patient that mutual understanding develops. With understanding comes more effective decision making about health care choices.

CONCLUSION

Nurses play a key role in the development and implementation of advance directives. Nursing values of mutuality, open and direct communication, caring, and health promotion and prevention support the use of advance directives for health care. The skill that nurses have in developing trusting relationships with patients can be used as a model for other health care professionals who are burdened with silence or unsupportiveness in their relationships with patients. The Patient Self-Determination Act of 1990[12] provides the impetus for nursing involvement with patients on the topics of living wills and durable powers of attorney for health care:

We help our patients speak.
We help them look deep within
For truth, conflict and decision.
Then we accept their paths
As we accept our own.

REFERENCES

1. Cate, F. H., & Gill, B. A. (1991). *The Patient Self-Determination Act: Implementation issues and opportunities* (pp. 65-73). Washington, D.C.: Annenberg Washington Program of Northwestern University.

2. *Choice in dying: Right-to-die case & statutory citations.* (1992, March 17). New York: Choice in Dying.

3. Crisham, P. (1990). Living wills—Controversy and certainty. *Journal of Professional Nursing, 6*(6), 321.

4. Cruzan v. Director, Missouri Dept. of Health, 110 S. Ct. 2841, 111 L. Ed. 2d 224, 58, USLW 4916 (U.S. Mo., June 25, 1990).

5. Faden, R. R., & Beauchamp, T. L. (1986). *A history and theory of informed consent.* New York: Oxford University Press.

6. Gamino, D. (1992, May 15). A living will fails to ensure dignified death. *Austin American-Statesman,* pp. A-1, A-12.

7. Johnson, R. A., & Weiler, K. (1990). Aid-in-dying: Issues and implications for nursing. *Journal of Professional Nursing, 6*(5), 258-264.

8. Katz, J. (1984). *The silent world of doctor and patient* (pp. xiv, 28-29, 47, 102-103, 228). New York: Macmillan.

9. Kjervik, D. K., & Grove, S. (1988). A legal model of consent in unequal power relationships. *Journal of Professional Nursing, 4*(3), 192-204.

10. Lange, A. J., & Jakubowski, P. (1976). *Responsible assertive behavior: Cognitive behavioral procedures for trainers* (p. 58). Champaign, Ill: Research Press.

11. Parker, R. S. (1990). Nurses' stories: The search for a relational ethic of care. *Advances in Nursing Science, 13*(1), 31-40.

12. Patient Self-Determination Act of 1990, 42 U.S.C.A. § 1395 cc (f)(1)(A)(i)(1991 Supp. pam.), PL 101-508 § 4206, 104 Stat. 1388-115 (1990).

13. Robertson, J. A. (1991). Second thoughts on living wills. *Hastings Center Report, 21*(6), 6-9.

14. Schloendorff v. Society of New York Hospital, 211 N.Y. 125, 129-30, 105 N.E. 92, 93 (1914).

15. Sehgal, A., Galbraith, A., Chesney, M., Schoenfeld, P., Charles, G., & Lo, B. (1992). How strictly do dialysis patients want their advanced directives followed? *Journal of the American Medical Association, 267*(1), 59-63.

16. Theis, E. C. (1990). Life-sustaining technologies: Ordinary or extraordinary? *Focus on Critical Care, 17*(6), 445-450.

17. Weber, G., & Kjervik, D. K. (1992). The Patient Self-Determination Act—The nurse's proactive role. *Journal of Professional Nursing, 8*(1), 6.

18. Weiler, K. (1989). Financial abuse of the elderly: Recognizing and acting on it. *Journal of Gerontological Nursing, 15*(8), 10-15.

CHAPTER 102

Tutor or tyrant?

MARTHA A. CARPENTER

The nurse makes decisions based on experiences, nursing knowledge, and the environment. Each of these components contains symbols to which the nurse gives meaning that is generated through interaction.[23] Interpretation of meanings, which forms the basis for action, involves both an internal process and external events.[2] This process, known as symbolic interactionism, suggests that actuality is the aggregate of objects and events existing in the shared world and reality is the meaning given to that world through the individual interactive process. When symbols are interpreted as tutorial, options for behavior are multiple and the way is open for ethical choice. When symbols are interpreted as tyrannical, options for behavior are limited and the outcome is likely to be unethical.

Human preference for the tutor, not the tyrant, is evident in both individual and global events. Recent national upheavals in Europe and South Africa exemplify mass objections to tyranny, while individual stories emerge reflecting the same objection. Elena Bonner[3] and Nadine Gordimer[11] represent a much larger number of women who elected to be tutored by their environment. Each of their stories tells of several decades of struggle. Elena Bonner stood against the entire communist government, including the KGB, preserving the right of free expression and quality health care for herself and for her husband. Nadine Gordimer also stood up in the face of a repressive government in her quest for the eradication of racial inequality. She worked not only for the rights of South African black men, but also for her own dignity, which she saw as diminished by her country's political system. These examples are important to nursing, as they represent women and women's capacity to reject the tyrannical for both personal and societal rights. Health care operates as a common concern at every level of this global picture; it shares and reflects the tutor-or-tyrant concerns.

Without nursing there would be no health care.[18] Nursing represents the largest number of care givers in any health care system. Care giving includes the sharing of information designed to enhance autonomous decision making. When done well, the educational role exhibits reciprocal aspects. Nurses and patients learn from each other, and nurses learn from both successes and failures. Professional progress thus demands growth as tutors in the educational role. The capacity of nurses to recognize that which is tutorial diminishes tyranny and makes growth possible. Learning contributes to growth, healing, and integration of individual personalities and of the professional aggregate, resulting in continually improving health care.

The tyrant is then identified as that which controls, subverts, and limits an individual or group in creative efforts of expression, growth, and progress. The values of the tutor include its support, recognition, and expansion of creative efforts. The tutor cherishes change and growth, which the tyrant abhors. The tutor searches for choice, learning, and negotiation, all of which endanger the tyrant.

NURSING ETHICS

Theories of nursing ethics represent a most recent concern in the long history of the search for understanding of the good. Historically, ethics has been the domain of the male-dominated, philosophical realm.[14] Linear Aristotelian logic was applied and universal answers reported. The resulting traditional ethical theories assume a distinct separation of mind and body. In that realm, the mind, most closely identified with the male, was considered superior to the body, identified as female and weaker. The superior mind would apply universal principles such as justice, beneficence, autonomy, and nonmaleficence to ethical questions and discover a single, best answer. If considered at all, women were relegated to inferior and invisible positions. The tyranny of the male perspective continues.

This limited historical framework serves as the basis of Kohlberg's "theory of moral development."[16] Using male subjects and the assumptions of traditional ethics, Kohlberg defined six stages within three levels of moral reasoning. The most advanced stage presumes ethical decisions based solely on universal principles. Related research including female subjects, sometimes nurses, suggested that woman failed to develop to the highest levels of moral reasoning. Despite the obvious tyranny of the male focus of this theory, nurse researchers, fascinated by Kohlberg's tidy developmental outline, used this hierarchy to produce many research projects that appear to support the inferiority of women, and thus nurses, in ethical decision making.[15]

This view of women as morally inferior has been challenged by Carol Gilligan.[10] As one of Kohlberg's graduate students, she was both literally and figuratively tutored by him and his ideas. She altered Kohlberg's multiple-choice research instrument to include open-ended questions about situations of ethical concern in people's lives. She found that women consider relationships and connectedness important in ethical behavior. Ethical decision making from the feminist perspective requires special consideration of each relationship and of the intervening variables of experience, knowledge, and environment. Gilligan's view of moral reasoning presents an alternative to the justice-focused, hierarchical theories. As feminist studies expand to include the ethics of care,[6,13] the influence on nursing ethics becomes clear and supportive of nursing ideals.

Theories that focus on the ethics of care identify most closely with nursing ethical issues. Caring involves receptivity, relatedness, and responsiveness.[20] The essence of caring lies in the relationship between the one caring and the one cared for. The ethics of caring also addresses the difficulty of caring for strangers when guidelines developed over time with family and friends are absent. Particular feelings and concerns gain importance in the ethical decision making of caring. Caring for strangers is a primary mission of nursing and central to nursing ethics.

Finally, a warning regarding dualistic thinking that sets the ethics of care in opposition to, as if entirely distinct from, the ethics of justice: Nursing can avoid the failings of gender-dominated ethical thinking evident in the history of ethical theory. A focus on the interpersonal would support a continuum between the subjective, personal caring and the objective, impersonal justice.[25] Defining justice as an obvious part of caring makes it a supportive partner rather than an opposing force.[9] It is within the domain of nursing ethics that the tyranny of dualism may submit to the tutor of continuums. Through such considerations, the particulars that tutor ethical behavior are partners with, rather than tyrannized by, absolute principles. Recognition of a common ethical perspective would serve to speed the long-awaited healing between nursing and the feminist movement.[12,22]

Commonly tyrants are clearly identified as external physical forces. Internal perceptions that shape our view of reality and our responses to it may well have a tyrannical hold. A consideration of that which appears to be tyranny within the nursing profession may be useful in efforts to redirect and use our energies toward more productive and growth-producing ends. Tyranny in ethical decision making appears in various forms in nursing. The following discussion includes the tyranny of emotions that paralyze the mind and eliminate any hope of movement toward ideal goals. This is followed by consideration of the tyranny of metaphors and images that control and limit thinking so as to preclude options that might lead to growth. Finally, the tyranny of the ease of habit is discussed as overshadowing the difficulty of change.

EMOTIONAL TYRANNY

The history of ethics has been written by those who would ignore the emotional component, viewing it as a lesser and purely negative part of the adult decision-making process.[4] The emotions may tutor the intellect and energize the ethical quest. The effective and cognitive aspects of the human psyche tutor in the sense that each serves to complement the other while bringing about reciprocal and corrective effects. Through our feelings, we peruse that which is recognized as injustice, maleficence, and dishonesty and correct these failings in ourselves, fellow workers, and the health care system. This capacity to recognize the unethical and to allow emotions to tutor rather than tyrannize behavior is as important to our humanity as the opposable thumb and the use of semantic abstraction.

The tyranny of the emotions in nurses' ethical decision making is evident in expressions representing emotional extremes.[5] These extremes are much like the extremes of acute and chronic illness. As with acute illness, the crushing, short-lived emotional response to unethical behavior may inflict damages that, if unrepaired, over time leave the victim in an incapacitating chronic state. Conversations with psychiatric nurses revealed expressions such as "blind rage" and "paralyzing fear" representing one extreme. The opposite end of the continuum is represented by the all-too-common "burned out," "really do not care," and "does not matter." This emotional continuum is represented by a variety of terms. DeWolf[8] finds that medical nurses use the terms *comfort* and *discomfort* to identify the emotions in nurses' ethical decision-making process. Whatever the terms, the result is the same: at times, nurses identify role models and other means that will allow them use of tutoring pursue ethical issues to satisfactory ends. More commonly the easier, but more devastating, venue of reduced ethical concern is selected.

Nurses report a wide range of reported events that appear to provoke emotional tyranny. Such events included physicians' persuading vulnerable patients to remain in a research study in which subjects had expressed intolerable suffering and from which they had asked to withdraw, as the research protocol had promised. In another example, hospital and nursing administrators chose to increase the number of beds on a unit despite federal regulations limiting the unit population. In yet another example, patients who had expressed wishes to be allowed to die were resuscitated. In the cases involving research protocol and do-not-resuscitate requests, the nurses allowed emotional tyranny to preclude alternative actions. In the case of the overcrowded unit, nurses elected to be tutored and to tutor each other as they persisted in their objections and ultimately reported the violation to a visiting Occupational Safety and Health Administration (OSHA) inspection team, thus provoking a return to the legal number of beds. Options for ethical resolution, such as insistence—on honesty of protocol and/or continued charting of patient wishes—were not evident to those helpless in the tyranny of emotion.

During any ethical decision-making process, nurses' emotions undergo change.[27] Change brings consequences. The nature and quality of the change dictates either continued quality patient care or reduced quality of care. If the change is toward the tyrannical, outcomes might include the lessening of personal congruity and integrity or a departure from the profession. Departure may be overt as in the pursuit of another profession, or more dangerously covert as individuals continue in nursing positions but fail in professional responsibilities. The latter case represents the nurse who identifies the lack of morality in others as a mechanism to reduce the anxiety of examining one's own unethical behavior. Such externalizing of ethical and emotional control represents one aspect of being our own worst enemy.

TYRANNY OF METAPHOR

While individual nurses chose between the emotional tutor or tyrant, the nursing profession chooses to accept a change of metaphor. The old metaphor of the handmaiden has given way to that of advocate.[28] The political and social advantages of this new metaphor are impelling. To represent patients who cannot represent themselves, to share one's knowledge in support of the less informed, and to be the voice for the voiceless moves nursing into the finest traditions of Western Judeo-Christian civilization and the true intent of the original Pythagorean professional.

Nursing's eagerness to take on this role of advocate displays some tyrannical aspects. Surely, at their best, all health case workers are patient advocates. Yet the nurse's role as advocate may put him or her in opposition to other members of the team.[1] Is it possible that the nurse is the only patient advocate and others are only pretending? More likely it is nursing's eagerness to assume this role that has blinded us to the advocacy aspects of other roles. Recent federal legislation on advance directives will have a yet-undefined influence on the advocacy role. Tyrannical acceptance of the advocate metaphor may well result in paternalism starting with an *m*. Thus nursing's supportive maternalistic role would be indistinguishable from paternalism's power and control.

Questions abound. Will nursing expend the time and energy required for introspection and change? Old games[21,24] will be replaced by responsible and direct behavior. Unlike the Cheshire cat, nursing will be constantly visible, as accountability requires a voice that is heard and demands respect. Advocacy implies accountability for shared knowledge and clarity in the pursuit of others' values. Such a position presupposes the development and delineation of nursing knowledge. In addition, the listening skills now rewarded in nursing will need to be balanced with rewards for giving voice to that which is heard. Change always challenges. As nursing emerges from the voiceless confines of its historically submissive role, a kinship with others who are struggling for recognition and acceptance will become evident. Coming out of the closet represents a variety of challenges.[17] However, the resultant freedom and growth far outweigh the alternative stagnation.

While the role of the advocate is more demanding than that of handmaiden, it represents only part of caring. Other professionals such as physicians, clergy, and lawyers appear to have rejected, if they ever thought of, the idea of a professional metaphor. Nursing might be tutored by other professions in rejecting the idea of an isomorphic metaphor for a multifaceted profession.

If advocacy were seen as a task shared by all members of the team and representing only part of the nurse's role, then nursing could be seen in a more expansive light. Nursing's history might tutor us to care not only for the individual but also for the environment.[19] Nursing would be more visible and accountable in the formation of public policy. Nursing can choose to be tutored to take on a more assertive, even aggressive, role in recognition of the need for advocacy without being tyrannized by a myopic view of nurses' role.

TYRANNY OF HABIT

Dewey's *Theory of Valuation*[7] suggests that every choice of action has an ethical component. Most of us fail to realize the values inherent in daily actions, as their worth was decided in the forgotten past. Conversations with intensive care nurses in both Sweden and the United States regarding ethical concerns in practice reveal that nurses frequently report events of a dramatic and singular nature. Repeated and routine activities seem to lie outside the realm of ethics. Only in the extreme, dramatic events do nurses recognize the patient's right to refuse medication, patients' and families' rights to knowledge of alternative treatments, and rights to dignity and truth. Yet nurses daily allow or deny these rights through habitual performance of duties. There is a clear relationship here between nursing's performance-oriented education and the task-oriented nurse. In both cases, the thinking time required for ethical consensus appears to be absent. The nurse is somehow compelled to administer all the medications, get all consent forms signed, and see that all patients are bathed and toileted. These are the things she or he has been taught to do. These patients' rights to refusal, options, and dignity are lost. "We've

always done it this way" becomes an even poorer excuse for continuation. Nurses need to unlearn habitual, nonproductive habits through reflection and change habitual meanings given to their surroundings.

A recent discussion with a colleague, J.C., revolved around the tutor-or-tyrant questions of habit. J.C. has earned her doctorate, and her office letterhead declares her equal status with physicians with whom she practices mental health care. However, these external symbols do not ensure equality. Being tutored by her own sense of inequality, she began examining her own thoughts and behaviors. The result of this examination included small but significant gestures resulting from assumptions based on images formed during years of education and practice in nursing. These assumptions include subservience, inferiority, powerlessness, and lack of respect. Not only did she recognize these as being her own but also presumed that they were held by her colleagues.

This projection of image resembles that reported by Weitzman[26] who recognized the error in her assumptions. Being tutored by this knowledge, J.C. has effected a change in her posture, her appearance, her degree of participation in discussions, and her choice of verbals and nonverbals. She reports that these changes have improved and increased her own personal sense of fairness and equality. In addition, she perceives herself to be increasingly influential in clinical and ethical decisions related to patient care. While avoiding the self-centered paternalistic extreme, J.C. has grown in her capacity to foster and support herself and others.

Nurses can learn subtle lessons from J.C.'s example. The always-important achievement of equality in title makes a lame substitute for equality in daily practice. The obvious lesson is that of concern for habitual, repeated behaviors that continue unnoticed in the face of the more dramatic, "sexy" ethical question. A careful look at those activities consistent with the values inherent in professional nursing would reduce the focus on the dramatic as unsolvable ethical dilemmas. As the ethical components of daily activities are recognized and adjusted for the good, responses to the tougher questions will be more readily found.

CONCLUSION

While there are remarkable forces outside nursing that would limit and suppress nursing's efforts, our concern here is with the internal barriers. The ideas presented here challenge nursing to dismantle those barriers. Recognizing this ownership is the first step toward change. Nurse administrators could develop support groups, nursing ethics committees, and formal policy channels for the recognition and management of ethical concerns. Nurse educators are encouraged to consider expanding the mechanisms that support and encourage student creativity and risk taking. Nursing's leaders are challenged to role model advocacy and its limits as essential to creating the ethical environment necessary for healing. Nursing must sacrifice the questionable ease of low profile and face the uncertain risks of visibility and change. Only by tutoring ourselves according to the noble ideals of nursing can we tutor others to heal.

REFERENCES

1. Bernal, E. W. (1992). The nurse as patient advocate. *Hastings Center Report, 22*(4), 18-27.
2. Blumer, H. (1969). *Symbolic interactionism: Perspectives and method.* Englewood Cliffs, N.J.: Prentice Hall.
3. Bonner, E. (1986). *Alone together.* New York: Alfred A. Knopf.
4. Callahan, S. (1988). The role of emotion in ethical decision making. *Hastings Center Report, 18*(3), 9-14.
5. Carpenter, M. (1991). The process of ethical decision making in psychiatric nursing practice. *Archives of Psychiatric Nursing, 12*(2), 31-37.
6. Code, L. (1989). Experience, knowledge, and responsibility. In A. Garry & M. Pearsall (Eds.), *Women, knowledge, and reality.* Boston: Unwin Hyman.
7. Dewey, J. (1939). *Theory of valuation.* Chicago: University of Chicago Press.
8. DeWolf, M. S. (1989). *Ethical decision making in the acute medical setting.* Paper presented at the 13th Annual Midwest Nursing Research Society Conference, Cincinnati, Ohio.
9. Friedman, M. (1987). Beyond caring: The demoralization of gender. *Canadian Journal of Philosophy, 13,* 87-110.
10. Gilligan, C. (1982). *In a different voice.* Cambridge, Mass: Harvard University Press.
11. Gordimer, N. (1989). *The essential gesture.* New York: Penguin Books.
12. Heide, W. (1973). Nursing and women's liberation. *American Journal of Nursing, 73*(5), 824-827.
13. Hoaglund, S. (1988). *Lesbian ethics: Toward new value.* Palo Alto, Calif: Institute of Lesbian Studies.
14. Hodge, J. (1988). Subject, body, and the exclusion of women from philosophy. In M. Griffiths & M. Witford (Eds.), *Feminist perspective in philosophy.* Bloomington: Indiana University Press.
15. Ketefian, S. (1981). Moral reasoning and moral behavior among selected groups of practicing nurses. *Nursing Research, 30*(3), 171-176.
16. Kohlberg, L. (1981). *The meaning and measurement of moral development.* Worcester, Mass: Clark University Press.
17. Kus, R. (1985). Stages of coming out: An ethnographic approach. *Western Journal of Nursing Research, 7*(2), 177-198.
18. McCloskey, J. C., & Bulechek, G. (1992). *Nursing interventions classification.* St Louis: Mosby.
19. Nightingale, F. (1980). *Notes on nursing.* New York: Churchill Livingstone.
20. Noddings, N. (1984). *Caring: A feminine approach to ethics and moral education.* Berkeley: University of California Press.
21. Roberts, J. (1986). Games nurses play. *American Journal of Nursing, 86*(7), 848-849.
22. Talbott, S., & Vance, C. (1981). Involving nursing in a feminist group—now. *Nursing Outlook, 29*(10), 592-599.
23. Thomas, W. I. (1931). The definition of the situation. In *The unadjusted girl.* Boston: Little, Brown.
24. Tisdale, S. (1986). *The sorcerer's apprentice.* New York: McGraw-Hill.
25. Walker, M. (1989). Moral understandings: Alternative "epistemology" for a feminist ethics. *Hypatia: A Journal of Feminist Philosophy, 4*(3), 15-28.
26. Weitzman, L. (1975). Sex role socialization. In J. Freeman (Ed.), *Women: A feminist perspective.* Palo Alto, Calif: Mayfield Publishing Co.
27. Wilkinson, J. M. (1987). Moral distress in nursing practice: Experience and effect. *Nursing Forum, 23*(1), 16-29.
28. Winslow, G. R. (1984). From loyalty to advocacy: A new metaphor for nursing. *The Hastings Center Report, 14*(3), 32-40.

CHAPTER 103 _____

What are the ethical issues from a worldwide viewpoint?

CONSTANCE A. HOLLERAN

DAILY DECISIONS

The decade of the 1990s had a turbulent start. The breakup of the U.S.S.R., severe famine in sub-Saharan Africa, and rampant inflation and currency instability in parts of Europe and Latin America are some of the situations that have had an impact on people's mental and physical health.

For nurses in those crisis situations, ethical issues frequently arise. Who can forget the pictures of the starving Somalians? How does a nurse working with those groups decide how to divide limited food and drugs?

In the work situation in Bosnia-Herzegovina, how does a nurse with a family meet her professional responsibilities during the war? In a graphic description, Louise Branson,[2] in London's *Sunday Times,* reported:

Rockets screaming overhead and mortar explosions shatter the nerves of those who have no choice but to stay and endure. Trapped and virtually abandoned, the women patients of the town's psychiatric hospital cowered, babbling nonsense amid the stench. One gurgled like a baby in a corner. Two others, one tattooed and dressed only in a vest, fought each other.

Most nurses have fled. Only 15 of 86 workers remain. Their job has degenerated into a single basic function: ensuring the survival of their charges. They feed the 309 inmates, prevent the violent from attacking the submissive, and attempt to clothe those who insist on wandering around naked. The intensity of the bombardment dictates the severity and frequency of the patients' epileptic fits.

Such a situation must have created tremendous internal conflict in everyone on that staff. Branson went on to say:

In Visegrad nobody was safe from "ethnic cleansing," at the hospital the Serbs transported 61 inmates of their own na-

tionality to safety. Those left—mostly Muslims, Croats, Slovenes and a few mislaid Bosnian Serbs—have been abandoned.

There was one heroic professional nurse who stayed with the psychiatric patients. Her name should be noted. It is Stoja Lugonja. She kept in touch with her teenaged children by phone but she stayed to oversee the care of all those patients.

Should ethical standards vary throughout the world? This is a controversial question that can be debated from a variety of perspectives. From a truly moral absolutist viewpoint, ethical standards should be the same everywhere, no matter in which culture one is born. From a cultural relativist viewpoint, there can be no one standard because philosophical traditions in different parts of the world have come to different conclusions regarding ethical conduct. In some Western Pacific cultures, it was ethically acceptable up to 100 years ago to eat human flesh. In 1992, one still reads of female circumcision, a culturally accepted practice that is considered ethical in societies in which it is practiced openly. Many people know about the ancient custom of allowing or even helping elderly to go to an isolated area to die a quiet death. They also may know of Americans in their 90s who have been kept alive though unconscious through the use of sophisticated equipment and drugs. Is one practice ethical and the other not, or do technology and resources make a difference? Recent publicity about a Michigan doctor openly assisting terminally ill people in committing suicide has caused discussions worldwide.

RAPID CHANGES AHEAD

Changes brought about by scientific advancement are having profound effects on the health field and on nursing. Developments that in the past were not seriously even dreamed about are today a reality—so much of a reality that in several developed or industrialized countries the citizens feel they must put limits on some types of scientific research to provide safeguards for the public. In some countries that means a requirement of extensive peer review. In one, the government may start requiring researchers to obtain a government license before even beginning certain kinds of projects.[9] Genetic engineering is moving so fast. The development of artificial insulin and genetic engineering to prevent arterial clogging are surely good steps. But what are the dangers?[2]

Aroskar[1] states "Dealing with ethical concerns in the world of nursing practice and service requires dealing with the political dimension as well. Ethics and politics interface and overlap. . . . Isn't ethics about right or good action and politics about power and manipulation?" From an international perspective, this is true— not that current politics changes the ethics of an issue, but that political changes can change the way a society sees and thinks. Take attitudes on abortion in the United States in 1950 compared to those in the 1990s, for example. Although many groups in that society have not changed their views, the court rulings and laws have changed dramatically, to such an extent that political careers are being built around the issue.

ETHICAL ISSUES OF INTERNATIONAL CONCERN

Are international ethical issues of concern to American nurses? Nurses need to raise this question in many settings. I personally continue to feel very strongly that U.S. nurses have a responsibility to speak out on several types of issues of concern to nurses worldwide, and I will discuss just a few of these.

Drugs: Usefulness and need

The lack of availability of drugs in developing countries leads to headlines that for a day or two spark heated discussions. Otherwise, things seem to go on as usual. Three topics that continue to cause major controversy in the 1990s are the export of outdated drugs, the export of drugs not yet certified as safe and effective for American distribution, and the promotion and aggressive sale of nonessential drugs. In countries facing grave financial crises, the expenditure on drugs can restrict the availability of needed health services. These are all issues that are decided by those with more power than hospital nurses. Yet hospital and community nurses see the results of decisions about such drugs, and they can have some influence on policies regarding them.

A few years ago, diplomatic pressure from the United States was reported to have been applied to one of the poorest countries in the world when the government of that country decided that it would import only the 200 drugs identified as being essential by the World Health Organization (WHO). Is this appropriate action to be taken by the government? Outdated drugs, the efficacy of which must be in doubt, are still being sent to developing (nonindustrialized) countries either as contributions or for sale. Is it safe and ethical to give such a drug to a dying child in Uganda but not in New York? Yet another situation arises when drugs not cleared for use in the United States are tested, tried, or used regularly in other countries so that the market can be developed. Is it ethically sound, for example, to export an experimental contraceptive when it has not yet been determined to be safe for use in one's own country? How about American women being denied a drug that is considered safe for use in France?

How can and should nurses make their ethical concerns known? To me, these are natural issues on which nurse teachers, students, the state nurses' associations, and the American Nurses Association should speak out. To do so they need to hear from their members, after which they can approach the appropriate policymakers. Individual members should contact their own elected officials to make their wishes known on those issues that are of international significance.

Infant formula and weaning foods

A few years ago the aggressive promotion of commercially prepared infant formula in poor countries made headlines in the United States and in the United Nations' agencies, prompting congressional hearings, lobbying by health professional organizations and others, and organization boycotts. A WHO code was developed and agreed to by the World Health Assembly (WHA), which meets in Geneva each May to set policy and the budget for the WHO. The only country voting against that code was the United States.

Eventually, the code was accepted by most of the companies involved and the controversy quieted down, although recently many people have expressed concern that costly weaning foods are now being promoted among people who can barely afford subsistence diets. Commercial trade is important to every country. Yet it is also important, in terms of moral responsibility, to see that people are not made to feel that they must buy costly imported foods when perfectly good and inexpensive local products are readily available. Wealthy people in all countries may wish to spend money on such things, but that is not the issue. The problem I see arises when parents feel that their children must eat, on a regular basis, the food that the hospital gave the mothers as free samples. And to provide these samples in areas where water may be unsafe, refrigeration unavailable, and costs high can lead to health and other problems for a family. I have seen mothers give very diluted formula to babies that resulted in malnourishment, illness, and even death. Nurses are usually the ones responsible for patient education. Are they giving out those samples?

The transmission of human immunodeficiency virus (HIV) through breast-feeding raises new questions of ethics that no one can yet answer. The United Nations Children's Fund (UNICEF) and the WHO continue to encourage breast-feeding in areas of limited resources where the child's health is more at risk from diarrhea and childhood diseases. These are not necessarily direct care-or-cure ethical issues, but I believe that they are international and ethical issues of nursing.

Cultural differences

Ethics evolve from the morals and values held by a society. Such values develop from religious, historical, and cultural traditions, and these may vary from country to country. For example, the rights of the individual versus the rights of society at large, and the right to know (e.g., information about illness, treatment, or outcomes) versus the right to withhold information are perceived very differently in different cultures. In other words, what is generally felt to be "right" in the West may not be "right" in some Eastern or other cultures. Currently, there is much discussion about rights of privacy versus the right to know because of the spread of acquired immunodeficiency syndrome (AIDS). Some countries say that the right to privacy requires that testing for the virus can be done only if a person requests it. Yet other countries require the testing of all foreigners and may test without an individual's consent. The clash centers on the rights of the many versus the rights of the individual. If ethics are seen as being universal, such issues create dilemmas that are not easily resolved.

Sources of organs for technology

The expansion of high technology in the health care system of the industrialized countries has raised many new issues for health care workers to consider. Some of the more controversial ones revolve around questions of when death occurs, how long people should be kept alive, and the quality of life of patients who are being kept alive by artificial means. I will not deal with those issues here.

But, have you considered the ethical implications of the sources of some organs for transplantation? Should you know? Should you raise the issue? In a newspaper report[10] early in 1988 it was said that children in Bangladesh were being kidnapped to make their organs available for transplants! Consider the implications. Do health professionals play a role in such situations? When transplants are done, do they ask about the source of the organs? Should poor children from poor countries lose their lives so that children in industrialized countries can live? There have been reports that this issue is being exploited for political reasons. Yet the article I mentioned was quoting a government official of the country involved. It is something to think about.

More recently it was reported that "the sale of kidneys from people who need money to people who need transplants has developed into a multimillion dollar business across India that is drawing recipients from Europe and the Middle East. . . . Agents seek people with healthy kidneys to supply those in need of them. Often, they find donors in the slums."[4]

In Argentina, a major investigation was initiated in early 1992 into the disappearance of many psychiatric patients from one hospital over a period of several years. Bodies have recently been found in various burial sites with body parts missing. It seems those parts had been sold for organ transplants by some of the medical staff.[8] (See the box on page 766).

Health workers at risk

Few health professionals, it is hoped, will ever have to help the wounded and suffering during an armed conflict, guerrilla war, or political or civil disturbance. But everyone should be prepared and know how to face such situations. The International Committee of the Red Cross (ICRC) constantly monitors the Geneva conventions.[5] Not all countries that have recognized those conventions abide by them. Everyone should be familiar with them, however.

```
┌─────────────────────────────────────────┐
│    NEWSPAPER HEADLINES ILLUSTRATING       │
│           UNETHICAL PRACTICES             │
├─────────────────────────────────────────┤
```

"India Seeks to Ban Human Organ Trade"
  International Herald Tribune
  August 1992
"Argentine: L'Hôpital de l'horreur—Les malades men-
  taux étaient utilisés comme banques d'organes"
  (Argentina: Hospital of Horrors—The Mentally Ill
  Have Been Used as Organ Donors)
  La Suisse
  March 1992
"Mentally Ill Are Pawns in Bosnia War"
  Sunday London Times
  August 1992

At the International Council of Nurses (ICN), we heard about several nurses and other health workers who were jailed and some who were physically tortured for providing emergency care to wounded people who were in opposition to the government. Also, nurses and other community workers have been jailed for helping to bring about social changes that would improve the health and well-being of the poor. Social action is seen as political opposition. There are dozens of armed conflicts going on around the world now.

Nurses working in prisons

Nurses working in prisons are often asked to do body searches on prisoners to look for drugs or weapons. Does this raise ethical issues? Does such a dual role jeopardize the confidentiality rights of the prisoner in the nurse-client relationship?

Some nurses believe that it does and that security personnel should be trained to do body searches. They asked the ICN to develop an official position on this issue.[6] However, nurses in some countries argue that nurses should do such searches to protect the patients from harm from nonexpert searches, so there is not universal agreement among nurses on this matter.

In addition to the body search problem, nurses who work in prisons face other issues involving confidentiality. They may have access to confidential information about a prisoner that could be important for others to know. How should such situations be handled?

ETHICS IN NURSING AND OTHER PROFESSIONS

A 1988 text on ethics by Joan Callahan[3] looks at similar ethical issues in a variety of professions. Again, the ethical implications of many of those topics will be viewed differently in different parts of the world. The recognition that nurses, lawyers, social workers, and others confront similar problems should encourage nurses to open lines of communication to colleagues in other professions.

The Council of International Organizations of Medical Sciences (CIOMS), to which the ICN belongs, has sponsored conferences on ethical issues. The most recent one was called "Ethics and Research on Human Subjects—International Guidelines," and the conference was held in Geneva. The proceedings were published in late 1992.

The ICN developed its first code of ethics in 1953. It has been revised and updated periodically. Its current format offers broad guidelines rather than specific suggestions for resolving individual issues. (See the box on p. 767.) This approach has proved to be advantageous when the national nurses' associations have needed to adapt the code to meet their specific needs. In 1988, it was agreed, after considerable discussion and review, to keep the current code to guide nurses as they deal with ethical issues worldwide, and that policy continues today.

CONCLUSION

The issues of morality, ethics, and legality at times are closely linked. At other times, the distinctions are difficult to understand.

Nurses must consider all of these aspects in situations in which they might be asked to withhold their services;[7] or in times of war, as was mentioned earlier; or in caring for or refusing to care for people with certain diagnoses, such as AIDS.

The pace of change is so rapid in these days of genetic engineering and technological advances that we all need to remind ourselves to stop to consider the ethics of some aspects of progress itself. No one chapter can deal with all ethical issues of a global or international nature—all we can hope to do is to broaden our awareness, recognize and respect our differences, and think and discuss together. The International Council of Nurses is in the process of publishing a book on ethics for nurses to help in this process.

CODE FOR NURSES, ICN
Ethical Concepts Applied to Nursing

The fundamental responsibility of the nurse is four-fold: to promote health, to prevent illness, to re-store health, and to alleviate suffering.

The need for nursing is universal. Inherent in nursing is respect for life, dignity, and rights of man. It is unrestricted by considerations of nationality, race, creed, colour, age, sex, politics or social status.

Nurses render health services to the individual, the family and the community and coordinate their services with those of related groups.

Nurses and people

The nurse's primary responsibility is to those people who require nursing care.

The nurse, in providing care, promotes an environment in which the values, customs and spiritual beliefs of the individual are respected.

The nurse holds in confidence personal information and uses judgement in sharing this information.

Nurses and practice

The nurse carries personal responsibility for nursing practice and for maintaining competence by continual learning.

The nurse maintains the highest standards of nursing care possible within the reality of a specific situation.

The nurse uses judgement in relation to individual competence when accepting and delegating responsibilities.

The nurse when acting in a professional capacity should at all times maintain standards of personal conduct which reflect credit upon the profession.

Nurses and society

The nurse shares with other citizens the responsibility for initiating and supporting action to meet the health and social needs of the public.

Nurses and co-workers

The nurse sustains a cooperative relationship with co-workers in nursing and other fields.

The nurse takes appropriate action to safeguard the individual when his care is endangered by a co-worker or any other person.

Nurses and the profession

The nurse plays the major role in determining and implementing desirable standards of nursing practice and nursing education.

The nurse is active in developing a core of professional knowledge.

The nurse, acting through the professional organization, participates in establishing and maintaining equitable social and economic working conditions in nursing.

Used with permission of International Council of Nurses.

REFERENCES

1. Aroskar, M. A. (1987). The interface of ethics and politics in nursing. *Nursing Outlook, 35*(6), 268.
2. Branson, L. (1992, August 30). Mentally ill are pawns in Bosnian war. *Sunday Times* (London).
3. Callahan, J. C. (1988). *Ethical issues in professional life.* New York: Oxford University Press.
4. Hazarika, S. (1992, August 18). India seeks to ban human organ trade. *International Herald Tribune* (New York Times Service).
5. International Committee of the Red Cross. (1983). *Basic rules of the Geneva conventions and their additional protocols.* Geneva: Author.
6. International Council of Nurses. (1986). *The nurses' role in the care of detainees and prisoners.* Geneva: Author.
7. International Council of Nurses. (1987). *Guidelines on essential services during labour conflict.* Geneva: Author.
8. Lucas, J. (1992, March 15). Argentine: L'hôpital de l'horreur. [Argentina: Hospital of horrors] *La Suisse* (Geneva), p. 7.
9. McKie, R. (1988, August 7). Designer baby ethics. *Observer* (London), p. 14.
10. Slave trade. (1988, April 17). *Sunday Times* (London), p. A19.

Concluding Notes and Future Directions

JOANNE COMI McCLOSKEY, HELEN KENNEDY GRACE

As we have said before in previous editions, there is no "ending" for a book on issues in nursing. Given the purpose of the book, "to provide a forum for knowledgeable debate on today's nursing issues so that intelligent decision making can occur," an ending is, in fact, inappropriate.

An issue is an issue for one of two reasons: (1) what is known is not well understood, or (2) not enough is known. What is needed is debate on what is known to foster understanding and ongoing search for knowledge about what is not known. Thoughtful debate and research are the keys to understanding a professional issue.

Yet, searching and debate are not enough for continued growth. Decision making also has to occur, and sometimes it has to occur in the absence of full knowledge. In this case, it is even more important to understand what is known and to be able to put this knowledge into a broader perspective.

The broader perspective requires that one keep current on the changes in the profession and health care field. Many things have changed since the first publication of this book in 1981. Recent changes in nursing include growing enrollments in schools of nursing following a severe decline, more opportunities for nurses to be employed outside of hospitals, more use of the computer and recognition of a standardized nursing language for documentation, more concern with costs and delivering a quality product, more push by more nurses for participation in policy-making, a growing effort to restructure hospitals to allow more nurses to have input into organizational decision making, more concern by all nurses with the care of the elderly and those with chronic illnesses, and more interest in nursing and health care in other parts of the world.

Yet, despite the many changes, the dilemmas faced by nursing remain much the same as in the past. Stat-

ing them in the debate format, the dilemmas are as follows:

- Unity versus diversity
- Standards versus access
- Quality versus cost
- Independence versus dependence
- Collaboration versus competition
- Inside control versus outside control
- Safety versus risk

Our previous recommendations to aid resolutions would be supported again by our authors. In alphabetical order, the recommendations are:

1. To clarify our mission
2. To get more involved professionally and politically
3. To produce more and better-prepared leaders
4. To promote flexibility and diversity
5. To realign education and service
6. To support nursing research
7. To take control of our own destiny
8. To widen our horizons to include relevant issues outside the profession

Our authors report that we are making progress on many of these suggestions. In addition, they offer some new recommendations, which build on the growing strength of nursing and in general have an optimistic tone about the future. Among these are the following:

9. To form partnerships among ourselves and with others to reform the health care system
10. To differentiate our practice so that patients are better served and nurses are better used
11. To implement nationwide, and even worldwide, a standardized nursing data set so that the impact of nursing can be studied and known

12. To participate in and encourage international exchanges to broaden our perspectives, learn from each other, and multiply our strengths

In general, the picture for nursing is good. Nurses are more involved and more influential in health care policy-making arenas. Nursing research is alive and healthy. More nurses are preparing for leadership positions. And education and service have closer ties than in the recent past. This is not the time, however, to sit back and congratulate ourselves. There is still much ignorance in the profession. The average staff nurse is still largely unaware of the bigger picture, and most are not professionally committed. And financial cutbacks and worries abound in education and in practice, which threaten to undo or at least slow recent gains. There are also large groups of underserved populations who need more and better nursing care. We need to continue to push forward, using the momentum that we have. We must continue to identify and work to resolve the important issues facing our profession.

We believe that continuous thought and debate on important issues can lead to effective decision making and professional growth, both for the individual and the profession as a whole. With our learning and growth will come important benefits for our patients and, we believe, for society in general. This book, now in its fourth edition, has been our contribution to that process.

Index

A

Abortion, 12
Access, issues of, and community nursing centers, 384
Accreditation, and external audit, 347-348
Acquired immunodeficiency syndrome (AIDS). *See also* HIV-AIDS;
  Human immunodeficiency virus
  in Russia, 598
Acute care, patient classification schemas for, 105-106
Adranvala, Tehmina, 52
Advance directives, 703, 752-756
  ethical aspects of, 753-754
  objections to, 754-755
  in relation to nursing practice, 755-756
  types of, 752-753
Advances in Nursing Science, 90
Agency for Health Care Policy and Research (AHCPR), 63, 137,
  225, 319, 511
  Clinical Practice Guidelines, 61
Aid to Families with Dependent Children (AFDC), 433
Alaska, health care reform in, 422
Alma Ata agreement, 383, 469
Ambulatory care, patient classification schemas for, 107
American Academy of Nursing, 391
American Academy of Physician Assistants, 635
American Assembly for Men in Nursing, 689-690
American Association of Colleges of Nursing (AACN), 390-391,
  678
American Association of Critical-Care Nurses (AACN), 391
  certification program of, 330
  on use of nursing research in practice, 63-64
American Association of Industrial Nurses, and consolidation
  issue, 608-609
American Association of Nurse Anesthetists, 186
  certification by, 328-329
American College of Nurse Midwifery, 186
American Health Care Association, 306
American Journal of Nursing, 89, 116
American Medical Association, 423
American Nurses Association (ANA), 366, 389
  Cabinet on Nursing Practice, 144
  Cabinet on Nursing Research, 95
  and consolidation issue, 608-609
  and definition of nursing, 7
  definitions related to ANA position statements on unlicensed
    assistive personnel (1992), 214
  quality standards and guidelines for, 285, 316-320
  size of, 607
  Standards of Home Health Nursing Practice, 311
  Task Force for Unlicensed Assistive Personnel (TFUAP),
    212-219
  on use of nursing research in practice, 62-63

American Nurses Credentialing Center (ANCC), 22, 329
American Nurses Foundation, 89
American Organization of Nurse Executives (AONE), 27, 391
American Society for the Prevention of Cruelty to Animals
  (SPCA), 731
American Society of Superintendents of Training Schools for
  Nurses, 607
Annual Review of Nursing Research, 66, 90
Applied Nursing Research (ANR), 66-67
A Relational-Knowledge Computer System (ARCS), 748
Artificial insemination, 742-743
Assisted reproductive technology
  artificial insemination in, 742-743
  concept of personhood in, 743
  gamete intrafallopian transfer in, 743
  influence of, on one's personhood, 743-744
  in vitro fertilization in, 742
  nurse's role in promoting personhood within technological
    context, 744-745
  surrogate mothering in, 743
Associate degree (AD) programs, 32, 154-155, 177
  enrollments in, 158-160
Association of Collegiate Schools of Nursing, and consolidation
  issue, 608-609
Association of Critical Care Nurses, and support for nursing
  research, 61
Association of Men Nurses of Berlin, 50
Association of Physician Assistant Programs (APAP), 635
Australia, health care financing in, 544
Automated patient chart (APC), 271

B

Baccalaureate degree nursing programs, 154, 155
  enrollments in, 158-160
Backus v. Baptist Medical Center, 690
BARRIERS scale, 70
Barrow, Nita, 53
Belgium, health care financing in, 542-543
Benedictine Institute for Long Term Care, 307, 308
Bias, toward unpopular patients, 656-657, 671-675
Biomedical technology, 746-747
Birth centers, 245-246
Bloodborne pathogens, costs of safety precautions to reduce risk of
  exposure to, 475, 515-520
Blue Cross/Blue Shield, 444
  in financing of medical care, 479
Brazil, impact of woman's roles on nursing services in, 606, 650-654
Breckinridge, Mary, 241
British North America Act, 467
Brown, Esther Lucille, 20

C

Canada Health Act (1984), 471
Canadian health care system, 419, 467-472, 543
  establishment of, 467-468
  future directions, 471-472
  issues in cost containment
    hospitalization, 470-471
    medical care, 469-470
  philosophical basis, 468-469
Candau, M. G., 52
Career development, 546, 549-557
  need for, 556-557
  possibilities of, 552-556
  review of literature, 549-592
Care management in long-term care, 503
CareMaps, 463
  background of, 254-255
  development of, 257-258
  documentation and responsibilities of, 258-259
  establishing goals and infrastructure in, 255, 257
  nurses and physicians in, 258
  ownership of, 259-260
Carnegie, Mary Elizabeth, 154
Case conferences, in measuring nursing practice quality, 345-346
Case management, 209-210, 254-260
  background, 254-255
  caremap development, 257-258
  documentation and responsibilities, 258-259
  establishing goals and infrastructure, 255, 257
  in hospital nursing, 224
  nurses and physicians, 258
  ownership of, 259-260
  and work redesign, 463
Cavell, Edith, 51
Chart/record audit, 338
Chief Nursing Officers (CNOs), 49
  in National Ministries of Health, 52
Child abuse, 703, 731-740
  background, 731-732
  nurse's role
    as mandatory reporter, 738
    in assessment of at-risk parents, 732-735
    in child abuse prevention, 738-739
    on multidisciplinary team, 737-738
    in recognizing, 735-737
    in specialty tracks in family abuse, 739-740
Child Abuse Potential Inventory, 733-734
Chisholm, Brock, 52
Civilian Health and Medical Program of the Uniformed Services (CHAMPUS), 439, 442
Classification of nursing interventions, 130
Client satisfaction surveys, in measuring nursing practice quality, 348
Clinical competence, 336-340, 386
  definition of, 336-337
  future measurement approaches to, 339-340
  measurement concepts in, 337
  objective testing in, 338-339
  performance testing in, 337-338
Clinical Conference Series, 93

Clinical nurse specialist (CNS), 19, 182
  comparison of nurse practitioner with, 19
  current mandates/challenges, 23-24
  functions of, 20-22
  historical origin of, 19-20
  regulation and reimbursement issues of, 23
  organizational placement of, 20
  profiles of, 20
  in transition, 23
Clinical Nursing Research, 67
Clinical specialist, 3
Clinical staff, cultural diversity of, 662-663
Cocaine (crack) exposure
  costs of, 475-476, 522-527
  effects on mother and infant, 523-524
  influencing factors, 526
  scope of problem, 522-523
  understanding cost levels, 524-526
Cockayne, Elizabeth, 52
Collaboration
  definition of, 24
  between nurses and physicians, 547, 580-583
  in nursing education, 172-173, 174
  and role conflict, 605, 638-642
Collective bargaining, 376-378
Colorado, health care reform in, 422
Committee for National Board for Nursing Specialties, 331
Committee on Allied Health Education and Accreditation (CAHEA), 635
Community-based education and practice
  multidisciplinary, 547, 586-594
    costs in, 594
    definitions in, 586-588
    reasons for changes in, 588-594
Community-based nurse-midwifery education (CNEP), 243
Community-based primary health care, 226
  barriers to success, 231
  building, 226-227
    community volunteer coalitions, 228
    continuous leadership development, 229-230
    factors critical to success, 228
    focus on issues that matter most, 229
    interagency council roles, 228
    participation in community celebrations, 230-231
    partnership case study, 228
    project staff roles, 227
    respect for individual and community values, 229
  philosophical admonitions, 231-232
Community care versus hospitalization, 221
Community college–nursing home partnerships in nursing education, 172-173, 177-180
Community Health Accreditation Program (CHAP), 293-294, 347
Community health nursing
  leadership for change in, 209, 233-239
    client's current condition, 233
    environmental determinants of health, 237-238
    human and biological determinants of health, 238-239
    medical/technical/organizational determinants of health, 235-237
    social determinants of health, 234

Community nursing centers, 358-359, 382-386, 429
    access issues in, 384
    cost issues in, 385
    definition of, 382-383
    history of movement, 382-383
    quality issues in, 384-385
    opportunities and challenges, 385-386
    and primary health care, 383-384
Community partnerships program, 173
Computer-based patient record, 210, 270-273
    effect of, on nursing practice, 273-275
Computerized clinical simulation testing, in measuring clinical
    competence, 339-340
Conduct and Utilization of Research in Nursing
    (CURN), 61
Consumer(s)
    demand for quality health care, 295
    involvement of, in measuring quality, 289-291
    passive role of, and health care costs, 479-480
Consumerism
    and nursing, 419, 450-458
        background, 450-452
        challenge, 452-453
        empowering communities, 453-454
        information and empowerment, 456
        promoting change, 453
        public health in community, 454-455
        steering toward consumer empowerment, 457-458
        targeted campaigns for health promotion, 455-456
Consumers for Choices in Childbirth, 451
Continuing education programs, 66
Continuous quality improvement, 290-291
    and job stress, 629
    in graduate nursing education, 199-200
Corporatization, implications of, 719
Cost, issues of, and community nursing centers, 385
Cost containment
    in Canadian health care system, 469-471
    in hospitals, 222
Council for Nursing Centers, 383
Council of International Organizations of Medical Sciences
    (CIOMS), 766
Council of Nurses in Advanced Practice (CNAP), 23
Council of Primary Health Care Nurse Practitioners, 437
Council on Certification of Nurse Anesthetists, certification
    program of, 330
Cruzan v. *Director, Missouri Department of Health,* 754
Cultural diversity
    and bias toward unpopular patients, 656-657, 671-675
    of clinical staff, 662-663
    in curriculum, 658-661
    and ethics, 765
    in faculty, 661-662
    and increasing pool of minority students, 657, 676-681
    and male nurses, 657, 683-690
    needs in, 663-664
    in nursing, 656, 658-664
    in student body, 656, 661, 665-669
    and women's health, 657, 692-699
CURN Project, 64

Curriculum
    changes in, for community college–nursing home partnerships,
      179-180
    in graduate education, 191-192
Curriculum Committee of the National League of Nursing
    Education (NLNE), 153

D

Data set development, 141
Decision making, and ethics, 703-704, 758-762
Delphi technique, 131
Developing countries
    costs of health care in, 541-544
    impact of woman's roles on nursing services in, 606, 650-654
    primary health care in, 210-211, 276-280
        community-based approach, 277-280
        selective approach, 277
        top-down approach, 277
    self-care in guiding quality nursing practice in, 350-355
Diagnostic-related group (DRG), 251, 295
    and costs of nursing care, 485-486
    effect of, on nursing education, 173
Direct nursing care costs, 483-484
Directory of Nurse Researchers of Sigma Theta Tau, 95
Diversity, in nursing education, 150-168
Dock, Lavinia Lloyd, 50
Dracup-Breu model, 61, 64
Drugs, and ethics, 764
Dumping, 621
Durable power of attorney for health care, 753, 754

E

Eating disorders, and women's health, 694
Economy, effect of, on men in nursing, 685-687
Effectiveness, in outcomes research, 137
Efficacy, in outcomes research, 137
Elderly
    meeting long-term obligations to, 209, 248-252
    rationing health care for, 707-708
        alternative to, 708-709
Electronic medical chart (EMC), 271
Electronic medical record (EMR), 271
Electronic patient chart (EPC), 271
Employer-mandated insurance, 421
Employment Retirement Income Security Act (ERISA), 445
Equal Employment Act (1972), 532
Ethics
    and advance directives, 703, 752-758
    and assisted reproductive technology, 703, 742-745
    and child abuse, 703, 731-740
    and decision making, 703-704, 758-762
    and health care rationing, 702, 705-709
    and HIV-AIDS pandemic, 702-703, 725-729
    implications of Oregon model for nursing practice, 702,
      711-717
    and indigent care, 702, 718-724
    and knowledge technology, 703, 746-756
    and nursing, 18
    worldwide viewpoint of, 704, 763-770
Expert system, 747, 748

F

Fair Labor Standards Act, 376
Federal Employees Health Benefits Program (FEHBP), 439, 443
Feminism, 547, 572-578
　economic realities, 574-575
　　public media, 576-577
　　science and research agendas, 576
　　women's health, 575-576
　ideologies
　　applying feminist ideology, 573-574
　　caring, 572
　　revisiting feminism, 573
　personal politics, 577-578
Fenwick, Ethel Bedford, 50
Fishbone diagram, 322
Flextime, 210, 262-263
　benefits of, 263
　difficulties with, 263-264
Florida, health care reform in, 422
France, health care financing in, 543
Friend, Phyllis, 52
Frontline nurse, role conflict for, 604, 616-622
Future of the Health Professions Project of the Pew Charitable Trusts, 188

G

Gamete intrafallopian transfer, 743
German Woman Suffrage Association, 50
Glasnost, in Russia, 598
Global Nursing Advisory Committee, 55
Goode model, 61, 64
Gorman Report, 184
Governance
　community nursing centers in, 358-359, 382-386
　faculty in, 359, 393-397
　International Council of Nurses in, 359-360, 407-410
　nursing organizations in, 359, 388-392
　power of nursing in changing health care system in, 358, 361-372
　shared, in nursing, 359, 398-405
　unionization in, 358, 373-381
　World Health Organization in, 359-360, 410-414
Graduate nursing education
　advanced practice roles in, 200
　changes in, 151-152, 188-194
　choosing program in, 184-186
　continuous improvement in, 199-200
　dual degrees in, 200
　emerging models for, 198-199
　history of, 182-183, 188-189
　issues in doctoral education
　　conceptions of doctoral education, 192
　　faculty, 193
　　monitoring program quality, 193
　　scientific integrity, 192-193
　　students, 193
　　substantive nursing knowledge, 192
　issues in master's education, 189-192
　　changing consumer demand, 190-191

Graduate nursing education—Cont'd
　　curricular content, 191-192
　　role of master's degree, 189-190
　making right choice, 151, 182-187
　minority students in, 680
　in nursing, 80
　personal considerations, 186
　　future directions in, 186-187
　postdoctoral training in, 193-194
　reasons for attending, 183-184
　reform in, 152, 196-206
　stimulus for change within, 197-198
　types of degrees in, 183
GRASP classification system, 484
Great Society, 718-719

H

Health care
　continuous quality improvement in, 290-291
　crisis in, 287-288
　financing, 288, 508
　growing consumer role in, 289-290
　improving quality through standard setting, 292
　involving consumer in measuring quality, 290-291
　limits of medical science in, 288-289
　private accreditation in, 292-294
　in Russia, 595-596
Health Care 2000, 35
Health care costs
　balancing quality and, 474, 490-499
　of cocaine exposure, 475-476, 522-527
　coinsurance in, 706
　and compensation for nurses, 476, 528-532
　containment of, 474, 477-482
　costing out nursing services, 474, 483-488
　deductibles in, 706
　factors accounting for rise in, 506
　　administrative costs, 507-508
　　aging population, 507
　　excess capacity of system, 507
　　financing, 506
　　lack of emphasis on primary care and prevention, 507
　　medical malpractice litigation, 507
　　relative price increase, 507
　　technology, 507
　in foreign countries, 476, 541-544
　inequitable financing of, 479
　for long-term care, 474-475, 501-505
　and need for reform, 321, 480-482, 510-512
　of nursing education, 476, 534-540
　overcapacity of hospitals in, 477-478
　passive role of consumer in, 479-480
　paying for, 475, 506-514
　rising number of uninsured, 509
　safety precautions to reduce risk of exposure to bloodborne pathogens, 475, 515-520
　state of American health care, 509-510
　surplus of specialized providers in, 478
　trends in, 506
Health care delivery system, in nursing education, 171, 174

Health Care Financing Administration (HCFA), 307
Health care policy, and implementation of nursing minimum data set, 116
Health care rationing, 702, 705-709
    and elderly, 707-708
        alternatives to, 708-709
    explicit rationing in, 706
    implicit rationing in, 706
    long-term care in, 505
    market rationing in, 705-706
Health care reform
    and Canadian health care system, 419, 467-472
    and changes in hospital nursing, 224-225
    and costs, 321, 480-482, 510-512
    employer-mandated insurance, 421
    and financing of health care, 418, 432-436
    and long-term care, 251-252
    and managed competition, 421
    and market-based reform, 421
    and nursing and consumerism, 419, 450-458
    nursing's agenda for, 418, 426-431
    proposals of professional organizations for, 423
    single-payer proposal for, 421
    solving dilemma of, 418, 420-425
    statewide initiatives, 421-422
        Alaska, 422
        Colorado, 422
        deficiency of statewide initiatives, 423
        Florida, 422
        Minnesota, 422
        Oregon, 422-423
        Vermont, 423
    third-party reimbursement issues for advanced practice nurses, 419, 437-448
    top-down approaches to, 421
    and work redesign, 419, 460-465
Health care system
    cyclical nature of, 296
    distribution of payment for, 508-509
    in Latin America, 350-351
    power of nursing to change, 358, 361-372
    standard setting, 292-294
Health insurance
    and demand for quality care, 295-296
    issues for advanced practice nurses in '90s, 419, 437-448
        design of strategies for reimbursement policy, 445-447
        financial survival for nurses in world of third-party reimbursement and managed care, 448
        history of, 437-439
        implementation of reimbursement legislation and negotiation with managed-care systems, 447-448
        private component, 443-445
        public component, 439-443
Health Insurance Association of America (HIAA), 446
Health maintenance organizations (HMOs), 433, 445, 706
Health workers at risk, and ethics, 765-766
Healthy People 2000, 196, 383, 384, 722
HELP model from Utah's Latter-Day Saints Hospital, 271
Henderson, Virginia, 53
    definitions of nursing, 8-9

Henry Street Settlement, 50
Hepatitis B and hepatitis B vaccination, 518
Hierarchical cluster analysis, 132
Hill-Burton program, 477
HIV-AIDS, 702-703, 725-729
    ethical challenges for nurses, 727
        personal and professional values, 728
        personal autonomy, 727
        research, 728
        treatment, 727-728
    stigmatization of persons with, 725-726
Home health care
    patient classification schemas for, 107
    quality assurance in
        accounting for individual differences among clients, 313
        comprehensive quality assurance system, 314
        measurement limitations, 313-314
        multidisciplinary care delivery models, 313
        multiple contextual factors, 313
        status of, 285, 310-314
Horn model, 61, 64
Hospital-based (diploma) education programs, 32, 153-154
Hospital Insurance and Diagnostic Services Act (1957), 467
Hospitals
    changes in nursing practice in, 208, 220-225
    overcapacity of, and health care costs, 477-478
    role of unlicensed assistive personnel in, 222
Human immunodeficiency virus. *See also* Acquired immunodeficiency syndrome (AIDS); HIV-AIDS
    and postexposure management, 518-519

I

Illness severity and health status measures, 107-108
Image, 69, 90
Incentive programs in quality improvement, 306
Independent Practice Association (IPA), 445
Indigent care, 702, 718
    access and equity in, 721-723
    and health and poverty, 720
    history of, 718-719
    payment for, 721
    priorities in, 720
    safety net in, 719-720
Indirect care costs, 484-485
Infant formula, and ethics, 764-765
Infections, 694-695
Information technology, 747
International classification of nursing, 60, 143-147
International Classification of Nursing Practice (ICNP), 116, 146-147
International Committee of the Red Cross (ICRC), 765
International Council of Nurses (ICN), 359-360, 407-414, 766
    blueprint for future action, 410
    continuing role of, 52-55
    leadership award of, 53-54
    leadership of, 4, 50-51
    organization and administration of, 359-360
    purpose and objectives of, 408-410
    and world health, 116, 414

International exchange models
  development of models, 204-206
  for nursing education, 202-203
  role of nursing and higher education, 203-204
International Journal of Nursing Studies, 95
International nursing leaders, 4, 49-56
In vitro fertilization, 742

J

Japan, health care financing in, 543
Job satisfaction of staff nurse, 16-17
Job stress, for nurses, 17, 623
Johnson, Robert Wood, and support for nursing research, 61
Joint Commission for Accreditation of Healthcare Organizations (JCAHO), 311
  accreditation visits of, 333
  Agenda for Change of, 322
  and bloodborne pathogen risks, 519
  on nurse executives, 27
  on nursing care plan, 267-269
  on quality assurance, 306
  refocus of, on quality, 299-300
  and support for nursing research, 61
  and total quality management, 490
Joint Task Force on Third-Party Reimbursement for the Services of Nurses, 437
Journal of Nursing Administration, 44
  1992 Directory of Consultants, 44

K

Karll, Agnes, 50
Kellogg, W. K., Foundation, 173
  Community College–Nursing Home Partnership
    curriculum change for, 179-180
    faculty development for, 179
    institutionalizing change, 180
    leadership for, 178-179
Kisseih, Docciah, 52
Knowledge technology, 703, 746-756
  biomedical technology, 746-747
  costs and benefits, 749-750
  ethical consideration, 748-749
  in expert system for nursing, 748
  implications in, 750-751
  information technology, 747
  literature-based knowledge-building system, 748

L

Labor-Management Relations Act, 376
Lambie, Mary, 52
Latin-American countries, self-care in guiding quality nursing practice in, 350-355
League of Red Cross Societies, 52
Lemmons v. City and County of Denver, 532
Literature-based knowledge building system, 748
Living will, ethical aspects of, 753-754
Long-term care, 209, 248-252, 501
  case management and cost effectiveness of, 503
  costs of, 249-250
  criteria for determining costs, 501

Long-term care—Cont'd
  current problems in, 250-251
  definition of, 209
  demography and old age in, 248-250
  directions for reform, 251-252
  financing, 250-251
  fluctuation of individual care needs, 502
  increasing complexity and deteriorating service, 502
  need for, 501
  patient classification schemas for, 106-107
  providing services appropriate to needs, 502-503
  quality assurance in, 285, 303-309
    association efforts in, 306
    decision making in, 304-306
    home environment, 303-304
    incentive programs in, 306
    nature of chronic illness in, 304
    peer review in, 306
    quality service in, 308-309
    regulatory efforts in, 306-308
  refocusing public health and community nursing, 503
    allocating costs, 504-505
    cost reduction through flexibility, 504
    proliferation of health workers, 503
    quality versus quantity in nursing homes, 503-504
    rationing care, 505
    respite care, 504
  role of nursing in, 252

M

Male nurses, 657, 683-690
  and American Assembly for Men in Nursing, 689-690
  effect of economy on, 685-687
  effect of military on, 685
  history of, 683-685
  and nursing as women's work, 687-689
  and organized nursing, 689
Managed care, 209-210, 436, 444-445
  background, 254-255
  CareMap development, 257-258
  documentation and responsibilities, 258-259
  establishing goals and infrastructure, 255, 257
  financial survival for nurses in world of, 448
  growth of, 451, 460
  implementation of reimbursement legislation and negotiation with, 447-448
  nurses and physicians, 258
  ownership of, 259-260
Managed competition, 421
Market-based reform, 421
Maternity Center Association (MCA), 241, 242, 245
Medicaid, 439
  effect of, on hospitals, 221
  in health care expenses, 432, 433, 719
  and payment for long-term care, 250, 251
Medical Record (Duke University), 271
Medical records, computer-based, 270-275
Medicare, 439, 442
  effect of, on hospitals, 220-221
  explicit rationing in, 706

Medicare—Cont'd
   and health care expenses, 171, 250-251, 432-433, 719
   Peer Review Organization (PRO), 490
Medicare Catastrophic Illness Protection Act (1988), 432
Military, effect of, on men in nursing, 685
Minimum Data Set (MDS), 307
Minnesota, health care reform in, 422
Minority students, recruitment and retention of, into nursing,
      160-162
   institutional commitment, 161
   retention mechanisms, 161-162
Mississippi University for Women v. *Hogan,* 691n
Moores, Yvonne, 52
Multidisciplinary team, nurse's role on, 737-738

N

National Association of Childbearing Centers (NACC), 245, 246
National Association of Colored Graduate Nurses, and
      consolidation issue, 608-609
National Association of Home Care, in measuring quality, 345
National Association of Insurance Commissioners (NAIC), 446
National Association of Pediatric Nurse Associates and
      Practitioners, and support for nursing research, 61
National Association of Transplant Coordinators, and support for
      nursing research, 61
National Center for Nursing Research (NCNR), 90
   establishment of, 35
   research priorities at, 187
   State-of-the-Science Invitational Conference of, 197
National Center on Child Abuse and Neglect (NCCAN), 739
National Certification Board of Pediatric Nurse Practitioners and
      Nurses, 22
National Certification Corporation for Obstetric, Gynecologic, and
      Neonatal Nursing Specialties, 22
National Citizen's Coalition for Nursing Home Reform
      (NCCNHR), 290
National Commission on Nursing, 210
National Council of State Boards of Nursing (NCSBN), 23, 391
National Demonstration Project (NDP) on Quality Improvement in
      Health Care, 323-325
National Federation of Specialty Nursing Organizations (NFSNO),
      331, 390, 611-612
National Health Grants Act, 467
National League for Nursing (NLN), 389-390, 451, 607
   accreditation criterion, 9
   health care reform of, 423
   and health care reform, 428-429
   and proliferation of nursing conceptual models, 88
   for research training, 89
National League for Nursing Education (NLNE), 607
   and consolidation issue, 608-609
National Organization for Public Health Nursing (NOPHN),
      450-451, 608-609
National Organization Liaison Forum (NOLF), 331, 391
National Organization of Nurse Practitioner Faculties
      (NONPF), 635
Neill, Grace, 51
Neural networks, 747-748
New Jersey relative intensity measure (RIM), 483-484
New York State Nurses Association (NYSNA), 6, 7

Nightingale, Florence, 3, 683-684
   challenges of, 49-50
   definitions of nursing, 8-9
   International Fund, 52
   perspective of nurse administrators, 26-27
Norrie, Charlotte Gordon, 51
North American Nursing Diagnosis Association (NANDA),
      97-98, 116
Nurse(s)
   in assessing child abuse, 732-740
   in case management, 258
   collaboration between physicians and, 547, 580-583
   independent practice of, 24
   job stress for, 623
      definition of, 624
      future directions, 628-629
      measurement, 626
      organizational behavior, 624
      recent changes, 626-628
      role theory, 624
      sources of, 623-624
   in primary public health care, 280
   professional role of, 588-591
   in promoting personhood, 744-745
   reimbursement for services, 3
   and unpopular clients, 656-657, 671-675
   values and qualifications of practicing, 69-70
Nurse administrators, 3. *See also* Nurse executive(s)
   as arbitrator, 28
   challenges for, 29-31
   as coordinator, 28
   flextime for, 262
   functions of, 27-28
   as guide, 28
   as image setter, 28
   and implementation of Nursing Minimum Data Set, 116
   as implementer, 28
   Nightingale's perspective of, 26-27
   as planner, 27-28
   roles of, 27, 28-29
      in strengthening nursing theory-practice bond, 79-80
   and use of unlicensed assistants, 212-219
Nurse-anesthetists, certification for, 330-331
Nurse entrepreneurs, 43-48
   challenges for, 46-47
   characteristics of, 44-46
   definition of, 43
   examples of services provided by consultants, 44
   functions of, 43-44
   risks in starting your own business, 47-48
Nurse executive(s). *See also* Nurse administrators
   and costing of nursing care, 486
   role of, in increasing use of nursing research in practice, 71
Nurse-initiated treatments, definition of, 130
Nurse-midwifery, 209, 241-247
   background of, 241-242
   in birth center, 245-246
   certification in, 330-331
   constraints on education, 242-243
   constraints to practice, 243

Nurse-midwifrey—Cont'd
  education for, 246
  future for, 246-247
  nursing prerequisite challenged, 243-245
Nurse practice acts
  legal definitions in, 6
  suggested language for, 7
Nurse practitioner (NP), 3, 10
  comparison of, with clinical nurse specialist, 19
  current mandates/challenges, 23-24
  education for, 22
  functions of, 22
  national certification for, 22
  origins of, 22
  and physician assistants, 634-636
  regulation and reimbursement issues, 23
  specific role issues for, 22-23
  in transition, 23
Nurse researchers, 38-41. *See also* Nursing research
  in building research program, 41
  and collaboration, 40-41
  definition of, 38
  nature of research, 38-39
  study design, 40
  study sample, 39
  and substantive content of research, 39-40
  utilization of findings, 41
Nurses' Associated Alumnae, 607
Nurses' Settlement, 50
Nurse staffing
  history of patient classifications for
    acute care, 105-106
    home and ambulatory care, 107
    long-term care, 106-107
  illness severity and health status measures, 107-108
Nurses United for Reimbursement of Services (NURS), 447
Nurses' voice
  and being colleague, 639-640
  and consequences of choice, 640-641
  definition of, 638
  silencing, 638-639
Nursing
  activities in, 130
  advanced practice as definitional problem, 10-11
  as academic discipline, 33
  building science of, 90-91
  conceptual models of, 77
  and consumerism, 419, 450-458
    background, 450-452
    challenge, 452-453
    empowering communities, 453-454
    promoting change, 453
  cultural diversity in, 656, 658-664, 676
    of clinical staff, 662-663
    in curriculum, 658-661
    of faculty, 661-662
    needs in, 663-664
    in student body, 661
  definition of, 3
  description of work in, 11-12

Nursing—Cont'd
  development of metasystem for classification, 101-102
  dictionary definitions of, 5-6
  example of expert system for, 748
  Florence Nightingale on, 8-9
  graduate education in, 80
  history in, 683-685
  impact of health care finance on, 418, 432-436
  legal definition of, 6-8
  in long-term care, 252
  men in, 657, 683-690
    and American Assembly for Men in Nursing, 689-690
    and nursing as woman's work, 687-689
    and organized nursing, 689
  metaparadigm, 76
  motivation for choosing as career, 15-16
  opportunities in, 3
  power of, to change health care system, 358, 361-372
  public health in community, 454-455
    information and empowerment, 456
    targeted campaigns for health promotion, 455-456
  quest for professionalism, 546, 559-565
    stages in, 559-564
    in Russia, 548, 595-601
    reform in, 598-601
  shared governance in, 359, 398-405
    definition of, 399-402
    implementation of, 402-403
    motives for, 402
    role and system effects of, 403-404
  steering toward consumer empowerment, 457-458
  strategies for changing image, 546-547, 566-570
    as factor in employment, 568-569
    recruitment, 566-568
    retention, 569-570
  strategies to improve ethnic mix in, 680-681
  theories and definitions, 9-10
  Virginia Henderson on, 8-9
  in World Health Organization, 412-413
Nursing '90, 69
Nursing: A Social Policy Statement (ANA), 7, 23
Nursing care plan, 210, 267-269
Nursing certification, 285-286, 327-335
  current situation, 328
    certification by institutions, 332-333
    certification by professional organizations, 328-331
    certification by state, 331-332
  goals of, 328
  self-regulation of profession, 327-328
Nursing Child Assessment by Satellite Training (NCAST), 61, 734
Nursing Consortium for Research in Practice at Stanford
  University Hospital on nursing research, 67
Nursing curriculums, redesign of, and indigent care, 723
Nursing diagnosis taxonomy development, 59-60, 123-128
  benefits of taxonomy, 123-124
  development of Taxonomy I, 124-126
  development of Taxonomy II, 126
  issues concerning NANDA taxonomy
    collaboration with American Nurses Association, 126-127
    communication between databases, 127

Nursing diagnosis taxonomy development—Cont'd
conceptual framework, 126
validating Taxonomy I, 126
Nursing education, 153-157. *See also* Graduate education
arguments against diversity, 155-156
arguments for diversity, 156
collaborative efforts in, 172-173, 174
community college–nursing home partnerships, 177-180
curriculum change, 179-180
faculty development, 179
institutionalizing change, 180
leadership, 178-179
costs of, 476, 534-540
increasing revenues, 535-537
reducing expenditures, 537-539
creating culturally sensitive learning environment, 668
cultural diversity
in curriculum, 658-661
in faculty, 661-662
in student body, 656, 661, 665-669
current status of minorities in programs, 676-680
curriculum change for primary public health care, 280
development of, 153-155
diversity in, 150-168
effect of population shifts on, 170-171, 173-174
effects of cost controls on, 173
enrolling minority students, 667-668
financial aid for students in, 159-160
health care delivery system in, 171, 174
imbalance in enrollments between ADN and BSN programs, 158-160
and implementation of Nursing Minimum Data Set, 115
and indigent care, 723
institutions of higher education in, 172, 174
international exchange
development of models of, 204-206
funding of international exchange, 206
international faculty exchange, 204-205
reasons for, 202-203
role of nursing and higher education, 203-204
mainstreaming student services, 668-669
minority faculty in, 669
multidisciplinary community-based, 547, 586-594
need for reform, 150-152
nontraditional admissions criteria for, 667
nontraditional learners in, 150-151, 163-168
new directions for new issues, 168
reflections and failures, 165-167
social, economic, and cultural realities, 163-165
for nurse-midwives, 242-243, 246
orientation and preceptorship programs for, 666
partnerships in, 151, 170-175, 177-180
physician's role in, 563
recruitment and retention of minority students into nursing
and retention barriers, 160
strategies, 160-161
recruitment in, 666-667
in Russia, 599
types of programs, 153
Nursing entrepreneurs, 3-4

Nursing faculty, 3, 32-37
challenges facing, 36-37
characteristics of, 32-33
for community college–nursing home partnerships, 179
cultural diversity of, 661-662
doctoral education for, 33
female dominance in, 34
functions of, 34-36
governance, 359, 393-397
autocratic model, 393
benevolent anarchy model, 393
collegial model, 393-394
political model, 394
in international education, 204-205
noncomparability of credentials, 33-34
qualifications of, 32
recruiting minority, 669
in research and scholarship, 35
in service, 35-36
in teaching, 35
Nursing-focused patient outcomes, 60, 136-141
conceptual issues, 138
definition of issues, 138-139
theoretical issues, 139-141
data set development, 141
evolution of, 136-137
effectiveness, 137
efficacy, 137
Nursing Grants and Fellowships Program, 89
Nursing Home Reform Act (1987), 290, 307
Nursing homes, quality versus quantity in, 503-504
Nursing Home Standards Guide of Public Health Service, 306
Nursing intelligentsia, differentiation between practicing nurse and, 617-618
Nursing intervention, definition of, 130
Nursing interventions classification (NIC), 60, 98-99, 129-134
definition of intervention terms, 130
arrangement of interventions in taxonomic structure, 132-133
refinement of intervention labels and defining activities, 131-132
validation of interventions and taxonomy, 133
development of, 129
generation of initial list of interventions, 130-131
identification and resolution of conceptual and methodological issues, 129-130
features of, 133-134
Nursing knowledge
nursing-focused patient outcomes, 136-141
Nursing Minimum Data Set, 113-120
nursing research in practice, 61-72
nursing theory–nursing practice connection, 76-80
nursing theory–nursing research connection, 87-91
patient classification schemas, 104-110
primary of practice, 82-86
reorganization of, 59, 92-102
Nursing Management, 69
Nursing Minimum Data Set (NMDS), 59, 113-120, 144
concept of, 114
development of, 114
elements of, 115-116

Nursing Minimum Data Set—Cont'd
  issues related to implementing and using, 117-118
  progress toward adopting and implementing, 115
    acceptance of, 120
    administration, 116
    appropriateness, 119
    clinical practice, 115
    documentation, computerization, and review of nursing data, 118
    health care policy, 116
    nursing education, 115
    research, 116-117
    testing, 119-120
  purposes of, 114
Nursing Organization Liaison Forum (NOLF), 23
Nursing organizations, 359, 388-392
  clinical specialty organizations, 390
  developing alliances among nursing organizations, 391
  early development of, 607-608
  early proposals for consolidation, 608-609
  Federation of Specialty Nursing Organizations, 611-612
  formation of professional organizations, 388-389
  functional specialty organizations, 390-391
  future of, 391-392
  interorganizational behavior, 612-613
  multipurpose organizations, 389-391
  need for unity, 614
  obstacles to consolidation, 613
    dues structure and union function, 613
    education and practice, 613-614
    membership, 613
  proliferation of specialty organizations, 609-611
  in Russia, 600
Nursing paradigm, fabrication of, 89
Nursing practice, 77-78
  advance directives in relation to, 755-756
  application of nursing theory in, 79
  as basis for nursing theory, 78
  case management in, 209-210, 254-260
  classification of, 96-101
  community partnerships in, 209, 226-232
  effect of computer-based patient record on, 210, 273-275
  flextime in, 261-264
  hospital changes in, 208, 220-225
  impact of biomedical technology on, 746-747
  and implementation of Nursing Minimum Data Set, 115
  leadership in, 209, 233-239
  measuring quality of, 342-348
    accreditation and external audit, 347-348
    adapting measurement to practice, 343
    barriers to, 342-343
    case conferences, 345-346
    client satisfaction surveys, 348
    models for practice, 343-348
    practice, documentation, and data management orientation, 344-345
    practice-based inservice education, 346-347
    record audit, peer review, and utilization review, 347
    shared evaluation visits and observations, 346
  multidisciplinary community-based, 547, 586-594

  and need for reforms in long-term care, 209, 242-250
  nurse-midwifery in, 209, 241-247
  nursing care plan in, 210, 267-269
  opportunities created in, 208-211
  primacy of, 58-59, 82-86
  self-scheduling in, 210, 264-265
  research in, 58, 61-72
  in Russia, 599-600
  unlicensed assistants in, 208, 212-219
  validation of nursing theory in, 78-79
Nursing professionalization, and conflict, 605-606, 643-648
Nursing Research, 61, 89-90, 93, 94, 95
Nursing research, 3. *See also* Nurse researchers
  advances in preparation of nurses to use, 65-66
  classification of, 92-96
  economic value of, 64
  emergence of, 89-90
  history of interface of nursing theory and, 59, 87
  and implementation of Nursing Minimum Data Set, 116-117
  minimizing barriers, dissemination and use, 66-67
  models for utilization of, 64-65
  strategies for increasing use of, 71
  using in practice, 58, 61-72
Nursing's Agenda for Health Care Reform, 171, 197, 418, 426-431, 454, 721-722
  managed care options encouraged, and mandated for uninsured, 429
  national debate, 430
  medical effectiveness testing, 429
  payment for services of nonphysician providers, 429
  public disclosure of vital health information, 429-430
Nursing services
  compensation for, 476, 528-532
    comparison of, with those of other professions, 530
    differentials, 529-530
    salary determination, 528
    salary levels, 528-529
  costing out, 474, 483-488
    dilemmas of, 486-487
    historical development, 483
    methods of, 483-485
    uses of, 485-486
  factors affecting worth of work, 531
    economic equity, 532
    nursing labor market, 531-532
Nursing shortage
  and health care reform, 427
  impacts of, 223
  and unionization, 378-379
Nursing staff, downsizing of, 222
Nursing theory, 76-77
  application of, in practice, 79
  emergence of, 87-89
  history of interface and nursing research of, 59, 87
  practice as basis for development, 78
  validation in practice, 78-79
Nursing theory–nursing practice connection
  interaction in, 78-79
  philosophical basis, 76-78
Nursing theory-practice bond, strengthening, 79-80

O

Objective testing, in measuring clinical competence, 338-339
Occupational health, and women's health, 697-698
Occupational Safety and Health Administration bloodborne pathogens standard, 518, 519
Omaha System, 99-100
    in measuring quality, 344-348
Omnibus Budget Reconciliation Act, 171, 311, 439, 442
Oregon Health Plan, 422-423, 702, 711-712
    decision-making model in, 713
    ethics in, 713-714
    legislative-administrative decision-making model, 712-713
    prioritization in, 714
        authority for nursing, 714
        data collection phase, 714-715
        ethical concerns, 716, 717
        implementation stage, 717
        ranking of health services, 715-716
        resource allocation stage, 716-717
Organs, sources of, for technology, 765
Outcomes research
    conceptual issues in, 138
        definitional issues, 138-139
        theoretical issues, 139-141
    evolution of, 136-137
    and health care costs, 511

P

Parenting Stress Index, 734
Pareto, 322
Partnerships, in nursing education, 151, 170-175, 177-180
Patient Care and Services (PaCS), 307
Patient classification schemas, 59, 104-110
    and costing of nursing services, 484, 486
Patient-focused care, and work redesign, 463
Patient-Focused Care Association, 463
Patient Management Problem (PMP), 339
Patient Self-Determination Act (1990), 252
Peer evaluations, in measuring clinical competence, 338
Peer review, in measuring quality, 306, 347
Perestroika, in Russia, 598
Performance testing, in measuring clinical competence, 337-338
Personal and professional assertiveness
    and career development, 546, 549-557
    and collaboration between nurses and physicians, 547, 580-583
    and feminism, 547, 572-578
    and multidisciplinary community-based education practice, 547, 586-594
    nursing in Russia, 548, 595-601
    and nursing's quest for professionalism, 546, 559-565
    strategies for changing nursing's image, 546-547, 566-570
Personhood
    concept of, 743
    influence of assisted reproductive technology on, 743-744
    role of nurse in promoting, 744-745
Perspectives in Psychiatric Care, 44
Petry, Lucile, 52
Pew Foundation Report, 196
Pew Memorial Trust, and support for nursing research, 61

Physician assistants
    areas of role conflict, 636
    background of, 633
    challenges for, 637
    current roles of, 633-634
    education of, 632-633
    gender issues for, 636-637
    national certification and state licensure for, 633
    similarities and differences with nurse practitioners, 634-636
    women in, 633
Physician dumping syndrome, 11
Physician-initiated treatments, 130
Physicians
    in case management, 258
    collaboration between nurses and, 547, 580-583
    in nursing education, 563
Pinheiro, Rosa, 52
Poole, Anne, 52
Practice-based inservice education, in measuring quality, 346-347
Advanced practice nurses
    third-party reimbursement issues for advanced, in 90s
        design of strategies for reimbursement policy, 445-447
        financial survival for nurses in world of third-party reimbursement and managed care, 448
        history of, 437-439
        implementation of reimbursement legislation and negotiation with managed-care systems, 447-448
        private component, 443-445
        public component, 439-443
Preferred provider organizations (PPOs), 433, 445, 451
Primary Care Health Practitioner Incentive Act, 442
Primary health care
    and community nursing centers, 383-384
    curriculum change for, 280
    in developing countries, 210-211, 276-280
        community-based approach, 277-280
        selective approach, 277
        top-down approach, 277
    nurse's role in, 280
Prison nurses, 674-675, 766
Private practice nurse, role of, 617
Professional literature, 66-67
Prospective pricing system (PPS), impact on hospitals, 220-221
Providers, surplus of specialized, and health care costs, 478
Public health nursing. *See* Community health nursing
Public Health Service
    Nursing Home Standards Guide, 306
    Task Force on Women's Health Issues, 196

Q

QAMUR model, 64
QualDex, 490-499
Quality
    balancing cost and, 474, 490-499
        compliance with budget, 496
        compliance with budget, 495
        compliance with staffing format, 495-496
        compliance with standards of nursing care, 491
        compliance with standards of nursing practice, 491
        cost-quality model, 490-491

Quality—Cont'd
    nursing hours race performance of patient day, 496
    occurrence of hospital-acquired infections, 492, 495
    occurrence of ontoward patient incidents, 492
    patient satisfaction, 495
    QualDex Process, 496-497
    significance of model and implications for practice, 497-499
    work load, 496
  defined, 296
  issues of, and community nursing centers, 384-385
Quality assurance
  in home health care, 285, 310-314
    accounting for individual differences among clients, 313
    comprehensive quality assurance system, 314
    measurement limitations, 313-314
    multidisciplinary care delivery models, 313
    multiple contextual factors, 313
  in long-term care, 285, 303-309
    association efforts in, 306
    decision making in, 304-306
    home environment, 303-304
    incentive programs in, 306
    nature of chronic illness in, 304
    peer review in, 306
    quality service in, 308-309
    regulatory efforts in, 306-308
Quality Assurance Model Using Research (QAMUR) model, 61
Quality care, measurement models for, 296-297
Quality improvement
  certification process in, 285-286, 327-335
  conventional approach to, 284, 287-294
  effect of standards and guidelines on, 285, 316-320
  in home health care, 285, 310-314
  importance of measuring quality, 284, 295-301
  in Latin American countries, 350-355, 386
  in long-term care, 285, 303-309
  multifaceted approaches to, 284-286
  ongoing processes for monitoring, 342-348, 386
  total quality management in, 285, 321-326
  validation of clinical competence, 336-340, 386
Quality outcomes, research in, 297-299
Quinn, Dame Sheila, 54

R

Raven, Kathleen, 52
Record audit in measuring quality, 347
Recruitment of nurses, 566-568
Regional Program for Nursing Research Development, 64
Registered care technologist (RCT), as response to nursing shortage, 223
Registered nurses, hospitals as primary work site for, 15
Regulatory efforts, in quality improvement, 306-308
Reimann, Christianne, 53
  Award, 53
Reiter, Frances, 20
Reproductive health, women's health in, 696-697
Research implementation, process of, 70
Research in Nursing and Health, 90, 95
Research Review: Studies for Nursing Practice, 66
Research training, nursing faculty role in, 35

Resident assessment protocols (RAPs), 307
Respite care, in long-term care, 504
Retention of nurses, 569-570
Revolution: The Journal of Nurse Empowerment, 369
RN, 69
Robert Wood Johnson Foundation Teaching Nursing Home Program, 172
Robert Wood Johnson University Hospital (RWJUH)
  development of QualDex at, 490-499
Role conflict
  and collaboration, 605, 638-642
  and frontline nurse, 604, 616-622
  and number of nursing organizations, 604, 607-614
  between nurses and physician assistants, 605, 632-637
  and nursing professionalization, 605-606, 643-648
  sources of stress for nurses, 605, 623-629
  and traditional roles of women in Brazil, 606, 650-654
Rural Elderly Enhancement Program (REEP), 226
Rural Health Clinic Services Act, 439
Russia
  health care system in, 595-596
  nursing in, 548, 595-601
  upheaval in, 595

S

Safety precautions
  costs of, to reduce risk of exposure to bloodborne pathogens, 475, 515-520
  defining safety precautions, 515-516
    costs of safety precautions, 516-518
    Hepatitis B and Hepatitis B vaccination, 518
    human immunodeficiency virus and postexposure management, 518-519
    using data to reduce injury-exposure risks, 519-520
Science, and primacy of practice in nursing, 82-86
Self care, in guiding quality nursing practice in Latin America, 350
Self-funded plan, 445
Self-managing work teams, establishment of, 380-381
Self-scheduling, 210
  benefits of, 264-265
  difficulties with, 265
Sermchief v. *Gonzales,* 7
Service, role of nursing faculty in, 35-36
Shared evaluation visits and observations, in measuring quality, 346
Shared governance in nursing, 359, 398-405
  definition of, 399-402
  motives for, 402
  in penetration of, 402-403
  role and system effects of, 403-404
Sigma Theta Tau, 61, 366
  and compilation of *Director of Nurse Researchers,* 95
  on use of nursing research in practice, 63
Singapore, health care financing in, 542
Single-payer proposal, 421
Skill inventories, in measuring clinical competence, 338
Snellman, Venny, 52
Snively, Mary Agnes, 51
Social Policy Statement (1980), 20, 366

Staff nurses, 15-18
  advanced degrees for, 3
  changing and expanding roles for, 16
  demographic data on, 15
  flextime for, 262-264
  future challenges for, 17-18
  level of job satisfaction, 16-17
  motivation for career choice, 15-16
  role and challenges, 3
  self-scheduling for, 264-265
  stressful work environment for, 17
Standard setting, in health care system, 292-294
State licensing laws, 6-8
Stetler-Marram model, 61
Students, in international education, 205
Summary Time-Oriented Record (STOR) system at University of
  California at San Francisco, 271
Supervisory Home Visit Tool, 346
Surrogate mothering, 743
Sweden, health care financing in, 544
Switzerland, health care financing in, 543-544
Symbolic interactionism, 758

T

Task Force on Nursing Practice in Hospitals of American Academy
  of Nursing, 210-211
Taxonomy of nursing interventions, definition of, 130
Team nursing, 19
THERESA system at Grady Hospital in Atlanta, 271
Third-party reimbursement. *See* Health insurance
Total quality management (TQM), 285, 321-326, 490
  foundations of, 322-323
  and job stress, 629
  and National Demonstration Project (NDP) on Quality
    Improvement in Health Care, 323-325
  and potential downside of quality, 325
  and work redesign, 463
Training of unlicensed assistive personnel, 216
Tri-Council, 391

U

Uniform Minimum Health Data Sets (UMHDSs), 144
Uninsured, rising number of, and health care costs, 509
Unionization, 358, 373-381
  challenges for profession, 380-381
  and changing nature of practitioner, 375
  and collective bargaining, 376-377
  consumer characteristics and societal demand, 374-375
  environment, 373-374
  growing autonomy of profession, 375-376
  historical perspective of employment, 376
  legal environment, 379-380
  model of collective relationship, 377-378
  nursing shortage, 378-379
U.S. Army Nurse Corps, 685
Unlicensed assistive personnel (UAP), 208, 212, 219
  ANA definitions related to ANA position statements on, 214
  basic problem in, 215-216
  criteria in deciding to use, 215
  practice, 216

Unlicensed assistive personnel (UAP)—Cont'd
  regulation of, 217
  role of, in hospitals, 222
  training, 216
  utilization of, 217
Unpopular clients, and nurses, 656-657, 671-675
Utilization review, in measuring quality, 347

V

Vermont, health care reform in, 423
Violence against women, and women's health, 695
Visiting Nurse Association (VNA) of Omaha in measuring quality,
  344-348
Voice, 638

W

Wald, Lillian, 50
Walter Reed Army Institute of Research, 89
Weighted ratios, 131
Western Interstate Commission for Higher Education
  (WICHE), 61
  on nursing research, 67
Western Journal of Nursing Research, 90, 95
WICHE Communicating Nursing Research, 93
Williamsburg Conference of nurse educators, 20
Women
  and nursing services in Brazil, 605, 650-654
  in Russia, 597
Women's health
  global perspective of, 657, 692-699
    changing agenda in, 698-699
    eating disorders and nutritional problems, 694
    illness experiences and responses, 693-698
    infections, 694-695
    occupational health, 697-698
    reproductive health, 696-697
    violence against women, 695
Work redesign, 419, 460-465
  case management, 463
  implications of national trends, 462
  national trends affecting hospitals, 460-462
  outcomes, 464
  patient-focused care, 463
  phases of, 464
  strategies for future, 464-465
  total quality management, 463
World Health Organization (WHO), 410-411
  Alma Alta Conference (1978), 383, 469
  and collaborating centers for nursing development, 413-414
  functions of, 411
  goal of, 411-412
  interaction with International Council of Nurses, 414
  nursing in, 4, 54-55, 412-413
  organization and administration of, 411